Crisis Intervention Strategies

Ninth Edition

Richard K. James

Professor Emeritus, University of Memphis

Julia Whisenhunt

Professor, University of West Georgia

Rick A. Myer

Professor Emeritus, University of Texas,
El Paso

 Cengage

Australia • Brazil • Canada • Mexico • Singapore • United Kingdom • United States

Crisis Intervention Strategies, 9e
Richard K. James, Julia Whisenhunt, Rick A. Myer

SVP, Product: Cheryl Constantini

VP, Product: Thais Alencar

Portfolio Product Director: Laura Ross

Associate Portfolio Product Director: Conor Allen

Product Assistant: Renee Bunszel

Learning Designers: Emma Guiton and Debra Myette-Flis

Content Manager: Mark Turner

Vendor Content Manager: Anupam Bose, MPS Limited

Content Project Manager, International: Ramkumar Palani

Digital Project Manager: Andy Baker

Senior Director, Product Marketing: Neena Bali

Content Acquisition Analyst: Deanna Ettinger

Production Service: MPS Limited

Designer: Erin Griffin

Cover Image Source: Michal Sikorski/Alamy Stock Photo

For product information and technology assistance, contact us at **Cengage Customer & Sales Support, 1-800-354-9706 or support.cengage.com.**

For permission to use material from this text or product, submit all requests online at **www.copyright.com.**

Library of Congress Control Number: 2023915848

Student Edition:
ISBN: 978-0-357-62269-8

Cengage
5191 Natorp Boulevard
Mason, OH 45040
USA

Cengage is a leading provider of customized learning solutions. Our employees reside in nearly 40 different countries and serve digital learners in 165 countries around the world. Find your local representative at **www.cengage.com.**

To learn more about Cengage platforms and services, register or access your online learning solution, or purchase materials for your course, visit **www.cengage.com.**

Printed at CLDPC, USA, 02-24

Dedication

Through the timeline of 37 years and nine editions of this book, we have never experienced an ecosystemic crisis that has affected people and first responders worldwide the way the COVID-19 pandemic has. The pandemic is an example of chaos theory in action, with a titanic struggle to find innovative ways to deal with the countless emergencies and challenges therein. But that is how we remain resilient and how we survive—by evolving to meet such horrific challenges. Accordingly, we would like to dedicate this ninth edition to the first responders who went directly into harm's way to provide services for a world in desperate need of support and assistance. From EMT's and fire personnel who transported sick people, to law enforcement officers and social workers who made wellness checks, to doctors and nurses who risked their lives and health during double and triple shifts, and to the grandparents, parents, brothers and sisters, and dear friends who stood vigil and cared for their loved one, this ninth edition of the crisis book is dedicated to you. This edition is also dedicated to my beloved daughter, Samantha Whitehawk, Nurse Practitioner at St. David's Hospital ICU in Austin, Texas, who was in the middle of that crisis tsunami and worried her dad every night she went to work. Thank you all for being there for us.

Dr. Dick James

2 Handling Specific Crises: Going Into the Trenches   167

3 On the Home Front: Crisis in the Human Services Workplace 511

Chapter 14
Violent Behavior in Institutions 512

Chapter 15
Human Services Workers in Crisis Burnout, Vicarious Traumatization, and Compassion Fatigue 554

4 No Man's Land: Facing Disaster 591

Rationale for the Book

The Primacy of Crisis Intervention

The Chinese characters embedded in the front of this book symbolize both "danger" and "opportunity!" Further, the lotus flower pictured on the cover roots in mud and grows out of murky water to blossom into a stunning symbol of purity and rebirth. This symbolism encapsulates the focus of this book while capturing the essence of **crisis**—the human dilemma that is common to all cultures. We believe that practically all counseling is initiated as crisis intervention. As much as the helping professions would prefer otherwise, people tend either to avoid presenting their problems to a helper until those problems have grown to crisis proportions or become ensconced in situational dilemmas that wind up in unforeseen crises. Our ideal objective, as human services workers, is to establish primary prevention programs so effective that crisis intervention will seldom be needed. Although recently a shift has occurred, still many people are not as quick to adopt preventive measures for their psychological health as for their physical health.

The Case for an Applied Viewpoint

The materials and techniques we promote in this book come from two sources: first, the authors' own experiences in teaching and counseling in crisis situations; second, interviews with people who are currently in the trenches, successfully performing counseling and crisis intervention. We have obtained input from many different individuals in the helping professions, whose daily and nightly work is dealing directly with human dilemmas, and we have related their views to the best of current theory and practice from the professional literature. Through many hours of dialogue, these experts have provided the most contemporary strategies and techniques in use in their particular fields. They have also reviewed the content on each crisis category and have provided much helpful commentary and critique of the ecology and etiology, tactics and procedures, terminology, and developmental stages of the specific crises with which they work. Therefore, what you read in the case-handling strategies comes directly from the horse's mouth.

Where controversies exist in regard to treatment modalities, this text attempts to present as many perspectives as possible. The authors have endeavored to incorporate, synthesize, and integrate the case-handling strategies of these resource people in a comprehensive, fluid, and dynamic way that will provide crisis workers with a basic set of tenets about effective crisis intervention. This book is not about long-term therapy or theory, nor is it a volume dealing with crisis from only one theoretical perspective, such as a psychoanalytic approach or a cognitive-behavior system. The book incorporates a wide diversity of therapeutic modalities and reflects our eclectic and integrated approach to crisis intervention.

Specific crises demand specific interventions that span the whole continuum of therapeutic strategies. The strategies present in this book shouldn't be construed as the only ones available for a particular crisis. They are presented as "best bets" based on what current research and practice indicate to be appropriate and applicable. Yet, these strategies may not be appropriate for all practitioners with all clients in all situations.

Good crisis intervention, as well as good therapy of any other kind, is a serious professional activity that calls for creativity and the ability to adapt to the changing conditions of the therapeutic moment. To that extent, crisis intervention at times is more art than science and is not prescriptive. Therefore, we would caution you that there are no clear-cut prescriptions or simple cause-and-effect answers in this book. We encourage you not to fall into the trap that since you have heard something before and the strategy you used worked to perfection, to simply use the same strategy again. Each crisis and person is unique, meaning the intervention strategy must be tailored for that situation.

The Case for an Experiential Viewpoint

The fact that no single theory or strategy applies to every crisis situation is particularly problematic to those who are looking for simple, concrete answers to resolve the client problems they will face. If you are just beginning your career in the human services, we hope that while reading and trying out activities in this book, you will suspend your judgment for a while and be open to the experience as you read about crisis workers attempting to implement theory into practice.

Moral Dilemmas. Another issue that permeates many of the topics covered in this book is the emotions they generate and the beliefs about what is morally "right" and what is morally "wrong" that pervades them. People have been willing to go to prison or die because of the strong beliefs they held about many of these topics. Where such moral issues and beliefs abound, we have attempted to deal with them in as even-handed a manner as possible. Although many of you will deal with crises in an office setting or possibly responding to a disaster, understand that not all crisis intervention takes place in those settings. A classic current example is the role law enforcement plays in crisis intervention. We spend a fair amount of time detailing how crisis intervention team officers play an important role in responding to crisis individually and as members of a crisis response team. This book is not about the morality of the issues covered, but rather about what seems to work best for the people who are experiencing the dilemma. We ask you to read the book with that view in mind, and for at least a while, suspend your moral view of the situation or problem as you read about crisis workers attempting to grapple with these heart- and gut-wrenching problems.

At times, we have been questioned and criticized for our use of regional cultural dialects and the use of profanity in our dialogues. That is not done to disparage or demean anyone or any group of people. We do this to portray, as realistically as we can, the way people in crises talk. Know that people in crisis are not necessarily politically correct and, even more important, they may use colorful language. When individuals experience crisis, their emotions are raw, behavior is uncharacteristic, and thought processes are altered. Crises create such disequilibrium that social and political filters may not be used. As such, to help prepare readers for the experience of crisis intervention, we attempt to present case vignettes that depict a relatively realistic crisis and the emotions, behaviors, and thoughts that most often are experienced with the crisis state.

Finally, because of a virtually unlimited supply of different crisis situations, we have had to make tough decisions about what kinds of problems to illustrate in the most *generic and comprehensive way possible* so as to reach the broadest possible audience. We understand and empathize very deeply with readers who may have suffered terrible crises that are not mentioned in this book and are puzzled, chagrined, and angry that we have not given space and time to the particular crisis that they have suffered through. For that we apologize. The space available means that we simply cannot include all situations. However, what we, the authors, would like you to do rather than rail at our callous treatment in ignoring a particular crisis situation is to imagine how the strategies and techniques you are reading about might apply to the particular crisis you have experienced. Hopefully, what we say about those crises may help you come to understand the dynamics of your own a bit better.

Basic Relationship Skills. The listening and responding skills described in Chapter 3 are critical to everything else the worker does in crisis intervention. Yet, on cursory inspection, these techniques and concepts may seem at best simplistic and at worst, inane. They do not appear to fix anything because they are not "fixing" skills. What they do is give the crisis worker a firm basis of operation to clearly explore the dilemma the client is facing. Basic listening and responding skills are the prerequisites for all other therapeutic modalities.

Our experience has shown us over and over that students and trainees who scoff at and dismiss these basic relationship skills are the ones who invariably have the most trouble meeting the experiential requirements of our courses and workshop training sessions. We feel very strongly about this particular point and thus ask you to read Chapter 3 with an open mind. Much the same can be said about Chapter 4, The Tools of the Trade. Students and veteran human service workers who operate out of a client-centered mode may find what we are proposing pretty close to heresy because a lot of these tools are directive and judgmental as to the action to be taken, particularly when client safety is concerned. Again, we ask you to suspend judgment and give these tools a good tryout in this new venture.

The learning objectives for each chapter are based on Bloom's Taxonomy but tend to focus on lower order skills. This is because reading a book cannot, in and of itself, prepare individuals for crisis work. In addition to gaining the knowledge of crisis intervention, one of two things needs to happen to move readers into higher order learning. First, the Mind-Tap supplement that goes with this book will do that admirably with the supplementary materials it provides. Second, instructors can put the knowledge, theories, and techniques to work in live classroom exercises that include critical demonstrations, role play, and discussion, to apply the knowledge to produce skill and technique in crisis intervention.

Role Play. If this volume is used as a structured learning experience, the case studies in each chapter are a valuable resource for experiential learning, as are the exercises your instructor will give you and the videos provided in MindTap. It is essential that you observe effective crisis intervention models at work and then follow up by actually practicing and enacting the procedures you have observed. Intensive and extensive role play is an excellent skill builder. A critical component of training is not just talking about problems but practicing the skills of handling them as well. Talking about a problem is fine, but attempting to handle a live situation enables the trainee to get involved in the business of calming, defusing, managing, controlling, and motivating clients. Role play is one of the best ways of practicing what is preached, and it prepares human services workers for developing creative ways to deal with the variety of contingencies they may face. Role play gives human services workers the chance to find out what works and doesn't work for them in the safety of a training situation and affords their fellow students and trainees an opportunity to give them valuable feedback.

A major problem in role playing is the perception of standing up in a class or workshop and risking making a complete fool of oneself. We want to assure you that in our classes and training sessions, we don't expect perfection. If our students and trainees were perfect at crisis intervention, they wouldn't be taking

instruction from us in the first place! Therefore, put your inhibitions on the shelf for a while and become engaged in role plays as if the situations were real, live, and happening right now. Further, be willing and able to accept critical comments from your peers, supervisors, or instructors. Your ego may be bruised a bit in the process, but that's far better than waiting until you are confronted with an out-of-control client before you think about what you are going to do. The bottom line is that the classroom is the safest place to do this, and as you will soon discern, safety is our most important product. Over and over, our students report that this component of instruction was the most profitable to them and was also the most fun!

Give the exercises that go with each chapter your best effort, process them with fellow students or trainees, and see what fits best with your own feelings, thoughts, and behaviors. Many times, our students and trainees attempt to imitate us. Although it is gratifying to see students or trainees attempting to be "Dr. J.," "Dr. W" or "Dr. M," it is generally an exercise in futility for them. What they need to do is view us critically as we model the procedures and then incorporate their own style and personhood into the procedures. We would urge you to do the same.

Some of these chapters are REALLY long. We didn't put all that "stuff" in there to bore you and put you to sleep with verbiage. We did it because the field of crisis keeps expanding rapidly, as does the knowledge base. Therefore you need to know "the stuff" to do your job effectively. If you just watch the PowerPoint presentations, you might get enough knowledge to pass your instructor's tests. However, you won't know enough to help your client or yourself when you get in a tight spot. So read, read, read.

Finally, if you are never, ever going to be a crisis interventionist but a "consumer," this book still can be very useful. Sad to say, but just through living, you are going to encounter a lot of crises in this book that are going to afflict you, your loved ones, your friends, your workplace, and the ecosystem in which you live. To that end, this book can give you the basic knowledge to deal with the crisis or know when it's time to get help.

Organization of the Book
Part One, Basic Training

Part 1 of the book introduces the basic concepts of crisis intervention as well as telephone and online crisis counseling. It comprises Chapters 1 through 6.

Chapter 1, Approaching Crisis Intervention. Chapter 1 contains the historical background, basic definitions, and the theoretical and conceptual information needed for understanding applied crisis intervention.

Chapter 2, Culturally Effective Helping in Crisis. Chapter 2 is concerned with how crisis and culture interact. Effectively helping people from diverse backgrounds who are undergoing a crisis or have survived a disaster mandates an understanding and sensitivity to culturally diverse issues. What are called "social locations" for both worker and client play a major role in crisis intervention work. A derivation of those social locations, called SAFETY locations, has been formulated to specifically to help a person in crisis. We have also introduced Relational Cultural Theory into this edition as a key operating system for integrating crisis with multicultural practice.

Chapter 3, The Intervention and Assessment Models. Chapter 3 introduces the task model for crisis intervention as well as the triage assessment system for rapidly assessing the severity of the crisis in a multidimensional way in real time. We have also introduced the LASER model as an ethical decision making model for crisis intervention.

Chapter 4, The Tools of the Trade. Chapter 4 introduces the basic communication techniques and skills applied to crisis intervention. It also details the strategies used to attack various kinds of problems that hinder individuals as they attempt to resolve the crisis and details how crisis workers operate on the directive–nondirective action continuum.

Chapter 5, Crisis Case Handling. Chapter 5 is an overview of how crises are handled. Long-term therapy is compared with crisis intervention. Different venues where crisis intervention operates are explored to give an overview of the general tactics and strategies that are used.

Chapter 6, Telephone and Behavioral Telehealth Crisis Counseling. The majority of crisis intervention is still done on the telephone by trained volunteers. However, with the advent of the Internet, social media, and the social exclusion brought on by COVID-19, more and more crisis intervention is being done online in behavioral telehealth formats. Chapter 6 explores the issues and techniques that are involved in these two mediums of crisis communication.

Part 2, Handling Specific Crises: Going into the Trenches

Part 2 (Chapters 7 through 13) addresses a variety of important types of crises. For each chapter in Part 2, the background and dynamics of the particular crisis type are detailed to provide a basic grasp of the driving forces behind the dilemma. Although some theory is present to highlight the therapeutic modalities used, comprehensive theoretical systems are beyond the scope of this book. For the sources of that information, turn to the reference section at the end of each chapter.

In Part 2, we provide scripts from real interventions, highlighted by explanations why the crisis workers did what they did. Throughout this section, techniques and cases are used to support live tryout, experiencing, and processing of the cases and issues in each chapter.

Chapter 7, Posttraumatic Stress Disorder. Chapter 7, Posttraumatic Stress Disorder (PTSD), is the linchpin chapter of this section. Many of the following chapters will have problems that may be the precursors of PTSD or, alternatively, represent the manifestation of it. This chapter examines both adults and children who have suffered traumatic experiences and are in crisis because of them.

Chapter 8, Crisis of Lethality. Chapter 8 focuses on strategies that crisis workers need in working with people who are manifesting lethal behavior. Suicidal and homicidal ideation flows through many other problems that assail the people the human services worker is likely to confront and is a consideration for all providers of crisis intervention services both in regard to the safety of those clients and keeping the interventionists safe.

Chapter 9, Sexual Assault. Chapter 9 addresses another societal crisis that practically every human services worker will eventually encounter—clients who have either experienced or been affected by sexual assault. People who have been sexually assaulted are a special population because of the negative moral and social connotations associated with the dehumanizing acts perpetrated on them. This chapter is in three parts. First, it details crisis intervention techniques in the immediate aftermath of sexual assault on adults. Second, the chapter examines the long-term traumatic wake impacting adult survivors of sexual abuse experienced in childhood. Third, the chapter details intervention techniques with children who have suffered sexual abuse and the family systems in which they live.

Chapter 10, Partner Violence. Chapter 10 deals with a crisis that many people in an intimate relationship face: being treated violently by their partner. This chapter provides strategies to help people who are suffering abuse in *any kind of intimate partner relationship*.

Chapter 11, Family Crisis Intervention. Chapter 11 deals with the whole family as they seek to navigate the family system through a crisis. The chapter describes the types or crises families experience as well as their path to resolution,

Chapter 12, Personal Loss: Bereavement and Grief. Chapter 12 presents a type of crisis that every person will sooner or later face: personal loss. Even though the phenomenon of loss has been with us as long as the human species has existed, many people in our contemporary culture are poorly prepared and ill-equipped to deal with it. This chapter examines a variety of loss models and looks at different types of losses. This chapter also provides models and strategies for coping with unresolved or complicated grief. We have woven into the chapter a discussion of the effects of the COVID-19 pandemic, particularly related to the altered grief experience.

Chapter 13, Crises in Schools. Schools have become a focal point for the violence perpetrated by gangs and disenfranchised and socially isolated children and adolescents. This chapter will examine crises as they impact schools from preschool through higher education. It will examine what crisis workers need to do in assessing, screening, and working with the potentially violent individual student who is estranged from the social mainstream of the school. It will also deal with what the crisis worker needs to know in dealing with suicide, a problem that has become endemic in youth. This chapter will detail how and what goes into making up a crisis response team for a school building and system and how and what they respond to when a potential metastasizing crisis occurs.

Part 3, On the Homefront: Crisis in the Human Services Workplace

Part 3 (Chapters 14 and 15) concentrates on the problems of crisis workers themselves and their employing institutions.

Chapter 14, Violent Behavior in Institutions. Chapter 14 tackles the little publicized and badly neglected type of crisis that workers in many institutions face daily: violent behavior within the walls of the institution. Regardless of the organizational settings in which they are employed, workers will find in this chapter useful concepts and practical strategies that they and the institution can put to immediate use with agitated and potentially assaultive clients.

Chapter 15, Human Services Workers in Crisis: Burnout, Vicarious Traumatization, and Compassion Fatigue. Chapter 15 is about you and all human services workers who are in the helping professions. No worker is immune to stress, burnout, and the crises that go with human services work. This fact is particularly true in crisis work. This chapter should prove invaluable information for any worker anywhere whose work environment is frenetic and filled with crisis intervention or whose personality tends to generate compulsive behavior, perfectionism, or other stressors that may lead to burnout.

Part 4, No Man's Land: Facing Disaster

Part 4 focuses on an ecosystem view of crisis and crisis intervention in large-scale disasters.

Chapter 16, Disaster Response. Chapter 16 explores the theoretical basis and operating paradigm for large-scale disasters through an ecosystemic viewpoint. This chapter introduces the concept of a megacrisis by describing the way these disasters change functioning on a day-to-day basis. The chapter details a family as they experience a natural disaster and how they interact with a variety of crisis workers and the services the workers provide for the family as they move through post-disaster events over the course of a year. Finally, the chapter highlights the personal impact of large-scale disasters and the experiences of crisis workers who were involved with them at the scene of the disaster.

Supplementary Materials

This text is accompanied by several supporting products for both instructors and students.

MindTap

MindTap for *Crisis Intervention Strategies*, 9th ed., engages and empowers students to produce their best work—consistently. By seamlessly integrating course material with videos, activities, apps, and much more, MindTap creates a unique learning path that fosters increased comprehension and efficiency.

For students:

- MindTap delivers real-world relevance with activities and assignments that help students build critical thinking and analytic skills that will transfer to other courses and their professional lives.
- MindTap helps students stay organized and efficient with a single destination that reflects what's important to the instructor, along with the tools students need to master the content.
- MindTap empowers and motivates students with information that shows where they stand at all times—both individually and compared to the highest performers in class.

Additionally, for instructors, MindTap allows you to:

- Control what content students have access to and when they access it with a learning path that can be used as-is or matched to your syllabus exactly.
- Create a unique learning path of relevant readings and multimedia and activities that move students up the learning taxonomy from basic knowledge and comprehension to analysis, application, and critical thinking.
- Integrate your own content into the MindTap Reader using your own documents or pulling from sources like RSS feeds, YouTube videos, websites, Google Docs, and more.
- Use powerful analytics and reports that provide a snapshot of class progress, time in course, engagement, and completion.

Ancillary Package

Additional instructor resources for this product are available online. Instructor assets include an Instructor's Manual, Educator's Guide, PowerPoint® slides, and a test bank powered by Cognero®. Sign up or sign in at http://faculty.cengage.com to search for and access this product and its online resources.

The Cengage Instructor Center is an all-in-one resource for class preparation, presentation, and testing. The instructor resources available for download include:

- **Instructor's Manual** Includes key terms with definitions, a chapter outline, and additional activities and discussion questions that may be conducted in an on-ground, hybrid, or online modality.
- **PowerPoint Slides** Helping to make lectures more engaging, these handy Microsoft PowerPoint slides outline the chapters of the main text in a classroom-ready presentation. The PowerPoint slides reflect the content and organization of the text and provide ample opportunities for generating classroom discussion and interaction.
- **Test Bank** A comprehensive test bank, offered in Blackboard, Moodle, Desire2Learn, and Canvas formats, contains learning objective-specific multiple-choice and essay questions for each chapter. Import the test bank into your LMS to edit and manage questions and to create tests.
- **Cengage Learning Testing, Powered by Cognero** This assessment software is a flexible, online system that allows you to import, edit, and manipulate test bank content from the *Crisis Intevention* test bank, or elsewhere, including your own favorite test questions; create multiple test versions in an instant; and deliver tests from your LMS, your classroom, or wherever you want.

Acknowledgements

In writing a book that covers so many diverse areas of the human condition, it would be extremely presumptuous of us to rely solely on our own expertise and theories of truth, beauty, and goodness to propose crisis intervention techniques as the one true path of enlightenment to dealing with crises. We decided that the only realistic way to present the most current, reliable, and practical techniques of crisis intervention would be to go straight to the people who do this work day in and day out. They are not "big names" but rather people who go methodically about the business of crisis intervention daily in their respective venues. They work in such diverse occupational roles as ministers, law enforcement officers, psychologists, social workers, psychiatrists, nurses, marriage and family counselors, correction counselors, and school counselors. They work in every kind of agency and institution that deals with people and their dilemmas. They range geographically from across the United States to across the world. They are an encyclopedia of practical knowledge, and we are deeply in their debt for the help, advice, time, interviews, and critique they have given us. This book would not be possible without their assistance, and we thank them one and all.

We would also like to thank the students in our crisis intervention classes at the University of Memphis. If you watch the videos that accompany this text, you are going to meet some of them up close and personal—both as crisis interventionists and wild and severely distressed clients! You will find that they are not perfect as rookies, but they are pretty darn good. They had fun doing the videos and hope you will have as much fun practicing these skills as they did. Thus, we want you to know we appreciate you deeply and have stood in awe and admiration in regard to how many of you have gone on to excel in this field.

Finally, we extend our grateful appreciation to the Cengage team members who provided support throughout this process.

Basic Training
Crisis Intervention Theory and Application

Part 1 introduces you to the fundamental concepts, theories, strategies, and skills needed to understand and conduct effective crisis intervention. Chapter 1 presents a brief historical overview of the field and introduces the conceptual dimensions of crisis work. Chapter 2 deals with the ecosystemic and multicultural considerations involved in providing crisis intervention. Chapter 3 serves as a key to the application of assessment and intervention strategies in crisis intervention. Chapter 4 describes the basic skills and techniques crisis interventionists use. Chapter 5 explains the major components of effective case management in crisis intervention. Chapter 6 discusses two of the main ways that crisis intervention is delivered—by telephone and internet.

Approaching Crisis Intervention

1

A Brief History of Crisis Intervention

LO1 We open the ninth edition of this book with a brief history of crisis intervention. While crisis itself has probably been in existence since the dawn of humankind, formal crisis theory, research, and intervention comprise one of the newest fields in psychotherapy. Most laypersons probably would think of formal crisis intervention as historically having to do with large-scale disasters, such as hurricanes or 9/11, and most typically performed by government agencies like the Federal Emergency Management Agency (FEMA) in the United States or by charitable organizations like the Red Cross. While

the Red Cross and the Salvation Army have been involved in disaster relief for approximately the past century, FEMA has been in existence only for about 40 years, and until quite recently, none of these organizations has had much to say or do about crisis intervention from a mental health perspective. But what we do know in 2023 is light-years ahead of what we knew when the first edition of this book appeared in 1987. If you could find the first edition in your library, it would look very little like this book does now.

The First Crisis Line. Suicide prevention is probably the longest-running intervention program in which an individual crisis is addressed from a mental health standpoint. The first identifiable crisis phone line was established in 1906 by the National Save-a-Life League (Bloom, 1984). Dr. Edwin Shneidman's (2001) landmark research into the causes of suicide, which started in the 1950s, has now spanned seven decades. Suicide has achieved such importance as a mental health problem that it has become an "ology" and has a national association devoted to its study and a national suicide and crisis hotline number, 988.

Cocoanut Grove Nightclub Fire. Most people who study the field would probably say the benchmark for crisis intervention was the Cocoanut Grove night-club fire in 1942, in which more than 400 people perished. Dr. Erich Lindemann (1944), who treated many of the survivors, found that they seemed to have common emotional responses and a need for psychological assistance and support. Out of Lindemann's work came the first notions of what may be called "common" grief reactions to a disaster. Dr. Gerald Caplan (1961) was also involved in working with the Cocoanut Grove survivors. Sometimes referred to as the father of crisis intervention, his experiences led to some of the first attempts to explain what a crisis is and to build a theory of crisis. However, not until the 1960s did the first attempts occur to provide a structure for what would become crisis intervention.

The Community Mental Health Act of 1963. This federal act completely changed the way mental health services were delivered in the United States by mandating the development of community mental health centers as primary providers for people with mental illness in the United States, who, prior to that act, were generally housed in large state insane asylums. As the large state "insane asylums" were closed down and replaced by community mental health centers, one of the primary mandates of those centers was to provide emergency services and crisis intervention 24/7. While the community mental health concept was laudable, the idealistic notion that patients would be docile, medication compliant, and fully functional proved to be problematic, and those problems would end up in homeless shelters and prisons.

The New Asylums—Prisons. Although the following statistics are dated, they are probably conservatively representative of the mental health problems of the United States. There are more individuals with serious and persistently serious mental illnesses in the Los Angeles County Jail, Chicago's Cook County Jail, or New York's Riker's Island Jail than any psychiatric

facility in the United States (Torrey et al., 2010). In 2006, more than one million two hundred thousand inmates in federal and state prisons and local jails could be identified as having a diagnosable mental illness. (James & Glaze, 2006). This grim statistical analysis of incarcerated people portrays a sad legacy of the Community Mental Health Act and what this country has done about it.

A follow up by the Department of Justice in 2012 into incarcerated people with mental illness found that 1 in 7 people imprisoned in state and federal institutions (14 percent) and local jail inmates (26 percent) met the criteria for serious psychological distress of some kind (Bronson & Berzosfsky, 2017). In 2014, about 10 times more individuals with serious mental illness were in prisons than mental health hospitals (Torrey et al., 2014). In a compiled report of policies and practices of prison mental health, the Prison Policy Initiative (2022) found that the number of prisoners had skyrocketed to 44 percent in local jails and 43 percent in prisons. Our own experience working in a prison mental health unit from 2012–2017 subjectively confirms that this is a fairly accurate estimate.

How could this happen with such good intentions of the Community Mental Health Act? One of the overarching tenets of crisis intervention that flows through every theoretical model is the concept of support. When familial supports either wear down and out or were never there in the first place, when no medical professional is there to monitor medication, when mental health clinics are underfunded and overwhelmed with clients, and when little vocational opportunities or rehabilitation counselors are available.

As a result of this evolution in mental health care (or the lack of it), it should not be surprising that a great deal of crisis intervention is now done on the streets and in the homes of local communities. What might surprise you is that a lot of it is being done by police officers.

Birth of the Police Crisis Intervention Team. Indeed, one of the major, serendipitous outcomes of deinstitutionalization has been the birth of the police Crisis Intervention Team. Faced with continuous interactions with individuals who experience psychological disorders and were off their medication, many confrontations with the police ended violently, with individuals with mental health issues forcibly being taken into custody. That interaction often resulted in the consumer or police officer being injured or being killed. These continuous confrontations culminated in the city of Memphis in 1987 when a man who was experiencing a mental health crisis related to his diagnosed schizophrenia was shot to death by the police. The resulting hue and cry from the citizens of Memphis resulted in a radical shift in police thinking and the establishment of the first **police Crisis Intervention Team** specifically trained to de-escalate and defuse people with mental health issues and who demonstrate dangerous behavior to themselves or others (James & Crews, 2009).

Word about what we were doing in Memphis soon spread, and other law enforcement jurisdictions that were grappling with the same problems across the country began asking for help in training their officers. What started out as a small group of mental health professionals, government officials, and police officers attempting to deal with a critical local political problem has now spread across over 2700 jurisdictions in the United States, Canada, Australia, Europe, and Africa and is now considered a "best practices" model for police departments (Rogers, et. al., 2019; Watson & Fulambarker, 2012), which we will thoroughly explore in Chapter 5, "Crisis Case Handling."

International Movement. The United States has not been alone in its endeavors to organize large-scale crisis intervention operations. Internationally, the United Nations Inter-Agency Standing Committee (IASC, 2007) has published guidelines for mental health provision in emergency situations. Europe has established the European Society of Traumatic Stress Studies (ESTSS, 2022) and their Traumatic Stress Network to develop evidence-based responses to large-scale disasters and provide assistance to those parts of the European Union that suffer from a lack of psychological resources. The **International Federation of Red Cross and Red Crescent Societies** has entered into the psychosocial facet of disaster relief by helping individuals and communities heal psychological wounds and rebuild social structures after an emergency or critical event. Its mission is to change people into active survivors rather than passive victims (International Federation of Red Cross and Red Crescent Societies, 2022).

Most notably, the Australians have been in the vanguard of dealing with the mental health issues of large-scale disasters particularly through the research and writing of Beverley Raphael (Raphael, 1977, 1986; Raphael & Wilson, 2000), determining early on whether crisis intervention procedures were effective (Bordow & Porritt, 1979), and staying on the cutting edge technologically in providing services to hard-to-reach populations (Williams et al., 2020).

Grassroots Movements

To really understand the evolution of crisis intervention, though, is to understand that several social movements have been critical to its development, and these did not start fully formed as "crisis intervention" groups by any means. Three of the major movements that helped shape crisis intervention into an emerging specialty were Alcoholics Anonymous (AA), Vietnam veterans, and the women's movement of the 1970s. Although their commissioned intentions and objectives had little to do with the advancement of crisis intervention as a clinical specialty, they had a lot to do with people who were desperate for help and weren't getting any. These groups all started as grassroots movements.

The need for crisis intervention services remains unrecognized by the public and by existing institutions until a critical mass of survivors comes together to exert enough legal, political, or economic pressure to cause the particular crisis category, malady, or social problem to become formalized. Until that time, it remains informal, nonprofessional, and unsubsidized. The problem is responded to or handled mainly through ad hoc, informal means by former victims, current victims, friends, or significant others who are affected by the problem. The free storefront clinics for Vietnam veterans that grew out of a refusal of the Veterans Administration to handle their problems, and the attempt by Mothers Against Drunk Driving (MADD) to deal with the crisis of drunk driving in the face of resistant state legislatures are excellent examples of grassroots responses to unmet needs.

Initiators of crisis intervention services are generally concerned with one particular crisis category that personally affects them in some way. Typically, the crisis gets far enough out of hand to cause noticeable community problems before remedial responses are initiated. At first, the initiators are mavericks who are starting a victims' revolt. The revolt is against an entrenched status quo or power structure that shows little awareness of or responsiveness to the problem. The victims' revolt somehow manages to get a fledgling crisis agency started despite the benign neglect and reluctance of mainstream society.

The fledgling crisis agency is initially funded by private donations, as with the many telephone call-in lines for victims of domestic violence that were started at local YWCAs in the 1970s. The services are often provided by volunteers who are loosely organized. The crisis agency gains access to public funding only after the agency has attained validation and some recognition by a substantial portion of the power structure. If, after a time, the crisis agency does not attain credibility sufficient to garner substantial private support or a modicum of public support, the agency begins to falter and eventually folds and ceases to operate. However, if it attains enough critical mass through consumer support, it can grow and become institutionalized as a legitimate entity.

In the 1970s, Vietnam veterans' efforts to get post-traumatic stress disorder (PTSD) categorized as a mental disease and get financial support for research and treatment were a classic example of this revolt and grudging acceptance by the mainstream. So were the efforts of the National Organization for Women and other women's groups in the 1970s to raise the curtain on domestic violence and child abuse in the United States and to get state legislatures to deal with them as criminal acts.

It is this grassroots influence that often captures the attention of the media, impels people to join as volunteers, and causes a greater number of clients and victims to seek the services of the agency. Initially, community leaders may deny that the crisis exists, minimize its seriousness, or express doubt that it represents a recurring problem. But when the crisis and agitation about it persists, they finally come to realize that someone must become proactive—someone must exert the leadership, energy, time, resources, and resolve to confront the crisis. Thus, the formation of an agency is sanctioned or even encouraged and if it succeeds and is publicly recognized as fulfilling a need, the quest to expand and mature begins.

As mainstream institutions, such as governmental structures, become aware of the problem and as volunteer centers reach the saturation point at which needs are obviously going unmet, some governmental or institutional funding is provided. Pressure politics, public relations, and public image building affect the course and growth of an organization and the problem it seeks to solve. For example, the plight of the Vietnam veterans afflicted with PTSD was largely ignored until the problem spilled over from the streets into the seats of power and authority—from personal crisis to politics. When the PTSD problem began to affect members of Congress, the power of the federal government and the resources of the Veterans Administration were brought to bear not

only to create a network of veterans centers throughout the country but also to slash bureaucratic red tape to ensure that services for Vietnam veterans were taken to where veterans with PTSD lived, which was sometimes on the streets, instead of requiring veterans to report to regular VA hospitals.

The activism of those veterans in the 1970s is present today in the comprehensive frontline treatment and exit programs of the armed services and the extensive use of veterans' outreach centers across the United States. Satellite outreach centers throughout the country have now been established by the VA to make it substantially easier for veterans of the Middle Eastern conflicts to access services that would otherwise require them to travel to mainstream VA hospitals.

The Importance of Volunteerism

Contrary to the popular misconception that paid veteran crisis workers descend on a large-scale disaster like smoke jumpers into a forest fire, most crisis intervention in the United States is done by volunteers. Volunteer workers perform all kinds of services in most crisis agencies—from menial chores to answering the phone to frontline crisis intervention with clients. Volunteerism is often the key to getting the fledgling crisis agency rolling. The use of trained volunteers as crisis workers has been a recognized component of many crisis centers and agencies for years (Clark & McKiernan, 1981; Roberts, 1991, p. 29; Slaikeu & Leff-Simon, 1990, p. 321). Probably the greatest number of frontline volunteers are used in staffing 24-hour suicide hotlines in major cities. Such hotlines require an enormous number of crisis workers because the crisis service never ceases—it must be provided 7 days a week, 52 weeks a year. Roberts (1991, p. 29) reported that more than three quarters of all crisis centers in the United States indicate that they rely on volunteer crisis workers and that such volunteers outnumber professional staff by more than 6 to 1. Typically, as the numbers and needs of the clientele increase, the agency reaches the point where compassion and volunteerism alone cannot handle all of the complex personal, social, economic, public relations, psychological, and political problems that assail it.

The Need for Institutionalism

As crisis agencies become well known and as their clientele are drawn from a wider segment of the community (to the point that the work cannot be handled by the communication system of grapevine, word of mouth, notepad, e-mail, and social media X (formerly know as Twitter)), the agency sees that if it is to continue to grow and serve its clients, it must institutionalize. The seeds of bureaucracy are thus born.

To manage all of its vital functions, the agency must centralize and formalize most aspects of its operation. It takes on a formal board of directors, establishes rigorous auditing and record-keeping functions, and requires more money, paid staff, and staff support. As crisis agencies become crisis organizations, they gain more power, prestige, and notoriety. They tend to attract the attention of the human services professions because they offer fertile fields for funded research, placement of practicum and internship students, and employment of graduates. Crisis agencies sometimes attain eminent success to the point that it becomes a vested interest of the human services professions to formalize the competencies of the personnel of such successful agencies through certification, licensure, and accreditation.

The progression from the humble origins of Alcoholics Anonymous as a support group formed by fellow individuals with alcoholism in the 1930s to the current classification of alcohol use disorder to the proliferation of thousands of treatment centers around the world, huge government funding for research and prevention, university courses on the subject, and the state licensure or certification of substance misuse counselors provides an outstanding example of the evolution from self-help by a group of people recovering from alcohol use disorder in crisis to the full institutionalization of the crisis of drug misuse.

As a specialty evolves, it develops its own empirical base, professional research, and writings. For example, for crisis intervention, we have publications such as *Crisis Intervention; Journal of Interpersonal Violence; Victimology, Violence and Victims,; Journal of Family Violence; Death Studies; Journal of Traumatic Stress; Suicide and Life Threatening Behavior; Child Abuse and Neglect; Journal of Child Sexual Abuse; Aggression and Violent Behavior;* and *Violence Against Women.* The amount of data and information in the field has expanded so much that the *Encyclopedia of Psychological Trauma* (Reyes et al., 2008) includes 720 large pages covering everything from A (Abuse, child physical) to W (Workplace violence).

Specialty areas may also attain a distinct level of recognition by building a base of national or regional affiliates, as with various topic- or malady-centered hotlines, chat rooms, and websites; AA chapters; spouse abuse centers; and victim assistance programs. Local, state, regional, and national conferences are organized to provide for the exchange of ideas and problem-solving strategies. These conferences range from specialty areas that bring together some of the greatest research minds in the field, such as the First Annual Conference on Trauma, Loss, and Dissociation in 1995, to "in the trenches" conferences such as the Crisis Intervention Team International (CITI) convention, which provides practical, hands-on programs for crisis intervention police officers who deal with the mentally ill.

The emergence of hundreds of crisis-oriented organizations in the 1970s, 1980s, and 1990s (Maurer & Sheets, 1999) and the realization of the role that immediate intervention plays in alleviating traumatic stress (Mitchell & Everly, 1995) attest to the dramatic transformation and professional acceptance of crisis intervention from a psychological backwater field to a pervasive specialty. It is worth noting that the main literacy magazine of the American Counseling Association ran as its featured article in the August 2021 edition of *Counseling Today* that crisis counseling had become every counselor's job (Bray, 2021). Probably the best testament to the center stage on which crisis intervention is now playing is the birth in 2006 of the American Psychological Association's newest division, Division 56, Trauma Psychology, along with the provision of counseling (Council for Accreditation of Counseling & Educationally Related Programs, 2009) and school psychology (National Association of School Psychologists, 2010) professional accreditation standards for training graduates in crisis intervention. One of the major players in the field of trauma, Christine Courtois (Courtois & Gold, 2009), has eloquently stated the critical need for the inclusion of psychological trauma training in all helping service curricula. Thus, like lots of other concepts in mental health that evolve and continue to grow to meet increased demands for crisis services, it is incumbent that beginners in the mental health field understand the processes and evidence-based practices associated with crisis intervention (Cutler et al., 2013) that this book is about.

The Media and the Societal Impetus for Crisis Intervention

Why, from the 1970s to the present, has the crisis intervention movement experienced such extraordinary growth? Probably no single factor alone can explain why. In the United States, the bombing of the

Murrah Federal Building in Oklahoma City, 9/11, the mega natural disaster of Hurricane Katrina, the mass shootings at Virginia Tech, Northern Illinois University, Columbine High School, the Sandy Hook and Uvalde elementary schools, and a variety of public massacres such as Las Vegas and El Paso have all given rise to the demand for crisis intervention. Yet, such natural and human-made disasters have been with us since the city of Pompeii was buried by Mt. Vesuvius and Rome was sacked and burned. What has changed public perception to the extent that the acronym PTSD—which in the first edition of this book was a brand-new term that lots of psychologists were unfamiliar with or didn't believe was a valid diagnostic—is now common parlance?

The media's role in creating awareness of crises and crisis intervention has probably generated the most profound change in public consciousness of what it means to be in crisis after a large-scale disaster. When Matthew Brady's pictures of the windrows of dead from the American Civil War Battle of Antietam were put on display in New York in 1863, this first use of photographic media changed forever how people would perceive wars and the psychological trauma that invariably comes with them. Public perception of war as glorious changed forever as its horror and carnage were brought to the American doorstep by Brady's harrowing pictures. Since that time, the ability of the media has advanced from the still-life daguerreotypes of Brady to real-time sound and video of the jumpers from the 9/11 Twin Towers, New Orleans citizens sitting on top of flooded buildings from Katrina, and of Kiev residents running from a drone bombing, all of which come into your living room in real time in graphic detail.

Charlotte Huff's article on the stress of media overload in negative news coverage in the November (2022) issue of *Monitor on Psychology* raises some interesting questions about how the mainstream media and social media affect the perception of viewers and readers and potentially contributes to negative mental health outcomes from negative news overload. It raises the question of how potent the media is in the creation of vicarious crisis associations and whether that has metastatic effects in the spread of it. She reports on the phenomena of *"doomscrolling"* or feeling impending doom when scrolling excessively through negative news.

Probably even more profound is the emerging role of social media with the good and ill it can bring into a crisis milieu and the questions it brings with it: How well are individuals able to separate fact from fiction and override misinformation transmitted through social media (Wang et al., 2022)? How does collective memory sway users' thinking and acting during a crisis? Does time spent involved in a crisis-related social medium lead to mental health impairment (El Frenn et al., 2022) and panic behavior (Dia et al., 2022)? There is some evidence that it does have deleterious effects on mental health (El Frenn et al., 2022; Price et al., 2022). Or is it, in fact, a positive outlet of personal catharsis and emotional and cognitive problem solving (Goode, 2022). It is still unclear exactly what impact such real-time media has on the public, but clearly, it does have an impact and changes our perception of the world as ever smaller, more interconnected, and certainly more dangerous, unsafe, and crisis prone (Marshall et al., 2007). At its best, it has brought acceptance of trauma and crisis intervention procedures into the public mainstream and raised consciousness that failure to navigate through them without help is not some character defect. An outstanding example is the following farm publication's outreach to its readers.

One would be hard pressed to find a publication more unlike the Illinois Farm Bureau weekly newspaper to be in the business of promoting good mental health for its readership, but as of this writing in April 2023, that is exactly the case (Sloup, 2023). American farmers day in and day out are besieged with multiple stressors in producing a crop. This often results in severe stress and opens a Pandora's box of mental health issues that are exacerbated by embarrassment, an unwillingness to obtain help, and particularly the lack of accessibility to mental health help in rural areas.

A very positive approach to this problem in Illinois has been launched by the University of Illinois Agricultural Extension service in conjunction with the Illinois Farm Bureau by coordinating and publicizing a United States Department of Agriculture (USDA) funded voucher program. It is designed to broaden access for agricultural producers and their families to mental health services and provides vouchers for up to three free mental health sessions. Conjointly, the Southern Illinois University School of Medicine Center for Rural Health and Social Service Development is offering free telehealth counseling sessions with up to six free sessions. No insurance backup is required for either program (Sloup, 2023). There are valid reasons for the widespread acceptance of crisis intervention as a therapeutic specialty, and media examples such as this has certainly played a part in that shift.

COVID-19 and the Rise of Telebehavioral Health

The COVID-19 pandemic changed the way the world operated, and it certainly changed the way a great deal of the format of psychotherapy and crisis intervention and how it had been provided (Myers, 2021). A historic shift from face-to-face to telebehavioral therapy occurred and reshaped the clinical skills therapy used to fit an online environment (Rhodes, 2023). Along with the legal ramifications of the provision of those services (Wheeler, 2023), practitioners had to be mindful and adhere to the new ACA (2014) internet usage standards. Further on the horizon but looming quickly is the role that technology (Phillips, 2019) and artificial intelligence will have in therapy (Giovannetti, 2023). This evolution of therapeutic provision will be discussed at length in Chapter 6, "Telephone and Online Crisis Counseling."

A Positive Shift in Attitude

As a result of such programs and publicity, people in general have become more positive in their acceptance of outreach strategies following a crisis and are more knowledgeable about its psychological ramifications, such as PTSD. There is less "blaming the victim" as somehow psychologically inadequate. Probably most important from a pragmatic point of view, it is cost effective (Roberts, 1991). People in human services and political leadership positions have discovered that when they either ignore crisis situations or leave solutions entirely to the experts who have little political clout, lasting solutions elude them, and the leaders themselves are blamed and held publicly responsible. Reactive responding has not worked very well.

Leaders have discovered that endemic crises will not easily go away and that reaction or no action may result in problems metastasizing out of control. In a sense, then, political expediency has dictated not only the widespread acceptance of effective crisis intervention strategies but also that crisis intervention become proactive, preventive, and integrated on the local, national, and international levels. One need go no further than the aftermath of Hurricane Katrina to understand the full impact of what this paragraph is about.

The Case Against Too Much "Helping"

With the rise of postintervention psychological assistance in the last 20 years, an interesting phenomenon has started to emerge. "Do-gooder" individuals and paternalistic bureaucracies appear on the scene and want to "straighten" things out and "help" people. Van den Eynde and Veno (1999) reported the case of an Australian community that literally had to kick government "help" out of town after the discovery of a case of long-term mass pedophilia in their midst. Even though the community clearly had the situation under control, the government authorities kept insisting they did not. What they had to do to get the government out of their town is interesting reading indeed.

In a worst-case scenario, crass commercialization, pseudoscience, vicarious thrills, and outright fraud mark the traumatic wake of a crisis (Echterling & Wylie, 1999; Gist, et al., 1999a; Gist, et al., 1999b; Lohr et al., 1999). Gist, et al., (1999) have coined the term "trauma tourism" to describe the burgeoning industry in postintervention psychological trauma replete with trade shows, trade publications, talk shows, and charitable giving and bus tours of trauma areas. Indeed, such tours became so acrimonious in New Orleans that tour companies were fined by city officials for bus tours through the devastated ninth ward of that city (Brown, 2012).

The assumption is that disaster invariably leads to psychopathology, and psychopathology sells. If people are perceived as incapable of caring for themselves and are traumatized and in a panic state after a disaster, it follows that they must be somehow infirm and unequal to the task and need assistance. A paternalistic government is then tasked with taking care of them. This view may be even more true with marginalized and disenfranchised groups who are seen as socially or technically unsophisticated and in need of benevolent and well-intentioned guidance and protection (Gist, Lubin et al., 1999a; Kaniasty & Norris, 1999; Ober et al., 2000). On the other hand, such groups of disenfranchised and dislocated persons, particularly if they are migrants or undocumented persons, may be given short shrift by the authorities and may be persecuted if they come to the attention of bureaucracies that are dealing with a crisis (Brown, 2009, pp. 215–226). It is with good reason that activists in the counseling field have proposed that social justice is the new benchmark against which crisis intervention and training should be measured (Espelage, 2022; Mamarosh, 2022; Rector, 2021;

Smith et al., 2022), and that is particularly true in the aftermath of disasters.

However, the fact is that in most instances, victims of disaster do not panic. They organize themselves in a collective manner and go about the business of helping one another and restoring equilibrium (Kaniasty & Norris, 1999). Called the "altruistic or therapeutic community," the typical immediate collective response to a disaster is characterized by the disappearance of community conflicts, heightened internal solidarity, charity, sharing, communal public works, and a positive "can-do" attitude (Barton, 1969; Giel, 1990). So, as of 2023, crisis intervention has emerged from a psychological backwater 40 years ago when we started writing the first edition of this book to a veritable tidal wave of interest, although at times controversial and full of heated debate, and that includes defining exactly what a crisis is.

Definitions of Crisis

LO2 This book is mainly about doing crisis intervention with individuals and microsystems such as families and workplaces. To a lesser extent, it is also about macrosystems in crisis and how the crisis interventionist functions within those systems, whether in institutions such as hospitals, schools, and mental health centers or as service providers after large-scale disasters. To that end, we start this book in a pretty boring way by giving you not only a history lesson but also a long list of definitions of crisis as it applies to both individuals and systems. We apologize for that, but we do this because we want you to understand that this business is still so new that the definition of an individual or a system in crisis is by no means fixed or absolute. As a matter of fact, as you are going to find throughout this book, there is a whole lot about crisis and crisis intervention that is not fixed or absolute! Consider, then, the following definitions of individuals in crisis.

Individual Crisis Definitions

1. People are in a state of crisis when they face an obstacle to important life goals—an obstacle that is, for a time, insurmountable by the use of customary methods of problem solving. A period of disorganization ensues, a period of upset, during which many abortive attempts at solution are made (Caplan, 1961, p. 18).

2. A crisis arises from a traumatic event that is unpredictable and uncontrollable. There is an inability to influence it by one's actions. The nature of the event changes values and priorities, and indeed changes everything (Sarri, 2005, pp. 19–24).

3. Crisis is a crisis because the individual knows no response to deal with a situation (Carkhuff & Berenson, 1977, p. 165).

4. Crisis is a personal difficulty or situation that immobilizes people and prevents them from consciously controlling their lives (Belkin, 1984, p. 424).

5. Crisis is a state of disorganization in which people face frustration of important life goals or profound disruption of their life cycles and methods of coping with stressors. The term *crisis* usually refers to a person's feelings of fear, shock, and distress *about* the disruption, not to the disruption itself (Brammer, 1985, p. 94).

6. Crisis is a temporary breakdown of coping. Expectations are violated and waves of emotion such as anger, anxiety, guilt, and grief surface. Old problems and earlier losses may surface. The event's intensity, duration, and suddenness may affect the severity of response to the crisis (Poland & McCormick, 1999, p. 6).

7. Crisis is a loss of psychological equilibrium or a state of emotional instability that includes elements of depression and anxiety which is caused by an external event with which individuals are unable to cope with at their usual level of ability (Kleespies, 2009, p. 15).

8. Crisis in a clinical context refers to an acute emotional upset arising from situational, developmental, or sociocultural sources, and results in a temporary inability to cope by means of one's usual problem-solving devices (Hoff et al., 2009, p. 4).

9. A crisis may be a catastrophic event or a series of life stresses that build rapidly and accumulate such that the person's homeostatic balance is disturbed and creates a vulnerable state, which, if not resolved, avoided, or redefined will cause self-righting devices to no longer be effective and plunge the person into psychological disequilibrium (Golan, 1978, p. 8).

It should immediately become clear that the term *crisis* has different meanings to different people and is used to describe a variety of incidents, settings, and situations and the adaptations, albeit less than adequate, that people attempt to make in response to them. To summarize these definitions, for an individual, **crisis** is the perception or experiencing of an event or situation as an intolerable difficulty that exceeds the person's current resources and coping mechanisms. Unless the person obtains relief, the crisis has the potential to cause severe affective, behavioral, and cognitive malfunctioning up to the point of instigating injurious or lethal behavior to oneself or others. At that point, the crisis becomes a behavioral emergency (Kleespies, 2009).

Behavioral Emergencies

A **behavioral emergency** occurs when a crisis escalates to the point that the situation requires immediate intervention to avoid injury or death to oneself or others, or the person is in imminent risk of serious injury or death by another. Direct or intentional behavioral emergencies fall into the general categories of engaging in self-injurious behavior, perpetrating violent interpersonal behavior, and being a victim of violence as opposed to a behavioral crisis, which may not necessarily be potentially lethal (Kleespies, 2009, p. 13; Kleespies, 2014, pp. 11–12). Suicides/homicides resulting from broken romances provide a classic example of these categories. One might suppose that behavioral emergencies only occur in hospital emergency rooms or CIT officer contacts with out-of-control mentally ill individuals who misuse substances and are otherwise cognitively impaired in some manner. While Pinkhasov and associates (2020) have found that to indeed be true in a significant numbers of cases that show up in hospital ERs, that is only a small percentage of behavioral emergencies. Take a guess where the large majority of them happen?

Chances are, it's going to be in the chair sitting opposite to yours in a counseling session. Behavioral emergencies occur dynamically when emotional dysregulation occurs and subsequent attempts to regain homeostasis are not successful. If unchecked, dysregulation continues to escalate and becomes a behavioral emergency with potentially life-threatening consequences that can have long-term, transcrisis outcomes, and those often happen in one-on-one or group counseling sessions (Ford, 2021). Very little had been said about our concept of transcrisis until Julian Ford did an excellent job detailing it in his *Crisis in the Psychotherapy Session* book (2021). You need to understand it is very real, and with the transcrisis points that exist in it, it is present in every human service worker's environment, and you need to be prepared to deal with it.

We believe that **indirect and noncommissioned behavioral emergencies** can also occur. Indirect behavioral emergencies occur when people make bad decisions and wind up placing themselves in potentially lethal situations. Indirect and noncommissioned behavioral emergencies are crises that happen with no directed purpose or intentionality to do something harmful to oneself or others. Drunk driving, boating, snow skiing, swimming, and project construction may all turn into behavioral emergencies that have the potential for injurious or lethal behavior and call for intervention. A parent who, after receiving a phone call informing her that her child has been seriously injured in a school bus accident, becomes hysterical, leaves her newborn at home with a pot of cooking oil boiling on the stove, and drives 90 miles an hour to the hospital is creating a behavioral emergency to put it mildly. Persons with borderline personality disorder are the archetype of people whose unstable lifestyles continuously set them up to fly into crisis after crisis and oftentimes move quickly into behavioral emergencies by impulsively deciding to complete suicide or engage in **parasuicide behavior** (accidentally doing something or going into a situation a reasonable person wouldn't and getting themself killed).

More often than we would like to imagine, not only crisis interventionists but also common, every day, human service workers and first responders will deal with people whose behavior has escalated to the point that they can be considered to be experiencing behavioral emergencies. For that reason, when you first make the acquaintance of the Triage Assessment Form in Chapter 3, "The Intervention and Assessment Models," you will note that scores of 10 (maximum) on the form's scales all have lethal feeling, behaving, and thinking as part of their assessment anchors.

Systemic Crisis Definitions

LO3 "Individual crisis" is really something of an oxymoron because as most crises unfold, they rarely remain confined to one person. They ripple out and affect numerous other people who interact with the person in crisis. To think that the crisis created by a date rape or a parent with alcohol misuse disorder affects only the person who was assaulted or the parent who drinks is to have a very wrong notion indeed about what a crisis is and what you may have to do and with whom you may work. Therefore, when we consider a definition of crisis, we are bound to examine how that crisis affects the system within which the individual operates. For most individuals, the first ripple effect of a crisis will be within the family system. Although you will meet numerous family members as they are affected by various kinds of crisis in this book, we have developed a new chapter that more closely examines the family system itself as it is impacted as opposed to the individual originally targeted by the crisis.

Systemic crises may come in many forms. They may be economically based, perhaps affecting only the families of a small produce chain that goes bankrupt when the refrigeration in their warehouse fails or when supply chains fail during the COVID-19 epidemic, and they cannot obtain produce or keep help. They may be natural disasters, as small as a tornado tearing up a small Kansas farming community or as large as a COVID-19 mega epidemic that kills millions. They may be human made, ranging from a structural failure that causes a building to collapse to wars that kill and displace millions of people. They may be psychologically based, ranging from fear of a school bully to an entire nation rendered paranoid by the terrorist attacks of 9/11. As you will see in the last chapter of this book, large-scale disasters that become systemic crises most generally fit the public perception of what crisis intervention is about. Indeed, the role of crisis interventionists as mental health service providers in that setting is becoming larger and larger. Consider, then, the following definitions of a system in crisis, in which the term *system* ranges across families, churches, businesses, neighborhoods, communities, large cities, geographical flood plains, and nations.

1. A crisis that threatens the organization is unexpected, demands a rapid response in a short time frame, and threatens its basic values (Hermann, 1963, p. 63).
2. Communities in crisis have several characteristics in common with individuals. Within the group there is an atmosphere of tension and fear. Rumors run rampant. Typical functioning is at a standstill, schools and businesses are closed, and health and emergency resources may be in short supply (Hoff et al., 2009, p. 209).
3. Communities in crisis go through chronological stages following a disaster that are known as the impact, heroic/rescue, honeymoon, disillusionment, and reconstruction/recovery phase. Each phase has identifiable characteristics and sequential timelines and depending on how the various systems in the community react, may move forward positively or not (Roberts, 2005, p. 205).

4. A systemic crisis is a negative event or outcome, which includes the element of surprise, disruption of operations, and is a threat to the property, financial and physical resources, well-being of individuals within the system, and the reputation of the system to provide for the well-being of its constituency (Zdziarski et al., 2007, p. 6).

Mega Crisis

The King Kong of a systemic crisis is a **mega crisis**. Whether you know it or not, you have all been involved in a mega crisis. Whether you were directly affected or tangentially so, the COVID-19 pandemic was a mega crisis (Parrott, 2020). Helsloot and associates (2012) very aptly characterize a mega crisis as, "Not just more of the same, but a crisis that defies boundaries, limits, neat demarcations, patterned connections, and linear consequences" (p. 5). Mega crises are threats to the very existence of the systems it affects. They generate unprecedented and apparently unmanageable challenges. Indecision is fatal in addressing them, particularly when real time tempo is speeded up and relying on past reaction models is fatal to positive outcomes as well (Lagedec, 2012, p.13).

There is no example we can think of short of the World Wars that exemplifies chaos theory at work better than the COVID-19 pandemic. Its onset brought dramatic changes to the culture and the ecosystem of the entire planet. It certainly did so to the operating systems and procedures of counseling and crisis intervention, and its effects on this discipline can be found throughout this new edition.

To sum up what we believe generally defines a **systemic crisis**: When a traumatic event occurs such that people, institutions, communities, and ecologies are overwhelmed and response systems are unable to effectively contain and control the event in regard to both physical and psychological reactions to it, the crisis has become systemic. The size of the system may range from a family to a mental health clinic, to a nation, to the world, but the main identifying factor is that the system is in disequilibrium and previous response systems and coping mechanisms no longer work. If adequate intervention doesn't occur, the potential exists for irreparable damage or termination of the system. Sandwiched between individual and systemic crises is another type of crisis with which the interventionist is likely to be faced, which we have called a "*metastasizing* crisis."

Metastasizing Crisis

A **metastasizing crisis** occurs when a small, isolated incident is not contained and begins to spread. The analogy to the spread of cancer is apt because what may start out as a focal and localized problem that could have been easily cured with early, preemptive intervention, if it is not diagnosed or remedied but is allowed to grow through benign neglect, it may suddenly become endemic within the system. At that point, it is anything but easy to excise or remedy. A school system's neglect in dealing with isolated cases of bullying can soon lead to a culture of bullying that moves out of the classroom and into cyberspace to pervade and wreak havoc on students' lives 24 hours a day. Predispositioning both personnel and resources can go a long way toward what is called *primary* intervention, which seeks to proactively handle problems before they metastasize and get out of control. From that standpoint, many crisis interventionists are also engaged in **primary prevention**, stopping a problem before it starts, as well as **secondary intervention**, minimizing the harmful effects that have already occurred (Caplan, 1964).

Characteristics of Crisis

The following discussion of characteristics of crisis represents an expanded definition of what *crisis* means.

Presence of Both Danger and Opportunity. Crisis is a *danger* because it can overwhelm the individual to the extent that serious pathology, including homicide and suicide, may result. Crisis is also an *opportunity* because the pain it induces impels the person to seek help (Aguilera & Messick, 1982, p. 1). If the individual takes advantage of the opportunity, the intervention can help plant the seeds of self-growth and self-realization (Brammer, 1985, p. 95). People can react in any one of three ways to crisis. Under ideal circumstances, many individuals can cope effectively with crisis by themselves and develop strength from the experience. They change and grow in a positive manner and come out of the crisis both stronger and more compassionate (Danish, 1977).

Others appear to survive the crisis but effectively block the hurtful effect from awareness, only to have it haunt them in innumerable ways throughout the rest of their lives. Yet others break down psychologically at the onset of the crisis and clearly demonstrate that they are incapable of going any further with their lives unless given immediate and intensive assistance (Rapoport, 1967).

Seeds of Growth and Change. In the disequilibrium that accompanies crisis, anxiety is always present, and its discomfort provides an impetus for change (Janosik, 1984, p. 39). Often, anxiety must reach the boiling point before the person is ready to admit the problem is out of control. One need look no further than the substance abuser for affirmation of this assertion. By waiting too long, for example, individuals with substance misuse disorder may become so entrenched that they may need a therapeutic jackhammer to break the addiction down into manageable pieces. Even here, however, a threshold point for change may be reached, albeit in last-ditch desperation, when the abuser finally surrenders to the fact that something must be done.

No Panaceas or Quick Fixes. People in crisis are generally amenable to help through a variety of forms of intervention, some of which are described as *brief therapy* (Cormier & Hackney, 1987, p. 240). For problems of long duration, however, quick fixes are rarely available. Many problems of clients in severe crisis stem from the fact that the clients sought quick fixes in the first place, usually through a pill. Such a "fix" may dampen the dreadful responses but doesn't change the instigating stimulus, so the crisis deepens.

The Necessity of Choice. Life is a process of interrelated crises and challenges that we confront or not, deciding to live or not (Carkhuff & Berenson, 1977, p. 173). In the realm of crisis, *not to choose is a choice,* and this choice usually turns out to be negative and destructive. *Choosing to do something* at least contains the seeds of growth and allows a person the chance to set goals and formulate a plan to begin to overcome the dilemma.

Universality and Idiosyncrasy. Disequilibrium or disorganization accompanies every crisis, whether universal or idiosyncratic (Janosik, 1984, p. 13). Crisis is universal because no one is immune to breakdown given the right constellation of circumstances. It is idiosyncratic because what one person may successfully overcome, another may not, even though the circumstances are virtually the same. It is foolhardy to maintain a belief that one is immune to psychic assaults, that one can handle any crisis in a stable, poised, and masterful fashion. Thousands of "tough" veterans of the Vietnam, Afghanistan, and two Gulf Wars suffering from posttraumatic stress disorder (PTSD), who have turnstiled through VA hospitals, veterans' centers, and other medical facilities, are convincing proof that when a crisis boils over, disorganization, disequilibrium, disorientation, and fragmentation of an individual's coping mechanisms can occur no matter how conditioned against psychological trauma the person may be.

Resiliency. Yet, the National Comorbidity Survey found that while their nationally representative sample had more than a 50 percent prevalence of traumatic events for both men and women, only about 5 percent of men and 10 percent of women developed PTSD (Kessler et al., 1995). One of the key jobs of the crisis interventionist is finding the right combination of support systems and coping mechanisms and forming them into action plans that will tap the reservoir of resiliency that most people have to move them through and beyond the crisis.

Perception. As paradoxical as it may seem, the precipitating event is not the major cause of the crisis. It is the *perception* of the event that plays a huge role in a crisis. How individuals interpret events has a great deal to do with how amenable the crisis will be to resolution (Callahan, 2009, p. 21). As the old adage states, "One man's fruit may be another man's poison." It is no accident that the Cognitive scale in the Triage Assessment Form that you will encounter in Chapter 3, "The Intervention and Assessment Models," is the most complex of the three scales. How people appraise precipitating events and what the interventionist can do to reframe and temper catastrophic interpretations of the event will have a great deal to do with how well and how quickly the crisis is alleviated.

Complicated Symptomology. Crisis is *not* simple; it is complex and difficult to understand, and it defies cause-and-effect description (Brammer, 1985, p. 91; Kliman, 1978, p. xxi). The symptoms that overlie precipitating crisis events become tangled webs that crisscross all environments of an individual. When an event reaches a flash point, there may be so many compounding problems that crisis workers must intervene directly in a variety of areas. Furthermore, the environment of people in crisis strongly affects the ease or difficulty with which the crisis can be handled. Families, individuals, partners, institutions, and employees may all directly affect problem

resolution and a return to stability. When large numbers of people are affected at the same time by a crisis, the entire ecological system of a neighborhood, community, geographical region, or country may need intervention. Unless you have been living in Antarctica or a cave in Nepal, there is no better example than living the experience of quarantine with the COVID-19 outbreak. It affected every aspect of daily existence and was a harbinger of every kind of crisis imaginable.

Transcrisis States

Crises have typically been seen as time limited, usually persisting a maximum of 6 to 8 weeks, at the end of which the subjective discomfort diminishes (Janosik, 1984, p. 9). That view is now changing, and the effects of the original crisis may extend a good bit beyond that time frame (Callahan, 1998; Ford, 2021; Salzer & Bickman, 1999). Indeed, the impact of a crisis may last a lifetime (van der Kolk & McFarlane, 1996). What occurs during the immediate aftermath of the crisis event determines whether or not the crisis will become a disease reservoir that will be transformed into a chronic and long-term state. Although the original crisis event may be submerged below awareness, and the individual may believe the problem has been resolved, the appearance of new stressors may bring the individual to the crisis state again. This emotional roller coaster may occur frequently and for extended periods of time, ranging from months to years. An adult who has unresolved anger toward a dead parent and transfers that anger to other authority figures, such as supervisors or employers, is in a **transcrisis state**.

A transcrisis state is all too common with many therapeutic problems and can become the bane of a psychotherapist. This state becomes a way of life rather than a single speed bump in life's road, and people in this state tend to redefine themselves in terms of that state and are stuck in it. This chronic "stuckness" can translated into a negative smorgasbord of feelings of rage, guilt, anger, depression, fear, hopelessness, and failure. It can appear in and outside of therapy through continuous, ongoing breakdowns. It manifests in a dysfunctional lifestyle mode that continuously gets clients in trouble. Dealing with a transcrisis state can become very frustrating for a therapist who can become callous and inured to repetitive "behavioral emergencies" and trivialize them (Ford, 2021, p. 28). The individual with Borderline Personality

Disorder is a therapist's benchmark for transcrisis states and points, and when those waypoints are hit, standard therapy gets suspended, and they need to be dealt with using a crisis intervention model.

The adult may have apparently attained functional and adequate mental health. However, this appearance is gained at the cost of warding off and repressing the "unfinished business" of making peace with the lost parent. Later, during the stress related to getting along with another authority figure, the person blames that authority figure and has no conscious awareness that the unfinished repressed material (submerged in a transcrisis state) is at the root of the problem. Although the person with the transcrisis state may come to identify the problem as poor relationship skills and enter counseling to improve those skills, this action is also a symptom of the psychological roller-coaster ride that started with the unfinished business. The relationship skills may be temporarily improved, but the source of the transcrisis state may not have been recognized or expunged. It has merely subsided, and a temporary state of equilibrium has been achieved, but the original trauma will usually reemerge and instigate a new crisis the moment new stressors are introduced. Dynamically, this pattern is defensive repression. Therapeutically, this transcrisis state calls for crisis intervention techniques.

Transcrisis Differentiated from Posttraumatic Stress Disorder

People familiar with PTSD may ask, "So how is a transcrisis state different from PTSD?" First, PTSD is identifiable as a trauma and stress related disorder (American Psychiatric Association, 2013) caused by an extremely traumatic event, and very specific criteria must be present for a diagnosis of PTSD to be made. Although a person who is suffering from PTSD may be in a transcrisis state, not all people who are in a transcrisis state suffer from PTSD. Indeed, it would probably be more appropriate to look at all the different kinds of anxiety and personality disorders found in the fifth edition of the *Diagnostic and Statistical Manual of Mental Disorders* (DSM-5, DSM 5-TR, American Psychiatric Association, 2013, 2022) as representative of transcrisis states because of the chronic kinds of thinking, feeling, and acting that keep these individuals constantly in psychological hot, if not boiling, water.

But it is not just people with anxiety and personality disorders who may be in a transcrisis state. A broad range of people, from so-called normal individuals who are constantly fired from jobs because of their uncontrollable tempers to those with psychoses who quit taking their medicine because it has unpleasant side effects, are also representative of individuals in transcrisis states. Armsworth and Holaday (1993), in their review of affective, behavioral, cognitive, and physiological-somatic effects of trauma, identified a number of factors that, although not found in PTSD descriptors, would probably be inherent in many transcrisis states. The key differentiating element of a transcrisis state is that, whether it is due to trauma, personality traits, substance misuse, psychosis, or chronic environmental stressors, the state is residual and recurrent and always present to some degree. Although people in a transcrisis state are generally capable of functioning at some minimal level, they are always at risk, and any single small added stressor may tip the balance and send them into crisis. Therefore, when we assess individuals in crisis, our focus is not only on the current clinical/diagnostic state of the individual, but also, and as importantly, on the repetitious cycle of problems and the historical precursors that may have caused the crisis to arise. A medical analogy would be a person experiencing a chronic sinus condition who continually takes nasal decongestant and so can function, although at a less than optimum level. However, if the person is exposed to a virus, the sinus condition may progress to an infection and eventually pneumonia.

Being aware that someone is operating in a transcrisis state also gives us important information regarding the kind and degree of therapeutic intervention to provide in both the short and the long term. We probably would deal far differently with the salesperson who just turned 45, lost her job with a company she had been with for 20 years, has been unemployed for 6 months, and is now clinically depressed and suicidal than we would with the salesperson who just turned 45, lost her job for the 20th time, has been unemployed for 6 months, and is now clinically depressed and suicidal. Although immediate intervention in regard to the suicidal ideation of both women might be very similar, our view as to what caused the depression, how we would treat it, and what transcrisis issues we might expect would be very different. Paradoxically, transcrisis states may be seen as strength-based barriers that shield individuals and allow them to continue to cope in the face of chaos and can be used by the human service worker to good advantage if the transcrisis states can be reframed in terms of resilience (Ford, 2021, pp. 28–29) when transcrisis points arise.

Transcrisis Points

Transcrisis points occur frequently in transcrisis states within the therapeutic intervention. These points are generally marked by the client coming to grips with new developmental stages or other dimensions of the problem. Transcrisis points do not occur in regular, predictable, linear progression. For example, an abused spouse may go through transcrisis point after transcrisis point talking to a crisis worker over the telephone before making a decision to leave the battering relationship, often calling crisis workers a dozen times in the course of a few days. The abused spouse may then make a decision to leave the battering relationship and go to a spouse abuse shelter, only to find that the necessity of making a geographic move or finding a job instigates a crisis almost as potent as the battering.

Human services workers who practice long-term therapy are often shocked, confused, and overwhelmed by the sudden disequilibrium their clients experience. Handling these transcrisis points can be the equivalent of standing in the middle of a Los Angeles freeway and attempting to stop traffic. Behaviorally, such clients may vacillate from a placid to an agitated state so fast that the worker puts out one brush fire only to be confronted by yet another. It is at these transcrisis points that standard therapeutic strategies and techniques are suspended, and the therapist must operate in a directive crisis intervention mode. In particular, transcrisis points can be seen as benchmarks that are crucial to progressive stages of positive therapeutic growth, and they need to be hammered home in positive, reinforcing ways.

> HSW: Look what you have come through, grappled with, and are now breaking away from. Sure, there's anxiety and some fear when you get to these change points, but that's just a sign that change, positive change, is occurring. Those old ways of behaving helped you get through hard time, and testing out these new tools is a little scary but exciting, too. I think, and I am really proud of you for starting to put them in operation.

These points are characterized by approach-avoidance behavior in seeking help, taking risks, and initiating action steps toward forward movement. So, when encountering these transcrisis points, a person will experience the same kind of disorganization, disequilibrium, and fragmentation that surrounded the original crisis event. Leaping one hurdle does not necessarily mean that the entire crisis is successfully overcome. Survivors of a catastrophe may expunge the event from memory and then be faced with repairing gaping wounds in personal relationships that have been torn apart by their long-term pathological behavior. People who have spinal cord injuries may be successfully rehabilitated physically but may retreat into substance misuse or become depressed and/or suicidal as they attempt to begin a new lifestyle from a wheelchair.

Therefore, it is not only the initial crisis with which the worker must contend but also each transcrisis point as it occurs if clients are not to slip back into the pathology that assailed them in the first place. Transcrisis points should not be confused with the jumps and starts that go with working through typical adjustment problems. Although these points may be forecast with some degree of reliability by workers who are experts in the particular field, their onset is sudden, dramatic, and extremely potent. In that regard, these psychological aftershocks can be just as damaging as the initial tremor and may require extraordinary effort on the part of the human services worker to help the client regain control. This book is also concerned with these transcrisis states and points; many of the cases portrayed represent both components.

Theories of Crisis and Crisis Intervention

LO4 No single theory or school of thought encompasses every view of human crisis or all the models or systems of crisis intervention. We present here a brief overview of theories relevant both to crisis (as a phenomenon) and to crisis intervention (as an intentional helping response). Janosik (1984) conceptualizes crisis theory on three different levels: basic crisis theory, expanded crisis theory, and applied crisis theory.

Basic Crisis Intervention Theory

The research, writings, and teachings of Erich Lindemann (1944, 1956) gave professionals and paraprofessionals a new understanding of crisis. Lindemann helped caregivers promote crisis intervention for many sufferers of loss who had no specific pathological diagnosis but who were exhibiting symptoms that appeared pathological. Lindemann's basic crisis theory and work made a substantive contribution to the understanding of behavior in clients whose grief crises were precipitated by loss. He helped professionals and paraprofessionals recognize that behavioral responses to crises associated with grief are normal, temporary, and amenable to alleviation through short-term intervention techniques. These "normal" grief behaviors include (1) preoccupation with the lost one, (2) identification with the lost one, (3) expressions of guilt and hostility, (4) some disorganization in daily routine, and (5) some evidence of somatic complaints (Janosik, 1984, p. 11). Lindemann negated the prevailing perception that clients manifesting crisis responses should necessarily be treated as "abnormal " or pathological.

While Lindemann focused mainly on the immediate resolution of grief after loss, Caplan (1964) expanded Lindemann's constructs to the total field of traumatic events. Caplan viewed crisis as a state resulting from impediments to life goals that cannot be overcome through customary behaviors. These impediments can arise from both developmental and situational events. Both Lindemann and Caplan dealt with crisis intervention following psychological trauma using an equilibrium/disequilibrium paradigm. The stages in Lindemann's paradigm are (1) disturbed equilibrium, (2) brief therapy or grief work, (3) client working through the problem or grief, and (4) restoration of equilibrium (Janosik, 1984, pp. 10–12). Caplan linked Lindemann's concepts and stages to all developmental and situational events and extended crisis intervention to eliminating the affective, behavioral, and cognitive distortions that precipitated the psychological trauma in the first place.

Differentiating Basic Crisis Theory from Brief Therapy. The work of both Lindemann and Caplan gave impetus to the use of crisis intervention strategies in counseling and brief therapy with people manifesting universal human reactions to traumatic events. While **brief therapy theory** typically attempts to remediate more or less ongoing emotional problems, **basic crisis theory**, following the lead of Lindemann and Caplan, focuses on helping people in crisis recognize and correct temporary affective, behavioral, and cognitive distortions brought on by traumatic events. Although brief or solution-focused therapy may be the equivalent of crisis intervention (in that it seeks to restore the person to a state of homeostasis or equilibrium), not all brief or solution-focused therapy is related to crisis intervention.

Perhaps the following example will clarify the difference between the two. A student fails one algebra test and concludes that they can never pass algebra and, therefore, cannot become an engineer (as the parents are perceived to expect/demand). The student progresses to a feeling of helplessness, then to hopelessness, and then contemplates suicide. Here, crisis intervention that focuses on suicide prevention is clearly indicated. Another student fails one algebra test and, feeling uncomfortable, disappointed, and confused, makes an appointment to see the school counselor. Here, the modality becomes a typical brief or solution-focused therapy situation in which the emphasis is on how to improve study habits and test-taking skills.

Differentiating between brief or solution-focused therapy and crisis intervention depends on how intensely the client views the problem as intolerable or on how much emotional disequilibrium the client experiences. Severe emotional disequilibrium over the event may escalate the person into crisis and the therapist into a crisis intervention modality.

Expanded Crisis Theory

Expanded crisis theory was developed because basic theory, which depended on a psychoanalytic approach alone, did not adequately address the social, environmental, and situational factors that make an event a crisis. As crisis theory and intervention have expanded, it has become clear that an approach that identifies predisposing factors as the main or only causal agent falls short of the mark. A prime example of this restrictive view was the erroneous diagnosis by practitioners who first encountered PTSD victims that pathology preceding the crisis event was the real cause of the trauma. While preceding factors can certainly create a fertile field for PTSD and other psychopathology, it has become apparent that, given the right combination of developmental, sociological, psychological, environmental, and situational determinants, anyone can fall victim to transient pathological symptoms. Therefore, expanded crisis theory draws not only from psychoanalytic theory but also from general systems, ecosystems, adaptational, interpersonal, chaos, and developmental theory. The following are synopses of the major theoretical components of the expanded view.

Psychoanalytic Theory. Psychoanalytic theory (Fine, 1973), applied to expanded crisis theory, is based on the view that the disequilibrium that accompanies a person's crisis can be understood by gaining access to the individual's unconscious thoughts and past emotional experiences. Psychoanalytic theory presupposes that some early childhood fixation is the primary explanation for why an event becomes a crisis. This theory may be used to help clients develop insight into the dynamics and causes of their behavior as the crisis situation acts on them (Safran & Hunter, 2020).

We have come almost completely full circle in our view of this approach. First thought to be the only valid way to view pathology resulting from trauma, then dismissed as patently false and an excuse for the government not to meet the medical needs of veterans suffering from PTSD, current treatment approaches see predisposing factors as one of the many factors that can contribute to PTSD and other psychopathologies.

Systems Theory. Systems theory (Haley, 1973, 1976; Hardy, 1997) is based not so much on what happens within an individual in crisis as on the interrelationships and interdependence among people and between people and events. Belkin (1984) adds that this theory "refers to an emotional system, a system of communications, and a system of need fulfillment and request" in which all members within an intergenerational relationship bring something to bear on the others, and each derives something from the others (pp. 350–351). Indeed, Slaikeu (1990, p. 6) defines crisis intervention as "a helping process aimed at assisting a person or a *family* so that the probability of debilitating effects is minimized, and the probability of growth is maximized."

Systems theory represents a turning away from traditional approaches, which focus only on what is going on within the client. A standard systems approach to crisis may be thought of in interpersonal terms. Systems theory is contextual in that it suggests that we look at the environment within which the person lives and the dynamic interactions the person has within that environment, which can provide information into the predisposing factors, onset, length, intensity, and resolution. It is not static but evolutionary, adaptable and flexible in its application and in defining what a "family system" is and how that fits in with the intervention (Fiese et al., 2019; Slaikeu, 1990). Normally the "environment" in basic systems theory can be thought of as the extended family unit, the neighborhood, school, job, social clubs, fraternal or civic organizations, beauty parlors, bars, church, and so on.

Ecosystems Theory. Ecosystems theory (Bronfenbrenner, 1995) broadens out the base of the system and looks at crisis in relation to the environmental context within which it occurs (James et al, 2003; Myer & Moore, 2006). Systemic interactions may occur from the microsystem (family and community) out to the macrosystem (nation) or vice versa. There is great value in looking at crises in their total social and environmental settings—not simply as one individual being affected in a linear progression of cause-and-effect events (Hardy, 1997; James & Gilliland, 2003, pp. 336–368). Cook (2012, pp. 6–7) proposes that an ecological counseling perspective operates with three fundamental propositions: First, while behavior is personal (the individual), it also contextual (the physical environment and the culture within which the individual operates); second, behavior is interactional in the sense that individuals influence and are influenced by the environments within which they function; third, individuals attempt to control and make sense of the environments they are engaging, which ranges from their romantic choices, their career preferences, the churches they decide to attend, or their recreational decisions to collect stamps as opposed to climbing mountains. Thus, people continuously attempt to make meaning of the multiple contexts in the environment so they can operate effectively, and that is no small chore. These three propositions take on added importance during a crisis because all the previous meaning making and sense of how one *has* operated effectively in a familiar environment may go flying out the window in a crisis environment where chaos calls for a whole new set of tactics and strategies.

The fundamental concept of ecosystems theory is analogous to "ecological systems in which all elements are interrelated, and in which change at any level of those interrelated parts will lead to alteration of the total system" (Cormier & Hackney, 1987, p. 217). The passage of time, proximity to the epicenter of the crisis, what develops over time, and the environment all contribute to the ultimate resolution of the crisis. Ecosystems theory comes into play most typically when large-scale disasters occur and affect very large **macrosystems (the total culture in which people live)**. The expanding role of communication systems and their ability or inability to link systems is a critical ingredient that will be explored in Chapter 16, "Disaster Response."

Adaptational Theory. Adaptational theory, as we use the term, depicts a person's crisis as being sustained through maladaptive behaviors, negative thoughts, and destructive defense mechanisms. Adaptational crisis theory is based on the premise that the person's crisis will recede when these maladaptive coping behaviors are changed to adaptive behaviors.

Breaking the chain of maladjusted functioning means changing to adaptive behavior, promoting positive thoughts, and constructing defense mechanisms that will help the person overcome the immobility created by the crisis and move to a positive mode of functioning. As maladaptive behaviors are learned, so may adaptive behaviors be learned. Aided by the interventionist, the client may learn to replace old, debilitating behaviors with new, self-enhancing ones. Such new behaviors may be applied directly to the context of the crisis and ultimately result in either success or reinforcement for the client in overcoming the crisis (Cormier & Cormier, 1985, p. 148; Meichenbaum, 2005; Sokol & Fox, 2020). People who have learned ineffective coping skills and continue to use them even though they continually wind up in psychological hot water best manifest this approach. Changing ingrained and entrenched behaviors and thoughts that create transcrisis invariably means changing maladaptive mechanisms and coping skills—not an easy job!

Interpersonal Theory. Interpersonal theory (Rogers, 1977) is built on many of the dimensions Cormier and Hackney (1987) describe as enhancing personal self-esteem: openness, trust, sharing, safety, unconditional positive regard, accurate empathy, and genuineness (pp. 35–64). The essence of interpersonal theory is that people cannot sustain a personal state of crisis for very long if they believe in themselves and in others and have confidence that they can become self-actualized and overcome the crisis. Rogers' (1961) person-centered approach's belief that people are resilient and can self-actualize and prosper under the toughest of circumstances fits well with crisis intervention. When people confer their locus of self-evaluation on others, they become dependent on others for validation of their being (Raskin & Rogers, 1995). Therefore, as long as a person maintains an external locus of control, the crisis will persist. Building deep, empathic relationships with clients is critical from a Rogerian perspective (1961) and is especially so in establishing initial contact with persons in crisis and providing support in allowing them to regain control of the situation.

Thus, the outcome goal in interpersonal theory is returning the power of self-evaluation to the person.

Doing so enables the person to once again control their own destiny and regain the ability to take whatever action is needed to cope with the crisis situation. In terms of crisis intervention, interpersonal theory is reflected in the initial tasks of Predispositioning, Problem Exploration, and Providing Support in our overall crisis intervention model to be introduced in Chapter 3, "The Intervention and Assessment Models."

Relational Cultural Theory. The major problem with interpersonal theory is that it gives little thought or credence to the tangled web of cultural, system, and ecological variables that play significant roles in how crises fulminate and what they mean in regard to attempts at intervention. **Relational Cultural Theory** evolved out of Jean Miller's (1976) book, toward a *New Psychology Of Women*, which was a feminist reaction to entrenched linear, individualistic, cognitive theories. Jordan (2000, 2018) seized on Miller's work and built a counseling theory that focused on developing empathic relationships that were deeply interwoven within the client's culture and its operating systems. This theory will be reviewed extensively as a bedrock theory for multiculturalism and crisis in Chapter 2, "Culturally Effective Helping in Crisis." A major axiom of their theory is that when crises arise, there is disconnection, in which individuals separate from their support system. In attempting to remove themselves from the crisis stimulus, support systems are often abandoned, and that is a critical component in fostering hopelessness and helplessness. Support systems and the need for them is a cornerstone of every crisis intervention model of which we are aware (Aguilera, 1998; Kanel, 2011; Roberts, 2005; Sandoval, 2013), including our own.

Another major tenet of RCT is its tolerance of *ambiguity*, which is a benchmark of the chaotic, cognitive processes of an out-of-control crisis (Duffy & Haberstroh, 2020). The ability to tolerate ambiguity and the muddled thinking and emotional pinballing that goes with it is the signature of an all-star crisis interventionist. Crisis workers must be able to have the patience and tolerance to wade through the client's ambiguity and not be dismissive, bored, or otherwise frustrated by it. Utility with RCT is a good yardstick to measure that ability.

Finally, RCT echoes a canon of Rogers, and that is *authenticity* (Jordon, 2018). The crisis worker does not come across as an all-seeing, all-knowing expert but rather another human being with all the strengths and weaknesses that being human entails, and that requires being genuine and transparent in the relationship.

The end goal of RCT is about developing mutual empathy. (Jordan, 2018) which is different than the one way, counselor-to-client empathy drilled into human service workers. This is important because in many crisis interventions, the client and interventionist are not acquainted and have no previous contact or working relationship. Thus, overcoming perceived cultural barriers is critical in bonding with clients, and being inauthentic is one of the fastest ways we know to exacerbate the crisis. We will spend a fair amount of time addressing this issue when you meet the SAFETY model in Chapter 2, "Culturally Effective Helping in Crisis."

Chaos Theory. Why is a meteorologist (Lorenz, 1993) who thinks a butterfly cruising along in a jungle path in the Amazon is capable of starting a hurricane in the Atlantic getting a reference in a crisis intervention book? Furthermore, what in the world do words like *fractals, bifurcations, intermittences, folded towel diffeomorphisms,* and *smooth noodle maps* have to do with crisis? These are all concepts that seek to capture the structural complexity underlying chaos theory, and Edward Lorenz, in his attempts to better predict weather patterns, is seen as its founder.

Not a lot has been written about chaos theory in the human services field, which is curious. The primary reason we include chaos theory is, as you may well imagine, that in most crises, there is a lot of chaos! But lo and behold, it turns out that chaos isn't random and that it has all kinds of ramifications for a range of other occupations, including psychotherapy (Haynes, 1995; Helby, 1995; Iwakabe, 1999; Miller, 1999), and that most certainly includes crisis interventionists who often find themselves in the middle of a dictionary definition of chaos.

Early conceptualizations of chaos theory by scientists in the fields of meteorology, mathematics, and physics viewed the theory as applying to systems or events that appeared random but, on closer inspection, revealed an underlying order (Gleick, 2008). Paradoxically, what happens in chaotic systems appears to be random and unpredictable, so there is no possibility of determining what future outcomes will be, but in fact, there is (Lorenz, 1993, p. 9).

Chaos theory is really sort of a theory of evolution when applied to human functioning such as crisis intervention. It is evolutionary in that it is essentially an open-ended, ever-changing, "self-organizing" system whereby a new system may emerge out of the crisis (Butz, 1995, 1997; Chamberlain, 1993, 1994). A chaotic (crisis) situation—which Postrel (1998, p. xv) calls "emergent complex messiness"—evolves into a "self-organizing" mode whenever a critical mass of people come to perceive that they have no way to identify patterns or preplan options to solve the dilemma at hand. Because the chaotic situation falls outside of known alternative solutions, both physicists and human services workers necessarily resort to spontaneous, trial-and-error experimentation to try to cope with the crisis. The "messiness" of the crisis lies not in disorder but in an order that is unknown, unpredictable, and spontaneous, an ever-shifting pattern driven by millions of uncoordinated, independent factors that necessitate experimentation yet may finally result in a global clarification of the crisis. Such experimentation may lead to false starts, temporary failure, dead ends, spontaneous innovation, creativity, improvisation, brainstorming, cooperative enterprise, and other "evolutionary" attempts to make sense of and cope with the crisis (Gleick, 2008, pp. 33–42).

The crisis intervention attempts in the wake of British Petroleum's Deep Horizon well blowout provide a vivid example of chaos theory at work—in both a positive and a negative sense. So, it is not just the "messiness" of an utterly new phenomenon like the blowout of the deep well in the Gulf of Mexico and the attempts to look at and fix the disaster at one fixed point, such as the wellhead. While that point is critical, it is also reductionistic in terms of chaos theory and doesn't look at the total gestalt, or "big picture," of the economic, ecological, and psychological costs of the crisis. All the tangled threads and points on the fabric of the crisis don't portray the underlying and interlocking patterns that provide information about the big picture and the potential ramifications of these dynamic systems on one another and on the total system after the crisis erupts.

Okay, so you didn't sign up for a course in higher mathematics or physics, which is where chaos's roots are, and the foregoing paragraphs are making your hair hurt! But a basic understanding of this exotic and esoteric theory should give you two important pieces of information. First, big crises call for a lot of different people working from a lot of different perspectives in a well-coordinated manner who can connect the myriad dots in a chaotic situation, see the underlying patterns, make sense of them, and change to meet changing conditions as new eddies and vortexes swirl out of the crisis. Myer and his associates have attempted to demonstrate what this theory looks and acts like when combined with ecosystemic theory after a disaster on a college campus (Myer et al., 2011).

Second, transcrises come close to manifesting chaos theory at work. Lots of times, transcrises don't make sense and don't appear to have any discernable pattern, but much like the theoretical mathematician, just because you don't have an equation to solve the problem doesn't mean that one doesn't exist. There is an underlying pattern, and that's why all professional crisis interventionists use the right side of their brain a lot because dealing with crisis calls for a lot of creative thinking. No other writers at present are discussing chaos theory as it applies to crisis intervention, but our guess is that they will as we attempt to unravel and understand the genetics that make up this field.

Developmental Theory. Because many crises have their bases in the developmental stages that humans pass through, developmental theory must play a part in crisis intervention. Developmental stage theorists such as Erikson (1963), Levinson (1986), Levinson and Levinson (1996), Sheehy (1984; 1996), and Blocher (2000) clearly believe that movement through various developmental life stages is critical. Developmental tasks that are not met and accomplished during particular life stages tend to pile up and cause problems. As individual needs and wants butt heads with the demands and expectations of society and the individual fails to move on to the next life stage, the potential for crisis arises. Neglected, abused, and bullied children; alienated and isolated adolescent drug abusers; people who lack education or lack vocational satisfaction or success; or those exposed to domestic violence, divorce, suicide, homicide, and a host of other problems may be unable to meet life stages effectively. When an external, environmental, or situational crisis feeds into preexisting developmental crises, intrapersonal and interpersonal problems may reach the breaking point.

Applied Crisis Theory

Brammer (1985, pp. 94–95) characterizes applied crisis theory as encompassing three domains: (1) normal *developmental crises,* (2) *situational crises,* and (3) *existential crises.* Given the ecosystem theory perspective, we have added a fourth domain, (4) *ecosystemic crises.*

Developmental Crises. Developmental crises are events in the normal flow of human growth and evolution in which a dramatic change or shift occurs that produces abnormal responses. For example, developmental crises may occur in response to the birth of a child, graduation from college, a midlife career change, retirement, or even the aging process. Developmental crises are considered normal; however, all persons and all developmental crises are unique and must be assessed and handled in unique ways.

Situational Crises. A situational crisis emerges with the occurrence of uncommon and extraordinary events that an individual has no way of forecasting or controlling. Situational crises may follow such events as terrorist attacks, automobile accidents, kidnappings, sexual violence, job loss, or sudden illness and death. The key to differentiating a situational crisis from other crises is that a situational crisis is random, sudden, shocking, intense, and often catastrophic.

Existential Crises. An existential crisis includes the inner conflicts and anxieties that accompany important human issues of purpose, responsibility, independence, freedom, and commitment. An existential crisis might accompany the realization, at age 40, that one will never make a significant and distinct impact on a particular profession or organization; remorse, at age 50, that one chose never to marry or leave one's parents' home, never made a separate life, and now has lost forever the possibility of being a fully happy and worthwhile person; or a pervasive and persistent feeling, at age 60, that one's life is meaningless—that there is a void that can never be filled in a meaningful way.

Ecosystemic Crises. Ecosystemic crises typically occur when some *natural* or *human-caused* disaster overtakes a person or a (large or small) group of people who find themselves, through no fault or action of their own, inundated in the aftermath of an event that may adversely affect virtually every member of the environment in which they live. Such crises may be the result of natural phenomena such as hurricanes, floods, tsunamis, earthquakes, volcanic eruptions, tornadoes, blizzards, mudslides, drought, famine, and forest or grassland/brush fires. Other instances of ecosystemic crises may be *biologically derived,* such as a disease epidemic like COVID-19 or the effects of a huge oil spill; *politically based,* as in war, a refugee crisis associated with war, or ethnic cleansing; or *severe economic depression,* such as the Great Depression of the early 20th century.

Crisis Intervention Models

LO5 Three basic crisis intervention models discussed by both Leitner (1974) and Belkin (1984) are the *equilibrium model,* the *cognitive model,* and the *psychosocial transition model.* These three generic models provide the groundwork for many different crisis intervention strategies and methodologies. Two newer models that target the ecological factors that contribute to crisis are the *developmental-ecological model* (Collins & Collins, 2006), and the *contextual-ecological model* (Myer & Moore, 2006). Two field-based practice models are *psychological first aid* (Raphael, 1977; U.S. Department of Veterans Affairs, 2006), which is used in the immediate aftermath of disasters and terrorist attacks, and Roberts' (2005) ACT model, which is more generic but primarily trauma based.

The Equilibrium Model

The equilibrium model is really an equilibrium/disequilibrium model. People in crisis are in a state of psychological or emotional disequilibrium in which their usual coping mechanisms and problem-solving methods fail to meet their needs. The goal of the equilibrium model is to help people recover a state of precrisis equilibrium (Caplan, 1961). The equilibrium model seems most appropriate for early intervention, when the person is out of control, disoriented, and unable to make appropriate choices. Until the person has regained some coping abilities, the main focus is on stabilizing the individual. Up to the time the person has reacquired some definite measure of stability, little else can or should be done. For example, it does little good to dig into the underlying factors that cause suicidal ideation until the person can be stabilized to the point of agreeing that life is worth living for at least another week. This is probably the purest model of crisis intervention and is most likely to be used at the onset of the crisis (Caplan, 1961; Leitner, 1974; Lindemann, 1944).

The Cognitive Model

The cognitive model of crisis intervention is based on the premise that crises are rooted in faulty thinking about the events or situations that surround the crisis, not in the events themselves or the facts of the events or situations (Ellis, 1962; Meichenbaum, 1977). The goal of this model is to help people become aware of and change their views and beliefs about the crisis events or situations. The basic tenet of the cognitive model is that people can gain control of crises in their lives by changing their thinking, especially by recognizing and disputing the irrational and self-defeating parts of their cognitions and by retaining and focusing on the rational and self-enhancing elements of their thinking.

The messages that people in crisis send themselves become very negative and twisted, in contrast to the reality of the situation. Dilemmas that are constant and grinding wear people out, pushing their internal state of perception more and more toward negative self-talk until their cognitive sets are so negative that no amount of preaching can convince them that anything positive will ever come from the situation. Their behavior soon follows this negative self-talk and begets a self-fulfilling prophecy that the situation is hopeless. At this juncture, crisis intervention becomes a job of rewiring the individual's thoughts to more positive feedback loops by practicing and rehearsing new self-statements about the situation until the old, negative, debilitating ones are expunged. The cognitive model seems most appropriate after the client has been stabilized and returned to an approximate state of precrisis equilibrium. Basic components of this approach are found in the rational-emotive work of Ellis (1982), the cognitive-behavioral approach of Meichenbaum (1977), and the cognitive system of Beck (1976).

The Psychosocial Transition Model

The psychosocial transition model assumes that people are products of their genes plus the learning they have absorbed from their particular social environments. Because people are continuously changing, developing, and growing and their social environments and social influences (Dorn, 1986) are continuously evolving, crises may be related to internal or external (psychological, social, or environmental) difficulties. The goal of crisis intervention is to collaborate with clients in assessing the internal and external difficulties contributing to the crisis and then help them choose workable alternatives to their current behaviors, attitudes, and use of environmental resources. Clients may need to incorporate adequate internal coping mechanisms, social supports, and environmental resources in order to gain autonomous (noncrisis) control over their lives.

The psychosocial model does not perceive crisis as simply an internal state of affairs that resides totally within the individual. It reaches outside the individual and asks what systems need to be changed. Peers, family, occupation, religion, and the community are but a few of the external dimensions that promote or hinder psychological adaptiveness. With certain kinds of crisis problems, few lasting gains will be made unless the social systems that affect the individual are also changed, or the individual comes to terms with and understands the dynamics of those systems and how they affect adaptation to the crisis. Like the cognitive model, the psychosocial transition model seems to be most appropriate after the client has been stabilized. Theorists who have contributed to the psychosocial transition model include Adler (Ansbacher & Ansbacher, 1956), Erikson (1963), and Minuchin (1974).

The Developmental–Ecological Model

Collins and Collins (2006) have developed a developmental-ecological model of crisis intervention that integrates developmental stages and issues with the environment within which the individual operates. In this model, the crisis worker needs to assess both the individual and the environment as well as the interrelationship between the two and then factor in the developmental stage within which the person is operating. Any situational crisis must always be considered in relation to the stage of development the person is in, and the potency of the crisis may depend on how well there has been stage mastery of the tasks affected by the crisis.

The Contextual–Ecological Model

Myer and Moore (2006) have developed an ecological model that focuses on contextual elements of the crisis. Their first premise is that contextual elements may be seen as layered. These layers are dependent on two elements: proximity to the crisis by physical distance and reactions that are moderated by perception and the meaning attributed to the event.

The second premise of this model is that reciprocal impact occurs between the individual and systems affected by the event. Understanding the reciprocal effect of the crisis involves the recognition of two elements: the interaction among the primary and secondary relationships and the degree of change triggered by the event. Primary relationships are those in which no intervening component (other individuals or systems) interacts with or mediates the connection. An example of a primary relationship would be between an employee and a company. If an

accident occurred and the company immediately took a number of steps to support employees and assure them that safety measures had been increased so such an accident would be unlikely to happen again, the employees might feel secure, safe, and satisfied with the company's efforts. A secondary relationship is mediated by at least one other individual or system. For example, if an employee's family members were so terrified for the safety of their loved one that no amount of assurances would satisfy them, then the primary relationship between the employee and the company would be affected.

The third premise is that time directly influences the impact of a crisis. The two major time elements are the amount of time that has passed and special occasions such as anniversaries and holidays following the event.

Myer and Moore (2006) propose a formula for gauging the impact of the crisis on the individual or system. The formula can be summarized as a function of proximity to the event, reaction to the event, relationship to the event, and amount of change caused by the event, which is then divided by the amount of time that has passed. What is critical in this formula is understanding that no single component can be considered separately. Close proximity alone may not have as much bearing on the impact of the crisis as the degree of change resulting from it. While this highly theoretical model as of yet has no empirical basis, nor does it yet have a great deal of utility for intervention, it poses questions and generates premises that can help us understand the impact of the crisis as it interacts between and within a variety of systems and individuals.

Psychological First Aid

LO6   Slaikeu (1990, p. 6) breaks crisis intervention into two parts: First-order intervention, or **psychological first aid**, seeks to address the immediate crisis situation and provide immediate relief, possibly to a wide range of individuals. Second-order intervention, or **crisis therapy**, seeks to resolve the crisis and is generally provided by trained, licensed human services professionals. In this book, most of what would be seen as psychological first aid and initial crisis therapy is what we define as crisis intervention. To attend to the mental health needs of survivors of large-scale disasters, public health personnel are now being taught to use empirically grounded, best practice techniques called psychological first aid that are designed to provide immediate, palliative mental health assistance to survivors (Parker et al., 2006).

The National Institute of Mental Health (2002) defines psychological first aid as establishing the safety of the client, reducing stress-related symptoms, providing rest and physical recuperation, and linking clients to critical resources and social support systems. Raphael (1977) first coined the term *psychological first aid* in her discussion of crisis work with an Australian railway disaster. She described a variety of activities that provided caring support, empathic responding, concrete information and assistance, and reuniting of survivors with social support systems. Paramount in psychological first aid is attending to Maslow's needs hierarchy and taking care of survival needs first. Many counselors, social workers, and psychologists helped meet the basic support needs of food, shelter, clothing, and other survival needs during the aftermath of Hurricane Katrina before they ever did any "counseling."

The National Center for PTSD (U.S. Department of Veterans Affairs, 2006) has published a field manual, *Psychological First Aid: Field Operations Guide*, that offers an evidence-informed modular approach for assisting people in the immediate aftermath of disaster and terrorism, to reduce initial distress, and to foster short- and long-term adaptive functioning. The manual states that it is for use by first responders, incident command systems, primary and emergency health care providers, school crisis response teams, faith-based organizations, disaster relief organizations, Community Emergency Response Teams, Medical Reserve Corps, and the Citizens Corps in diverse settings. This approach to psychological first aid includes the following eight core actions (U.S. Department of Veterans Affairs, 2011, p. 18):

1. **Contact and Engagement**
   Goal: To respond to contacts initiated by survivors, or to initiate contacts in a nonintrusive, compassionate, and helpful manner.
2. **Safety and Comfort**
   Goal: To enhance immediate and ongoing safety and provide physical and emotional comfort.
3. **Stabilization** (if needed)
   Goal: To calm and orient emotionally overwhelmed or disoriented survivors.
4. **Information Gathering**: **Current Needs and Concerns**
   Goal: To identify immediate needs and concerns, gather additional information, and tailor psychological first aid interventions.
5. **Practical Assistance**
   Goal: To offer practical help to survivors in addressing immediate needs and concerns.
6. **Connection with Social Supports**
   Goal: To help establish brief or ongoing contacts with primary support persons and other sources of support, including family members, friends, and community helping resources.
7. **Information on Coping**
   Goal: To provide information about stress reactions and coping to reduce distress and promote adaptive functioning.
8. **Linkage with Collaborative Services**
   Goal: To link survivors with available services needed at the time or in the future.

Psychological first aid provides the bare-bones basics of crisis intervention. It is designed to be palliative. It is not designed to cure or fix anything but rather to provide nonintrusive physical and psychological support. Social workers would be very comfortable with this model because a great deal of it resembles social work services. If we consider the first four tasks (Predispositioning, Problem Definition, Providing Support, Safety) of the model of crisis intervention you will meet in Chapter 3, "The Intervention and Assessment Models," as being close to what is meant by psychological first aid, then psychological first aid is clearly necessary. Whether it is also *sufficient* in providing immediate crisis intervention services is another matter, although there is some evidence it does have lasting effects on psychological wellbeing (Ironson et al., 2021; McCart et al., 2020). Certainly, not all people need immediate psychological assistance, nor should they have it forced on them, but the high adrenal moments of a lot of crisis intervention make us believe that something more than psychological first aid is needed to defuse emotional volatility, de-escalate life-threatening behavior, and reframe and cool the insane, irrational, hot cognitions that typify many crisis situations.

The ACT Model

The ACT model proposed by Roberts (2005) is an acronym:

*A*ssessment of the presenting problem, including emergency psychiatric and other medical needs and trauma assessment

Connecting clients to support systems
Traumatic reactions and posttraumatic stress disorders

The model has seven generally linear stages: crisis assessment, establishing rapport, identifying major problems, dealing with feelings, generating and exploring alternatives, developing plans, and providing follow-up (pp. 104–106). This model has been designed to deal with the onset of a traumatic event and, probably even more appropriately, with what Kleespies (2009) calls behavioral emergencies.

Playbook/Game Plan Model

As you will see in detail in this book, specially trained police officers called Crisis Intervention Team (CIT) officers are playing a larger and larger role as first-line responders to the mentally ill and other emotionally distraught individuals who come to the attention of law enforcement. Major Sam Cochran (retired former coordinator of the Memphis Police Department CIT) has developed a crisis intervention model based on coaching, which has a great deal of face validity given that most police officers have engaged in some kind of team sport, so a playbook/game plan makes perfect sense, and there is ready acceptance in trying to learn it. It is specifically tailored to diffuse and de-escalate angry, distraught, out-of-control, potentially lethal individuals who are in the middle of a crisis and who come to police attention through 911 "mental illness" calls (Kirchberg et al., 2013). It trains first-line responders through a game plan strategy that teaches them how to assess individuals' verbal and nonverbal behavior and develop a game plan that uses a combination of verbal de-escalation techniques (plays) to defuse individuals who may be manifesting lethal behavior toward themselves or others. We will visit some of these "plays" in Chapter 4, "The Tools of the Trade."

Eclectic/Integrated Crisis Intervention Theory

In current psychotherapeutic theory, the term "eclectic" has taken on a somewhat negative connotation as a sort of an "anything goes, try and see if it works" approach and has generally been replaced with the term "integrated," which critics of "eclecticism" believe implies a more purposeful and planful treatment methodology. As far as we're concerned, it's a "rose" by any name, so call it what you will; we believe it's a best bet on how to go about doing the business of crisis intervention. Eclectic/integrated crisis intervention involves intentionally and systematically selecting and integrating valid concepts and strategies from all available approaches to helping clients. Eclecticism/integrated theory is thus a hybrid of all available approaches. It operates from a task orientation instead of concepts. Its major tasks (James & Gilliland, 2003, p. 374; Lazarus, 1989; Thorne, 1973, p. 451) are (1) to identify valid elements in all therapeutic systems and integrate them into an internally consistent whole that does justice to the behavioral data to be explained; (2) to consider all pertinent theories, methods, and standards for evaluating and manipulating clinical data according to the most advanced knowledge of time and place; and (3) to identify with no specific theory, keep an open mind, and continuously experiment with those formulations and strategies that produce successful results. This theoretical approach would find favor with current multicultural and social justice approaches to counseling because the workers enter into the relationship with no preconceived notion of the "right" therapeutic approach but rather allow the social and cultural factors that contribute to the client's problems to unfold before making a decision on what the "best bet" approach to take might be (Ratts & Pedersen, 2014, p. 7).

Throughout this book, you will find an eclectic/integrated approach to the interventions presented. Much of what happens will depend on the situation in which we find ourselves. "Situation" may be defined as including the type of crisis, the physical and ecological setting in which it occurs, individual characteristics, cultural background, and significant others who may be directly or indirectly involved. Probably more important than all the factors that affect clients are the knowledge, strength, and skills that interventionists bring to the crisis and meld into the client's world.

The eclectic/integrated approach fuses two pervasive themes: (1) all people and all crises are unique and distinctive, and (2) all people and all crises are similar. We do not see these themes as mutually exclusive. All people and all crises are similar in that there are global elements to specific crisis types. The dynamics of bereavement are generic and provide us with general guidelines for intervention. However, treating individual cases of bereavement is anything but generic. How a family perceives the impact of the death of a member depends on a number of factors: the deceased member's place in the family, what each member of the family does in response to the death, and how the changed family system now operates. The treatment of surviving family members who have lost a child after rearing five others, compared to those who have lost their only child, born late in the parents' life, who had become the focus of existence for the couple, may call for far different intervention strategies, even if bereavement is the generic issue.

An eclectic/integrated approach does not mean throwing any theory or technique at the crisis. Using an eclectic approach means not being bound by and locked into any one theoretical approach in a dogmatic fashion. Rather, it means being well versed in a number of approaches and theories and being able to assess the client's needs so appropriate techniques can be planned and fitted to them. Many human services workers avow an eclectic/integrated approach but actually use the word to rationalize not being able to do anything very well. Being a true eclectic/integrated interventionist means doing lots of hard work, reading, studying, experiencing, and being supervised and critiqued by other professionals. It also means taking risks and being willing to abandon an approach that on first inspection might seem reasonable and proper but, once entered, proves fruitless for the particular situation.

Eclectic/integrated therapy performed well is equal parts skill and intuition. Paying attention to your feelings as much as to your cognition about the situation is crucial. Changing to a more effective intervention is often based on nothing more scientific than a feeling that something is amiss. Although having a "gut" feeling is little justification, in the scientific sense, for doing something, it can nevertheless be a sound basis for action. There is no known formula for deciding when to move from a nondirective to a highly directive stance with a client in crisis, nor is there an equation that tells a therapist that mental imagery may be more effective than confrontation as an intervention technique. An eclectic approach done well is the zenith of the performing art of crisis intervention.

Characteristics of Effective Crisis Workers

LO7   Almost everyone can be taught the techniques in this book and, with practice, can employ them with some degree of skill. However, the crisis worker who can take intervention to the performing art level is more than the sum of techniques read about and skills mastered. A master of this art is going to have not only technical skill and theoretical knowledge but also a good deal of the following characteristics.

Life Experiences

Workers handle a crisis or not to the extent that they are a whole person or not (Carkhuff & Berenson, 1977, pp. 162–163). A whole person has a rich and varied background of life experiences. These life experiences serve as a resource for emotional maturity that, combined with training, enables workers to be stable, consistent, and well-integrated not only within the crisis situation but also in their daily lives. However, life experiences alone are not sufficient to qualify one to be a crisis worker and can be debilitating if they continue to influence the worker in negative ways.

This issue is central to crisis intervention because many people who work as volunteers, support personnel, and professionals are products of their own crisis environments. They have chosen to work with people experiencing the same kind of crisis they themselves have suffered, and they use their experiential background as a resource in working with others. For example, people recovering from an alcohol or substance use disorder may work in alcohol and drug units, survivors of Intimate Partner Violence (IPV) may work in spouse abuse centers, and PTSD victims may counsel in veterans' centers. These professionals have had firsthand experience with the trauma their clients have experienced. Does this background give them an edge over other workers who have not suffered the same pain?

The answer is a qualified yes—qualified in that the person who carries emotional baggage into the helping relationship may be even less effective than the person who has had few, if any, life experiences. One sees examples of emotional carryover into the intervention process in the proselytizing of persons with alcoholic misuse disorder who vilify others to assuage their own insecurities and fears about "falling off the wagon" and in the child abuse worker, themself a former victim of sexual abuse, who castigates parents for their failure to confront the abusers.

Such human services workers may have tremendous difficulties because they mingle many of their own problems with those of their clients. The workers alternate among feeling states characterized by sympathy, anger, disappointment, and cynicism, which are detrimental both to themselves and to their clients. We do not believe crisis workers must have "lived in the crisis" to be able to understand and deal with it effectively. We do believe that interventionists who have successfully overcome some of life's problems and have put those problems into perspective will have assets of maturity, optimism, tenacity, and tough-mindedness that will help them marshal their psychological resources to assist their clients.

You should also be cautioned that on-the-job training in this business is a very arduous way to win one's spurs, particularly for a worker who has led a sheltered, constricted life and decides through misguided idealism to become a Florence Nightingale and fix the problems of the world. This rose-colored view does little for clients in general and may do considerable harm to workers as their good intentions pave the road to **burnout**. We hasten to add that chronological age has very little to do with having or not having self-enhancing life experiences and a broader, more resilient viewpoint. We know people ranging in age from 21 to 65 who are emotional adolescents. When threatened by face-to-face encounters with the real world, they may be characterized by rigidity, insularity, and insecurity. The ideal crisis workers are those who have experienced life, have learned and grown from those experiences, and supports those experiences in their work by thorough training, knowledge, and supervision. This individual constantly seeks to integrate all these aspects into their therapeutic intervention in particular and into living in general.

Personal Characteristics

Poise. The nature of crisis intervention is that the worker is often confronted with shocking and threatening material from clients who are completely out of control. Probably the most significant help the interventionist can provide at this juncture is to remain calm, poised, and in control (Belkin, 1984, p. 427). Creating a stable and rational atmosphere provides a model for the client that is conducive to restoring equilibrium to the situation. Effective crisis workers are as steady and well-anchored psychologically as the Rock of Gibraltar. This does not mean that effective crisis workers are made of stone and are not frightened, tense, anxious, and at times unsure of themselves. However, in the very act of making self-disclosing owning statements of their frailties and shortcomings, the worker models the assuredness, transparency, and congruency that are prized professional assets in any professional human service worker (Carkhuff, 1987; Rogers, 1961).

Creativity and Flexibility. Creativity and flexibility are major assets to those confronted with perplexing and seemingly unsolvable problems (Aguilera & Messick, 1982, p. 24). In our courses and training workshops, students and trainees often have difficulty conducting role plays with peers because they have no formula for getting the "right" answer. Although practice in tough role-play situations builds confidence, how creative individuals are in difficult situations depends in large measure on how well they have nurtured their own creativity over the course of their lives by taking risks and practicing divergent thinking.

Energy and Resiliency. Functioning in the unknown areas that are characteristic of crisis intervention requires energy, organization, direction, and systematic action (Carkhuff & Berenson, 1977, p. 194). Professional training can provide organizational guidelines and principles for systematic acting. What it cannot do is provide the energy requisite to perform this work. A crisis worker must also be resilient. By its very nature, crisis work has many "downs" when, no matter how capable, no matter how committed, no matter what was tried or done, "success" was not achieved. Crisis workers must have "bounce back" potential. They take care of themselves physically and psychologically and make wise use of their available energy.

Quick Mental Reflexes. Crisis work differs from typical therapeutic intervention in that time is a critical factor. Crisis intervention requires more activity and directiveness than ordinary therapeutic endeavors usually do. Time to reflect and mull over problems is a rare commodity in crisis intervention. The worker must have fast mental reflexes to deal with the constantly emerging and changing issues that occur in the crisis. The worker who cannot think fast and accurately is going to find this business very frustrating indeed.

Assertiveness. One of the major problems that interventionists who have been trained in formal professional programs experience in attempting to apply the skills in this book is their reticence at times to be proactive, assertive, and directive. These therapeutic stances run counter to what has been hammered into them with regard to not being judgmental, not breeding client dependence, not imposing their values on the client, being accepting, and unconditionally positively regarding their clients as human beings of worth. While we believe wholeheartedly in those dictums and employ them whenever possible, crisis intervention has different rules.

Many clients who are in crisis do not talk or act nicely. For that reason, you need to be able to assertively set limits to behavior, both in regard to maintaining your own integrity and keeping the client stabilized so intervention can occur. Clients are likely to have exhausted their repertory of coping skills and drained their psychological resources to the point that their ability to act, think constructively, or control their feelings is gone. At such times, crisis interventionists cannot be passive. You are the expert on the scene, you have the fund of knowledge needed, and you need to employ your skills, knowledge, and abilities in as clear and directive a manner as you possibly can. The nine intentional helping strategies described in Chapter 4, "The Tools of the Trade," are predominately interventionist driven and have little passivity or reactivity. Much like competitive athletics, if you are going to do this well, you need to get your game face on and get actively involved.

Spirituality.   We are not talking about whether you hug a redwood tree, light candles at an altar, bow before a deity, take communion, observe holy days, or read and pray from a holy text to satisfy you spiritual needs. That's organized religion, which is all well and good and, indeed, may play a significant part in your spiritual growth. When we speak of spirituality, this is how many people make sense of and meaning of their lives and find peace and purpose for it, and in so doing, it is how one makes meaningful connections with others. There is a good deal of evidence that spirituality plays a meaningful role in the resiliency of individuals after a disaster and is critical in empowering them to move forward (Arkin et al., 2022; Lee et al., 2022; Sato et al., 2022; Zhang et al., 2022).

Crisis workers who short change or are dismissive of their clients' spiritual beliefs are likely going to be grossly ineffective. The same can be said in regard to the workers themselves if they do not have a belief system and a spiritual basis to fall back on and support them when faced with clients with horrific problems (Hersh, 2022). Rather, it is critical that the worker forge a way of being with clients in their religious/spiritual struggles such that a therapeutic environment is created to reconnect clients with their spiritual foundations (Campbell, 2021). To that end, Sandage and associates (2020) have developed a Rational Spirituality Model (RSM) that is a creative clinical process that engages spiritual, existential, religious, and theological concerns that can pervade their clients' struggles and triumphs.

Spirituality may not be for everyone, but it is incumbent, then, that crisis workers have a support source of their own, know when to seek nourishment from that support source, and if that is a spiritual support (Akin, et al., 2022; Lee et al. 2022), know when to let that higher power take over for them (Hardiman & Simmonds, 2013; Naz et al., 2012). If you don't have that spiritual support to fall back on, or other support source, you are missing a critical piece of self-care (Barton, 2020) and frankly, you need to read the Burnout chapter pretty closely. Suffice it to say, this is not easy stuff to master, and it takes a lot of self-introspection as you move into the business. It is a topic one of your authors spends a lot of time with when in supervision.

Other Attributes.   Crisis workers have found the following attributes to be of utmost importance to themselves and their clients: tenacity, the ability to delay gratification, courage, optimism, a reality orientation, calmness under duress, objectivity, a strong and positive self-concept, an appropriate sense of humor, and abiding faith that human beings are strong, resilient, and capable of overcoming seemingly insurmountable odds. Poll yourself: Do you have these attributes? We also want you to understand that admission into the inner circle of the profession is not reserved solely for a few super heroes. Most interventionists we know, certainly including ourselves, are at times perplexed, frustrated, angry, afraid, threatened, incompetent, foolish, vain, troubled, and otherwise unequal to the task. We allow ourselves and our students and trainees at least one mistake per day and go on from there. We would very much like you to remember that cognitive billboard, "You get one free, learn from it!" and place it squarely in the forefront of your mind.

Rewards

Standing up to the intense heat of the crisis situation to help people through seemingly unsolvable problems is some of the most gratifying and positively reinforcing work you can do in the psychotherapy business. The intense personal rewards that accrue to crisis workers lead us to believe that this work would be high on Glasser's (1976) list of positive addictive behaviors.

Now consider for a moment yourself as a client. Everyone is at times subject to the whims of a randomly cruel universe, and the kinds of crises that are dealt with in this book are apt to be visited on us all. Understanding how to navigate through these constellations of problems is a valuable resource. How well we live depends on our ability to handle the problems that confront us when we least expect them. As you read through the material, you may find yourself "living into" some of these problems and asking yourself, "I wonder how I'd fare if I were a client?" We believe that this, too, is a worthwhile perspective if you can look beyond the dilemmas to the coping techniques and bank them for future reference and use.

Summary

Historically, crisis intervention has developed and evolved in about the last 60 years. Its origins have typically been in grassroots organizations, groups of people who came together to solve a specific crisis that was assailing them. Through both natural and human-made crises and the influence of the media, crisis intervention has moved from a backwater psychological specialty into the mainstream of helping skills.

Our composite definition of *individual crisis*, derived from the sources given at the beginning of this chapter, is *a perception or experiencing of an event or situation as an intolerable difficulty that exceeds the person's current resources and coping mechanisms. Unless the person obtains relief, the crisis has the potential to cause severe affective, behavioral, and cognitive malfunctioning up to the point of instigating injurious or lethal behavior to oneself or others.* Because systems play an equally important part in the business of crisis intervention, we define *systemic crisis* as follows: *When a traumatic event occurs such that people, institutions, communities, and ecologies are overwhelmed and response systems are unable to effectively contain and control the event in regard to both physical and psychological reactions to it, the crisis has become systemic.* These general definitions are enhanced by considering several important principles and characteristics of crisis as follows:

1. Crisis embodies both danger and opportunity for the person experiencing the crisis.
2. Crisis is usually time limited but may develop into a series of recurring transcrisis points.
3. Crisis is often complex and difficult to resolve.
4. The life experiences of human services workers may greatly enhance their effectiveness in crisis intervention.
5. Crisis contains the seeds of growth and impetus for change.
6. Panaceas or quick fixes may not be applicable to many crisis situations.
7. Crisis confronts people with choices and the negative or positive consequences they accrue.
8. Emotional disequilibrium and disorganization accompany crisis.
9. The resolution of crisis and the personhood of crisis workers interrelate.

Understanding transcrisis states and transcrisis points helps in understanding many crises. Clients experiencing crises rooted in their transcrisis states or transcrisis points show recurring trauma like symptoms derived from earlier traumatic events. Transcrisis states and points have parallels with and differences from PTSD.

Basic crisis theory views crisis as situational or developmental rather than pathological in nature. *Expanded crisis theory* adds to and enhances basic theory by incorporating and adapting components from psychoanalytic, general systems, ecosystems, adaptational, interpersonal, relational, chaos, and developmental theory.

Five fundamental crisis intervention models are equilibrium, cognitive, psychosocial transition, developmental-ecological, and contextual-ecological. The *equilibrium model*, probably the most widely known model of the five, defines equilibrium as an emotional state in which the person is stable, in control, or psychologically mobile. It defines disequilibrium as an emotional state that accompanies instability, loss of control, and psychological immobility. The *cognitive model* views the crisis state as resulting from faulty thinking and beliefs about life's dilemmas and traumas. The *psychosocial transition model* assumes that people are products of both hereditary endowment and environmental learning and that crisis may be caused by psychological, social, or environmental factors. The *developmental-ecological model* considers developmental stages in relation to the ecological system within which the individual develops. A *contextual-ecological model* looks at layers, relationships, and time when it examines a crisis. The *psychological first aid* and *ACT* models are both practice-based field models that deal with disasters and trauma-related crises. The *playbook/game plan* model is targeted toward police officers and other first-line responders who deal with potentially lethal, out-of-control clients. An eclectic/integrated theoretical position incorporates and integrates all valid concepts of crisis intervention.

Effective crisis workers share a number of positive personal characteristics. They maintain poise, quick wittedness, creativity, tenacity, assertiveness, and resiliency, among a host of other attributes, while confronting the difficult issues of clients in crisis.

Culturally Effective Helping in Crisis

2

Multicultural Perspectives in Crisis Intervention

LO1 Laura Brown is a past president of Division 56, Trauma Psychology; she is a diplomate (recognized as knowing a lot and contributing a lot) in clinical psychology, has received numerous awards, and

has authored what we believe is the best book on cultural competence when it comes to doing trauma therapy, *Cultural Competence in Trauma Therapy: Beyond the Flashback* (2008). So, we can pretty much assume she knows what she's talking about when she says, "After three decades of working intentionally with trauma I can say with utter certainty that I know that

I have no idea of how any particular person will have experienced and made sense, or not, of [their] traumatic experiences" (Brown, 2008, p. 16). Therefore, as you read this chapter, understand that one of the best minds in this field is confessing to her lack of understanding when it comes to ferreting out all the ways that culture affects her clients. The message is that we're a long way from knowing all we need to know to effectively weave multicultural competence into crisis intervention. However, we do know more than we did in the last edition of this book, and the way research is moving (Cunningham, 2000; Duffey & Haberstroh, 2022; Kress et al., 2018; Stone & Conley, 2004), we're going to know more and more. So please understand that this chapter isn't a global positioning system (GPS) for multicultural competence in crisis intervention that will precisely target your destination but more like a compass that will point you in the right general direction.

The 21st century United States, as in most countries worldwide, is culturally diverse, and it is incumbent on mental health professionals to enhance our multicultural competence. So just what is this abstract and amorphous thing called "culture"? And how does it become "multi"? Furthermore, what makes it important in the crisis business? Bernal and Rodriguez (2012, p. 4) propose that **culture** is an intergenerationally transmitted system of meaning shared by a group of people and may have concrete objects such as buildings and art, subjective components such as social norms, and beliefs that define it as separate and distinct from other cultures. Adler (1997) defines culture as "that complex whole which includes knowledge, beliefs, arts, laws, morals, customs, and capabilities acquired by a person as a member of society. It is a way of life of a group of people, the configuration of all the more or less stereotyped patterns of learned behavior which are handed down from one generation to the next through the means of language and imitation" (p. 14). Members of a given culture hold all of the foregoing to be pretty much self-evident truths to live by as a way of making order and sense out of their lives. Thus, they are generally able to live with one another in an overall peaceful, profitable way with some sense of control over their lives and the community within which they reside. The "multi" part emerges when individuals of various cultures co-exist in a shared community. In so doing, individuals of those various cultures bring with them the aforementioned culturally based assumptions, values, beliefs, and biases.

Vontress (as cited in Shallcross, 2013) explains that we are all multicultural beings. As such, understanding others' worldview is critically important, but recognizing shared aspects of humanity is also necessary to developing multicultural competence. To that end, Sue et al. (2022) discuss the concepts of **culture-specific** and **culture-universal** orientations, sometimes referred to as cultural relativism and cultural universality (p. 27). Sue and colleagues explain that professionals who assume a culture-universal orientation focus on the treatment issue (i.e., diagnosis) and adjust their intervention to address the specific diagnosis or treatment issue. Conversely, individuals who assume a culture-specific approach understand the role of culture in the development, presentation, and treatment of any mental health condition. Therefore, those assuming a culture-specific approach adjust their intervention to match the client's culture and, thereby, address the treatment issues (Sue et al., 2022). Sue et al. explain that most modern mental health professionals adopt an approach that is "**culturally adaptive**" rather than practicing from either extreme of a culture-specific or culture-universal orientation (p. 27). This adaptive or **culturally responsive** approach takes into account the client's diagnosis or treatment issues while honoring the "premise that race, ethnicity, and culture are powerful variables in influencing how people think, behave, and define events" (Sue et al., 2022, p. 32). This is highly important because the manifestations of various psychological states and disorders may differ based on culture-specific *idioms of distress* (or cultural constructs of distress), which can be described as "socially and culturally resonant means of experiencing and expressing distress in local worlds" (Nichter, 2010, p. 405). Rather than pathologizing a client's experience or reaction, it is important to explore the underlying social-embedded narratives that contribute to the client's present experience. As such, Sue et al. presume that cultural competence is prerequisite to counseling competence (p. 27), and we believe the same can be said for crisis intervention.

Pulling these concepts all together, a related construct is multicultural counseling and therapy (MCT), which Sue and Torino (2005) describe as

> Both a helping role and a process that uses modalities and defines goals consistent with the life experiences and cultural values of clients, utilized universal and culture-specific helping strategies and roles, recognizes client identities to include

individual, group, and universal dimensions, and balances the importance of individualism and collectivism in the assessment, diagnosis, and treatment, of the client and client systems (p. 6).

The fundamental aspects of MCT hold true for crisis intervention. Throughout this chapter, we will expound on ways in which key aspects of a MCT approach are reflected in crisis intervention. Additionally, we will introduce you to **Relational Cultural Therapy** (RCT), which is a culture-centered counseling theory that can be used to help the counselor and client explore the intersection of intrapersonal, interpersonal, and social-embedded experiences (Jordan, 2017) that are interwoven in crisis intervention. Let's begin exploring the application of MCT principles to crisis intervention, starting with early conceptualizations of culture.

Powerful lessons were learned over 50 years ago, in 1973, when Billig and Tajfel discovered innate tendencies for humans to engage in social categorization. They discovered the ingroup/outgroup effect that occurs when categorizations are implied among groups of individuals: "the mere mention of 'groups' by the experimenters was sufficient to produce strong intergroup discrimination" (Billig & Tajfel, 1973, p. 48). Broad social categorization without considering the multitude of variations within a given group can be problematic, particularly when considering diversity categorizations. The ingroup/outgroup effect can also promote alliance with one's perceived ingroup to the exclusion of one's perceived outgroup. Relatedly, the concept of "othering" is used to denote those instances in which we conceptualize others as inherently different based on some group membership. In so doing, we fail to recognize the universal aspects of humanity and, instead, focus on group membership (that may be arbitrarily defined) to conceptualize and explain the differences between us, which, if you are in the crisis business, may become particularly difficult to navigate when individuals' cultural backgrounds are different from yours.

The role that culture plays in crisis intervention has to do with what Savicki (2002) has termed uncertainty avoidance—and, as you will learn in this book, attempting to avoid uncertainty and get back in control of a situation gets a lot of attention. **Uncertainty avoidance** has to do with the degree to which cultures feel threatened by uncertainty and ambiguous situations and, as a result, rules, procedures, rituals, and laws may be formulated to buffer uncertainties of

individual judgment (Savicki, 2002, p. 27). What this means in crisis intervention is that a crisis worker who ventures into a different culture had better be aware that the residents of that culture are basing their ability to get though the crisis on their own set of cultural survival standards, and those don't necessarily square up with the crisis worker's cultural standards.

Miller (as cited in Bray, 2019) stated the following regarding the process of joining clients in a way that is multiculturally sensitive and therapeutically effective. "My clients needed me to always remain human, real and compassionate with them so they felt safe and cared for, thereby inviting a genuine, healing dialogue" (para. 54) and that is not easily done in crisis intervention when chaos reigns supreme and you may appear as a stranger with strange and different ideas. This statement poignantly encapsulates the application of multicultural competence to crisis intervention; our work is not likely to be effective if clients do not trust us, and trust is contingent upon clients feeling safe, seen, and respected. Therefore, understanding and being culturally competent in the heat of a crisis event is critical because few clients will mirror the crisis worker's cultural images. Thus, culturally competent crisis workers should be aware of their personal beliefs, values, biases, and attitudes (Ford, 2021); have an awareness of and knowledge of the world view of culturally diverse individuals and groups; and have the ability to employ culturally appropriate intervention skills and strategies with a diverse clientele (Sue et al., 2022). A tall order, indeed, and not easily done!

Core Multicultural Attributes

LO2 Kiselica (1998) identifies four attributes that are widely accepted as necessary for crisis workers and other mental health workers who intervene with clients from various cultural backgrounds. These four attributes include the following: (1) self-knowledge, particularly an awareness of one's own cultural biases; (2) knowledge about the status and cultures of different groups; (3) skills to effect culturally appropriate interventions—including a readiness to use alternative strategies that better match the cultures of crisis clients than traditional strategies; and (4) actual experience in counseling and crisis intervention with culturally different clients (Kiselica, 1998, p. 6).

Sue (1992, p. 12; 1999a, 1999b) reminds us that failure to understand clients' worldviews may lead human services workers to make erroneous interpretations, judgments, and conclusions that result in doing serious harm to clients, especially those who are culturally different. Despite the fact that the world is culturally pluralistic, many of our books, professional teachings, research findings, and implicit theories and assumptions in the field of counseling and crisis intervention are specific to North American and European cultures. Such theories and assumptions are usually so ingrained in our thinking that they are taken for granted and seldom challenged, even by our most broad-minded leaders and professionals (Pedersen, 1999; Ponterotto et al., 2006; Ridley, 2005). As an example, critics of "culture-blind" crisis interventionists propose that their reductionistic and outmoded logical positivism (based solely on observable scientific facts and their relationship to each other and the natural laws of nature) has no place in dealing with widespread violence and social upheaval in large, ethnically different populations caught in long-term wars, rebellions, or other social disasters. They further believe that Western traumatologists adopt a naive view that trauma leads in linear fashion to posttraumatic stress disorder (PTSD) in all people in all cultures. Social constructivists, in particular, rail at this normative view of trauma. They believe it may be much more appropriate to consider trauma, and the crisis intervention that follows it, in much broader social terms, such as safety, grief, injustice, and faith, as opposed to distinct clinical categories of PTSD and depression (Silove, 2000).

There is also a great deal of debate on the validity of any measures that are used to assess the various aspects of crisis that are dealt with in this book because cultural bias and cultural artifacts can skew results to make clients look very different from what they actually are, and this can lead to erroneous treatment decisions (Brown, 2008; Cokley, 2007). Further, the biggest mental health assessment measure of all, the *Diagnostic and Statistical Manual* of the American Psychiatric Association (2022), has come under fire for its limited inclusion of social and cultural factors in the diagnoses of mental disorders. Although the DSM 5 demonstrated some marginal improvements over previous DSM editions in the integration of culture into the diagnostic paradigm (Tomlinson-Clarke & Georges, 2014), the DSM 5 was harshly criticized for failing to critically examine the role of cultural and systemic factors (Ecks, 2016) in the conceptualization, manifestation, and diagnosis of psychological disorders. As such, in the development of the newest version, the DSM 5-TR (American

Psychiatric Association, 2022), efforts were made to address the underlying truth that "the experience of mental illness is influenced by a patient's cultural background, and the risk of mental illness is significantly associated with social determinants of health and mental health" (Moran, 2022, para. 1). Time will tell how effective these shifts are in addressing the multifaceted ways in which culture and mental health intersect.

Ivey (1987) and Arredondo (1999) emphasize that counseling and therapy should begin with counselors' awareness of their own assumptions, values, and biases regarding racial, cultural, and group differences before considering individual variations on those themes. Ivey (1987) states that "only by placing multicultural counseling at the core of counseling curricula can we as counselors truly serve and be with those whom we would help" (p. 169). That statement is probably exponentially true for crisis workers. Specifically in regard to crisis, Brown (2008, p. 167) believes that, more than any other form of distress, persons who live with complex trauma do so in relation to their psychosocial cultural context, and to deny the social identities they bring out of that culture is a pretty effective way to stop intervention before it starts.

Culturally Biased Assumptions

LO3 As Brown (2008) notes, no measure of training in trauma-informed practices can make mental health professionals effective in the absence of a keen understanding of their own cultural lens and the client's cultural identity. Brown attributes much of this to the centrality of the therapeutic relationship and the inherent challenges of forming a strong therapeutic rapport when the mental health professional does not demonstrate cultural competence. She states that trauma has the power to alter clients' identity so fundamentally that it can be difficult for therapists to comprehend and understand how clients perceive themselves (Brown, 2008), but it is incumbent on therapists to seek to understand with heightened awareness and intentionality. Those statements hold doubly true for crisis workers given the profound nature of the crises to which they respond, the multiculturally rich state of the world, and the likelihood for large-scale (sometimes international) disaster relief. The following culturally biased assumptions taken from Pedersen (1987) and Martín-Baró (1996) are ones that crisis workers would do well to remember so as to avoid the related pitfalls these tend to create:

1. People all share a common measure of "normal" behavior (the presumption that problems, emotional responses, behaviors, and perceptions of crises are more or less universal across social, cultural, economic, or political backgrounds and theories and concepts can be modified to fit all groups). Although there are clearly differences and nuances based on culture, the ways in which individuals initially respond to crises have some relatively universal manifestations. This does not mean, though, that crisis workers should treat all clients exactly the same. To do so would mean to completely ignore the overarching assumption of this chapter—that multicultural competence is prerequisite to effective crisis intervention.

2. The definition of problems can be limited by the academic discipline's boundaries (the ways in which crisis workers conceptualize the client's response and the ways in which they should respond is different from the way a professional from a related field may respond, such as how a medical doctor, psychiatrist, or spiritual figure may conceptualize the crisis and their tasks). In fact, successful crisis intervention often requires the use of multiple supports and resources so individuals are provided holistic care. Indeed, when possible, collaboration is typically a best practice in crisis intervention.

3. Western culture depends on abstract conceptualizations and designations for crisis workers (presumptions that others understand the crisis worker's role and intent and that they value the role of mental health support in crisis response). Each culture may have nuanced assumptions or definitions for what crisis workers do, or they may have no similar occupation against which to compare crisis workers. To presume that others buy into the idea of mental health support from a complete stranger would be a massive overstep.

4. Formal counseling is more important than natural support systems surrounding a client (the presumption that clients will be better off with the support offered by professionals over the support of family, peers, and other support groups). This assumption completely disregards the role and effectiveness of informal supports such as family, friends, and peers.

5. Everyone depends on linear thinking (the presumption that each cause has an effect, and each effect is tied to a cause—to explain how the world works—and that everything can be measured and described in terms of good or bad, appropriate or inappropriate, and/or other common dichotomies, and there are no gray areas). Anyone who has been through a crisis or trauma-causing event can readily speak to the often-irrational nature of their thought processes as they try to make sense of the event. Rationality has little room in the initial crisis reaction, which is one reason why we use multiple skills that help clients make some sense of their thoughts and feelings, focus on the problem at hand, and identify a strategy to move forward.

6. Individuals need to fit into the system (the presumption that the system does not need to change to fit the individual). Although it can, at times, be difficult to work with clients whose needs are highly unique, crisis workers are tasked with meeting clients where they are and helping support clients in meeting their individual needs. Admittedly, this can be challenging when crisis workers are tired and overworked, and resources are limited. However, effective crisis workers are able to differentiate their intervention to match the client's needs.

7. The client's past (history) has little relevance to contemporary events (the presumption that crises are mostly related to here-and-now situations and that crisis workers should pay little attention to the client's background). This one is tough. Although the primary focus in crisis intervention is on the present crisis event, the past certainly affects the client's present reaction. As such, although crisis workers do not dig up the past unnecessarily, to ignore the past is also to overlook key aspects of the client's current distress.

8. The belief that knowledge should be based on logic, facts, and empirical evidence alone (the presumption that society operates much like the laws of physics and qualitative measures such as community attitude should be rejected). Feelings may or may not be rooted in facts. When individuals are faced with overwhelming circumstances of which they cannot make sense, logic and fact will have little bearing. Feelings can be absolutely overwhelming and, when this happens, logic tends to fly out the window. When crisis workers try to employ logic to nullify or reject clients' reactions, they will likely be seen as cold, rejecting, and ineffective.

9. The belief that all humans seek pleasure and happiness over pain and sorrow and these negative emotions should be avoided or sublimated (the presumption that human growth can never occur through the suffering that is a natural aspect of all human development). It is probably true that, for the most part, humans seek pleasure over pain. However, to discredit the growth-inducing nature of trauma would be a major oversight. To ignore the potential power of posttraumatic growth (Tedeschi & Calhoun, 2004) would minimize the way in which trauma can transform individuals in sometimes profoundly meaningful and enriching manners.

10. Independence is valuable and dependencies are undesirable (the presumption of Western individualism that people should not be dependent on others or allow others to be dependent on them). Hopefully, at this point in your training, you are keenly aware of the cultural biases implicit in this statement and the high likelihood of those biases to cause harm or, at the very least, limit the development of therapeutic rapport.

11. Individuals are the basic building blocks of all societies (the presumption that crisis intervention is directed primarily toward the individual rather than units of individuals or groups such as the family, organizations, political groups, or society). This assumption is particularly problematic for large-scale disaster response or systemic crises, in which entire communities are affected by the crisis event. Bronfenbrenner (1981) taught us about the importance of recognizing the interaction between multiple ecological systems to understand the individual's development and navigation through life. To ignore the impact of these systems in the development of, response to, and healing from crises would be negligent.

12. Psychological homeostasis and balance must be maintained so people sail through life on an even keel (the presumption that disequilibrium, change, and crisis are always bad and cannot have seeds of growth in negative life events). It is often through suffering, challenges, and disequilibrium that we grow. Although we may strive for psychological homeostasis, we should not rule out the opportunity for growth that comes along with suffering. And crisis workers should be prepared to face the reality that clients will rarely achieve psychological homeostasis following our intervention; rather, crisis workers strive to increase stabilization to the point that the client can make self-determined decisions in response to the crisis event.

13. Human services workers already know all their assumptions (the presumption that if workers were prone toward reacting in closed, biased, and culturally encapsulated ways that promote domination by an elitist group, they would be aware of it). Multicultural competence is a continual pursuit. Crisis workers should engage in a lifelong process of discovering themselves as a means of improving their effectiveness, enhancing their relationships, and engaging in personal growth (Ford, 2021).

All of the foregoing assumptions are flawed and untenable. Hackney and Bernard (2017) describe counseling as "a multicultural experience" that "affects all aspects of process" (p. 6). In order to understand their clients as cultural beings, mental health professionals must first discover their own cultural identity and worldview (Hackney & Bernard, 2017). Mental health professionals who do not understand their own cultural biases and the cultural differences and values of others may misinterpret the behaviors and attitudes of clients from other cultures. Such workers may incorrectly label some client behavior as resistant and uncooperative. They may expect to observe certain client behaviors (such as lack of self-disclosure) that are contrary to the basic values of some cultural groups (Cormier & Hackney, 1987, pp. 256–258). Specifically, in the field of crisis intervention, there has been criticism of the Western-based trauma model and particularly the elevation of PTSD as a pathological entity that has been coined in self-serving ways by survivors' groups, politicians, and profiteering lawyers and therapists when there is little empirical evidence to support such an assumption (Silove, 2000; Summerfield, 1999).

Universal Versus Focused Views

LO4 There are both universal and focused views on multicultural counseling. A **universal view** considers not only racial and ethnic minorities but other minority or special populations as well. A **focused view** looks at multicultural counseling in relation to "visible and racial ethnic minorities" (Sue et al., 1992). We agree with Brown (2008, p. 12) that using racial designation, ethnic labels, or any one characteristic, trait, preference, or other category to identify people may have little or nothing to do with the crises they are encountering and is probably a pretty poor unimodal cultural lens through which to view a person who has been traumatized. To view culture from such a narrow perspective is, we believe, asking for a lot of trouble in crisis intervention.

Working on the Individualist/Collectivist–High/Low-Context Continuum

LO5 From a multicultural perspective, we may generally look at communication along an individualist/collectivist continuum. **Individualism** is a worldview that centralizes the personal—personal goals, personal uniqueness, and personal control—and peripheralizes the social group or social context within which the individual operates. **Collectivism** is based on the assumption that groups bind and mutually obligate individuals, that the personal is simply a component of the larger social group or context and subordinate to it (Oyserman et al., 2002).

These concepts are important because they tend to dictate how the client sees themself in relation to self-concept, sense of well-being, emotional control, and relational and attributional styles (Williams, 2003), which are all critical components in how crisis intervention strategies are formulated and applied to individuals who are in crisis. For instance, a person who lives in a collectivist culture or subculture and who experiences a traumatic event may find that the entire family unit reacts conjointly to the crisis event. Now, consider the implications when that traumatic event is perceived to have some tone of shamefulness. One such example comes from Ecuador, when one of your authors met a woman whose family had all but disowned her following a miscarriage. Although the woman had not done anything to purposefully endanger the unborn child, her family believed she was responsible for the unborn child's death and, as a result, she was treated as though she was at fault for the miscarriage. She carried that shame and self-hatred for years without even questioning the legitimacy therein. Although one can easily assert that the family unit in individualistic cultures tends to react when a family member experiences a crisis, there are some notable differences that we can observe through a cultural lens.

In a meta-analysis of 170 studies on the individualist/collectivist worldview, Oyserman et al. (2002) found that individualism centers on one's self-concept

rather than one's family life, compared to collectivism, in which the opposite is true. In regard to "sense of well-being," individualists view well-being as related to a sense of personal control; collectivists do not. Even more important in terms of crisis intervention, individualism proponents tend to view the event in terms of their own personal preferences, while collectivist proponents interpret the event in relation to what they believe the expectations of others might be. A rather startling discovery contradicts the accepted belief that people who are collectivist consider the group, and particularly the family, as taking precedence and obligation over individual well-being. They found essentially no difference between individualists and collectivists regarding "sense of family obligation." When a dilemma was presented, collectivists responded by identifying themselves as part of a cooperative group, and individualists considered themselves to be individuals participating as part of a team effort.

Finally, Osyerman and associates (2002) discovered that communication and conflict resolution styles varied in relation to individualism and collectivism. Individualism consistently predicted goal-oriented, low-context, direct communication; collectivism opted for indirect, high-context communication. In confrontational situations, individualists adhered to a confrontational and arbitrational approach; collectivists preferred an accommodation and negotiation approach.

But how do people in a collective society operate under stress and traumatic conditions? The Heppners and their associates (2006) conducted research in establishing the Collectivist Coping Styles Inventory (CCSI) that attempted to discern how stressful and traumatic events are handled from an Asian perspective. Indeed, the 3,000 Taiwanese college students in the study endorsed coping strategies very different from those of their Western counterparts. Their acceptance, fatalism, efficacy, and interpersonal harmony strategies when faced with stressful events are unlike any other factors endorsed on traditional coping strategy inventories in the Western world. Family support and religious and spiritual resources are also different from their Western counterparts. Filial piety and elder support are important, and advice is generally sought within the sanctity of the family (Heppner et al., 2006). The authors determined that the CCSI "contained constructs that appear quite different than Western coping inventories and provide new information about collectivistic styles of coping with stressful and traumatic life events" (p. 114).

The Chinese kanji characters of crisis and opportunity that appear on the cover of this book are evident in the Taiwanese students' approach to coping with crisis. The Confucian and Buddhist philosophies that one endures suffering, looks for positive meaning, and exercises control and restraint predominate in their responses. Finally, their avoidance and emotional detachment from the stressful event and private emotional outlets are also different. Whereas in the United States, we might expect an outpouring of emotion and immediate public support and grief following a traumatic event (Halpern & Tramontin, 2007, p. 98), the results from this study suggest that these students seek outside help as a last resort, and when they do, it is most often in a confidential and anonymous manner. Their coping strategies revolved around avoiding shame and seeking help in safe, anonymous ways. The Heppners and their associates (2006) suggest that these students might go to a mental health professional who was unknown to them or their families or go into a chat room on the internet to discuss their problems. The point is that, at least for these Taiwanese students who participated in the study, when under stress or traumatized, they might seek mental health help very differently than would their American counterparts.

High/Low-Context Approaches. To put the foregoing analysis in operational terms useful to the crisis worker, the individualist/collectivist continuum uses what Hall (1976) calls a high/low-context approach. In low-context cultures, one's self-image and worth are defined in personal, individual terms. In high-context cultures, one's self-worth and esteem are tied to the group. In low-context cultures, information is generally transmitted explicitly and concretely through language; in high-context cultures, information is transmitted in the physical context of the interaction or internalized in the person. In high-context cultures, facial expressions, gestures, and tone of voice are as important as the meaning of words that are said. Thus, in high-context cultures, the individual will expect the other person to know what the problem is so that the person who is trying to communicate distress does not have to talk directly about the issue (which could be embarrassing or shameful). This communication style can be very problematic for a crisis worker who operates from a low-context style in which specific and concrete

information is sought to determine what is needed to address the problem.

From the high-context client's standpoint, the low-context worker's attempt to gather specific information about the client's personal and social status in relationship to the crisis may be seen as intrusive, rude, and offensive. A high-context culture uses stories, proverbs, fables, metaphors, similes, and analogies to make a point (Augsburger, 1992). Thus, a high-context crisis worker might be very delicate, ambiguous, sensitive, and somewhat circumlocutory in discussing personal and social issues related to the crisis. In trying to help a low-context client, a crisis worker using such a communication style might be viewed as not being remotely aware of the frustrated client's needs.

As a result, one of the major challenges in crisis intervention with culturally diverse individuals lies in both sending and receiving communication that is understandable and clearly communicates what we are attempting to do while not exacerbating an already potentially volatile situation. While it is impossible to know the nuances of every culture and the subtleties of the client's native language, one of our rules of the road in crisis intervention in which cultural differences are pronounced is that there are these two broad groups (high context and low context), and we need to find out which one the client is operating in so that we can respond accordingly. In other words, we need to adjust to the client rather than asking the client to adjust to our communication style.

Crisis worker: (speaking to an East African man, a recent immigrant, who has been injured in a train wreck and doesn't know what has happened to his family) I understand you are from Somalia. I don't know a lot about your country or customs, so please let me know if what I am saying doesn't agree with what you think is right. I will do my best to explain our processes here in the United States, and we can explore how we might be able to proceed in a way that respects your cultural background. Our common goal is to find out about your family and get you the medical help you need.

We also need to clearly own that we may be culturally ignorant and, thus, appear to be insensitive to the crisis client's needs. Such admissions early on go a long way in letting the client clarify their needs. Those owning statements are true whether we are dealing with survivors of a natural disaster, survivors of sex trafficking, war refugees from Ukraine, or survivors of mass shootings. There is no place for ego in crisis intervention; it is more important to help your client than to hold fast to appearances of expertise.

High/Low Uncertainty Avoidance Approaches.

High- and low-context cultures get a lot of space in professional human service publications. What doesn't, and is particularly appropriate to crisis intervention, is understanding whether the culture one is entering into is operating on high or low uncertainty avoidance principles (Savicki, 2002, p. 27). High uncertainty avoidance cultures develop a broad range of rules, regulations, and procedures to cover a multitude of contingencies. In other words, if you are entering a high uncertainty avoidance culture, you had better understand they have a playbook of what is right and proper that will rival that of a playbook from the National Football League (if you are not a football fan, those books are huge and enormously complicated). If you don't understand and operate within it, you'll wind up butting your head against a very large cultural wall. On the other hand, if you are entering a low uncertainty avoidance culture, you may well be frustrated by a "Relax! Be happy! We're all alive! We have food and water! Hurricanes come and go! We'll rebuild tomorrow!" view. That sort of a "chill out" worldview can sabotage the herculean efforts of highly motivated disaster workers who are operating on short timeframes and deadlines, leaving them embittered and burned out from the experience.

Meet the Super Multiculturally Competent Crisis Worker.

Here's an abridged definition of what Sue and Sue (2013, p. 46) believe a multiculturally competent human services worker should be. They should actively engage in a reflective process to become aware of and monitor their own "values, beliefs, assumptions . . . preconceived notions, personal limitations" about others (Sue et al., 2022, p. 33). Second, they should work to understand their client's worldview and the sociocultural context in which their client lives. Third, they approach their work with enhanced intentionality so they are utilizing practices that are culturally responsive and conducive to their clients' development (Sue et al., 2022). That's a whole lot of "shoulds" and sounds like a human services worker straight out of Marvel comics. As of yet, we have not discovered that superworker, so how can a human services worker at least get close to what Sue and Sue are proposing? We believe workers can come closest

to that high standard when they operate from what cultural anthropologists call an *emic* model (Kottak, 2006) and what Brown (2008) calls *social location* when applied to people in trauma.

Emic Versus Etic Models of Multiculturalism

LO6 An **emic** model encompasses the smorgasbord of components that make up individuals from their subjective view of who they are, not just what their individual parts are, but more the total Gestalt of how they come together. Conversely, an **etic** model describes traits and factors common to all within the group that can be objectively identified by outside observers (Friedman & Schustack, 2010; Kottak, 2006). While both are important in obtaining what cultural and contextual factors are operating in the crisis, when face-to-face for the first time with a person in crisis, finding the parts of the individual that make up the total Gestalt of the crisis and fitting those to the worker are of critical importance. Why is this so?

There is a great deal of research that, more than anything else, the strength of the therapeutic alliance or working relationship that is created between the worker and the client will determine, to a large degree, therapeutic effectiveness (Leibert & Dunne-Bryant, 2015; Wampold, 2010, 2012), and that may be particularly true with individuals experiencing psychotic behaviors (Owens et al., 2013). One of the critical training components of the Memphis Police Department CIT training program is how the CIT officer makes initial contact with a client because those first few moments of contact have profound ramifications on the building of a working bond between the officer and the consumer and the ultimate positive resolution of the crisis (Kirchberg, 2014).

So please meet the emic model of Dr. Dick James, an 80-something cisgender man who is mostly happy about still being above ground; concerned grandfather; husband who thinks he's been married longer than he's been alive sometimes; former construction worker (He had to pay for school somehow) who is now hard of hearing because of too many days on an air hammer and gets yelled at for not wearing his hearing aid; fisherman and hunter who pals around with one of his daughters doing those activities; White guy who grew up in a university town but had blue-collar parents; 1960s era gourmet who now has digestive trouble eating pizza and drinking beer; trainer for police officers to deal with individuals with a mental health issue and who are severely agitated; former baseball player and track runner in an integrated high school in the 1960s, where he developed lifelong friends; former school counselor in a blue-collar Midwestern town; Presbyterian who goes pretty regularly to church but has been a Baptist and a Methodist and has a lot of friends who are Catholic and Jewish; author of books like this one instead of the great American novel he always imagined he would write; and jokester whose sense of humor leaks out and sometimes gets him in trouble; and survivor of a crisis at age 21 when he got shot in the chest while with a girl who he would have probably married . . . if he hadn't gotten shot, and so on.

These are what Laura Brown (2008, p. 24) calls **social locations,** the individual identifiers that go far beyond, race, sex, and skin tone that make us specific and unique individuals that reside in a cultural group. Both she and we believe they are important from a multicultural standpoint when you are doing this work. So, if you compare all that to just Dr. James older adult, or Dr. James professor, or Dr. James White guy, or any other unitary, focused etic view of Dr. James, you surely aren't getting the view you got a couple of sentences ago, and our guess would be you might not respond in quite the same way if you were doing crisis intervention with him. Thus, we take a universal/emic view rather than a focused/etic view in crisis intervention. Therefore, when we speak of cultural diversity, we are speaking in the broadest possible terms in regard to all factors that somehow make clients "different" from the interventionist. Hopefully, the following analogies illuminate what is meant by a universal/emic view.

Your worldview, if you are a New York City social worker and you have spent your entire life in the city and are now trying to help a Midwestern farmer who has just lost everything in a flood, is going to be as different from his worldview as his suspiciousness may be directed toward you when you make reference to his "pinto" cows (Holstein breeds and not mustang horses). Similarly, our worldviews would likely be different from that of an Ecuadorian or Turkish survivor of an earthquake who we are attempting to help. Or, how about your first attempt at crisis intervention with a Christian Scientist who may have a very different view of healthcare and how it is delivered than you do? Does that mean you will be ineffective and should not try to assist in large-scale disaster response or a different religion? Certainly not! What it does mean is that multicultural differences are not always obvious, and multicultural competence is an ongoing pursuit. In a statement that absolutely captures the essence of what is meant by a universal view, Halpern and Tramontin (2007) quote New York regional mental health officials: "In the large and diverse state of New York, when you know one county in the state you know one county" (p. 316). So how in the world do you do this business if there is that much diversity, not just in the world, but in one state?

Laura Brown (2008, p. 12) has used Hays' **ADDRESSING model** (2001, 2008) as one of the bases for her book on multiculturalism and trauma. The ADDRESSING acronym encompasses Age, acquired and Developmental Disabilities, Religion, Ethnicity, Social class, Sexual orientation, Indigenous heritage, National origin, and Gender. D'Andrea and Daniels (2005) have developed a comparable model called **RESPECTFUL** (Religious/spiritual, Economic class, Sexual identity, Psychological development, Ethnic/racial identity, Chronological age, Trauma and threats to well-being, Family, Unique physical issues, and Language and location of residence). From our own experience, we would add geographic locale, living area (urban, suburban, rural), occupation, education, and marital or partner status. We believe these variables are major components that start to capture the essence of how the crisis interventionist needs to think about clients and work with the multiple identities that intersect with the crisis.

However, Brown is about the business of doing trauma therapy, and while crisis may certainly occur in the delivery of trauma therapy, it isn't the same as doing crisis intervention with an out-of-control female client who is experiencing suicidal/homicidal thoughts and who has just been dumped by the love of her life and is now standing on the guardrail of the I-40 Hernado De Soto bridge over the Mississippi river. We believe that when such a crisis occurs, a more specific model to operationalize social locations is warranted.

LO7 **The SAFETY Model.** To that end, Dr. Kristi Nobbman has developed a further iteration of social locations that we believe applies more specifically to the work of crisis intervention. Nobbman has developed the **SAFETY model** (Stability, Affect, Friction, Environment, Temperament, and Yearning) (Nobbman et al., 2014). The SAFETY acronym is not happenstance. Safety is the overriding task for everyone involved in a crisis. Myer et al. (2022) provide more detail of the SAFETY model in their book, *Crisis Intervention Ethics Casebook*. Here, we will try to introduce the model and explain how it applies to crisis intervention.

In terms of the SAFETY model, here is a short definition of the acronym:

Stability: Stability refers to consistency, logic, and strength of purpose in terms of thinking and behaving. Achieving stability in a crisis is the primary goal.

Affect: Affect is observed emotions, both verbal and nonverbal. The intent is to move the client from agitated or blunted locations to calm and tranquil ones.

Friction: Friction is identified by the triggers that escalate the situation, whether they are intrapersonal, interpersonal, or systemic. Finding friction points/locations and easing them is critical to developing stability.

Environment: Environment refers to the physical and/or personal setting as well as the social aspects of what/who is involved. Changing the environment by physically moving locations or removing individuals or other noxious stimuli that may agitate the individual are often critical. The environment can have major implications for physical and psychological safety.

Temperament: Temperament is our natural way of being. However, in this context, temperament also addresses how the crisis worker and the client generally act based on all of their cultural experiences and knowledge. For the crisis worker, temperament may also have something to do with their experience handling crises and ability to handle the demands of multiculturally competent crisis work.

Yearning: Yearning refers to what drives clients into crises and their attempt to alleviate it. It may be a physical, psychological, social, and/or spiritual desire/longing. Most often, clients yearn to ease frustrated attempts to obtain something that has been lost, such as drugs, a loved one, or their pre-trauma self.

Compounding the issue even more is the fact that you, the interventionist, are bringing all these social locations into the equation, too. Consider Figure 2.1 and how Dr. James' social locations fit (or not) with Leron, an individual you will meet in Chapter 3, "The Intervention and Assessment Models," who is having a really bad day. Dr. James will do a quick assessment of Leron's affective, behavioral, and cognitive functioning and immediately start identifying his social locations, which he believes may affect his intervention with Leron. By owning who he is, he is attempting to engage the client, which is the first task of the crisis intervention model you will meet in Chapter 3, "The Intervention and Assessment Models." Besides dealing with the very obvious social locations that differ between crisis workers and their clients, you need to be aware of *all* the baggage you carry into this particular environment that may hinder your efforts. Thus, Dr. James' social location of hearing impairment may not be visible, but on a noisy street, it can be problematic, to say the least, if he misinterprets what he hears and is too proud not to mention this fact early on to a client who may see him as a whole lot of other things that are not helpful if he can't respond clearly and correctly. So, he needs to be very aware of his own **friction** and the **environment locations** in the SAFETY model.

Likewise, he needs to be sensitive to the fact that one of Leron's present social locations is intoxication, and it may be more the whiskey than the man doing the talking in regard to his **temperament location**. So, while our crisis interventionist may or may not have trouble because of his own social locations, he needs to be cognizant that those factors may indeed be operating and may exacerbate the friction Leron is already feeling toward authority figures and the government. Thus, for the master practitioners of crisis intervention, it is critical to their success that they are sophisticated enough to know when social locations they inhabit may become the major dynamic they are dealing with (Brown, 2009, p. 40) and what they need to do about it.

It is of more than passing interest that in workshops we have conducted with three different groups of counselors (Nobbman et al., 2014), counselor educators (James, 2013b), and CIT police officers (James et al., 2013a) that involved identifying their social locations with videos of persons in crisis, the CIT officers were able to name more of their social locations than either the counselors or counselor educators. Why do you suppose that is so? We believe it has a good deal to do with CIT officer training and their experience and ability to quickly assess clients' social locations and to broach the gap between their own locations and the client's/consumer's to bond with them.

Broaching. To that end, crisis workers need to practice what Day-Vines and her associates (2007) called

Dr. James' Social Locations

Born and raised in Illinois

Lives in Memphis

Past middle age

Family raised, lives with wife

Employed as professor

Earned a Ph.D.

Upper middle class

Caucasian cisgender man

Mentally alert

Intoxicated

Generally good health

Police consultant

Angry with housing authority

Crisis interventionist

Depressed over loss of family
and inability to find work

Hearing impaired,
especially with
background noise

Counseling Psychologist

Crisis setting

Born in Mississippi

Middle of a major thoroughfare
in rush hour traffic

Lives in Memphis

Middle-aged

Threatening, armed with
two broken bottles

Black
cisgender man

Drinking heavily

Health deterioration

Police on the scene,
traffic stopped

Family left him

Homeless

Out-of-work forklift operator

Three years of high school

Lower middle class, moving to lower class

Poor history with Police

Leron's Social Locations

Figure 2.1   ADDRESSING Social Locations: Dr. James and Leron

broaching. Broaching refers to the crisis worker's consistent display of openness to invite the client to explore issues of diversity and a recognition that race, ethnicity, or some universal trait may be contributing to the crisis. Being able to assess for those individual social locations, fit them with the worker's and rapidly tap into the client's social locations is critical in establishing an empathic working alliance. Let's look at one example. Remember, as we mentioned in the Preface, there is some strong language in this book and some terms that we do not personally endorse. This is crisis intervention, though; the last thing clients are

concerned about is your feelings. Raw emotions and unfiltered thoughts are to be expected. When clients start using directing words toward you that make you uncomfortable, you have to respond with professionalism and maintain your helping stance. So, give that a try in the following brief exchange.

Leron: What the hell you doin' out here, you nosey ass White guy? Unless you from Channel Five, I ain't got nuthin' fo' you. I want the whole world to know about them Nazis down at the housin' authority done kicked me out fo' no good reason.

Dr. James: I realize that I'm a White guy who isn't homeless and furthermore that I have a police T-shirt on that says I work for the man. I understand that may affect your ability to trust me, but the T-shirt also says CIT, which means I am a person who trains police officers to deal with folks who have problems that frustrate them and cause them to take actions they normally wouldn't do unless they felt they had no other options. That seems to be about where you are right now. So, if you have questions about who I am, I'll be glad to answer them. By the way, one of the "Who I ams" is that I'm a little hard of hearing and it's noisy out here so I'd appreciate it if you could speak up a bit so I am sure I get everything you are saying. So, I wonder if you might trust me enough to tell me what got you out here in the middle of one of the busiest streets in Memphis to get the attention you seem to need.

While making a number of owning statements to let Leron know what his social locations are both professionally and physically, our sweat-drenched doctor immediately attempts to intervene. Dr. James finds what Leron is *yearning* for and what *friction* he is currently suffering that is critical enough to put his life at risk by standing in one of the busiest streets in Memphis at rush hour.

To make things even more problematic, it isn't just "culture" that factors into this increasingly complex picture but the "ecology," or setting, you are working in as well. By setting, we mean the living environment in which the intervention occurs. It is 98 degrees Fahrenheit (36.6 C) out on that street where Leron is standing. Do you suppose that adds to the problem? Your intervention will change and be influenced by a number of variables that are specific to the setting. Are you working in a nice, air-conditioned office with one person or in a packed evacuation center with the power going on and off, that is full of people 24/7 who haven't had a bath in a while, and you haven't either? Are you working in the panhandle of Oklahoma in 100-degree weather in July with a blast furnace wind blowing all the time and you are from Minnesota? Or perhaps you are from an Iowa farming community where the tallest building is a grain elevator, and you find yourself on Michigan Avenue in Chicago buried in the canyon of skyscrapers. So, it isn't just culture by itself; it is also the ecological landscape you are operating in that is going to affect how and what you do.

Awareness of Both Ecology and Multicultural Competencies

LO8   Figure 2.2 is a diagram of the effects of ecology/culture on client–worker interactions. Notice that the "crisis" triangle has a component at each corner: the crisis worker, the client, and their ecological/cultural determinants. The two-way arrows connecting the three corners indicate the mutual and dynamic interaction that constantly occurs among all the possible ecological/cultural factors that affect both crisis worker and client: family, race, religion, locale, physical ability, sex, economic class, vocation, physical needs, social affiliations, and so on. The triangle itself represents the environment in which you are working and the ecological background and cultural attitudes, beliefs, and heritages you and the client bring into that setting. Thus, for a therapy to be ecologically valid or appropriate, it needs to correlate with clients' ethnocultural and linguistic experiences that they bring into therapy and the cultural structure of the therapy provided for them (Rodriguez & Bernal, 2012). For this to happen, Rodriguez and Bernal (p. 25) propose that a complex constellation of language, persons, metaphors, content, concepts, goals, methods, and context need to be in place. Now, add attempting to carry out all these in a crisis, and you may begin to understand how daunting ecologically/culturally valid crisis intervention can be.

A study by Norris and Alegria (2006) exemplifies this concept. The relationship of age to PTSD is an outstanding example of the effect of cultural context. Norris and Alegria (2006) report that among three samples of disaster survivors, manifesting PTSD occurred at higher rates in younger Mexicans, middle-aged Americans, and older Poles. Clearly, there was no one consistent effect of disaster by age. Rather, the cultural context of the country and the

Figure 2.2   The Dynamic Effect of Ecology/Culture on Client–Crisis Worker Interactions

variation in historical social roles that are dictated in those countries would seem to have a great deal of influence on how the crisis will unfold when age is a factor (Norris & Alegria, 2006). So, if you are in the PTSD treatment business, it ought to become apparent that culture can have some profound effects on the emergence of post-trauma symptoms and what clients bring into the therapeutic setting. Moreover, a singular treatment approach will not be sufficient to address their varied needs.

Locus of Control. When the crisis worker is factored into the equation, the intervention becomes even more complex. Internal versus external locus of control is a particularly aggravating problem that may bedevil crisis workers. Most crisis workers have a high internal locus of control and believe that through personal effort, one can start to regain psychological homeostasis and equilibrium (Atkinson et al., 1998). Understand, then, that no therapy is done in a sterile vacuum, free from the multiple effects of the ecological/cultural background. That statement is even truer in the highly charged emotional context of crisis intervention.

The wise crisis worker understands this complexity and, when faced with an out-of-control client whose ecological context and background may be extremely different from the crisis worker's, goes slowly and carefully. The wise crisis worker is highly sensitive to and asks questions about the person's preferred mode of receiving assistance. As an example, Weisaeth (2000) reports on deciding *not* to do critical incident stress debriefing (CISD) with a UN peacekeeping battalion of Fiji Islanders who were doing duty in South Lebanon. After an artillery attack that left many dead and wounded civilians they had been sheltering in their compound, the Fijis worked through their stress by using a very intense and emotional group ceremonial ritual that involved a mildly intoxicating drink called *kawa*. Weisaeth wisely decided to drop any attempt at a standard CISD because it was apparent the Fijis had their own quite adequate way of dealing with the trauma. Any attempt to shoehorn CISD into the Fiji cultural tradition might have caused a great deal of resistance and done more harm than good.

Particularly in crisis intervention, we seldom have the freedom to choose which clients we will get or take, and we generally do not have the luxury of making referrals simply because the client's ecological/cultural background does not fit nicely into our own. What we can and must do is be acutely sensitive to the client's emerging needs and, in Carl Rogers' terms (Raskin & Rogers, 1995), prize that person in regard to their distinctive individuality in the context of the crisis situation. Above all else, research on the outcomes of therapy tells us that establishing a relationship built on trust and credibility is far and away the most important condition for a successful outcome of any kind of therapeutic endeavor (Capuzzi & Gross, 1995, pp. 12–25).

Toward Culturally Effective Helping During a Crisis

The plain and simple truth is that we don't know a lot about how culture, crises, and crisis intervention interact (Brown, 2008, pp. 256–257). Very little research has been done in the area, although progress has recently been made by key leaders, such as Duffey and Haberstroh (2022). Certain cultures don't even have words for trauma (Silove, 1998)! However, we do know that deeply held cultural beliefs and previously learned ways of dealing with the world rapidly surface when individuals are placed in a crisis situation (Dass-Brailsford, 2008). When a traumatic event occurs, there is a high probability that people will revert to their long-held cultural beliefs no matter where they live and work at the moment (Brown, 2009, p. 154).

Certainly, much human-made crisis revolves around lack of cultural understanding and conflicts between cultures. Eidelson and Eidelson (2003) have documented how distorted beliefs may produce excessive death, suffering, and displacement as a result of conflicts among and between groups regarding ethnicity, nationality, religion, or other social identities and issues. These researchers focused on five core belief domains that propel both individuals and groups to make dangerous assumptions about people who are different from themselves. The domains are identified as revolving around assumptions regarding superiority, injustice, vulnerability, distrust, and helplessness. Deeply entrenched patterns for understanding, perceiving, and interpreting events appear to govern and produce emotions and behaviors that may ultimately lead to conflicts and problematic and destructive crises. Distorted and dysfunctional beliefs appear to be at the core of many of the problems that crisis interventionists and other helping professionals face.

An example of such a distortion is the widespread belief among New Orleans Black people that levees were blown up to save White residential districts from Hurricane Katrina's floodwaters. There is, in fact, a historical precedence for blowing up New Orleans' levees to save parts of the city. The fact that it did not happen in Katrina's case makes little difference to those people who lost everything but the shirts on their backs. How do you think you would be received if you attempted to do crisis intervention with these individuals—particularly if you were White, and more particularly if you told them you didn't believe that the levees were intentionally blown up? Do you give up before you start? Not hardly!

Past history and experience may play a pivotal role in how recipients of service perceive crisis intervention. Mexican American families whose homes had been damaged in the 1989 Northern California Loma Prieta earthquake refused to go to mass shelters in schools and auditoriums. They continued to live in tents and also refused to go back to their damaged homes. The same was true after the 1995 Northridge earthquake near Los Angeles, even after authorities assured the Mexican Americans that it would be safe. The reason for their refusal was that aftershocks from the 1985 earthquake in Mexico City had killed and injured many people who had gone to such shelters or had returned to damaged homes. It finally took bicultural, bilingual "assurance teams" of crisis workers to convince the recent immigrants in California to go to shelters or return to their homes (Myers & Wee, 2005, pp. 59–60).

Culturally Effective Helping

LO9 As the field grows and expands and as mental health professionals progressively develop multicultural competence, we will see numerous shifts in what is considered a best practice when working with individuals who are culturally diverse. However, as you will find throughout this book, the rules of the road and intervention strategies used in a traditional therapeutic setting can be quite different from what transpires in crisis intervention. When there is no time for the initial development of therapeutic rapport and having well-thought-out conversations about diversity, the crisis worker must respond to the best of their ability in a way that maximizes safety while honoring and respecting diversity. This is no small feat. Indeed, the application of multicultural counseling competencies to crisis intervention continue to emerge. To

that point, the multicultural approaches to crisis intervention described here do not have universal support among helping professionals whose focus might be on a traditional therapeutic setting in which there is time to explore cultural identities. In this book, we are hoping to demonstrate our sincere belief that all therapeutic intervention, regardless of the setting, must be conducted from a multiculturally competent stance. However, the way multicultural competence manifests will be different when faced with critical, time-sensitive incidents like those found in crisis intervention work. The most elegant therapeutic application of multicultural competence in crisis intervention we have found was developed by Duffey and Haberstroh (2020).

Relational Cultural Counseling (RTC). In their book, *Introduction to Crisis and Trauma Counseling,* Duffey and Haberstroh (2020) propose an application of Jordan's (2018) Relational Cultural Therapy (RCT) to both crisis intervention and trauma therapy. RCT, originally developed in 1981, is based on fundamental principles as described by Jordan (2018): (a) we grow through relationships and are inevitably interdependent, connected, as a core condition of our being; (b) engagement in "growth-fostering" (p. 7) and reciprocal relationships allow individuals to exercise "relationship differentiation, rather than separation" as a natural part of development (p. 6); (c) mutual empathy is a prerequisite for growth-fostering relationships, and mutual empathy "involves mutual impact, mutual care, and mutual responsiveness" (p. 7); (d) growth can occur in profound ways when there is conflict or "differences in connection" when those differences are handled with openness and a willingness to own one's role in the conflict or difference (p. 8); and (e) the RCT therapist must have a "responsive presence" that demonstrates a profound respect for the client and openness to change rather than reliance on a specific set of skills (p. 8). These basic tenets are not taken lightly and require intensive, ongoing effort on behalf of the therapist and vulnerability and trust on the part of the client. Those are graces not easily extended by individuals who are in acute distress and whose past relationships might not have set the stage for them to be open to the prospect of a complete stranger being trustworthy or even able to help.

Further, RCT provides a highly interactive conceptualization of growth and relationships. As Jordan explains, "connection is the goal of RCT" and "disconnection is the challenge it seeks to overcome" (p. 8).

Various isms (e.g., racism, sexism, classism) and social stigmatizations can lead to chronic disconnections. And, although RCT therapists can work with clients to address chronic disconnections, doing so requires a mutual experience of vulnerability that can be highly threatening to individuals who have been oppressed and marginalized (Jordan, 2018). Indeed, working to overcome internalized thoughts and beliefs about oneself, whether those thoughts and beliefs are rooted in oppression or trauma, is an arduous process. RCT therapists recognize the inherent presence of power and privilege in the therapeutic relationship, and they seek to address it through a genuine encounter characterized by vulnerability and mutual empathy.

Through meeting clients where they are, without hiding behind facades and enforcing unnecessary power differentials in the therapeutic relationship, therapists can connect with clients in a reciprocal and mutually beneficial manner. In so doing, clients and therapists both grow through the relationship.

Perhaps this sounds really hard, and maybe a little intimidating. Let's explore what Jordan (2018, pp. 28–29) defines as the core concepts of RCT, which can help operationalize your understanding of this therapeutic approach.

1. "People grow through and toward relationship throughout the lifespan." (Relationships are the cornerstone of human experience, and it is innate for humans to seek relationships. Likewise, we learn and grow through our relationships. Maintaining, rebuilding, or forming new relationships are critical components of crisis intervention).
2. "Movement toward mutuality rather than separation characterizes mature functioning." (As we mature into life and our relationships, we should ideally seek connection with others. However, that process can be disrupted, particularly when a crisis occurs, causing the prospect of connection with others to be overwhelming and even threatening. That's why early bonding, openness to the client, and building trust to form a mutual working relationship are critical).
3. "Relationship differentiation and elaboration characterize growth." (Learning to effectively navigate relationships is a significant characteristic of personal growth. Attempting as hard as you can to see why something seems to make sense to the client and acknowledging that to the client goes a long way toward dealing with communication problems in crisis intervention).
4. "Mutual empathy and mutual empowerment are at the core of growth-fostering relationships." (Relationships that are growth-promoting are characterized by the experience of reciprocal empathy, vulnerability, and empowerment of both individuals. Surprising as it may be, every crisis interaction has within it the power of growth, not only for the client but also for the interventionist).
5. "Authenticity is necessary for real engagement and full participation in growth-fostering relationships." (Being true to oneself is necessary to the establishment of growth-promoting relationships. Simply put, don't be a fake. You can't be Dr. Myer, Whisenhunt, or James. Be your decent self).
6. "In growth-fostering relationships, all people contribute and grow or benefit. Development is not a one-way street." (Relationships that are truly growth-promoting are not one-sided; both individuals grow as a result of the relationship. Whether success or failure, we learn from and take something away from the exchange with the client).
7. "One of the goals of development from a relational perspective is the development of increased relational competence and capacities over the lifespan." (As we mature, we ideally become more adept at fostering healthy relationships. We have probably learned more from our mistakes than our successes, but doing so requires humility and an openness to learning).
8. "Mutual empathy is the primary means through which we grow. Placing mutual empathy at the core of human development not only affects the individual but also contributes to the growth of a just society. Social justice is the outcome of the practice of mutuality in which the needs and experience of both people in any given interaction are respected and honored." (The experience of empathizing with others and allowing them to empathize with you, which takes some measure of vulnerability, is the key to developing healthy relationships. Moreover, through feeling *with* others and allowing them to feel *with* us, we promote a relationship that is inherently respectful. If you get really good at the practice of mutual empathic understanding while doing crisis intervention, we believe you will be upholding the principles of social justice in action).

Jordan writes extensively about each of these concepts and their therapeutic application, and we highly encourage you to thoroughly review her work. However, as you are learning about RCT, you might be wondering how RCT can be operationalized for use in such a short-term context. Enter Duffey and Haberstroh (2020).

It probably goes without saying that a pure application of RCT to crisis intervention is highly difficult, if not impossible. However, Duffey and Haberstroh (2020) propose the application of the aforementioned core concepts of RCT in crisis work. Through joining the client in an authentic, mutually empathetic, and respectful manner, rapport can be developed, and support can be provided. That is a pretty simplistic explanation. So, let's examine some of Duffey and Haberstroh's (2020) applications of RCT to crisis work.

First, remembering that RCT is a way of being with a client more than a specific set of skills, Duffey and Haberstroh talk about the importance of being authentic with clients who are in crisis and allowing them to exercise authenticity as "a source of direction, hopefulness, and relief" (p. 5).

Second, in addition to an authentic and sincere presence in the relationship, this also includes non-judgement for the client's statements, behavior, feelings, and thoughts. Second, crisis workers consider context (e.g., the situation, setting, triggers, behavioral cues) and avoid perpetuating stereotypes or beliefs that are detrimental to growth. Rather, using RCT as a guiding framework, crisis workers conceptualize clients through a "strengths-based, relational lens" to understand their reaction and the underlying factors may contribute to their reaction (Duffey & Haberstroh, 2020, p. 6).

Third, crisis workers strive to reduce the presence of "power-over" and, instead, strive to establish a "power-with,"(egalitarian) approach (p. 6), which can be seen as a shared sense of power between the crisis worker and the client. Fourth, crisis workers understand the inherent need for connection and seek to join the client but recognize the client's patterns of disconnection. Fifth, and relatedly, crisis workers recognize clients' patterns of acute disconnection, they understand the inherently protective nature of those patterns (i.e., survival), and they do not take offense to the client's efforts to protect self through keeping the crisis worker at a distance. Sixth, utilizing an RCT framework, crisis workers help clients build "relational resilience" through connection and mutuality, thereby equipping clients to manage relational stress in a healthy manner that does not result in chronic disconnection.

Finally, RCT crisis workers utilize a relational model for ethical decision-making that requires them to put the crisis worker-client relationship at the center of the decision-making process and that accounts for situational context, including awareness of diversity factors and the client's unique needs (Duffey & Haberstroh, 2020). Summed up, RCT practitioners are compassionate, responsive, and empathic (Duffey & Haberstroh, 2020). Simple words, but hard-earned skills. Regardless of the skills we use in our work, if we do not meet the client where they are and demonstrate a keen respect for their worldview, we are highly unlikely to be effective. RCT provides a compass through which to connect with clients while challenging ourselves to learn and grow through the process as we cultivate power-with.

Positive Aspects of an Effective Multicultural Counselor

LO10 Sue (1992) states that multicultural helping is enhanced when the human services worker "uses methods and strategies and defines goals consistent with the life experiences and culture values of the client" (p. 13). Belkin (1984) points out that cross-cultural counseling need not be a negative experience, that it may effectively resolve client problems as well as provide a unique learning experience for both client and helper, and that the main "barrier to effective cross-cultural counseling is the traditional counseling role itself, which is not applicable to many cross-cultural interactions" (p. 527). Belkin further states that the principal cross-cultural impediments are (1) language differences, (2) class-bound values, and (3) culture-bound values (p. 534). Belkin concludes that perhaps the most positive discovery and/or belief of the effective cross-cultural counselor is that humans everywhere are more alike than they are different (p. 543).

Cormier and Hackney (1987) cite several strategies that culturally effective helpers use. For instance, such helpers (1) examine and understand the world from the client's viewpoint, (2) search for alternative roles that may be more appealing and adaptive to clients from different backgrounds, and (3) help clients from other cultures make contact with and elicit help from Indigenous support systems (p. 259). Cormier and Hackney also specify that to be culturally effective, helpers should not (1) impose their values and expectations on clients from different backgrounds, (2) stereotype or label clients, client behaviors, or cultures, or (3) try to force unimodal counseling approaches upon clients (pp. 258–259).

As an example of such unimodal expectations, Sue (1992) notes that traditional helpers may tend to emphasize the need for clients to verbalize their emotions. He points out that some clients (such as traditional Japanese) may have been taught as children not to speak until addressed; that many cultures highly value restraint in expressing strong feelings; and that patterns of communication, contrary to ours in the United States, may "tend to be vertical, flowing from those of higher prestige and status to those of lower prestige and status" (p. 12). The unenlightened worker seeking to help such a client may perceive the client to be inarticulate, unintelligent, lacking in spontaneity, or repressed (p. 13).

School crisis worker: (speaking softly to a recently immigrated Japanese family whose son has just been severely injured in a high school football game and is going to be out of school for an extended period) I would like to be helpful to your family in this difficult time for you, not knowing how well your son will recover from his injuries and what that means as far as his academic work and chances of going on to college are. I have had experience in dealing with these kinds of issues with a number of students and their parents and could certainly act as your advocate if you would like someone from the school to do that. It is what I do, and it would be my pleasure and honor to do it for you if you so desire. I'll leave my business card, and you may call me at any time.

At the other end of the continuum, Dass-Brailsford (2008) notes that Black culture, particularly in the South, uses physical contact to establish connections, so hugging, ritual handshakes, demonstrative grieving, and joyful exclamations all have healing and bonding power.

School crisis worker: (speaking with displays of emotion and warmth to an Black family whose son has just been severely injured in a high school football game and is going to be out of school for an extended period) (Gives mother a heartfelt embrace and then shakes father's hand and grasps his forearm) I hate this for you and Rashad. It is a terrible blow, not knowing how this will affect his football career and chances for college. You must be really scared and anxious to know how this will all play out. If you would let me be the point man on this with the school, I'd appreciate the opportunity to help you. I've done this with a lot of kids. I know Rashad and can get things coordinated with his teachers and see that the college applications go out like they're supposed to. I'll get on that tomorrow, or if you want to think on it, I'll wait for your call, but understand you and Rashad are important to this school, and we'll be with you. You are part of the Arlington High School family and that's how it is.

If the parents of our football player happen to be Hispanic, and the parents don't speak English and you took French in high school, you are going to need a translator you can trust who has the cultural background to know exactly how to put your words in tone, decibel level, gestures, body language, and directed to mom, dad, or both so you convey your intent as closely as possible (Zalaquett et al., 2010). That means you are going to have to do a little planning ahead if you are counseling individuals who don't speak the language that most people in your country do.

So now you are thinking, "This is impossible. I can't begin to know the words and the culture of everyone I meet, so I'm bound to mess up." Not so! If you pay attention to Cormier and Hackney's points a few paragraphs back, you are going to be pretty much on course. The major themes in both of the foregoing examples are that the worker demonstrates empathy, caring, and positive regard while searching for a role that is compatible with the client's worldview and offers to act as advocate without injecting their own values or conditions into the situation. While at times we do make mistakes in entering into clients' cultural worlds, there are very few clients who do not respond positively when these general facilitative conditions are in operation. In other words, most clients will give you grace if they know your intent is sincere.

When in Rome, Italy . . . or Georgia

Understanding the cultural milieu in which they operate is of critical importance to crisis workers who perform fieldwork or outreach services. Crisis interventionists' notions of what kind of help is needed and what is or is not appropriate help is a manifestation of their own cultural and societal upbringing, education, and views (Kaniasty & Norris, 1999). Cultural differences are particularly problematic when the worker is transported to and works on the client's "turf" and has little time to become attuned to the cultural and ecological framework within which the client operates.

We are not simply talking about work abroad or with specific racial, ethnic, or religious groups. Within the United States, survivors of the California blizzards of 2023 or wildfires that destroy everything in their wake, individuals who lived through the massive Texas flooding in 2022, Georgia residents who face outbreaks of tornadoes on almost an annual basis, or survivors of the 2017 hurricane that devastated Puerto Rico may each have views about what constitutes helpful intervention that are very different from the crisis worker's. Such individuals may take umbrage at the crisis worker's attempts to assist (Silva & Klotz, 2006).

When responding to crises that affect large groups of people who might have very different social locations from the crisis worker, it is imperative that crisis workers remain attuned to culturally embedded patterns of responding to crisis events, emotional expression, help-seeking behaviors, grief and loss customs, and natural support systems and tread softly as they attempt intervention (Silva & Klotz, 2006). Indeed, exercising multicultural competence in crisis intervention requires high levels of self-awareness, observation, sensitivity, and humility.

Language Barriers

LO11 Although it may be difficult enough to work with people in crisis from the same generic cultural background and who speak the native language as a first language, the manifestation and communication of first-generation Americans' or immigrants' personal problems may be very different from what the crisis worker is used to handling. As a result, assessment and intervention become more complex and difficult.

Confidentiality issues are also problematic because translators or children of parents who do not speak English have to act as interpreters. People in the United States with "green cards" or student visas run the risk of having information about their mental health status given to government agencies, which may then make negative evaluations about their immigration status. This issue is further compounded by language problems that make communicating clients' needs and crisis workers' offers of services subject to misinterpretation. Particularly for foreign students, having to leave school because of

"mental health problems" may cause tremendous loss of face in their families and in their home countries. If not handled sensitively, the worker's attempts to provide help may exacerbate rather than mollify the crisis (Oropeza et al., 1991).

If the crisis worker is not fluent in the native language, how can information be conveyed? While not the ideal, a good translator is critical to this endeavor, as opposed to using a family member as translator, particularly since the children, who because of their schooling know more English than their parents do, would probably serve as family translators. The need to discuss intimate details and preserve family roles makes it paramount that third-party translators be available (DeWolfe, 2000).

Crisis worker: (speaking through a translator to a Pakistani family who lost all their belongings in a house fire and whose only members who are fluent in English are their children) Please tell Mr. and Mrs. Maqsood that I apologize for not speaking Urdu. I can either speak through you or through their children, and I would like to know which they might prefer.

Religion and Spirituality

LO12 Religion and spirituality are so loaded with emotionality that many human services workers regard it as an exposed electrical wire, not to be touched on pain of death for fear they will be seen as either proselytizing for their religion or insensitive to other spiritual beliefs. However, to deny or act as if religion, faith, and spirituality are not part of any crisis is to neglect a large part of a crisis response for most people. With the exception of pastoral counseling, it is interesting that little space is given to the effects that religion has in the counseling business and particularly in traumatic events and the crises that flow from them (Schlosser et al., 2010). Yet for most people, trauma is the ultimate challenge to meaning making, and for most people, that meaning making is attached to some kind of faith (Brown, 2009, p. 228). If you have read any of Viktor Frankl's (2006) work on logotherapy and his experiences in Nazi concentration camps, you will start to understand just how powerful attempts at meaning making is in one's life can be and the part that spirituality plays in the process. This is particularly true in the context of a crisis. Audate (2021) makes an eloquent argument that although spirituality is esoteric, and obscure, it is indelibly intertwined with our culture, traditions and way of life and is critical in exploring its meaning and providing an avenue of posttraumatic growth and, at a deeper feeling level, endeavoring to make both ourselves and the world better (pp. 274–275). While some people may not be spiritual, many people are spiritual, and here are a few examples of where spirituality enters the crisis business.

Perilla and associates (2002) found that after Hurricane Andrew, besides being exposed to more of Andrew's wrath because of their low-income-earning state, Latinos and non-Hispanic Black survivors showed **differential vulnerability** to traumatic effects compared to White survivors. That is, they were more traumatized than White survivors, and at least part of this difference related to their fatalistic view that they had little control over the situation. They believed that whatever God willed would happen. Crisis workers who face such fatalism do themselves and their clients no service when they attempt to persuade clients to change their worldview from an external to an internal locus. In fact, the crisis workers would do far better to use the religious and spiritual beliefs that minorities have to guide their intervention (Myers & Wee, 2005, pp. 60–61).

There is a reason that the triage assessment system you will encounter in Chapter 3, "The Intervention and Assessment Models," has a spiritual/moral component. Religious and spiritual beliefs play a huge role in the outcome of a crisis as people attempt to make sense of events that seemingly make no sense at all. Faith plays a large part in how people try to come to terms with a randomly cruel universe that crashes down on the notion of a supreme being that runs a just and moral world. As Bingham (2010) states for Black people, "What is difficult to understand is that the church is far more than family" (p. 22), and if you are not attuned to the importance of their church and faith for many Black people (Grills, 2004) and numerous other ethnic minorities (Taylor et al., 2004), you are probably going to have trouble helping them through the crisis. And yes, this applies to all groups of individuals who are guided by religion or spirituality, regardless of majority or minority membership.

It should not be surprising that recent immigrants who have seemingly adapted to the culture of their new country rapidly revert to old and customary ways of behaving in a crisis (Augsburger, 1992) just as the Caribbean and Latin American clients of Shelby and Tredinnick (1995) did after Hurricane Andrew struck south Florida. Shelby and Tredinnick spent considerable space reporting on the cultural differences they encountered doing disaster relief work in the aftermath of Hurricane Andrew. The large Caribbean and Latin American populations they dealt with had punitive religious interpretations of the disaster and punitive child-rearing practices, particularly under stress, that differed greatly from what the crisis workers believed to be ethically and morally right. The workers had to be very sensitive in not challenging these deeply held beliefs. In short, while it may appear to you to be superstition without basis, if it is bringing solace and respite, crisis workers need to put their own beliefs on the shelf and encourage spiritual coping behaviors that help people heal (Dass-Brailsford, 2008).

So just what do you do when you are confronted with spiritual issues? What the workers did with Andrew survivors was allow them to process feelings of guilt and responsibility in line with their religious interpretation of the event without passing any judgments on the merit of those beliefs. Furthermore, educating parents with ethnically different views of child rearing about the ways children generally respond after a trauma, along with the normal developmental issues they face, may indeed be a tall order given the brevity of crisis intervention. Such interventions, although needed, may be something the crisis worker wishes to consider very carefully.

To offload this tricky issue by merely suggesting that persons consult with their minister, priest, rabbi, or imam is to abdicate your responsibility as the crisis worker. Further, while you may certainly seek advice and counsel from a religious leader of a particular person's faith, that by no means guarantees that you will be congruent with that particular individual's sense of meaning making. There is also no way in the world you can become an expert in all the religions and practices of people in crisis that you will encounter. What we believe is that you can do what Schlosser and his associates (2010) propose and what has worked for us by making an owning statement that directly addresses the issue.

Crisis worker: (working with a client whose family members have just been killed and injured in a landslide) You have not mentioned your faith or religious affiliation. When I have been involved in similar situations with people who have lost loved ones, for many people, faith is an important part of how they deal with such terrible tragedies. Even though one's faith is a deeply personal matter, and I may know very little about your religious faith,

I am wondering if you would like to talk about that with me, or perhaps I can find a leader of your faith with whom you can talk if you would prefer that. One way or the other, I want you to know that I am going to be here with you to help you work your way through this difficult time.

After that, you generally need to practice the listening and responding skills you will encounter in Chapter 4, "The Tools of the Trade." For people who are in a transcrisis state due to a loss of faith and who have unresolved grief, we will have more to say about spirituality and faith in Chapter 12, "Personal Loss: Bereavement and Grief."

Support Systems

LO13 As you will soon see, providing support is so critical that we designate it as a separate task in our crisis intervention model (Chapter 3, "The Intervention and Assessment Models"). Social supports, such as family, friends, and peers, and professionals when no other supports are there or those former social support systems have been abandoned, are critical because they work (Taylor, 2007)! However, how people in crisis utilize social support systems is not always linear or direct. Shelby and Tredinnick (1995) found that Black individuals and Hispanic populations tended to rely on extended support systems much more heavily than European Americans. Dass-Railsford (2008) had a number of conversations with social service authorities, convincing them that children whose biological parents were missing post-Katrina were not abandoned but in the care of other competent adults who would care for them and keep them safe. For some cultures, "family" means a lot more than the residents of the house at 708 S. Grove Street. Therefore, the workers' efforts needed to focus more on systemic approaches that dealt with extended family networks rather than individuals.

As helpful as social support may be, for some people, the cultural prohibitions against opening oneself up to receive social support may be like going from the frying pan into the fire. In their research on Asians and Asian Americans, Kim et al. (2008) found that the college students they studied were far more hesitant than their European American counterparts to seek any support systems because their inability to handle the crisis would bring shame not only on themselves but on their families as well. One reason for this reluctance, they suggest, may be that the very act of seeking support would require the students to self-disclose personal issues, which would put even more stress on them. Reframing such support in more culturally acceptable terms may be one way of allowing individuals to receive help. Organista and Munoz (1996) suggest using manuals and homework assignments, much like a teacher and a classroom assignment, to avoid the stigma of being seen by a mental health worker and receiving psychotherapy.

Crisis worker: (working with a female Asian college student who is thousands of miles from home and who has been sexually assaulted and is largely noncommittal or oblique in her response to the assault) Li Mai, suffering and enduring what you have is hard for any woman. It is very difficult to speak of such personal violations for almost every woman I have encountered who has undergone what you have. It is very common to not want to talk about a sexual assault because of all the negative emotions that go with it—particularly the guilt for thinking you were not cautious enough or the shame if it becomes known. To be clear, I firmly believe this was not your fault. Period. But I can appreciate the complex feelings you might have right now. I also know there are some things that you need to know about and could use some help with. You might wish to think of me more as a teacher who can give you important information which you can then use as you see fit. Or perhaps a coach who can help you make adjustments, just like a soccer player or a figure skater so they are able to perform better. I hope you will think about what I have said and perhaps frame this incident in that manner and see me as that teacher or coach.

The shame of self-disclosure about a perceived moral or personal failing is not to be taken lightly. One of the hallmarks of domestic violence is the embarrassment and shame if word gets out that the person is being physically abused. Certainly, no Jewish women are ever beaten by their spouses because that does not happen in the Jewish religion/culture. Whoa! Unless the city of Memphis has a different Jewish population than most other places in the world, the domestic violence reports that flow into our Family Trouble Center would indicate otherwise. However, such myths have a powerful social influence and pressure people not to seek support (Zimberhoff & Brown, 2006). Myth busting is part and parcel of a lot of the crises in this book, and providing education is a primary task for the crisis worker.

Crisis worker: I want you to be aware that there's a notion that Jewish women do not get beaten by their husbands. Or at the very least, good Jewish wives and mothers don't get beaten. Yet, the fact is that we have many, many reports that in Memphis, Tennessee, Jewish women do suffer abuse at the hands of their partner, and I don't think there are that many bad Jewish wives and mothers around. So, I want you to understand that is a myth, and you are not the only Jewish wife who has experienced abuse. In fact, I would like you to come to a group of women in a support group who are coming out of the kind of abusive relationship you have been in. It may interest you to know that there are three women in the group I am thinking of that are also Jewish.

Occupation as a Cultural Barrier

LO14 The ecological model in Chapter 1, "Approaching Crisis Intervention," may also be applied to the "culture" of particular occupations. It is interesting that most multicultural counseling experts, with the exception of Laura Brown (2008, p. 25), give little or no acknowledgment to occupation as a major social location. An occupation is inextricably tied to most of our lives and is how we identify ourselves. Go to a party, meet a stranger, and after some initial pleasantries, we'll bet that somewhere in there will be a "So what do you do?" or "Where do you work?" question.

The occupational culture of agriculture of Chandler Mountain, Alabama, is far different from the financial culture of Wall Street, New York. We believe that to not take occupation into consideration as a defining part of one's culture and ecosystem is to be absolutely oblivious to a major contributing factor in how one lives. Police work is an excellent example. Police officers might be thought of as psychologically at-risk due solely to the high stress and potentially lethal situations they face. However, that is far from true.

Any crisis worker who proceeded to deal with a law enforcement officer (LEO) based on the erroneous notion that high stress caused by exposure to lethal situations was the sole factor contributing to a crisis would be very mistaken. LEOs constitute a distinct occupational culture and closed ecosystem because of their paramilitary structure, irregular work schedules, constant exposure to life-threatening situations, brotherhood, and general reticence to help-seek (Rufo, 2016). Indeed, LEOs live in a constant state of

survival, and their training and work experience tend to have lasting effects on their worldview, such as pervasive threat-based assessments and heightened sensitivity to risk (Rufo, 2016). They have high rates of exposure to stress (Jetelina et al., 2020) and trauma-inducing stimuli, such as suicide (Cerel et al., 2015), which can leave permanent marks on them and even contribute to the development of PTSD (Cerel et al., 2015). And, in recent years, there have been increasing levels of intentional and targeted attacks against LEOs (Schouten & Brennan, 2016) as members of an institution that is aggrieved by many. In addition to the constant stress of the job, a major issue that bedevils LEOs is their romantic life. They do not usually talk about their jobs or their feelings because they sense their partners are uncomfortable hearing about such matters, or they may be trying to protect their partners. Additionally, LEOs may experience marked family stress due to financial concerns and needing to work overtime or take on extra jobs to meet financial needs or due to conflicts between the family unit and their work (e.g., missing important events, being too tired to engage in family tasks [Karaffa et al., 2015]). These multiple dimensions of law enforcement compound stress reactions to crisis events and should be considered in crisis intervention.

It is not to seek thrills that trainers of the Memphis Police Department Crisis Intervention Team (CIT) ride patrol shifts with CIT officers. Although those rides provide us with valuable on-the-scene experience, they also help us appreciate the ecosystem within which the officer operates. The alliance with CIT officers that emerges from riding the Saturday night shifts with them helps break down occupational barriers and establish our own "bona fides" as being "culturally aware" of what the officers are going through. No amount of reading or expertise that we know of compensates for lack of knowledge and sensitization to this cultural milieu.

Geographic Locale as a Cultural Barrier

LO15 Lenihan and Kirk (1999) have developed a rural, community-level crisis intervention plan for very small towns and rural areas that lack the typical crisis infrastructure and support systems available to even medium-sized communities. Many small communities and isolated rural areas are assailed by crises, yet these crises are not large enough to call for federal responses. However, the state emergency management agency may send crisis workers from neighboring counties and state agencies to assist the target community. Or, the community itself may request volunteer help from universities, charities, civic groups, and local governments in close proximity. People in these areas may be very suspicious of outsiders, even those from neighboring communities, attempting to "tell them what to do." Yet collective fear, rumor, parochialism, and inaccessibility to services can keep the community traumatized and immobile without such help. Lenihan and Kirk propose that intervention strategies must absolutely address the cultural issues that will exist between outside service providers and recipients of service before any meaningful work can be done. They advocate an immediate assessment of the traumatic event's effect not only on individuals but on the culture as well. In a sense, they are "triaging" the whole community. They propose that no outside crisis response team can do an adequate job if it does not first seek out, identify, and consult with a broad cross section of community leaders about how and with whom crisis intervention should proceed.

Particularly important is ascertaining what the community's belief systems are and if there are subcultures within the system that may have different responses from those of the community at large (Chemtob, 2000). Any crisis response must be integrated into the community leadership and organizations such as social clubs, churches, civic groups, and fraternal organizations. Providing sensitive consultation for community leaders without "ramming it down their throats" is imperative. The same is true of using basic listening skills in hearing what the community has to say instead of a bull-in-a-china-shop, officious, expert, "we know what's best for you" approach (van den Eynde & Veno, 1999).

Evaluating and finding the natural leaders of the community and teaming up with them are important in forming workable alliances and providing the citizens an anchor of familiarity, security, and control at the scene. Any action plans should be developed cooperatively and should be concrete, doable, and manageable considering the available community financial and human resources (Lenihan & Kirk, 1999). In short, outside interventionists in such communities do best when they function as guides and helpers who operate along a continuum of directive to nondirective intervention. That is, the interventionist should be only as directive as the degree to which the client (the community) is immobilized.

The Dilemma of Local Consultation

A real dilemma occurs in consulting and working with the local authorities. On the one hand, they know best the infrastructure and needs of the community. Involving community representatives and leaders as intermediaries and consultants can give workers much easier access to the population and can provide helpful tips in regard to local taboos or cultural artifacts that can interfere with service delivery (Chemtob, 2000).

On the other hand, because outside workers are not invested in the local infrastructure and are not enculturated, they may blithely go about their business and, in the process, attempt to redress a variety of long-held social injustices and practices (Golec, 1983). The wise crisis worker who goes into a different geographical area needs to understand that this dilemma *always* exists, whether the location is Kabul, Afghanistan, or Atlanta, Georgia. We are *absolutely not* proposing that crisis workers go about the business of changing and redressing all the perceived evils and shortcomings they may run into. However, as with Shelby and Tredinnick's (1995) report on the cultural reactions of their clients to a disaster, we are not so sure that one should stand passively by while victims project their frustrations by beating their children. What we do urge is that crisis workers *absolutely* need to be aware of this dilemma.

So, should crisis workers leave well enough alone? Certainly, the ability of a community to take care of itself is paramount. Members of the community understand the political, religious, and cultural roots and infrastructure far better than outsiders. Yet when a disaster strikes and the community's resources are exceeded, there is a good deal of research that indicates such altruism does not extend to low income earners, older adults, the less educated, and ethnic minorities. Such groups may be disenfranchised and denied a part in the "democracy of a common disaster" (Kaniasty & Norris, 1995). Although older adults, in particular, may be seen as needing assistance with physical complaints or illness, such attention does not necessarily extend to dealing with property damage or keeping a roof over their heads, food on the table, and medicine in their cabinets (Kaniasty & Norris, 1997; Kaniasty et al., 1990).

Kilijanek and Drabek (1979) coined the term "pattern of neglect" in regard to the lack of aid received by older adults in their study of a Kansas tornado's devastation of Topeka. The "squeaking wheel gets the grease" is probably even more true in the wake of a disaster. **YAVIS clients**—those Young, Attractive, Verbal, Intelligent, and Socially well-connected clients from higher socioeconomic backgrounds—get better service because they have the power, influence, technical savvy, and verbal articulation to get help. People whose social locations differ from those of YAVIS clients tend to do less well and are not knowledgeable enough, not verbal enough, not able enough, not young enough, not technologically sophisticated enough, and not assertive enough to get the help they need (Brown, 2009). Crisis interventionists need to be acutely aware of this pattern and take pains to ensure that all individuals who seek and desire assistance in the traumatic wake of a disaster obtain it.

The Necessity of Acting

LO16   When we are in the heat of the moment in a crisis, observing the "niceties" of another culture that tends to deal obliquely and subtly with problems may not be in the best safety interests of those clients. The foregoing statement is made very conditionally. That is, whenever possible, we want to take as much time as we can to understand the client's issues and perceptions, and that holds true of the collective populace as well. Certainly, being sensitive to the clients' cultural and ecological background is part of a patient and thorough problem exploration.

We further believe that one of the worst therapeutic errors a worker can make is to attempt to "hurry" the process. Crisis intervention should never be hurried. Although it may seem paradoxical, the fastest way to resolve a crisis is to take your time to understand what is going on. Still and all, if we have a client who is "running amok" (a Filipino cultural term for being absolutely, violently out of control), their cognitive processes are going to be seriously impaired, their behavior is going to be threatening, and their emotions will be out of control. What that means in the reality of the situation is acting rapidly and in a very concrete manner to assure their own and others' safety. Finally, helping anybody, no matter how culturally different, is complex in a crisis. So, take your time.

Many culturally diverse families have years of coping with crisis and are extremely resilient. If a person from a different cultural background is a recent immigrant, these successes may be minimized in the immigrant's new country or territory and seen as irrelevant or inconsequential. They are not! The astute crisis worker will attempt to recognize and marshal these past successes to the current dilemma. Normalizing the crisis experience is particularly important for the culturally diverse who may already be isolated socially and believe no one else is having similar responses. Empowerment, particularly for the culturally diverse, is the watchword in crisis intervention (Congress, 2000).

There is a delicate balance between helping and interfering. This is a constant bipolar dilemma for both recipients and providers of service after a disaster. On the one hand, the recipient appreciates the help, good intentions, and sincere concern. On the other hand, those same providers may be met with confusion, skepticism, and perceived psychological threat by the same recipients (Wortman & Lehman, 1985). Our experience has been that this bipolar dilemma can occur not only on the same day, but even in the same hour!

Training

The American Red Cross training for mental health disaster relief certification has course work in diversity training and cross-cultural differences. And the U.S. Department of Health and Human Services (n.d.) has developed a training program for disaster and crisis response workers: *Cultural Competency Program for Disaster Preparedness and Crisis Response.* The National Institute of Mental Health (2002) report and recommendations for dealing with the traumatic wake of mass violence cautioned practitioners that disaster mental health training needs to incorporate cross-cultural training because variations in understanding the meaning of thoughts, behaviors, and feelings by ethnically different persons can influence the validity of assessments, treatment protocols, and general interaction with survivor populations. Whether the crisis worker is going to Kobe, Japan, or Long Beach, Mississippi, understanding that it is culturally alien turf is critical to crisis work. The U.S. Department of Health and Human Services' *Developing Cultural Competence in Disaster Mental Health Programs: Guiding Principles and Recommendations* (2003) contains a variety of helpful suggestions for working with people in a large-scale disaster.

Where It Stands Now . . . Sorta

Multicultural counseling, as it's applied to crisis intervention, has evolved markedly over the past 30 years, although much is left to be learned and the application to crisis intervention remains in its infancy. What seems reasonable and shows some success is **cultural adaptation** that modifies evidence-based treatments to accommodate the cultural beliefs, attitudes, and behaviors of the cultural group to whom one is providing services (Whaley & Davis, 2007). To that end—and this is certainly easier said than done in the field of crisis where chaos theory tends to run rampant when service delivery is most critical—carefully controlled studies need to occur that measure both traditional therapeutic approaches against well-described cultural adaptations of those therapies and cultural-specific practices that look nothing like our current intervention models. Rodriguez and Bernal (2012) have compiled and reported on a variety of models that are attempting to culturally adapt evidence-based treatments. It will be interesting to see which, if any, of these models emerge as valid and if they have transferability to crisis intervention. It would also be very interesting to see what effect client–interventionist congruency, in terms of Brown's (2008) social locations hypothesis, has on treatment. To this point, we have still been unable to find any research that asks the most essential question arising from this chapter: "How sensitive was the interventionist in regard to your social locations, and was it helpful the crisis worker was sensitive to your social locations?"

Summary

While not a great deal is yet known about exactly how ecological/cultural determinants interact with crisis, it is clear that they do. This interaction has significant implications for crisis interventionists as they work with people from different cultural backgrounds. One of the major differences interventionists need to recognize is the different methods of communication and allegiances between individualist/collectivist–high/low-context systems. Social locations, the many facets that make up each person's life, are as important "within" culture/ethnicity variables as the "between" variables that differentiate one group from another. This chapter espouses a more universal/emic view instead of a focused/etic view in defining multicultural counseling and cautions the reader to be a discerning consumer in regard to what prevailing multicultural views may hold for the practice of crisis intervention. We have generated a new SAFETY social locations model that we believe seems to fit the specific environment of a crisis setting. We also discussed the application of Relational Cultural Therapy to crisis intervention as a means of promoting culturally competent crisis intervention work. Particularly important to crisis interventionists is disabusing themselves of tunnel vision perspectives, assumptions, and unconscious biases they may have about people from different cultures.

The Intervention and Assessment Models

3

Learning Objectives

After studying this chapter, you should be able to:

1. Apply the concepts of equilibrium/disequilibrium and mobility/immobility to stabilizing an individual in crisis.
2. Know how the hybrid model of crisis intervention is used, what its component parts are, and apply them in practice.
3. Know and apply the Triage Assessment System (TAS) and its affective, behavioral, and cognitive components in doing real-time assessment of an individual in crisis.
4. Practice assessment protocol for substance misuse, misuse of illicit and prescription

drugs, and drug interaction contributors to crisis.
5. Determine if lethality is present by assessing for its potential.
6. Explain how the interaction of the duration of time, the degree of emotional stamina, the developmental stage of the client, and the ecosystem contribute to the crisis and its resolution.
7. Employ the LASER model in making ethical decisions in crisis settings.

Introduction

LO1 The purpose of this chapter is to present an applied crisis intervention model that describes in detail the major tasks involved in dealing with a crisis. The TAS is introduced as a rapid but systematic technique for the crisis worker to use to adjudicate the severity of a client's presenting crisis situation and gain some sense of direction in helping the client cope with the dilemma. Finally, this chapter details how to use the LASER model in operating ethically in a crisis environment. This chapter and Chapter 4, "The Tools of the Trade," are a prerequisite for learning and using effective intervention models and techniques for succeeding chapters, and we urge you to consider this foundation material carefully.

The model of crisis intervention you are about to encounter emphasizes an immediacy mode of actively, assertively, intentionally, and continuously assessing, listening, and acting to systematically help the client regain as much precrisis equilibrium, mobility, and autonomy as possible. Two of those terms, **equilibrium** and **mobility**, and their antonyms, **disequilibrium** and **immobility**, are commonly used by crisis workers to identify client states of being and coping. Because we will be using these terms often, we would like to first provide their dictionary definitions and then give a common analogy so their meaning becomes thoroughly understood.

Equilibrium. A state of mental or emotional stability, balance, or poise in the organism.

Disequilibrium. Lack or destruction of emotional stability, balance, or poise in the organism.

Mobility. A state of physical being in which the person can autonomously change or cope in response to different moods, feelings, emotions, needs, conditions, and influences; being flexible or adaptable to the physical and social world.

Immobility. A state of physical being in which the person is not immediately capable of autonomously changing or coping in response to different moods, feelings, emotions, needs, conditions, and influences; inability to adapt to the immediate physical and social world.

A person not in crisis is in a state of approximate psychological and behavioral equilibrium, like a motorist driving with some starts and stops down the road of life—for both the short and the long haul. The person may hit some potholes but does not break any axles. Aside from needing to give the car an occasional tune-up, the person remains more or less equal to the task of making the drive. In contrast, the person in crisis, whether it be acute or chronic, is experiencing serious difficulty in steering and successfully navigating life's highway. The individual is at least temporarily out of control, unable to command personal resources or those of others to stay on safe psychological pavement.

A person not in crisis is capable of negotiating hills, curves, ice, fog, stray animals, wrecks, and most other obstacles that impede progress. No matter what roadblocks may appear, such a person adapts to changing conditions, applying brakes, putting on fog lights, and estimating passing time. This person may have fender benders from time to time but avoids head-on collisions. The person in a dysfunctional state of equilibrium and mobility has failed to pass inspection. Careening down hills and around dangerous curves, knowing the brakes have failed, the person is frozen with panic and despair and has little hope of handling the perilous situation. The result is that the person has become a victim of the situation, has forgotten all about emergency brake, downshifting, or even easing the car into guardrails. They fly headlong into catastrophe and watch transfixed as it happens. The analogy of equilibrium and mobility applies to most crisis situations. Thus, it becomes every crisis worker's job to figuratively get the client back into the driver's seat of the psychological vehicle. As we shall see, sometimes this means the client must temporarily leave the driving to us, sometimes it means sitting alongside the client and pointing out the rules of the road, and sometimes it means just pretty much going along for the ride!

All of that being said, the crisis worker will meet a number of individuals who were having difficulty maintaining psychological equilibrium before the crisis. Many people who were displaced by Hurricane Katrina, for example, were physically and psychologically fragile before the hurricane due to a combination of intra-, inter-, and ecosystemic factors. We will have more to say about such people, who are more typically in a state of transcrisis, in Chapter 5, "Crisis Case Handling."

A Hybrid Model of Crisis Intervention

LO2 Gerald Caplan's (1964) pioneering work on crisis resulted in his development of a four-stage model of crisis. Those stages are: (1) exposure to a stressor(s) and attempts to restore homeostasis, equilibrium, and mobility; (2) failure to restore homeostasis, equilibrium, and mobility; (3) a behavioral emergency occurs with correlative affective and cognitive dysfunction and dysregulation; and (4) a breakdown of physical health and psychosocial functioning then occurs. There are numerous models for crisis intervention (Aguilera, 1998; Flannery & Everly, 2000; Ford, 2021; Kanel, 1999; Kleespies, 2009; Lester, 2002; Roberts, 2005; Slaikeu, 1990) based on Caplan's four-stage model. All of these models depict crisis intervention in some linear, stage, or stepwise fashion, although Ford's (2021) model, because of its setting in individual therapy sessions, is adaptable and flexible to the idiosyncratic needs of the specific client. Indeed, through 30 years of publishing this book, we did much the same, with the admonition that changing conditions might well mean that the interventionist would have to recycle and move back to earlier steps. We no longer believe that a stage or purely step model captures the way crisis intervention works, and here's why.

The problem that we have struggled with as we try to teach students like you about crisis intervention is that, at times, crisis is anything but linear. Many times, crisis intervention absolutely epitomizes chaos theory—with starts, stops, do-overs, and U-turns. At times, doing crisis work is a lot like being a smoke jumper, controlling a psychological brush fire on this side of the mountain only to be faced with a new one on the other side of the valley. Fighting those psychological fires according to a neat, progressive, linear plan is easily said but not so easily done. Therefore, we have combined our former linear model with a systems model we helped develop (Myer et al., 2011), resulting in what could more appropriately be called a hybrid model for individual crisis intervention that is generally linear in its progression but can also be understood in terms of tasks that need to be accomplished. While some of these tasks certainly would usually be done in the beginning, middle, or end of a crisis, changing conditions may mean you have to accomplish some tasks you would normally do later, first. Or indeed, a task you thought was already accomplished comes apart and has to be done over not once, but multiple times.

A further problem with a strict linear model is that each step should be discrete, following from step one to step two and so on, with particular techniques to employ in each of those steps. In crisis intervention, issues suddenly erupt that defy discrete, stepwise techniques. Focus on getting a commitment from a person to do something, which would normally come at the end of a crisis session, may need to happen immediately if that person is standing out in the middle of a busy intersection at rush hour! Likewise, gaining that commitment to get out of the street may call for assertion techniques that are anything but what we might normally do when making initial contact with a client. Consider the following analogy.

Picture yourself as a linesperson on the cross arm of a power pole, hard hat on, heavy insulated clothing, leather over-insulated gloves, dug in with your climbing spikes, attempting to repair a high-voltage (crisis) transmission line in North Dakota in January with the wind blowing sleet in your face at 20 miles an hour. On your utility belt are a variety of tools. You know the steps required to get the transformer hooked back up and the sequential manner in which you will employ the tools on your belt to get the job done. The problem is, Mother Nature is not happy, the wind picks up, and a coupling breaks loose, or a new fuse you just put in blows, and you have to start all over again! If you can picture this analogy in your mind's eye, you are well on the way to understanding how crisis intervention works. As we describe the model, we will give you some examples of when you

have to change tools to meet the changing conditions up on that pole.

The model you are about to examine is the hub around which the crisis intervention strategies in this book revolve, and the tasks/steps are designed to operate as an integrated problem-solving process (Myer et al., 2013). It is not complex but rather is designed to be simple to implement, easy to use, and adaptable to just about any crisis we can think of that you would likely encounter.

Task 1. Predispositioning/Engaging/Initiating Contact

Predispositioning may be seen as first and foremost getting ready to do something. It is usually the first step in a crisis model: placing oneself, or something, in a position to be of use in some future occurrence. Typically, systems such as the armed forces and government agencies such as Federal Emergency Management Agency (FEMA) use predispositioning to get supplies, equipment, and personnel ready to meet some future emergency. Indeed, in Chapter 16, "Disaster Response," you will see predispositioning in operation on a very large scale. In the counseling literature, predisposition was originally studied by Prochaska, DiClemente, and Norcross (1992) in regard to what motivated people experiencing substance dependency to decide to change. Since their seminal work, the concept of predisposing clients to get them ready for counseling has become widespread.

In crisis intervention, predisposition is somewhat different. It means predisposing individuals to be receptive to our intervention when, in many instances, they may not be at all enthused about our presence or be so out-of-control that they are only vaguely aware of us. Therefore, predisposition has a lot to do with the attitudinal set and predisposition of how the crisis worker enters the situation. A number of clients the crisis worker will meet do not act, talk, or look nice or necessarily have good hygiene. The ability to convey empathy and be authentic as to who and what you are doing without pretense is critical (Kleespies & Richmond, 2009).

Particularly with a first contact, predispositioning the client about what to expect is paramount. Along with letting the client know what is going to occur, it is important to make contact in such a way that the client can see the interventionist as an immediate ally and support and not another in a long line of people, representative of bureaucracies and institutional authorities, who have been anything but helpful in resolving their problems. One of the most critical initiating components of crisis intervention is how workers introduce themselves to a client who has never met a crisis interventionist—which is a fairly common occurrence in this business. It is not just to fill time that our practicum training with aspiring crisis intervention team police officers now devotes an initial session specifically to how officers introduces themselves to a recipient of services (Memphis Police Department, 2010). Our primary objectives in predisposing an individual to accept crisis intervention are twofold: (1) to establish a psychological connection and create a line of communication, and (2) to clarify intentions about what is going to happen.

Establishing a Psychological Connection. First and foremost, you need to introduce yourself in a way that is nonthreatening, helpful, and assumes a problem-solving as opposed to an adversarial approach.

Leron: (standing in the middle of a main city street in five o'clock rush hour traffic waving two broken whiskey bottles) The God damned house authority. NO place to live. Kicked me out, the rotten bastards. Everybody needs to know them for the crooks they are.

CIT officer: (slowly approaching the subject from a distance with hands visible, empty, and open) Man! You really are angry with them to make this kind of statement out in the middle of Union Avenue during rush hour. My name's Scott Lewis, a CIT officer with the Memphis Police Department. I didn't catch your name. Mind telling me?

One of the most important elements in making **first contact** is getting the client's name and introducing yourself in a nonthreatening manner. Note that Scott approaches the subject slowly, not only because he is armed with two whiskey bottles (which has to do with another task that is pretty important here, providing for the client's safety and your own), and responds to his current affective and behavioral state of being. Before he ever asks a question about why this has happened, he immediately states his name and asks for the client's. Also note that his full name, not his rank or the police department, comes first.

Another advantage with the approach used by Scott is that he allows Leron to maintain some control over the situation. The housing authority has already taken his home and barred him from his belongings. Imagine if Scott rolled onto the scene

and immediately began demanding that Leron get out of the street and put down the whiskey bottles. Scott would likely get the response "Screw you, cop." Scott would be seen as just another authority figure who doesn't listen. By establishing a problem solving helpful connection, Scott allows Leron to maintain momentary control of the situation. By reflecting Leron's anger and using a limited catharsis strategy, the crisis worker immediately attempts to convey empathic understanding of the extreme measures the client has taken in attempting to problem solve and allows the client to emotionally ventilate about his dilemma.

Clarifying Intentions. Clarifying intentions means informing the client about what the crisis intervention process is and what the client can expect to happen. For many clients who are in crisis, this will be their first contact with a crisis interventionist, and they will have little if any idea of what is going to happen or how it is going to happen. Leron most likely has had experiences with the police that will lead him to believe that nothing positive is going to happen with Officer Lewis. Thus, the CIT officer needs to quickly apprise him of what will happen.

CIT officer: Okay I can see right off you clearly have some issues with the housing authority. Right now, I am going to listen very closely to what got you out here. I may ask you some questions, so I get a clearer notion of the problem. We've got some time, and I am going to take the time to hear you out. I'll also probably kinda sum up what you're saying so I'm sure I heard you right. So, I wonder if we could move this over underneath that shade tree cause it's hot and not very safe out here.

Leron: (weaving unsteadily and sweating profusely) No! As soon as I do that, those other cops will bum rush me. Long as I'm out here they got to pay attention and that News 5 chopper stays up there. Lost my job through no fault of my own and now kicked out.

CIT officer: Okay. I hear what you're saying about keeping the evil stuff the housing authority has done to you in the public's eye. However, sooner or later we're going to need to get out of the street. I'd like that to be sooner since it is 98 degrees out here and my guess is you're getting thirsty and would like to get it settled and get out of the sun. Nobody's going to bum rush you. It's between you and me right now. That's the way I'd like to keep it.

Officer Lewis uses basic listening and responding statements that own what is going to happen in the next few minutes. He also states the immediate end goal of the crisis resolution for him as "getting out of the middle of the street." He clearly states his intention to listen, gets the client's perspective, and does no harm to him while this is going on. While the client's end goal may be completely different—bringing the housing authority to justice in some manner—the interventionist states from the outset in pretty clear terms what he is going to do. In clear, concise statements, the interventionist creates a line of communication by using open-ended questions, reflection of feelings, and owning statements (all of which you will learn about in the next chapter) that reinforce and encourage the client to tell his story. The major intentional strategy here is allowing the client to cathart but also keeping the client in real time and not allowing the interaction to degenerate into all the perceived injustices ever perpetrated on him.

This introduction "stuff" may sound pretty simplistic, but in the heat of the moment, it is surprising how that can go by the wayside. It may also seem like a "one and done" deal, but even for a client who has known the interventionist for a long time and is currently out of touch with reality, anchoring the client by stating who the interventionist is, clarifying intentions, and stating what needs to happen are a critical ingredient for a successful intervention.

Task 2. Problem Exploration: Defining the Crisis

A major initial task in crisis intervention is to define and understand the problem from the client's point of view. This is particularly difficult in the middle of a chaotic situation where there are complex biopsychosocial contributors interacting with one another (Kleespies & Richmond, 2009). Unless the worker perceives the crisis situation as the client perceives it, all the intervention strategies and procedures the helper might use may miss the mark and be of no value to the client. Intervention sessions begin with crisis workers practicing what are called the **core listening skills**: empathy, genuineness, and acceptance or positive regard (Cormier & Cormier, 1991, pp. 21–39).

The problem definition of a crisis does not mean going on a psychological archaeological dig to dredge up and sift every artifact of the client's past. Defining the crisis does mean attempting to identify the precipitating event across the affective, behavioral, and cognitive components of the crisis. This task serves two purposes. First, the interventionist sees the crisis from the client's perspective. Second, defining the crisis gives the interventionist information on the immediate conditions, parties, and issues that led to the eruption of the problem into a crisis.

CIT officer: I understand that the housing authority screwed you over somehow. So, tell me what got you so mad and frustrated you needed to get everybody's attention.

As Leron angrily expounds on the housing authority's injustices toward people and himself, Officer Lewis uses an expansion strategy to broaden the client's view of the problem without letting the problem escalate. He restates the client's complaint and follows with an open lead.

Inevitably, other issues will surface as the interventionist attempts to define the crisis. In the case of Leron, Officer Lewis may suspect that Leron is dependent on alcohol, given the fact that he has two empty whiskey bottles in his hands and is having trouble keeping his balance. He also is now aware that Leron has recently been laid off from his job. While these issues need attention, at the moment, the interventionist needs to remain focused on the crisis—getting Leron out of the street and assisting him in accessing the resources needed to address the eviction from his apartment. The other issues should be placed on the back burner and may well be discussed after the crisis has been resolved.

CIT officer: So they lost your application for delayed payment while you wait for unemployment to kick in, then said you hadn't filed and kicked you out. I understand how that could make you so mad. So how about putting those bottles down and stepping over to that shade tree. I see you're sweating pretty hard out here in the hot sun and bet you could use some water. I just happen to have some bottles in my lunch cooler. I've got a couple of ideas about how to get you out of this predicament.

Task 3. Providing Support

The third task in crisis intervention emphasizes communicating to the client that the worker is a person who cares about the client. Workers cannot assume that a client experiences feeling valued, prized, or cared for by the worker. In many crisis situations, the exact opposite will be true. The support step provides an opportunity for the worker to assure the client that "here is one person who really cares about you." We believe that providing support occurs in three ways.

Psychological Support. First and most immediate is providing psychological and physical support. Deep, empathic responding using reflection of feelings and owning statements about the client's present condition serve as a bonding agent that says emphatically, "I am with you right here." In Task 3, the person providing the support is the crisis worker. This means that workers must be able to accept, in an unconditional and positive way, all their clients, whether the clients can reciprocate or not. The worker who can truly provide support for clients in crisis is able to accept and value the person no one else is willing to accept. While Officer Lewis is attempting to get Leron out of the street, he also offers genuine support and help in getting the client out of his predicament with the housing authority.

Logistical Support. In a more general sense, support may be not only emotional but also instrumental and informational (Cohen, 2004). At times, the client may not have money, food, clothing, or shelter. Little psychological support will be desired or progress made until the basic necessities of living and surviving are met. Physical support means giving clients concrete assistance to help weather the crisis. This support comes in many forms, ranging from providing pamphlets to arranging the transportation of clients to organizations that have the resources needed to help them to simply giving them a drink of water.

CIT officer: I can't imagine what it's like not to have a job or a roof over your head. Where's your family in all this?

Leron: Tormeda and the kids done went to her momma's in Arkansas. Nothin' to eat and no place to live ceptin' the street. Momma took her back cause I ain't no account and cain't feed 'em or put a roof over dere heads.

CIT officer: The words "terrifying" and "hopeless" come to mind. I can see why this might come down to the only solution you can think of. I really do want to help you out with this and get you back on your feet, and I do maybe have an idea or two about how to do that. But I don't want to see you arrested, and if we don't move this out of the middle of the street so I can share some of my ideas with you, nothing will happen except you going to jail. So, you have a choice. What's your wish? Help getting this resolved or jail?

Leron: Jail don't sound good . . . been there, done that.

CIT officer: I hear that. I don't want to see you in jail either, so come on over here and let's look at some options.

Leron: (walks slowly over to the curb and sets the bottles down) Okay, I be done. I be givin' you a shot at dis. I guess I be needin' some hep.

In this exchange, Officer Lewis forms a bond with Leron. Officer Lewis does not judge Leron; instead, he encourages him to stay out of jail. This encouragement helps Leron regain a belief that the situation is not as dire as it seems and maybe, with help, a solution can be found. Encouragement is a critical component in crisis intervention because, for most clients, what they are going through is anything but encouraging. Catching clients' even feeble attempts to problem-solve gives them a chance to regain some hope, validates that they still have capabilities, and starts reframing thinking toward a proactive, problem-solving mode (Courtois & Ford, 2009, pp. 86–87).

Social Support. Third, providing support means activating clients' primary support system: family, friends, coworkers, church members, and so forth. For many people in crisis, this primary support system may be absent (a car accident 600 miles from home), fed up with their behavior (lying and stealing from them to subsidize an addiction), or unequal to the task of providing support as a result of the crisis (symptoms of posttraumatic stress disorder). Conversely, clients may feel too embarrassed or guilty to ask for help from their immediate support system, such as Sunday school members (loss of job and inability to contribute to their church financially). At such times, the interventionist is not only the initial point of contact and immediate psychological and physical anchor but also the "expert" who provides information, guidance, and primary support in the first minutes and hours after the initiating event (Aguilera, 1998; Cohen, 2004).

Informational Support. At other times, clients do not have adequate information to make good decisions. The need for informational support is particularly critical in the next step, examining alternatives. One of the best techniques a crisis interventionist can be in command of is the ability to provide information on where, how, who, and what resources clients can access to get out of the predicament they are in. That is particularly true of people who, after a disaster, are trying to access the basic necessities of living (Ruzek, 2006).

Default Task: Safety

Safety is a default task that is *always* operational. Safety is a primary consideration throughout crisis intervention for a variety of reasons that are both physically and psychologically based. The task of assessing and ensuring the client's and others' safety is always part of the process, whether it is overtly stated or not. When we speak of safety, we are concerned about the physical safety not only of the client but also of those who may interact themselves and, just as importantly, about keeping ourselves safe. Whether by commission or omission, clients often put themselves in hazardous situations as a result of their affective, behavioral, and cognitive reactions to the crisis. Leron's attempt to publicize his plight clearly puts him, the general public, and the officer at risk. While Leron's crisis is with the housing authority, the immediate crisis of Leron in the middle of a main street with two broken whiskey bottles in his hands is a safety issue. Nothing is more paramount in a crisis than ensuring safety.

We have personally known three human services workers who have been killed at the hands of clients in crisis. One of your authors could very easily have been added to that list early in his career when he talked a violent teenager into handing over a gun pointed a foot from his face. He didn't think the weapon would work. After the youth was taken into custody, blanks were loaded into the gun, and it fired very well, to the shock of a shaken 24-year-old junior high school counselor who thought he was immortal! There are no dead heroes in this business, only dead interventionists. We will have a great deal more to say on the subject of the interventionist's safety in Chapter 14, "Violent Behavior in Institutions."

Generally, when we think about safety in a crisis, we assume that someone is engaging in lethal behavior toward themself or others. But limiting the task of ensuring safety to issues of life and death overlooks many clients whose safety is in jeopardy. The fact is that in much crisis intervention, people do not intend to cause harm to themselves or others but engage in activities that have a high potential for that to happen. You can extend the task of ensuring safety to include meeting the daily needs of clients such as finding shelter and food.

CIT officer: Leron, I want to keep you safe, man, and the middle of Union Avenue at rush hour is anything but that. I can get you some help not only as far as the housing authority is concerned but also in regard to getting some food in your belly and a roof over your head, but that has to start happening over in my squad car. Otherwise, the TAC team will come and take you in to custody and none of that will happen. When did you eat last?

Leron: Don't remember . . . yesterday maybe . . . no, a couple of days ago, I think. Got some stuff out of the back of one of them restaurants on Beale Street.

Officer Lewis is working to protect Leron from inadvertently being injured. Food and the offer of shelter are used to entice Leron off the street. This offer makes a clear point that all crisis interventionists need to heed: If a person's basic physical needs are not being met, it is unlikely that the crisis will diminish until those needs are met.

Safety also includes assuring clients that they are psychologically safe. As we shall see in Chapter 9, "Sexual Assault," many clients who have been subject to vicious assaults by sexual perpetrators have suffered secondary victimization, being revictimized by authority figures, government bureaucracies, religious entities, social service agencies, and, yes, incompetent therapists (Ochberg, 1988). Making it safe for a client in crisis to trust the interventionist comes before everything else and is a critical part of creating the trust and bond necessary to move forward (Courtois & Ford, 2009). Safety is a default task that is merged and subsumed in all the other tasks in the model, from predispositioning to follow-up.

Tasks 1, 2, 3, and the safety task involve a lot of listening activities, although they are not necessarily passive or devoid of action, particularly when safety issues are involved. Taken together, these four steps most nearly represent what has become known in the field as *psychological first aid* (refer to Chapter 1, "Approaching Crisis Intervention").

Task 4. Examining Alternatives

Examining alternatives addresses an area that both clients and workers in crisis intervention often neglect—exploring a wide array of appropriate choices available to the client. In their immobile state, clients often do not adequately examine their best options. Some clients in crisis actually believe there are no options. Clients may develop tunnel vision and become stuck in an endless merry-go-round of attempting to engage in the same futile behavior.

Alternatives can be viewed from three perspectives: (1) **Situational supports** are people known to the client in the present or past who might care about what happens to the client. (2) **Coping mechanisms** are actions, behaviors, or environmental resources the client might use to help get through the present crisis. (3) **Positive and constructive thinking patterns** on the part of the client are ways of reframing that might substantially alter the client's view of the problem and lessen the client's level of stress and anxiety. The effective crisis worker may think about an infinite number of alternatives pertaining to the client's crisis but discuss only a few of them with the client. Clients experiencing crisis do not need a lot of choices; they need appropriate choices that are realistic for their situation. Some of these coping skills may already be present in the client, but under the stress of the crisis, they may be forgotten or dismissed as ineffective because they were used "back when" or "back there" and are no longer workable in the here and now.

Leron: Used to have money in ma pocket. Had me a car 'n' a house 'n' food on de table. Fok lift op . . . e . . . ray . . . tore and damn good. Could figger stuff out. Fo'man on ma crew. Lotsa ideas 'bout movin' on up, din da compnee go bust. No mo'! Ain't got no job, no skills, no family, no nuthin' ceptin' damn housin' a-tho-it-tee.

CIT officer: Leron, it sounds like right now you're out there all alone against this big monster called MHA. I've got an idea. Okay, so your application for rent reduction got lost in the bureaucracy when you got laid off and they made it sound like it was your fault and blamed you for not submitting it when in fact you did. Your gripes to them haven't gotten you anywhere, and now you want everybody to know that they are trying to weasel out of their mistake. I've got one idea that might help, and that's the pro bono law student advocacy association of the Memphis University Law School. They take on stuff like this. I can take you down there and introduce you to somebody I know there, but I've got another concern. I wonder when was the last time you had something to eat and a place to lay your head down where you felt safe, could get some sleep and get some energy back?

By offering to physically transport Leron to the law school, Officer Lewis indicates that he is involved with Leron beyond him being a nuisance to get off the street. He also makes a hunch about Leron's physical condition, and that hunch segues into one of the most important tasks of crisis intervention, which is safety.

Examining alternatives is literally a "right here, right now" activity. Rapidly changing conditions may mean discarding old options that worked a half hour ago for completely new ones. One of the hallmarks of a world-class crisis worker is the ability to be resilient and rapidly brainstorm new ideas and implement them in a hurry.

CIT officer: (noticing Leron's unsteady gate) Leron, how much have you had to drink today?

Leron: 'Bout most of them two bottles.

CIT officer: I can understand why you'd need all that liquid courage to do this. Okay! Maybe we need to think about getting you sober before you talk to anybody down there. What about me taking you out to the Bartlett Salvation Army halfway house, getting some food in your stomach, cleaned up, some sleep so you got it all together and can talk real straight to the folks at the advocacy center.

Task 5. Planning in Order to Reestablish Control

A hallmark of people in crisis is the feeling of loss of control. Chaos reigns, and every effort to manage the situation has failed. Reestablishing control means helping clients create a plan to guide them in the resolution of the crisis. Such a plan needs to consider what options are available to the client and what choices need to be made in regard to those options. One of the primary strategies in planning to reestablish control is mobilizing the client.

The fifth step in crisis intervention, making plans, flows logically and directly from the Task 4 alternatives. Much of the material throughout this book focuses either directly or indirectly on the crisis worker's involvement with clients in planning action steps that have a good chance of restoring the client's emotional, behavioral, and cognitive equilibrium. A plan should (1) identify additional persons, groups, and other referral resources that can be contacted for immediate support, and (2) provide coping mechanisms—something concrete and positive for the client to do now, definite action steps the client can own and comprehend. The plan should focus on systematic problem solving for the client and be realistic in terms of the client's coping ability.

While it may be that crisis workers have to be very directive at times, as much as possible, it is important that planning be done in collaboration with clients so clients feel a sense of ownership of the plan. At the very least, explaining thoroughly what is about to occur and gaining client acquiescence is extremely important. The critical element in developing a plan is that clients do not feel robbed of their power, independence, and self-respect. The central issues in planning are clients' *control* and *autonomy*. The reasons for clients to carry out plans are to restore their sense of control and to ensure they do not become dependent on support persons like the worker. It should be emphasized that planning is not what clients are going to do for the rest of their lives. Planning is about getting through the short term and getting some semblance of equilibrium and stability restored. Most plans in crisis intervention are measured in minutes, hours, and days, not weeks, months, or years.

CIT officer: I can't give you much more time. I gave you a choice. Those alternatives are to do something about the issue rather than going to jail. What do you want to do? I need for you to put those bottles down and walk over here and get in the car. Are you willing to do that and get some help for your problem and some food in your stomach?

Leron: (hesitates and shrugs; puts bottles down and walks over to the car) Okay . . . maybe you can get me some help.

(Next afternoon at the legal aid office.)

Legal aid worker: Mr. Brown, I believe we can exert some leverage on the housing authority and can make a case for you. This will take at least a couple of weeks, though, and I understand you have nowhere to stay.

(Officer Lewis, before dropping Leron off at the Salvation Army, has made a promise to pick him up and take him to the legal aid office.)

Officer Lewis: Leron, have you thought perhaps you might go over to Arkansas?

Leron: Man, I don't want to be beholden to my mother-in-law. She don't care much for me no how.

Officer Lewis: Well, you don't have a job, so you could go back out to the Salvation Army new halfway house. You'd qualify to get in it based on being out of work and the fact that you were intoxicated helped get you into that predicament.

Leron: Man, I ain't no charity case.

Officer Lewis: I hear that and understand you got your pride, but what about using their job counseling program out there to help you get back to work? I mean it's not like you're going there forever, and you'd be right there if anything comes in. They'd also do some job counseling.

Leron: Well, when you put it that way, could be okay.

Many times, in crisis the alternatives are not what the client wants but what is necessary. When Officer Lewis reframes the stay at the Salvation Army as not charity but a way of getting Leron back to work, it becomes much more palatable and makes the alternative a much more positive and desirable one. Being able to reframe the alternative is empowering and one of the key ingredients in getting clients involved and energizing them to move forward.

Psychoeducation. At the time of the first edition of this book in 1987, there was not a great deal of information about many of the maladies in this book. Thus, interventionists didn't have a lot of information to give clients about the psychological course of the aftermath of a crisis. However, in the intervening 36 years, a tremendous amount of reliable and valid information has been discovered about the course of the crises discussed in this book. Giving clients this information, called *psychoeducation,* can be of tremendous benefit in helping them understand what is going on with them psychologically and allay the pervasive anxiety that may paralyze them into not taking action.

Psychoeducation means providing information to victims and survivors about what is happening and is probably going to happen to them psychologically in the aftermath of a traumatic event. Psychoeducation has become an extremely important treatment component in helping people in crisis get control back in their lives, not only in preemptive work such as educating people about suicide, domestic violence, and sexual assault but also in understanding what happens in the traumatic wake of a crisis, such as the terrifying flashbacks and nightmares of posttraumatic stress disorder (PTSD) (Briere & Scott, 2006; Courtois et al., 2009; Kleespies, 2009). Psychoeducation is a task in and of itself. However, for the present, we have put it under planning because of the critical part it plays in helping to mobilize the client. Psychoeducation means providing clients with information about their condition, what they can expect in the way of affective, behavioral, and cognitive dimensions of it, and how they can develop coping skills to alleviate it.

We would not expect a first grader to have much knowledge or many psychological resources to deal with bullying, so we would be pretty directive in providing the child with information and strategies to deal with it. Likewise, for a person who knew nothing about how to deal with housing bureaucracies, options to get out of an unemployment line, and the common depressive symptoms that might exacerbate those problems into a full-blown crisis, the crisis worker's best treatment option is to start providing information and instructing the client about what needs to be done and how to take care of oneself psychologically while doing it.

Rehabilitation counselor: (at Salvation Army Treatment Center a week later) Leron, we have a lot of information that I believe will help you as far as getting employable is concerned. We also found out that you are most likely clinically depressed. That's important information because it goes a lot toward answering why you have been in such a rut, unable to do much about your problems, and why you wound up in the middle of the street a frustrated and angry man. We're going to set you up with an appointment to get some medication for that and also to get some counseling. I am going to give you a lot of information on why we think this is a good plan, so if you have any questions, stop me and I'll try and answer them.

Task 6. Obtaining Commitment

The sixth task, obtaining commitment, flows directly from Task 5, and the issues of control and autonomy apply equally to the process of obtaining an appropriate commitment. It may seem like overkill to devote a specific task/step to commitment as opposed to just making it a part of planning. However, getting a specific commitment from a client in crisis to do something differently than what has not been working is a big deal. The commitment step is clear, concise, and behaviorally specific. As a result, it is clear to clients what they are going to do and what the worker will do.

CIT officer: So tell me what we're going to do.

Leron: We gonna get out to the Salvation Armee and get me sobered up, din two' morro you gonna come git me 'n' tak me dow to legal aid 'bout 4:30, if'n I git in de polelesse car now and don't be givin' you no mo' trouble.

If the planning step is done effectively, the commitment step is apt to be easy. Many times, the commitment step is brief and simple, consisting of asking the client to verbally summarize the plan.

Sometimes, a handshake may be used to seal the commitment. In some incidents where lethality is involved, the commitment may be written down and signed by both parties. The objective is to enable the client to commit to taking one or more definite, positive, intentional action steps designed to move that person toward restoring precrisis equilibrium. The worker is careful to obtain an honest, direct, and appropriate commitment from the client before terminating the crisis intervention session. No commitment should be imposed by the worker. Commitments should be free, voluntary, and believed to be doable. The core listening skills are as important to the commitment step as they are to the problem definition or any other step. Any hesitation on the part of the client to commit to the plan of action should be reflected and queried by the worker. A worker-imposed plan or commitment will not work.

Task 7. Follow-up

When we speak of follow-up in crisis, we are not talking about days, weeks, or months. Long-term follow-up after a disaster is a special condition we will deal with in Chapter 16, "Disaster Response." We are generally speaking of following up in a time frame of minutes, hours, and days. Follow-up in crisis intervention has to do with keeping track of clients' success in maintaining precrisis equilibrium, not whether they are maintaining long-term goals or changing deep-seated personality traits.

CIT officer: (stopping by Salvation Army halfway house the next day) Leron, glad to see you. You look lots better today. Clean and sober. I checked with the coordinator, and they have you set up for some vocational evaluation. While I'm not your social worker, I did stop by the U of M law students' pro bono advocacy service, and they are willing to look into your problem with MHA. I think you can get a voucher here to get a bus down there. You've got my card, let me know if I can do anything for you.

Short-term follow-up is also important as a reinforcing event that tells clients you are still in this with them. Engaging in follow-up is extremely important when clients have little other social support system.

As a postscript to the foregoing scenario with Leron and Officer Lewis, we want to speak to our use of Leron's Memphis street language while inebriated. In past editions, we have received some critical comments from students questioning the use of that vernacular as demeaning. Nothing could be further from the truth. Leron's language usage has nothing to do with his value as a human being. If you were put off by it, you need to step back and consider your own social locations and the biases they may carry into the situation. We use specific vernaculars at times throughout the book to make the scenarios as realistic as possible. We will do that with other characters you'll meet in the book. We apologize if that's off putting, but that's the real world of crisis intervention and one component of the different social locations you will encounter as you do this work.

The model of crisis intervention we have been describing in some detail is summarized briefly in Figure 3.1.

Assessment in Crisis Intervention

LO3   Assessment is a pervasive strategy throughout crisis intervention. This action-oriented, situation-based assessment is the basis for systematically applying our task model. Thus, the entire task process is carried out under an umbrella of assessment by the crisis worker. Because many of the assessments

Assessment

Overarching and continuous throughout the crisis:
Evaluating the client's present situational crisis in terms of the client's coping ability, mobility, support systems needed, physical resources required, and degree of threat to self and others. Making judgments as to type and kind of action needed, based on the crisis worker's action continuum.

Tasks

Overarching default task: Ensuring safety. Continuous assessment of how safe the client, others in the environment, and the worker are throughout the crisis. Putting in place and implementing procedures that will ensure the safety of *all* those involved in the crisis, including the crisis worker.
1. **Predispositioning/engaging/initiating contact.** Making initial positive contact with the client. Setting the stage for what the worker is going to do, what the client can expect from the worker, and how the worker will operate throughout the crisis.
2. **Exploring the problem.** Defining the problem as it currently manifests itself across the affective, behavioral, and cognitive domains of the individual. Exploring the intrapersonal, interpersonal, and systemic effects of the crisis as it operates in the current environment within which the person operates.
3. **Providing support.** Determining what kinds of support systems have worked in the past, what support systems are currently available, and what support systems will be needed. More

specifically, determining how much the worker will need to function as the main support system during the crisis and indicating to clients how that will happen.
4. **Examining alternatives.** Considering immediate short-term options to de-escalate the crisis and defuse the situation. Examining the choices the client currently has available in a realistic and time-efficient manner; includes finding situational supports, installing coping mechanisms, and reframing thinking to be more positive and solution focused to generate achievable short-term goals.
5. **Making plans.** Generating a short-term plan from the alternatives that are positive and doable, and translating into immediate action steps the client can comprehend, own, and implement.
6. **Obtaining commitment.** Obtaining a verbal or written commitment to a plan that can be comprehended, owned, and put in operation by the client.
7. **Follow-up.** Immediate, short-term follow-up by the worker to ensure that the plan is working and that the client and others are safe.

Crisis Worker's Action Continuum

Crisis worker is nondirective   Crisis worker is collaborative   Crisis worker is directive

(Threshold varies from client to client)   (Threshold varies from client to client)

Client is mobile   Client is partially mobile   Client is immobile

The crisis worker's level of action/involvement may be anywhere on the continuum according to a valid and realistic assessment of the client's level of mobility/immobility.

Figure 3.1   Model of Triage Assessment Form for Crisis Intervention CIP-Solutions, June, 2009

in crisis situations occur spontaneously, subjectively, and interactively in the heat of the moment, we are not dealing here with formal techniques such as DSM 5-TR (American Psychiatric Association, 2022) diagnostic criteria or assessment instruments that are typically used in ongoing clinical evaluations. Kleespies and Richmond (2009) have a laundry list of mental status exam questions that cover everything from orientation/memory to visual/spatial organization. While these may be extremely useful in a set-piece intake assessment session at a hospital, a lot of times, there is neither the time nor the setting to engage in even a verbal comprehensive mental status examination.

Assessment is critically important because it enables the worker to determine (1) the severity of the crisis; (2) the client's current emotional, behavioral, and cognitive status and the client's level of mobility or immobility in these three areas; (3) the alternatives, coping mechanisms, support systems, and other resources available to the client; (4) the client's level of lethality (danger to self and others); and (5) and how well the worker is doing in de-escalating and defusing the situation and returning the client to a state of equilibrium and mobility.

Assessing the Severity of Crisis

It is important for the crisis worker to evaluate the crisis severity as quickly as possible during the initial contact with the client. Crisis workers generally do not have time to perform complete diagnostic workups or obtain in-depth client histories. Therefore, a rapid assessment procedure, such as the Triage Assessment System (Myer, 2001; Myer et al., 1991, 1992) and its assessment siblings—the Triage Assessment Checklist for Law Enforcement (TACKLE; James et al., 2006), the Triage Assessment System for Students in Learning Environments (TASSLE; Myer et al., 2007), and the Triage Assessment Form: Family Therapy (Myer, 2015)—are recommended as a quick and efficient way of obtaining information relevant to the specific crisis situation. These triage systems enable the worker to gauge the severity of the client's current functioning across affective, behavioral, and cognitive domains. The degree of severity of the crisis may affect the client's mobility, which, in turn, gives the worker a basis for judging how directive to be. The length of time the client has been in the present crisis will determine how much time the worker has in which to safely defuse the crisis.

The ABCs of Assessing in Crisis Intervention

Crisis is time limited; that is, most acute crises persist only a matter of days or weeks (the exception being large-scale disaster events) before some change—for better or worse—occurs. The severity of the crisis is assessed from the client's subjective viewpoint and from the worker's objective viewpoint. Objective assessment is based on an appraisal of the client's functioning in three areas that may be referred to as the ABCs of assessment: *affective* (feeling or emotional tone), *behavioral* (action or psychomotor activity), and *cognitive* (thinking patterns).

Affective State. Atypical or impaired affect is often the first sign that the client is in a state of disequilibrium. The client may be overemotional and out of control or severely withdrawn and detached. Often, the worker can assist the client to regain control and mobility by helping the client express feelings in appropriate and realistic ways. Some questions the worker may address are: Do the client's affective responses indicate that the client is denying the situation or attempting to avoid involvement in it? Is the emotional response normal or congruent with the situational crisis? To what extent, if any, is the client's emotional state driven, exacerbated, or otherwise influenced by other people? Do people typically show this kind of affect in situations such as this?

Behavioral Functioning. The crisis worker focuses much attention on *doing, acting out, taking active steps, behaving,* or any number of other psychomotor activities. In crisis intervention, the quickest (and often best) way to get the client to become mobile is to facilitate positive actions that the client can take at once. That said, if a client is having a hyperactive or hysterical reaction, slowing down with an admonishment to take a deep breath and doing nothing for a moment while getting back into control is paramount with a client who can't maintain behavioral control. People who cope with crisis successfully and later evaluate their experiences favorably report that the most helpful alternative during a crisis is to engage in some concrete and immediate activity. However, it is important for the worker to remember that it may be very difficult for immobilized people to take independent and autonomous action, even though that is what they need to do most.

These are appropriate questions that the worker might ask to get the client to take constructive action:

"In cases like this in the past, what actions did you take that helped you get back in control? What would you have to do now to get back on top of the situation? Is there anyone who, if you contacted them right now, would be supportive of you in this crisis?" The fundamental problem in immobility is loss of control. Once the client becomes involved in doing something concrete, which is a step in a positive direction, an element of control is restored, a degree of mobility is provided, and the climate for forward movement is established.

Cognitive State. The worker's assessment of the client's thinking patterns may provide answers to several important questions: How realistic and consistent is the client's thinking about the crisis? To what extent, if any, does the client appear to be rationalizing, exaggerating, or believing part-truths or rumors to exacerbate the crisis? How long has the client been engaged in crisis thinking? How open does the client seem to be toward changing beliefs about the crisis situation and reframing it in more positive terms of cooler, more rational thoughts, or is the client engaged in a downward spiral of catastrophic thinking with no hope of ameliorating the crisis?

The Triage Assessment System

Because rapid and adequate assessment of a client in crisis is one of the most critical components of intervention (Hersh, 1985), assessment has a preeminent place in the crisis intervention model as an overarching and ongoing process. Constant and rapid assessment of the client's state of equilibrium dictates what the interventionist will do in the next seconds and minutes as the crisis unfolds (Aguilera, 1998). Unhappily, many assessment devices that can give the human services worker an adequate perspective on the client's problem are unwieldy and time consuming and require that the client be enough in control to complete the assessment process or be physically present while undergoing evaluation. Although we might gain a great deal of helpful information with an extensive intake form, a background interview, or an in-depth personality test, events often occur so quickly that these are unaffordable and unrealistic luxuries.

What the interventionist needs in a crisis situation is a fast, efficient way of obtaining a real-time estimate of what is occurring with a client. Such a tool should also be simple enough that a worker who may have only rudimentary assessment skills can use the device in a reliable and valid manner. It should enable the assessment to be performed rapidly by a broad cross-section of crisis workers who have had little if any training in standardized testing or assessment procedures. What you are about to encounter (see Figure 3.2) is a composite of several forms of the Triage Assessment Form (TAF), which we believe admirably fits the foregoing criteria.

The Triage Assessment Form

Variations of the general TAF have been tested with police officer trainees, veteran crisis intervention team police officers who deal with the mentally ill, school counselors, community agency workers, secretaries, undergraduates, agency and crisis line supervisors, volunteer crisis line counselors, university professors, residence hall staff, and counselors-in-training (Blancett, 2008; Conte, 2005; Logan et al., 2006; Myer, 2001; Myer et al., 1991, 1992; Pazar, 2005; Slagel, 2009; Watters, 1997). Before training, none of the groups had any familiarity with the TAF.

The ratings of these groups were compared with expert triage ratings in a variety of different crisis scenarios (Minimal Impairment, Moderate Impairment, and Severe Impairment). These researchers found that police officer trainees tended to overrate and label the Moderate Impairment scenario as Severe Impairment (probably because they were very sensitive to not underrating the severity for fear of criticism or making a mistake that could cause a fatality). Veteran crisis intervention team police officers' ratings almost replicated the expert ratings (Logan et al., 2006; Pazar, 2005). The most problematic area of the scale appears to be the Moderate Impairment range (Watters, 1997). Veteran mental health workers either underrated or overrated Moderate Impairment scenarios. When queried, those veteran mental health workers who gave lower ratings than the experts indicated that they had seen, heard, and handled far more problematic behavior and felt Moderate was too high a rating. Conversely, other veteran mental health workers interpreted subtle responses in the Moderate scenarios to imply a greater threat than what was being portrayed and thus gave higher ratings than the experts. Overall, the ratings of all the other groups, such as the school counselors and volunteers, were deemed reliable and comparable with the ratings of the experts. All groups were congruent with the Minimal Impairment and Severe Impairment range (Blancett, 2008; Logan et al., 2006; Pazar, 2005; Watters, 1997). What the research seems to imply is

Client Name: _____ Time/Date: _____

Crisis Worker: _____ Contact Type: _____ Phone: _____ Office: _____

Field

Crisis Event:

_____

_____

_____

Disposition:

_____

_____

_____

Severity Scales
Check those that apply

	1 No Impairment	2/3 Minimal Impairment	4/5 Low Impairment	6/7 Moderate Impairment	8/9 Marked Impairment	10 Severe Impairment
A F F E C T I V E	○ Stable mood, control of feelings.	○ Affect elevated but generally appropriate.	○ Evidence of negative feelings pronounced and increasingly inappropriate.	○ Feelings are primarily negative and are exaggerated or increasingly diminished.	○ Feelings are negative and highly volatile or may be nonexistent.	○ Feelings are extremely pronounced to being devoid of feeling.
	○ Feelings are appropriate.	○ Brief periods of slightly elevated negative mood.	○ Duration of feeling intensity longer than situation warrants.	○ Efforts to control emotions are not always successful.	○ Extremely limited control of emotions.	○ No ability to control feelings regardless of potential danger to self or others.
	○ Emotions are under control.	○ Emotions are substantially under control.	○ Emotions are controlled but focused on crisis event.	○ Emotions not under control but remain focused on crisis.	○ Emotions start to generalize from crisis event to other people and situations.	○ Emotions of the crisis are generalized to other people and situations.
	○ Responses to questions/ requests are calm and composed.	○ Responses to questions/ requests are emotional but composed.	○ Responses to questions/ requests vary from rapid and agitated to slow and subdued.	○ Responses to questions/requests are emotionally volatile or beginning to shut down.	○ Responses to questions/ requests noncompliant due to interference of emotions.	○ Cannot respond to questions/requests because of interference of emotions.

Figure 3.2   Triage Assessment Form for Crisis Intervention.

Source: Compiled from Triage Assessment Form (TAF), Triage Assessment System for Students in Learning Environments (TASSLE), Triage Assessment Checklist for Law Enforcement (TACKLE). Crisis Intervention & Preventions Solutions Inc. Pittsburgh, PA.

	1 No Impairment	2/3 Minimal Impairment	4/5 Low Impairment	6/7 Moderate Impairment	8/9 Marked Impairment	10 Severe Impairment
B E H A V I O R S	○ Behaviors are socially appropriate.	○ Behaviors mostly effective, outbursts if present are inconsequential.	○ Behaviors are somewhat ineffective, yet not dangerous.	○ Behaviors are maladaptive but not immediately destructive.	○ Behaviors are likely to intensify crisis situation.	○ Behaviors are totally ineffective and accelerate the crisis.
	○ Daily functioning unimpeded.	○ Can perform tasks needed for daily functioning with minimal effort.	○ Performing tasks needed for daily living minimally compromised.	○ Performance of tasks needed for daily living is noticeably compromised.	○ Ability to perform tasks needed for daily functioning seriously impaired.	○ Unable to perform even simple tasks needed for daily functioning.
	○ Threat or danger nonexistent.	○ Behavior demonstrates frustration, but is nonthreatening.	○ Behaviors minimal threat to self or others.	○ Behavior is a potential threat to self or others.	○ Impulsivity has the potential to be harmful to self or others.	○ Behaviors are highly destructive possibly to cause injury/death to self or others.
	○ Behavior is stable and non-offensive.	○ Behaviors mostly stable and non-offensive.	○ Behavior becoming unstable and offensive.	○ Upon request, behaviors can be controlled with effort.	○ Behaviors are very difficult to control even with repeated requests.	○ Behavior is out of control and nonresponsive to requests.
C O G N I T I V E	○ Decisions are considerate of others.	○ Decisions may not be considerate of others.	○ Decisions are inconsiderate of others.	○ Decisions are offensive and antagonistic of others.	○ Decisions have the potential to be harmful to self or others.	○ Decisions are a clear and present danger to self and others.
	○ Decisions are logical and reasonable.	○ Decisions becoming indecisive but only with respect to crisis.	○ Decisions becoming illogical, unreasonable, and generalized beyond crisis.	○ Decisions about crisis beginning to interfere with general functioning.	○ Decisions are illogical, have little basis in reality, and general functioning is compromised.	○ Decision making frenetic or frozen and not based in reality and shuts down general functioning.
	○ Perception of crisis event substantially matches reality.	○ Thinking influenced by crisis, but under control.	○ Thinking focused on crisis but not all consuming.	○ Thoughts are limited to crisis situation and are becoming all consuming.	○ Thoughts about crisis have become pervasive.	○ Thoughts are chaotic and completely controlled by crisis.
	○ Able to carry on reasonable dialog and understand and acknowledge views of others.	○ Able to carry on reasonable dialog, understand and acknowledge views of others.	○ Ability to carry on reasonable dialog restricted and problems in understanding and acknowledging views of others.	○ Responses to questions and requests are restricted or inappropriate and denies understanding views of others.	○ Defiant to requests and questions and/or inappropriate with and antagonistic of others.	○ Requests and questions are believed as threat and responded to aggressively.
	○ Problem solving intact.	○ Problem solving minimally compromised	○ Problem solving limited.	○ Problem solving blocked.	○ Problem solving ability absent.	○ Problem solving not observable with no ability to concentrate.

Figure 3.2   (continued)

Digital Download   Download at Cengage.com

CRISIS EVENT

Identify and describe briefly the crisis situation: _____
_____
_____

AFFECTIVE DOMAIN

Identify and describe briefly the affect that is present.
(If more than one affect is experienced, rate with #1 being primary, #2 secondary, #3 tertiary.)

ANGER/HOSTILITY: _____
_____
_____
_____

ANXIETY/FEAR: _____
_____
_____
_____

SADNESS/MELANCHOLY: _____
_____
_____
_____

FRUSTRATION: _____
_____
_____
_____

BEHAVIORAL DOMAIN

Identify and describe briefly which behavior is currently being used.
(If more than one behavior is utilized, rate with #1 being primary, #2 secondary, #3 tertiary.)

APPROACH: _____
_____
_____

AVOIDANCE: _____
_____
_____

IMMOBILITY: _____
_____
_____

COGNITIVE DOMAIN

Identify if a transgression, threat, or loss has occurred in the following areas and describe briefly.
(If more than one cognitive response occurs, rate with #1 being primary, #2 secondary, #3 tertiary.)

PHYSICAL (food, water, safety, shelter, etc.): _____
_____
_____

Transgression_____ Threat_____ Loss_____

Figure 3.2 (continued)

Crisis Event (continued)

PSYCHOLOGICAL (self-concept, sense of emotional well-being, ego integrity, self-identity, etc.): _____
_____
_____

Transgression_____ Threat_____ Loss_____

SOCIAL RELATIONSHIPS (positive interaction and support, family, friends, coworkers, church, clubs, etc.): _____
_____
_____

Transgression_____ Threat_____ Loss_____

MORAL/SPIRITUAL (personal integrity, values, belief system, spiritual reconciliation): _____
_____
_____

Triage assessment   (X = Initial assessment/O = Terminal assessment)

Affective   **Behavioral**

___ Anger ___ Fear ___ Sadness   ___ Approach ___ Avoidance ___ Immobile

1 2 3 4 5 6 7 8 9 10   1 2 3 4 5 6 7 8 9 10

Cognitive

___ Transgression ___Threat ___Loss

1 2 3 4 5 6 7 8 9 10

_____ Physical _____ Psychological _____ Relationship _____ Moral/spiritual

Initial total score: _____ Terminal total score: _____ (if used)

Transgression_____ Threat_____ Loss_____

Describe the observations that led you to check the characteristics above:
_____
_____

that the scales should be taken at face value, and the less interpretation made of what the affect, behavior, and cognition imply, the more congruent ratings will be. In other words, trying to read too much or too little into what is being observed appears to invalidate the instrument when clients are operating in the moderately impaired range.

Although simple to use, the TAF is also elegant in that it cuts across the affective, behavioral, and cognitive domains, or dimensions, of the client; compartmentalizes each dimension as to its typical response mode; and assigns numeric values to these modes that allow the worker to determine the client's current level of functioning. These three severity scales represent mechanisms for operationally assigning numeric values to the crisis worker's action continuum, as shown in Figure 3.2. The numeric ratings provide an efficient and tangible guide to both the degree and the kind of intervention the worker needs to make in most crisis situations. Perhaps more important, they not only tell the worker how the client is doing, but they also tell the worker how they are going in attempting to de-escalate, defuse, and help the client regain control. The rationale and examples for each of the scales are discussed on the following pages. Because the original TAF scales were not parallel across numerical ratings with different numbers of anchors, workers reported having difficulty with assessment. As a result, Myer (2014) has developed a more efficient parallel set of ratings for each dimension.

The Affective Severity Scale. No crisis situation that we know of has positive emotions attached to it. Crow (1977) metaphorically names the usual emotional qualities found in a crisis as yellow (anxiety), red (anger), and black (depression). To those, we would add orange (our students chose this color) for frustration, which invariably occurs as clients attempt to meet needs. These needs range all across Maslow's (1954) needs hierarchy, from inability to get food, water, and shelter (Hurricane Katrina) to interpersonal issues (attempts to regain boyfriend/girlfriend) to intrapersonal issues (get rid of the schizophrenic voices) to spiritual concerns (God can't let this happen). Frustration of needs is often the precursor of other negative emotions, thoughts, and behaviors that plunge the client further into crisis. Even more problematically, some very famous psychologists have investigated the relationship between frustration and aggression and found that aggression is always a consequence of frustration (Dollard et al., 1939, p. 1). That outcome particularly does not bode well when the client is in crisis.

Undergirding these typical emotions may lie a constellation of other negative emotions such as shame, betrayal, humiliation, inadequacy, and horror (Collins & Collins, 2005, pp. 25–26). Clients may manifest these emotions both verbally and nonverbally, and the astute crisis worker needs to be highly aware of incongruencies between what the client is saying, how the client is saying it (voice tone, inflection, and decibel level), and what the client's body language says, or, if for either psychological or physical reasons, the person does not communicate at all.

Invariably, these negative emotions appear singularly or in combination with each other when a crisis is present. In their model, Myer and associates (1992) have replaced the term *depression*, because of its diagnostic implications, with *sadness/melancholy*.

When any of these core negative emotions become all-pervasive such that the client is consumed by them, the potential for these emotions to motivate destructive behavior becomes extremely high.

The Behavioral Severity Scale. While a client in crisis is more or less behaviorally immobile, immobility can take three different forms. Crow (1977) proposes that behavior in a crisis approaches, avoids, or is paralyzed in the client's attempts to act. Although Crow's proposal may seem contradictory, it is not. A client may seem highly motivated but be acting maladaptively toward a specific target or acting in a random, non-goal-directed manner with no specific target discernible. Alternatively, the client may attempt to flee the noxious event by the fastest means possible, even though the immediate threat to the client's well-being is gone. While in many instances, taking stock of the situation before acting is an excellent plan, clients transfixed in the face of immediate danger need to flee or fight. Although a great deal of energy may be expended and the client may look focused, once the crisis goes beyond the client's capacity to cope in a meaningful and purposeful manner, we would say that the client is immobilized, stuck in the particular approach, avoidance, or static behavior in a continuous loop no matter how proactive they may seem to be. At the severe impairment end of the continuum, maladaptive behavior often takes on a lethal aspect in regard to either the client or others.

The Cognitive Severity Scale. Ellis has written at length about the part that thinking plays in emotions and behavior (Ellis, 1971; Ellis & Abrahms, 1978; Ellis & Grieger, 1977; Ellis & Harper, 1975). In a crisis situation, the client's cognitive processes typically perceive the event in terms of transgression, threat, loss, or any combination of the three. These "hot" cognitions, as Dryden (1984) calls them, can take on catastrophic dimensions at the extreme end of the continuum.

Such highly focused irrational thinking can cause the client to obsess about the crisis to the extent that little, if any, logical thinking can occur within or beyond the boundaries of the crisis event. The event itself consumes all of the client's psychic energy as the client attempts to integrate it into their belief system. The client may generate maladaptive cognitions about intrapersonal, interpersonal, or environmental stimuli. Transgression, threat, or loss may be perceived in relation to physical needs such as food, shelter, and safety; psychological needs such as self-concept, emotional stability, and identity; relationship needs such as family, friends, coworkers, and community support; and moral and spiritual needs such as integrity and values.

To differentiate between transgression, threat, and loss, think of these dimensions in terms of time. *Transgression* is the cognition that something bad is happening in the present moment, *threat* is the cognition that something bad will occur, and *loss* is the cognition that something bad has occurred. When cognitions of the crisis move to the severe impairment end of the continuum, the perception of the event may be so extreme as to put the client or others at physical risk. Sometimes, the client's thinking moves from "It's a pain in the neck that this is happening, but I'll get over it" to "It's absolutely intolerable, I will not stand for this, and I'll never get over it." This kind of shift, from cool to hot cognitions (Dryden, 1984), is setting the client up to make some bad decisions. Such decisions most probably will result in even worse behavioral consequences for the client and others.

Certainly, the innate intellectual capacity of clients has much to do with how they respond cognitively to a crisis and how the crisis worker should respond to them. Given the same crisis, a client with borderline intelligence may perseverate on the need to obtain basic nurturance, while a person with average intelligence might brood on the existential issue of whether a higher power had a hand in the crisis.

There are four basic areas of cognitive functioning that are likely to become involved in a crisis: physical, psychological, social relationships, and moral/spiritual beliefs. These look a lot like Maslow's (1954) needs hierarchy, and in some ways, they are, and in some ways, they aren't. In a disaster, as you will see in Chapter 16, "Diaster Response people are pretty much concerned with getting food in their bellies and a roof over their heads first and worrying about other things second. On the other hand, it is not uncommon for all of these dimensions to come into play at once. Physical: "I am hungry, cold, and don't know how much longer I can stand it on top of this roof." Psychological: "I screwed up by not listening and preparing for the hurricane." Social: "Where is my family? Have they survived?" Moral/Spiritual: "How could God have done this to us?"

Some of you who are reading this book may take issue with the moral/spiritual component, but we believe, as others do, that spirituality is a key component in the crisis business (Arkin et al., 2022; Lee et al., 2022). We like Pargament and Sweeney's definition (2011) of spirit in their work developing the spiritual fitness component of the new U.S. Army's Comprehensive Soldier Fitness Program. They define *spirit* as "the essential core of the individual, the deepest part of the self, and one's involving human essence" and *spirituality* as "the continuous journey people take to discover and realize their essential selves." Pargament (2007) adds that it is looking for the *sacred* in one's life. If you think that people who are in crisis don't get down to the core of their being and, at times, try feverishly to figure out what is sacred, morally right, and how their spirit and spirituality tie into this business, and that this is not really worthy of your consideration, you would be dead wrong.

Comparison With Precrisis Functioning. Although it may not always be possible, the worker should seek to assess the client's precrisis functioning with the TAF as a guide to determine how effectively the client functioned prior to the event. Comparing precrisis ratings with current ratings lets the worker gauge the degree of deviation from the client's typical affective, behavioral, and cognitive operating levels. The worker can then tell how atypical the client's functioning is, whether there has been a radical shift in that functioning, and whether that functioning is transitory or chronic. For example, a very different approach would be used to counsel someone with chronic schizophrenia experiencing auditory hallucinations compared to an individual experiencing similar hallucinations from a prescription drug. Such an assessment can be made in one or two questions without having to ferret out a great deal of background information.

Rating Clients. In rating clients on the TAF, we move from high to low. This backward rating process may seem confusing at first glance, but the idea is that we rule out more severe impairment first. So, if we were rating affect, we would consider whether the client fits any of the descriptors under Severe Impairment. If not, we would then consider the descriptors under Marked Impairment. If we were able to check off at least two of those descriptors, the client would receive a rating of 9. If we could identify only one of the descriptors, the client would receive an 8. We would repeat this rating process across all three dimensions to obtain a total rating. Based on the total rating, which will range from 3 to 30, we generally group clients into three categories. A 3–10 rating means minimal impairment; these clients are generally self-directing and able to function effectively on their own. A rating of 11–19 means that clients are more impaired; they may have difficulty functioning on their own and need help and direction. This midscore range is the most problematic as far as the disposition of clients is concerned. Low teen scores (11–15) call for at least some guidance and directiveness from the worker to get the client on course as opposed to a single-digit score where the client can be pretty much self-directed with minimal guidance and information. High teen scores (16–19) are indicative of clients who are losing more and more control of their ability to function effectively and call for a good deal more than passive and palliative responses from the worker so they do not escalate into 20 territories. Clarity in setting boundaries and finding specific and continuous support systems for the immediate future is generally called for when scores fall into this range. Clients with a total score of 20 or above are moving deeper into harm's way; they are likely to need a great deal of direction and a secure and safe environment so they do not escalate into the lethal range. Scores in the high 20s almost always mean that some degree of lethality is involved, whether it is premeditated or clients are simply so out of control that they cannot stay out of harm's way.

Rating clients on the triage scale also means rating the crisis worker! How is this so? If the worker is effective in stabilizing a client, the triage scale score should go down. If it does not, then the worker probably needs to shift gears and try another approach. While the TAF is not absolutely precise and is not intended to be, it does give a good numerical anchor that the crisis worker can use in making judgments about client disposition and the effectiveness of the intervention. Our students very quickly become skillful at making these ratings on sample cases, and so will you.

Severity. One rating issue that constantly arises is the question, "What do you mean by severe? Shouldn't a mother who just got news that her son was badly injured in a school bus accident be pretty hysterical and out of control?" That is certainly true. However, what puts the mother into a crisis category and allows us to rate her as "severely impaired" on the TAF is threefold. First, even though the feelings, thoughts, and behaviors may seem reasonable responses given the horrific situation, what kind of potential trouble does that get the mother into? Are her feelings, thoughts, and actions liable to exacerbate the situation further? Second, it is not just the **intensity** but also the **duration** of the feelings, thoughts, and actions and how well clients can **control** themselves as time moves forward and the context of the crisis changes. We might reasonably expect an initial response that is highly volatile, but if, after 8 hours, that same degree of emotional energy was still present, it would be obvious that the client was out of control, in crisis, and in need of assistance. Conversely, if this situation would normally elicit an intense reaction but none was forthcoming and emotions were stone-walled, behaviors paralyzed, thinking frozen, and positive action conspicuously absent, we would elevate our TAF as well. Correlative with intensity is how long that intensity has existed. Extended duration and inability to control feelings, behavior, and thinking invariably indicates a deepening of the crisis and an elevated TAF. That being said, most assessment beginners want to know how we measure intensity. Likewise, what's the time frame or duration before we escalate our rating? We wish we could give you a pounds, yards, hours answer. But that's where Kleespies' (2014) notion of clinical expertise and experience come into play. There is no formula for those variables except your own clinical experience that the situation is progressing to a point where a decision to get the individual to a safe place with adequate supervision is warranted.

A typical example that generally does not require crisis intervention, but down the road may warrant marriage counseling, is Dr. and Mrs. James' escalating discussion about closely watching their discretionary funds now that both are retired, and those funds and a cruise trip down the Rhine river not being compatible with financial resources in the parsimonious doctor's view and the aesthetics of riding the river from Holland to Switzerland being worth every penny to Mrs. James.

That discussion is not quite up to arming themselves with kitchen utensils, but the decibel level of the discussion is starting to annoy the neighbors, and we could easily triage both in the middle TAF range. Fortunately, the telephone rings as the TAF is moving into the high teens. Their youngest daughter is on the line with news of the latest escapades of the grandkids. Mrs. James immediately warms her tea in the microwave, settles on her easy chair, and when asked how things are going, sweetly answers, "Oh your father and I were just having a conversation about that Rhine River trip we talked about, and so how are my babies doing?" With that break in the action, Dr. J. exits to his shop and starts shaping up a fishing tackle box. While the dialogue may resume and become heated again, this husband-and-wife team has learned over fifty years how to cool things down and are now back in the TAF single digits (Mrs. James) and low teens (Dr. J). Their intensity has been high, but duration was short, and control was readily available. Contrast that same financial discussion among numerous other couples that results in kitchen utensils being picked up, phone calls ignored, police response, resulting domestic violence charges, and adjudication in family court to the Memphis Police Department Family Trouble Center for anger management. That is a pretty common example of how intensity and duration can stoke a smoldering domestic fire to white hot.

As our prior description of TAF research has indicated, ratings in the teens are the most difficult to determine in regard to how much directive action on the part of the worker needs to be taken. That is particularly true during the course of intervention when the client bounces between low and high teen ratings or oscillates back and forth between high teens and low twenties. Our rule of thumb is that if the client continues to cycle between ratings and we are unable to de-escalate to a consistent lower rating, more directive action needs to be taken, and the client informed that if control cannot be maintained, we are going to take action to keep the individual safe. We could be mistaken, and we could make the client angry, but the overriding ethical standard in play is, "Do no harm!"

Alternate Forms of the TAF

The TAF has been modified for use with police departments (Logan et al., 2006), higher education/ student affairs personnel (Armitage et al., 2007), and disaster relief workers (James et al., 2007) and has also been adapted to families (Myer, 2015) based on the increased interaction with and need to provide services or actions for mentally ill and emotionally distraught individuals in each of these venues. All these alternate forms of the TAF have been developed because of the expanding needs of a variety of workers who do not have a mental health background yet who come in contact with emotionally disturbed individuals for whom they are expected to render service of some kind. All of the following variations of the TAF have been modified for ease and simplicity of use and have or are undergoing field testing.

The second section of the TAF form is titled "Observations" (see Figure 3.3). This section is divided into three columns, listing some of the behaviors that

Observations (Check all that apply)

___ off medication*	___ aggressive gestures	___ hysterical*
___ hallucinating[†] (___smells ___sights ___sounds ___touch)	___ physically violent[†]	___ confusion*
	___ verbal threats to self or others	___ unable to follow simple directions*
___ bizarre behavior/appearance	___ suicidal/homicidal thinking/ verbalizing*	___ unable to control emotions
___ poor hygiene		___ cannot recall personal information* (phone, address)
___ absurd, illogical, nonsensical speech	___ suicidal/homicidal gestures/ behaviors[†]	___ situation perceived as unreal* (spectator)
___ paranoid/suspicious thoughts	___ suicidal/homicidal plan clear[†]	
___ flashbacks, loss of reality contact*	___ uncooperative	___ nonresponsive*
___ intoxicated/drugged*	___ reckless behavior	
___ possible developmental disability	___ impulsivity	

*Support services recommended.
[†]Protective custody recommended.

Figure 3.3   Triage Assessment System for Students in Learning Environments (TASSLE): Observational Checklist.

Source: Myer et al., 2007.

may be seen with an individual in crisis. Several of the items have been identified as critical for either getting clients support or removing them to a place of safety. A general guideline is the more items you check, the more likely a person will either need support or should be removed. Most often, checking numerous items means the individual's rating on the severity scales will also be high. High scores on the severity scales generally mean an increased need for support services and an increased potential for hospitalization.

The first column addresses psychological problems. Check appropriate descriptors in this section based on your observations and questioning of individuals. You may not be able to gather all this information because clients may be uncooperative or simply unable to respond to questions. A good source for some of this information is other people who may know the client. Asking them about the individual may give you the information needed to check the appropriate descriptors in this column.

The second column focuses on clients who are dangerous to themselves or others. They may be only threatening harm or actually making suicidal or homicidal gestures. If they are simply threatening harm, you will need to make a judgment as to whether the person is an immediate danger to self or others. Simply making threats to harm oneself or others does not automatically mean the client needs support services or removal. A standard guideline is if a person has a plan formulated and if the means to carry out the plan are available, that person is a threat and needs to be monitored in a safe place by qualified mental health workers until the threat has abated.

The third column relates to the severity scales most directly. Listed in this column are feelings, behaviors, and thoughts persons may experience when in a crisis. These correspond to characteristics on the severity scales. Generally, you can complete this section based on your observations and experience with students. Four of the descriptors have been identified as being critical: (1) hysterical, (2) confusion, (3) unable to follow simple directions, and (4) nonresponsive. Individuals who fit these descriptors are vulnerable, mentally fragile, and unable to care for themselves.

In summary, the TAF and its derivative alternate forms provide multiple three-dimensional combinations of the domains of assessment regarding the degree of impairment the crisis is causing, target specific areas of functioning, and let the crisis worker evaluate the client quickly and then construct specific interventions aimed directly at the areas of greatest immediate concern.

Default Drug Assessment

LO4 Both legal and illegal substances and drugs have a major effect on mental health and commonly provide fuel to stoke a crisis. Although the ways illegal drugs change brain chemistry and behavior has gained wide attention, legal drugs may promote adverse psychological side effects in just as dramatic a manner. In particular, combinations of non-psychotropic drugs are routinely given to combat several degenerative diseases in older adults. At times, these drugs may have interactive effects that generate unanticipated psychological disturbances. One has to read no further than the consumer trade books on prescribed drugs to obtain a rather frightening understanding of the psychological side effects prescription drugs can cause.

Therefore, the human services worker should attempt to assess prior trauma, psychopathology, and use, misuse, or abuse of legal and illegal drugs in an effort to determine whether they correlate with the current problem. "Talking" therapies do little good when neurobiological substrates are involved. If the human services worker has reason to suspect any of the foregoing problems, an immediate referral should be made for a neurological/drug evaluation. Given the foregoing, Officer Lewis's question about how much Leron had been drinking is a default question in regard to use or misuse of both prescription and nonprescription medications or intoxicants. Do not assume that only individuals who have been consuming alcohol, using illegal drugs, or being treated for mental illness and off their drugs are the only recipients of crisis services. Two classic examples are secondary psychosis due to diabetes and bad drug interactions for older people who may be on a veritable smorgasbord of drugs for medical reasons.

The following questions are practically mandatory during initial exploration activities with a person in crisis and should be asked in a non-accusing way.

Our own default questions, which you should feel free to adopt as your own, go something like this.

CW: I am going to ask you some questions about drug use. Understand I am not concerned about legal issues. What I am concerned about is whether taking drugs of any kind or changes in those drugs are affecting you and perhaps accelerating the crisis. Lots of times people have a reaction to medication or changes in medication. Are you on any medication right now? Is it for emotional problems? Have you stopped taking it? Perhaps it has cost too much or maybe it has some bad side effects? Are you on any medications for other physical problems? Have you stopped taking or changed medications? Did you have any alcoholic beverages with your medication? Has there been any way you feel like you have changed or felt different since you went on or changed or went off a medication?

If there is reticence or embarrassment on the individual's part about responding to the request for drug use, repeat as sincerely as possible that you have no interest in illegal use or wish to cause embarrassment for use of certain drugs.

CW: I sense you may be a little hesitant to tell me what drugs you have been using but let me assure you I have no interest in legal issues with them or connection with any drug enforcement. Practically everyone uses some kind of drugs today, but sometimes there are bad interactions, and they can cause some of the problems you're having, so if you could remember or have a list, I'd like to hear or see what they are.

Default Lethality Potential Assessment

LO5 Not every crisis involves the client contemplating suicide or homicide. However, in dealing with crisis clients, workers must always explore the possibility of harm to self or others because destructive behavior takes many forms and wears many masks. Crisis workers need to be both wary of and competent in their appraisal of potential suicidal and homicidal clients. What may appear to the crisis worker as the main problem may camouflage the real issue: the intent of the client to take their life or someone else's life. Contrary to popular belief, most suicidal and homicidal clients emit definite clues and believe they are calling out for help or signaling warnings. However, even the client's closest friends may ignore those clues and do nothing about them. For that reason, every crisis problem should be assessed as to its potential for suicide and homicide. The most important aspect of suicidal/homicidal evaluation is the crisis evaluator's realization that suicide and

homicide are always possible in all types of clients. A complete and comprehensive number of lethality protocols are discussed in Chapter 8, "Crisis of Lethality."

Assessing the Client's Current Emotional Functioning

LO6 Four major factors in assessing the client's emotional stability are (1) the duration of the crisis, (2) the degree of emotional stamina or coping at the client's disposal at the moment, (3) the ecosystem within which the client resides, and (4) the developmental stage of the client.

The duration factor concerns the time frame of the crisis. Is it a onetime crisis? Is it recurring? Has it been plaguing the client for a long time? A onetime crisis of relatively short duration is called *acute* or *situational*. A long-term pattern of recurring crisis is labeled *chronic, long-term,* or *transcrisis.*

The degree factor concerns the client's current reservoir of emotional coping stamina. During typical periods of the client's life, the coping reservoir is relatively full, but during crisis, the client's reservoir is relatively empty. Assessing the degree factor, then, involves the crisis worker's determination of how much emotional coping strength is left in the client's reservoir. Has the client run out of gas, or can the client make it over a small hill?

The ecosystem is a very large extraneous variable that can dramatically influence client coping (Collins & Collins, 2005; Halpern & Tramontin, 2007; James et al., 2003; Myer & Moore, 2006). Geographic region and accessibility, communication systems, language, cultural mores, religious beliefs, economic status, and social micro- and macrosystem interactions are only some of the ecosystemic variables that may have subtle or profound effects on a client's emotional coping ability. No individual's crisis can be taken out of the ecosystemic context in which it occurs, and to believe it can be somehow treated separately without considering that context is to make a grave intervention error.

Developmental stages (Collins & Collins, 2005) certainly play a part in the client's emotional functioning during a crisis. Merely transitioning from life stage to life stage has its own potential for crises (Blocher, 2000; Erikson, 1963). Understanding the developmental tasks of different life stages, which may frame a client's view of a crisis and how the client responds to it, is critical for crisis workers. Further compounding the issue, developmental tasks are sometimes not accomplished at a particular life stage, and developmental crises occur (Levinson, 1986). It does not take much imagination to foresee that adding a situational crisis may have a tremendous impact on a "stuck-in-stage" individual's emotional coping skill.

The Client's Current Acute or Chronic State.

In assessing the crisis client's emotional functioning, it is important that the crisis worker determine whether the client is a normal person who is in a *onetime* situational crisis or a person with a *chronic,* crisis-oriented life history. The onetime crisis is assessed and treated quite differently from the chronic crisis. The onetime crisis client usually requires direct intervention to facilitate getting over the specific event or situation that precipitated the crisis. Having reached a state of precrisis equilibrium, the client can usually draw on normal coping mechanisms and support people and manage independently.

The chronic crisis client usually requires a greater length of time in counseling. That individual typically needs the help of a crisis worker in examining available coping mechanisms, finding support people, rediscovering strategies that worked during previous crises, generating new coping strategies, and gaining affirmation and encouragement from the worker and others as sources of strength by which to move beyond the present crisis. The chronic case frequently requires referral for long-term professional help.

The Client's Reservoir of Emotional Strength.

The client who lacks emotional strength needs more direct responses from the crisis worker than the client who retains a good deal of emotional strength. A feeling of hopelessness or helplessness is a clue to a low reservoir of emotional strength. In some cases, the assessment can be enhanced by asking open-ended questions for the specific purpose of measuring that reservoir. Typically, if the reservoir is low, the client will have a distorted view of the past and present and will not be able to envision a future. Such questions can reveal the degree of emotional stamina remaining: "Picture yourself after the current crisis has been solved. Tell me what you're seeing and how you're feeling. How do you wish you were feeling? How were you feeling about

this before the crisis got so bad? Where do you see yourself headed with this problem?" In general, the lower the reservoir of emotional strength, the less the client can get hold of the future. The client with an empty reservoir might respond with a blank stare or by saying something like "There are no choices" or "No, I can't see anything. The future is blank. I can see no future." The worker's assessment of the client's current degree of emotional strength will have definite implications for the strategies and level of action the worker will employ during the remainder of the counseling.

Strategies for Assessing Emotional Status.

The crisis worker who assesses the client's total emotional status may look at a wide array of social locations (Brown, 2008) that affect both the duration (chronic versus acute) and the degree (reservoir of strength) of emotional stability. Some factors to be considered are the client's age, educational level, family situation, marital status, vocational maturity and job stability, financial stability and obligations, drug and/or alcohol use, legal history (arrests, convictions, probations), social background, level of intelligence, lifestyle, religious orientation, ability to sustain close personal relationships, tolerance for ambiguity, physical health, medical history, and past history of dealing with crises. A candid look at such factors helps the crisis worker decide whether the client will require quick referral (for medical treatment or examination), brief counseling, long-term therapy, or referral to a specific agency.

Ordinarily, no one factor alone can be used to conclude that the client's reservoir of emotional coping ability is empty. However, some patterns can often be pieced together to form a general picture. A person in middle age who has experienced many disappointments related to undereducation and subsequent underemployment would be viewed differently from a young person who has experienced a first career disappointment. A person who has experienced many serious medical problems and hospital stays would feel differently from a person who is having a first encounter with a medical problem. The foregoing example is a *facilitative* affective assessment of the individual. By "facilitative assessment," we mean that data gleaned about the client are used as a part of the ongoing helping process, not simply filed away or kept in the worker's head.

Assessing Alternatives, Coping Mechanisms, and Support Systems

Throughout the helping process, the crisis worker keeps in mind and builds a repertoire of options, evaluating their appropriateness for the client. In assessing alternatives available to the client, the worker must first consider the client's viewpoint, mobility, and capability of taking advantage of the alternatives. The worker's own objective view of available alternatives is an additional dimension.

Alternatives include a repository of appropriate referral resources available to the client. Even though the client may be looking for only one or two concrete action steps or options, the worker brainstorms, in collaboration with the client, to develop a list of possibilities that can be evaluated. Most will be discarded before the client can own and commit to a definite course of action. The worker ponders questions such as: What actions or choices does the client have now that would restore the person to a precrisis state of autonomy? What realistic actions (coping mechanisms) can the client take? What institutional, social, vocational, or personal (people) strengths or support systems are available? (Note that "support systems" refers to people!) Who would care about and be open to assisting the client? What are the financial, social, vocational, and personal impediments to client progress?

Assessing for Legal and Ethical Issues

LO7 If you've gotten the idea that we think assessing is a big deal in crisis intervention, you are absolutely right! That said, we have one more biggie left to cover, and this is important from the standpoint of keeping you out of legal trouble in a courtroom and ethical malfeasance that can get you in front of a licensing board. It also does not leave "ethics" as a stand alone, somehow separate, concept but ties it directly into your therapeutic efforts. You can fill a bookcase with the legal and ethical dilemmas of providing psychotherapy, but if you were to search for literature dealing with the legal and ethical issues of crisis, you'd find only a couple we know of, and yes, we wrote them (Myer et al., 2022; Zanskas et al., 2017). Why we wrote them is both simple and complex.

It is simple from the standpoint that ethical guidelines are regularly encroached upon during crisis intervention. In an office setting, providing procedural informed consent is a standard of practice and among the first items of business for mental health professionals initiating a therapeutic relationship. Can you imagine telling people in a crowded reception center crisis after a tornado wiped their home and grandmother off the face of the earth to calm down and not to say anything until you have obtained their informed consent? Try asking a person in crisis to sign a form stating that they understand the limits of confidentiality while standing on a bridge railing. So, turn to the ethical codes of the helping professions for help, right? Not so fast.

Ethical codes do not specifically address the unique circumstances surrounding the provision of crisis intervention services (Hanson et al., 2005; Welfel, 2013). In fact, the American Counseling Association, National Association for Social Work, American Association for Marriage and Family Therapy, and American Psychological Association do not even mention the word *crisis* in their ethical codes. These ethical codes as well as others do not speak directly to the ethics of conduct expected in crisis intervention or disaster situations (Thoburn et al., 2012). So does that mean ethical standards do not apply in a crisis situation? Not hardly. Licensed mental health practitioners in crisis or disaster contexts need to recognize that providing counseling-related services can be considered treatment and the basis for ethical and legal culpability (Kleinman & Stewart, 2004), and their supervisors along with them (Remley & Herlihy, 2020).

The major ethical conundrum in crisis intervention has to do with the five moral principles at the foundation of ethical decision making (Kitchener, 1984). They are autonomy, beneficence, fidelity, justice and nonmaleficence. Veracity was subsequently added to the 2014 ACA COE's code. The typical friction point in crisis intervention occurs when autonomy butts heads with the other moral principles. The principle of **autonomy** refers to a client's right to self-determination (ACA, 2014) and is seen as a preeminent ethical standard as ultimately, clients are responsible for their own decisions. Under this standard, informed consent and confidentiality are fundamental client rights supported by the principle of autonomy.

A particularly vociferous professional debate occurs with psychologists between prioritizing autonomy versus beneficence (Drogin, 2019). Drogin (pp. 272–273) proposes that most psychologists rank beneficence before autonomy because it gives them greater control over clients in regard to such issues as involuntary commitment and the inability to refuse psychotropic medication. Counterpointing that stance, Drogin proposes that the government's overriding goal should be to promote human dignity and individual autonomy and not have that autonomy overridden by the state or its agents. We should have the right to make mistakes and determine our own fate, even when it goes against the public grain.

Drogin quotes a famous statement in a dissenting opinion by Justice Brandeis to make his point. "Experience should teach us to be most on our guard to protect liberty when government's purposes are beneficial (*Olmstead v. United States*, 1928, p. 479). What do you think about this argument?

With all due respect to Eric Drogin, the trouble is that lots of times, individuals in crisis do not have much control over their thinking and acting such that their autonomy needs to have strictures put on it. Put in plain words, they can't control themselves, and somebody else needs to keep them out of harm's way. Birrell and Freyd (2006) maintain that, in fact, autonomy does not rest with the client when ethical decisions have to be made. Given that fact, autonomy flies directly into the face of nonmaleficence and beneficence, which emphasizes avoiding actions that could cause harm (ACA, 2014).

Consultation, review of ethical codes, knowledge of jurisdictional laws, and use of ethical decision-making models are methods intended to ensure that helping professionals allow sufficient time to process and consider the implications of a decision and develop a best course of action, but therein lies the problem. Most crisis situations do not allow the leisure of timely use of those actions. Adding to the dilemma, Tarvydas and Ng (2012) propose that cross-cultural counseling (which there is a lot of in crisis intervention) is particularly vulnerable to ethical conflict and dilemmas. The ethical decision-making models, assumptions, assessments, and interventions of individuals engaged in crisis intervention have been developed from one cultural perspective but are often implemented within the worldview of another culture and can cause conflicts. (Pedersen & Marsella, 1982).

So, what's a possible solution? Kleespies (2014) advocates the use of naturalistic decision-making

models (NDMs). These types of models emphasize clinician experience and long-term memory as the tools facilitating the crisis interventionist's ability to "think on one's feet" to make decisions while under time pressure and constraints. Situational awareness and the ability to rapidly gather, analyze, and synthesize information are all considered essential abilities to make decisions under stress. Accrued situational experience and the ability to rapidly conceptualize the context of the current crisis situation are characteristics of these models. That wealth of experience is all well and good for a veteran interventionist, but what about beginners like most of you reading this book?

We think that the best way to integrate crisis intervention, except in special circumstances that involve mandated reporting of legal issues, is through the basic philosophical principles on which ethical standards are developed, but employed in a hierarchical manner. These principles are a common thread through all ethical standards (Drogin, 2019; Pope & Vasquez, 2016; Remley & Herlihy, 2020; Stone, 2017; Wefel, 2016). Interestingly, most discussions of these ethical standards are presented as being separate from actual counseling activities (Birrell & Bruns, 2016), handed down by professional organizations and interpreted by licensing boards with little thought about tying them into the actual therapy being provided. We disagree with that concept and believe they should be highly integrated, particularly when used in crisis intervention when the potential to do harm is high (Myer et al., 2022, pp. 70–71). Therefore, as we interact with clients, we are mentally ordering the ethical standards that will best fit their needs and will be tied to the theoretical approach, clinical techniques, and assessment tools we employ.

For this purpose, we propose the LASER protocol as a legal and ethical decision-making model for crisis intervention (Myer et al., 2022). This model is different from other ethical models in that it operates in real time. It allows interventionists to make immediate decisions on how best to ethically abide by standards and still provide optimal service to the client. Particularly important in this model is the utilization of each component as it applies to and changes with the dynamics of the situation. There are five linear components to the LASER model summarized here (For a complete description, see Myer and associates (2022) (Crisis *Intervention Ethics Casebook*).

Legal, the first step of the LASER protocol, considers legal responsibilities. What immediately comes to mind for this step are crises that involve harm to self or others and situations concerning the abuse of vulnerable populations. From the landmark Tarasoff (1976) California Supreme Court decision, there is firm legal precedent that mental health professionals have a duty to provide reasonable care to protect intended victims or notify law enforcement if they are aware an individual poses a serious danger to the intended victim (Wheeler & Bertram, 2019). Problematically, there is no federal law that provides guidance on this issue, and each state has its own particular definition of how that standard is put into practice (Kenny et al., 2017). Issues such as time limitation to report and what "reasonable suspicion" means are examples of state variance (Kenny et al., 2017; Wheeler & Bertram, 2019). Then, add those two to a variety of bumble bees that can come flying out of Pandora's legal box such as licensure requirements, privileged communication, client abandonment, competence, and documentation (Wheeler & Bertram, 2019). Given the multitude of legal issues, you need to know how the state you live in or practice in handles them before anything in the way of any kind of therapy, crisis intervention included happens.

Assessment

Assessment is the lynchpin for making appropriate decisions, not just for intervention but also for ethical choices in crises. The Triage Assessment Form (TAF) is uniquely suited for making these decisions. This assessment form was developed specifically for crisis intervention and has received national and international acceptance as a practical tool for crisis intervention (Bonynge & Thurber, 2008). The TAF can be combined with other on-the-spot assessment devices such as specific lethality tools to form an intervention plan that has good ethical grounding. The following are *general* guidelines for hierarchical ordering of the ethical standards and not chiseled in stone.

Single digit to low teens on the TAF suggests that the autonomy of individuals should rarely be violated. Fidelity, nonmaleficence, and veracity are still a factor when TAF ratings are low but generally stand aside when the client is capable of making good decisions and acting on them in a rational manner.

Individuals who have reactions in the TAF high teens will typically have trouble making autonomous decisions and will need more directive and supportive guidance from the interventionist. Beneficence, fidelity, and veracity are key moral standards at this juncture. The whole notion is that "We are in this together, and we'll work it out and see it through."

For individuals with total ratings in the twenties or a score of 10 on any of the three subscales, do no harm and nonmaleficence is the gold standard ethical principle in operation. No matter what protestations come from the client or significant others, safety is an overriding concern for the client and perhaps others. Meeting whatever a state's requirements are on reporting lethality should be a given. There should be no ethical waffling on your part. Angry exhortations and threats aside, when the TAF is that high, your direct action to avoid malfeasance is mandated to get the client under close, safe personal supervision.

Setting

The setting and context of crisis intervention has a major impact on the ethical decision-making process, and those range across in-house private practice, walk-in clinics, mental health institutions, emergency rooms in hospitals, school buildings, and standoff street crisis negotiations with CIT officers. Each of these settings have participating entities that have policies that define procedures to be used in legal and ethical situations, which they believe to be reasonable and proper and also cover them in regard to legal actions (Wheeler & Bertram, 2019).

Context. Environmental context also plays a significant role in how ethical decision-making plays out. Stone (2015) makes a strong case about how urban, suburban, and rural school settings play a differential role in ethical decision making. Subsumed under setting and context, three major factors have the potential to shape ethical decisions. The factors are **Procedures**, **Policies**, and **Politics** (Myer et al., 2022).

Procedures. First, procedural issues in a specific setting influence which ethical principle takes precedence. For example, the use of veracity in dealing with the death of a relative may be very different with a child in an elementary school than that of a spouse in a work setting. On the one hand, beneficence may be the overriding principle, while veracity is tempered with a child, while with the surviving spouse, fidelity and beneficence may go hand-in-hand with veracity. A similar situation in an agency might mean the principle of fidelity is critical and is demonstrated by empathically informing the individual of a death and providing beneficent support, trust, and bonding in the therapeutic relationship. Familiarizing yourself with your institution's protocols, particularly when a loss has occurred, is excellent preparation to avoid getting blindsided when you are tasked with delivering bad news. If you don't know about bad news protocols, don't be afraid to ask. If there isn't one in place, get busy and construct one because sooner or later you will need it.

Policies. Second, institutional policies affect the application of ethical principles in crises. The policies of school systems, mental institutions, and police departments are, by necessity, radically different in keeping the system smoothly running. This is particularly true of record keeping that may be dictated by both federal and state legal requirements along with the institution's professional business operating requirements (Bertram & Wheeer, 2019; Pfefferbaum et al., 2012; Stone, 2017). Paying close attention to what those requirements are can keep you out of legal, ethical, and occupational hot water.

Politics. Finally, politics generated both within and outside the institution can have an influence on decisions involving ethical principles. Time and time again, institutions that are resistant to the political ramifications of their actions attempt to sweep bad news under their institutional rug to preserve the "good" name of individuals or institutions and not bring negative publicity down on them. Classic examples of that are Megan's Law (1994) (not keeping track of sexual offenders) and the Jeanne Clery Act (1990) (not keeping track of crimes on college campuses).

You need to understand that no school superintendent, hospital administrator, or mayor swears to uphold the counselor, psychologist, or social worker ethical standards, particularly when their job is at stake, and they are receiving political heat from political interest groups bent on maintaining a positive image. So, the politics of a situation may run very counter to what the ethical standards of your profession and your personal integrity can tolerate.

It could be argued in a rather hypocritical, rationalizing sense that playing the political game is engaging in nonmalfeasance and beneficence to the institution, but then one has to live with the lack of veracity when looking in the mirror every morning. Make no mistake about it. If you stay in the human

service business very long, politics will rear its ugly head and you'll have to make some hard ethical decisions yourself on where you stand. Our best advice is that when politics start to surface in conflict with your ethical stance, you need to make a thorough written record of everything you have done, being particular in regard to persons, settings, and times that were involved. You would also be well advised to consult with a trusted other professional and make thorough notes of their recommendations as soon as the dilemma arises and not after it happens if at all possible.

Ethical Principles

Selecting the ethical principle or principles that are most important for crises is not simple because crisis situations can change very quickly and result in the need to adjust which ethical principle is important. This shift is based on legal issues suddenly surfacing and needing to be considered, the reactions of individuals quickly becoming more or less severe, and issues related to the setting that involve the three "Ps" (i.e., policies, procedures, politics) (Myer et al., 2022).

Autonomy is seen as the foundation stone of the ethical principles of psychotherapeutic practice. However, when a crisis occurs, autonomy often butts up against beneficence and malfeasance in that therapists are caught between what is best for the client and what may be best for society if the client begins to trample on others' rights. The best and most objective solution to the autonomy dilemma is what the individual's TAF score is showing. The higher the score, the more nonmalfeasance and veracity predominate and the less does autonomy.

The ethical concept of justice is another thorny issue that often has more to do with the interventionist's biases than anything else. The principle of justice concerns fairness, equality, and nondiscriminatory care (ACA, 2014). It is easy to mouth those words, but the potential for bias and prejudice to arise in a crisis is ever present when clients have failure after failure to get better. In CIT officer language, these are the "Pete" and "Repeats" they see over and over in their patrol areas. These individuals who perpetually cycle through the mental health system can wear an interventionist's patience and empathy out.

Given this possibility, the TAF can also be applied to the interventionist. What do you suppose needs to happen when your own TAF score zooms into high teens and, heaven forbid! the twenties when making contact with a resistant client who doesn't look, smell, talk, or act good? Think that won't happen? Think again when your stress bucket is overflowing and spilling out all over you. While that happens to the very best of us, it still is a nonstarter. Crisis workers must find a way not to allow their emotions and resulting actions based on frustration, anger, guilt, or embarrassment to interfere with appropriate ethical decisions. If that happens, probably not much "justice" is going to come that person's way until you get good supervision, which is a sine qua non in the crisis business (Brucia et al., 2020; Pope & Vasquez, 2016; Stone, 2017; Welfel, 2015; Wheeler & Bertram, 2019).

Resolution

Stop! Pause a moment. Are you sure of the legal ramifications of what you're going to do? Okay! What does the triage assessment tell you about how directive you're going to be to get this settled? Is your setting stable? Is backup consultation available if possible? Are significant others that may give you trouble out of the way? Is it safe to proceed? Are significant others who may be supportive within reach? Is the general environment and setting peaceful enough without outside interference? Have you done a hierarchical ordering of your ethical standards?

Good enough! You're ready to attempt to resolve this situation. Resolution is not formulaic but indeed relies on Kleespies' (2014) concept of "thinking on your feet." Fine words, but what does that mean in practice? It means you are going to use the techniques and strategies in this book as a foundation on which to build your armory of skills.

You will make mistakes. We all do. Thankfully, clients are pretty resilient even in crisis and can survive us. You will learn to be resilient and bounce back. You'll learn to be flexible and adaptable and change when things aren't working, and you'll be able to do it surrounded by chaos. You'll learn from your mistakes by processing with supervisors and trusted others. You will learn that individuals do not come out of a molding machine with a DSM 5-TR diagnosis stamped on their foreheads but are idiosyncratic and bring their own personal story like no other to you. You will gain knowledge from it and incorporate it to be more effective because of that contact the next time out. To lift a phrase from Nathan Berryman, a Memphis police detective and all-star CIT officer, "Working with an unknown consumer (client) is like cracking a safe. You roll the combination a little too fast and nothing happens. You roll it a little slower and, darn, nothing happens. But you keep rolling and then click! You've got 'em!" Indeed, given practice, you too will know when "You hear that click and you got 'em!"

Summary

The hybrid model in this chapter has to do with tasks to be accomplished during a crisis that do not always move in a stepwise linear progression. Overarching all tasks is safety—not only for the client but for others and the worker as well. Making initial contact in a crisis is not always easy. That's why we have designated predispositioning, engaging, and initiating contact as a new primary task that is critical in laying the groundwork for the intervention to follow. Problem exploration includes affective, behavioral, and cognitive dimensions of the current crisis; it involves finding out what got the immediate crisis going and generally does not delve into all the past issues of the client. Providing support means finding what human resources are available to help the client and what role the crisis worker will play in either finding or being part of the support system. Examining alternatives and options, making plans, obtaining commitments, and following up are neither extensive nor long-term. They are target-specific attempts to find short-term solutions to restore pre-crisis equilibrium.

A major difference between crisis intervention and other human services endeavors, such as standard counseling, social work, and psychotherapy, is that the crisis worker generally does not have time to gather or analyze all the background and other assessment data that might normally be available under less stressful conditions. A key component of a highly functioning crisis worker is the ability to take the data available and make some meaningful sense out of it. This may be somewhat unsettling to those human services workers who are accustomed to having complete social and psychological workups available to them before they proceed with an intervention. However, the ability to quickly evaluate the degree of client disequilibrium and immobility—and to be flexible enough to change your evaluation as changing conditions warrant—is a priority skill that students should seek to cultivate. That's why you have been introduced to the hybrid task model and the Triage Assessment Form.

From onset to resolution of the crisis, assessment is a central, continuous process. Substance abuse and drug interactions, along with assessment of potential lethality, are default assessment areas that need to be covered when using the TAF. The crisis worker must not assume that because the crisis appears on the surface to have been resolved, assessment is no longer

needed. The balance sheet of assessing the client's crisis in terms of severity, current emotional status, alternatives, situational supports, coping mechanisms, resources, and level of lethality is never complete until the client has achieved their precrisis level of mobility, equilibrium, and autonomy. Only then are the psychological debts of the client reconciled. The resumption of precrisis equilibrium does not imply that the client needs no developmental or long-term therapy or medical treatment. It does mean that the crisis worker's job is done, and the acute phase of the crisis is over.

Ethical standards are an integral component of the assessment process and need to be fully integrated with intervention. The LASER model has been developed as a tool to satisfy that requirement and keep the interventionist on safe legal and ethical ground.

The Tools of the Trade

4

Learning Objectives

After studying this chapter, you should be able to:

1. Employ the use of open-ended leads in responding to people in crisis.
2. Employ the use of closed-ended questions in responding to people in crisis.
3. Employ the use of restatement and summary clarification in responding to people in crisis.
4. Employ the use of owning statements in responding to people in crisis.
5. Use techniques of facilitative listening in crisis intervention.
6. Employ the nine basic strategies of crisis intervention.
7. Describe the basic facilitative conditions of empathy, genuineness, and acceptance to promote human growth and how they are used with a person in crisis.
8. Use the facilitative listening techniques and basic crisis intervention strategies as they are employed in the field.
9. Determine levels of crisis worker acting on the directive, collaborative, nondirective action continuum.
10. Employ action strategies to mobilize individuals in crisis.

Introduction

Accurate and well-honed listening skills are necessary and indeed sometimes sufficient skills that all therapists, but particularly crisis interventionists, must have. For that reason, listening skills are a major component of the crisis intervention model. Our preferred conceptual model for effective listening comes from person-centered counseling (Egan, 1982, 1990; Rogers, 1977). Those skills will be familiar to even neophyte human services workers. However, using them effectively in the heat of a crisis may become daunting. That said, there are a variety of other basic verbal techniques you will meet in this chapter with which many human services workers will probably not be familiar. Many of these verbal sets are much

more directive, action oriented, and judgmental and may take some getting used to by veteran workers when first tried out.

Listening in Crisis Intervention

Open-Ended Questions

LO1 Often, human service workers are frustrated by a client's lack of response and enthusiasm. Workers may make statements such as "All my clients ever do is grunt or shake their heads yes or no." We can do something about getting fuller, more meaningful responses if we ask questions that are not dead ends. **Open-ended questions** usually start with *what* or *how* or ask for more clarification or details. Open-ended

85

questions encourage clients to respond with full statements and at deeper levels of meaning. Remember that open-ended questions are used to elicit from clients something about their feelings, thoughts, and behaviors and are particularly helpful in the Problem Exploration phase of intervention in the Task model. Here are some guidelines for forming open-ended questions.

1. **Request description:** "Please tell me . . . " "Tell me about . . . ," "Show me . . . ," "In what way does . . . ?"
2. **Focus on plans:** "What will you do . . . ?" "How will you make it happen?" "How will that help you to . . . ?"
3. **Expansion:** "Tell me more." "Could you give me some more details?" "How about expanding on that a bit?" "So then what happened?"
4. **Assessment:** "How is that different from before?" "What are you doing about that?" "When that happened, how did you handle it?" "Who might you get to help you?"
5. **Stay away from "why" questions.** From an outsider's perspective, beginners in the crisis intervention business may be intrigued by the seemingly illogical things people in crisis think, feel, and do. As a result, beginners feel compelled to find out why a person thinks, feels, or does the illogical things that are characteristic of individuals who are in crisis. It is our contention that "why" questions are generally poor choices for obtaining more information. Even though they may provide the client with an opening to talk more, they also make clients defend their actions. Notice Jake's response in the example below as the crisis worker queries him about the reasons for his behavior toward his wife, Rita. "Wife" is included in the latter part of this sentence in relation to Rita as there is more information that makes the nature of their relationship key to further understanding the situation you will meet later in this chapter, as the crisis worker queries him about the reasons for his behavior.

CW: Why do you continue to beat your wife?

Jake: Hey! If she'd be a little more affectionate, I wouldn't have to beat her up! It's her fault!

As this example demonstrates, what generally happens is that clients become defensive and attempt to intellectualize about the problem or externalize it to somebody or something else without taking responsibility for or ownership of the problem.

Closed-Ended Questions

LO2 **Closed-ended questions** seek specific, concrete information from the client. They are designed to elicit specific behavioral data and yes or no responses. Closed questions usually begin with verbs such as *do, did, does, can, have, had, will, are, is,* and *was.* Contrary to what typically occurs in long-term therapy, closed-ended questions are often used early on in crisis intervention to obtain specific information that will help the crisis worker make a fast assessment of what is occurring. In most counseling programs, closed-ended questions are a "no-no!" because they indeed tend to close off interaction rather than facilitate dialogue. Thus, using closed questions is problematic for many graduate students whose instructors have harped at them, "Keep it open!" While in long-term therapy, the formulation of a plan of attack on the problem might be weeks or months in the making, crisis intervention often calls for instigating plans of action immediately. Closed-ended questions are particularly suited to obtaining commitments to take action. Closed questions also work when clients are so distraught that they do not have the verbal or cognitive capacity to speak to details about the crisis. "Yes" and "No" answers may be the best you can get. They are also highly appropriate in regard to safety issues. We don't mince words about safety issues, and we are not interested in circuitous responses. "Are you going to kill yourself?" may seem insensitive, coarse, and callous. It is not! We'll have a great deal more to say about this issue in Chapter 8, "Crises of Lethality."

Here are some guidelines for forming closed-ended questions.

1. **Request specific information:** "When was the first time this happened?" "Where are you going to go?" "Are you thinking of hurting her?" "Have you gone back there?" "Does this mean you are going to kill yourself?"
2. **Obtain a commitment:** "Are you willing to make an appointment to . . . ?" "Will you confront him about this?" "Do you agree to . . . ?" "When will you do this?"
3. **Increasing focus:** "Do you understand what I am saying?" "Can you do this for me now?" "Are you on track with me?"
4. **Avoid negative interrogatives:** A negative interrogative is a closed question often used as a subtle way to coerce the listener into agreeing with the speaker. *Don't, doesn't, isn't, aren't,* and *wouldn't*

all tend to seek or imply agreement. The negative interrogative statement "Don't you believe that's true?" really is a camouflaged exclamatory statement saying, "I believe that's true, and if you have an ounce of sense, you'll agree with me!"

CW: Don't you think it'd be a good idea if you stay away from Rita?

Such statements generally have little place in a crisis interventionist's repertoire of verbal skills. A far better way of asking for compliance is with an assertive owning statement.

CW: Jake, I understand how difficult it is for you, but for the sake of both you and Rita, I'd really like you to continue to build on last week's success by agreeing to the "stay away from her" contract again this week.

Restatement and Summary Clarification

LO3 Restatement and summary clarification are critical ingredients in crisis intervention. Clients in crisis may have difficulty expressing themselves because of their disjointed thought processes or the chaos that is going on around them in the environment. By restating what the client is saying in the crisis worker's own words, the crisis worker can gain agreement from the client on what the client is attempting to say, feel, think, and do. Further, good **restatement** is particularly important in crisis intervention because it tells the client that "Somebody is listening to me!" Restatement generally has to do with the content of the crisis event rather than the underlying feelings and thoughts about it. A sort of default way of looking at this technique is using a famous line coined by Sgt. Joe Friday in the old TV series *Dragnet*, "All we want are the facts," and then giving those facts back in your own words. Restatement can also serve as an effective break point for a client who is freewheeling in an ideational flight of emotions or thoughts.

CW: Time out a second, Jake. You've put a lot out here and my memory banks are getting pretty full. Let me summarize what you've said, and let's see if we are on the same track.

Restatement sounds simple. It is simple if the crisis worker focuses totally on the client's world. Restatement is not simple if the crisis worker is distracted by environmental stimuli or becomes preoccupied with their own thoughts, questions, evaluations, agenda, biases, or stereotypes about what the client is saying. So be wary! There are usually lots of environmental stimuli in a crisis, and it is easy to become distracted. Finally, **summary clarification** ribbon-wraps the dialogue. That is, it packages the preceding dialogue and lets both client and crisis worker know they are on the same wavelength. Particularly at the commitment stage of intervention, the crisis worker or, better yet, the client may be asked to summarize what the plan is and how they are going to go about doing it.

CW: I want you to summarize what the game plan is, then, when the urge starts to overtake you to go see Rita.

Jake: OK, so I do this thought-stopping thing when the urge to give her a call or cruise by her house starts going off in my head. I don't go to my favorite bar because that just adds to it. Instead, I go to the driving range and start hitting golf balls or go get on my game console and kill aliens. When I get settled down, I write down all my thoughts and feelings and bring them to you next session. As a last resort, I call the crisis line.

Owning Feelings

LO4 **Owning** means communicating possession: "That's mine." Often in conversation we avoid specific issues by "disowning" statements with phrases such as "They say . . . ," "I heard the other day that you . . . ," "It's not right for you to . . . ," and "Don't you think you ought to . . . ?" Whether intentional or not, such verbal manipulation functions to avoid ownership of responsibility for what's being said or to avoid awareness of one's own thoughts and feelings concerning an issue.

Using owning or "I" statements is probably more important in crisis intervention than in other kinds of therapy because of the directive stance the crisis worker often has to take with clients who are immobile and in disequilibrium. It is further important in creating a direct bond between client and worker, particularly when a behavioral emergency is occurring, and the worker wants the undivided attention of a client who is having trouble maintaining behavioral control. Therefore, we illustrate a number of different types of owning statements the crisis worker may find useful for particular problems that occur during intervention.

Although used more often in crisis intervention than in normal therapeutic settings, owning statements should nonetheless be employed sparingly because the crisis worker's main job is to focus on the client and not on themselves. Given that admonition, when working with clients in crisis, it is very important to own your feelings, thoughts, and behaviors because many clients are using you as a model. So if you imply, "We think this way" (meaning I and the director of the clinic, the school principal, the chief of police, the population of North America, the world, or higher power), then the client does not have much of a chance against that awesome cast and is liable to become dependently compliant or defensively hostile as in the following example.

CW: (authoritatively) You know that the Family Trouble Center is a branch of the police department, and we can have you arrested, don't you?

Jake: (defiantly) Yeah, well, so what? I might as well be in jail anyway.

Collaborative Owning Statements. Early on in crisis intervention, the use of "we" is generally not advised because it implies not only the interventionist's thoughts but a host of others' as well. The only parties we are concerned about are the person in crisis and the interventionist. Everybody else can get put on the bench and stay out of the game, at least for the time being. That being said, at some point "we" are going to strike a deal and make movement toward a short-term goal if at all possible. A critical component in eliciting cooperation and compliance from people who are sometimes less than cooperative is to build here-and-now relationships that emphasize a collaborative approach that says "you" are not alone, but "we" are in this together, using what Weiner and Mehrabian (1968) term **relational markers.** Relational markers shorten the psychological distance between the client and the worker through the use of such words as "this," "these," "we," "our," "here," and "now" as opposed to "that," "those," "mine," "there," and "then." Notice the difference between the two words "this" and "that" in the crisis worker's response to Jake's statement that it is really hard to change.

CW: Jake, I know it is tough, but *this* (**right now, right here**) is something we can work out. While I can't do much about *that* (**past time, out there**) stalking behavior, we can start on *this* (**right now, right here**) self-monitoring anger management model.

Using this language sets the stage for examining alternatives, making plans, undertaking commitments, and engaging in safer behavior. It distances the stalking and jealous behavior and brings the new concept up close and personal. It also acknowledges Jake's attempts and desire to change and how tough it is to do that all alone, but it indicates that now help has arrived. The crisis worker's response hooks "we" together with "this" thing right here in front of us, as opposed to "you" and "that" thing way out there that is much harder to get a handle on.

Disowned Statements. Many of us chronically disown many human qualities that indicate we are less than perfect! Beginning crisis workers are particularly vulnerable to this fallacy because they do not want to be seen as inadequate, insecure, or otherwise unequal to the task. Small wonder that clients learn to distrust or become dependent on such all-knowing, well-integrated individuals. Let us take, for example, my feeling of confusion.

If I pretend I understand when, in fact, I am confused, the client who is listening to me is going to be doubly confused. Being willing to own my confusion or frustration and attempt to eliminate it is a trust-reinforcing event for two reasons: (1) both client and worker can reduce the need to pretend or fake understanding of one another and begin to see more clearly where communications are getting crossed, and (2) the client can begin to become actively involved with the worker in an attempt to work together.

CW: Right now I don't know what to think. You say you love her, yet your actions do everything to drive her away.

Jake: I know 'cause it confused me too! Well, it's like I want her to love me, and then I get jealous and paranoid, and like a switch gets flipped, and then I lose it. It frustrates me. I'm my own worst enemy, and I hate myself for it.

Conveying Understanding. Clients in crisis often feel that no one understands what they are going through. The **"I understand"** statement is an owning statement that clearly conveys to the client that you do understand that what is happening right now is causing the client distress. This does not mean that you understand what the client is going through because you don't. I cannot understand what it is like to have prostate or breast cancer. I can understand the fear and anxiety that the client is presently demonstrating and acknowledge that. The "I understand" statement may have to be combined with what is commonly called a "broken record" (repeated) response because the individual may be so agitated or out of touch with reality that they do not hear what is being said the first time.

CW: OK, Jake, I do understand it's frustrating when she gives you the cold shoulder, and all the ways you try to win her affection don't work.

Jake: (pounding his fist on the table and yelling) Every damn thing I do anymore is wrong!

CW: I understand right now that it's so frustrating the only thing that seems to work is lashing out at her physically.

Value Judgments. At times, the crisis worker has to make judgment calls about the client's behavior, particularly when clients are in danger of doing something hurtful to themselves or to others. Owning statements speak specifically to the worker's judgment about the situation and what they will do about it.

Jake: (making threatening gestures and with a trembling voice) I . . . I . . . just caaann't taaake much more . . . of this. I'll huuurt her . . . huuurt her real bad.

CW: (making a judgment) The way you say that really concerns me. I believe that would not be in your best interests and wouldn't get you what you want, which is back with Rita. I'd have to call the police to see that you are both kept safe.

However, using owning statements does *not* generally mean making value judgments about the client's character, because such judgments are putdowns and do nothing to change behavior.

CW: (sarcastically) Yeah, you're a really big man to have to punch your wife out because you aren't as smart as she is. That really shows me a lot. I think maybe a stint out on the county work farm might take some of that energy out of you.

Positive Reinforcement. To be genuine in crisis work is to say what we feel at times. When a client has done well and we're happy and feel good about it, we say so. However, such positively reinforcing statements should always be used in regard to a behavior and not some personal characteristic. Positive reinforcement is used a great deal in crisis intervention to gain compliance. Many times, taking mini-steps to get a client to calm down or stop engaging in a dangerous behavior is tied to positive reinforcement.

CW: (Jake is standing up and pounding his fist on the table, swearing.) I need you to take a deep breath and let it out gently. (With difficulty, Jake complies.) Great! That shows me you can get control of your emotions.

We often use positive reinforcement to successively approximate a client toward a mini goal we are seeking to achieve in the real time environment of the crisis session. Every approximation toward the goal of compliance and de-escalation of emotions and behavior should immediately get a "Way to go!" in chaining positive behaviors together.

CW: Good! You were able to take a deep breath. Now, could you cue yourself that every time you start pounding your fist, you will take at least three deep breaths, lower your arms, and allow yourself to relax and picture that tranquil lake scene? Just do that now. Excellent, I see you are starting to relax. Can you feel the tension draining out? Terrific! Just continue to do that and feel the difference. See how great that feels and how you have gained mastery over your emotions? It shows me you have the guts to handle your emotions.

Positive reinforcement is also used as a launching pad to move the practice of new, alternate, proactive behaviors out of the session and into the field.

CW: Jake, I know this is about the last place you'd like to be, and I think it took a lot of guts to come in here and admit to me you've got some problems. You've had a lot of tough steps to take, but you've made progress and I think are ready to take the next one to watch for ALL the cues you have learned and combine them into the new improved "Serenity Now, Jake" (both laugh).

However, the use of positive reinforcement is also a double-edged sword. Many times in crisis intervention, reinforcing a client for a behavior may breed dependency or be seen as anything but reinforcing by the client. So, be careful about what behavior gets reinforced. That is particularly true of clients with borderline personality disorder who may constantly try to solicit positive comments from the worker to feed their need for approval and acceptance.

Jake: (sneeringly) Guts, my ass! If it weren't for the cops, I sure as hell wouldn't be in this stink hole with a jerk like you doing this crap.

CW: (owning feelings) I'm sorry you feel that way, but I meant what I said.

Personal Integrity and Limit Setting. When a client starts to browbeat, control, or otherwise put us on the hot seat, it does little good to try to hide our anger, disappointment, or hurt feelings. Furthermore, it is important to set clear limits with clients who are starting to get out of control or are trying to manipulate the crisis worker.

Jake: (sneeringly) What do you know? You're nothing but a snot-nosed girl! I don't have to take this crap!

CW: (calmly, owning feelings and setting limits) I don't appreciate the demeaning comments, the language, or your attitude toward me. I'd like an apology, and I'd also like you to be civil. If you can't, I'll assume you'd rather explain your problems to your probation officer, and we'll terminate the session.

Assertion Statements. Finally, because crisis intervention often calls for the crisis worker to take control of the situation, requests for compliance in the form of owning statements are often very directive, short, and point specific. These owning statements, also known as **assertion statements,** clearly and specifically ask for a specific action from the client. Remember your middle school grammar lesson: Subject, verb (action), direct object and repeat as needed. Use the KISS protocol (Keep It Simple Stupendous).

CW: I want you to commit to me and yourself that you'll stay away from her for the next week. I want you to sign this contract that you'll do that for your own safety and hers as well.

Jake: (wistfully wringing his hands) I dunno, that's a long time. I really miss her right now.

CW: I understand it's hard, particularly when you'd like to do something, but I need for you to sign this paper so you can both stay safe by staying away from her. I need to be sure you're committed to doing this.

Facilitative Listening

LO5 In summary, listening is the first imperative in crisis intervention. When the word *listening* is used, the term is being applied broadly to several important behavioral and communications skills discussed in this chapter. To function in a facilitative way, workers must give full attention to the client by:

1. Focusing their total mental power on the client's world.
2. Attending to the client's verbal and nonverbal messages (what the client does not say is sometimes more important than what is actually spoken).
3. Picking up on the client's current readiness to enter into emotional and/or physical contact with others, especially with the worker.
4. Emitting attending behavior by both verbal and nonverbal actions, thereby strengthening the relationship and predisposing the client to trust the crisis intervention process.

One important aspect of listening is for the worker to make initial owning statements that express exactly what they are going to do. These **predispositioning** statements are extremely important in crisis intervention because many times, the client is making contact with the worker for the first time and has no idea what is going to happen or what the worker may do in a threatening, chaotic environment.

CW: Rita, I can see you're really hurting. To fully understand what's going on and what needs to be done, I'm going to focus as hard as I can on what you're saying and how you're saying it. As well as listening to what you say, I'm going to be listening for those things that aren't said, because they may have some bearing on your problems, too. So, if I seem to be really concentrating on you, it's because I want to fully comprehend in as helpful and objective a way as possible what the situation is and your readiness to do something about it.

The second important aspect of listening is to respond in ways that let the client know that the crisis worker is accurately hearing both the facts and the emotional state from which the client's message comes. Here, we are searching for both the affective and content dimensions of the problem. The crisis worker combines the dilemma and feelings by using restatement and reflection.

CW: As you lay the problem out—the abuse by your husband, the job pressures, the wonderful yet guilt-ridden times with Sam—I get the feeling of an emotional juggling act with everything from bowling pins to hand axes being juggled and now a burning baton has just been tossed into the mix. Now you're just sitting paralyzed wishing you'd never taken the job, wondering how you can get out, wanting answers, but having so many problems that you don't even know the right questions to ask.

The third facet of facilitative listening is facilitative responding. It provides positive impetus for clients to gain a clearer understanding of their feelings, inner motives, and choices. Facilitative responses enable clients to feel hopeful and to sense an inclination to begin to move forward, toward resolution, and away from the central core of the crisis. Clients begin to be able to view the crisis from a standpoint of more reality or rationality, which immediately gives them a sense of control. Here, the crisis worker targets an action.

CW: So, given all the things you are juggling, which ones do you want to throw out and which ones do you want to keep juggling? You've given me all kinds of information about how well you've handled the business up to this crisis point. Think back on how you handled that particular piece of juggling. What worked then that might work now? Using that as an example, can we sort each one of these out and get the act cleaned up and just say that particular ball isn't important right now and throw it out for at least awhile?

The fourth dimension of facilitative listening involves helping clients understand the full impact of the crisis situation. Such an understanding allows clients to become more like objective, external observers of the crisis and to refocus on it in rational ways rather than remaining stuck in their own internal frame of reference and emotional bias.

Rita: I feel like the whole world is caving in on me. I wonder if I'll ever be able to get out from under all the mess I'm in now.

CW: You're sounding emotionally frozen by what is happening. I'm wondering what would happen if we could step back for a moment and look at it as if we were third-party observers to your situation—as if you were someone else in a soap opera. What would you say to that person?

Rita: Well . . . **(moment of thought)** . . . I'd say she's not the first or only one to experience lots of trouble—that things may look horrible now, but that eventually things get worked out—especially if she's lucky and can bear up long enough.

CW: Then looking at it from outside yourself does give you an additional view.

Helping clients refocus is not a solution in itself. It is an extension of the art of listening that may facilitate forward movement when clients are emotionally stuck.

These four aspects of listening don't operate in a fragmented or mechanical way. Such listening requires skill, practice, an emotionally secure listener, and both physical and emotional stamina on the part of the listener. The following dialogue gives a brief but comprehensive demonstration of how facilitative listening is combined in its many dimensions. The client now is Jean, Rita's daughter. Don't be perplexed at the shift in clients. One person in crisis may well also put a significant other into a crisis situation as you will observe in Chapter 11, "Family Crisis Intervention." In this instance, Rita's problems have boiled over into her 13-year-old daughter's life.

Jean: I feel put down and ignored by my mother. Every time anything is mentioned about Sam—that's her secret boyfriend—she gets mad and leaves the room. Everything has changed. It's like I'm no longer important to her. I don't know what's happening or what to do.

CW: You're feeling hurt and disappointed, and you're also bewildered by her responses to you.

Jean: **(crying and very upset)** I . . . I feel like I no longer count. I'm feeling like I'm in the way. Like I'm suddenly no good. . . . I feel like now I'm the problem.

CW: You're blaming yourself even though you're trying to understand what has happened and what you should do.

Jean: **(crying is slowing down)** By Sunday night I felt like killing myself. I planned to do it that night. I was feeling abandoned, alone, and hopeless. I just wanted to find some way to end the hurting. I didn't think I could go on another day. I felt like I was no longer her daughter—like she had either disowned me or had been living a lie. I don't know if I can go on.

CW: Even though you were feeling like you were at the brink of death, you somehow managed to pull out of it. What did you do, and what are you doing now to keep from killing yourself?

Jean: **(not crying—pondering the crisis worker's last response)** Well, Marlene and her parents came by. I spent the night with them. That really helped. It was lucky for me that they came by and invited me. They were so kind and understanding. I had a bad night. Worrying about all that stuff. But they, especially Marlene, helped me so much.

CW: Let's see if you can tell me what you have learned from that experience that can help you the next time you feel like killing yourself.

Jean: (pause, as if studying the crisis worker's response) To get away . . . with someone who cares and understands.

CW: Tell me someone you can contact whenever you feel hopeless and lonely and suicidal so that next time, you won't have to depend on luck.

Jean: Well, I'd call Marlene again . . . or my uncle and aunt. They'd be quick to invite me over . . . and there are several friends at school I could call. (Dialogue continues.)

This segment of dialogue contains several of the elements of listening that have been described. It contains accurate reflective listening, open-ended questions, and attention to the client's safety (without asking closed questions, giving advice, or encroaching on the client's prerogatives and autonomy). Also, the crisis worker keeps the focus right on the central core of the client's current concerns, paving the way for the client's forward movement from the immediate crisis toward safer and more adjustive actions. The worker's selective responses are geared toward enabling the client to become aware of and pursue immediate short-term goals. The worker does not digress into external events, past events, the mother, the secret boyfriend, gathering background information, or conducting long-term therapy.

Basic Strategies of Crisis Intervention

LO6 Myer and James (2005) have formulated nine strategies used in crisis intervention. The basic core listening and responding skills already discussed are the foundation of these strategies. There is no formula for using these strategies. They may be used singly or in combination. Their use depends a great deal on the crisis context, the triage level of the client, and on what task of the crisis intervention model the interventionist is working. Here are the nine strategies.

Creating Awareness. The crisis worker attempts to bring to conscious awareness warded off, denied, shunted, and repressed feelings, thoughts, and behaviors that freeze clients' ability to act in response to the crisis. **Creating awareness** is particularly important for Task 2, Problem Exploration.

CW: It would be easier to just put it out of your mind, but I wonder what shoving it back will get you?

You came here, so I'm pretty sure you want to get this out in the open and get some resolution. What would all this mess look like if it were sitting out there on the table?

Allowing Catharsis. Catharsis means simply letting clients talk, cry, swear, berate, rant, rave, mourn, or do anything else that allows them to ventilate feelings and thoughts; it may be one of the most therapeutic strategies the crisis worker can employ. To do this, the crisis worker needs to provide a safe and accepting environment that says, "It's OK to say and feel these things." By so doing, the crisis worker clearly says they can accept those feelings and thoughts no matter how bad they may seem to be. A word of caution here! Allowing angry feelings to continue to build and escalate may not be the wisest course of action. This strategy is most often used with people who *can't* get in touch with their feelings and thoughts as opposed to those whose feelings are already volcanic. This strategy is most likely to be used for Task 2, Problem Exploration, and Task 3, Providing Support.

CW: It's tough to talk about it. After all, it is an affair you are having. Perhaps you think I'll pass moral judgment on to you for that. I won't! What I would most like you to do is to open up those push-pull feelings. Tell me more about being scared and angry at the same time.

Providing Support. Often, the crisis worker is the *sole* support available to the client. As such, the crisis worker attempts to validate that the clients' responses are as reasonable as can be expected given the situation. Many times, clients believe they must be going crazy, but they need to understand that they are not "crazy" and that most people would act in about the same way given the kind, type, and duration of the crisis. Oftentimes in crisis, in an attempt to calm clients, workers state that it is "normal" to have such and such reactions. Nothing could be further from the truth. There is nothing "**normal**" at all about stress reactions associated with a sexual assault. Such attempts are at best placating and at worst discounting of the client. A far better description, we believe, is the word "**common**." Clients need to understand that while there is nothing "normal" about their feeling, acting, and thinking in a crisis situation, it is certainly "common" to most people. This kind of affirmation is particularly critical to clients who feel they have no support system available to them. That being said, the crisis worker *never* supports clients' injurious or lethal feelings, thoughts, or actions toward themselves or others.

Providing support is particularly useful when the client is attempting to move into action. In standard therapy, supervisors often express a great deal of concern about breeding dependence on the therapist. It should be clearly understood that when we are dealing with clients in crisis, they may well need to be dependent on us for a short while. That doesn't mean we are going to adopt clients and take them home with us! It does mean that when the client is drained of emotional, cognitive, or behavioral resources, we are supportive, and we provide a shoulder to lean on.

Rita: I don't know which way to turn, what to do. This is not me! I am so confused and so alone. My God! How did I ever get in this awful mess?

CW: Right now you may feel that way, but I am in this with you, and I am going to stay in it until we get some control and direction back for you.

Rita: I don't know how there can ever be any control. **(Starts sobbing.)**

CW: We are going to get some control, and I am going to stay with you until that happens.

Promoting Expansion. The crisis worker engages in **expansion** activities to open up clients' tunnel vision of the crisis. Oftentimes, clients are so wrapped up in the crisis and are continuously engaging in self-defeating thoughts and behaviors that they are unable to see other perceptions and possibilities. Increasing expansion helps clients step back, reframe the problem, and gain new perspectives. This strategy is primarily used to help clients resolve stuck cognitive reactions. By confronting clients' narrow and restrictive views, crisis workers help clients consider other perspectives. This strategy is particularly effective with clients who are not able to recognize environmental cues that may help them perceive alternate meanings of events and possible solutions to them.

CW: This may be distasteful, but I want you to think about this. You know one possibility would be to get a restraining order. That is pretty common in most partner violence situations, but it is used in other instances too.

Emphasizing Focus. Conversely, at times, the problem is that clients are too expansive and need to **focus** their freewheeling, out-of-control flights of ideation about the crisis that have little basis in reality. The crisis worker attempts to partition, compartmentalize, and downsize clients' all-encompassing, catastrophic interpretations and perceptions of the crisis event to more specific, realistic, manageable components and options. This strategy has utility across all tasks of the crisis intervention model.

CW: Given this huge mess, what is the one thing you need to do right now to get some relief? What could you focus on that would tell you immediately that some pressure was off rather than trying to take care of everything and everybody?

Providing Guidance. The term *guidance* has come to have somewhat of a negative connotation in the field of counseling because it implies that clients are incapable of helping themselves. However, many times, clients in crisis do need **guidance** and direction. They don't have the knowledge or resources available to make good decisions. Thus, the crisis worker provides information, referral, and direction in regard to clients' obtaining assistance from specific external resources and support systems. For example, one of the handiest tools that crisis workers have is a directory of all the social services available in their catchment area. This strategy is used almost exclusively to respond to clients' behavioral reactions.

Rita: I have no idea how to go about getting a restraining order.

CW: Up until now, you would have had no reason to. However, the staff at the Family Trouble Center can do that for you and would be glad to help you do it. I can give you that number if you want.

Promoting Mobilization. The crisis worker attempts both to activate and marshal clients' internal resources and find and use external support systems to help generate coping skills and problem-solving abilities so they become **mobilized** and do not remain stuck in the crisis situation.

CW: There is a support group of women I know of that meets regularly at St. Michael's Catholic Church. They all struggle with some of the same relationship issues that you are having. Hearing and interacting with them might give you some new ideas on how to go about solving this knotty problem. You have some good ideas and are pretty geared up to act on them, but it might not hurt to get their perspectives.

Implementing Order. The crisis worker provides **order** and methodically helps clients classify and categorize problems to prioritize and sequentially defuse the crisis in a logical and linear manner. Too often, clients see the crisis as a mountainous tidal wave washing over them when what they need to do is grab a metaphorical life jacket and float along until it dissipates or build a small dike and let it rush by them. These actions, while apparent to an outside observer, are oftentimes missed by client in the maelstrom of a crisis.

CW: It seems overwhelming, but let's put it into pieces you can manage. Break it down. If this were your business instead of your love life, how would you parcel the problem out, and what order of priorities would you give to each part? What's the first thing you would do? While it might not make it perfect, what would it take to make this situation more tolerable?

Providing Protection. Providing **protection** is paramount in crisis intervention; it is so important that it is its own overarching task in our intervention model. The crisis worker safeguards clients from engaging in harmful, destructive, detrimental, and unsafe feelings, behaviors, and thoughts that may be psychologically or physically injurious or lethal to themselves or others.

CW: I want to make the clearest personal statement I can to you Rita. I really fear for your safety. I would not confront Jake alone after work at the garage. I understand you don't want a big scene in front of other people, but to do that alone with nobody around seems to me a really dangerous thing to do.

When these nine strategies are used with the basic verbal crisis intervention skills in this chapter, they form the backbone of crisis intervention techniques. By using them with the Triage Assessment Form, crisis interventionists should have a comprehensive, real-time assessment of how they are doing as they move the client through the model.

Climate of Client Growth

LO7 According to Rogers (1977), the most effective helper is one who can provide three necessary and sufficient conditions for client growth. These conditions he named *empathy, genuineness,* and *acceptance* (pp. 9–12). These therapeutic conditions are particularly critical to doing effective crisis intervention. To create a climate of **empathy** means that the crisis worker accurately senses the inner feelings and meanings the client is experiencing and directly communicates to the client that the worker understands how it feels to be the client. The condition of **genuineness** (also called *realness, transparency,* or *congruency*) means that the worker is being completely open in the relationship; nothing is hidden, there are no facades, and there are no professional fronts. If workers are clearly open and willing to be fully themselves in the relationship, the client is encouraged to reciprocate. The term **acceptance** (also referred to as *caring* or *prizing*) means that the crisis worker feels an unconditional positive regard for the client. It is an attitude of accepting and caring for the client without the client necessarily reciprocating. The condition of acceptance is provided for no other reason than that the client is a human being in need. If these conditions of empathy, genuineness, and acceptance can be provided for the client, then the probability that the client will experience positive emotional movement is increased.

Communicating Empathy

In describing the use of empathy to help clients, we will focus on five important techniques: (1) attending, (2) verbally communicating empathic understanding, (3) reflecting feelings, (4) nonverbally communicating empathic understanding, and (5) silence as a way of communicating empathic understanding (Cormier & Cormier, 1991; Gilliland & James, 1998, pp. 116–118). First, however, it is necessary to differentiate empathy from sympathy and distancing.

Sympathy. Beginners in the field confuse empathy with sympathy. Sympathy is fine at the right time and conveys support, but it means essentially taking on the person's problems and feelings rather than attempting to experience and convey what the person is feeling. Mostly, we think of sympathy as a sad feeling with tears attached to it. It can just as well be righteous indignation and anger. Particularly when we are attempting to do exploration with a client in crisis, we will do better to put sympathy on the shelf for a while. Dr. Whisenhunt has a great line worth remembering when the interventionist starts to get too wrapped up in the story line. "Don't chase the tears!" as demonstrated below.

CW: You poor thing. That's terrible! Nobody should be allowed to get away with that kind of behavior. How about I call the police right now!

The behavior, indeed, may be terrible, but the crisis worker will do better to make a deep, reflective response that captures the client's feeling. That statement conveys empathic understanding and does not lead the interventionist down a dead-end road that may wind up in a countertransference swamp (the interventionist's own issues).

CW: You seem really torn—condemning yourself for being a fool, but still wanting and hoping the relationship to be something and go somewhere. It sounds like you know it is over, but you don't quite know what to do yet.

Distancing. At times, crisis workers may be so overwhelmed and frightened by what they are confronted with that they seek to distance themselves from the overwhelming affect by engaging in what we call "funeral home counseling." Here are a few examples of what people say when they have no idea what to say but feel they need to say something. These attempts to be palliative are generally not helpful and can, in fact, hinder intervention. Lots of times these statements are centered on a religious/spiritual theme: "It's God's will." "God works in mysterious ways." "Heaven wouldn't be heaven if it were only filled with old people." "They are in a better place." Another way of distancing is by rationalizing, discounting, and minimizing: "Well, you still have your health." "It could have been worse." "Don't feel guilty about it." "Try to get your mind off it." "Just try and relax a little." "It's tough, but you need to calm down." These statements probably say more about the *worker's* crisis state than they do about the client's. A far better way, when aspiring crisis workers don't know what to say, is to say nothing or to own the feeling of what they are experiencing. At times, owning our own inability to find words to convey the depth of feeling is probably one of the best ways to indicate that you do feel for the client.

CW: (reaches out and, with permission, touches Rita's arm and says nothing for a few moments) I wish I had something to say that would take this pain and confusion away and make this all right, but right now I just don't.

Attending. The first step in communicating empathy has little to do with words and a lot to do with looking, acting, and being attentive. The foregoing crisis worker's response is much more about attending than saying or doing. In most initial counseling and therapy sessions, the client enters with some anxiety related to the therapy itself in addition to the stress brought on by the crisis. In crisis situations, such anxiety is increased exponentially. Shame, guilt, rage, and sorrow are but a few of the feelings that may be manifested. Such feelings may be blatant and rampant or subtle and disguised. Whatever shape or form such feelings take, the inattentive crisis worker can miss the message the client is attempting to convey. Worse, an inattentive attitude implies a lack of interest on the part of the worker and does little to establish a trusting relationship.

Mehrabian (1971) reports that 55 percent of emotional output and communication occurs through the face and body, while 38 percent comes from voice tone and only 7 percent from words used. Whether these percentages of overwhelming nonverbal communication are precise or not, one thing is for sure in the crisis business, the effective worker focuses fully on the client, both in facial expression and in body posture. By nodding, keeping eye contact, smiling, showing appropriate seriousness of expression, leaning forward, keeping an open stance, and sitting or standing close to the client without invading the client's space, the crisis worker conveys a sense of involvement, concern, commitment, and trust. Vocal tone, diction, pitch, modulation, and smoothness of delivery also tell clients a great deal about the attentiveness of the crisis worker. By attending closely to the client's verbal and nonverbal responses, the crisis worker can quickly tell whether they are establishing an empathic relationship or exacerbating the client's feelings of distrust, fear, and uncertainty about becoming involved in the relationship.

Attentiveness, then, is both an attitude and a skill. It is an attitude in that the worker focuses fully on the client right here and now. In such moments, the crisis worker's own concerns are put on hold. It is a skill in that conveying attending takes practice. It is just as inappropriate for the crisis worker to look too concerned and be in too close proximity as it is to lean back with arms folded and legs crossed, giving a cold stare. Here is an example of an appropriate blend of both verbal and nonverbal skill in attending to a client empathically.

Rita: (Enters room, sits down in far corner, warily looks about the room, crosses her legs and fidgets with her purse, and avoids direct eye contact, manifesting the appearance of a distraught woman who is barely holding together.)

CW: (rises behind desk and observing the behavior and physical appearance of the client, moves to a chair a comfortable distance and a slight angle from Rita's, sits down, leans forward in an open stance, and with an appearance of concern and inquisitiveness looks directly at Rita) I'd like to be of help. Where would you like to start?

The crisis worker sees the apprehension in the client and immediately becomes proactive. The crisis worker moves close to the client but does not sit directly in front of her in what could be construed as a confronting stance. The worker inclines forward to focus attention—eyes, ears, brain, and whole body—onto the client's world. The whole posture of the crisis worker is congruent with the verbal message of offering immediate acceptance and willingness to help. In summary, effective attending is unobtrusive, natural, and without pretense. It is a necessary condition for empathic listening.

Verbally Communicating Empathic Understanding. When you can accurately hear and understand the core emotional feelings inside the client and accurately and caringly communicate that understanding to the client, you are demonstrating effective listening. The deeper your level of listening (understanding), the more helpful you will be to your clients. For instance, reflecting a client's message at the interchangeable level is helpful.

Rita: I'm thinking about just walking in and telling Jake I want a divorce—regardless of what Sam is ready to do. I don't think I can go on much longer. My ulcer is beginning to act up, I'm an emotional wreck, and everyone is expecting more of me than I can give.

CW: You sound like you are feeling a sense of urgency because it's adversely affecting your physical and emotional well-being.

A deeper level of listening and communicating empathic understanding to Rita might be expressed thus:

CW: Rita, your sense of urgency is getting to the point where you seem about ready to take a big risk with both Jake and Sam. I sense that your physical and emotional stresses have about reached their

limits, and you're realizing that no one else is going to act to give you relief—that you are the one who is going to have to decide and act.

The second response is more helpful because it confirms to Rita a deeper understanding than the first response. Both responses are helpful because they are accurate and neither add to nor detract from the client's verbal, nonverbal, or emotional messages. While the first response is considered minimally helpful, the second response is more facilitative because it lets the client know the worker heard a deeper personal meaning (risk) and a personal ownership of possible action. A word of caution to the worker, however: Beware of reading into the client's statements more than the client is saying, and take care to keep your response as brief as possible.

Reflection of Feelings. Reflection of feelings is a powerful tool to get at shunted or denied affect. In standard therapy, we constantly hammer at uncovering affect because of client resistance to dealing with threatening and warded off feelings. However, in crisis intervention, the desire to uncover feeling is not always the therapeutic best bet. A client who is scoring an 8, 9, or 10 on the Affective Scale of the Triage Assessment Form probably does not need to have a crisis worker attempt to elicit even more feelings. It is not the job of the crisis worker to tell the client what they are feeling. The following dialogue moves from a reflection to a judgment and tells the client how she feels.

CW: You are bitter and resentful about being in this dead-end marriage. You can't figure a way out.

Rather, what the crisis worker should do is make an educated guess using conditional statements that allow the client to accept or reject the worker's guess. Conditional words such as "Could it be," "I'm wondering if," "Seems like," "Perhaps you could consider," "Sounds as though," are all couched in terms that leave clients free to accept or reject the interventionist's guesses toward feeling states.

CW: It *seems* that you are pretty bitter and resentful about this dead-end marriage and are frustrated that you can't figure a way out.

Effective communication of empathic understanding to the client means focusing on the client's expressed affective and cognitive messages. The worker deals *directly* with the client's concerns and does not veer off into talking *about* the client's concerns or some tangential person or event. That distinction is important.

Rita: I'm afraid Jake might attack me even worse if I tell him I want a divorce.

CW: He did beat you pretty badly. Sam would probably go bananas at that. Your husband Jake has such a violent temper. **(talking about the situation and tangentially focusing on Jake)**

CW: You're feeling some reservations about telling Jake because you really don't want to be beaten up again. **(dealing with Rita's current feelings and concerns)**

The latter response is preferred because it stays on target with Rita's feelings and concerns in the here and now and because it avoids getting off onto Jake, Sam, or any other third party or issue.

The central issue in empathic understanding is to hone in on the client's current core of feelings and concerns and communicate to the client (in the worker's own words) the gist of what the client is experiencing.

Nonverbal Communication. Empathic understanding means accurately picking up and reflecting more than verbal messages. It involves accurately sensing and reflecting all the unspoken cues, messages, and behaviors the client emits. Nonverbal messages may be transmitted in many ways. The worker should carefully observe body posture, body movement, gestures, grimaces, vocal pitch, movement of eyes, movement of arms and legs, and other body indicators. Clients may transmit emotions such as anger, fear, puzzlement, doubt, rejection, emotional stress, and hopelessness by different body messages without using the words that go with those feelings.

Crisis workers should be keenly aware of whether nonverbal messages are consistent with the client's verbal messages. "Keenly aware" means that you are always monitoring body language for signs of aggression—particularly toward you! While this may sound like harping, throughout this book, we will continuously be talking about safety—both the client's and yours. In fact, Chapter 14, "Violent Behavior in Institutions," is specifically designed to keep you out of the hospital or mortuary. Thus, a part of empathic understanding is the communication of such inconsistency to the client, who may not be consciously aware of the difference. For example:

CW: (observing the way Rita's face lights up whenever she speaks or thinks about Sam) Rita, I notice you

are talking about all the trouble it is for you to continue your relationship with Sam. But your body tells me that those are the moments you live for—that right now, your only ecstasy is when you're with Sam.

The crisis worker's main concern with nonverbal communication also involves the worker's own body messages. All the dynamics of the client's body language apply to the worker as well. Your nonverbal messages must be consistent with your verbal messages. It would not be empathic or helpful if your words were saying to the client, "I understand precisely what you're feeling and desiring," but your body was saying, "I don't care," or "I'm bored," or "My mind isn't fully focused on what you're saying." Your voice, facial expression, posture—even the office arrangement and environment—must say to the client: "I'm fully tuned in to your world while you're with me. I want to give my total mental and emotional energy to understanding your concerns while you're here. I will not be distracted." If your body can communicate such messages so they are unmistakably understood by the client, then you will have effectively communicated empathy to the client nonverbally, and you will stand a better chance of being helpful.

Silence. Silence is golden. Beginning crisis workers often feel compelled to initiate talk to fill any void or lapse in the dialogue because they believe they would not be doing their job otherwise. Nothing could be further from the truth. Clients need time to think. To throw out a barrage of questions or engage in a monologue says more about the crisis worker's insecurity in the situation than it does about resolving the crisis. Silence gives the client thinking time—and the crisis worker too.

Indeed, at such times, verbiage from the crisis worker may be intrusive and even unwelcome. Remaining silent but attending closely to the client can convey deep, empathic understanding. Nonverbally, the message comes across: "I understand your struggle trying to put those feelings into words, and it's OK. I know it's tough, but I believe you can handle it. However, I'm right here if you need me."

Rita: The last beating . . . I was so ashamed, yet I couldn't seem to do anything except go back to him.

CW: It hurts you not only to get beaten but also that others might find out—which seems even worse. As a result, you don't see any alternatives.

Rita: (thinks hard, eyes focused into the distance for more than a minute) Yes and no! I see alternatives, but I guess until now I haven't had the guts to do anything. I rationalized that something must be wrong with me or that the situation would get better, but it hasn't for five years. It has gotten worse.

CW: (silence; looks at Rita for some 30 seconds while collecting thoughts) A couple of things strike me about what you said. First, you've decided to quit blaming yourself. Second, by the fact that you're here now, you've chosen at least one alternative to that five-year merry-go-round of abuse.

In this scene, silence is allowed to work for both the client and the worker. The client needs time to work through her response to the worker, and she is unconditionally allowed to do this. The same is true of the crisis worker. The client's comment is synthesized and processed for its full meaning. By reacting immediately, the crisis worker might make less than a potent response. Taking time to digest both the content and the affect of the client enables the worker to formulate a response that is more likely to be on target and helpful.

Taking Time. Cochran (2014) proposes that we have "time." At the point that a crisis erupts, clients often have tapped out their human supports; people are tired of them and don't want to waste any further time with them. It is critical that you are not hurried and that you take your time and that the client gets a clear sense that you are taking time to carefully understand what's going on.

CW: I know things are hectic, but I want to take time to understand your side of it as it played out today. We have plenty of time, so I'm going to sit down and listen. Start wherever you'd like because we do have time.

Communicating Genuineness

Contrary to the thinking of most beginning human services workers, as evidenced by their behavior, being fully oneself and not some pseudotherapist or mimic of a particular therapist one has heard or seen is an absolutely necessary condition, particularly in crisis intervention. Rogers (1969, p. 228) puts it in clear, simple, and succinct terms:

When I can accept the fact that I have many deficiencies, many faults, make a lot of mistakes, am often ignorant where I should be knowledgeable, often prejudiced when I should be open-minded, often have feelings which are not justified by the circumstances, then I can be much more real.

Rogers' statement means putting on no false fronts but rather being oneself in the relationship and communicating what "oneself" is to the client. In short, it is being honest.

The advice to be honest is not simply a platitude. To be honest is to be congruent; it means that the crisis worker's awareness of self, feelings, and experience is freely and unconditionally available and communicable, when appropriate, during intervention in a crisis. Egan (1975, 1982, 1986, 1990) has listed essential components of genuineness that would serve the beginning crisis worker well.

1. **Being role free.** The crisis worker is genuine in life as well as in the therapeutic relationship and is congruent in both experiencing and communicating feelings (Egan, 1975, p. 91).
2. **Being spontaneous.** The crisis worker communicates freely, with tact and without constantly gauging what to say, and behaves freely, without being impulsive or inhibited, rule bound or technique bound. Worker behavior is based on a feeling of self-confidence (p. 92).
3. **Being nondefensive.** Crisis workers who behave nondefensively have an excellent understanding of their strengths and weaknesses. Thus, they can be open to negative, even hostile, client expressions without feeling attacked or defensive. The crisis worker who is genuine understands such negative expressions as saying more about the client than the worker and tries to facilitate exploration of such comments rather than defend against them (pp. 92–93).
4. **Being consistent.** People who are genuine have few discrepancies between what they think, feel, and say and their actual behavior. Crisis workers who are consistent do not think one thing and tell a client another or engage in behavior that is contrary to their values (pp. 93–94).
5. **Being a sharer of self.** When it is appropriate to the situation, people who are genuine engage in self-disclosure, allowing others to know them through open verbal and nonverbal expression of their feelings (p. 94).

The following dialogue between the crisis worker and Rita demonstrates comprehensively the points both Rogers and Egan make.

Rita: Just what the hell gives? Here I am going crazy, and you put it back on my shoulders. You're supposed to help get me out of this mess!

CW: I can see that you're really mad at me because I don't behave the way you think I ought to.

Rita: Well, how can you be such a caring person if you let me hang out there, pushing me to take such risky chances? I could lose everything.

CW: You see me as being a real hypocrite because I'm pushing you to take some action rather than sympathizing with you.

Rita: God knows I could use some . . . and when you act so callously (**cries**) . . . you're like every other damn person!

CW: What would I be doing if I were acting in the most helpful way I possibly could, in your opinion, right now?

Rita: Well, I know you can't solve this for me, but I'd sure as hell like for you to point the way or help me solve this.

CW: So, what you're really wanting is to be able to solve this dilemma on your own, and what you're wanting from me is to help you find your own inner choices that are best for you. What I want to do is to help you find those choices. Let's look at your current options right now.

The dialogue aptly depicts the crisis worker owning feelings, using "I" statements, and focusing on the client's emergent concerns rather than allowing the focus to shift to tangential matters or defensive responses by the worker. Such statements allow the crisis worker to retain integrity, squarely face client hostility without becoming hostile in turn, and model a safe and trusting atmosphere in which clients see that it is all right for them to demonstrate angry feelings and still be accepted by the crisis worker. At the same time, the crisis worker stands by and is consistent with a therapeutic approach without being intimidated by or defensive with the client. The crisis worker, above all, has the self-confidence and congruence to make such statements in a way that is facilitative for the client.

Communicating Acceptance

The crisis worker who interacts with complete acceptance of clients exudes an unconditional positive regard for clients that transcends clients' personal qualities, beliefs, problems, situations, or crises. The worker is able to prize, care for, and fully accept clients even if they are doing things, saying things, and experiencing situations that are contrary to the worker's personal beliefs and values. The worker is able to put aside personal needs, values, and desires and does not require clients to make specific responses as a condition of full acceptance. That is not easily done with clients in crisis. There is a preferred client acronym in therapy named YAVIS for the young, attractive, verbal, intelligent, and sociable therapist dream client. In most crisis situations, the YAVIS client is not going to magically appear. By the time many clients in crisis get to the worker, they have severe communication problems, disheveled appearances, and have not maintained good hygiene practices. Thus, acceptance is easily said and less easy to manifest.

Rita: (**disheveled, clothes look slept in, underarm deodorant has failed, makeup is smeared**) I hate to bother you with all my problems. I know you're married and have never been divorced. You must think I'm a screwed-up mess. I look a mess and probably smell like it too. I was so scared I didn't go home, sent Jean to her aunt's, and slept in my truck at the state park.

CW: I hear your concern, and I want you to know that what has happened to you, or even how you look and what you choose to do have nothing to do with my regard for you. What I'm really hoping we can do is to help you arrive at those choices that will best help you get through this crisis and successfully get back in total control of your life.

Rita: I appreciate that very much. But sometimes I wonder whether my running around with Sam doesn't strike you as unwise and immature.

CW: I hope I'm not giving off negative vibes to give you that impression, because your personal preferences have nothing to do with my caring for you. It seems like you really have a concern about my feelings about how you should act.

Rita: Not really. It's just something inside me—that if I were you, I'd be wondering.

CW: So, a source of concern inside you is whether I may evaluate you negatively. What I want you to know is that my esteem for you is not based on what you do.

Even when clients persist in projecting onto the crisis worker negative evaluations or notions such as those expressed by Rita, the worker doesn't have to buy into such notions. If the worker can truly feel an unconditional positive regard for the client, there will be no need for denial, defensiveness, or diversion from the reality of the worker's true feelings. If the worker demonstrates caring and prizing of the client, regardless of the client's situation or status, the client will be more likely to accept and prize himself or herself. That is the essence of acceptance in crisis intervention.

In the Field

LO8 The foregoing scenarios all occur in an office where there is time to think, formulate responses, and make thoughtful comments, all with knowledge about the client's history. As such, it is more crisis therapy for a client in a transcrisis state and at a transcrisis point. What happens when the worker is in the field, has little knowledge about the clients or their problems, and the crisis is escalating by the minute? Above anything else in this situation, the crisis worker's initiating techniques are critical to bonding with an out-of-control client who is unknown to the responder (Kirchberg et al., 2014). While Major Sam Cochran, retired, has formulated the following coaching plan and plays specifically for CIT officers (Cochran, 2014), these four plays can be used by any crisis worker in the field. These are simple, initial steps in creating trust and quick bonds that are critical to de-escalation. Interestingly enough, in the heat of the moment, when we are training mental health workers or police officers, they sometimes *forget to use them!*

1. Introduce yourself in a way that says, "I am here for you, and I am no threat." CW: "Hi, I'm Dick James, I'm part of the mobile crisis team. I can see you are really frustrated. I'd like to help if I can."
2. Obtain the person's name and personalize it if possible. CW: "It must be pretty serious for you to have run everybody out of the house, got a can of gas, and are considering blowing the house apart. I am sorry I didn't get your name. Could you tell me your name, please?"
3. Express what you are seeing across affective, behavioral, and cognitive dimensions, and use "I" statements to do it. CW: "So first off you are really angry and frustrated that your boss wouldn't listen to your plan to save money and blew you off. As a result, it was the last straw and you kicked everybody out of the shop and now won't let anybody back in. Seems like you're thinking this will finally get his attention. I can see how

physically and emotionally wrung out you are from trying to stem that tidal wave of stuff washing over you.
4. Summarize the information you have obtained and feed it back so both parties are on the same page. CW: "Is that about right what I said? Let me know if there is something I missed because I want to be sure we are clear between each other."

From a theoretical standpoint, these four opening plays are the ground work of Relational-Cultural Theory (RCT) by seeking to establish mutual empathy, therapeutic authenticity, and real engagement in bonding with previously unknown recipients of service (Jordan, 2007, p. 1007).

Safety in the Field. Setting limits is part of safety procedure, and that involves determining the degree of threat a person is feeling and how they intend to protect themselves from it (Cochran, 2014). It is not uncommon to meet people in crisis in the field who are armed with some kind of a weapon that they are not displaying. They are armed not necessarily to hurt someone else but rather to try to protect themselves. Therefore, if the person is acting in a defensive manner and your triage rating on them is high, assume a person may have a weapon, and ask to see it. CW: "Lots of times, people in your situation have good reason to believe someone might hurt them and so have a weapon of some kind. If you do, I'd like you to just lay it down beside you. I want to help you out, but I need to feel safe too."

If the person is noncompliant or seems not to hear you, back off and get law enforcement help.

Assessing for Medical Problems in the Field. Many of the people the crisis worker will meet in the field have medical problems that are contributory to the crisis. Finding medical staff who have worked with clients is often critical in de-escalating a crisis by getting clients to their medical support system. Many of the clients are well known as repeaters by police officers, EMTs, and 911 operators. Getting them to medical staff and facilities that know them and are their care providers is a first priority. After making initial contact with clients, potential medical issues, both physical and psychological, need to be checked out.

CW: You look a bit pale and fatigued to me. Have you been having some medical problems lately?

If the person doesn't acknowledge any medical issues, don't just dismiss the issue. Query them in regard to any medical staff they have seen.

CW: So, OK, no major medical problems then. What about the small ones? Have you seen any doctors, nurse practitioners, chiropractors, or counselors lately for the day-to-day stuff?

Drugs in the Field. Just a gentle reminder because we spoke to assessing for drug use in Chapter 3, "The Intervention and Assessment Models." This is a default area that must be covered, and in the heat of the moment, people forget it. Next to weapons, gathering information on drug use and misuse for both illegal and prescription drugs is critical in planning action steps (James, 2014). It does little good to attempt to de-escalate a person who has misused drugs or, as frequently is the case in mental illness, has stopped taking psychotropic medication, and the illness has resurfaced. It is also not uncommon, particularly in geriatric clients who are taking a variety of drugs, for bad drug interactions to occur when a new drug is introduced into the client's regimen.

CW: (suspected mental illness) You said you are smelling bad things. Have you been taking any medicine for those bad smells? When was the last time you took it?

CW: (suspected bad drug interaction) Mrs. Smith, your children tell me you have really been down in the dumps the last few days since you last visited the doctor. What did the doctor tell you and did he change your medication at all?

Support in the Field. Finding out what human support systems are available, what systems have ceased to exist, and what the client has done to access these systems, if any, are primary to any intervention plan and the disposition of where the client is physically going to go.

CW: Is there anyone available now to give you some support? By "anyone" I mean family, friends, ministers, human service workers, boss, coworkers.

Meeting Basic Needs in the Field. If the basic needs of food, water, clothing, medical care, and shelter are not being met, then little resolution to the crisis will occur, or, at the very least, helping the client get some of these needs met will go a long way toward gaining trust and compliance.

CW: I wonder when the last time it was you had a decent meal. So, I wonder if getting something in your stomach wouldn't at least start to feel like you had some control back.

Using Cochran's (2014) basic plays and immediately checking out safety, drug use, support systems, and basic needs are typically the precursors to any other techniques used when you are in the field, and it is your first meeting with the client.

Acting in Crisis Intervention

LO9 As shown in Figure 4.1, the crisis worker's level of action and involvement in the client's world, based on a valid and realistic assessment of the client's level of mobility/immobility, may be anywhere on a continuum ranging from nondirective through collaborative to directive. The appropriateness of alternative coping mechanisms hinges on the client's degree of mobility. Thus, assessment of client mobility is a key concept governing the degree of the crisis worker's involvement. One of the first things the worker must determine is what event precipitated the crisis. What brought on the disequilibrium?

Crisis worker is directive.	Crisis worker is collaborative.	Crisis worker is nondirective.

Client is immobile.	Client is partially mobile.	Client is mobile.

From the initiating crisis event to resolution, counseling should move from left to right on the directive–nondirective worker continuum as the client moves from immobile to mobile.

Darker shading indicates a more directed approach to counseling when the client is assessed as immobile.

Lighter shading indicates the crisis worker becoming more nondirective and the client becoming more mobile.

Figure 4.1   The Directive–Nondirective Action Continuum

The answer may not be very clear in the client's complex and rambling story. So, the worker may have to ask, early in the interview, "What *one event* brought you to seek counseling today?" When you discover the major precipitating event that took away the client's autonomous coping ability, it will likely signal your primary focus with the client.

Directive Intervention

Because the gold standard for beginning training in long-term psychotherapy has been to learn the practice of person-centered or nondirective therapy, we find that our students have difficulty transiting into an active, assertive, directive stance as they start to practice crisis intervention. Yet Allen and associates (2014) report that when clinicians received training in trauma-focused cognitive-behavioral therapy, their beliefs changed toward the utility of structured/directive approach to treatment. Directive intervention is *not* about passing moral judgments or general character appraisal on an individual.

Directive intervention is about providing the specific information and guidance clients need to make decisions, setting limits on behaviors that range from inappropriate to lethal, and apprising them of the consequences of their affective, cognitive, and behavioral responses to the crisis based on the interventionist's expert clinical judgment and the self-same lack thereof in the client. The directive approach is necessary when the client is assessed as being too immobile to cope with the current crisis. A triage score in the high teens or twenties typically calls for a good deal of directiveness from the worker. The crisis worker is the principal definer of the problem, searcher for alternatives, and developer of an adequate plan and instructs, leads, or guides the client in the action. Directive counseling is an "I" approach. This is an example of a worker-directed statement: "I want you to try something right now. I want you to draw a deep breath, and while you are doing it, I want you to just focus on your breathing. Don't let any other thoughts enter your mind. Just relax and notice how your tensions begin to subside." By using a very directive stance, the worker takes temporary control, authority, and responsibility for the situation.

Rita: I don't know which way to turn. My whole world has caved in. I don't know what I'll do tonight. It's all so hopeless. I'm scared to even think about tonight. (**Rita appears stunned and in a state of panic.**) I don't know what to do.

CW: I don't want you to go home in the state you're in now. I'm going to call Domestic Abuse Services, and if they have room for you at their shelter, I want you to consider spending at least one night there. Keep Jean at your sister's house for the time being. Domestic Abuse Services has offices and a counseling service at one location and a shelter at a different address, which is unlisted. I don't want you to worry. We have a van that can take you to the shelter. In the morning, you can leave the shelter and go talk with the Domestic Abuse Services counselors, or you can come back and talk with me; but right now, my main concern is that you are safe for today and tonight.

There are many kinds of immobile clients: (1) clients who need immediate hospitalization because of chemical use or organic dysfunction, (2) clients who are suffering from such severe depression that they cannot function, (3) clients who are experiencing a severe psychotic episode, (4) clients who are suffering from severe shock, bereavement, or loss, (5) clients whose anxiety level is temporarily so high that they cannot function until the anxiety subsides, (6) clients who, for any reason, are out of touch with reality, and (7) clients who are currently a danger to themselves or others. Immobile clients are more apt to be suicidal or homicidal than clients who are ready to respond to collaborative or nondirective counseling. Or, because of their inability to function effectively, they are more likely to engage in activities that put themselves or others at risk for serious injury. The worker must be able to make a fairly accurate and objective assessment of the client's level of mobility.

However, if the worker makes an error of judgment (believing a client to be immobile when, in fact, they are not), no harm is usually done because the client may simply respond by refusing to accept the worker's direction. In most cases of this sort, the worker can then shift into a collaborative mode and continue the helping session. Many times, a worker will begin in a directive mode and then shift into a collaborative mode during the session. For example, with a highly anxious client, the worker may begin by directing the client in relaxation exercises, which may lower the client's anxiety level to the point where the worker can make a natural shift into a collaborative mode to continue the counseling.

Collaborative Counseling

The collaborative approach enables the crisis worker to forge a real partnership with the client in evaluating the problem, generating acceptable alternatives, and implementing realistic action steps. When the triage assessment indicates that the client cannot function successfully in a nondirective mode but has enough mobility to be a partner in the crisis intervention process, the worker is collaborative to that degree. When a client has a triage score that is in the high single digits to middle teens, the crisis worker can typically operate in a collaborative mode. Many crisis interventions operate in this mode. Collaborative counseling is a "we" approach, in contrast to the "I" approach of directive counseling and the "you" approach of nondirective counseling. Consider some typical worker statements in the collaborative mode: "What 'they' are going to do sounds overpowering as you say it, but we haven't really considered what 'we' can do if we come up with a plan." "You've come up with a lot of good ideas, but you sound a little confused about which one to act on. Could we put our heads together and make a priority list of alternatives?"

The collaborative client is a full partner in identifying the precipitating problem, examining realistic alternatives, planning action steps, and making a commitment to carrying out a realistic plan. The collaborative client is not as self-reliant and autonomous as the fully mobile client but does have enough ego strength and mobility to participate in resolving the problem. The worker is needed to serve as a temporary catalyst, consultant, facilitator, and support person. Here is an example of a collaborative response to a client. This collaborative approach is a hallmark of Relational Cultural Therapy (RCT) in attempting to reconnect disconnected, isolated, and abandoned recipients of crisis service with a support system, albeit at the moment perhaps only the interventionist (Duffey & Haberstroh, 2020; Jordan, 2018).

Rita: I've thought about going to my mother's or going to the emergency women's shelter or even calling my school counselor friend for a place to stay tonight.

CW: Let's examine these three choices, and maybe some others available to you that I know of, and we'll see which one will best meet your requirements.

Nondirective Counseling

The nondirective approach is desirable whenever clients are able to initiate and carry out their own action steps. While the crisis worker will want to be as nondirective as possible and give the client as much control as the client can handle, in the initial stage of a crisis, the worker is seldom nondirective because of the high level of ratings on the Triage Assessment Form (see Chapter 3, "The Intervention and Assessment Models"). With the "you" approach of nondirective counseling, the worker uses a great amount of active listening and many open-ended questions to help clients clarify what they really want to do and examine what outcomes various choices might produce. These are some possible questions: "What do you wish to have happen?" "What will occur if you choose to do that?" "What people are available now who could and would assist you in this?" "Picture yourself doing that—vividly see yourself choosing that route. Now, how does that image fit with what you're really trying to accomplish?" "What activities did you do in the past that helped you in situations similar to this?" The worker does not manage, manipulate, prescribe, dominate, or control. It is the client who owns the problem, the coping mechanisms, the plan, the action, the commitment, and the outcomes.

The worker is a support person who may listen, encourage, reflect, reinforce, self-disclose, and suggest. Nondirective counseling assists clients in mobilizing what already is inside them—the capacity, ability, and coping strength to solve their own problems in ways that are pretty well known to them already but that are temporarily out of reach. Here is an example of a nondirective response.

Rita: This is it. I've had the last beating I'm going to take from that jerk! I'm simply going to get myself out of this hell!

CW: You've made a decision to choose a different life for yourself, and you've decided that you are the one who is going to start it.

Action Strategies for Crisis Workers

LO10 A number of action strategies and considerations may enhance the worker's effectiveness in dealing with clients in crisis. However, before committing to doing anything with the client, consider the following "rules of the road."

Recognize Individual Differences. View and respond to each client and each crisis situation as unique. If you really believe you are multiculturally sensitive, this is the essence of an emic multicultural view where both your and the client's social locations will play a big part in what will happen. Even for experienced workers, staying attuned to the uniqueness of each person is difficult. Under the pressures of time and exhaustion and misled by overconfidence in their own expertise, workers find it all too easy to lump problems and clients together and provide pat answers and solutions. Treating clients generically is likely to cost the worker and the client a great deal more in the long run than it saves in time and effort in the short run. Stereotyping, labeling, and taking for granted any aspect of crisis intervention are definite pitfalls.

Assess Yourself. Ongoing self-analysis on the part of the worker is mandatory. At all times, workers must be fully and realistically aware of their own values, limitations, physical and emotional status, and personal readiness to deal objectively with the client and the crisis at hand. Crisis workers need to run continuous perceptual checks to ascertain if they have gotten in over their heads. (Go to Chapter 15, "Human Services Workers in Crisis Burnout, Vicarious Traumatization, and Compassion Fatigue," for a thorough description of the phenomenon called "burnout.") If for any reason the worker is not ready for or capable of dealing with the crisis or the client, the worker must immediately make an appropriate referral.

Show Regard for Client Safety. The worker's style, choices, and strategies must reflect a continuous consideration of the client's physical and psychological safety as well as the safety of others involved. The safety consideration includes the safety of the worker as well as the ethical, legal, and professional requirements mandated in counseling practice. The greatest intervention strategies and tactics are absolutely useless if clients leave the crisis worker and go out and harm themselves or others.

The golden rule is "When in doubt about client safety, get help." If you aren't sure what to do, consult with another crisis worker. Consultation does not mean you are inadequate. What it does mean is that you are a professional practitioner who is seeking a second opinion to validate your own, or you realize that this problem is not an area of your expertise, so you are conferring with a person who does have the expertise. Thus, concern for a client's safety may mean appropriate referral interventions, including immediate hospitalization. You need to understand that when you do this, clients may be extremely angry at you; they may say you are unethical, have violated their trust and confidentiality, and even threaten to sue you for unprofessionalism.

Provide Client Support. The crisis worker should be available as a support person during the crisis period. Clients may need assistance in developing a list of possible support people, but if no appropriate support person emerges in the examination of alternatives, the worker can serve as a primary support person until the present crisis is over. A warm, empathic, and assertive counseling strategy should be used with clients who are extremely lonely and devoid of supports. For example:

CW: I want you to know that I am very concerned about your safety during this stressful time and that I'm available to help. I want you to keep this card with you until you're through this crisis and call me if you feel yourself sliding back into that hopeless feeling again. If you call either of these numbers and don't get an answer or get a busy signal, keep trying until you get me. You *must* make contact with *me*. I will be very disturbed if you are in a seriously threatening situation again without letting me become involved with you. I really want to impress on you my genuine concern for you and the importance of making an agreement or contract to call me whenever your safety is threatened. Will you give me that assurance?

Define the Problem Clearly. Many clients have complicated and multiple problems. Make sure that each problem is clearly and accurately defined from a practical, problem-solving point of view. Many clients define the crisis as someone else's problem or as some external event or situation that has happened. Attempting to solve the crisis of some third party (who isn't present) is counterproductive. Pinpoint the client's own problem with the event or situation and keep the focus on the client's central core of concern. Also, attempt to distill multiple problems down into an immediate, workable problem and concentrate on that problem first. We cannot overemphasize the tenacity with which the worker must avoid being drawn off on tangents by some highly emotional or defensive clients with difficult problems.

Consider these exchanges with Rita's husband, Jake.

Jake: You don't seem to like me much.

CW: Right now, that's not the issue of importance. What I'm trying to do is help you identify the main source of your problem.

Another example:

Jake: Haven't you ever hit your wife, too?

CW: No, but that's not what we're working on now. I'm trying to help us figure out a way for you to avoid fighting with her when you first get home each evening.

In both instances, the worker stays focused on the client and does not get caught up on side issues such as worker competency, beliefs, and attitudes. Now, the worker is ready to work on Task 4, "Examining Alternatives."

Consider Alternatives. In most problem situations, the alternatives are infinite. But crisis clients (and sometimes workers) have a limited view of the many options available. By using simple, open-ended questions and open-ended leads, the worker usually can elicit a surprising number of choices from the client of which they were previously unaware. Then, add your own list of possible alternatives to the client's list. For example, "I get the feeling that it might help if you could get in contact with a counselor at the Credit Counseling Bureau. How would you feel about adding that to our list?" Examining, analyzing, and listing alternatives to consider should be as collaborative as possible. The best alternatives are ones that the client truly *owns*. Take care to avoid imposing your alternatives on the client if at all possible.

The alternatives on the list should be workable and realistic. They should represent the right amount of action for the client to undertake now—not too much, not too little. The client will generally express ownership of an option by words such as "I would really like to call him today." Worker-imposed options are usually signaled by the worker's words, such as *"You need to* go to his office and do that right away." Beware of the latter! An important part of the quest for appropriate alternatives is to explore with the client what options have worked before in situations like the present one. Often, the client can come up with the best choices, derived from coping mechanisms that have worked well in the past. But the stresses created by the immediate crisis may keep clients from identifying the most obvious and appropriate alternatives for them. Here, the crisis worker facilitates the client's examination of alternatives.

CW: Rita, you say you're feeling frightened and trapped right now, and you don't know where to turn. But it sounds like you'd take a step in a positive direction if you could get some of your old zip back. What are some actions you took or some people you sought out in previous situations when you felt frightened or stuck?

Rita: Oh, I don't know that I've been in a mess quite this bad before.

CW: Well, that may be true. But what steps have you taken or what people have you contacted before in a mess like this, even if it wasn't this bad?

Rita: Hmm . . . Well, one time or two I did go talk to Mr. Jackson, one of my auto mechanics instructors when I was at the Area Vo-Tech School. He's very understanding and helpful. He always seemed to understand me and believe in me.

CW: How would you feel about reestablishing contact with him whenever you're down again?

Plan Action Steps. After developing a short, doable list of alternatives, the worker needs to move on to making plans. In crisis intervention, the worker endeavors to assist the client in developing a short-term plan that will help the client get through the immediate crisis as well as make the transition to long-term coping. The plan should include the client's internal coping mechanisms as well as sources of help in the environment. The coping mechanisms are usually brought to bear on some concrete, positive, constructive action that clients can take to regain better control of their lives. Actions that initially involve some physical movements are preferred. The plan should be realistic in terms of the client's current emotional readiness and environmental supports. It may involve collaboration with the worker until the client can function independently. The effective crisis worker is sensitive to the client's need to function autonomously as soon as feasible.

Rita: Right now I'd like to just be free of the whole mess for a few days . . . just get off this dizzy merry-go-round long enough to collect my thoughts.

CW: It sounds to me like you really mean that. Let's see if together we can examine some options that might get you the freedom and breathing space you need to pull the pieces back together.

Rita: I can't really let go. Too many people depend on me. That's just wishful thinking. But it would be wonderful to get some relief.

CW: Even though you don't see any way to get it, what you're wanting is some space for yourself right now—away from work, kids, Jake, Sam, and the whole dilemma.

Rita: The only way that would happen is for my doctor to order it—to prescribe it, medically.

CW: How realistic is that? How would that help you?

Rita: It would call a halt to some of the pressures. The treadmill would have to stop, at least temporarily. Yes, I guess that kind of medical reason wouldn't be so bad.

CW: Sounds like consulting your doctor and laying at least part of your cards on the table might be one step toward getting medical help in carving out some breathing space for yourself.

Rita: I think so. Yeah, that's it! That's one thing I could do.

CW: Let's together map out a possible action plan—for contacting your doctor and requesting assistance in temporarily letting go. Let's look at *when* you want to contact your doctor, *what* you're going to say, and *how* you're going to say it—to make sure you get the results you must have right now.

The crisis worker is attempting to work collaboratively with Rita and to facilitate Rita's real ownership of her plan. The worker also implies a view of Rita as competent and responsible.

Use the Client's Coping Strengths. In crisis intervention, it is important not to overlook the client's own strengths and coping mechanisms. Often, the crisis events temporarily immobilize the individual's usual strengths and coping strategies. If they can be identified, explored, and reinstated, they may make an enormous contribution toward restoring the client's equilibrium and reassuring the client. For example, one woman had previously relieved stress by playing her piano. She told the worker that she was no longer able to play the piano because her piano had been repossessed. The crisis worker was able to explore with her several possible places where she could avail herself of a piano in times of stress.

Use Referral Resources. An integral aspect of crisis intervention is the use of referral resources. A ready list of names and phone numbers of contact people is a necessity. It is also important for the crisis worker to develop skills in making referrals as well as in working with a wide variety of referral agencies. Many clients need to be referred early to sources of help regarding financial matters, legal assistance, long-term individual therapy, family therapy, substance misuse, severe depression, or other personal matters. Here are suggestions we have found to be useful in working with a variety of agencies. Generally, we find that a breakdown in communication with agencies follows our having overlooked a few obvious and simple cautions. So do as we say, not as we sometimes do! It's a long list, but keeping it handy and using it will save you lots of headaches in the long run. A particular admonition is: Be nice to secretaries and receptionists so they remember you as a really nice person. They can make your access a lot easier to both people and materials.

1. Keep a handy, up-to-date list of frequently used agencies. Keep up with personnel changes.
2. In communities that publish a directory of human services, have available the most recent edition.
3. Cultivate a working relationship with key people in agencies you use frequently. Get on community boards, join organizations, and become integrated into the provider system.
4. Identify yourself, your agency, and your purpose when telephoning. Know secretaries and receptionists by name and use their names when you call. Treat them with dignity, respect, and equality, and thank them for helping you.
5. Follow up on referrals you make—within 24 hours if at all possible.
6. Don't assume that all clients have the skills to get the services they need. Be prepared to assist clients who may be unable to help themselves avoid runaround and bureaucratic red tape.
7. Whenever necessary, without engendering dependency, help clients make contact with the referral agencies to assist and to ensure that effective communication takes place.
8. Write thank-you messages (with copies to their bosses) to people who are particularly helpful to you and your clients.
9. Don't criticize fellow professionals or the agencies they represent, and don't gossip about either workers or agencies.
10. Keep accurate records of referral activities so you have a paper trail.
11. Know frequently used agencies' hours, basic services, mode of operation, limitations, and, if possible, policies such as insurance and sliding scale fees.
12. Be aware of any agency services the client is already using so services don't get duplicated.
13. Use courtesy and good human relations skills when dealing with agency personnel. Put yourself in their shoes and treat them as you would like to be treated.
14. Avoid expecting perfection of other agencies. Give agencies feedback on how they did and obtain feedback from them.
15. Be aware of sensory impairment in clients, especially in older adults, and make those impairments known in referrals.

16. If the agency has an orientation session, seek to attend and participate in it.

17. Practice honesty in communicating with referral agencies regarding the status or needs of clients. (Honest and ethical portrayal of the client's needs will build credibility with other agencies.)

18. Don't be afraid to use web-based or geographically distant agencies that you have checked out as legitimate. It can bring a wealth of agencies and people to your electronic doorstep, and they may have the resources that you don't have locally.

Develop and Use Networks. Closely allied with referral is a function called networking (Haywood & Leuthe, 1980). Networking, for crisis workers, is having and using personal contacts within a variety of agencies that directly affect our ability to serve clients effectively and efficiently. Although each person in your network is a referral resource, it is the relationship you have with that individual that defines it as a network. Effective crisis workers can't sit behind a desk and wait for assistance to come to them. They must get out into the community and personally get to know the key individuals who can provide the kinds of services their clients require. A personal relationship based on understanding and trust between the worker and vital network people is invaluable in helping the worker cut through bureaucratic red tape, expedite emergency assistance, and personalize many services that might otherwise not be available to clients.

As crisis workers, we do not operate alone in the world. We are interdependent. Networking permits us to spread the responsibilities among other helping professionals. We mean "helping professionals" in the broadest possible context: lawyers; judges; parole officers; ministers; school counselors; federal, state, and local human services workers; directors and key people in crisis agencies; prison staff; business and civic leaders; medical doctors; dentists; police; and political leaders may play important roles in the networking process. The development and use of effective networking are indispensable functions of the successful worker.

Get a Commitment. A vital part of crisis intervention is getting a short-term commitment from the client to follow through on the action or actions planned. The crisis worker should ask the client to summarize verbally the steps to be taken. This verbal summary helps the worker understand the client's perception of both the plan and the commitment and gives the worker an opportunity to clear up any distortions. It also provides the worker with an opportunity to establish a follow-up checkpoint with the client. The commitment step can serve as a motivational reminder to the client and also encourage and predispose the client to believe that the action steps will succeed. Without a definite and positive commitment on the part of the client, the best of plans may fall short of the objectives that have been worked out by the worker and the client.

CW: So, Rita, it seems to me that what you've decided to do is to reinitiate some kind of meaningful contact with Mr. Jackson. So we're both very clear on what you've committed yourself to doing, would you please summarize how and when you're going to proceed?

Rita: I'm going straight to my office today and phone him at school. I'll either talk to him or leave a message for him to call me. As soon as I talk to him, I'll set up a definite day and time to meet with him.

CW: And when you've set up . . .

Rita: Oh, yes! And when I've set up my appointment with him, I'm going to phone you and let you know how it went.

CW: Good. And in the meantime, you have my number on the card if you need me—especially if the safety of either you or your children becomes jeopardized.

Rita: That's right, and I'll call if I lose my nerve with Sam. I've got to get some space for myself there—at least some temporary space.

Experienced crisis workers are generally able to sense how far and how fast the client is able to act. Usually, the client is encouraged to commit to as much action as feasible. If we cannot get the client to make a giant leap forward, we'll take one small step in a positive direction. The main idea is to facilitate some commitment that will result in movement of the client in a constructive direction.

Summary

Crisis intervention from a practitioner's standpoint incorporates a number of fundamental counseling skills that are specifically tailored to crisis intervention. Listening is fundamental to all successful counseling, including crisis intervention, and includes such techniques as restatement, reflection, owning statements, and open- and closed-ended questions. Essential components of effective listening and communication include effective attending, empathy, genuineness, and acceptance. Action skills range across nondirective, collaborative, and directive worker strategies. These strategies may include helping the client focus or expand awareness, providing guidance and information, allowing cathartic release of emotions, providing support and protection, and mobilizing the client to action. As opposed to doing crisis therapy with a client with whom the worker has a working history, field work often means meeting a client for the first time. Thus, basic introduction and attending skills, along with an assessment of client weapon and drug use, availability of support systems, and whether basic food, water, shelter, clothing, and medical needs are being met, are critical to de-escalation and stabilization. Finally, the worker is not an island unto himself or herself. Building human services provider resources and establishing working relationships with them is critical to any crisis work.

Crisis Case Handling

5

Learning Objectives

After studying this chapter, you should be able to:

1. Describe the differences between handling long-term therapy and crisis intervention and when they are applied.
2. Explain how a walk-in mental health facility handles crises.
3. Explain what a mobile crisis response team is and how it operates.
4. Explain what a police Crisis Intervention Team is, how it is trained, what it does, and how it is integrated with mental health service providers.
5. Describe what "suicide by cop" means and why it occurs.
6. Determine the generic types of transcrisis in long-term therapy.
7. Identify persons with borderline personality disorder who are in a constant state of transcrisis.
8. Describe the rules of therapy for counseling difficult clients.

Handling Crisis Cases Versus Long-Term Cases

LO1 To understand crisis case handling, we need to distinguish between what crisis interventionists and long-term therapists do, the principles that underlie the two modes, and their objectives, client functioning, and assessment procedures. On first glance, typical models for long-term therapy do not look radically different from a crisis intervention model. Our own long-term, eight-step systematic counseling model (James & Gilliland, 2003, pp. 376–381) incorporates predisposition, exploration, examining alternatives, planning courses of action, and obtaining client commitment in much the same operational format as crisis intervention.

What is radically different is that in long-term therapy, defining problems, identifying alternatives, and planning are much broader in scope, more methodological, and rely on continuous feedback loops to check the effectiveness of the intervention. A typical counseling session with a long-term client reviews progress since the previous session, collaboratively refines the plan of action if needed, processes the content of the session and the client's feelings about it, and then proposes a new homework assignment to be tried out before the next meeting. Crisis intervention models do not operate with such liberal time dimensions or problem scopes. In crisis intervention, exploring the problems, identifying alternatives, planning, and committing to a plan are all much more compressed in time and scope. They may also not progress in a linear, sequential order. What may occur in long-term therapy in a rather leisurely fashion over a period of weekly sessions may occur in crisis intervention in a half-hour to 2 hours.

While in long-term therapy, a great deal of background exploration may provide the therapist with a panoramic view of client dynamics, the crisis worker's exploration typically is narrow, starting and stopping with the specific presenting crisis. The long-term therapist's view of alternatives and planning a course of action commonly incorporate psychoeducational processes that seek to change residual, repressive, and chronic client modes of thinking, feeling, and acting. In contrast, the crisis worker seeks to quickly determine previous coping skills and environmental resources available to the client and use them in the present situation as a stopgap measure to gain time and provide a modicum of stability in an out-of-control situation. While crisis workers use psychoeducational techniques a great deal, they typically do so to solve immediate short-term problems that evolve from the crisis itself by providing specific information about what is going on with the client, such as posttraumatic stress disorder (PTSD) symptoms, or specific information on how to access resources, such as getting help from Federal Emergency Management Agency (FEMA) for a housing loan after a tornado.

While the long-term therapist would view comprehensive personality change as a necessary part of the therapeutic plan, the crisis worker endeavors to change personality only to the degree necessary for restoring precrisis functioning. A long-term therapist would look toward an evidence-based methodological manipulation of treatment variables, assess those variables on a variety of dimensions, and process the outcomes with the client. A crisis worker often uses a "best guess" based on previous experience with what does and does not work with a particular problem (Kleespies, 2014).

Protocols for treatment in long-term therapy are typically evidence based and involve many tryouts as the protocol is fine-tuned to the individual's particular needs. Crisis intervention is a good deal more creative. Although it attempts to operate from evidence-based techniques, due to a myriad of logistical and tactical problems in obtaining hard research, the best that can be said about crisis intervention is that it operates from a "best practice" modality. That "best practice" modality further adapts and changes quickly as conditions warrant and may circle back through its intervention model if needed and wind up being radically different than the original game plan.

Finally, feedback and assessment of outcome measures in long-term therapy typically involve a great deal of processing between client and therapist as to the efficacy of treatment. If treatment outcomes are not as expected, a feedback loop is integrated into the model that will allow a return to any of the previous steps. Feedback and assessment in crisis intervention typically occur on a here-and-now basis, with an emphasis on what changes have occurred in the previous minutes and what the client will do in the next few hours.

It should be clearly understood that in long-term therapy, when a transcrisis state or point emerges, the therapist now becomes a crisis worker (Ford, 2021), and all the principles of crisis intervention are applied as crisis therapy until the client is stabilized. Beginning therapists often do not recognize such transcrisis events and freeze as they try to get back to baseline operating mode when "normal" went flying out the window and there is little chance of getting it back until the crisis is contained. Such events may particularly occur when therapy has been successful, the client is to be terminated, the client is frightened to death at the prospect of going out to face the world alone, and quickly deteriorates to the shock and chagrin of the therapist.

There are many approaches to long-term therapy. Although Thorne's (1968, pp. 11–13) approach is more than fifty years old, it is a classic representation of one of the most comprehensive and integrated systems to be found. To provide a clear delineation between crisis intervention and long-term therapy, we have compared our model of crisis intervention with Thorne's *principles, objectives, client functioning,* and *assessment* of case handling. Tables 5.1 through 5.4 summarize the contrasts.

Case Handling at Walk–In Crisis Facilities

Types of Presenting Crises

LO2 Clients who present themselves for crisis counseling at walk-in facilities generally fall into one of three categories: those who are experiencing (1) chronic mental illness, (2) acute interpersonal problems in their social environment such as drug addiction, domestic problems, or financial loss, or (3) a combination of the two. Most clients who avail themselves of community mental health clinics suffer from financial problems that prohibit them from seeking private therapy.

Table 5.1   Principles Compared Between Long-Term Therapy and Crisis Intervention

Long-Term Therapy Mode	Crisis Case-Handling Mode
1. **Diagnosis:** Complete diagnostic evaluation with observation; background of social, educational, and work history; intellectual, personality, and malady-specific psychological testing.	1. **Diagnosis:** Rapid triage crisis assessment face-to-face.
2. **Treatment:** Focus on basic underlying causes; on the whole person with continuous individual and group work over an extended time.	2. **Treatment:** Solution-focused on the immediate trauma/crisis component of the person to stabilize and restore psychological equilibrium.
3. **Plan:** Personalized comprehensive prescription directed toward fulfilling long-term needs across work, academic, and social environments.	3. **Plan:** Individual problem-specific prescription focused on immediate needs to alleviate the crisis symptoms in the current environment.
4. **Methods:** Knowledge and use of a variety of techniques to systematically effect a wide array of short-term, intermediate-term, and long-term therapeutic gains.	4. **Methods:** Knowledge of time-limited brief therapy techniques used for immediate control and containment of the crisis/trauma.
5. **Evaluation of results:** Systematic behavioral validation of therapeutic outcomes in terms of the client's total functioning through testing, long-term observation, and supportive reports from significant others in work and social environments.	5. **Evaluation of results:** Target crisis-specific behavioral validation by client's return to precrisis level of equilibrium through observation of client actions.

Table 5.2   Objectives Compared Between Long-Term Therapy and Crisis Intervention

Long-Term Therapy Mode (Listed in No Particular Order, But Global in Scope)	Crisis Case-Handling Mode (Listed in Linear Order with a Crisis-Specific Focus)
1. **Prevent problems:** More basic than cure. Use preventive procedures whenever possible. Explore comprehensive future needs based on current assessment of intra- and interpersonal skills and social, vocational, and financial resources.	1. **Ensure client safety:** Always assess client lethality and provide for the physical and psychological safety of the client and significant others.
2. **Correct etiological factors:** Involves comprehensive, evidence-based treatment of broad-based psychological and environmental factors in both the past and present.	2. **Predisposition.** Facilitate conditions for client–worker bonding. Reduce threat level.
3. **Provide systematic support:** Comprehensive measures directed toward improvement of the state of psychological and physical health and well-being of the individual across social and work environments.	3. **Define problem:** Clarify in concrete terms the issues that precipitated the crisis.
4. **Facilitate growth:** Treatment should ideally facilitate rather than interfere with natural environmental and developmental processes.	4. **Provide support:** Establish conditions, by either the crisis worker or significant others, so the client feels secure and free of threat or abandonment as the current crisis is resolved.
5. **Reeducate:** Treatment seeks to reeducate and teach new models of adjustment for lifelong coping.	5. **Examine alternatives:** Provide options for alleviating the immediate situational threat in relation to the crisis.
6. **Express and clarify emotional attitudes:** Major emphasis is on methods of securing emotional release and expression in a permissive and accepting environment.	6. **Develop a plan:** Formulate a stepwise procedure using client coping skills, crisis worker expertise, and systemic measures to energize the client to take immediate action.
7. **Resolve conflict and inconsistencies:** Therapy aims to help the client achieve insight and understanding into the causation and dynamic roots of the behavior and change.	7. **Obtain commitment:** Obtain agreement as to specific time, duration, and number of activities required to stabilize the client and/or crisis situation.
8. **Accept reality:** Help the client to accept what cannot be changed. Move forward into new realities and discard problematic histories.	8. **Follow-up.** Short-term follow-up to determine if crisis intervention strategies continue to work.
9. **Reorganize attitudes:** Move the person toward exhibiting a more positive view of life and more effective social integration.	
10. **Maximize intellectual resources:** Improve the functions of sensing, perceiving, remembering, communicating, thinking, behavior management, and self-control.	

Table 5.3   Client Functioning Compared Between Long-Term Therapy and Crisis Intervention

Long-Term Therapy Mode	Crisis Case-Handling Mode
1. Client shows sufficient *affect*; manifests some basis for experiencing and understanding their emotional state.	1. *Affectively*, the client is impaired to the extent that there is little understanding of their emotional state.
2. Client shows some ability to *cognitively* understand the connection between behavior and consequences and between what is rational and irrational.	2. *Cognitively*, the client shows an inability to think linearly and logically and formulate strategies to alleviate the crisis. Irrationality is the norm.
3. There is some modicum of *behavioral* control.	3. *Behaviorally*, the client is out of control and may pose a danger to self or others.

Table 5.4   Assessment Compared Between Long-Term Therapy and Crisis Intervention

Long-Term Therapy Mode	Crisis Case-Handling Mode
1. **Intake data:** Client is stable enough to provide in-depth background regarding the problem. Lengthy intake form may contain details of the client's total history: family, medical history, drug use, education, therapy background, and social history. Comprehensive personality and intellectual tests may be given.	1. **Intake data:** Client may not be able to fill out an intake form because of instability or time constraints; a verbal and/or visual evaluation of the current maladaptive state may be the only data available.
2. **Safety:** Client safety is not the primary focus unless there are clues pointing toward imminent danger to self or others.	2. **Safety:** Crisis worker's first concern is client's and others' safety; determining whether client is suicidal, homicidal, or otherwise a danger or threat to someone by intentional or unintentional acts.
3. **Time:** The therapist has time to procure a variety of assessment data to confirm or contraindicate the hypothesized problem. Total case diagnosis and workups are gathered before the treatment plan is developed. Personality assessment indexes are generally gathered to compare client functioning against norm groups on standard pathology measures.	3. **Time:** The crisis worker has no time for administering formal instruments. Workers must rely on immediate verbal and nonverbal cues emitted by the client to make an assessment of the degree of pathology.
4. **Reality testing:** The therapist assumes the client is in touch with reality unless assessment data or other clues indicate otherwise.	4. **Reality testing:** Using simple questioning procedures, the crisis worker must determine whether the person is in touch with reality and how effectively the person is functioning in real time.
5. **Referrals:** Referral resources have implications for long-term development. Examples of referrals might be to family services, mental health centers, vocational/educational assistance, and job placement services.	5. **Referrals:** Referral resources have implications of immediacy in terms of getting the client to safety and some degree of stability. Examples of referrals might be to the police, hospital emergency room, psychiatric or medical evaluation, or immediate support people.
6. **Consultation:** Consultants and other backup resources are available as needed. Collaboration is normally initiated after consultation with the client and/or the therapist's supervisor.	6. **Consultation:** Professional consultants who are trained in the diagnosis of pathology may be on call for backup purposes. Police and mobile crisis teams are sometimes available. Most likely, the worker is on their own.
7. **Drug use:** The therapist relies on data from the intake material and on information developed in the normal course of the therapy to ascertain the level and type of prescription medication or illicit drug or alcohol use.	7. **Drug use:** The crisis worker relies on verbal and visual responses to ascertain the level and type of prescription medication or illicit drug or alcohol use.
8. **Disposition:** Client typically starts and finishes with the same therapist over a course of months. May occasionally be referred to adjunctive therapeutic specialization during the course of therapy. Clients come and go voluntarily and return to the home environment.	8. **Disposition:** Client typically starts and stops with the same worker over a course of hours or days. May be referred permanently to long-term treatment with a therapeutic specialization once stabilized. Client may be involuntarily held for observation, arrested and jailed, or released back to supervised care of custodians, guardians, or significant others.

Chronic Crisis. Since the enactment of the federal Community Mental Health Act of 1963, the major responsibility for the treatment for people with mental illness has fallen on community mental health centers. Although in theory the act was designed to deinstitutionalize patients and return those who are able to functional living, in fact, the act has placed many people in chronic crisis.

In addition, increased drug misuse, a rise in crime, fragmentation of families, social isolation due to the COVID-19 pandemic, and a host of other societal ills have caused a tremendous upsurge in the need for mental health services. Originally focused on reintegrating long-term hospital patients into the community, mental health centers have tended to assign chronic cases a less-than-priority status. The unspoken reason is that these clients are extremely frustrating to mental health providers because they show little progress and are a constant financial and emotional drain on the resources of the agencies that come in contact with them. Many community mental health centers have de-emphasized this role and moved more toward dealing with common developmental problems (Slaikeu, 1990, p. 284). Perhaps more ominously, funding cutbacks have forced community mental health centers to look more closely at a client's ability to pay as a precondition for treatment, which means that people who may most need service may be relegated to a waiting list. Furthermore, because of legal ramifications and funding problems, people with severe mental disturbance such as schizophrenia who are committed to state hospitals typically have very brief stays and are turnstiled back onto the streets.

The result is that a host of chronically mentally ill people who have difficulty functioning, who are experiencing impoverishment, experiencing homelessness, and who may be victims or perpetrators of crime, and without support systems of any kind are left to fend for themselves. These people often have multiple problems besides a primary diagnosis of psychopathology. They may be noncompliant with treatment, disregard their medication, misuse alcohol and drugs, have other severe physical problems, and be victimized financially, physically, and psychologically by others and, as the references indicate, these are long standing problems endemic to public mental health (Bender, 1986; Krupski et al., 2015; Linn et al., 1990; Nurius, 1984; Pepper et al., 2000; Toolis et al., 2022). It is easy to understand why such people often wind up in crisis when understaffed and underfunded mental health clinics (Roberts, 1991, p. 31) and other social services agencies cannot care for them, and this is particularly true of the provision of services for individuals from minoritized and/or marginalized groups.

Ethnic and Minority Access. The need for mental health care among minoritized and/or marginalized groups has increased significantly since the advent of the COVID-19 pandemic, yet a variety of obstacles such as a lack health insurance, mobility, and easy access; lack of provider racial and ethical diversity; and firsthand experience of racial discrimination and negative perceptions of mental illness militate against the use of services (Centers for Disease Control and Prevention, 2023) by many ethnic and racial minority and disenfranchised groups. A recent significant development to this problem for at least one minority group has been the advent and push in the United States of LGBTQIA+ community centers in providing walk-in mental health crisis services for sexual and gender minorities and their idiosyncratic concerns (Pachankis et al., 2021). Because of a lack of services, the chronically mentally ill are often on a first-name basis with local police and personnel in emergency rooms, mental health clinics, and social services agencies.

Social/Environmental Crises. People with chronic mental health issues are not the only people who avail themselves of, or are brought to, walk-in facilities. People who have run away, with substance misuse, those experiencing domestic abuse, people with physical disabilities, crime victims, survivors of violent events, sexual abuse survivors, people with terminal illnesses, veterans, people who are unemployed, and relatives of people with chronic physical and mental illnesses are some of the many participants in a drama of social crisis that is played out every day and night in mental health clinics, emergency rooms, student counseling centers, social services agencies, and police stations across the country. Many precipitating events may be unexpected and sudden and may have an impact far beyond the individual on families and communities, leaving these systems disorganized and out of control. Crises that are generated in the social environment are some of the most potent for mental health workers because of their ramifications across systems and the heightened emotionality and immediacy that accompany them for both clientele and workers.

Combination of Types. The foregoing crisis types rarely occur as discrete categories. Overlapping among types and problems that face crisis workers is the rule rather than the exception. Attempting to stabilize someone with chronic schizophrenia without providing food and shelter, treating a trauma survivor without first working on a drug addiction, or considering vocational exploration without handling the depression of a middle-aged executive who has just lost her job is a waste of valuable time. Handling multiple crises with the same client is the rule rather than the exception.

Case Handling at a Community Mental Health Clinic

Center City is a generic representation of how clients who walk into or are brought to a community mental health facility are taken care of. This clinic's catchment area includes a number of housing projects, the downtown area, a state university medical facility, the city hospital, a Veterans Administration Hospital, a state psychiatric hospital, the county jail, several halfway shelters for people who misuse substances and who are experiencing homelessness, and a variety of other social services agencies. Furthermore, its catchment area has the highest crime rate and incidence of domestic violence in the city, a high percentage of school dropouts, and some of the most impoverished areas of the city. In essence, it is a poster child for the rough and tumble world of inner-city mental health provision.

Entry. Clients may come to the mental health clinic on their own, be brought by relatives or social services agencies, or be taken into custody by the police. At the moment of entry, disposition of the case begins. A person in crisis who walks in or is brought to Center City may range across the triage scale from mildly to severely disturbed. If the person is severely disturbed, a senior clinician is summoned. An attempt is made to remove the client to an isolated office to reduce environmental stimuli and calm the client so an assessment can proceed. The clinician tries to obtain a case history. If this is not possible, the clinician makes a visual and verbal assessment in regard to information-processing problems, tangential thinking, hallucinations, disassociation, threats to self or others, or severe drug misuse. If any of these symptoms are present, a psychiatrist is called to evaluate the client and decide whether hospitalization is warranted.

Involuntary holds. If the client is so mentally fragmented that they are clearly out of touch with reality or deemed an imminent danger to self or others, they are admitted to an inpatient mental health facility for a period of observation. The person is asked to voluntarily commit to hospitalization. If they are unwilling to do so, a physician may write an involuntary hold order. An officer of the Crisis Intervention Team, a special unit of the police trained to deal with the mentally ill, is then called to transport the patient. Under no circumstances do mental health workers become involved in transportation because of safety concerns and the possibility of stigmatizing themselves as punitive agents in the patients' eyes. If patients are financially able, they may be transported to a private psychiatric facility. If they are unable to pay, they are taken to the city hospital psychiatric emergency unit for evaluation and, depending on diagnosis, may be adjudicated to subsequent placement at the state hospital or other mental health facility. It should sadly be noted that, particularly in rural areas, the foregoing protocol may be the exception rather than the rule where there is little if any secure mental health infrastructure. When that occurs, jail is the mental health facility of last resort.

Intake Interview. If the individual is coherent enough to provide verbal and written information, an intake interview is started. Following closely the crisis intervention model in Chapter 3, "The Intervention and Assessment Models," the intake worker first attempts to assess for client safety, define the problem, and apprise the client of their rights. In a patient and methodical manner, the intake worker goes through a standard intake interview sheet. Through open-ended questions and active listening, the worker tries to obtain as comprehensive a picture of the client as possible. The worker also attempts to determine the precipitating problem that brought the client to the clinic. The intake worker must be nonjudgmental, empathic, and caring and must also obtain concrete and specific information from a client who may not be able or willing to reciprocate.

Two critical components are always appraised in this initial assessment: degree of client lethality and drug use. It is a given that crisis situations either involve or have the possibility of acting-out behavior. Therefore, the intake worker evaluates clients in relation to their plans or intent to do harm to themselves or others. Because of the widespread use and misuse of prescription and illicit drugs, the worker checks to determine if drugs are involved in the presenting problem. Thus, intake workers need to have familiarity with the **Prescriber's Digital Reference (PDR)**, which was known as a hard copy book called the *Physician's Desk Reference* until it was changed to its present online form in 2017. The intake worker must also have a working knowledge of the side effects of "street drugs" because of the high incidence of their use in the Center City area.

Disposition. After the intake has been completed, the worker constructs and writes a proposed diagnosis and treatment recommendations. The intake worker discusses the treatment recommendations and possible services with the client. It is then the client's decision to accept or reject services. If services are accepted, the intake worker introduces the client to the therapist who will most likely be in charge of the case. A full clinical team meeting is held to confirm or alter the initial diagnosis and treatment recommendations. At that time, a primary therapist is designated and assumes responsibility for the case.

Anchoring. On their initial visit, clients are never left alone. From their intake interview to disposition to a primary therapist, workers help clients feel that a personal interest is being taken in them and their problems. The worker takes and hands over the client to the therapist who will be in charge of the case. The therapist gives the client a verbal orientation about what is going to occur. The idea behind this methodical orientation is to demystify the world of mental health, familiarize clients with what their treatment will be, and provide them with a **psychological anchor** in the form of a real person who will act as their advocate, support, and contact person. Quickly establishing rapport with the primary therapist is helpful in forestalling future crises and is extremely important to unstable clients, given the threatening implications of entering a mental health facility, possible loss of freedom, and the bureaucratic maze of the mental health system. It is also designed to immediately empower clients and make them feel they have taken a step in the right direction.

Short-Term Disposition. Many crises relate to the basic physical necessities of living. If that's the case, the intake worker makes short-term provisions for food, clothing, shelter, and other necessities while setting in motion the wheels of other social services agencies to provide long-term subsistence services. If clients are unable to care for themselves, the state department of family services is appointed as a conservator to handle their money and look after their basic needs. Thus, it is very important that the intake worker and other staff thoroughly understand and can access the local social services network.

Long-Term Disposition. An interdisciplinary team reviews and evaluates the intake worker's diagnosis and recommendations. In some facilities, there is an in-house Crisis Resolution interdisciplinary team specifically tasked with comprehensive crisis intervention. This is a fairly new response to crisis intervention that we will introduce to you in the next section of this chapter. If the team considers it necessary, a psychiatrist and a pharmacist conduct a psychiatric and/or pharmacological evaluation of the client. If a psychological evaluation is required, a psychologist evaluates the person on standardized personality and intellectual measures. Depending on the client's needs, people from various specialty units join the team. Once the team is complete, it formulates objectives and goals, and an evidence-based therapeutic plan is put into operation. The team reviews this plan on a regular basis and changes it if necessary.

Twenty-Four-Hour Service. Center City operates 24 hours a day/seven days a week. After regular working hours, telephone relays are linked into the crisis hotline. Telephone workers there evaluate the call and make a decision about who should handle it. That may be a mobile crisis team or, in Center City, the police department crisis intervention team, which we will examine at length later in this chapter.

Mobile Crisis Teams (MCTs). MCTs have become an integral part of emergency psychiatric services (Ng, 2006), and Crisis Resolution Teams (CRTs) have been an outgrowth of that program. Mobile crisis teams (MCTs) operate for two distinct reasons. For certain clients, particularly older clients or clients with physical disabilities, it may be necessary to make home visits to provide services. In other cases, when a client is out of control and unwilling or unable to go to the clinic, crisis workers go wherever the client is.

The Community Mental Health Act of 1963 mandated that those clinics receiving federal funds provide 24-hour emergency services. The mobile crisis team has been one answer to that mandate. In many cities, these mobile teams are on call and often follow up either along with or after local police departments have contained the situation.

Typically, a hotline or 911 mental disturbance call will ask for assistance. Either a police car with a mental health worker riding along will go to the scene, or mental health workers will follow up after the police. These teams are typically equipped with sophisticated communication and information retrieval systems that can call up client mental health files or criminal records. In some instances, psychiatric nurses may be members of these teams and can administer psychotropic medication in consultation with psychiatrists (Ligon, 2000).

Depending on state statutes, either the police or licensed mental health workers in these mobile units have the power to take clients into protective custody and transport them to a hospital rather than to jail. There are three problems associated with this approach. First, most such units operate in urban areas; many rural counties in the United States have little provision for such emergency services in regard to either staff, a mental health facility to transport a client to, or the ability to administer on-site crisis intervention (Aron et al., 2009; Bain, 2011; Rouse, 1998; Rural Health Hub, 2021; Yang, 2018). Second, no local police jurisdiction is going to transport someone 100 miles if it takes that police officer out of service for any length of time. The bottom line is that the mentally ill wind up in the place most convenient to put them—and that is usually jail, the very last place they need to be. Finally, although it has been proposed that MCTs are cost efficient and can reduce hospitalization (Bengelsdorf et al., 1993), there is little current research on their ability to do "on the scene" emergency psychiatric services.

The Crisis Resolution Team. CRT has been an outgrowth and evolution of the MCT. It may be in-house or it may be mobile. Developed in England in 2000 and adopted in many European countries, the United States, and Australia (Gimenez-Diez, 2022; Happell, 2009; Holgersen et al., 2022; Martin-Inigo et al., 2022; Reinke et al., 2022), it is composed of a specialized mental health team that provides rapid assessment and intensive treatment in the homes of individuals with severe mental illness experiencing a mental health crisis that is likely to require hospital admission. It is designed to operate 24/7 and provide onsite, at home services with a multidisciplinary team including psychiatrists, nurses, case managers, and other support personnel. A range of interventions include medication, crisis intervention psychotherapy, resiliency interventions, psychological and psychoeducational support for families, and help with everyday tasks of living (Aliouche, 2022; University of Cincinnati Center for Police Research and Policy, n.d.-b; Wheeler et al., 2015).

As with other approaches in the cloudy empirical statistical world of crisis intervention, outcomes are equivocal (Holgerson et al., 2022; Wheeler et al., 2015). They do appear to reduce hospital admissions and short stays after hospital discharge. However, there also appear to be variations in reduced admissions depending on geographical locale, community resources, threshold admission standards, and whether admission is voluntary or involuntary (UC Center for Police Research & Policy, n.d.-b). There are positive consumer outcomes in regard to feelings of accessibility, support, and psychoeducation in dealing with mental illness (Griffiths et al., 2020; Vasquez, 2023) and a range of treatment plans and flexibility beyond just medication (Hassellberg et al., 2021).

While a grand endeavor, one of the major problems, at least in England, is the lack of staff to implement the program. Lloyd-Evans and associates' (2018) survey of 218 English CRTs found almost no teams adhered fully to government guidelines for implementation and nurses were the only professional group employed in all the teams. There also was wide variability in implementation from a treatment stand point, and that holds true for a Spanish report on CRT implementation as well (Vasquez, 2023). Lamb et al. (2020) surveyed 75 English CRTs and found no teams received high fidelity in providing comprehensive, integrated staff and care. There also appear to be conflicts between traditional approaches with stand-alone professionals when brought together in multidisciplinary teams with new ways of thinking and delivering services (Klevan et al., 2018). While it is easy to cast critical stones at these endeavors, it should be understood that this is some of the most grueling, intense, and sometimes dangerous work and ground on which crisis intervention is delivered. Do you think you'd want to make this a career path, or perhaps turn away and leave it to the police?

Police and Crisis Intervention

It may seem odd to many of you reading this section that we are going to spend a lot of time talking about police officers and crisis intervention since crisis workers generally fall into counseling, social work, psychology, nursing, and other medical and social service professions. So why cops? What do they know about empathic responses to people in crisis, right? Just look at Ferguson, Missouri; New York City; St. Paul; Memphis; and a host of other places where cops hurt and killed people for no good reason.

Certainly, bad cops exist, but so do good ones. We would now like to introduce you to a different kind of law enforcement officer who has been specially trained to support individuals who are experiencing crisis.

Changing Role of the Police

The role of the police is rapidly changing and expanding. In most communities, police departments are being tasked with more and more responsibilities in addition to traditional law enforcement. Increasingly, crisis work with the mentally ill and emotionally disturbed is one of those responsibilities. Because of the dearth of mental health services in the United States, police officers have become the de facto mental health service providers to the mentally ill (aka street psychiatrists) (Savage & Moribto, 2020). It is commonly thought that patrol officers concern themselves mainly with **instrumental crimes** such as theft, robbery, and assault. The fact is that police officers deal with a multitude of **expressive** kinds of crime, in which individuals pose a serious threat to themselves or others because of their own anger, fear, vulnerability, depression, or lack of emotional control. Even though police departments do not relish investing much of their time away from providing for public safety and enforcing the law, they have found themselves more and more in a modality of law enforcement/crisis intervention (Borum, 2000; Miller, 2006; Saunders, 2010).

Police and People with Mental Health Crises

LO3 The problem has been ongoing and increasing since the advent of the Community Mental Health Act of 1963 and the changes it brought in releasing many mentally ill persons back into the community. That change meant that the first institutional authority likely to have interaction with persons with mental illness would not be a mental health professional but a police officer (Lamb et al., 2002; Watson & Fulambarker, 2012). As a result, sadly, for many mentally ill individuals, release into the "community" has actually meant release to jail as a holding facility. Survey research has revealed that among people who are incarcerated, approximately 15 percent of men and 30 percent of women meet the criteria for a mental health disorder (Steadman et al., 2009). The latest statistics are somewhat dated, listing over 350,000 inmates with mental illness (OMI) in 2012 (Treatment Advocacy Center, 2014). The report found that mental illness among inmates is

pervasive, with 64 percent of jail inmates, 54 percent of state prisoners, and 45 percent of federal prisoners reporting mental health concerns. Substance misuse is also rampant and often co-occurring (American Psychological Association, 2014). They are locked up because essentially there is no other place to house them, and their first mental health contact when in crisis is usually a law enforcement officer who put them there. Our own work in prisons indicates that is probably not an over estimate.

Gillig and associates (1990) studied a sample of 309 police officers in Cincinnati and Hamilton County, Ohio and found that during a 1-month period, almost 60 percent of the officers had responded to at least one call in which a presumably mentally ill person had to be confronted. Almost half of the officers had responded to more than one such call during the 1-month period. This response rate is not high and has remained constant, with approximately 20 percent of 911 calls related to mental health issues (Abramson, 2021). Livingston's (2016) meta-analysis of 85 studies of police response to mental illness calls found that one in four of those calls results in an arrest and one in ten people will have the police involved along their pathway to mental health help.

This dilemma puts a heavy responsibility on the shoulders of law enforcement officers, and although many dislike spending their time on crises of a social service nature, they are accepting encounters with the mentally ill as an appropriate aspect of modern police work and are more empathic to their illness (Bahora et al., 2008; Lakey, 2023; Watson et al., 2010; Watson & Fulambarker, 2012). They are also requesting more information, training, and collaboration with mental health and crisis intervention agencies (Compton et al., 2006). The foregoing has highlighted a need to develop training models that include police crisis intervention training with the mentally ill (Compton et al., 2006; Erstling, 2006; Gillig et al., 1990; Luckett & Slaikeu, 1990; Vermette et al., 2005). Indeed, if one looks at the training the Boston Police Department and the Boston Emergency Services Team has put together, it starts to look more like the start of a degree in crisis intervention (Savage & Morabito, 2020).

Because of that ongoing need, the Memphis Police Department developed the **Crisis Intervention Team** (CIT; James, 1994; James & Crews, 2014). CIT was developed specifically to train patrol officers to deal with the mentally ill and emotionally disturbed. One of the authors of this book was fortunate enough to be involved in that initial, innovative endeavor, which started in Memphis in 1987. Little did we realize at the time that this program, with its humble beginnings attempting to resolve a local problem, would catch fire nationally. Today, the program has come to be known as the Memphis Model for police crisis intervention with the mentally ill. In 2005, the first national convention for Crisis Intervention Team police officers was held in Columbus, Ohio. More than 1,000 police personnel came to that program from all over the country. CIT has become an annual international convention since its original gathering. And it now draws police officers and mental health professionals from all over the world. It is with a good deal of pride that one of your authors had a hand in training many of those officers who came to Memphis from such diverse jurisdictions as Anchorage, Alaska; Ft. Lauderdale, Florida; Montgomery County, Maryland; Hutchinson, Kansas; Canada; Sweden; and Australia. Currently, in over 2,700 jurisdictions across the United States, law enforcement is establishing CITs, and thousands of police officers are being trained along the lines of what you are about to read in the next few paragraphs (Addy & James, 2005; CIT International, 2014).

The Crisis Intervention Team (CIT) Program

Because budget constraints, economic factors, and social problems have generated enormous numbers of homeless people and patients with mental illness dumped onto the streets who formerly would have been hospitalized as inpatients, many more mentally disturbed people now come into contact with the general public than ever before. Consequently, the Memphis city government, the mental health community, and the police department realized that incidents of police involvement with the mentally ill had resulted in the mentally ill themselves being vulnerable to serious harm and the increased possibility of police officers, untrained in dealing with the mentally ill, getting seriously injured or even killed. Why can't mental health workers take care of the enormous numbers of emotionally out-of-control people on the streets? Because it is a physical and fiscal impossibility to put enough mental health workers onto the streets to monitor and serve the needs of these out-of-control people and to do so in accordance with the "least restrictive environment" movement in a democratic society.

Spearheaded by the local affiliate of the National Alliance on Mental Illness, the Memphis Police Department, the mental health community, the city government, and the counselor education and social

work departments of two local universities formed a unique and creative alliance for the purpose of developing and implementing proactive and preventive methods of containing emotionally explosive situations in the streets that frequently lead to violence. Because the police were the first and often the only responsible officials on the scene of an out-of-control situation, calling in outside consultants proved unworkable. Therefore, the unique and cohesive alliance of several important community groups determined that highly trained and motivated police officers were the logical personnel to form a frontline defense against the crisis of dangerously expressive, out-of-control persons in the streets. This massive alliance effort resulted in the CIT program becoming an example of how a successful program can work to accomplish the objectives of public safety and welfare, economic feasibility, and police accountability (James & Crews, 2014).

It is a bad error in judgment, though, to assume that CIT is just 40 hours of training. There has been a good deal of criticism that CIT has not lived up to its promise (Roger et al., 2019; Seo et al., 2021; Westervelt, 2020) and is merely a face-saving attempt by police departments and city administrators to cover their tracks when police violence toward the metal ill is uncovered. There is some merit in that argument. While Seo et al. (2021) in their meta-analysis found that, while CIT officers attitudes toward the mental ill and how they perceived the mentally ill should be handled by the justice system changed, little changed in regard to arrests and use of force. They concluded that CIT-type interactions with the mental ill were moderately effective, but outcomes were variable and depended on the model used. Koziarski et al. (2021) examined both CIT and Crisis Co-response teams in Canada and found that both types are dogged with a variety of challenges that can impede their success. Rogers et al.'s (2019) overall analysis indicates many of the same failures, although they found that where smaller jurisdictions adhered to the Memphis model, the outcomes were good.

Ron Bruno, the immediate past executive director of CIT International quoted in Westervelt's critical analysis, states that cities and counties too often fail to carefully integrate the program into the wider behavioral mental health care system and route calls away from the police. Put succinctly, CIT is not just training but a concept that entails a cooperative relationship between consumer organizations such as the local National Alliance on Mental Illness, local mental health care providers, and police departments working in an integrated and conjoint fashion. We have seen first hand that when that concept is not in operation, the approach will likely falter. However, in response to detractors, when it is an integrated community effort, it will be successful, and there is hard evidence to show that it is.

Our own experience in consulting with communities who wish to establish CIT programs and training police departments is that successful programs had complete buy in from the community and mental health providers and that those providers worked hand-in-hand in consulting, training, and evaluating, and following up and refining their programs. Regrettably, we have seen other communities that consider CIT to be a politically expedient way to appear to have face validity in dealing with the mentally ill but with little content validity behind it, and, as a result, they have poor outcomes that garner severe criticism and tarnish the image of CIT. All that being said, there is a good deal of evidence that if program quality is high and community commitment is also, outcomes will be good. Given the foregoing qualifiers, here is what typical training looks like.

The Concept. To comprehend what a difficult and delicate task it has been to bring to fruition a successful and workable CIT program, one must understand how the alliance network functions. If your community does not have such a program and you think it would be a good idea to get one started, read the following very carefully. The pervasiveness of mental illness, particularly those with mental illness who experience homelessness, is endemic and pervades all jurisdictions that attempt to establish CIT programs. Major Sam Cochran, who was the longtime coordinator of the Memphis CIT program and has been instrumental in helping disseminate the Memphis Model all over the country, puts it very well when he says, "It is not just a program to train police officers to deal with the mentally ill. It is a concept that brings all kinds of interest groups together in a network, and if that concept is not nourished, the program will fail."

The network behind the Memphis CIT program consists of the Memphis city government and the Memphis Police Department (hereafter just referred to as the police); the Alliance for the Mentally Ill; five of the six local community mental health centers; the emergency room components of public hospitals; academic educators from the Department of Counseling,

Educational Psychology and Research at the University of Memphis and the School of Social Work at the University of Tennessee; the YWCA Abused Women's Services; the Sexual Assault Resource Center; and several private practice psychologists and private mental health hospitals (hereafter referred to as the mental health community). The power, force, and success of the alliance derive from the process and fundamental working relationship that the police and mental health community have used to both form and maintain the CIT program. The alliance was formed because both the police and the mental health community realized that the problem of crisis in the streets was too severe for either to handle alone and that working together would make life much easier and safer for both as well as provide improved and safer service for clients and the community (James & Crews, 2014).

The alliance conducted a great many collaborative, systematic, and democratic meetings over a period of several months to hammer out a workable CIT blueprint. As a result of these meetings, key individuals from all segments of both the police and the mental health community developed effective working relationships with one another and learned a great deal about each other's problems, competencies, rules, and boundaries.

Police were brought into mental health facilities for an orientation into the world of mental health. Mental health personnel were brought into the police academy and accompanied police on patrols to learn about the problems, procedures, competencies, roles, and boundaries that law enforcement officers face in their everyday work. Then, formal training was developed to ensure that not only the CIT officer selectees but also all supervisory-level police personnel understood the problems, objectives, and operational procedures of the CIT program (James, 1994, p. 187; James & Crews, 2014). The development and training phases provided some essential attitudinal and professional understanding between the police and the mental health community. As a result, CIT officers and their superiors know precisely what training and consultation resources the mental health community can provide. And the mental health professionals know what competencies and resources the police in general and the CIT officers in particular have to offer.

This model is not just about training cops but developing collaborative efforts among police, the mental health community, and consumer advocates to provide first response mental health help to acutely ill individuals (Kasick & Bowling, 2013; Watson & Compton, 2019). Concomitantly, all sides develop mutual respect, understanding, trust, and cooperation. A CIT officer intervening with a distraught mental patient will likely listen empathically to the patient's feelings and concerns, be familiar with the mental health services available (will possibly know the patient's caseworker personally), and will, within the boundaries of professional ethics, communicate to the patient an understanding of the short-term needs of that person as well as a desire to provide for the immediate safety and referral requirements to contain and stabilize the patient's current crisis.

The mental health center caseworker will also understand and have confidence in the CIT officer's ability to be a stabilizing and safe influence on the patient and will, if needed, likely call on the CIT officer for emergency assistance with a particular client. The mental health caseworker may collaborate with the CIT officer in obtaining anecdotal information needed to enhance the patient's treatment plan and prevent the recurrence of that particular patient's crisis in the streets (James, 1994, p. 191). All of the foregoing happens with consumer advocates such as the local Alliance for the Mentally Ill playing a critical advisory role in the process.

Based on the trust and confidence built through the powerful and cohesive alliance just described, the police department opted to select experienced police patrol officers to receive training and then serve in the dual role of police officers and Crisis Intervention Team specialists. Volunteers for the program had to have good records as officers, pass personality tests for maturity and mental stability, and be recommended, interviewed, screened, and selected to receive CIT training. The police department committed itself to putting trained CIT officers on duty in every precinct in the city, 24 hours every day. All upper-echelon supervisory officers received a formal orientation about the role and function of CIT officers so whenever a call involving a suspected mentally disturbed person anywhere in the city is received, the CIT officer is the designated responsible law enforcement official at the scene—regardless of rank—and all other officers at the scene serve as backups to the CIT officer who handles the case (James, 1994, p. 194; James & Crews, 2014).

CIT Training Using Mental Health Experts and Providers. An integral part of the CIT program is the special preservice training provided for the officers.

The importance of effective training by competent, committed, motivated professionals cannot be overemphasized (Lavole & Alvarez, 2022). We also insist that they ride with experienced CIT officers on a Friday or Saturday evening shift prior to the scheduled training of each new group of CIT officers. As Erstling (2006) states, spending 8 hours in a patrol car together goes a long way toward learning to trust and understand one another.

The following topics are covered in the 40 hours of CIT training:

1. Cultural awareness of the mentally ill, including social locations awareness
2. Substance misuse and co-occurring disorders
3. People with cognitive and physical disabilities
4. Treatment strategies and mental health resources
5. Patient rights, civil commitment, and legal aspects of crisis intervention
6. Suicide intervention
7. Using the mobile crisis team and community resources
8. Psychotropic medications and their side effects
9. Verbal defusing and de-escalating techniques
10. Borderline and other personality disorders
11. Family and consumer perspectives
12. Fishbowl discussion on-site with patients with mental illness on patient perceptions of the police

The foregoing areas are largely subject matter information based. These educational sessions are supplemented with a group meeting with inpatients at a local mental health hospital, which is used to create a positive interaction of police and patient views of one another and hopefully facilitate understanding of each other's roles as providers and recipients of service. These sessions are all preparatory to progressive, step-wise more complex verbal de-escalation and defusing practicums over the last three days of training.

De-escalation and Defusing Techniques. Verbal de-escalation and defusing techniques are taught throughout the weeklong training. These skills are considered so critical that four different trainers are used for 12 hours of training. Basic introductory techniques are taught first. How do you introduce yourself? What is the nonverbal message you convey by your body posture and language? What voice tone do you use? These skills are taught on the second day of training.

Next come basic exploratory skills and establishing a relationship. Skills taught include (1) how and when to use open-ended and closed-ended questions, (2) what owning statements are and why they are important, (3) how to keep clients secure without cornering them (for more information, go to Chapter 14, "Violent Behavior in Institutions"), (4) officer and client safety, (5) crowd control, (6) when and when not to use reflection of feelings or thinking, and (7) summary recapping techniques and restatement for client and officer understanding and communication (Memphis Police Department, 2014). These skills are taught on the third day of training.

The training is also greatly enhanced if it can skillfully integrate the conceptual with the experiential. Realistic role play by veteran CIT officers and honest critique of trainees is essential. On the fourth day, four hours of training are devoted to role plays of actual police–client encounters. Veteran CIT officers role-play clients. These officers bring many valuable firsthand experiences into the learning environment that heighten interest, enhance motivation, and provide realism (James, 1994, p. 187). Trainees are divided into teams of four, and each member of the team is given 4 minutes onstage to attempt to defuse and de-escalate the client. The rest of the trainees (there are usually about 24–30) watch all of the teams perform and hear their critiques. The idea is that by watching others perform, trainees learn from the others' successes and failures. Scenarios range from clients with dementia chasing the devil out of the house with ammonia to consumers with schizophrenic episodes believing demons are coming out of the telephone to a person with diabetic psychosis who believes they are being poisoned by family members to enraged, jilted, suicidal spurned lovers to intoxicated veterans with PTSD diagnoses and hallucinating in the middle of a main street with five o'clock traffic. The only information trainees are given is a 911 operator's summary of the call before interaction with the role players starts. The role players escalate or de-escalate their aberrant behavior depending on how and what trainees do. After all four trainees have performed, a panel of veteran CIT officers and experienced mental health workers comment honestly and objectively on both positive and negative aspects of trainees' performance.

On the fifth day of training, complex CIT scenarios are demonstrated. All of the verbal skills used in preceding sessions are integrated to deal with very difficult clients. Such difficult scenarios as suicidal and clients with severe psychosis are demonstrated, and intervention techniques are broken

down and analyzed as to appropriate and inappropriate responses by a panel of veteran CIT officers and mental health workers. Instant replay is used after corrective support comments are made so positive outcomes occur and new skills are learned. At the end of the week, trainees have the basic skills necessary to intervene with the mentally ill. Like most beginners, the new CIT officers are a little unsure of themselves. However, one of our most rewarding experiences in this business has been seeing these officers come back to aid in training, having developed some of the most outstanding crisis intervention skills we have seen in the 50-plus years we have been doing this work.

Fishbowls With Clients. Fishbowl discussions are unique and powerful sessions for CIT trainees. During this component of the training, trainees are brought to an inpatient mental health facility to meet in a discussion group circle with selected mental health patients. A mental health professional, who also serves as an instructor in the CIT training program, sits in the center of the circle with the patients surrounded by the CIT trainees. The professional engages in interviews and dialogues with the mental health patients, in the "fishbowl," so to speak. CIT trainees observe and hear what patients with mental illness have to say about their own personal needs and about their prior interactions, experiences, and perceptions of the police. After the fishbowl interview and dialogue, trainees who had been observing the professional–patient dialogue have an opportunity to ask questions and interact directly with the patients. The fishbowl discussion has been described by CIT trainees as profoundly motivational and an essential part of their learning, orientation, and training.

The Success of CIT. In more than four decades since its start in Memphis, CIT has grown exponentially, with training centers now located throughout the country and thousands of police officers trained in its protocols (Saunders, 2010). It is noteworthy that the CIT concept is now international, with its own newsletter and convention. *The Team News*, the newsletter of CIT International, is available at http://www.citinternational.org. CIT programs can now be found across the United States, Canada, Australia, and Sweden. But is there any evidence it really works?

In its first 16 months of operation in 1987–1988, Memphis CIT officers responded to 5,831 mental disturbance calls and transported 3,424 people to mental health facilities without any patient fatalities.

Wright-Carrier (1992) conducted a pre- and post-16 months baseline analysis start-up of the Memphis Police CIT operations. She found significant differences in the increase of mental health calls, increased transport to mental health facilities, a decrease in the number and length of barricade situations where people with emotional disturbance refuse to come out of their domiciles, and a decrease in officer injuries post start-up. Both calls and transports have increased significantly over the 35-plus years the program has been in operation. This increase in "mental disturbance" service calls happens in other jurisdictions as well (Kisely et al., 2010; Teller et al., 2006) and is most likely attributable to increased awareness by the public of the CIT program. That increased awareness is particularly true of relatives and others responsible for the care and well-being of the mentally ill. Publication and support by the National Alliance on Mental Illness (2011) for CIT officers has led to the belief that caregivers' loved ones will be handled in a sensitive manner and not be killed or injured by the police.

Along with increased calls, there appears to be a reduction in the use of force. (Compton et al., 2008; Wills et al., 2023), more diversion from jail to hospitals (Compton et al., 2014b; Lamb et al., 2004; Ritter et al., 2011; Skeem & Bibeau, 2008), decreases in time spent on each call, and increased cooperation between mental health service providers and police (Kisely et al., 2010). In a comprehensive review of research outcomes, Compton and associates (2008) found that, along with a reduction in the use of force by CIT officers, officers had more sensitivity toward the mentally ill with commensurate diversion instead of arrest, fewer officer injuries, and reduced hostage team callouts. Schriver (2021) examined the introduction of CIT officers on 76 college campuses and found that 10 percent of calls were for mental health issues that encompassed suicidal ideation, substance misuse, homelessness, and violence toward others. Over half of the officers in the departments had CIT training, and the number of CIT officers was related to the perceived effectiveness of handling calls and diffusing the crisis. Khalsa et al. (2018) examined 6,353 mental illness calls to Colorado police. Their findings included SWAT use less than 1 percent, injuries less than 1 percent, and use of force less than 5 percent. Transfer for treatment was significantly higher for psychiatric illness, suicide threat or attempt, psychiatric illness and drug use, and violence potential. These findings occurred even in the presence of a weapon or threat of violence. Perhaps as significant, they found that the risk of suicide reduced the odds of transfer to jail.

From those positive hard data outcomes, Watson and Compton (2019) argue that when the total concept of CIT's community involvement with police is followed, there is enough evidence to move CIT from a "best practices" designation to "evidenced based."

A footnote is warranted here. There is a dearth of hard, evidence-based outcomes in the whole field of crisis intervention given it is nonconductive in any way, shape, or form to controlled experimental study. For all the criticism garnered by law enforcement, it is one of the few arenas in which hard data outcomes are being retrieved and studied. In summary, given this writer's inherent positive bias having been one of the original founders in Memphis, if done in a comprehensive way that involves high community involvement and support, there is enough empirical evidence to support its continued use.

Co-respondent Teams. A variation on the CIT program is the co-response team program, which teams a mental health professional with a police officer (Abramson, 2021; Lakey, 2023; Savage & Morabito, 2020; Semple et al., 2020; University of Cincinnati Center for Police Research and Policy, n.d.-a; Westervelt, 2020). These setups are different than a mobile crisis team, which would have only a mental health practitioner making a crisis intervention call. The model pairs a trained police officer with a mental health professional to respond to individuals having behavioral health crises. The purpose is to de-escalate the crisis, keep the respondent out of the criminal justice system, and connect them to appropriate health providers. There are wide variations to this model with funding, geographical issues, personnel resources, and specific fit to the community. Responses may be primary, initial, contacts, secondary follow-ups, or both. Mental health professionals may physically be "ride alongs" or "rides separate" or be "remote and on call." Hours of operation vary greatly but generally are available late afternoon and evening hours when incident calls are greatest. Given these variations, it is difficult to determine specific outcomes, but the University of Cincinnati Center for Police Research and Policy (n.d.-a) has garnered these potential outcomes from a comprehensive review of the programs:

1. Limited evidence suggests that co-responder teams de-escalation efforts result in fewer incidents where force is used and lower rates of injury compared to when either police or mental health professionals are working alone.

2. Research suggests better and more efficient referral to behavioral health systems.

3. It appears there are lower arrest rates with co-responder teams.

4. Lower rates of police retention for mental health problems appear to occur.

5. Officer time spent on these calls appears to be reduced. That outcome is critical in getting officers back into service with officer shortages and backed-up calls.

6. There is limited evidence that they may be cost effective to police departments.

7. They appear to reduce pressure on the behavioral health care system with fewer hospitalizations and emergency department visits.

8. Stronger interagency collaboration appears to strengthen greater communication and trust between police and mental health agencies.

9. Advertising the positive and true of the apparent alliance with the community in an age of paranoia and suspicion of police seems to be a major achievement.

10. Outlining policies and procedures appears to allow for greater consistency and accountability in the delivery of services. Note that all of the foregoing findings have "limited" and "appear" as qualifiers.

There are major advantages to this approach. Clearly, one of the primary ones is worker safety. As with police entering domestic violence situations, there is nothing more dangerous than making a home visit when a crisis is occurring. The second is consultation. The two heads are better than one concept when de-escalation breaks down can serve both CIT officers and mental health workers well. Further, the "ride alongs" specifically serve to break down cultural barriers and foment a "We are in this together team approach," and occupational barriers and cultural stereotypes come down.

There is not a lot of outcome data on co-responder units given their variability of implementation. Marcus and Stergiopulus (2022) reviewed 1,018 articles on both CIT and co-responder studies and summarized that the reports are largely observational, low or moderate quality, and lacking control groups (2022). Three Canadian studies (Ghelani et al., 2022; Koziaerski, 2021; Semple et al., 2020) found varying degrees of success and challenges in implementation. Semple and associates' study found significant differences between co-response teams and regular police units in time spent on calls, reduced cost of service, an increase in community resources, and a decrease in involuntary apprehensions. Ghelani and associates reviewed eight studies and found reduced involuntary hospital transport, improved referral, and reduced emergency department wait times. An Australian study (Meehan et al., 2019) also reported reduced emergency department use and successful resolution of the crisis in the majority of cases No outcomes in regard to use of force or client or responder injuries were detailed. Systemically, a number of co-responder programs are the zero-baseline start point of the Sequential Intercept Model (SIM).

Sequential Intercept Model (SIM)

The Sequential Intercept Model (SIM) was developed to create an interface and integration between criminal justice systems and mental health systems in an attempt to decriminalize mental illness contacts with the police (Munetz & Griffin, 2006) in the twenty-first century. The model has gained traction as a viable alternative to putting the mentally ill in the U.S. biggest mentally ill holding facilities—jails and prisons. Since its inception, the SIM's credence has grown tremendously and is now included in the 21st Century Cures Act. The model is designed as an effective framework for systematically assessing available community resources, finding service gaps between mental health and justice systems, identifying and locating opportunities for diversion from the criminal justice system, and implementing reforms at six distinct justice decision points or "intercepts." (Substance Abuse and Mental Health Services Administration, 2022).

The six points (Substance Abuse and Mental Health Services Administration, 2022) start with emergency services and health services providers at point 0. The co-responder team is a good example of a 0-point contact or initial impact with criminal justice system personnel who answer 911 calls for emotional disturbances from specially trained dispatchers. At intercept point 1, co-responders make contact and attempt to de-escalate the crisis. At intercept point 2, a court hearing occurs, and attempts are made to match services with individuals and provider services. Pretrial supervision and diversion services are put in place to reduce sentencing to jail. Initial assessment and screening for mental disorders and substance misuse issues occurs.

Intercept point 3 involves adjudication to specialized courts such as adult drug, mental health, and veterans treatment courts. And, if jailed, a provision to provide behavioral health and medical treatment to detainees is made. Point 4 involves pre-release transition planning for release from incarceration. Medication and prescription access are set up for post-release. Case managers are closely involved with prerelease planning. Intercept point 5 occurs with follow-up by specialized community case managers with close supervision of parolee caseloads with mental disorders. Those services would include medication compliance assistance and checks for medical assistance to prevent relapse. Access to recovery supports, benefits, and employment is facilitated by supervisors.

The SIM is a laudable and viable model. However, our own personal experience in a number of years in corrections work makes us reserved in passing judgment on its overall success because of the current lack of funding and support to deal with the huge population of mentally ill individuals currently incarcerated in the United States and the critical infrastructure and support staff to implement SIM. Hopefully, as SIM takes further hold and evolves, this will change. While SIM has a financial cost, that cost is insignificant when keeping a mentally ill individual in jail in Shelby County, Tennessee cost about 60,000 dollars a year.

LO4 **Suicide by Cop.** Indeed, it is extremely significant that the death toll is so low when CIT officers and co-responders make the scene of a crisis event such as a shooting, hostage, or barricade situation. A fairly common phenomenon called "suicide by cop" has been well established (Lord, 2015). In essence, people who do not quite have the courage to kill themselves engage in some activity that gains the attention of the police. Once the police arrive, they engage the police in a threatening manner and succeed in getting themselves shot. In short, the cops complete the suicide (Lindsay & Lester, 2004). Police are highly aware of this dangerous phenomenon and are also very interested in learning how to handle it (Lindsay & Lester, 2004; Vermette et al., 2005). Indeed, the research suggests that tighter bonds and coordination between police and mental health providers, such as what occurs in CIT and co-responder programs, can reduce this phenomenon (Dewey et al., 2013).

Why is this so? A number of studies (Bonfine et al., 2014; Compton et al., 2006, 2014a; Ellis, 2014) have examined a number of variables of CIT officers immediately before and after undergoing CIT training. After training, those officers demonstrated much-improved attitudes, more support for treatment, more knowledge, less social distancing, more confidence in dealing with the mentally ill, and less stigmatization of them. In summary, besides their increased skill at defusing and de-escalating the violent mentally ill and emotionally disturbed, CIT police officers have become some of the most caring and concerned crisis workers the mentally ill have. Indeed, it is much more difficult to get a cop to kill you when that police officer is doing everything they can to diffuse and de-escalate the situation and prevent any kind of suicide from occurring. Given the foregoing, Perrou (2019) has detailed fifteen indicators of suicide-by-cop potential. These indicators closely parallel those found in the suicide chapter, except when they are occurring in a law enforcement situation, the triage rating will typically be in the high twenties lethal range. The 15 indicators are that the subject:

1. is barricaded and refuses to negotiate,
2. has just killed someone, particularly a close relative, his mother, wife, or child,
3. says that he has a life-threatening illness,
4. demands of police do not include negotiations for escape or freedom,
5. has undergone one or more traumatic life changes —(death of a loved one, divorce, financial devastation, etc.),
6. before the encounter, the subject has given away all of his money or possessions,
7. has a record of assaults,
8. says he will only surrender to the person in charge,
9. indicates that he has thought about planning his death,
10. has expressed an interest in wanting to die in a "macho" way,
11. expresses interest in "going out in a big way,"
12. expresses feelings of hopelessness or helplessness,
13. dictates his will to negotiators,
14. demands to be killed, and
15. sets a deadline to be killed.

So if you are a co-responder working a potential suicide-by-cop situation, Perrou (2019) has also listed indicators that you are de-escalating the situation and progressing toward a peaceful resolution. If these indicators are occurring, you are on the right track and should stick with what you are doing. These are also good indicators you are making progress with hostile, violent clients in Chapter 14, "Violent Behavior in Institutions." So, along with Perrou (2019), here are our own indicators:

1. There is less interactive tension. The safety, social location or friction is markedly diminished.
2. There is a lower voice tone, with more modulated and tempered conversation and less anger, profanity, and threats of violence.
3. There is diminished aggressive body language, particularly less hypervigilance and agitated movements and gestures with calmer, more controlled body language.
4. There is less pronouncement of hopelessness and helplessness and more vocalization of a possible future.
5. There is a greater willingness to listen to co-responders' suggestions, interact, and consider suggestions.
6. There is an honorable, face-saving solicitation to a solution, i.e., "We'll go out the back door and back the crowd out front away so they won't see you."

Transcrisis Handling in Long-Term Therapy

LO5   Clients in long-term therapy are not immune from crisis (Ford, 2021). Therapy tends to move in developmental stages with psychological troughs, crests, and plateaus. Even though clients have success in meeting therapeutic goals, each new stage brings with it what are seen in many instances to be even more formidable obstacles. The beginning therapist who has seen a client make excellent progress is often in for a rude awakening when the client's progress comes completely undone, and behavior regresses to pretherapeutic functioning—or worse!

Anxiety Reactions

A puzzling aspect of therapy occurs when clients are highly successful in achieving tremendously difficult goals and then are completely undone by a task that, to the objective observer, does not seem all that difficult. Although it seems cognitively irrational, the fear of failure to achieve this minor goal becomes a self-fulfilling prophecy. The client fears that others will see through their sham of competence and irrationally thinks that any real progress is a delusion. At such times, clients engage in various types of flight behavior. Severe anxiety is one

way of escaping the threatening situation. Consider Melanie's present dilemma. Melanie has escaped from a marriage to a physically abusive ex-husband with alcohol misuse disorder and subsequently completed two years of secretarial science at a community college, but she has fallen apart when faced with an interview for a job she desperately wants. She has done a lot of work with her community college counselor in developing a resume and role-playing job interviews, plus working through a poor self-concept and failure identity after escaping a failed abusive marriage.

Melanie: (extremely anxious and agitated, calling her Adult Vocational School counselor at 1 A.M.) I hated to call you, but I'm so scared. I've thrown up twice, and I've got the shakes. This hasn't happened since I walked out on Bill over three years ago. God, I can't get a grip, and I need to do my best tomorrow. I know I'll just blow it. I can't think straight, and I can't remember a thing about interviewing. Everything's just running together.

The vocational counselor, now turned crisis interventionist, puts Melanie at a 5 on the triage scale for cognitive and behavioral threat and a 6 for affective anxiety/fear. If the therapist does not help diminish the anxiety, the potential is that Melanie may move upward to 8–9 on these scales by the time she goes for her job interview.

CO: Just do this for a minute, Melanie. Take a deep breath, and let it out slo-o-owly. That's right! Now take another! OK, again. (Continues in a patient, calm voice for about 2 minutes, taking Melanie through a brief deep-breathing exercise to calm her anxiety attack.)

After the deep-breathing exercise, when Melanie has regained some semblance of control, the counselor paces with her through the role play they had conducted the previous session, has her write down her blunders and strong points, discusses those with her, determines that her attack is receding, and assesses her as now being between a 2 and a 3 on the subscales. A quick review of the client's other successes reinforces and further buttresses the positive change in current functioning.

CO: Now notice the change in your voice. I'll bet you've also calmed down to where you aren't shaking. Did you notice how much more you're in control now? Remember what you're there for. Although a lot depends on this for you, you've also done even bigger, more threatening and scary things in your life like getting the hell out of that malignant marriage. Remember! You've become very good in secretarial science. They need you as much as or more than you need them. I want you to put that up as a big signboard in your head, in Day-Glo pink: THEY NEED YOU JUST AS MUCH AS YOU NEED THEM!

By role-playing the scene, the counselor puts Melanie back on familiar ground and puts the problem back into context—getting a job as opposed to having a free-floating anxiety attack. By marshaling the client's resources and very specifically and objectively reminding her of what her strengths are, the therapist concretizes the vague dread she feels at having to face the interview. The therapist's exhortation about who needs whom is not placating here. It is realistic. Melanie's ego needs to be reminded of these facts so she will have a positive mental set toward both her personhood and her skills as she enters the interview. Finally, the therapist offers her the opportunity to have a safety net.

CO: Melanie, I think you're ready to get some sleep and go knock their socks off tomorrow. However, if you wake up tomorrow morning and really have some questions or think you need to role-play that interview once more, give me a call. I've got some free time before your interview, and we can go over it once more. Now go to bed, get some sleep, and dream about that Day-Glo pink billboard.

By leaving her with a positive injunction and making time for her the next day, the therapist continues to provide a support system and a security net for Melanie.

Regression

The risk of taking the next step in therapeutic development may become too overwhelming, even though clients have been highly successful in attaining prior goals. When clients are overwhelmed, they may regress in their behavior, retreating to maladaptive but familiar ways of behaving, feeling, and thinking (Stewart, 2012).

Melanie: (somewhat embarrassed and mumbling in a childlike voice) I know what you're going to say, but I was thinking I really couldn't cut this, and Bill made that offer even after I got him arrested that

he still loved me and was getting help, and I know he doesn't drink much anymore.

CO: (interpreting the dynamics) What you're really saying is the prospect of that interview is scaring the hell out of you, and it's so scary that you'd give up 3 years of hard work and sacrifice to go back to a really lousy, not to mention dangerous, way of living, when you're about to get the gold ring. I'm wondering why you've decided to sabotage yourself now.

By interpreting the client's dependency needs of the client, the therapist welds regressive thinking to the current threat of becoming independent as manifested in the job interview. Although the client's behavior and affect are not blatant, she is moving insidiously higher on the triage cognitive loss subscale. Left alone, that negative self-talk could convince the client to give up her new self-identity and go back to the long-dead and dangerous marriage.

The interventionist is really working hard on a major component of Ford's (2021) FREEDOM acronym and is recycling back to client safety and refocusing on present functioning (pp.116–117). If Melanie continues in her reactive emotional set, she could move further into Caplain's (1964) crisis stage 3 toward a behavioral emergency. The therapist needs to get Melanie to recognize her emotional and cognitive triggers that are propelling her toward complete emotional dysregulation and refocus her on the present, real time and reassess herself in light of her new strengths and skills.

Melanie: Oh, I just knew you'd say that, but I'm not sure I can do this. I mean a big outfit like United Techtronic.

CO: (in a cool, clear, no-nonsense, but not condemning, voice) Big or small, United Techtronic is not the question. The question is, are you going to choose to blow this before you even see if you can cut it? That's one way of never finding out if you're good enough. You can make that choice, although you've now been making a different one for 3 years. I'd hope you wouldn't do that—I believe you are good enough—but then, it's your choice.

This reality-based approach (Glasser, 1965) directly confronts the client with the underlying and unwarranted irrational decision she is about to make and vividly points out how she is trying to delude herself into buying back into a dependent status and revictimizing herself.

Problems of Termination

When clients have met their goals for therapy, are fully functioning, and are ready to get back to the business of living their own lives, they may suddenly produce terrible problems that only their therapist can solve. Whatever these problems are, it is an excellent bet that they have been told that it's time to terminate, or they have figured out that termination is about to happen. At such times, it is a common occurrence for dependency issues to arise. These problems generally can be resolved by successively approximating the client to termination. For example, instead of every week, the counselor schedules the student every 2 weeks, then once a month, and then for a 6-month follow-up. The other option is to clearly discuss the possibility that this issue will arise (Norcross et al., 2017).

CO: Melanie, I think it's time we discussed you spreading your wings and flying away from here. You landed that job and . . .

Melanie: (interrupts) But I couldn't have done that without you. You give me the courage to try those things. You've been so wonderful. I just couldn't have done any of this without you. And there's still the problem with the kids and . . .

CO: (gently interrupting) I appreciate those compliments. They mean a lot to me. Yet although we've worked together on those things, it's been you who's done it, not I. What I want to talk about with you now is some of those fears and really being on your own, like what you just said. That's pretty common to have those feelings; lots of people do. Sort of like when you left home the first time. I want you to know I'll be here if you need me, but I want you also to know that I think it's time for you to be on your own. I'd like to discuss this with you in today's session. You're a different person than when you walked into the adult ed center two years ago. You have a high school diploma; you've even got some community college credits. Your word processing skills are excellent and so is your organizational ability, real concrete assets you didn't have, plus determination and staying power in tough times. I take pride in helping you accomplish those things, but it's you who did it and this is just the start of a great career path. I'll miss our time together, but that's the whole idea about school and, for that matter, counseling. Moving forward. Sure there'll be pot holes in life, and you may need to get a tune up once in a while, but that's life and we pretty much don't grow if we don't run into and get out of those, and you've sure shown that.

Norcross et al. (2017) examined the responses of 65 therapists representing an eclectic array of different therapeutic modalities in regard to their terminating behaviors. They found a surprising number of commonalities.

The general findings were:

1. Reflect on the client's growth and on how they plan to continue that growth.
2. Discuss the therapeutic process—both what went well in therapy and what could have been better.
3. Discuss any feelings of grief or anxiety about ending the treatment relationship.
4. Talk about personal growth as an ongoing process and give the client guidelines for when it might be appropriate to return to therapy.
5. Urge the client to use the new skills learned in therapy.
6. Frame personal development as unfinished and ongoing.
7. Express pride in the client's progress and the relationship.
8. Prepare explicitly for termination.

Crisis in the Therapy Session

One of the scariest times for a therapist occurs when a technique has done its job exceedingly well, and the client gains insight or release from a deeply buried traumatic experience—and then completely loses control. This unexpected turn of events can unsettle the most experienced therapist. As this wellspring of affect emerges, it may go far beyond cathartic insight and leave the client in a severe state of disequilibrium.

At this point, it is absolutely mandatory to stay in control of the situation and take a firm and directive stance, no matter how frightening the client's actions or how personally repulsive the uncovered material may be. Our own admonition to students is, "You may feel physically sick, start to break out in a sweat, and wish to be anyplace else but in that room. After the session is over, you can have a world-class anxiety attack if you wish—you probably deserve it—but right now, you are the therapist, and you are going to stick with the client." By demonstrating cool levelheadedness to the client, the therapist is modeling behavior that the client can emulate. Further, there is the legal, ethical, and moral issue of client abandonment, and that is not a character-building experience you want to have on your record or conscience in any of those three venues.

CO: I'm just wondering if the reason you ever got into that abusive marriage is that sometimes your father might have abused your mother, and that's what was modeled as the way a marriage ought to be.

Melanie: (recoils in a shocked state) He never did have intercourse with me.

CO: (taken aback) I'm not quite sure what you said— "intercourse"?

Melanie: (breaking down and sobbing) For 12 years, that bastard would mess with me and my sister, and Momma knew. She knew and wouldn't do anything about it. (completely breaks down) I . . . God . . . he beat us if we didn't do . . . he'd make us masturbate him . . . oh Lord . . . how could he . . . I've kept this secret . . . I can't handle this. I should have done something . . . killed him . . . (uncontrolled and wracked sobbing and shaking).

CO: (recomposing herself and gently touching Melanie's arm and quietly talking in a consoling and affirming voice) I am truly sorry for uncovering that old wound, but you *can* handle it. You've finally got it out. You lived with that hell as a child and another hell as an adult. You are a survivor. I'm sorry I triggered that buried hell, but I think it is good you were able to trust me enough to speak to it. That takes a great deal of courage. I am angry and sad that happened. Yet here you are. A survivor and moving forward with your life, and I appreciate your tenacity and sheer guts and determination.

Ford (2021) writes a great deal about emotional dysregulation not only in the client but in the therapist as well. That is particularly true when the therapist is blind-sided by unknown material that launches the client into crisis. Staying the course with her, the therapist owns her feelings honestly and uses a broken record to reaffirm and reaffirm the client's strengths.

Psychotic Breaks

Staying calm and cool is even more important when a person is having a psychotic break from reality. No matter how delusional or dissociative the client becomes, the central thesis is that if the client can maintain contact with reality and take at least a modicum of constructive action, then stay in the game.

Manuel: (walks into the therapist's office unannounced and unknown) I need help, and they recommend you. But no telephones, they listen to me through the telephone. (Picks up the telephone in a threatening manner.)

CO: (in a slow, even voice) I need for you to put that telephone down before we go any further. I will help you, but I want you to put the telephone back on the stand. We've never had the pleasure of meeting. What is your name?

Manuel: It's Manuel. (hesitates) I'm just coming apart. They won't leave me alone.

CO: I understand that, but I need you to put the phone down and keep it together so you can tell me who's after you. Go ahead and sit down and tell me what's bothering you.

The counselor immediately dropped into crisis intervention mode with this unknown but clearly extremely agitated person. She institutes Cochran's (2014) game plan—get a name, make contact, ask an open-ended lead, but attempt to get some behavioral compliance by calmly asking who the person is, and invite him to tell his story but on the condition that he sit down and do so in a calm manner.

Manuel: It's my on-site intern supervisor. He wants to fire me and catch me stealing, so he listens in on my phone conversations. They'll kick me off the intern site and out of school. He's in league with Satan, and he's probably in this room. I can smell the brimstone. Can't you? (Starts to become agitated and mumble about hell.)

CO: (calmly but in an assertive voice) No, I can't. If you think it's coming from the phone, move away from it so we can concentrate on the problem with your supervisor. OK! You're having trouble with your supervisor. Now we're getting somewhere. That's good, but stay with me. I personally guarantee Satan is not here. I want to know about your supervisor and how long this has been going on. The community college is not going to kick you out. I'll be acting as your advocate so put that idea out in orbit with Mars. I also want to get you to a safe place where nobody can hurt you, but to do that I need your help, and I need you to stay in contact, so I can help you.

Manuel: OK. (Sits down and starts to talk about his supervisor.)

The community college counselor's humdrum day of going over student resumes comes to a screeching halt, and she is now in full crisis interventionist mode with initial TAF ratings of: Affective is 8/9 (feeling negative and highly volatile with limited control of emotions and situation generalizing to other areas). Behavior is 10 with daily functioning impaired and impulsivity likely to be harmful and intensify the situation. Cognitive is 10+ with decision making frozen and not based in reality with thoughts that are hallucinatory and delusional and are completely controlled by the crisis.

She immediately seeks to establish contact by obtaining the client's name, while at the same time establishing ground rules for conduct in the counselor's office. When the young man starts to dissociate and talk incoherently, the counselor is directive and seeks to keep Manuel in contact with reality by focusing the discussion on his grievance with his supervisor. While she validates the client's fear, the only acknowledgment she gives to evil spirits is her concern for the client's safety. A cardinal rule is that you may acknowledge the client's duress from the hallucination, but you never side with it. The counselor reinforces the client for staying in contact with her and repeats her request to put the telephone down. Because clients with psychosis may have difficulty hearing others because of the intrusive hallucinations assailing them, the therapist slowly and clearly repeats her requests for compliance (broken record). By staying in control, the therapist turns a potentially violent situation with an unknown client into a satisfactory resolution.

It would be easy to become unhinged with the olfactory hallucination and the agitated paranoia the client is manifesting. A first major consideration is safety, and that means the worker's physical safety, which will be discussed at length in Chapter 14, "Violent Behavior in Institutions." If the decision is made to stay with the client, and this is indeed risky since his triage is clearly in the high twenties, then she will need to be very aware of safety issues and read Chapter 14, "Violent Behavior in Institutions," on how to do that. If she stays with this client who is in Caplain's (1964) Stage 4, which is a breakdown of health and psychosocial functioning, then it may seem paradoxical, but focusing on strength and resilience is critical in Stage 4. She is going to need to put on her best Carl Rogers counseling cloak on and communicate empathic and nonjudgmental understanding and focus on any positive behaviors she can glean from the client (Ford, 2021, pp. 27–28).

CO: So if I understand correctly, the stress from your supervisor has gotten so severe that it has started manifesting itself in evil smells. Yet, as bad as it has become, you've had the strength and sharpness of mind to come to counseling seek some answers. I think that takes a lot of courage and foresight, and if you can stay calm and collected as you are doing now, we'll work through this until we get some help. Can you do that?

People With Borderline Personality Disorder (BPD)

LO6 Most clients try to manipulate their therapists during the course of therapy for a variety of reasons. These reasons may range from avoiding engagement in new behaviors to testing the therapist's credibility. Clients with personality disorders are the ultimate test of the therapist's ability to handle manipulative behavior and can create severe crises for themselves and the therapist if not dealt with in very specific ways (Kocmur & Zavasnik, 1993). At the top of that list is the person diagnosed with borderline personality disorder (BPD). In 1938, Adolph Stern, an American psychotherapist, described a group of clients who did not respond well to treatment and, in fact, generally got worse. He labeled them as a "borderline group" that lay somewhere between neurosis and psychosis (Stern, 1938). While that notion is no longer deemed valid (Paris, 2008, p. 3), no one has yet come up with a better way to describe clients who have some of the most intractable, stubborn character pathology imaginable, and it has been named borderline personality disorder (BPD), although there are critical current views of it as a stigmatizing label and whether it even exists as an identifiable diagnoses!

So in a more contemporary view, Napal-Femandez (2019) characterizes BPD as "at the border" in regard to behaviors society perceives as "mad" and places them on the edge and at variance with Western binary stereotypes and "on the border" between culturally defined masculine and feminine behavior. Napal-Femandez proposes it is no surprise that the diagnosis is more frequent in women, LGBTQIA+ persons who don't fit the standard universal "subject" built from the male model. Masland et al. (2023) take this criticism a step further and propose that BPD is one of the most gender stigmatized of psychological disorders, and there is research to support this conjecture (Modeste, 2021).

This feminist view is one part of an ongoing controversy surrounding BPD as a viable diagnosis. Zanders et al. (2019) argue that BPD is fraught with conceptual difficulties in differentiating it from other major mental illnesses and may be only a variation of those maladies, although at present, it is generally listed as comorbid with them.

BPD's controversial nature is international as well. With the addition of it in the *International Classification of Diseases 11th Revision* (ICD-11) (WHO, 2019), the pressure to include the plethora of these challenging patients conflicts with the lack of an evidence-based and credible diagnostic system (Gutierrez et al., 2023). Gutierrez and associates (2023) conducted research on 1,799 identified BPD subjects by comparing them with the *ICD-11* domains for the borderline pattern. Statistical analysis did not differentiate BPD as a distinct construct and found it undifferentiated from general negative affectivity. Their caustic conclusion was that the BPD pattern is superfluous and even misguiding.

So with this introductory understanding that not only are the people who manifest a BPD diagnosis controversial and full of contradictions but so is the disorder itself, here's what you are likely to see when meeting a person diagnosed with BPD and why they take center stage as individuals in transcrisis.

- Current estimates are that about 2.7 percent of the adult population in the United States are candidates for a BPD diagnoses and also are likely to have co-occurring mood, anxiety, and substance misuse disorders (Tomko et al., 2014). The keystone for BPD is emotional dysregulation (Bud et al., 2023). Linehan's (1993) DBT biosocial model is the theory of how these emotionally dysregulating symptoms arise and are maintained.
- Carpenter et al. (2013) have extrapolated Linehan's (1993) original biosocial model of emotional dysregulation into four parts: emotion sensitivity, heightened and labile negative affect, a deficit of appropriate regulation strategies, and a surplus of maladaptive regulation strategies. Those are appropriate clinical descriptors, but they hardly describe how a person with borderline personality will manifest those psychological characteristics.

An individual's normal personality construct implies stable and enduring patterns of thinking, feeling, and acting across time and situation (Reyes et al., 2008). The person with borderline personality disorder is the antithesis of that construct, and this particular disorder of personality is a handmaiden to many of the crises in this book—particularly if the traumatic event occurred during childhood (Schultze, 2023; Godbout et al., 2019; Zanarini, 2000). Indeed, a whole field of therapy called **mentalization** (Bateman & Fognagy, 2006; Kvarstein et al., 2015; Kvarstein et al., 2019; Harpoth et al., 2020) has developed that specifically targets trauma in childhood and the lack of attachment to significant positive parenting figures as a major precursor to "getting" BPD.

Probably the best way to describe this disorder is through the title of Kreisman and Straus' (2010) classic book for people attempting to live and deal with borderline personalities: *I Hate You—Don't Leave Me*. There is good reason for this ambivalence. Indeed, there is a good deal of evidence that many individuals with borderline personality disorder have had a rogues' gallery of childhood horrors of physical and sexual abuse and long-term parental neglect (Allen, 2001; Brown, 2009; Herman et al., 1989; Schultze et al., 2022; Sroufe et al., 2005; Stalker & Davies, 1995). The rate of childhood sexual assault has been estimated to be a staggering 75 percent in people with borderline personality disorder (Battle et al., 2004). As a result, persons with BPD may be diagnosed as have co-occurring disorders of PTSD and BPD (Harned & Sloth, 2022; Kleindienst et al., 2021; Oshodi et al., 2020) and are likely candidates for what many practitioners and researchers refer to as "complex PTSD" (Briere & Scott, 2006; Courtois & Ford, 2009).

Complex PTSD can be loosely described as symptoms of PTSD coalescing with those of BPD into a veritable psychological swamp of bad affective, behavioral, and cognitive outcomes. Diagnosis can be extremely problematic because persons with BPD may manifest antisocial personality disorder (Falcus & Johnson, 2018), depressive and bipolar disorder (Mneimne et al., 2018; Woodard, 2023), schizophrenia, and attention deficit hyperactivity disorder (Paris, 2018) along with drug misuse and about anything else in the DSM 5-TR (American Psychiatric Association, 2022) depending on the highly idiosyncratic nature of the presenting problems.

The DSM 5-TR (2022) requires that for a diagnosis of BPD, the individual must manifest five of the nine identifying criteria, which are: fear of abandonment, unstable or changing relationships, unstable self-image, stress-related paranoia, anger management including temper tantrums and physical fighting, self-injury, suicidal ideation and suicidal behavior, frequent mood swings, and impulsive behaviors such as excessive spending, sexual practices that are unsafe, reckless driving, substance misuse, and binge eating. Given the foregoing characteristics and behaviors, it should not be surprising that there is a behavioral kaleidoscope of presenting problems. Indeed, one of the major problems of diagnoses is that no two persons with BPD are cut out of the same bolt of psychological cloth and may present very differently. That warning given, the following mnemonic IMPULSIVE (Senger, 1997) with descriptors (Biskin & Paris, 2012) followed by our own warning signs is a good yardstick for meeting BPD criteria:

1. **I**mpulsiveness in two damaging areas such as unsafe, promiscuous sex, excessive shopping/spending, eating disorders, drug use, and on and on.

2. **M**ood instability with excessive, dramatic, and rapid mood swings ranging from euphoria to depression triggered by external events and extreme sensitivity to them.

3. **P**aranoia or dissociation when under real or imagined stress. This particularly includes suspicions involving relationships and feeling of disconnect from oneself or that the world is unreal (derealization).

4. **U**nstable self-image of who and what the patient is.

5. **L**abile, intense relationships with extreme possessiveness and trust issues. The "I hate you, don't leave me" conundrum.

6. **S**uicidal thinking, gestures, and self-injury. Lots of BPD is first identified by emergency room admission for suicide attempts.

7. **I**nappropriate anger beyond acceptable social boundaries, including temper tantrums, rage events, and even fighting over inconsequential matters.

8. **V**ulnerability to abandonment with frantic efforts to avoid real or imagined abandonment and continuing paranoia that it will happen, which becomes a self-fulfilling prophecy and wrecks relationships.

9. **E**mptiness in a profound, existential way that life is pretty much meaningless, which can lead to the hopelessness of suicidal ideation and "I don't give a damn" behavior.

Whether BPD actually exists as an identifiable stand-alone malady is open to question. Paris (2018) puts it well, though, stating that even when all of these other maladies are comorbid, they cannot account for the complexity of the disorder. So while they are tough customers and can be extremely trying, there are some pretty good reasons

that persons with borderline diagnoses act the way they do and are the hallmark of the client who is in transcrisis.

Because of these early experiences with trusted others who could not be trusted, the person with a borderline personality has serious attachment problems that can rapidly surface in therapy. There is evidence that these individuals also harbor a deep sense of betrayal (Kaehler & Freyd, 2009). As you can readily see, there is good reason for this mistrust, sense of betrayal, and thus the constant vigilance, testing of the relationship, and paranoia that mark therapy with these individuals.

All-pro, all-star, and all-world therapists have trouble dealing with these individuals, so why in the world are we exposing you rookies to them? First of all, they provide a good example of how manipulative clients can work you over and lead you into being a case example in our chapter on burnout. More importantly, perhaps, they are clients you will run into that manifest many of the crises in this book. Among other maladies, they misuse drugs, become violent, are suicidal, are involved in sexual practices that can become both emotionally and physically imperiling, practice self-mutilation, experience sexual assault, have PTSD, and on and on, so here is a snapshot of a client who can utterly confound you if you are not careful. The saying goes that "You haven't won your spurs as a therapist until you have dealt with a person with BPD."

The BPD is an open Pandora's box of intractable crises in terms of the presenting problems and issues that occur in therapy, as graphically described by the following researchers over a long period of time and topics (Bagge et al., 2004; Beck & Freeman, 1990; Belling et al., 2014; Borschmann et al., 2013; Borschmann & Moran, 2011; Brockian, 2002; Chatham, 1989; Drapeau & Perry, 2004; Fonagy et al., 2011; Falcus & Johnson, 2018; Freidel, 2004; Harned & Sloan, 2022; Jimenez, 2013; Kleindienst et al., 2021; Kreisman & Straus, 2004; Kroger et al, 2014; Lachkar, 2011; Lawrence et al., 2011; Leichsenring et al., 2011; Mneimne et al., 2018; Paris, 2008; Sansone et al, 2011; Wirth-Cauchon, 2001; Zeigler-Hill & Abraham, 2006) and summarized below.

Presenting Problems. People with borderline personality disorder have problems like no other client has. They often include the following in therapy:

1. A wide variety of presenting problems that may shift from day to day and week to week

2. Unusual combinations of symptoms ranging across a wide array of neurotic to subpsychotic behaviors

3. Continuous self-destructive and self-punitive behavior ranging from self-mutilation to suicide attempts

4. Impulsive and poorly planned behavior that shifts through infantile, narcissistic, or antisocial behavior

5. Intense emotional reactions out of all proportion to the situation

6. Confusion regarding goals, priorities, feelings, sexual orientation, and so on

7. A constant feeling of emptiness with chronic, free-floating anxiety

8. Unstable and low self-esteem and high and unstable negative affect

9. Poor academic, work, and social adjustment

10. Extreme approach and avoidance behavior to social relationships

11. Chronic suicidal and/or homicidal ideation

12. Paranoid ideation

13. Depersonalization and hallucinations

14. Drug misuse including alcohol

15. Indiscriminate sexual behavior and sexual victimization

16. High dropout rate from therapy and poor therapeutic alliance.

Therapeutic Relationship. People with borderline personality disorder do everything in their power to turn the therapeutic relationship upside down. They have:

1. Frequent crises such as suicide threats, misuse of drugs, sexual acting out, financial irresponsibility, and problems with the law

2. Extreme or frequent misinterpretations of the therapist's statements, intentions, or feelings with strong transference issues that can illicit even stronger countertransference issues in the therapist

3. Unusually strong, negative, acting-out reactions to changes in appointment time, room changes, vacations, fees, or termination in therapy

4. Low tolerance for direct eye contact, physical contact, or close proximity in therapy

5. Unusually strong ambivalence on issues

6. Fear of and resistance to change with an inability or resistance to carry out therapeutic assignments

7. Frequent phone calls to, spying on, and demands for special attention and treatment from the therapist

8. Inordinate hypersensitivity to significant others including the therapist.

People with borderline personality disorder vacillate between autonomy and dependence, view the world in black-and-white terms, are ever vigilant for perceived danger, have chronic tension and anxiety, are guarded in their interpersonal relationships, and are uncomfortable with emotions (Beck & Freeman, 1990, pp. 186–187; Lachkar, 2011; Linehand, 1993; Paris, 2008). Because of these personality traits, they are apt to continuously test the therapeutic relationship to affirm that the therapist, like everybody else, is untrustworthy and not capable of living up to their expectations, while at the same time, they desperately crave attention, love, and respect (Brockian, 2002; Freidel, 2004; Kreisman & Straus, 2004; Lachkar, 2011; Linehand, 1993; McHenry, 1994; Paris, 2008; Yeomans, 1993). Do you start to get the picture of why they can become psychological albatrosses around therapists' necks?

When dealing with someone with borderline personality disorder, it is important to set clear limits, structure specific therapeutic goals, provide empathic support, validate the client's actions as understandable, model a safe environment, provide psychoeduction, actively confront maladaptive emotional dysregulation and distorted thinking, caringly confront manipulative and maladaptive behavior, and rigorously stick with these guiding principles (Briere & Scott, 2006; Chatham, 1989; Groth et al., 2021; Kreisman & Straus, 2004; Lachkar, 2011; Linehan, 1993; Paris, 2008). This is easier said than done because of the dramatic kinds of problems and emotions that these people display. The following dialogue with Tommy, a college student, depicts such problematic behavior.

Tommy: (calling the therapist at 2 A.M.) I can't take this any longer. Nobody cares about me. I think I'm going crazy again—all these weird voices keep coming into my mind. It'd just be easier if I got a gun and blew myself away.

TH: I can understand the belief that nobody cares about you, considering how you were put in foster care as a kid and how that uncaring attitude of others seems to follow you wherever you go. If that's the case that those abandonment fears are driving you to this point, then I'm concerned enough about your welfare to call 911 and get the police there immediately to take you to the hospital. (Wise in the ways of people with borderline personality disorder, the therapist immediately confronts Tommy's statement while validating his fears.) If things are that serious, a phone conversation won't get the job done.

Tommy: Well, I didn't say I was going to kill myself right now! You always jump to conclusions. I just couldn't sleep or study because of all these voices, and I really need to talk about them.

TH: I'm willing to talk for 15 minutes, but if I don't see you calmed down and functional by that time, I'll feel warranted in calling 911.

Setting limits and monitoring client safety is critical (Kreisman & Straus, 2004; Paris, 2008). By voicing legitimate concerns about the client's safety and setting a specific time limit on the conversation, the therapist reaffirms therapeutic control and does not become engaged in a rambling dialogue. The latter would serve nothing other than to reinforce maladaptive client behavior and cause a sleepless therapist to be angry and irritable the next day! No special considerations other than those normally given to any other clients should be given to those with borderline personality disorder. The therapist is immediately empathically active in engaging Tommy's confrontational behavior (Groth et al., 2021). Part of dialectical behavior therapy is encouraging check-up calls (Linehan, 1993) or phone coaching (Chapman, 2019). The question is, do you make yourself available for 2:00 A.M. calls unless you are working a night shift on a crisis line? At least the therapist sets time limits with Tommy as recommended by Chapman (2018). With all due respect to the providers of DBT, we think if you do that, particularly if you are a neophyte dealing with a tough customer, you are playing into the manipulative hands of the client. The writer of this chapter is not a DBT expert and has gotten trapped into a lengthy 2:00 A.M. phone conversation with a male with borderline personality disorder and only succeeded in reinforcing "Don't you dare leave me behavior!" and making himself a candidate for the burnout chapter. That said, Chapman (2018) does make an eloquent case for phone coaching and how to handle clients when clients go off the rails, but he seems to be mainly speaking to therapists who are experts in DBT and have the availability of other expert DBT therapists for consultation and support.

Tommy: But Dr. James, I really need to change the appointment and see you tomorrow. I've got this research presentation, and my group's meeting during our appointment time. Can't you move somebody else around?

TH: I have an appointment with another client at that time, Tommy. As I told you, to reschedule I need to know 48 hours in advance. It wouldn't be fair to him anymore than it would be fair to you if I did that to your regular time.

Tommy: (sarcastically) You just really don't give a damn about me, do you?

TH: The fact is, I do give a damn, and that's why I'm not going to cave in and change the appointment time. We're not talking about rejection here; we're talking about a reasonable policy that I use on everybody. I know lots of times it would be easy for you to believe I'm blowing you off. At times you certainly aren't the easiest client to deal with, but I knew that going in, and I committed to see this through with you. I'll expect you at our regular Thursday time.

The therapist owns both his positive and his negative feelings about the client and directly interprets and confronts the client's underlying fear of rejection (Chatham, 1989). The therapist directly confronts his all or none, "You don't care about me!" abandonment issues (Groth, 2021) using Glasser's (1965) consequences of actions (1965) with a clear owning statement. Finally, by reminding the client of his regular appointment, the therapist targets behavior rather than affect. Focusing on behavior is far less problematic than dealing with relational issues, either inside or outside therapy, because of the client's low tolerance for intimacy (Beck & Freeman, 1990; Drapeau & Perry, 2004; Freidel, 2004).

Treatment noncompliance is par for the course with clients with borderline personality disorder.

TH: So how did your assignment go in thought stopping and not arbitrarily categorizing women as saints or prostitutes?

Tommy: Well, I was real busy this week. Besides which, you didn't really make that thought stopping stuff very clear. And then the rubber band reminder on my wrist broke.

TH: (frustrated, voice raised, and becoming agitated) This is the sixth week I've gone through this with you. You continuously put women in those one-up or one-down positions. Yet you continuously complain that no women are interested in you. How do you ever expect to have an equitable relationship unless you change your thinking?

Tommy: (flushed and shouting) Oh yeah? You're so perfect? I'll bet your supervisor would like to know the way you verbally harass your clients. Screw you! Who needs therapy or bitches, anyway? They're all sluts anyway. (**Storms out of the room and slams the door.**)

Maintaining professional detachment and keeping one's cool are critical and difficult (Kreisman & Straus, 2004). The therapist's frustration may turn to anger if the therapist ascribes malicious intentions to the client's nonperformance, particularly when trying to change the client's black-and-white thinking. Overt frustration often results in reciprocal acting out by the client. The client's passive noncompliance is a balancing act between fear of change and fear of offending the therapist through outright refusal to comply with therapeutic requests. When noncompliance is consistently the normative response, the therapist needs to step back from the situation, seek outside consultation, confront these issues openly, and acknowledge freely the client's right to refuse an assignment rather than doggedly proceeding (Beck & Freeman, 1990).

TH: Tommy, I feel really frustrated right now. We've been going at this one assignment for six sessions. Maybe I'm the problem—pushing too fast. On the other hand, I feel you maybe don't want to make me disappointed, so you go through the motions. You've always got the right to say no to an assignment, and we can certainly discuss the pros and cons of that. What do you want to do about this assignment?

People with borderline personality disorder and other dependent types of clients display the behavior of externalizing and project their problems onto others. They then attempt to get the therapist to intercede for them by acting as an intermediary or otherwise "fixing" the problem.

Tommy: If you could just write my econ professor a note telling him I'm under your care. I've only missed five classes, and he's threatening to flunk me.

TH: School and therapy are separate, and I won't get into that.

Tommy: (whining and pleading) But you know how bad off I've been.

TH: If you are sick enough to miss class, perhaps you should consider an academic withdrawal for medical reasons.

Tommy: Well, I'm not that bad off that I need to quit school.

TH: How has getting others to make excuses for you helped in the past?

In refusing to be used by the client, the therapist avoids a pitfall that would invariably lead to more dependent behavior and the continuation of cyclical, self-reinforcing, dependent, and manipulative behavior. Finally, the watchword with people with borderline personality disorders and other clients who consciously or unconsciously seek to manipulate the therapist is: Remain calm throughout therapy, and do not respond to each new crisis as an emergency. The key question therapists must ask themselves is, "Who's doing the majority of work here?" If the answer is, "Not the client!" then there is a good chance the therapist is being manipulated.

Counseling Difficult Clients

LO7 Crisis workers must be prepared to deal with many different types of clients, some of whom are "difficult." To assist in coping with such clients, here are some examples of appropriate ground rules as well as suggestions for confronting difficult clients.

Ground Rules for Counseling Difficult Clients

Workers who must deal with difficult clients regularly may wish to print a set of ground rules to place in the hands of clients at the initial session or before the first meeting. The following are our rules garnered over many years of practice. They may be used with individuals, couples, or groups:

1. We start on time and quit on time. If couples are involved, both parties must be present; we will not meet unless both parties are present.
2. There will be no physical violence or threats of violence.
3. Everyone speaks for themselves.
4. Everyone has a chance to be fully heard.
5. We deal mainly with the here and now; we try to steer clear of getting bogged down in the past and in blaming others.
6. Everyone faces all the issues brought up—nobody gets up and leaves just because the topic is uncomfortable, and everyone stays for the entire session.
7. Everyone gets an opportunity to define the current problems, suggest realistic solutions, and

make at least one commitment to do something positive. At least one positive action step is desired from each person present.

8. Limits to graphic descriptions, abusive language, and swearing and cursing need to be clear as to what will and will not be tolerated.

9. Everyone belongs, because we are all human beings and because we are here.

10. The crisis worker will not take sides.

11. There will be no retribution, retaliation, or grudges over what is said in the session. Whatever is said in the session belongs and stays in the session.

12. The time we spend together is for working on the concerns of the person or people in the group—not for playing games, making personal points, diversion, ulterior purposes, or carrying tales or gossip outside the session.

13. When we know things are a certain way, we will not pretend they are another way—we will confront and deal with each other as honestly and objectively as we possibly can.

14. We will not ignore the nonverbal or body messages that are emitted—we will deal with them openly if they occur.

15. If words or messages need to be expressed to clear the air, we will say them either directly or with role playing—we will not put them off until later.

16. We will not expect each other to be perfect.

17. Being drunk or otherwise drug intoxicated is not acceptable in therapy. We do not work with "wet" clients.

18. In the event the ground rules are broken, the consequences will be discussed by the persons involved immediately with the therapist. People who comply with the rules will not be denied services because one person disobeys the rules.

Along with detailing what therapy will entail, the therapist should initially go over the ground rules, in person or over the phone, before the first session so the potential client understands what will be expected. This procedure goes a long way toward averting in-session crises. Anecdotally, in the writer's work with prison inmates housed in a special mental health unit who could be oppositional defiant at times, discussion of these rules and acknowledgment verbally on individual intake for group therapy made sessions go much more smoothly. If this is not possible, a brief orientation that includes the ground rules is advisable at the start of the first meeting. Continuous breaking of rules is indicative of noncompliance and grounds

for termination of therapy. While the foregoing may sound punitive, particularly when dealing with difficult clients, clear limits need to be set and imposed. It is noteworthy that DBT practitioners will terminate clients for four successive absences from therapy as noncompliant. They also will not respond to phone calls for 24 hours after a suicide or self-injury attempt in the belief that it is only reinforcing maladaptive behavior (Chapman, 2018).

Confronting Difficult Clients

In dealing with difficult clients, the worker may have to *confront* such behavior directly. We must be able and ready to use confrontation, assertion, and directive tactics, such as saying, "I will not permit you to violate our ground rules by attacking her that way." There is a possibility that a client may be so difficult that the session may have to be terminated. (This should happen very, very infrequently.) In such a rare case, the worker would openly admit, "We're getting nowhere, so let's adjourn and see if we can figure out a way to try again." Consultation with a professional colleague for suggestions would be one of the first steps the therapist would take after such an adjournment (Chapman, 2018).

Confidentiality in Case Handling

One benchmark of crisis is the dramatic onset of potentially violent behavior. Further, that violent behavior may occur outside individual therapy setting anywhere from a street corner to a hospital waiting room. It is noteworthy that the ethical standards of all the mental health professions have little to say about crisis other than breaking confidentiality when lethal behavior is apparent. Interactions between crisis workers and clients are unlike standard therapy sessions, and applying standard ethical codes and practices means taking that into account (Myer et al., 2022). A particular admonition to the crisis interventionist is appropriate here in discussing case handling. That admonition involves the issues of confidentiality and privileged communication and the legal and moral dilemmas that swirl within many crisis settings. Dealing with those issues invariably means the interventionist will be faced with ethical standards that appear to conflict with one another (Beauchamp & Childress, 2019). In particular, the ethical principles of beneficence and nonmaleficence often conflict with client autonomy

(Myer et al., 2022, p. 86). As part of a standard therapeutic procedure, the concept of informed consent concerning the client's rights and limitations of therapy is typically discussed prior to the start of counseling (Welfel, 2016). When crises occur, that may not be possible for a variety of reasons, including (Myer et al., 2022, p. 87):

1. Individuals not being able to comprehend or understand informed consent due to their shock over the severity of the crisis
2. Needing to tell their "story" without interruption or rejoinders that they are treading on thin ice regarding the limits of confidentiality

3. Changing content may eradicate the original promise of confidentiality and client autonomy and charge the interventionist with prioritizing nonmaleficence as a first priority.
4. The context and environment where intervention is happening may militate against confidentiality and autonomy.

Given these conditions, it is critically important that crisis interventionists understand and use the LASER protocol (Myer et al., 2022), defined in Chapter 3, "The Intervention and Assessment Models," in making sound ethical decisions while providing sound crisis intervention.

Summary

Case handling in crisis intervention differs from long-term therapy. Although crisis intervention deals with many of the same components as long-term therapy, crisis work can be differentiated by its emphasis on expediency and efficiency in attempting to stabilize maladaptive client functioning as opposed to a fundamental restructuring of the client's personality. Case handling in crisis intervention emphasizes concern for client safety, brevity in assessment, rapid intervention, compressed treatment time, and termination or referral once equilibrium has been restored. Case handling in crisis intervention can occur both at walk-in facilities and in long-term therapy settings.

Since the Community Mental Health Act of 1963, the major responsibility for treating the mentally ill has fallen on community mental health centers. Such centers, along with a wide variety of other community social services agencies, are on the front lines in dealing with crises of chronic mental illness, severe developmental problems, and the social and environmental issues that afflict individuals. Because of the wide variety of clientele seeking services, walk-in facilities must have close linkages with other social services agencies, the legal system, and both short- and long-term mental health facilities. Mental health workers who staff such facilities must have a broad background in dealing with a wide variety of psychological problems and be ready and able to deal with whatever crisis walks in the door.

Because of the consequences of the Community Mental Health Act of 1963, police departments have assumed greater and greater responsibility for initial contact and disposition of the mentally ill. The creation of the Memphis Model of the Crisis Intervention Team (CIT) has resulted in the development and use of regular patrol officers to defuse and de-escalate the mentally ill and other emotionally violent clients. Variations of this model are now in use throughout the United States and may include co-response teams composed of police officers and mental health providers working together. These responders are the baseline point for the Sequential Intercept Model.

Clients in long-term therapy may also experience transcrises as they move through the therapeutic process. These crises may be instigated by situational events in the client's environment; by attempts to engage in new, more adaptive behaviors; or by past traumatic material that is uncovered in the therapy session. When such transcrises occur, therapy may degenerate to the point that clients undergo severe traumatic stress and revert to pretherapeutic functioning levels. At these points in therapy, long-term work must be suspended, and the therapist must concentrate on the emergent crisis until the client has achieved success in overcoming the current stumbling block. Borderline personality disorder is probably the archetype of difficult and transcrisis-prone clients with which the therapist will work in long-term therapy. Delivering rules of conduct for long-term therapy is important in diminishing in-session crises.

Telephone and Online Crisis Counseling

6

Learning Objectives

After reading this chapter, you should be able to:

1. Identify the reasons for the popularity of crisis lines.
2. List the steps for handling different types of clients at crisis line centers.
3. Describe that no one is perfect in doing crisis line intervention and mistakes are repairable.
4. Recognize ways crisis line interventions handle difficult callers.
5. List strategies for handling extremely distressed callers.
6. Identify the administrative rules for handling difficult callers.
7. Identify the different types of hotlines and their uses.
8. Describe the influence of tele-behavioral health in crisis intervention.

Introduction

By far, the vast majority of crisis counseling is handled by volunteers on the telephone; however, as we move further into the 21st century and the aftermath of the COVID-19 megacrisis, other technologies such as the internet, smartphones, and so on are playing an increasing role in real-time crisis counseling (Glass & Bickler, 2021; Mazzar et al., 2020; Reinhardt, 2019; Vitiello, 2022). Whether the service provider using the various technologies will be a professional with credentials, a well-meaning volunteer with little to no training, a charlatan out to steal your money, or a computer programmed to do crisis intervention is an interesting question (Gross & Anthony, 2003; Hsiung, 2002; James & Gilliland, 2003, pp. 417–428).

This chapter focuses on telephone use in crisis counseling, but clearly, the use of other technologies in crisis intervention has arrived (Gould et al., 2021). The growth of technologies other than the telephone is occurring at such a staggering rate that numerous books specifically targeted for training in tele-behavioral health are being published (Gilbertson, 2020; Luxton et al., 2016; Magnavita, 2018; Mahmoud, 2022; Robertson, 2020). In addition, organizations such as Mental Health America (https://www.mhanational.org/) and the American Tele-health Association (https://www.americantelemed.org/) that have a specialty area for tele-behavioral health have also come into existence. The final section of this chapter addresses the new, cutting-edge technologies used in tele-behavioral health (Madigan, 2020). Here is a quote from the noted physicist Max Planck: "A new scientific truth does not triumph by convincing its opponents and making them see the light, but rather because its opponents eventually die, and a new generation grows up that is familiar with it" (as cited in T. S. Kuhn, 1962). What do you think of it? You might want to think carefully about

Planck's quote because these new technologies are going about the business of how the whole notion of therapy is carried out. Only recently are professional programs playing catch-up in training therapists on the use of these new technologies rather than focusing on face-to-face encounters. Norcross et al. (2021) describe the different technologies for using tele-behavioral health with the therapist at the center of the technology. So the question becomes one of, "Will you be at the center of this new technology, or will you still be twiddling your thumbs waiting for clients to come to your office in person?"

Case Handling on Telephone Crisis Lines

LO1 The telephone has long played an integral role in crisis work. The old Bell Telephone advertisement "Reach out and touch someone!" is a slogan that is particularly appropriate to crisis counseling. Slaikeu (1990, pp. 105–141) refers to emergency telephone help as a "first-order intervention" or "psychological first aid." Indeed, the telephone is the most prevalent medium for the initial contact in most crisis service delivery. There are several reasons for the popularity of the telephone in solving psychological problems.

Convenience. Convenience is paramount (Lester, 2012; McCoun et al., 2020). Cell phones especially have become such an easy way of communicating that calling for psychological assistance is a natural extension of "taking care of business." The tremendous upsurge in the use of cell phones allows a person to call a crisis line from anywhere, including the site of the crisis as it is happening in real time. Further, with the new "smart" phones, not only can clients avail themselves of a crisis hotline or their therapist, they can also access a variety of self-help groups in chat rooms, computer-assisted therapy, and psychoeducational materials (Boschen, 2009; Gross & Anthony, 2003; Preziosa et al., 2009). As in the case of domestic violence, most crises do not occur during normal business hours. When help is needed in a crisis, it is needed immediately, and mobile phones make 24/7 assistance even more available.

Client Anonymity. Guilt, embarrassment, shame, self-blame, and other debilitating emotions make face-to-face encounters with strangers very difficult, particularly in the immediate aftermath of a traumatic event. Opening oneself to another is an act of vulnerability. The ability to hide one's identity may facilitate greater openness and freedom from inhibition (Keasar et al., 2022; Lester, 2012). This is particularly true of adolescents (Christogiorgos et al., 2010; Tolmach, 1985), those who are socially isolated or psychologically desperate, and the relatively stable person who has a one-shot crisis (Lester, 2012). Telephone counselors understand that clients have such feelings and are generally not concerned about identifying a client unless a life-threatening emergency is involved. Conversations usually are on a first-name-only basis for both the worker and the client. Thus, a survivor of date rape may call a rape hotline and freely discuss their emotions without having to muster the courage to face what may be perceived as a judgmental human services worker.

Control. A great deal of fear, anxiety, and uncertainty occur when a client's life is ruptured by a crisis (Williams & Douds, 2012). The concept of secondary victimization by institutions (Ochberg, 1988) is well known to victims of a crisis who have sought assistance from a social agency and then been victimized by its bureaucratic callousness. Going in person for help may be positively humiliating. In telephone counseling, the client decides when and if assistance is to be sought. At any time during a dialogue on a crisis line, the client may terminate the conversation without fear of recrimination (Williams & Doud, 2012). Finally, looks don't matter in phone counseling. Anybody who is self-conscious about how they look finds the phone a wonderful way to obtain counseling (Wark, 1982).

Immediacy of Access. Crisis intervention can occur any place a telephone, or for that matter, a computer, is available (Hoffberg, 2019). Today, most people always carry a smartphone. Most institutions and clinics and many private practitioners use smartphones as a primary means of communication.

For example, a harried residence hall supervisor who is trying to deal with a distraught, suicidal student hurting from severe homesickness and academic failure can call the school's counseling center crisis hotline. The clinician on call for that evening immediately responds to the request for assistance. While procedures may differ based on policies at the school, generally, the clinician will check with the residence hall supervisor on the current mental status of the student and then come to the residence hall.

The clinician may also talk to the student over the phone. If the clinician determines additional help is needed, a request may be made for the police to transport the student to the city crisis stabilization unit. In case of an imminent threat such as a tornado or the presence of a potential assailant on campus, text and computer messages can go out to all the students and university staff.

Cost Effectiveness. Crisis lines are inexpensive for both the client and the community (Moroz et al., 2020). Clients who cannot pay for private therapy or afford transportation can usually avail themselves of a phone. Most community agency hotlines are staffed by volunteers and are paid for by funded grants, the United Way, or other charitable funds. Reese et al.'s (2006) study of telephone counseling strongly implies that, for people of limited financial means, face-to-face counseling where money is a factor is not an option. Instead, a free community crisis line is a viable option.

Therapeutic Effectiveness. Volunteers who staff crisis lines have probably been the single most important discovery in the history of suicide intervention (Dublin, 1969). Volunteers have few pretensions about their "professional role" and are often seen by callers as having more credibility than a paid professional because they "do it out of the goodness of their hearts." Although the idea of obtaining counseling from a volunteer may seem no better or worse than talking to a bartender or hairdresser, volunteers typically go through a good deal of training in initial point-of-contact mental health counseling (Derkx et al., 2009). Phipps et al. (2007) found that volunteers who went through training specifically designed to deal with trauma showed a significant gain in knowledge and skills from pre- to post-training. Mishara and his associates (2005) found that less than 0.3 percent of 2,611 calls they monitored at 14 participating call-in centers were found to be blatantly unacceptable in helper responses and could possibly put the lives of the callers at risk. In similar research conducted in 2016, Mishra again found no significant difference between the effectiveness of volunteers vs. professionals in responding to callers in crisis with suicidal ideations.

While some professionals may still have concerns about the effectiveness of crisis hotlines, research consistently indicates that they are probably as good as other types of face-to-face counseling and are particularly attractive to young people, older adults, and people who do not have financial access to professional therapists (Bryant & Harvey, 2000; Day & Schneider, 2002; Evans et al., 1986; Fukkink & Hermanns, 2009; Lester & Brockopp, 1973, p. 86; Mishara, 2016; Reese et al., 2002, 2006; Rohland et al., 2000).

Access to Support Systems. One of the major reasons people call hotlines is for social support (Watson et al., 2006). Many people who are lonely, anxious, or isolated by physical illness need support (Burgess et al., 2008). Whether you are a shut-in, shy, think you are ugly, recently divorced, widowed, abused, or addicted or you have leprosy, panic attacks, bad thoughts, or any of the issues of problem callers you are about to meet in this chapter, the need for social support and an empathic ear and voice is the common thread that runs through most crisis lines. Beyond the support of the line itself are the telephone and online support systems to which you can be referred or gain access on your own.

Support groups make extensive use of telephone networks (Lester & Brockopp, 1973). From A (Alcoholics Anonymous) to Z (Zen) support groups, telephone support networks provide constant links to group members between organized meetings. A Google search conducted on April 8, 2023, identified over 57 million sites for support groups. The bottom line is that if you can't find a support group out there somewhere for your problem, you are probably an alien escapee from Roswell's Area 51, and this book isn't going to be a lot of help to you.

Avoidance of Dependency Issues. A user of telephone crisis lines can't become dependent on a particular human services worker who may not always be readily available. Standard practice in most crisis lines discourages workers from forming lasting relationships with clients so dependency issues do not arise (Lester, 2012).

Worker Anonymity. The fact that workers are anonymous has as many benefits as client anonymity. The absence of body language, facial expressions, and a visual image allows clients to project whatever idealized view they may conjure up for the appearance of the therapist. By facilitating the development of transference, within limits, the client can make positive changes. The point here is that not only can clients make of the therapist what they will, they can make of them what they need (Lester, 2012; Williams & Douds, 2012).

Availability of Others for Consultation. Crisis lines are seldom staffed by one person. When someone encounters a difficult client, other staff at the agency are available for consultation. Furthermore, at least one phone line is reserved for calling support agencies when emergency services are needed.

Availability of an Array of Services. A vast array of information, guidance, and social services is quickly available via telephone linkages. The specialized services of different agencies and the expertise they offer can provide on-the-spot guidance for emotionally volatile situations. Many an angry parent or guardian has received "5-minute parenting sessions" from the staff of a "parenting line," thus short-circuiting potential child abuse (National Parenting Helpline, 2023). Any crisis hotline should have readily available a list of phone numbers of specialized agencies to which they can refer callers. The LINC, or Library and Information Network for the Community, is available in most large metropolitan areas and is standard reference for most telephone crisis lines.

Service to Large and Isolated Geographic Areas and Populations. Many rural areas that have no after-hours mental health facilities or staff are tied in to toll-free crisis lines that cover huge geographic areas. These crisis lines, in turn, are tied into emergency service staff such as police, paramedics, and hospital emergency rooms that serve those rural areas and can respond to a crisis line call for assistance that may be 150 miles away. Certainly, populations that are home-bound, such as older adults, physically disabled, or agoraphobic, have a lifeline they would not otherwise have (Lester, 2012; Riding & Werth, 2014; Schueller et al., 2019; Williams & Douds, 2012).

Telephone Counseling Strategies

LO2 Conducting crisis intervention over the telephone is a double-edged sword. Although phone counseling offers the advantages just listed, for generating responses, the crisis worker is entirely dependent on the content, voice tone, pitch, speed, and emotional content of the client. Telephone counseling, and internet counseling for that matter, isn't for everyone, and that includes both clients and interventionists (Eckardt, 2011). For many human services

workers, it is unsettling to deal with ambiguous client responses and not be able to link body language to verbal content. Furthermore, crisis workers depend entirely on their own verbal ability to stabilize clients and have little physical control over the situation. It takes only one experience of having a suicidal client hang up on a worker to understand how frustrating and emotionally draining crisis intervention over the telephone can be. Consequently, a great deal of care and effort needs to be taken in responding to clients. The following section outlines some effective telephone counseling strategies.

Making Psychological Contact

First, psychological contact needs to be made, and this endeavor takes precedence over anything else the phone worker does. Making psychological contact is different than establishing rapport. You were probably taught that establishing rapport takes several therapy sessions, yet in crisis intervention, you do not have this luxury. Rapport must be assumed (Kleespies & Richmond, 2009; Myer et al., 2013). Psychological contact means that the worker attempts to establish as quickly as possible a nonjudgmental, caring, accepting, and empathic relationship with the client that will give the worker credibility and elicit the client's trust. Therefore, *providing support* becomes the first order of business because many times, if not most, it is safe to assume that people who use crisis lines have exhausted, worn out, or are separated from their support systems. If the client feels no trust in the relationship and hangs up the phone, the crisis worker cannot make an astute dynamic analysis, synthesize material, diagnose the problem, and prescribe a solution! In establishing psychological contact on the phone, providing support is a first priority and is highly integrated with defining the problem through active listening and responding skills.

The following dialogue is an example of making contact with callers. Understand that each situation is unique. We know of no set formula for making contact. In the commentary, we use the Triage Form to assess the caller and explore the strategies being used.

CW: (Two A.M. on Monday morning. Phone rings.) Metro crisis line. This is Chris. Can I help you?

Telephone caller (TC): (Silence with soft muffled sobs.)

CW: (Waits patiently.) I understand it's pretty hard to talk sometimes, especially when things seem so overwhelming, but if you could, just take a deep breath and then let it out. I wonder if you could just do that?

TC: (Takes a deep breath and exhales. Sobs less frequently.)

CW: (in a soft, modulated, soothing tone) That's good! Just do that a few more times. Just relax. I'll stay right on the line until you feel like talking. We've got plenty of time. I'd like to know your name when you feel ready.

The phone worker must be able to react in a calm and collected manner. Thus, the worker's voice must be well modulated, steady, low key, with an adequate decibel level but not high pitched. Neither should the content of the worker's response be deprecating, cynical, cajoling, or demeaning. Although the foregoing criteria may seem obvious, few people realize how their voice sounds or are aware of what happens to their voice level and pitch when they are caught up in a rapidly escalating and evolving emotional event. Furthermore, when the person on the other end of the line is acting out, angry, intoxicated, or otherwise demanding of the worker to "fix things right now," the worker needs a great deal of self-discipline and emotional security to refrain from becoming caustic, judgmental, and demanding.

While crisis line counseling is on a first-name basis only, making initial contact means getting a name out to the caller and attempting to get one back. As simple as this sounds, in the heat of the initial moments of a call, neophyte workers forget to do this. Chris the veteran does not and patiently queries the caller for their name.

Defining the Problem

Once psychological contact is established, the worker attempts to define the problem by gaining an understanding of the events that led to the crisis and by assessing the client's coping mechanisms. Open-ended questions on the *what, how, when, where, who* continuum usually let the worker get a clear picture of the event itself. However, in assessing the coping mechanisms of the client over the phone, it may be hard to get a clear picture of the client's affect. Thus, it behooves the worker to become more sensitive to the underlying emotional content and to try to reflect the implied feeling content more than might be required in a face-to-face encounter. Reflecting feelings is a tough job for most beginning mental health workers and is even more difficult on the phone. Yet, the worker absolutely must try to reflect feelings because there is no way to visually assess the client.

One real plus of phone counseling is that the beginning crisis worker can have supportive aid readily at hand without detracting from the counseling session. One useful tactic is to have a reference list of feeling words that cover the gamut of emotions. A second tactic is to have at hand a list of standard questions the counselor can check off to be sure that all areas typically pertinent to the problem are covered. A third tactic is to keep handy a notepad on which the worker can jot down the salient aspects of the events and coping mechanisms the client has used and make a rapid assessment on the triage scale.

TC: (timorously) O . . . O . . . O . . . K. I just don't know where to start, it's just an avalanche. I've got no place to turn, so I thought this was my only chance, so I called.

CW: I'm glad you did call. Sounds like right now you're really overwhelmed, so perhaps you could just take it from where you felt like things fell apart and tell me about that. And I want you to take your time. Take plenty of time and tell me what's going on. We've got all the time in the world, and I'm here to listen until you say everything you need to and we get a real clear picture of what's going on and what needs to happen. Can you tell me your name?

TC: It's Cicily.

The client goes on to explain she has just moved to town from out of state in an attempt to reconcile with her estranged husband. The husband indicated that he wanted nothing more to do with the marriage and was filing for divorce. She indicates that she was pretty much in denial about the failed marriage and had taken a last chance on getting it back together. The denial has now been given a rude reality check. The job that was supposedly waiting for her has also fallen through. She is currently at a friend's house with her 4-year-old son, less than $200, and a car on its last wheels. She has no relatives or support system besides her friend from college days.

The crisis worker, Chris, listens intently to the client's story. He interrupts only to clarify and summarize what's going on with the client. Chris deeply reflects the feelings of aloneness, hopelessness, and helplessness that wash over her. Using the strategy of Allowing Catharsis, the crisis worker allows the client to grieve and ventilate over her failed marriage When the client's emotional behavior starts to escalate, the crisis worker uses calming techniques such as asking the client to take a deep breath or reinforces the concept that they have plenty of time to work through this problem. The goal of this tactic is to help the client re-establish a sense of control. As Chris listens to her, he is rapidly jotting notes down and making an assessment on the triage scale. Her predominant emotion is anxiety, which is free-floating into all areas of her life. She is having a lot of difficulty controlling her emotions.

Cicily's score on the Affective Severity scale is 7. She indicates that she has been essentially frozen in time for the last 4 days after her meeting with her estranged husband. Her friend has been taking care of her son while Cicily has either sat paralyzed staring aimlessly at TV or been hysterically sobbing in bed. Finally, at the urging of her friend, she called the crisis line. Her score on the Behavioral Severity scale is 7 because her daily functioning is clearly impaired. She is immobilized and frozen. As she relates her problems, her thinking seems linear, and she is able to put her story together logically. However, she has been perseverating on the crisis to the exclusion of anything else. There is a lot of wishing and hoping for things to get better and that somehow her husband will have a change of heart. She is filled with self-doubt and cannot make a decision about what to do. Her score on the Cognitive Severity scale is an 8.

Overall, her triage scale score is 22. This woman is clearly in crisis and may need more help than the crisis line can provide over the phone. Chris's immediate concern is with a statement Cicily made that "this was my only chance." A strategy that may be helpful as the dialogue continues is Increasing Expansion, helping the caller understand other options and choices, or Providing Guidance might also be useful.

Ensuring Safety and Providing Support

During problem definition, the phone worker must be very specific in determining the client's lethality level. If the crisis worker detects the potential for physical injury, the strategy of Providing Protection may be used. Determining if this strategy is needed comes by asking closed-ended questions that obtain information specific to the safety of the client, not only without hesitation but also with empathic understanding that clearly depicts the worker's overriding concern for and valuing of the client. These questions typically start with *do, have,* and *are,* and in phone dialogues, they should be put directly and assertively to the client. (For example, one might ask, "Do you have

the pills there with you now?" or "Are you alone, or is someone there who might help you before you do it?") The phone counselor should check what support systems are available to ensure the client's safety. For many phone clients, there will be no support system—the phone counselor is the immediate and sole support system.

CW: I can really hear the hurt and fright in your voice. It's scary being all alone, seeming to have nobody to lean on. I'm concerned about your saying this was your "last chance." Do you mean by that you're thinking of suicide?

TC: (**somewhat emphatically**) I had, but I just couldn't bear to see that bastard and his new girlfriend get custody of Jimmy.

CW: OK. That's good! I needed to check that out. Now you said you were staying with an old college friend, and she asked you to call. Is that where you are now?

TC: Yes, but I hate putting her out like this. But I don't have any other place to go. (**Starts sobbing heavily again.**)

CW: But she's OK with you staying there?

TC: Yesssss. But I hate being a burden on her.

CW: But that's what friends are for. Would you do the same for her if things were reversed?

TC: Well, sure, no question.

CW: So for the time being you've got a roof over your head, something to eat, and are safe?

TC: Yes, I guess so, but I don't know how long this can go on.

CW: What we're going to do is see if we can get some stuff done that will allow you to get back on your own. OK? Are you willing to do that? (**Cicily acknowledges she'll try.**) Good! Although I can't get your husband back, and I know that really left you feeling hopeless and all alone, I can find out about the job problem and perhaps see if we can't do something about that. So let's start with that if it's OK with you. We've got a number of referral sources here that might be able to match your skills, education, and abilities with a job. Would you be willing to tell me a little bit about yourself in that area—education, employment background, desired kind of work? I could pass that on to some of our referral sources and see what we could do. (**Chris listens while Cicily goes through her background, education, and other pieces of**

pertinent information, reinforcing her for staying on task, mobilizing her thoughts, and keeping her terrifying emotions in control.)

Based on the above dialogue, the triage rating decreases to probably the higher teens with Affect and Behavioral rating being both at a 6 and Cognitive being a 7 for a total of 19. The crisis worker partners with the caller, offering to work with her to get access to the resources she needs. In doing so, he uses the strategies of Providing Guidance and Promoting Mobilization by helping her identify strengths such as employment history and education.

Considering Alternatives and Making Plans

Creating alternatives and formulating a plan are integral to one another in any crisis situation but are even more closely tied together in phone counseling. To alleviate the immediate situational threat, the phone counselor needs to jointly explore alternatives that are simple and clear-cut. Without the benefit of an eyewitness view or an in-depth background of the client, the worker needs to be cautious about proposing alternatives that may be difficult to carry out because of logistical or tactical problems of which the worker is unaware. Alternatives need to be explored in a slow, stepwise manner with checks by the worker that the client can do the physical and psychological work necessary to complete the task. Role play, verbal rehearsal, and having the client recapitulate objectives are vital ingredients of a functional plan. No plan should be accepted until clients can reassure the worker that they thoroughly understand the plan and have the means and ability to put it into action.

CW: OK! I've got that information. I'll pass it along to the day shift, and they'll pass it along to the JOBS Council and a couple of employment agencies that work with us. I want you to call back to our number tomorrow about 1 P.M. and we'll have some information for you. Can you do that?

TC: Well yes, I can do that. (Cicily has calmed down and is only occasionally sniffling and lamenting her outcast state. Her triage scale score has moved down to about 15. Chris now approaches other areas of her crisis.)

CW: I wonder what you did when you got into predicaments beforehand? Maybe there was nothing quite like this, but I'm guessing there were other times when you were overwhelmed.

TC: Well, nothing like this, but I did take care of my mother before she died, kept a job with a printing company, and worked on my degree. Sometimes that was pretty overwhelming.

CW: So what did you do to take care of being overwhelmed?

TC: I'd make a list and set down my goals of what I was going to do and what I had to do. Like Alcoholics Anonymous, one day at a time, you know. It worked pretty well, but I just have got so many things now, I don't know if I can get it all lined out.

CW: But that worked before, and I understand there are lots of things going on like never before, but if it worked then, how about giving it a try now? (Chris immediately seizes on her past coping technique and attempts to put it to work. He acknowledges her belief that this is indeed different than before and doesn't discount the fact that it may be tough. He methodically helps her develop a game plan for tomorrow, not the rest of her life.) So we've got day care for Jimmy taken care of, and you don't really need the car for a while; you can get a bus or streetcar and go anywhere you need to. Even though you've only got 200 bucks cash, you could cash in that $3,000 worth of U.S. savings bonds your mother gave to Jimmy if you had to until you get back on your feet. You could then repurchase them, so you won't feel like you're robbing your son of his inheritance. So you've written those things down that you can do tomorrow, right? So we're just managing this, like you say, one day at a time, not worrying much beyond that and doing what can be done. Do you feel like we're making progress?

TC: I guess I do. I can do those things.

During this part of the intervention, the caller's triage rating continues to decrease now into the mid-teens. The crisis worker is still partnering with the caller while moving toward offering suggestions almost as a consultant. He uses Providing Guidance and Promoting Mobilization so the caller starts moving in a positive direction to resolve the crisis.

Obtaining Commitment

Commitment to a plan of action generated over the phone should be simple, specific, and time limited. If at all possible, the worker should try to obtain the client's phone number and call the client back at a preset time to check on the plan or, if the agency accepts walk-in clients, the worker should try to have the person schedule an appointment as soon as possible. If the worker is linking with other agencies, then a phone call should be made to the referral agent to check whether the client has completed the task. Although it is preferable to have the client take the initiative in contacting other agencies so dependence on the worker is not created, conditions may block the client from doing so. In that case, the worker should have no hesitation in offering to make the call.

CW: So there are three things you're going to do tomorrow. First you're going to call the day care number I gave you and get Jimmy in there. Second, you're going to go to the bank and open an account and cash in the bonds. Third, you're going to call back here at 1 P.M. and ask for the information on the job hunt. Those places I told you about will probably want you to come down, so you'll call them and make an appointment. Will you call back tomorrow night and ask for me? I come on at 11 P.M. I know this has been a pretty upsetting deal, so could you kinda repeat that to me and write down that stuff?

TC: Yes. I've got it. (**Cicily repeats to Chris the steps he has outlined.**) And I'll call back. Thanks a lot. You're a real lifesaver.

CW: You're welcome. Now get a good night's sleep. It's a fresh day tomorrow, and you'll get through it fine with that attitude. (**Chris judges Cicily now to be at a total triage rating of about 8. Affectively, she is in control of her emotions. She is thinking clearly enough to help establish a plan in a collaborative manner with the crisis worker and has committed to act on it the next day. Chris judges her to be mobilized enough that he can let her go off the line and reinforces her for getting back into equilibrium.**)

The call has taken more than an hour and a half, but in that time, a woman who is in a severe developmental and situational crisis has been able to grieve away some of the lost relationship with her husband, work through her terror of being all alone and jobless in a strange city, and start to make specific plans on how she'll get out of the dilemma. She still has many issues and a long road ahead of her, but she has returned to being a functional human again. A variety of strategies have been used to help the caller reestablish control of her life and be able to see a future

for herself. By any criterion of therapy, the crisis worker has done a good night's work!

Errors and Fallacies

LO3 For students or first timers who volunteer for crisis line duty, to say that they are incredibly nervous on their first shift is putting it mildly! Lamb (1973, 2002) has listed a number of irrational ideas that beginners indoctrinate themselves with as they start their careers as phone counselors. We list them here as a way to calm those of you who are about to start on this grand adventure.

First, you are not omnipotent! You are not there to be the instant expert. Your thoughts of "if only I were a psychiatrist, licensed social worker, counseling supercomputer, I could help this person" are doomed to failure. Nobody is an expert on everything that comes into a crisis line. There is no specific piece of information, if found, that will magically transform the caller into a paragon of good mental health.

Second, talking about "it," whatever "it" is, from suicide to getting a hair replacement, will not make "it" happen, and you will not be the instigator of causing "it" to happen. Callers are resilient and need somebody to talk honestly and openly about "it." Particularly in regard to suicide, tiptoeing around the topic generally indicates to the client that "it" is indeed scaring the daylights out of you too! If you can get an inkling of what "it" is, bring it out into the light of day, specify "it," and talk about "it."

Third, if you feel at times you are being manipulated, you probably are, and that is okay too—within limits. Understand that the caller's need to manipulate you is serving a purpose. As long as that purpose results in restoring the caller to psychological equilibrium without harming anyone, you are doing what you need to do. On the other hand, you are not a doormat to be walked over.

Fourth, not all callers are loving human beings, and you do not have to be Mother Teresa, loving and caring and sharing to all. Many people call exactly because they are *not* loving human beings! They are often overbearing, boring, nasty, insulting, hateful, and a pain in the neck! Having made that assessment, you now know why the caller is facing rejection from others and can directly speak to how their actions affect you and reflect on how those actions must be problematic when dealing with others.

By the same token, some callers like to gripe about the incompetence of other agencies, therapists, and significant others who have failed miserably to help them and have made their lives worse. They may be right. Agencies, therapists, and significant others are composed of human beings who get tired of being manipulated and taken advantage of. Questioning your credentials is really more of a question of "Can I really trust you? Can you understand what I am feeling?" Defending yourself and your credentials is pointless. Dr. James, licensed psychologist, licensed professional counselor, National Certified School Counselor, licensed English teacher, licensed school administrator, licensed real estate agent (retired), licensed fisherman, and world-renowned author of crisis textbooks can't! So why should you think you can? Don't get caught up in defending yourself, but rather turn the question back on the caller: "I don't think that is really what you are concerned about, but maybe you are wondering whether you can trust me. Why not run it by me, and let's see?"

Finally, there is the delusion of fixed alternatives. The beginner believes either "If I can't think of it, there must be no answer" or "If that's all I can think of, it must be the only answer." Or, alternatively, "I'll call a consultant. Surely they will know." None of these is correct. When you fall under this delusion, crisis intervention is stopped dead in its tracks. Crisis intervention is one part inspiration and nine parts perspiration. You muddle through this together. Solutions are created, not found. Further, you need to understand that you can't palm this caller off on another agency just because the problem is a tough one and you are at a loss as to what to do. Calling the police department's Crisis Intervention Team or the emergency Crisis Response Team from the local mental health authority may be appropriate or it may not. You need to know what other agencies can or cannot do. If you don't know, find out before you embarrass yourself.

What in the world can you do then? The best thing to do is be yourself. Trying to mimic Drs. James, Myer, or Whisenhunt, your instructor, or even Carl Rogers will likely cause complications. You got into this because you think you have some pretty good human qualities and sense of empathy for others. You undoubtedly do, so use them. You are there to listen. Few beginners ever believe this, but sometimes, a lot of times in fact, listening is more than enough. You can help the caller come up with alternatives and solutions or suggest some resources to pursue. You won't know *all* the resources available, but as time goes on, you will learn more. You will also learn your own limits and to acknowledge

when you are tired, confused, lacking in knowledge, or downright irritated with the hateful way the caller is acting. You are a pretty good human being doing your best under some trying circumstances. That's it! End of omnipotence!

Regular, Extremely Distressed, and Abusive Callers

LO4 The foregoing dialogue is a textbook example of telephone crisis line work. The problem is that the real world seldom functions in such neat and tidy ways. Many callers use the crisis line for reasons other than its intended use. When this happens, the overriding questions telephone workers must pose to themselves are: What is the person getting out of using the crisis line at this time, and is it helpful to the person? How is this person's use of the crisis line currently affecting its operation (McCaskie et al., 1990)? Crisis lines should not cater to a caller's every whim, fantasy, deviant behavior, or self-indulgence.

Chronic callers can be a plague to crisis lines and devour the time and energy of staff, which legitimate callers may desperately need (Lester et al., 2012; Spittal et al., 2015). Chronic callers can also be very frustrating to telephone workers because they do not improve (Lester, 2012). These callers can pose a serious morale problem for the volunteers and staff who receive such calls, particularly when the calls become sexually explicit and the sexually dysfunctional fantasies of callers are directed at the crisis worker (Brockopp & Lester, 2002; Lester et al., 2012).

A counterpoint to this negative view is the approach of the staff at the Lawrence, Kansas, Headquarters Crisis Center, who believe that "chronic" is a negative term and implies that these callers will never improve (Sicafuse et al., 2012). All behavior is purposive. If seen in that light, no matter how aberrant or weird the content of the call is, it is important to remember that those who regularly use the crisis line do so for a reason—it helps them make it through the day. For these clients, the call becomes part of their lifestyle and method of coping. Indeed, Spittal and associates' (2015) research on Australia's largest crisis line found that undergirding these regular callers were legitimate problems that ranged across suicidality, mental health issues, crime, child protection, and domestic violence issues, which all predicted being a frequent caller. Bassilios et al. (2015) found from a large national representative survey of Australians that they had a poor clinical profile with an increased risk of suicide. Repeat calls were associated with anxiety disorders, receipt of mental health care from general practitioners, and social disadvantage.

Middleton and associates (2014) reviewed research into frequent caller problems and how they were handled by a large sample of call-in centers. The composite solutions they found for responding to frequent callers included: limiting the number and duration of calls allowed, assigning a specific counselor to the calls, implementing face-to-face contact with a mental health or human services agency, initiating contact with the caller instead of waiting for callers to contact the service, providing short-term anxiety and depression treatment by telephone, and creating a specific management plan for each frequent caller.

Therefore, although the term *chronic* is often used in telephone crisis work, we believe it to be somewhat pejorative and agree with the staff at the Headquarters Crisis Center that "regular" better captures the essence of this clientele. If the caller's dynamics are reframed as lonely, isolated, and reaching out, then the response may be very different from one of mere aggravation (Brockopp & Lester, 2002). By setting limits of 10 to 20 minutes for **regular callers**, workers acknowledge their needs but also do not become controlled by the regular callers (Lester, 2002).

Understanding the Regular Caller's Agenda

Helping people in crisis is different than being nice to them. The agenda of regular callers places the crisis worker in a dilemma. Although the worker may feel ethically bound to respond to the caller, and the agency's protocol dictates that all calls must be taken, that does not mean that workers need to suffer the abuse and invective leveled at them by such callers. A very real difference exists between what callers may want and what they may need, and helping a caller is generally predicated much more on needs than wants. Often what these regulars want is a reaffirmation that their problems are unsolvable. Thus, they become dependent on the telephone worker to sustain their problem. The worker therefore needs to recognize such patterns and not support them when this blocks progress (Lester et al., 2012). Telephone workers do themselves and their callers a service when they show that they are not willing to be manipulated or abused and that they value their own needs as highly as they value those of the caller. Generally, if a telephone worker spends more than 15 to 20 minutes with a caller, the client's crisis becomes the worker's crisis (Knudson, 1991).

Given the foregoing admonition, the telephone worker needs to remember that the sameness of the material and the dependency these clients demonstrate day in and day out make it easy to forecast their repetitive behavior and treat them as bothersome, inept, boring, and unimportant clients. Many of these are "Yes, but . . ." callers. Although they seem highly receptive to the suggestions and plans that crisis workers make with them, in the end, they find all kinds of excuses and explanations to not follow through on what they promised to do—which makes them extremely exasperating (Waters & Finn, 1995, p. 269). Regular callers may tend to be placed in a stereotypical catchall category because they represent an aggravation to the crisis line. However, the reasons these people call are diverse. Identifying specific types is at least as important as identifying the specific caller (Lester et al., 2012). To this end, identifying some of the more typical regular callers, their outward behavior, inner dynamics, and strategies for counseling them is good to know. McCaskie et al. (1990) briefly described chronic callers that have identified mental health disorders. These remain relevant even many years later.

Paranoid. People with paranoia are guarded, secretive, and can be pathologically jealous. They live in logic-tight compartments, and it is difficult if not impossible to shake their persecutory beliefs. They see themselves as victims and expect deceit and trickery from everyone. The counseling focus is to stress their safety needs.

Schizoid. Those with schizophrenia have extremely restricted emotional expression and experience. They have few social relationships and feel anxious, shy, and self-conscious in social settings. They are guarded, tactless, and often alienate others. The counseling focus is to build a good sense of self-esteem through acceptance, optimism, and support.

Schizotypal. People with schizotypal behavior have feelings of inadequacy and insecurity. They have strange ideas, behaviors, and appearances. The focus of counseling is to give them reality checks and to promote self-awareness and more socially acceptable behavior in a slow-paced, supportive manner.

Narcissistic. Narcissists are grandiose, extremely self-centered, and believe they have unique problems that others cannot possibly comprehend. They see themselves as victimized by others and always need to be right. The focus of counseling is to get them to see how their behavior is seen and felt by others while not engaging in a "no-win" debate or argument with them.

Histrionic. People with histrionic personality disorder move from crisis to crisis. They have a shallow depth of character and are extremely ego-involved. They crave excitement and become quickly bored with routine and mundane tasks and events. They may behave in self-destructive ways and can be demanding and manipulative. The focus of counseling is to stress their ability to survive using resources that have been helpful to them in the past.

Obsessive–Compulsive. Those with obsessive-compulsive disorder are preoccupied by and fixate on tasks. They expend and waste vast amounts of time and energy on these endeavors. They often do not hear counselors because of futile attempts to obtain self-control over their obsessions. The focus of counseling is to establish the ability to trust others and the use of thought stopping and behavior modification to diminish obsessive thinking and compulsive behavior.

Bipolar I. The extreme mood swings of these callers range from superhero ideation when in a manic or hypomanic episode to "born loser" ideation when experiencing a major depressive episode. If they feel thwarted in their grand plans, they may become very aggressive toward those who would stop them. At the other end of the continuum, their depressive "doom, despair, and agony on me" outlook puts them at risk for suicidal behavior. Slowing down and pacing these callers in the manic episode is difficult but needs to be done and can be the precursor to or followed by a hypomanic or major depressive episode. Figuring out a way to put a psychological governor or safety valve on their runaway behavior in a manic episode is critical. However, confrontation about their grandiose plans only alienates them. In a depressive episode, suicide intervention is a primary priority.

Bipolar II. While similar to Bipolar I, people with this diagnosis experience only hypomanic and major depressive episodes. The hypomania episodes are not due to legally prescribed medication, street drugs, or other medical conditions. The medications that may have side effects that mimic hypomania episodes may be legal and either prescribed (e.g., Fentanyl) or over the counter (e.g., **Dextromethorphan**) or street drugs (e.g., meth or ecstasy, also known as molly). In hypomania episodes, people generally feel the need for decreased sleep and have an overabundance of energy, possibly affecting their cognitive functioning. Again, finding a way to slow down hypomanic behavior is vital. During a major depressive episode, attention should be given to potential suicidal ideations and behaviors.

Dependent. People with dependent personality disorder have trouble making decisions and seek to have others do so—often inappropriately. Feelings of worthlessness and insecurity and a fear of abandonment predominate. They are particularly prone to becoming involved and staying in self-destructive relationships. The focus of counseling is to reinforce strengths and act as a support for their concerns without becoming critical of them or accepting responsibility for their lives.

Self-Defeating. Those with self-defeating behavior choose people and situations that lead to disappointment, failure, and mistreatment by others. They reject attempts to help them and make sure that such attempts will not succeed. The focus of counseling is stressing talents and the behavioral consequences of sabotaging themselves.

Avoidant. People with avoidant personality disorder are loners who have little ability to establish or maintain social relationships. Their fear of rejection paralyzes their attempts to risk involvement in social relationships. The focus of counseling is the encouragement of successive approximations to meaningful relationships through social skills and assertion training.

Passive-Aggressive. Those with passive-aggressive behavior cannot risk rejection by displaying anger in an overt manner. Rather, they engage in covert attempts to manipulate others and believe that control is more important than self-improvement. The focus of counseling is to promote more open, assertive behavior.

Borderline. Borderline personality disorder is so named because such people are chameleon-like and at any given time may resemble any of the foregoing mental disorders. Also, they are always on the "borderline" of being functional and dysfunctional. One of the most challenging of callers, they are dealt with at length in Chapter 5, "Crisis Case Handling."

Handling the Extremely Distressed Caller

LO5 Calls from severely disturbed callers can be especially harrowing for neophytes and, if they would admit it, many experienced crisis workers. Extremely distressed callers often are "frequent flyers" calling crisis hotlines. On the neophyte phone counselor's first meeting with the disorganized and disjunctive thought processes of individuals with jumbled thoughts processes, all the training the crisis worker has ever received is likely to fall by the wayside.

These callers represent a cornucopia of mental illnesses. They may be delusional and hallucinatory; be unable to remotely test what they are doing, believing, or thinking against reality; be emotionally volcanic or conversely demonstrate the emotionality of a stone; lack insight or judgment about their problems and be unable to relate any linear or logical history of these problems; be so suspicious in their paranoid ideation that they believe even the phone worker is out to get them; be manipulative, resistant, and openly hostile and noncompliant to the simplest requests; not have the slightest idea of appropriate interpersonal boundaries with significant others or the crisis worker; demonstrate obsessive behavior and compulsive thoughts that they continually focus on to the exclusion of any effective functioning; have no meaningful interpersonal relationships with the possible exception of crisis line workers; impulsively place themselves in problematic and dangerous situations over and over; and present themselves in childlike or even infantile ways (Grunsted et al., 1991). Additionally it is not uncommon for the foregoing behaviors to be fueled by the intake of illicit drugs, which further accelerates the psychological fires raging within them.

Whether these behaviors are biochemically or psychologically based makes little difference. These people are so distanced from reality and so threatening that the beginning phone counselor's immediate reaction is likely to be to get off the line! However, if the worker pictures the disturbed client as a person whose developmental processes have gone terribly awry, then the call may take on structure and sense and become less intimidating. No matter how bizarre

the call may be, these primary axioms apply to the caller's behavior (Greenwald, 1985a, p. 1):

1. Behavior is always purposeful and serves motives that may be either conscious or unconscious.
2. Behavior is comprehensible and has meaning even though the language used may not.
3. Behavior is characteristic and consistent with personality even though it is exaggerated.
4. Behavior is used to keep a person safe and free of anxiety.

The following rules for dealing with disturbed callers are abstracted from a number of crisis hotlines (Epstein & Carter, 1991; Greenwald, 1985a, 1985b; Knudson, 1991; Lester & Brockopp, 1973; Tuttle, 1991).

Slow Emotions Down. Although disturbed callers have many feelings that have been submerged from awareness, the best strategy is not to attempt to uncover these feelings. The caller is being besieged by too many feelings and needs to find a way to get them in control. Focusing on here-and-now issues that are concrete and reality oriented is the preferred mode of operation. Do not elicit more feelings with open-ended questions such as "Can you tell me more about that?" Eliciting more feeling may result in feelings becoming more out of control and difficult for the crisis worker to deescalate. Instead, use calming interventions that force the person to order their thinking in small, realistic bits of detail.

CW: I understand how scary those thoughts are that keep creeping into your mind and the "things" you think are in the room. What I want you to do right now is look around the room and tell me what is there. Then, tell me what happened to start this thinking.

The idea is to slow emotions down and re-establish control. Although the worker may acknowledge the feelings, they are not the focus of attention. By breaking up freewheeling ideation into discrete, manageable pieces, the telephone worker gives the caller a sense of regaining control. The worker may also bring the caller back to reality from a flashback by asking the client what they are doing. Closed questions also help callers re-establish control.

CW: You say you're in that alley and he's assaulting you. Were you smoking a cigarette then? I know you just lit a cigarette a minute ago. I want you to slowly inhale, smell that smoke, and tell me where you are. Now blow the smoke out and see where it goes around the room.

Refuse to Share Hallucinations and Delusions. If a caller is hallucinating or delusional, the telephone worker should never side with the psychotic ideation.

Caller: Do you see, hear, smell, feel those things?

CW: No! I'm sorry, I don't. I understand right now you do, and that's terrifying, but what I want to do is get you some help. So stay with me. What is your address so we can get some support for you?

Little, if any, good ever comes from participating in such thinking, and as the delusion increases, it becomes difficult to extricate oneself from it. Yet grandiose thinking, no matter how bizarre, should not be denied.

CW: (inappropriate and sarcastic) Come on, now. The CIA isn't really listening to an auto mechanic by electronic eavesdropping. Certainly they've got better things to do than that. Why do you believe that?

CW: (appropriate and empathic) It's pretty clear that you really believe the CIA is listening to you. When did this start?

The worker affirms the paranoid delusion is real without agreeing to its veracity. By asking a *when* question, the worker can start eliciting information that will allow an assessment of the scope and extent of the paranoia. A *why* question is never appropriate because of the defensive reaction it may elicit in any caller.

Determine Medication Usage. The default questions on medication usage still hold whether intervention is face-to-face or by telecommunication (refer to Chapter 4, "The Tools of the Trade"). If at all possible, the crisis worker should obtain information about the use of any medication, the amount and time of dosage, and particularly, the stopping of medication without consulting the attending physician. Changing, forgetting, or disregarding medication is one of the most common reasons that people become actively psychotic (Ammar & Burdin, 1991). The crisis worker might also ask about medications being added recently in case interactions might be causing adverse effects. Furthermore, having this information will give the worker a better idea of the type of mental disturbance for which the caller is being treated. Regardless of the reasons or excuses clients give for not taking medicine, the worker should endeavor to get them to their prescribing physician so medication can be adjusted or reinstituted.

CW: Lemuel, I want you to call up your doctor as soon as we get off the phone. I understand that the medicine gives you a bad taste in your mouth and makes you feel queasy. However, your doctor needs to know that, and you need to let her know you're not on your meds.

Becoming familiar with the major tranquilizers, antidepressants, and antipsychotic drugs is important for this work (Patterson et al., 2021). However, given all the different kinds of drugs and their numerous generic and trade names, keeping track of them all is extremely difficult. In the past, the *Physician's Desk Reference (PDR)* was the go-to resource for information on what these drugs do, how much is generally given, and what the side effects are. However, given the constant influx of new medications, the PDR becomes dated quickly. Now, the internet is faster, more up-to-date, and easily accessed from any computer. Simply using a search engine to find information on a medication generally provides all you need including the scientific name, brand name, dosage, common side effects, rare side effects, and interactions with other medications. In other words, the information you need.

Keep Expectations Realistic. The telephone worker should keep expectations realistic. The caller did not become disturbed overnight. No crisis worker is going to change chronic psychotic behavior during one phone call. The crisis worker is buying time for the caller in a period of high anxiety and attempting to restore a minimum amount of control and contact with reality. If the caller is trying to "milk" the worker through an interminable conversation, confronting the problem in a direct manner will generally determine whether the caller is lonely or needs immediate assistance.

CW: It seems as if this can't be solved, and you say you can't wait until tomorrow to go to the clinic. I'm concerned enough that I think we ought to make arrangements to transport you to the hospital right now.

Maintain Professional Distance. Calls from severely disturbed individuals may evoke all kinds of threatening feelings in phone workers, leaving them feeling inadequate, confused, and in crisis themselves! Maintaining professional distance when exceedingly painful and tragic stories are related is difficult for even the most experienced phone worker. When these feelings begin to emerge, it is of utmost importance for workers to make owning statements about their own feelings and get supervision immediately. Passing the line to another worker in no way indicates inadequacy.

CW: Frankly, I'm a bit confused as to what to do. I've done everything I know, and I'm tapped out. I'd like to connect you with Irma, who may have some other ideas, while I talk to our director.

As confused and disoriented as disturbed callers may be, they seem to have a sixth sense about sensitive areas in others. **Countertransference** (the attributing to clients of the therapist's own problems) is not uncommon, and disturbed callers can sometimes unearth the worker's own hidden agendas and insecurities. A worker's strong reactions, either positive or negative, to these callers should alert the hotline worker that processing and feedback with a coworker or supervisor are needed.

Caller: (paranoid) I know who you are, when you work on the hotline, and where you live.

CW: (inappropriately responding to the threat in a shaky voice) What have I ever done to you? I'm trying to help you, and you get bent out of shape. I've got a good mind to hang this phone up right now or even call the police. We can trace these calls, you know!

CW: (appropriately responding to the implication in a clear, firm, but empathic voice) Jacques, those things are not important to what's going on with you right now. What is important is making you feel safe enough to go back to your apartment tonight and go to the doctor in the morning. I understand why you might get upset over me suggesting you see the doctor, but I also want you to clearly understand it's your safety I'm concerned about. So what's making you angry with me?

By deflecting the caller's paranoia and refocusing the dialogue back on the client's issues, the telephone worker's directive forces the caller, in an empathic manner, to respond to his own emotional state.

Avoid Placating.

Placating and sympathizing do little to bolster the caller's confidence or to help move the client toward action.

Caller: (depressed) I'm just not any good to anybody, much less myself.

CW: (inappropriately sympathetic) From all you've told me, you've had a really rocky road. Nobody should have to suffer what you have, but things can only look up.

Rather, by empathically responding and exploring past feelings and coping skills when life was better, the telephone worker not only acknowledges the dilemma but also focuses on the client's strengths.

CW: You do sound pretty hopeless right now, but I wonder how you were feeling when things weren't this way, and what you were doing then that you aren't doing now.

Assess Lethality.

Assessing for lethality is the other default area of inquiry, whether face-to-face or by telecommunication (see Chapter 4, "The Tools of the Trade"). Many clients who call crisis lines have active suicidal or homicidal ideation. It may seem puzzling that such people would call a crisis line when they seem so bent on harming themselves or others. Regular callers, in particular, should be assessed for suicidal or homicidal ideation because they are very prone to underscore the critical nature of their problems and "prove" their need for help by threatening lethal behavior (Brockopp, 2002a). Although telephone worker skills at assessing lethality vary, research finds that assessing lethality is effective as a preventive measure (Tyson et al., 2016). What suicidal callers are doing is trying to put distance between their thoughts and the actions that might result from those lethal thoughts. As much as the callers may avow intentions of lethality, they are still in enough control of themselves to attempt to place a buffer (the telephone worker) between thinking and acting (McCaskie et al., 1990).

Caller: If I can't have him, she sure as hell won't. I'll kill them both, and you, the police, or nobody else can stop me.

CW: Yet you called here, for which I'm glad. Something is holding you back, and I'd like to know what that something is.

Caller: Well, I'm a Christian, but their sins go beyond redemption.

CW: So as a Christian, you probably think the commandment "Thou shalt not kill" is pretty important. What you're saying is you're about to commit sin, just as they did. How will that help you, and how will it look in the eyes of God?

Although it may be construed that the telephone worker is manipulating the spiritual philosophy of the caller to achieve an end, the major goal of the crisis worker is to disrupt the irrational chain of thinking that is propelling the client toward violence. In that regard, when dealing with the disturbed caller, the overriding thesis is "Save the body before the mind" (Grunsted et al., 1991). Crisis intervention over the telephone with those who are severely disturbed is clearly not meant to be curative. It is a stopgap measure designed to be palliative enough to keep action in abeyance until help arrives.

Although no crisis line staff members that we know of would ever instruct their workers to give out their full names or home phone numbers, at times, callers can be very seductive in their attempts to extract personal information from crisis line workers. Rookies on the crisis line may be very taken with the heartbreaking stories they hear or feel very gratified by the strokes that dependent callers can give them. Under no circumstances should a crisis line worker ever give out their full name or other personal information, nor should the worker ever agree to meet the caller for social or professional reasons. The crisis line's credibility is built on anonymity, and that works both ways. In addition, serious ethical problems may arise when that anonymity is breached. Finally, crisis line workers who do not observe the foregoing run the risk of putting themselves in physical harm's way.

Given all that we have said about severely disturbed callers, our admonition is still to treat these clients not as types, but as individuals with their own idiosyncratic problems. However, those who are severely disturbed are not the only regular or problem callers.

Other Problem Callers

Telephone crisis workers must sometimes deal with covert callers, pranksters, silent callers, manipulators, sexually explicit callers, or even callers presenting legitimate sexual problems. It must be remembered and accepted that every call is an attempt by the caller to fulfill some need or purpose. The following are several types of problem callers and suggestions that should help workers understand and cope with such callers.

Rappers. Some callers may just wish to chat or talk. The question becomes whether time should be spent listening to someone who only wants to talk, with no seemingly pressing issues. However, if "lonely" is tacked onto the description of the person, this may change the telephone worker's perception of the problem. It may also be that the caller is having trouble bringing issues into the open and is testing the waters to get enough courage to jump in. By allowing some leeway in approaching issues while at the same time gently confronting the caller's loneliness, the worker sets reasonable limits on the conversation and still provides a supportive forum (McCaskie et al., 1990).

Third Party Callers. Some callers take the initiative to call on behalf of someone else (Draper et al., 2015, p. 264). Often, but not every time, these callers (third party callers) call seeking advice about a family member or close friend who is suicidal (Gould et al., 2022). The National Suicide Prevention Lifeline (2019) published tips for working with these callers. The tips include: (1) gather enough information to gauge the safety and risk of the suicidal person, (2) obtain contact and identification, if possible, (3) coach the caller on helping the person, (4) attempt to reach out to the person, and (5) contact 911 if the risk is imminent or other solutions are not possible.

Covert Callers. On the other hand, some callers who ask for help for another individual may actually be asking for help for themselves. As a result, always assume that the call is about the caller but never attempt to prove the call is about someone else (Brockopp, 1973a, p. 164; Brockopp, 2002a, pp. 171–175). Other callers may act surprised, "Oh, I thought this was a recording." The response is to affirm that it is not. "No, it isn't. I am Joe, and this is the crisis line. How can I help you this evening?" Yet others may make humorous jests as a test. "You must be really crazy to work there. I'll bet there are some real nuts who call up." The response to these calls is to avoid the "test" and respond empathically by saying, "I wonder if you're concerned that calls are handled seriously here?" These are most likely ways that timid and embarrassed callers have of checking out the crisis line to see what the opening response is and whether it is safe to talk. Intellectual types, on the other hand, tend to be know-it-alls who probably do have more expertise than volunteers. On their own intellectual ground, they always "win." In actuality, these callers are often very insecure and unsure of themselves under their self-assured exterior. The key to dealing with individuals that intellectualize is to immediately let them defeat you. "You're right. I am a volunteer here, and I don't know as much as you do about bipolar disorder. What I do know is you sound pretty concerned about it and seem to be looking for some help." Other callers may call and be silent or say they have the wrong number. Particularly at a suicide center, there are no wrong numbers. "May I help you?" or "What number were you calling?" are default responses to "wrong numbers."

Pranksters or Nuisance Callers. Teenagers who are bored at an overnight party may call the line just to bedevil the workers. If the prank call is treated seriously, they will probably hang up and not call back. If they are hung up on, they will continue to call (Brockopp 1973b; Waters & Finn, 1995, p. 270). Many calls may appear to be of a nuisance nature. However, any person making a nuisance call should be considered to have a problem. Therefore, it is important that calls not be arbitrarily seen as pranks. The crisis line must answer all calls in a straightforward, no-nonsense manner. The crisis line must clearly convey that they are not playing games with people but that callers will be listened to honestly and responded to directly no matter what the purpose (Brockopp, 1973b, pp. 206–210). By so doing, the crisis line builds the perception in the community that the line is serious about what they do (Brockopp, 2002a, pp. 187–190). The teenager who is a prankster one night may be the suicidal teenager another night.

CW: Is it a prank or a dare you're playing or maybe something else that you really do need to talk about?

CW: I do wonder if there is something you might like to talk about. If you do, feel free to call back.

Silent Callers. One of the most frustrating callers is the person who is silent. Silent callers are ambivalent. Either through embarrassment or hurt, they are reticent, or from previous negative experiences, they fear rejection and are just plain unable to muster the courage to talk. Workers must overcome their initial reaction to hang up, demonstrate acceptance, and attempt to remove any impediment that may keep the person from communicating (Brockopp, 2002b). For the silent caller, an appropriate response would be, "I'll be here when you feel you can talk."

CW: Sometimes it is really difficult to say what you need. Maybe it hurts so much you can't find words. Maybe you are not sure you can trust me. Whatever the reason you feel unable to talk, I am going to wait a little bit before I take another call.

Even if you can't talk now, understand that this line is open for you when you need to talk.

If there is still no response, after a minute or so you could say, "I guess it is difficult to talk about this right now. I'll stay on the line for another minute, and then I'll have to go to another call. Call back when you feel ready to talk."

Manipulators. A variety of callers achieve their unmet needs by playing games with telephone workers. Typical manipulative games include questioning the worker's ability, role reversal in which the worker is tricked into sharing details of their personal life, and harassment. Redirecting the manipulative ploy and focusing on the unmet needs of manipulators force them to look at the reasons for their manipulative behavior (Brockopp, 2002a, p. 174; Waters & Finn, 1995, p. 269).

CW: You certainly know a great deal more about that subject than I do. How does it feel to be in control like that?

CW: When you question my integrity or try to get me to share intimate details, I wonder if you realize that is trying to meet some of your own needs for control. I wonder if you have considered what those needs to control and manipulate others are getting you?

Sexually Explicit Callers. The primary purpose of the sexually explicit caller is to masturbate while talking to someone. The sexually explicit caller is a particular millstone hung on the crisis line because many female volunteers become angry, embarrassed, and afraid and resign out of frustration with frequent sex calls (Baird et al., 1994; Brockopp & Lester, 2002, pp. 133–135; Fenelon, 1990). Brockopp and Lester (2002, p. 136) propose staying on the line and tolerating the behavior while attempting to build a more trusting relationship without condoning the behavior itself. That is a very idealistic way of treating the problem and, in the opinion of your authors, is a great way to lose a lot of volunteers in a hurry! We will take a stand here and state that the crisis line is just not the place for that behavior to occur. An option is to switch the caller to another worker whose gender is different than the original one and reframe the call in a context suggesting that the caller needs help to put a severe damper on such calls.

Callers With Legitimate Sexual Problems. However, many people who have serious sexual or sexually related problems call crisis lines because of the anonymity allowed to frankly discuss their most private issues. These calls may embarrass workers who are not psychologically prepared for such intimate details, feel shocked at what they hear because of the criminal or exploitative nature, or do not have the technical expertise to handle them. Telephone workers must have education in dealing with sexual concerns and training in legal and ethical knowledge about what to do if the caller is a danger to a third party (Horton, 1995, p. 292). The very nature of calls dealing with sexual matters places crisis workers in a potentially value-laden, belief-centered moral and religious arena in which the worker's own opinions come into play. Although in most instances, the major role of the worker is to *not* let their opinions hold sway and influence clients, avoiding these hot areas may also mean denying the caller much-needed information (Horton, 1995, p. 307). Providing options and information about "responsible" sex is a viable approach, although it should be understood that a very fine line runs between the worker's own biases and providing balanced information and must be monitored carefully.

Even though the preceding types of callers are striving to fulfill their needs, they often pose problems for telephone workers. The following are some techniques to help prepare crisis workers to deal with this sometimes-difficult clientele.

Handling the Problem Callers

Pose Open-Ended Questions. Appropriate use of open-ended questions can help defuse the problems generated by frustrated callers (Epstein & Carter, 1991).

TC: You people don't know anything. Everything you've told me is a bunch of crap.

CW: What did you expect to gain from this call, then?

TC: Just to tell you what I think of your lousy service.

CW: If you were me, what would you be doing or saying right now?

These questions refocus the problem back to the caller and force movement toward problem solving rather than keeping the worker subjected to condemnatory statements.

Set Time Limits. When it is apparent that attempts to refocus the problem to the caller are futile, then a time limit should be set (Knudson, 1991).

TC: You ought to be congratulating me on getting my act together, no thanks to you.

CW: I'm glad you've done something positive since you last called. Now, we can talk about your current situation for 5 minutes. Then I'll have to take another call.

Terminate Abuse. When the caller's behavior escalates to what the worker perceives as abusiveness, the call should be terminated in a clear and firm manner (McCaskie et al., 1990).

TC: You bitch! Don't you dare hang up this goddamned phone!

CW: (assertively) I'm sorry, but that is language we do not tolerate, so I'm going to another caller now. When you can talk appropriately, feel free to call back.

Switch Workers. Particularly with a sexually explicit caller, switching the call to another worker not the same gender as the original worker takes the stimulus thrill out of the situation and makes it very difficult for the caller to bring masturbation to orgasm, which is usually the end goal of such a call (Knudson, 1991).

TC: I'd love to cover you with honey and lick you all over.

CW (female): (calmly and coolly) Given your specific problem, I'm going to switch you to Ralph. (Signals to Ralph.)

CW (Ralph): (assertively) I understand you have a problem. How can I help you?

If another worker is not available, the call should be shifted to a supervisor and terminated. The caller should be told that the worker will hang up and that action should be taken immediately (McCaskie et al., 1990).

CW (supervisor): (authoritatively and firmly) We are *not* here to answer demeaning remarks while you masturbate. You need to know that our calls are recorded, and obscene calls and using this service to masturbate are illegal. I am going to hang up. You may call back when you are ready to discuss this problem.

To bait a telephone worker and hold TC on the line, sexually explicit callers often externalize their fantasies by reporting some hypothetical significant other's problem in florid detail. When the first hint of this ploy *occurs*, the worker should interpret the behavior as the caller's own and make the switch (Knudson, 1991). Legal and ethical concerns emerge like the one above. Chapter 3, "The Intervention and Assessment Models," describes the LASER protocol to help in the decision-making process for this type of call (Myer et al., 2021). Crisis workers must question callers to determine reasonably the veracity of the information.

TC: I'm really worried about my uncle and his 10-year-old daughter. She's a little doll, and he's always giving her these massages in her bedroom and I . . .

CW: (**Interrupts.**) That's out of my area of expertise; please hold the line and let me switch you to our child abuse expert. Before I switch you over, I want you to know he is going to ask some questions to confirm what you just told me. His name is Ralph, and I am transferring right now. If the call is dropped please, please call back.

In this short exchange the crisis worker is predispositioning the caller to let her know what to expect. This process helps the caller not to be caught by surprise by what may seem to be intrusive and possibly intimate questions when individuals talk to another person. The caller is also asked, almost pleaded with, to call back if something happens when the call is transferred.

Use Covert Modeling. Covert modeling or conditioning (Cautela, 1976; Kazdin, 1975) has been used by Baird et al. (1994) to extinguish repeated calls, particularly by sexually explicit clients. In covert modeling, the client is asked to use mental imagery to picture either reinforcing or extinguishing a particular behavior. The following worker response is abridged from their technique.

CW: As you're talking, I'm wondering if you recognize your real problem and want help with it. I know this would be pretty difficult to give up. But sometime soon, I'm not sure exactly when, as you reach for the phone, you'll think to call a therapist instead. And this notion that you'll call a therapist and get help will get stronger every day as you think of it. You'll also start to feel better as you realize the crisis line isn't fulfilling your needs like therapy will. I'm going to hang up now and let you think about getting help with your real problem.

By suggesting that the need to call the therapist will grow, the worker plants the seed for anxiety about the caller's present behavior to grow along with the

need to change. Both negative and positive reinforcers are used in the image: the need to seek help and the good feeling that will come from doing so. The worker also speaks of seeking help for the "real problem." This unspecified problem allows the worker to respond emphatically without accusing the caller of terrible, deviant behavior but still clearly states that the caller needs help. The worker does not continue in a dialogue with the client but instead hangs up to let the seed start to grow.

LO6 **Formulate Administrative Rules.** Administratively, crisis lines need to set specific rules to extinguish abusive behavior by doing the following (Knudson, 1991; McCaskie et al., 1990; Middleton et al., 2014):

1. Limiting the number and duration of calls from any single caller
2. Limiting the topics that will be discussed
3. Requiring that only specific workers versed in handling abusive callers take such calls
4. Using speaker phones for on-the-spot consultation
5. Requiring the caller to establish a face-to-face relationship with an outside worker and allow communication between the therapist and crisis line personnel
6. Allowing the staff to prohibit calls for a day, a week, or more if physical threats are made
7. The service initiating contact with the caller instead of waiting for caller contact and coordinating short-term treatment programs for anxiety and depression by telephone
8. Creating a specific management plan for each caller

The Headquarters Crisis Center of Lawrence, Kansas, uses a tracking log for regular callers that lists their name, phone number, address, style of interaction, major and tangential issues, effective and ineffective response modes, their physician/therapist, medications, support groups, and lethality levels. The log is kept current and available to staff, saving them a great deal of time and energy. This center also has an internal messages notebook labeled "Client Concerns." It contains information about regular callers that workers can quickly read to become updated on the caller's circumstances. It is an effective method to keep staff current and can be used to offer feedback and suggestions to clients (Epstein & Carter, 1991). Staff should be brought together on a regular basis to discuss these callers, plan a strategy for them, make suggestions, and voice personal concerns (McCaskie et al., 1990). Finally, supervisors need to be acutely aware of the impact that such callers can have on personnel. Crisis center administrators should be ready, willing, and able to process the debilitating emotions that such calls often evoke in workers in a caring, empathic, and supportive manner through regularly planned supervision and emergency debriefing sessions when necessary. Crisis intervention over the telephone is tough, grueling work, particularly when clients such as the foregoing emerge. Crisis calls are frequently one-time events with very little opportunity for positive feedback. Particularly because crisis lines are run chiefly by volunteers, they need to be aware that not everyone can be helped (Waters & Finn, 1995).

Hotlines

LO7 As noted in Chapter 1, "Approaching Crisis Intervention," the first telephone crisis hotline was established in 1906 by the National Save-a-Life League to prevent suicide (Bloom, 1984). Indeed, the growing suicide prevention movement in the 1950s adopted the telephone as the primary mode of treatment because of its immediacy (Lester & Brockopp, 1973), and over the course of time, it has been the most often used method of suicide intervention (Lester, 2001; Mishara et al., 2005; SAMSHA, 2023; Seely, 1997a, 1997b; Slaikeu & Leff-Simon, 1990) with dedicated suicide hotlines in many countries, states, provinces, and cities. Other crisis-related hotlines include ones for domestic violence, addiction, sexual assault, veterans' concerns, and child abuse to name a few.

In 2022, the new national suicide prevention hotline of 988, formerly known as the Suicide Prevention Lifeline, was opened for callers experiencing suicidal ideations (Pope et al., 2022). The remaking of this hotline is to make it easier for callers to make contact rather than using the original ten-digit number (SAMSHA, 2022). The ten-digit number still works, but 988 is much easier to remember and call when in crisis. Veterans can use this hotline to access crisis workers with knowledge and experience with individuals who are familiar with their experience. This hotline also accepts calls from anyone in crisis due to a mental health issue or substance misuse. Another special component of this hotline that will be discussed in the next section of this chapter is that the hotline is also set up to receive text messages and conduct chats for individuals in crisis.

Generic crisis phone lines are typically open 24 hours a day, 365 days a year, while more specialized services may operate during regular business hours. People who are lonely, have panic attacks, gamble or drink to excess, abuse partners, grieve, are depressed, experience psychotic breaks, or experience a whole smorgasbord of crises that could qualify for Ripley's "Believe It or Not" call crisis lines. Hotlines developed for specific types of crises may have a more limited timeframe. In these situations, callers may be transferred automatically to another hotline, or a recording will encourage callers to contact another hotline or go to the closest emergency room for assistance.

Time-Limited Hotlines. A time-limited hotline is one that is put into operation for a specified period of time; it is typically used to deal with a specific problem or to engage a special client population, such as immediately before a potential disaster or after a disaster. These hotlines are useful to offer brief supportive therapy and for information or referral resources.

An example is when the State of Texas utilized a couple of specialized hotlines for victim assistance and victim compensation after the El Paso Walmart shooting on August 3, 2019. Another example is when Emergence Health Network, the local mental health authority in El Paso, created a specialized hotline during the COVID-19 pandemic. Volunteers for this hotline received specialized training to assist individuals needing emotional support and assistance to locate resources including medical, financial, housing, and food during the pandemic (Emergence Health Network Administrative Staff interview, March 2023).

Specialized Hotlines. Specialized hotlines deal with specific topics, such as troubled youth, parenting, veterans' issues, or farmers with concerns. Although brief supportive therapy may occur on such hotlines, generally, the major purpose is to provide crisis intervention by volunteers or professionals with an understanding and knowledge of the topic. These lines cut across all cultural groups and socioeconomic classes and may be located in urban, suburban, and rural regions. Some specialized hotlines are national, while others are regional. The National Runaway Hotline (1-800-RUNAWAY) not only spends time talking to runaways about their problems but also encourages them to get off the streets and into the nearest runaway shelter (National Runaway Safeline, 2023). The national domestic violence hotline (1-800-SAFE) is available to any victim of domestic abuse in the

United States (National Domestic Violence Hotline, 2023). The **Trans Lifeline** (877-565-8860) offers peer support and crisis intervention services for trans individuals who need resources 24/7. The National Football League even has a hotline. This hotline is available to call for players, coaches, team league staff, and their family members who may be in crisis (NFL Lifeline, 2012). These are a few of the national call centers that specialize in every kind of imaginable human dilemma. Because of the numerous attempts to jump off the Golden Gate Bridge, a unique direct hotline to crisis intervention call centers is placed on bridges (Jacobs, 2010). Another regional hotline is the Farm Family Resource Initiative in Southern Illinois (Farm Family Resource Initiative, 2023). This hotline (833-FARM-SOS [833-327-6767]) is part of a grant funded research project through the Southern Illinois University School of Medicine. Callers who own or work on farms in Illinois can call or text to receive support and crisis intervention. Many, if not most, of these specialized hotlines also now include the ability for real-time chat and texting, which will be discussed later.

Tele–Behavioral Health Growing Role in Crisis Intervention

LO8 Let's take a step back in time and suppose you are the first students to have access to the first edition of this book published in 1988. Land line telephones were the only technology readily available from the 40s to the 70s. You would find nothing about the technologies available today. Flash forward to the present, and those of you who were born after 1990 may find that unbelievable because the internet has always been a part of who you are and the way you communicate with others. Winston Churchill said, "Take change by the hand, because if you don't it will take you by the throat!"

The arrival of the COVID-19 pandemic caused counseling services to switch to the internet (Rhodes, 2023). The megacrisis of the COVID-19 pandemic certainly accelerated the use of other technologies in crisis intervention. Key to this growth is continuing advances in software, along with the proliferation of more advanced computers and smartphones. Gluekauf reported in 2018 that many therapists were skeptical of tele-behavioral health, citing critical reasons such as the lack of training, ethical concerns, lack of professional association direction, and licensure issues. The COVID-19 outbreak steam rolled those objections because of the urgent need to provide epidemic-based crisis counseling that was not face-to-face. Now that restrictions resulting from the pandemic have mostly lifted, face-to-face counseling has returned. Yet, tele-behavioral health has taken root and is here to stay, and it will continue to be important in the delivery of therapy and particularly crisis intervention (Glass & Bickler, 2021; Norcross et al., 2022).

While the telephone remains the most frequent way to connect remotely with crisis workers, the emergence of a variety of communication technologies linked to the internet and smartphones may reduce reliance on the telephone for crisis intervention. The emergence of video conferencing along with texting, mobile apps, email, chat rooms, and social media is changing crisis intervention, and all of these are now used to extend services. Cutting-edge technology-based modalities such as artificial intelligence are thought to be useful in offering counseling services (Giovannetti, 2023). For some populations, virtual reality is another possibility for crisis intervention.

Video Conferencing. Video conferencing became a necessity during the COVID-19 crisis. Business meetings, classes, visits with friends, and numerous other gatherings were held using video conferencing. Organizations and private practitioners providing mental health counseling joined in and were pretty much forced to switch service delivery in a matter of weeks if not days to remain in business (Garcia et al., 2022). The Emergence Health Network in El Paso, Texas, was one of those organizations. In-person, on-site services became minimal, with video conferencing services skyrocketing to over 90 percent (Emergence Health Network Administrative Staff interview, March 2023).

The rapid shift to tele-behavioral health resulted in several issues surfacing that are relevant for crisis intervention. A major concern is confidentiality regarding the platform and physical location the crisis worker uses. Care must be taken to ensure the platform is shielded from intrusion, eavesdropping, or hijacking by a third party. The issue regarding the location is that listening is restricted to approved individuals; that is, not family members, friends, or neighbors of the crisis worker. Think about during the pandemic when many work meetings were conducted via video conferencing and a family member unintentionally "photo bombed" an important discussion. Therefore, having a private room with possibly a locked door may be prudent to secure the location.

The second issue for video conferencing involves making contact with and observing individuals' reactions during the intervention process (Rhodes, 2023). The primary issue is the limitations of the camera being used by individuals in crisis. You will always see faces and sometimes maybe just below the shoulders of individuals. What you do not see is if individuals are wringing their hands or fidgeting with their legs. Although this information may seem miniscule, seeing the full body language of individuals in crisis is useful in making and maintaining contact.

The third issue involves assessing individuals in crisis. More and other questions may be needed than when the intervention is in person. Depending on the crisis, questions may include if individuals have a safety plan, the availability of weapons, who else is in the room, changes in medications, and so on. The point is that questions need to be tailored to the crisis at hand to complete a Triage Form as discussed in Chapter 3, "The Intervention and Assessment Models."

Texting. Texting via smartphones using various apps has become part of crisis intervention (Mazzer et al., 2021). Many, if not most, hotlines now have a texting option to contact crisis workers. A key issue in the use of texting is expectations for private practitioners. The primary issue with respect to expectations using texting is boundaries (MacMullin et al., 2020). This issue can be a real concern for private practitioners. Clients in crisis may expect an immediate response to a text regardless of the time or even if it is a holiday. What if you are driving, or your smartphone is not charged, or, heaven forbid, you forgot your phone? You may not be able to respond instantaneously. Providing clear parameters of availability is critical. Also, automatic replies can be used to guide clients to use other resources when in crisis. Organizations providing crisis intervention probably do not have a problem with availability. All these organizations will have a 24/7 with no holidays policy to respond immediately to calls for help.

Mobile Apps. Apps available to be downloaded on smartphones are another growing means to deliver crisis intervention (Parrish et al., 2022). Three strategies you might be using when referring individuals to apps are providing support, providing guidance, and encouraging mobilization. Each of these are helpful regardless of the Triage Form rating. For low to low-moderate triage ratings, these apps can be used as a psychoeducational tool to help individuals find information. For high-moderate to severe triage ratings, referring individuals to apps can help them access information and support 24/7.

If you have not done so already, go to the app "store" where you download apps on your smartphone. Select a crisis intervention topic (e.g., child grief, domestic violence, sexual assault, pet loss, and so on) and do a search. Several, if not many, apps will appear. Probably the majority of these apps are legitimate with the developers or sponsoring organizations really wanting to help. However, some may not be. Some apps may be endorsing a world view that may or may not be beneficial. Other apps may be designed to trick users into gathering personal information that can be sold or even trick you into sending money. Therefore, before referring individuals to one of these apps, make sure you have thoroughly checked it out. Never ever refer individuals to an app you have not inspected and do not consider on the up and up.

Chat Rooms. Synchronous live chat is additional support for telephone crisis intervention and is used for different types of crises (Cipolletti et al., 2021). As with mobile apps, helping individuals access chat rooms provides support, guidance, and mobilization. These three strategies are well suited for chat rooms because these can be used in concert not just to inform but also to give encouragement and assistance in accessing resources. The remainder of the nine strategies discussed in Chapter 4, "The Tools of the Trade," also are applicable in chat rooms.

Chat rooms for crisis intervention are generally hosted by websites. The websites offer information, but many also have the ability for real time synchronous chats. People log into these chat rooms for support groups by the millions to discuss health issues including mental health and crises. These websites may be more general, offering a variety of educational information and several hotline numbers, while some are dedicated to a specific type of crisis. As with smartphone apps, never ever refer someone to a website unless you have fully screened the site. Some websites, although likely well-meaning, may have an underlying second agenda that promotes ideas and beliefs that could be harmful to individuals who are vulnerable due to being in crisis.

Email. Similar to chatting via a website, websites may offer individuals the opportunity to contact crisis workers via email. This method is asynchronous and may not be the best method for individuals in crisis.

The obvious example is an individual who is actively suicidal, but other situations might occur immediately after a natural disaster in which the loss of life was great, such as the 2023 earthquake in Turkey and Syria. People in these two examples need immediate support without having to wait until someone logs into an email account. Yet in some instances, email can be extremely effective for guiding individuals to resources. And, you guessed it, we cannot emphasize this enough, do not refer individuals to a website offering email assistance without fully investigating the site or organization sponsoring the site.

Social Media. Finally, social media can also be useful in crisis intervention (Keasar et al., 2022). Regularly, and rightly so, social media is identified as being at the root of a crisis, too often suicide. Children through young adults are many times the target of cyberbullying, sadly resulting in suicide (Sedgwick et al., 2019). Yet, social media is useful in suicide prevention through the posting of positive messages (Keaser, 2022; Sedgwick et al., 2019). These researchers found that when messages suggesting suicidal ideations were responded to by trained volunteers, a decrease in the ideation was experienced. The decrease does not mean that all individuals who used social media to express suicidal ideations were helped, but many were.

Artificial Intelligence. AI is in its infancy with respect to providing counseling services in general and crisis intervention specifically (Giovannetti, 2023). AI involves the use of chat boxes that carry on conversation through texting and, in some cases, speech. Giovannetti states that chat boxes such as ChatGPT and Wysa are already being used. According to Giovannetti, AI has many advantages, such as being more attentive to individuals and less distractable. AI is also instantaneously available 24/7, which is a real advantage in crisis intervention. However, more research is encouraged before fully embracing this modality.

Virtual Reality. Another promising modality for crisis intervention is virtual reality (VR). Many computer programs available today perform assessment and self-help psychoeducational and therapeutic functions that are seen as effective and reliable (Christensen et al., 2014; Egan et al., 2014; van Ballegooijen et al., 2014; Twomey et al., 2014). The other great potential use of computer technology in tele-behavioral health is simulation and interactive VR

(Wiederhold & Wiederhold, 2005). VR can be defined as a set of computer technologies that, when combined, provide an interface to a computer-generated world (Wiederhold & Wiederhold, 2005, p. 5). Many of these programs are designed as games. Called "serious games," they are designed to reduce negative behavior or promote positive behavior change for a wide range of mental health concerns. Examples include panic attacks, posttraumatic stress disorder (PTSD), anxiety, obsessive compulsive disorders, and many more (Cann et al., 2014; Quero et al., 2014; Swirsky et al., 2014; Yin et al., 2014). They are reported to have a high level of acceptance by clients, and outcomes are comparable with those obtained when working with face-to-face therapists (Castro et al., 2014; Golomb et al., 2011; Li et al., 2014; Moritz et al., 2014; Park et al., 2015; Reger et al., 2011; Tortella-Feliu et al., 2011; Wuang et al., 2011). More will be discussed about VR in the next chapter addressing PTSD.

The Appeal of Online Counseling

Clearly, technological advances in hardware and software are much like the telephone in having the potential to provide a great deal of help to people who are geographically or psychologically isolated from specialized crisis services; have a physical or mental disability that does not permit them to travel to those services; are shy and do not want to meet face-to-face; need anonymity; have time management problems; are unavailable during normal working hours; or find it convenient, cost-effective, or simply natural to their way of life (MacMullin et al., 2021; Norcross et al., 2022).

Feedback. When it comes to direct therapeutic intervention, not all aspects of tele-behavioral health may be seen as better than face-to-face interaction, but there are many aspects of it that are. In crisis intervention, immediate and timely periodic feedback is critical. Periodic texting through mobile apps can serve this function well. Once the client's emotional control has been reestablished, asynchronous e-mails to check on how well the client is maintaining homeostasis and following through with efforts to resolve the crisis are at times indicated and helpful to support clients. Feedback at appropriate intervals varies but might include several times a day, every other day, or once a week. Clients that are suicidal/homicidal or survivors of domestic violence might need more follow up than clients who have just experienced a divorce or been in an automobile accident. Clients can also initiate contact when they feel the greatest need. Regular and frequent e-mail reports require the client to constantly monitor and report behavior, which is critical in crisis intervention (Castelnuovo et al., 2003). However, as the crisis interventionist, would you really want to sit at your computer all day long or constantly using your smartphone, checking emails? Imagine eating at a nice restaurant with your family and having to continuously check your smartphone for messages to see any clients who are in crisis. Or even worse, receiving an email at 5:07 in the morning when you are barely awake, or worse at 2:21 am with clients expecting an immediate response. As stated earlier, care must be taken to set expectations and boundaries with clients to preserve interventionists' personal lives. These expectations might involve letting clients know the times of day and the amount of time you read emails.

Disinhibition. A phenomenon that Suler (2004) named the **disinhibition effect** has appeared in e-therapy. What this effect means is that people tend to open up earlier with more distressing issues than they would normally in an F2F (internet acronym for face-to-face) therapy session. It is not clear why this effect happens, but it may be due to the absence of visual cues that might be perceived as judgmental or merely not having to look the therapist in the eye and tell individuals about the seamier side of one's life. The depersonalization and distance involved seem to make it safer to share intimate information (Keaser et al., 2022). This appears particularly true for men, who may be reticent to come for face-to-face counseling or even telephone counseling but will use e-mail at least as much as women (Wilson & Lester, 2002).

Whether this phenomenon changes with the increased use of Skype, where there is synchronous F2F, is another interesting e-therapy question. There is also some evidence that there is greater depth of emotional processing when people have to read something as opposed to listening (Hiltz, 1992). There may also be greater depth to cognitive processing, and that includes both client and worker. Certainly, it takes a great deal more time and thought to compose a written response; a cursory "hmmmm" probably won't be satisfactory (Wilson & Lester, 2002).

Problems of Legal and Ethical Issues in Tele-behavioral Health

Along with this potential and given some unique advantages over traditional and telephone interventions, there are some major areas of concern that cloud this new electronic horizon. As the flat worlders said to sailors who they thought were going over the edge of the world, "Be wary, there be demons and dragons out there!" While it is one thing to chat casually with another person half a world away, it is quite another to have people providing therapy or interventions about whose credentials you know nothing more than what they tell you. The reverse may also be true because clients may not be who they say they are. At their most malevolent, clients could attempt to infect the crisis interventionists' computers with viruses or other "malware" that could compromise their files (Maheu, 2001, 2003).

Legal and Ethical Issues. Certainly, any crisis worker or agency moving into this venue needs to know professional ethical standards and state and federal regulations and laws. The technological advances of caller identification, call blocking, and call tracing pose some complex legal and ethical dilemmas for the telephone hotline. Given the ability to screen and identify calls, is it right to deny services to problem clients? Furthermore, given the expectation and the safety callers feel due to the anonymity of call-in services, using these technologies could easily put confidentiality on a collision course with the duty to warn. Could other agencies demand the logs of such hotlines when involved in legal proceedings? Would the hotline workers be held civilly or criminally liable for their actions, given knowledge of who they were working with and what they might have said?

Because most telephone hotline workers are volunteers, they receive minimal training, and the agencies they work for are not bound by state or federal supervision or legislation in comparison to licensed mental health personnel (Seely, 1997a, 1997b). These issues further compound the problems of how to ethically use these new technologies. There are no clear answers to these dilemmas at present, but they are issues that need to be addressed at every level of government and most certainly within the agencies that provide such services. It clearly behooves social services agencies and professional preparation programs to develop policies and procedures for tele-behavioral health methods. Determining the role these will play in crisis intervention and therapy in general is still evolving (Glueckauf et al., 2018; Mazzer et al., 2021; Norcross et al., 2022).

Confidentiality. As stated earlier, one of the major issues of tele-behavioral health is confidentiality. Excellent encryption programs are used by ethical therapists to keep information. However, there is no such guarantee if you are using an internet service at public locations such as a café, laundromat, airport, and so on. Most, if not all, of these locations warn users when signing in that others may be able to see what you are doing. VPN services are most often safe with respect to providing privacy but before signing into any server, be careful to ensure confidentiality.

No matter what firewalls, antivirus programs, or malware prevention packages are being used through internet service provider, or that you have purchased, hackers can likely find ways to break through. In addition, even though websites may guarantee anonymity, once a message goes out, there is no absolute guarantee that it cannot be pulled out of the ether by people or agencies that you might not be too thrilled to have read your thoughts and pictures. An e-mail message is less like a letter and more like a postcard (Barnett & Scheetz, 2003). Text messages and chat rooms are similar. These are sometimes sent without much thought and sometimes to the wrong number. So! Do you really want to talk about your sexual inadequacies on a postcard? Additionally, the possibility of violating client confidentiality and the Health Insurance Portability and Accountability Act (HIPAA), which carries severe penalties for violations, are real concerns for practicing mental health professionals (Fisher & Fried, 2003).

It may also be argued that online therapy is problematic because of identity verification in emergency situations involving homicide, suicide, or other life-threatening events. In most telephone crisis intervention, there is usually some way to access emergency help for the individual. But if the client is in Vilnius, Lithuania, and the crisis interventionist is in Brisbane, Australia, this may be more difficult. Sandra DeJong's (2014) book *Blogs and Tweets, Texting and Friending: Social Media and Online Professionalism in Health Care* is a must read if you are going to venture into online therapy.

Charlatans. Sad to say, the field is ripe for electronic snake oil salespeople and nefarious individuals who may have somewhat less character and goodness in their hearts than Florence Nightingale. In his review of internet sites that purport to provide "crisis counseling," as early as 1999, Myer reported that not only are some of the fees exorbitantly high, but they are also based on the questionable claims of their promotional advertisements. Individuals might be putting themselves at risk for even more traumatization through secondary victimization at the hands of some very incompetent or outright charlatan "service providers." Clearly, although this venue holds much promise, it is a "buyer beware" situation. A cursory review of 227,000,000 hits returned by a search for "crisis intervention therapy" in June 2023 leads us to believe things haven't changed a lot since Myer's study; likely not all of the 227,000,000 are on the up and up.

There are countless counseling therapy apps out in the ether, and there are a great many that can be very helpful and, indeed, are available 24/7 when you may not be. You have reviewed an app and believe the site to be legitimate, the app is a helpful adjunct to your work with PTSD, and you recommend it to your clients. However if that app was from a company as reported in the May 2023 issue of Counseling Today, that company shared confidential mental health data on Facebook, Snapchat, and Pinterest for advertising purposes and is now under a proposed order from the Federal Trade Commission (FTC) to pay consumers back 7.8 million dollars (Wheeler, 2023). Although you as the health service provider who recommended that app may not be directly liable, don't bet on it that a personal injury lawyer might not come knocking on your door.

Technology Failure. The possibility of technology failure is always a concern, both for crisis workers and clients (MacMullin et al., 2020). What happens if your computer suddenly freezes in the middle of an intervention? What happens if either of you loses service due to power failure or the service provider hiccups, and you lose the connection? These issues and probably a dozen others have happened to everyone who is online. The most effective way to plan for technological glitches is to have alternative plans to reestablish communication. Of course, this may result in a barrier because of the loss of anonymity. Still, it is better to be safe than sorry should a technology failure occur in the middle of an intervention.

Licensing and Insurance. There are other demons that abound in the legal world of tele-behavioral health. Questions have been asked about the type of professional indemnity insurance needed, even if you are a volunteer at a crisis line (Glueckauf et al., 2018). What happens when you do therapy across state lines or countries? Do you need a license in that state or country, and what can happen if somebody commits suicide or homicide on your watch? How do you know your data are encrypted? How secure is the password used to protect your files? Do you know how to download/upload files safely, how to keep the files secure, how to back them up, and how and where they are stored? Are you familiar with the Online Therapy Institute's Ethical Framework for the Use of Technology in Mental Health (Nagel & Anthony, 2011b) and, for disaster responders, an ethical framework for the use of technology in disasters (Nagel & Anthony, 2011a)? The Online Therapy Institute's Ethical Framework for the Use of Technology in Mental Health (2023) offers a wealth of information and training on these and other topics. You also have to consider ethical standards of professional organizations you might be a member of and follow those. If you don't, you are jeopardizing clients and your professional credibility, and legal issues may materialize.

Technological Competence. If you are going to operate in tele-behavioral health, you need to be technologically competent and savvy about browsing the internet. You also need to be competent at identifying misleading websites, phishing emails, and other efforts to compromise your efforts at providing services. Some very "official" sounding websites, tests, emails, and so on are designed to lure you in to steal information and, frankly, cost you your hard-earned money. Things to watch for include but are not limited to misspelled words, grammatical mistakes, capital letters that are out of place, and deceptive web addresses to name a few. Taking a course in cyber security is probably a good idea if you provide tele-behavioral health services. The foregoing is especially true for crisis intervention. In an electric, chaotic world of crisis intervention, your caring and good intentions may distract you to being tricked into some form of a scheme to cheat and deceive you. Before you know it, you are caught in a whirlpool of problems just because you wanted to help.

Learning the Language. Understanding the language and communication styles is critical. Those of you who are part of the Gen X and Z generations probably already know this. The reason for knowing the language is to help to avoid misunderstandings and miscommunication (MacMullin et al., 2020) These individuals and sites are replete with their own language and **netiquette** (civil and appropriate rules of discourse when operating on the internet, particularly in synchronous time with other netizens). Anthony and Nagel (2010, pp. 5–6) contend that real life and online life are not separate but are more and more blended, to the point that, for millions of people, virtual life and real life are one and the same! For many individuals, the virtual world they surf through *is* the real world, so it is not hard to see how they would perceive the internet as the most viable way to access crisis intervention services.

Netiquette

As yet, there is no "Miss Manners" to rule on netiquette. However, Jenicus (2013) has compiled a list of websites that cover netiquette in regard to general rules, e-mails, listservs, business, Twitter, and netiquette for kids. Following are some basic netiquette rules you need to observe if you are working on the internet (Anthony & Nagel, 2010; Jones & Stokes, 2009):

1. A typo or two, particularly in synchronous time, is okay. Sloppy writing with lots of typos and grammar problems is not okay and indicates you don't care much about your client.
2. Emoticons can be helpful in conveying an emotion. They also can be too cute! Check with your client before you use them.
3. Lots of tweeters who use the internet have their own expansive set of acronyms. You need to be clear about what those are; don't hesitate to ask if you don't know an abbreviation.
4. Keep your text neutral by using a simple black font; 12-point Times New Roman, for example, is easy to read and even bland. Other fonts and colors can get pretty outlandish. Your clients can give you a lot of information through what they use.
5. You know what you mean when you write something. But as people read words (a novel is a good example), they attribute their own meaning and subsequent emotional response. So be careful as you construct your responses.
6. Stay cool! Use standard counseling skill responses to do exploratory work. Let the client talk. Brevity in written responses is a good thing.
7. Keep flame wars (intentionally written inflammatory remarks or misinterpreted ones) under control. If you make a mistake, discretely and quickly apologize for it. If you are running a group online, they need to know the limits and that they will be called on their inappropriate behavior.

Congruent with overall netiquette are some basic ways of enhancing text to make it more conversational and add emphasis (Anthony & Nagel, 2010, pp. 51–55). On the negative side, conflict seems to occur more online than in face-to-face intervention, so it appears that communications need to be constantly clarified so they do not get muddled (MacMallen et al., 2003). Even when emoticons, such as keyboard symbols that look like facial expressions, e.g., :), or emotional bracketing (e.g. worried, angry, scared) or altered text formats like different type sizes and fonts for emphasis are used, it may be very difficult to tell when and to what degree emotions are being displayed.

Predispositioning/Making Contact

Because of the nature of tele-behavioral health in crisis intervention, miscommunication can occur even when using video conferencing (MacMullin et al., 2020). You do not have the luxury of observing body language, voice intonation, rate of speech, or places with texting and email. With chat rooms, you have all that except body language, and with video conferencing, you also have limited body language. That means the first contact with clients and predispositioning is vital to create the potential for the successful resolution of a crisis. It is also important to get across to the client how crisis intervention takes place on each type of technology and that it is different from everyday emails, tweets, texting, and chat room dialogue.

Being culturally aware is important in that first contact. Cultural awareness in this situation is three tiered. These tiers include your culture and the client's culture, which has long been considered a must in any type of intervention. The third tier in crisis intervention is, as we have stated earlier, the culture of communicating via technology. The following is a case in which a chat room is used in the crisis intervention process.

Chat room crisis center: I'm Featherlite. I've got a problem at home. I'm a 16-year-old girl and I need some help with it. I've never done this before. I'm thinking about running away because I can't take much more of my parents climbing my frame because of my boyfriend. So where do we go from here? Can u help?

Dr. J: (synchronous chat room) Featherlite, I'm glad you messaged us. Call me Dr. J. Pleased to make your acquaintance, Featherlite. Interesting online name. I am curious. Are you as light as a feather?

While it may seem tangential, the interventionist seeks to establish psychological contact by querying her internet name.

Featherlite: Pretty much I guess. Especially when I dance. I'm on the modern dance team at my high school. Anyways that's what Dad used to say when I was a little kid and he'd pick me up on his shoulders and it kinda stuck. Right now, I'd like to pick him up and drop him off the Hernando De Soto Bridge.

Dr. J: Okay. I'd like to read what you have to say. Note I said "read" so that is a bit different from listening. There are some different rules of the road here and I'd like to go over them with you so things don't get messed up. First, we can't see each other, so a lot of what passes for nonverbal communication won't happen. Also, I can't catch the tone of your voice nor you mine. We might use emoticons to convey an expression, and I use things like brackets and boldface and some other ways of attempting to make clear what I am hearing and asking so there are some ways of using the computer to get meanings across, but there's still room to misread stuff and I don't want that to happen. I'm not going to worry too much about misspells and grammar, although I might ask you to clarify something if I don't understand it and you can do the same with me. I want us to be really clear on what's going on, so I won't try to read your mind and misinterpret the issues. So please don't be offended if I ask for clarification, okay? Even though we are working in real time, I may take some time to think about what you are saying. I'll let you know that by using some dots . . . so that you know I haven't stopped and there is more to come. If you like you can do the same. This is a crisis intervention website, so it is not long-term therapy. My whole purpose is to get you back on level ground so you can make some good, realistic short-term decisions about your problem and act on it. If you think you need more extensive help down the line, we can discuss that. I'll be asking you a lot of questions to get the problem really clear in my mind. I'll probably restate what you say so we are both in agreement on what's going on. To do that I may cut out your words and paste them back into my response in boldface. I'll take some guesses at what you are feeling and thinking. If I am wrong, just tell me so, and I'll try again. So this is a no-fault deal okay? Now, Featherlite, if you would, think a moment . . . and then tell me the one main thing that caused you to write in tonight. I do see you are pretty put out with your dad right now. You said "it" and that "you'd never done this before." Can you tell me what "it" means and what it is that you haven't done?

This opening statement is designed to give Featherlite an idea of how tele-behavioral health works and to get an idea of what the initiating problem is and the subtext underlying the initial query (Glueckauf et al., 2018; Jones & Stokes, 2009, pp. 14–16). This rather long introduction gives the client at least a thumbnail sketch of how the interventionist will operate. A lot of owning statements are used to convey who and what the interventionist is and what he will and will not do. Not engaging in this preliminary discussion is likely to put the intervention in peril from the start, particularly with a client who has never engaged in crisis intervention, let alone done so using tele-behavioral health. The interventionist's focus is on the immediate precipitating factors that got her to go online.

Throughout the remainder of the conversation, watch how culture influences and, at times, interferes in the intervention process. Culturally, Dr. J is much older than Featherlite, making cultural differences between them likely based on age alone. Yet, their social locations are more than simply age and are entirely different, such as gender, socioeconomic status, and marital status, to name a few. Dr. J must be careful not to let these differences creep into and sabotage the conversation. For example, Dr. J's views on teens who run away or do not respect parents' discipline may bias his approach, contributing to countertransference if he has issues with his own daughters. Featherlite, seeing Dr. J's name may think older people just do not understand. The client's name implies a possible technological cultural issue. Is Featherlite the client's real name, and if not, does this pose a possible ethical issue if Dr. J needs to do something to ensure her safety? It appears Featherlite is her user name and there's not much he can do if it becomes a safety issue other than ask for her real name, address, or phone number and then call for help.

Featherlite: Well "it" is like my parents y'know. They 4bid me to see my boyfriend, Arley, who is out of high school. They don't like him because they think he is like 2 old for me and they think he does dope and wants me to do it 2 y'know. We really got in it tonight. I'm down at the city library and just serched u up so I haven't done this crisisline thing ever before. I also haven't run away from home, but Arley says we can go to Kentucky and gt married there without my p's consent. I don't want to gt married right now. I want to finish h.s., but I love Arley and don't know how I can go home. I kinda slapped my mom and then my dad really slapped me and I took off.

Dr. J: SO YOU'VE BEEN FIGHTING WITH YOUR P'S BECAUSE THEY THINK YOUR BOYFRIEND IS SUPPLYING YOU WITH DOPE AND YOU'RE SO IN LOVE WITH HIM YOU CAN'T SEE ALL THE FAULTS THEY SEE. RIGHT?

Featherlite: Why are you SHOUTING. You sound like my father. Always critical. YOU THINK I M CRAZY TOO! Am I that bad? Maybe I will run off with him.

Dr. J: Oops $#%$#%%! I accidentally hit the caps lock. Sorry. Not shouting, just old arthritic fingers LOL [laugh out loud]. No I don't think you're crazy. The "right" was just asking if I was on the money not whether you are right or wrong about your feelings.

While lots of shorthand and acronyms get used by clients, the interventionist needs to be careful in this regard. The word *right* in the above example can have many implications. Is our well-intentioned interventionist just seeking acknowledgment, or is he implying somebody is "right," and if so, is it Featherlite, her parents, or somebody else? So it might be a bit better if he were to make things clearer by saying "Am I right?"

Adlington (2009, pp. 8–40) uses a variety of text formats to build rapport with clients. Bracketing and boldfacing serve to indicate that the interventionist is listening closely and thinking about what has been said (pp. 13–14). Adding dots conveys some time spent pondering the issue and that the writer is going to continue with the thought.

At this point in the conversation, the Affective rating seems to be around a 5, while the Behavioral Scale rating is a 6 and the Cognitive Scale is a 7. These ratings may be a little high based on the minimal information, but being a little high with the rating at first is better than being too low. The total rating suggests that Dr. J should partner with Featherlite to Provide Support and Allow Catharsis. Yet, care must be taken since Featherlite is equating Dr. J with her father.

Dr. J: Man! That really struck me about comparing me to your dad. Let me think on that a moment....

As in F2F, it is easy, perhaps even easier, to get lost in all the verbiage and, as a result, come back to the client with a whole flock of issues that get the client lost trying to determine which ones are important. A better way is to think of the core issue you want to cover and, as Adlington (2009) suggests, direct one central issue back to the client in boldface.

Dr. J: Featherlite, I get the sense this is more than me just sounding like your dad and being critical of your love life that's making you think of running away with Arley. Could you think a bit and tell me some of the long-term issues between you and your parents? I am guessing there may be a bit more than a boyfriend. Although right now **I do understand that the major issue is your wanting to be with Arley and your folks against it and that's what we will work on right now**.

Using the client's own font is one possible way of clearly restating what is being said in the client's own words.

Dr. J: So it seems right now you are so sensitive to your parents constant criticism that my goof up puts you on edge and I sound like your dad.

It should also be of interest what type of font the client uses (Adlington, 2009, p. 15). Would you respond differently if Featherlite were using **Braggadocio**, 𝕱𝖊𝖙𝖙𝖊 𝕱𝖗𝖆𝖐𝖙𝖚𝖗, or *Edwardian Script* rather than Comic Sans MS? Or, for that matter, if the message came with certain words in color (Adlington, 2009, p. 17)? Do you suppose it would make a difference in your interpretation if anger came back in red, purple, blue, or green?

Featherlite: I am so mad [crimson]. They're just jealous [green] because they were never in love like I am with Arley.

Dr. J: OK. I see the feelings. I have a series of questions to ask. They'll come one at a time. First, do you feel safe to go home tonight?

Featherlite: I don't know. The library closes at 11. I don't want to be on the streets then.

Dr. J: Do you have a friend or relative's house you could go to?

Featherlite: Maybe my aunt. Although my p's would be mad if I went there. Mom doesn't get along with her sister well. Arley would come and take me to his apartment if I called him. He gets off at 11.

Dr. J: You are probably not going to like my response, but right now that might not be your best option. I can get you on the line to run away. They would get you transportation there, then contact your Ps. That is escalating the situation some because

there would have to be a meeting between them and you and your parents and social services would be involved. Right now it is important for you to stay safe. We can continue messaging and set up some longer-term plans, but I want to see you under cover tonight.

Featherlite: U R probably right. I guess I could call my aunt.

Dr. J: Please do that and then either call into the crisis line phone number or e-mail me back . . . say 10 minutes. OK?

Featherlite: OK. I appreciate u. Pretty kul for an old ((((((gy)))))))) ! ! ! [The parenthesis denotes hugs.]

While this conversation is representative of what most crisis interveners would do in any format, there are some notable exceptions. First and foremost, triaging Featherlite is difficult because it is hard to triage her affect or cognition without seeing her facial expressions and hearing her voice. The intervener has to make a best guess based on what he actually knows. As with the initial triage assessment, the default approach is to make best-guess ratings that may be high to be on the safe side. You do not want to give individuals a low to moderate rating, pat them on the back, and say they are good to go when, in fact, they should have been rated higher. The intervention would be totally different for a low to a high-moderate or marked rating. The fact this is a 16-year-old girl about to be on the streets of Memphis alone at night gets her a 9 on the behavioral scale to be on the safe side and dictates most of the worker's actions in getting her to a safe place. Affective and cognitive would likely be in the moderate range (i.e., 6 to 7). The total score range is from 20 to 23, indicating Dr. J should be moving to a directive approach but also working to partner with Featherlite using Providing Protection and Providing Guidance strategies. These strategies would serve as a prevention tactic to safeguard her. Second, until practice makes the intervener unconsciously competent with the technology, he will have to be very cognizant of operating and conversing in this new system. Invariably, then, some focus is taken away from the client to deal with system conversance, as is demonstrated by Dr. J's poor fine motor coordination in hitting the caps lock key.

Need for Training

This brief chat is meant to give you a snapshot of how crisis intervention works in real time on the internet. It is not meant to make you an internet-competent crisis interventionist. Also, reading this brief section in a book is not going to make you a tele-behavioral health interventionist. Crisis workers engaging in this work and employing supportive computer programs need to have training beyond standard computer skills to deal with the inevitable technical problems and computer glitches. Understanding how the new medium integrates traditional and tele-behavioral health is critical (Norcross et al., 2022). Further, cultural diversity and linguistic differences make understanding "multiculturalism" as it applies to crisis intervention paramount for tele-behavioral health (Anthony & Nagel, 2010, p. 63). Issues revolving around social locations, as discussed in Chapter 2, "Culturally Effective Helping in Crisis," are particularly important when using technology as a modality for crisis intervention. The possibility of misunderstanding and miscommunication is always present.

The worker also needs to be comfortable in the medium (Glueckauf et al., 2018; MacMullin et al., 2020). Writing counseling responses using instant messaging or in chat rooms is altogether different from saying them over the telephone or in a face-to-face dialogue. Recognizing when clients are in trouble by their chat message content is very different from doing a visual assessment of clients face-to-face. Knowing how to obtain backup, use referral services, and contact emergency services over vast geographic distances is paramount. Even more important is getting supervision while doing the foregoing (Anthony & Nagel, 2010, pp. 127–141). Finally, the worker needs to educate clients about the limitations of tele-behavioral health and gain their informed consent (Glueckauf et al., 2018).

Does It Work?

That is a good, simple question; the answer is not so simple. Research looking at various forms of telephone and other technologies used in crisis intervention strongly suggests that it does work (Keasar et al., 2022; Mazzer et al., 2021; Sinyor et al., 2022). These reports also state that the field is ripe

for additional research that will help fine tune the intervention process. Areas to examine include training effects, differences between outcomes with volunteers and professionals, and the different technologies being used, to name a few. Maybe you are an aspiring researcher and reading this book will inspire you to generate a question to conduct research.

Parrish et al. (2021) identified two other issues that are needed to ensure technology is effective, specifically for mobile apps, when being used in crisis intervention. The first is to integrate crisis language in sites to help clients select ones that will be the most beneficial for their crisis. An example is using generic language such as behavior services being offered rather than referring to specific problems such as domestic violence, child abuse, suicide, and so on. Second, "best practices" need to be developed, tested, and disseminated to be used as a centralized resource for the development of apps used in crisis intervention. Developing these resources will help crisis workers refer clients or assist clients to understand and select appropriate resources.

The bottom line for any therapeutic endeavor is how well it works. Conducting rigorous controlled-outcome studies is difficult and basically not possible in crisis intervention. Determining the level of expertise and skillful intervention is equally problematic given that the vast number of crisis workers are volunteers. However, a number of studies have been done that sampled users of phone and electronic intervention services (Beebe et al., 2014; Chiang, 2012; Dalgin et al., 2011; Evans et al., 1986; Farrer et al., 2014; Gonzales et al., 2014; Mishara et al., 2005; Padach, 1984; Reese et al., 2002, 2006; Rhee et al., 2005; Swirsky et al., 2014; Tolmach, 1985; Wuang et al., 2011; Wark, 1984). Overall, they consistently rated electronic crisis intervention as helpful, there was a reduction in presenting issues, and a number stated they preferred this method to face-to-face counseling. The question remains: Do telephone and internet counseling work? The answer to that, whether it is done by volunteers working crisis lines or professionals working with their own clientele, is pretty much "Yes."

Summary

Telephone counseling and tele-behavioral health account for most crisis intervention work done in the world. Typically, local crisis lines field all kinds and

varieties of calls, while national hotlines field special, problem-specific issues such as runaways. Special crisis lines that are time limited may be set up immediately after major disasters. These services are staffed mainly by volunteers, who are generally seen as effective helpers by the people who call them. However, there are problem callers who can bedevil crisis lines. Some callers may use crisis lines for their own sexual gratification. Others may constantly call and tie up phone lines because of their loneliness.

A challenge is expanding and/or creating a more cohesive network of hotlines that allow transferring calls between hotlines, especially for transferring calls directly to hotlines that were developed for specific issues as discussed earlier. For example, a caller with suicidal ideations contacts the national 988 number, and when the crisis interventionist discovers the person is a farmer, they can appropriately transfer the call to someone with an understanding of and maybe even with experience in farming. Creating this network would involve more than having an extensive list of various hotlines and giving callers the numbers but would instead allow crisis interventionists to transfer calls seamlessly to specialized hotlines.

Tele-behavioral health crisis counseling is playing a larger and increasing role in crisis intervention. As the role of tele-behavioral health continues to unfold, professional training programs must keep up with the use of technology with increased training. Still, some questions about its use and the ethical safeguards that need to be part of it remain unanswered. Although professional organizations are catching up and integrating ethical standards designed to guide members in the use of tele-behavioral health, this training needs to become part of training standards.

Handling Specific Crises
Going Into the Trenches

Part 2 focuses on applying intervention strategies to several of the currently most prevalent types of crises in the human experience. The purpose of Part 2 is to provide crisis workers with information about the background, dynamics, and intervention methodologies needed to effectively help individuals or groups in various kinds of crises.

Part 2 contains a wide array of crisis case illustrations to enhance descriptions of not only the usual and accepted intervention practices for various types of crises but also many innovative and cutting-edge strategies for intervention. Indeed, some of these strategies are controversial, but they have gained enough treatment notoriety and preliminary research to be included. Part 2 examines posttraumatic stress disorder (PTSD), suicide, sexual assault, domestic violence, personal loss, crises in schools, and families in crises. The following three central themes pervade these chapters:

1. Some crises are *time limited,* and some are *transcrisis,* in that the person in crisis may progressively experience severe problems, either deal with or suppress them, and then experience and exhibit repeated responses and symptoms of the same crisis over a period of many years.

2. No one set of theories, assumptions, strategies, or procedures is appropriate for intervening in all crisis situations; rather, a systematic and integrative approach is recommended and demonstrated as the preferred mode of helping in a broad assortment of crisis problems and settings. The techniques employed in these chapters are "best bets" for the particular kind of client in the particular environment. They are, however, not the only "bets." They are meant to give you a variety of approaches and situations that will start to help you form your own "Gestalt" of an effective crisis worker.

3. Crisis intervention is hallmarked by elastic, fluid situations that change in seconds and minutes and may move from very benign to volatile situations in that time. Many of the case illustrations model such dynamics to give you a flavor of what the crisis worker must do to respond quickly and effectively.

Posttraumatic Stress Disorder

Learning Objectives

After studying this chapter, you should be able to:

1. Describe the history and evolution of posttraumatic stress disorder (PTSD) into a classified psychological diagnostic.
2. Explain the differences among peritraumatic, acute traumatic, posttraumatic, and complex PTSD terminology.
3. Describe the current diagnostic PTSD criteria for adults.
4. Classify the basic neurophysiology of PTSD.
5. Contrast the incidence of different trauma types and their effects on PTSD.
6. List the different phases of recovery in PTSD.
7. Explain the maladaptive coping patterns of PTSD.
8. Classify the different types of assessments used in the diagnosis and treatment of PTSD.
9. Explain the risks of treatment for PTSD.
10. Describe the use of different types of adult treatment protocols for PTSD.
11. Identify the role of psychotropic medication in the treatment of PTSD.
12. Define how trauma-focused therapy is operationalized throughout the recovery phases of PTSD.
13. Define the connection of crisis intervention and PTSD.
14. Describe group therapy in treating PTSD.
15. Explain how eye movement desensitization and reprocessing (EMDR) therapy is used to treat PTSD.
16. List the diagnostic criteria for PTSD in children.
17. Characterize the importance of support systems for children in combating PTSD.
18. List differences between Type I and Type II (complex) trauma in children.
19. Contrast differential treatment methods for PTSD in children.
20. Explain the potential for hope and growth after trauma.

Introduction

Part 2's discussion of the more common types of crises that you, as a mental health worker or consumer of mental health care, are likely to encounter opens with **posttraumatic stress disorder (PTSD).** The reason for beginning here is that PTSD can be the catalyst for other crises such as suicide (Stanley et al., 2020), partner violence (Semiatin et al., 2017) and substance misuse (Wilson et al., 2017). Other crises discussed in the book, (i.e., sexual assault or abuse, partner violence, loss, physical violence, hostage situations, and large-scale natural and human-made disasters) can set the stage for the development of the disorder (Carthy et al., 2023; Cusack et al., 2023;

Domino et al., 2021; Goodman-Williams et al., 2022; van de Ven et al., 2022). Going one-on-one with PTSD is tough enough, but to make matters worse, lots of times, PTSD turns into a tangled quagmire with a host of other comorbid (occurring along with it) problems that make it even harder to deal with as individuals bounce in and out of transcrisis (Masino & Norman, 2015). Complicating the issue, PTSD-like symptoms may appear in the very people who attempt to alleviate the mental and physical suffering of people in crisis (Casas & Benuto, 2022; Feldman et al., 2021; Henning & Brand, 2019; Meckes et al., 2021; Sprang & Steckler, 2023) and have become known as compassion fatigue (Figley, 2002) and vicarious traumatization (Pearlman & Saakvitne, 1995).

This chapter will probably touch on material you have been exposed to in other courses and might be somewhat redundant. Yet, we believe discussing the material in relationship to crisis intervention is important. Stick with it, and you will read that a background for understanding not only what PTSD is about, but what occurs in treating the other crisis and transcrisis topics in this book is critical. What we knew about PTSD in the first edition of this book in 1987 and what we know about it now—particularly the neurobiology and just how complex it is in manifesting the various traumatic responses that occur in humans—is like the difference between writing with a goose quill, inkwell, and papyrus scroll and word processing or the earliest version of dial phones, to push button phones, to cell phones and to the smartphones almost all of you use today. Bear with us! If you nail this chapter down, the other chapters will make a whole lot more sense as to how "all this stuff" goes together. In summary, PTSD has moved from the psychological backwaters and from the grassroots movement stemming from the Vietnam War to now being so central to treatment issues in mental health that now there is the National Center for PTSD (http://www.ptsd.va.gov) and the National Child Traumatic Stress Network (NCTSN) www.nctsn.org.

History

Terminology

LO1 LO2 Psychic trauma is a process initiated by an event that confronts an individual with an acute, overwhelming threat (Freud, 1917/ 1963). When the event occurs, the inner agency of the mind loses its ability to control the disorganizing effects of the experience, and disequilibrium occurs. The trauma tears up the individual's psychological anchors, which are fixed in a secure sense of what has been in the past and what should be in the present (Erikson, 1968). When a traumatic event occurs that represents nothing like the person's experience of past events, and the individual's mind is unable to effectively answer basic questions of how and why it occurred and what it means, a crisis ensues. The traumatic wake of a crisis event typically includes immediate and vivid reexperiencing, hyperarousal, and avoidance reactions, which are all common to PTSD. The event propels the individual into a traumatic state that lasts as long as the mind needs to reorganize, classify, and make sense of the traumatic event. Then, and only then, does psychic equilibrium return (Kramer et al., 2020).

The typical kinds of responses that occur immediately after the crisis may give rise to what are called **peritraumatic** (around, or like, trauma) symptoms. These are common responses as the mind attempts to reorganize itself and cope with a horrific event. For many people, these responses will recede after a few days. Most people are amazingly resilient in the aftermath of a traumatic crisis and quickly return to mental and physical homeostasis, but if the symptoms are persistent and continue for a minimum of 3 days to a maximum of 4 weeks and occur within 1 month of the traumatic event, then those time frames will meet the criteria of **acute stress disorder (ASD)** (American Psychiatric Association (APA, 2022)). Acute stress disorder diagnostic criteria are similar to the criteria for PTSD, which is discussed later in the chapter, except that the diagnosis can only be given in the first month after a traumatic event. ASD is somewhat different than PTSD because **dissociative symptoms** such as memory loss, a sense of detachment from the world, belief that things and people are unreal, a blurred sense of identity, and a general disconnect from reality may also be present (International Society for the Study of Trauma and Dissociation, 2015). As we will discover, tackling ASD symptoms immediately and head on is important, because these tend to be valid predictors for "catching" PTSD. Percentage rates for ASD vary a great deal depending on the trauma type, from vehicle accidents that range in the teens, to victims of robbery in the twenties, and to rape which skyrockets to the nineties (Gibson, 2015).

If the person can effectively integrate the trauma into conscious awareness and organize it as a part of the past (as unpleasant as the event may be), then homeostasis returns, the problem is coped with, and the individual continues to travel life's rocky road. If the event is not effectively integrated and is submerged from awareness, then the probability is high that the initiating stressor will continue to assail the person and become chronic PTSD. It may also disappear from conscious awareness and reemerge in a variety of symptomatic forms months or years after the event. When such crisis events are caused by the reemergence of the original unresolved stressor, they fall into the category of delayed PTSD (APA, 2022).

PTSD is a newborn compared with the other crises we will examine, at least in regard to achieving official designation. In 1980, PTSD found its way into the third edition of the APA's (1980) *Diagnostic and Statistical Manual of Mental Disorders* (DSM-III) as a classifiable and valid mental disorder. However, the antecedents of what has been designated as PTSD first came to the attention of the medical establishment in the late 19th and early 20th centuries.

Two events serve as benchmarks in the history of PTSD. First, with the advent of rail transportation and subsequent train wrecks, physicians and early psychiatrists began to encounter trauma in accident survivors with no identifiable physical basis. Railway accident survivors of this type became so numerous that a medical term, **railway spine**, became an accepted diagnosis. In psychological parlance, the synonymous term **compensation neurosis** although no longer used, was utilized for invalidism suffered and compensated by insurers as a result of such accidents (Trimble, 1985, pp. 7–10).

Concomitantly, Sigmund Freud formulated the concept of **hysterical neurosis** to describe the trauma cases of young Victorian women with whom he was working. He documented symptoms of warded-off ideas, denial, repression, emotional avoidance, compulsive repetition of trauma-related behavior, and recurrent attacks of trauma-related emotional sensations (Breuer & Freud, 1895/1955). However, what Freud found and reported on the pervasive childhood sexual abuse of these women as the traumatic root of their emotional distress was anathema to a puritanical Victorian society, and he was forced to disavow and then reject his findings (Herman, 1997, pp. 13–17).

Second, the advent of modern warfare in World Wars I and II, with powerful artillery and aerial bombardment, generated terms such as **shell shock** and **combat fatigue** to explain the condition of traumatized soldiers who had no apparent physical wounds. As early as the American Civil War, soldiers were diagnosed with **neurasthenia**, a state of mental and physical exhaustion. This malady was also termed **"soldier's heart"**

because of the belief that nerves at the base of the heart were somehow affected by combat. The term **nostalgia**, a 19th-century military term coined by physicians for combat soldiers with extreme homesickness, would be seen as combat-induced PTSD in current terms. The thought was that soldiers became nostalgic for home and thus started to manifest a variety of physical symptoms that would relieve them from combat and allow them to go home (Kinzie & Goetz, 1996). Various hypotheses such as the foregoing were proposed to account for such strange maladies (Trimble, 1985, p. 8), but Freud (1919/1959) believed that the term **war neurosis** more aptly characterized what was an emotional disorder that had nothing to do with the prevailing medical notion of neurology-based shell shock, the idea that concussion from the massive shelling common in World War I injured the brain's neurological systems. The U.S. Medical Service Corps came to recognize combat fatigue (being on the front line too long) in World War II and the Korean War as a treatable psychological disturbance. The treatment approach was that combat fatigue was invariably acute and that treatment was best conducted as quickly and as close to the battle lines as possible. The idea was to facilitate a quick return to active duty. The prevailing thought was that time heals all wounds and that little concern needed to be given to long-term effects of traumatic stress. Such has not been the case (Archibald et al., 1962). Indeed, a notable proponent of establishing the Vietnam Veterans Centers, Arthur Blank, ruefully commented that when he was an army psychiatrist in Vietnam, he believed there would be no long-term difficulties for veterans (MacPherson, 1984, p. 237).

Although PTSD can and does occur in response to the entire range of experiences, combat experiences are a significant cause of this disorder (Armour et al., 2017; Barr et al., 2019). The Vietnam War clearly brought PTSD to the awareness of both the human services professions and the public. Through a combination of events and circumstances unparalleled in the military history of the United States, veterans who returned from that conflict began to develop a variety of mental health problems that had little basis for analysis and treatment in the prevailing psychological literature. This combination of events and circumstances had insidious and long-term consequences that were not readily apparent either to the individuals affected or to human services professionals who attempted to treat them. Misdiagnosed, mistreated, and misunderstood, military service personnel became known to a variety of social services agencies that included the police, mental health facilities, and unemployment offices (MacPherson, 1984, pp. 207–330, 651–690).

As the war continued to grind on, more and more veterans started having psychological problems. Rebuffed by the Veterans Administration, these veterans formed self-help groups to try to come to terms with their psychological issues. These "rap" groups rapidly coalesced and became a political force that pushed the federal government to come to grips with their problems. One major result of their lobbying efforts was the establishment of the Vietnam Veterans Centers, where alienated veterans could seek help for a variety of readjustment problems. An informal network of mental health professionals became interested in the veterans and started to classify their symptoms and compare them to the work Kardiner (1941) had done on war neurosis. Their review of clinical records led them to generate 27 of the most common symptoms of the Vietnam veterans' "traumatic neurosis" (van der Kolk et al., 1996, p. 61). Interestingly, many of the physical or somatic complaints resemble those of a large retrospective archival study on the medical records of American Civil War Union veterans (Pizarro et al., 2006)!

At the same time, researchers in the growing women's movement were looking at psychological issues that occurred after domestic violence, rape, and child abuse. What they were finding in the individuals who had suffered from these civilian assaults closely paralleled the difficulties that Vietnam veterans were experiencing. Their research rediscovered what Freud had found 80 years before and had dismissed: that victims of physical and sexual assault suffered long-term effects of the psychological trauma (Herman, 1997, p. 32). These different research avenues culminated in combining the "Vietnam veterans syndrome," the "rape trauma syndrome," the "abused child syndrome," and the "battered woman syndrome" into one diagnostic category—posttraumatic stress disorder—in the third edition of the APA's *Diagnostic and Statistical Manual* in 1980 (van der Kolk et al., 1996, p. 61).

Although the Vietnam War may be no more than a reference in a high school history book, the wall memorial in Washington, D.C., or "crazy old Uncle Harold" who continues to wear combat fatigues and a headband with a ponytail, the war's effects are a crucial history lesson in mental health provision (or the lack thereof) that any aspiring mental health worker should learn. For that reason, the psychological lessons learned from the Vietnam War continue to play a major role in the discussion of PTSD in the eighth edition of this book. It should be clearly understood that, even 50 years after the fact, the events that caused the trauma in many of these approximately 1 million veterans who suffered and suffer from PTSD are as alive for them today as they were then (Price, 2011). What is perhaps even more ominous in regard to the Vietnam veterans is their "graying." Mounting evidence indicates that World War II and Korean War veterans have manifested delayed onset or worsening of posttraumatic complaints as they have grown older. Aging, with its subsequent loss of social supports through death, increased health problems, declining physical and mental capabilities, and economic hardship appears to put older veterans at increased risk (Lee et al., 2022; Palgi et al., 2015). Thus, it would appear that as this population ages, the mental health professions are a long way from being done with the legacy of Vietnam.

The conflicts in Iraq and Afghanistan have eerily similar parallels to Vietnam. There are no front lines, the enemy fades into the population, everyone in the theater of operations is essentially in combat. As a result, vigilance must be constant, 24/7, throughout one's entire rotation. Degree of combat exposure has been found to be one of the major predictors of PTSD (Miller et al., 2008; Smith et al., 2008), and anybody that goes into the "sandboxes" as they are now called can expect just that.

Two major differences are present in these conflicts. So far, there is general public support for the troops, whereas in Vietnam, there was not. A support group is critical in any crisis, and this is particularly true of troops in an increasingly unpopular war. Lack of support and outright hatred of returning troops was a major contributing factor for PTSD in Vietnam veterans. However, while the armed forces in the current conflicts are all volunteers and not 18-year-old draftees, there are a tremendous number of reserve units in combat action, and there are also huge differences in the number of women involved in direct combat action. The question, then, becomes what the use of reservists and women in combat portends for the onset of PTSD. Preliminary results regarding mental health problems in veterans returning from Iraq and Afghanistan have ranged from 19 to 44 percent of the samples examined (Hoge et al., 2006; Lapierre et al., 2007).

Summary of Diagnostic Criteria

LO3 PTSD is complex and can be a diagnostically troublesome disorder. To be identified as having PTSD, a person must meet the following conditions and symptoms as specified in the Diagnostic and Statistical Manual of Mental Disorders, Fifth Edition, Text Revision *(DSM-5-TR)* (APA, 2022). The DSM 5-TR also revised the language for clarity in the subcategory for children under 6 years of age.

Exposure. The first criterion states the individuals must have been exposed to a trauma in which they were confronted with an event that involved actual or threatened death or serious injury or actual or threatened sexual violence. One key word in the above sentence is "exposure." Exposure is not limited to being directly involved but also includes witnessing an event, indirectly learning about an event that exposed a person important to them to threatened death or injury (e.g., mangled bodies, serious injuries, and/or death) or repeated exposure to aversive details of an event associated with their occupation such as law enforcement, EMTs, firefighters, and so on. Therapists also fall into this category, especially those who work in areas such as child abuse, domestic violence, provide services at disasters, and, you guessed it, crisis intervention. Note that vicarious exposure of nonprofessionals seeing or hearing about these events via the media does not meet the bar for developing PTSD. This means PTSD is not the most appropriate diagnosis for individuals watching a disaster or traumatic event on a newscast.

Intrusive Thoughts. A second criterion is that the trauma intrudes into individuals' lives in one or more of several ways. One way is through intrusive recurrent thoughts with little or no control over them (APA, 2022). The issue with this criterion is control. The intrusive thoughts are different than getting a line of a song running through your head where you just cannot seem to get it out. But over a few hours or maybe even a day, you are able to stop singing the song in your head. An example of an intrusive thought is a person who was on an airline flight and, while landing, a tire blew out that caused the plane to skid off the runway. When the person watched the recent near misses of planes colliding on runways in early 2023, the person had thoughts pop into their mind about the event they experienced. For children the reexperiencing may occur through repetitive play such that it shows they are reliving the traumatic event.

This symptom can be observed by the emergence of nightmares. The nightmares typically occur on a regular basis and repeat the traumatic event. An example of this might be seeing the planes crash into the World Trade Center (WTC) on 9/11. Or having a nightmare about seeing people jump out of the windows and hearing the thump as they hit the sidewalk. Crisis workers providing intervention to these individuals might also develop similar nightmares, even though they were not physically in lower Manhattan on 9/11. For children, the nightmares may not appear to be related to the traumatic event but nonetheless occur regularly after the event.

A dissociative reaction or flashback is another way the traumatic event is reexperienced (American Psychiatric Association, 2022). This symptom may be the most well-known way by the public that PTSD is identified. This reaction could be brief to prolonged with individuals becoming unaware of their behavior. The dissociative state can occur anytime but may be more likely when awakening or intoxicated. During these times individuals may misinterpret common sounds as something they heard during the traumatic event. For example, veterans returning from Afghanistan might mistake the backfire of a car as the explosion of an Improvised Explosive Devise (IED). Reenacting a traumatic event may be the way children demonstrate this symptom. If in a car accident, they may crash cars together as they play or possibly draw pictures of cars crashing.

The traumatic event may also be reexperienced through an intense reaction when individuals feel a situation is the same or similar to the initial trauma (APA, 2022). The event does not have to be exactly the same, but it sparks an intense response because individuals associate it with the traumatic event. The intense reactions could involve excessive worry to prolonged anxiety or a panic attack with no history of those disorders.

Another way this symptom might be observed is when individuals who have survived a tornado or hurricane may have a physiological response such as violent shaking when a storm is predicted. Just seeing a cloud in the sky may cause individuals extreme anxiety. Children may not want to leave home or be away from primary caregivers in this situation. These reactions are far beyond what would be expected in the situation by most people who have had similar experiences.

Avoidance. The third diagnostic criterion involves individuals actively and persistently avoiding situations that remind them of the trauma. The key issue for this symptom is the active avoiding of stimuli or situations that trigger memories of the trauma to the point these efforts restrict individuals' functioning on a day-to-day basis (APA, 2022). Many people avoid stimuli or situations from time to time. They do not like going to a store to return items because they know it will be a hassle. Or, some people might not travel to certain places because they feel uncomfortable for one reason or another. Maybe you can think of a time when you experienced something like that. You might have taken a deep breath and gone to the place anyway or just put it off for a few days until you were in the right frame of mind, then went anyway. However, individuals diagnosed with PTSD become almost immobile, incapable of participating in situations being in or close to conditions that remind them of the trauma. Individuals might avoid memories, thoughts, or feelings associated with the trauma. When something reminds them of the trauma, they might change the topic or leave the room. They could also just tune out and not process what is happening. The manifestation might also involve dodging external stimuli that could include people, places, activities, or objects. Understand this list is not comprehensive because different stimuli spark memories for each individual. Below is a dialogue that shows the way crisis intervention might unfold with an individual when this symptom surfaces.

Mood Alteration. The fourth criterion involves negative cognitions and changes in mood after surviving a traumatic situation. The expression of this symptom is observed as individuals' negative thoughts about themselves or the world in general because of distorted beliefs (APA, 2022). You have to differentiate this indicator from people who have negative self-esteem or are just simply pessimistic. Other ways this symptom might be observed include blaming themselves for the trauma, feelings of detachment or estrangement, being alive, or the lack of feeling happiness. These indicators might be expressed by avoiding important events and the lack of feeling love or satisfaction. Because most everyone has passing feelings like these, again these indicators must block day-to-day functioning.

Hyperarousal. The next criterion involves a heightened startle response and hypervigilance. This symptom is not the same as being on edge, having drunk too much caffeine, or being overly nervous because you have to go to the dentist. A startle response and hypervigilance are much more dramatic. Individuals are exceptionally, persistently irritable and not able to concentrate because of being preoccupied thinking about the trauma (APA, 2022). They might have angry outbursts or be reckless, getting into fights both verbally and physically with others. These symptoms have the tendency to generalize indirectly to similar situations. The individual who was in the plane when it skidded off the runway might associate that trauma with riding in a car and see a car in front of it start to slow down, causing them to immediately become a back seat driver slamming on the imaginary brakes on the passenger side of the front seat.

In summary, not all these symptoms and indicators will be seen in everyone diagnosed with PTSD. Individuals experience and express them in unique ways. The symptoms must also be present for more than one month and, as we said previously, obstruct their ability to function on a day-to-day basis. The symptoms might also subside for a period of time then reemerge. The following dialogue illustrates the way the symptoms and indicators may resurface unexpectedly, resulting in a crisis.

The following case involves a man named Carlos who works as an Emergency Medical Technician (EMT). He has been working in his current position for the past 15 years. During that time, he has responded to hundreds of accidents and other medical emergencies. Most of the emergencies he has responded to were run of the mill and not serious. However, some were gruesome, involving mangled bodies after car accidents. While first on the job, the car accidents caused him discomfort and stress. However, after responding to so many, Carlos has become desensitized and reacts as a professional providing whatever medical assistance is needed. That was until a little over four weeks ago when he was the first EMT on the scene of a car accident in which every member of a family was killed after being hit head on by a drunk driver who survived. He immediately rushed to the mangled car and had to crawl inside to pull out the people that included a man, a woman, and three children. All were badly injured, and he started providing medical treatment on a girl aged between 10 and 15. She stopped breathing even though he did his best. Other first responders were at the scene by that time and attempting to provide treatment. When he was finally off work that evening and returned home, his wife could see he was visibly shaken. She asked what happened, and he simply said, "it will be in the news." After a few days, Carlos seemed to be back to his old self but a little on edge. Over the next four weeks, Carlos became increasingly protective of his family, including his wife and two daughters, ages 14 and 17. During the four weeks, Carlos began having terrible dreams and became very moody with exploding anger at unexpected times. Carlos' wife finally pressured him into talking to someone.

Carlos: (He and his wife walk up to the reception desk at the local community mental health center)

Receptionist: Hi, may I help you?

Carlos: (Shrugs) She says I need to get help or else. (Takes a deep breath and looks at his wife). See, I am trying, is that good enough?

Gabriella: (Looks at him with a scowl. Then at the receptionist) Thank you. Can you please help?

Receptionist: Okay, what's your name and what's the problem?

Carlos: My name is Carlos, and she thinks I am going crazy or something.

Receptionist: Okay I see, let me look at the schedule. (Two minutes go by.) I can schedule you next week on Thursday.

Carlos: What! Fuck. (Said under his breath.) I need to talk to someone right now. PLEASE or she is going to kick me out of the house.

Gabriella: (Looks at him and then the receptionist again) Calm down, let's figure this out. Please can you do anything? He needs to be seen immediately. He is not sleeping, tries to boss everyone around, and, well, just not himself.

Receptionist: Okay when did all this start?

Gabriella: It kind of started a month ago after that terrible accident when the family was killed. He was the EMT first on the scene (Looks at Carlos.) But a couple of weeks ago things got worse.

Receptionist: You waited how long? What has changed?

Carlos: Yeah, I just thought it would go away.

Receptionist: Okay I understand but this does not sound like an emergency at the moment. I'm sorry, the earliest appointment is on Thursday. We do have a hotline you can call. I can give you the number.

Carlos: (Becoming visibly agitated and takes a breath) YOU DON'T FUCKING UNDERSTAND. I don't want no hotline, she wants me to talk with someone right now. Not call someone.

Gabriella: There must be something you can do. PLEASE, just for me and our kids.

Receptionist: Okay, okay, okay, let me see what I can do. Please can you sit down?

Carlos: (Looks around the room) NO, I think I will wait right here. (Paces around in front of the desk)

Gabriella: (Walks over and sits down.)

At this point in the conversation, several statements and Carlos' behavior indicate that he is experiencing issues that have developed over several weeks after responding to a car accident with multiple fatalities. Indicators of a possible diagnosis of PTSD are present, such as becoming easily irritated, not sleeping, and not behaving in a typical manner. These indicators were mostly described by Gabriella, his wife, which in crisis situations is not unusual. Carlos may not even be aware he is having problems, at least not to the extent his wife observes. However, Carlos is in crisis and needs some type of intervention. At this point, Carlos' affect is clearly angry and is barely under control. Rating him is difficult because his feeling seems to fluctuate between 5 and 8 on the TAF. His pacing may indicate his TAF behavior is at least a 5, although it could be higher and is immobile or avoiding. Cognitively, Carlos feels threatened, and again, he is at least a 5 or possibly a 6 on the TAF.

Receptionist: (Makes a phone call which lasts three to five minutes) Carlos, if you can please sit down, Betty, one of our counselors will come and get you in a few minutes.

Carlos: (Shrugs and mumbles.) Okay thanks. (Sits down but continually scans the room.)

After about five minutes, a door opens, and a woman walks behind the reception desk and speaks to the receptionist who points toward Carlos. The woman walks over.

Betty: Hi, you must be Carlos. My name is Betty.

Carlos: (Looks over at his wife.) I need help. She thinks I am going crazy. I can't sleep, I am scared. I am......

Betty: (Interrupts.) Hold on Carlos, let's go back to my office. Is that okay with you? Is she your wife? Would you like her to come back with us?

Carlos: (Still appears agitated and scanning the room) NO, I am a big boy I can do this all by myself.

Gabriella: (Looks at him and says very softly.) It will be okay. Make sure you say something about drinking more.

As they leave the room, Carlos glances over his shoulder, looking angrily at his wife. As they walk to her office, Carlos is very watchful and several times flinches.

Betty: Here is my office; please go in and sit down,

Carlos: (**Walks in and scans the room and looks around.**) I don't know about this. It is really small. I am only doing this because my wife said she would kick me out if I didn't.

Betty: (**Smiles and softly chuckles.**) Yea, I know, all the offices are kind of small. You can't set up house in here that's for sure. Are you sure you do not want her to be here too?

Carlos: (**Clenches his teeth.**). YES, I already said that. Don't ask again. (**Voice lowers.**) Besides, she just doesn't understand.

Betty: (**Starts to close the door.**)

Carlos: Do you have to close the door?

Betty: Is closing the door a problem? I am not sure leaving it open is a good idea. Everything is confidential, and you probably are not wanting other people to listen in. Carlos (**Shrugs.**) Okay I guess but don't lock okay. I get kind of scared in closed spaces. (**Pauses and whispers**)

Betty: I won't lock it. And see, you have a clear path out if you want, (**Points to the door.**) Is that okay? I want you to feel safe.

In this brief exchange, another symptom of PTSD has surfaced, avoidance of stimuli that remind him of the crisis event. With the symptoms and responding to a horrific car accident reported by his wife earlier, Betty may be suspect that Carlos has developed PTSD. Betty also noted that Carlos appeared unusually vigilant walking back to her office again and was easily angered. In the first few moments in her office, his discomfort was apparent. According to his wife, the PTSD symptoms seemed to have been building over a few weeks. Carlos may not be aware of these symptoms or probably discounts them. At this point, his affect ranges from a low of 5 to likely closer to an 8 when he becomes angry mixed with fear. Behaviorally he seems to be avoiding, with the ratings going from a 5 to maybe a 7. The cognitive rating is 5 to 6, and he is experiencing a threat based on not

wanting the counselor to close or lock her door. Overall, that means ratings range from a low of 15 to 21 or a high moderate overall rating, suggesting Betty needs to use a "we" approach. Possible strategies to use at this point are Providing Support and Creating Awareness. Carlos needs support as he struggles to manage the aftermath of responding to a fatal car accident and awareness of the ways this is affecting his day-to-day functioning.

Carlos and Betty continue talking for over an hour. During that time Carlos seems to relax but remains cautious. Betty uses the strategies of Providing Support and Creating Awareness as she talks with him. We will return to this case study at the end of the chapter to conclude the crisis intervention session. We shift now to discussing other aspects of PTSD. This information is valuable when doing crisis intervention with individuals who have this disorder.

Complex PTSD

Although the DSM 5-TR (2022) does not include a diagnosis for complex PTSD, the ICD 11 does include this as a diagnosis (World Health Organization, 2018). Complex PTSD was introduced in 1992 by Herman (1992b). Since that time, debate has ensued whether or not it is a distinct diagnostic label (Dyer & Corrigan, 2021). Whether or not complex PTSD should be a distinct diagnosis is beyond the scope of this book. However, there is agreement among clinicians that complex PTSD is a result of repeated exposure to traumatic situations. Exposure normally involves interpersonal victimization and commonly occurs across key developmental stages where there is an actual or perceived inability to escape, for example, childhood sexual abuse (Courtois & Ford, 2020; Dyer & Corrigan, 2021).

A basic understanding of complex trauma or PTSD helps in crisis intervention. The reason is that, at times, individuals in crisis will suddenly take a 90-degree turn and start talking about something that seems totally unrelated to the presenting problem. You might say that this cannot happen, but believe us, it happens. We have been there and done that. Many times, these 90-degree turns are related and/or due to complex trauma. When the crisis worker is aware that these unexpected shifts might happen, it helps to avoid getting sidetracked. Kumar et al. (2022) makes the case that complex trauma is so widespread that clinicians should receive training to understand and treat individuals who are struggling after being exposed to multiple traumas. Kumar et al. (2022) state that treating individuals who have experienced multiple traumas is different than treating someone who has a one-time trauma. As we stated earlier, many times in crisis intervention, PTSD, or in this case, complex trauma, plays a real part in and influences individuals' reactions while in crisis.

Individuals with complex trauma histories often display greater complications involving cognitive (including dissociative), affective, somatic, behavioral, relational, and self-attributional problems beyond the symptoms of the "classic" form of PTSD (Courtois & Gold, 2009; Karatzias, 2019). The three cardinal symptoms of complex trauma are **somatization** (physical problems, associated pain, and functional limitations), **dissociation** (division of the personality into one component that attempts to function in the everyday world and another that regresses and is fixed in the trauma), and **affect dysregulation** (alterations in impulse control, attention and consciousness, self-perception, perception of perpetrators, relationships to significant others, and systems of meaning) (Courtois et al., 2009, pp. 85–86; Ford & Courtois, 2021).

Given the wide variety of maladaptive behaviors associated with complex trauma, making a differential diagnosis and understanding the symptoms, such as anxiety, depressive, organic mental, and substance use disorders, is complicated (APA, 2000; Kumar et al., 2022; Møller, 2021). In fact, it is probably more common to have **comorbidity** (the presence of two diagnosable disorders such as major depression and substance misuse) (Rutherford et al., 2021). Further, because of presenting symptoms, PTSD may be confused with adjustment, paranoid, somatic, and obsessive compulsive disorder, and personality disorders (Luciano et al., 2022; Møller et al., 2021; Pinciotti, 2023; Rutherford et al., 2021).

There are few "pure" cases and few symptoms are unique to the disorder (Masino & Norman, 2015). Thus, *no matter what the diagnosis, assessment in crisis intervention should always attempt to determine if there has been exposure to prior trauma,* particularly when the crisis seems to have occurred spontaneously, with no clear, immediate, precipitating stimulus.

The Question of Preexisting Psychopathology

For a variety of political and social reasons, society has been hesitant to perceive (and has not perceived) being a victim of war, domestic violence, or other types of human cruelty as the equivalent of having a mental health condition. Although this perception has changed, the common belief continues that individuals who have experienced these types of trauma should just "get over it." Vietnam veterans, who early on sought help from Veterans Administration (VA) hospitals, were misdiagnosed or thought to have some preexisting psychopathology or character disorder. As a result, they were revictimized by a bureaucratic and rigidly conservative mental health system that added psychic insult to psychic injury (Ochberg, 1988, p. 4). Survivors of partner violence fared no better and were often seen to have a "masochistic" personality that subconsciously enjoyed physical assaults (Herman, 1997, p. 117). Such revictimization and discounting by supposedly "caring" professionals exacerbate the trauma survivor's problems exponentially. Fortunately, that perception has mostly dissipated for professionals, but unfortunately, among the general population, some people still hang onto the belief that victims of partner violence must like it because they stay with the person doing the victimizing.

The DSM 5-TR (2022) identifies three pretraumatic factors that contribute to the development of PTSD. These include temperamental factors such as childhood emotional problems by the age of 6 and early mental health disorders (e.g., panic disorder, depressive disorder, and obsessive compulsive disorder). Environmental factors include low socioeconomic status, lower education, lower intelligence, minority racial/ethnic status, family psychiatric history and social support prior to exposure. The third factor is genetic, and physiological factors including being a woman, younger age at the time of trauma exposure as well as some genotypes that may increase or, in some cases, decrease the risk of developing PTSD. These are described in more detail below. However, and this is important, the DSM 5-TR states that matching any of the factors does not predict that individuals will develop PTSD.

Researchers have found evidence of a heritable component to the transmission of PTSD (Danielson et al., 2021; Sheerin et al., 2020; Wolf et al., 2023) and to one's ability to be resilient to its assaults (Southwick & Watson, 2015). Undoubtedly, some people, because of a previous psychiatric history, are more predisposed to breaking down under stress than are others (Boehm-Tabib & Gelkopf, 2023; Stuke et al., 2023). Furthermore, the number and magnitude of the trauma will predict higher potential for PTSD (Stuke et al., 2023). Exposure to multiple rapes, being held in a concentration camp, extended child abuse, the loss of loved ones, or prolonged frontline combat typically puts the individual at far greater risk for PTSD than a one-time physical assault by a parent or an auto accident in which no one was killed. Additionally, lack of education, community support, chronic child abuse, low economic status, increased number in family, gender (women are seen as at greater risk), age (younger age at time of event), marital status (not married), and lack of family support systems have all been seen as contributing factors for developing PTSD (Cross et al., 2018; Madnick & Spokas, 2022; May & Wisco, 2016; Southwick & Watson, 2015; Zalta et al., 2021).

However, no absolute factors guarantee that one person as opposed to another will develop PTSD. Brewin (2005) found that although there are a number of risk factors for PTSD, their effect sizes tend to be small and vary according to the nature of the trauma. Research conducted by Dewar et al. (2023) reports similar results, finding that many factors contribute to the development of PTSD, but several factors also help shield individuals from developing the disorder. Given the right conditions, it appears *anyone can be a candidate.* The collapse of a concrete walkway in a crowded hotel gives us a prime example of how one event may suddenly produce PTSD symptoms. Biographical data gathered following the Kansas City Hyatt Regency skywalk disaster revealed that few survivors had character disorders before the event. Yet 6 months after the event, many were experiencing a variety of presenting symptoms (Wilkinson, 1983). The overwhelming majority of these individuals had no previous psychiatric history.

Probably the best summary statement about who will and who will not manifest PTSD was made by Grinker and Spiegel (1945) in their study of World War II veterans. They concluded that no matter how strong or mentally stable a person might be, if the stress were sufficient to cross that particular individual's threshold, a "war neurosis" would develop. It should also be clearly understood that PTSD is not culture-bound (Madnick & Spokas, 2022). While there are variations on the theme cross-culturally, there is a great deal of evidence that PTSD is a cross-cultural phenomenon common to all people (Whealin et al., 2022). In summary, susceptibility and ability to be resilient to PTSD is a function of several factors: genetic predisposition, ecological factors, constitution, personality makeup, previous life experiences, state of mind, cultural artifacts, phase of maturational development at onset, spiritual beliefs, social support system before and after the trauma, and

content and intensity of the event (Greene-Cramer et al., 2021; Gutirrez et al., 2023; Southwick & Watson, 2015; Whealin et al., 2022).

Neurophysiological Responses

LO4   In the last 25 years, a tremendous number of psychobiological studies have conclusively demonstrated that trauma affects the individual in a variety of physical ways. Researchers have discovered that neurotransmitters, hormones, cortical areas of the brain, and the nervous system play a large role in PTSD (Daniels et al., 2013; Girgenti & Duman, 2018; Herringa et al., 2013; Lanius et al., 2013; Lu et al., 2013; Macdonald et al., 2012; Schore, 2013; Tyrka et al., 2013; Wolf et al., 2023). Putting this complex neurobiological puzzle together has tremendous ramifications about what kinds of drug therapies might be used in its treatment.

When a person is exposed to severe stress, neurotransmitters, neuromodulators, hormones, endogenous opioids, and specific cortical functions designed to deal with the emergency are activated (Grinker & Speigel, 1945; Santa Ana et al., 2006; Selye, 1976; Siegel, 1995; van der Kolk, 1996a, pp. 215–234; Vermetten & deArellano, 2002). Although cessation of the traumatic event may remove the person from danger and no longer require the body's system to function on an emergency basis, if the stress is prolonged, the nervous system may continue to function in an elevated and energized state as if the emergency were still continuing (Burgess-Watson et al., 1988; van der Kolk, 1996a, pp. 214–234).

Furthermore, evidence that intense and continuous stress can cause permanent physical changes in the brain has been reported Daniels et al., 2013; Malizia & Nutt, 2000; Vermetten & Bremner, 2002). These changed physiological states are important because they not only cause individuals extreme physical and psychological duress long after the traumatic event but also help explain why people do not "get over" PTSD.

In their study and review of the neuroanatomical correlates of the effects of stress on memory, Bremner and associates (1997) and Gurvitz et al. (1995) found significant decreases in the hippocampal area of the brain in combat veterans where explicit memory encoding, memory consolidation, and organization take place, as did Stein and associates (1994) in women who had experienced severe child sexual abuse. Whether the smaller hippocampus is a causal factor for PTSD or PTSD causes the hippocampus to become smaller is not known. However, Astur and associates' (2006) study of identified PTSD experimental subjects versus non-PTSD controls supports these findings of decreased hippocampal activity.

A great deal of psychophysiological assessment evidence indicates that stimulus presentation to PTSD sufferers of sights, sounds, and smells associated with the long-past traumatic event will immediately send the neuroendocrine system into overdrive and cause physiological responses such as increased heart rate, blood pressure, and triglyceride and cholesterol levels, along with decreased blood flow to the skin and gastrointestinal and renal areas. These psychophysiological responses are not evinced in control subjects who are presented with the same stimuli (Lating & Everly, 1995). One way to think about the chemical changes is that, in a manner of speaking, the traumatic event "rewires" your brain to send messages to function the same way in situations individuals perceive as similar.

Affective-State-Dependent Retention

Evidence is clear that physiological changes occur in the presence of trauma (Friedman, 2015; Khayyat-Abuaita et al., 2019) and are exacerbated when the trauma becomes ongoing and complex (Ford, 2009). Changed physiological functioning due to traumatic stimuli is important as a building block in Bower's (1981) hypothesis of *affective-state-dependent retention*. Bower has proposed that because the traumatic event was stored in memory under completely different physiological (increased heart rate, higher adrenal output) and psychological (extreme fright, shock) circumstances, different mood states markedly interfere with recollecting specific cues of the event. A meta-analysis by Karl et al. (2006) supports the hypothesis that changes in memory processing accompany PTSD. Therefore, the important elements of the memory that need exposure to reduce anxiety are not accessible in the unaroused state (Keane et al., 1985, p. 266) and can be remembered only when that approximate state of arousal is reintroduced by cues in the environment (Keane, 1976). Indeed, there is evidence that the release of neuromodulators such as norepinephrine when an individual is in a stressful situation leads to a pathological response to recall of previous traumatic events for which the individual has no previous memory (Bremner et al., 1997).

To the contrary, the classic dissociative, numbing response and "forgetting" of the traumatic event may be caused by excessive endogenous opioids secreted during prolonged stress (van der Kolk, 1996a, p. 227). Thus, the notion that a victim of PTSD can "just forget" or adopt a "better, more positive attitude" does little to effect change in the individual (Keane et al., 1985, p. 266). This proposal has important implications for treatment, particularly with respect to returning the person to as close an approximation of the event as possible. These neurological issues are even more ominously true for children.

Children and Neuropathology

When children in early childhood experience continuous traumatic events, conditions are created to develop neuropathology (Lu et al., 2013; Rogel et al., 2020; Ryan et al., 2017). If the trauma occurs during early developmental stages, a dramatic shift in the brain's functioning from an inquisitive, exploring, learning mode to a reactive, defensive, surviving mode takes place. When the Cross et al. (2017) stress response survival systems of the child's brain are operating in overdrive, the learning systems take a back seat. As a result, a wide array of typical developmental activities are placed on hold, with potentially catastrophic consequences across social and educational environments (Spinazzola et al., 2018). In plain language, operating systems in the child's brain get damaged.

Damage occurs in three areas: emotional dysregulation, which may be characterized by emotional emptiness or constant distress; dissociation, which manifests as mental disorientation and confusion; and hyperarousal, which physically drains the body to the point of exhaustion. The potential for these devastating outcomes to occur is particularly enhanced if the trauma comes at the hands of a caregiver who is supposed to be nourishing the learning brain of the child rather than activating the survival system (Lippard & Nemeroff, 2020). You will meet some of the characteristics of these neurological damaged children later in this chapter and in Chapter 9, "Sexual Assault." The foregoing paragraphs should give you a fair idea of why treating childhood PTSD and survivors of extended childhood trauma is so difficult and why transcrisis states are so common with these individuals.

Incidence, Impact, and Trauma Type

Incidence

LO5 If PTSD has been with us for so long, what made it finally surface with such profound impact? The DSM 5-TR (APA, 2022) reports that by age 75, the projected risk for PTSD is 8.7 percent.

Adults in the United States develop this mental health disorder at a rate of 3.5 percent, while adults in most other areas in the world have a much lower rate at between 0.5 and 1.0 percent. According to the DSM 5-TR, rates are higher among veterans and occupational first responders such as individuals working in law enforcement, firefighters, and emergency medical personnel. Individuals who have been victims of sexual assault, experienced military combat, captivity and ethnically or politically motivated internment, and genocide also have a high risk of developing PTSD. The DSM 5-TR suggests that research is not conclusive regarding the development of PTSD for individuals in different developmental stages from early childhood to older adults. So, in the common course of events, the chances of "catching" PTSD are fairly small.

But what do all these numbers mean? How is this information relevant for crisis intervention? The short answer is that only a small number of individuals develop full-blown PTSD symptoms. One takeaway from this fact is that crisis interventionists should not be alarmists by immediately labeling individuals after a traumatic event. We understand this is like preaching to the choir, but understand the choir has a responsibility to educate the general public, especially anyone in the media or other position to influence thought. Another takeaway is for you to find ways to support individuals to recognize internal and external resources. Internal resources include ways they have responded to, persevered, and overcome previous traumatic events. Crisis interventionists can also use the strategies of Providing Support, Promoting Motivation, and Providing Guidance with individuals to help them access external resources that deliver more extensive treatment. Yet, as you will find out, this is easier said than done in many situations. Taking time and being with individuals in the moment is critical. An important aspect of activating internal and accessing external resources involves exercising caution in focusing solely on the negative presentations (e.g., nightmares, hypervigilance, avoidance) following a traumatic event. Although these cannot be ignored in extended treatment, crisis intervention should work to deescalate the immediate episode and help individuals reestablish a sense of control. Once control is reestablished, you can focus on getting someone to the treatment that will help them long term. The classic at-risk example is the Vietnam veteran. The numbers of returning Vietnam veterans who were having some kind of personality disorder far exceeded what statistics would predict. It is estimated that 26 percent, or 960,000 Vietnam veterans, have had episodes of PTSD (Kukla et al., 1990). This massive number of veterans in severe psychological trouble was simply too large to ignore.

Mass shootings in the United States have risen to new heights. As of April 2023, more mass shootings have occurred than the number of days in the year. Mass shootings are defined as taking place in a public space in which four or more deaths occur (Bjelopera et al., 2013). Survivors experience a number of negative effects, developing fear, horror, and anxiety as well as PTSD (San Roman et al., 2019; Santilli et al., 2017). The case of Carlos is used to illustrate crisis intervention with someone who has PTSD.

Residual Impact

People's basic assumptions about their belief in the world as a meaningful and comprehensible place, their own personal invulnerability, and their view of themselves in a positive light account to a great extent for their individual manifestations of PTSD (Kira et al., 2020; Szabo et al., 2022). Even in the most well-integrated people who have excellent coping abilities, good rational and cognitive behavior patterns, and positive social support systems, the residual effects of traumatizing events may linger. An outstanding example of such residual effects is the experience of a retired Marine captain who had seen extensive field duty as a combat infantryman in Vietnam in 1968. The anecdote he relates typifies the residual effects in an individual who is psychologically well integrated, is securely employed in a professional job, has a tight-knit extended family support system, and, on the whole, enjoys life and has a positive outlook on it.

Chris: I had just gotten home from work late one summer evening. The kids had decided to camp out in the woods down by the creek. A thunderstorm was rolling in and I decided I'd better go down and check on them to see if they were packed in for the night. It had started to rain pretty heavily, and there was a lot of thunder and lightning. I pulled on a poncho and got a flashlight, crossed the road, and went into the woods. I don't suppose it was 200 yards to where the kids were camped. Now, I'd grown up running those woods, so I knew it like the back of my hand.

However, once I got into the woods, things kinda went haywire. I immediately thought, "Get off the trail, or you'll get the whole platoon zapped."

I slipped off the path and became a part of the scenery. Every sense in my body went up to full alert. I was back in Nam again operating with my platoon, and I was on a natural adrenaline high. Time and place kinda went into suspended animation, and I eased through the woods, kinda like standing off and watching myself do this, knowing it was me, but yet not me too. The last thing I remember before walking into the clearing where the kids had their tent set up was that we could have ambushed the hell out of that place. I don't harp and brood on Nam, put it behind me after I got out of the Corps, but that night sure put me in a different place than central Indiana, July 1984. I just couldn't believe that would ever happen. It's a bit unnerving.

Importance of Trauma Type

Catastrophes, when viewed by the public, tend to fall into one category: bad. However, one of the interesting phenomena around PTSD is that there is a marked distinction between natural and human-made catastrophes. Acts of God create far fewer instances of PTSD than human-made catastrophes. As an example, the volcanic eruption of Mount St. Helen's incident rate of PTSD was a very low 3 to 4 percent (Shore et al., 1986). However, peritraumatic reactions are present among many survivors of natural disasters (Massaazza et al., 2021). Schneider et al. (2019) report that survivors after Hurricane Sandy experienced a variety of mental health disorders but also that many people, after time, experienced post traumatic growth. Post traumatic growth involves five consistently occurring changes including: (1) improved sense of self, (2) more positive relationships, (3) greater appreciation of life, (4) emergence of new possibilities, and (5) improvement of spiritual and/or religious life (Tedeschi & Calhoun, 2021).

Human-made acts of trauma create even more instances of PTSD when the trauma directly affects the social support system of the family. Holocaust survivors, hostages, survivors of sexual assault, children of murdered parents, and survivors of incest are all strong potential candidates for PTSD. Survivors of both uncommissioned human-made disasters, such as the breaking of the Buffalo Creek dam, and commissioned trauma, such as the Chowchilla bus kidnapping, carry high potential for PTSD. The Buffalo Creek disaster occurred in 1972 when a coal company retainer dam broke during a series of heavy rainstorms; the resulting flood wiped out the residents of the Buffalo Creek valley in West Virginia. The bus kidnapping occurred in 1976 when a Chowchilla, California, school bus carrying elementary and secondary school children was hijacked at gunpoint. The children were taken from the bus and forced into a truck buried underground; eventually they were able to tunnel out. The distinction between the two types of human-caused traumatic events is that one is a "sin of omission" and the other is a "sin of commission." While the human acts of omission such as oil tank car derailments and explosions in towns can certainly cause PTSD, mass shootings such as Sandy Hook Elementary School and Columbine High School are potentially far more toxic because they are unpredictable, trust within the community is broken, and people are in shock and disbelief that such a heinous and nonsensical act can happen in their peaceful community (Jurgersen et al., 2013; Sullivan et al., 2018).

What makes these events so particularly terrible is that they seem to be tragedies that should not have happened, responsibility for them can be readily assigned, and they clearly violate accepted standards of moral conduct (Figley, 1985, pp. 400–401). As a result, there exists in any human-made catastrophe the likelihood of more severe posttraumatic psychological problems compared to natural disasters. The problem is that the line between the two is becoming less clear. More and more people look at technology as a means of controlling nature. Thus, for example, Mother Nature makes the rain, but the Army Corps of Engineers builds dikes and opens floodgates (Kaniasty & Norris, 1999), and when things go wrong, individuals (and lawyers) start looking for culprits.

Vietnam: The Combat Archetype

Why did Vietnam mark the birth of what was to become PTSD? Although any war could be construed to produce many PTSD symptoms, the rules of war changed in Vietnam and continued in the conflicts in Iran and Afghanistan (Lee et al., 2022). In Vietnam, the average age of the soldier was 19.2, compared with 26.0 in World War II (Brende & Parson, 1985, p. 19). A psychologically immature 19-year-old soldier was not mentally prepared for the psychic trauma that awaited him in Vietnam (MacPherson, 1984, pp. 62–63). Although many lessons were learned from the conflict in Vietnam, soldiers deployed in Iran and Afghanistan still faced many of the same combat situations. The result is that, even though preventive education is provided and post deployment care offered, veterans still develop PTSD at a high rate (Hale et al., 2021).

In a comparative analysis of PTSD among various trauma survivor groups, Wilson et al. (1985) isolated

10 variables that were hypothesized as predisposing to PTSD: degree of life threat; degree of bereavement; speed of onset; duration of the trauma; degree of displacement in home continuity; potential for recurrence; degree of exposure to death, dying, and destruction; degree of moral conflict inherent in the situation; role of the person in the trauma; and the proportion of the community affected. They compared these variables in a variety of trauma survivor groups: Vietnam combat veterans as well as survivors of rape, auto accident, armed robbery, natural disasters, divorce, life-threatening illness of a loved one, family trauma, death of a significant other, multiple traumas, and a control group.

Veterans were significantly affected in 7 of the 10 dimensions, survivors of sexual assault a distant second in terms of the number of predisposing variables present. When the data were transformed to fit precise PTSD criteria, all trauma groups were significantly different from the control group (Munsey, 2009, pp. 142–172). In plain words, the data suggest that one could not experience a catastrophic event more likely to produce "complex" PTSD than Vietnam—with one exception. With the expanded inclusion of women in combat roles, if sexual assault and combat are combined, such as occurred in Iraq and Afghanistan, then people who have been in combat and have also been sexually assaulted are one-and-a-half times more likely to be diagnosed with a mental health condition than those who have not been assaulted (Munsey, 2009).

Hypervigilance. In the most recent military conflicts, there are no front lines and no relief from constant vigilance. A 365-day combat tour was exactly that in Vietnam. In comparison to World War II troops, who might be in acute combat situations for a few days or weeks and then be pulled off the line, Vietnam "grunts" spent extended periods of time in the field, and even when they were in a base camp, they had to be alert for rocket attacks and combat assaults on their position. Hypervigilance became an ironclad rule of survival.

Learn from Billie Mac, a composite character of many combat veterans Dr. James has interviewed. Following is his writing as part of a **narrative therapy exposure** component (Mørkved et al., 2014; Mott et al., 2015) of cognitive processing therapy (Resick et al., 2008; Resick et al., 2007; Resick & Schnicke, 1993). Narrative therapy is designed to encourage recall through writing (Mott et al., 2015) and has been

found to be effective (Wei & Chen, 2021). The goal of this approach is to help individuals get unstuck (Monson & Shnaider, 2014) from the endless cycle of attempts to avoid the trauma yet continuously perseverate on it. The purpose in his written narrative is twofold.

First, the primary goal of trauma-focused therapy (TFT) is to help survivors thoroughly examine and unpackage traumatic memories so they can reappraise and reframe those events for healthier living. While TFT will work on here-and-now trauma-related problems the survivor is confronting, initial therapy focuses on the historical feeling, behaviors, cognitions, and contexts that are hypothesized to play a central role in the onset of PTSD (Monson & Shnaider, 2014).

Second is the concept of **meaning making**. Meaning making is both *global* and *situational* (Liao Siling et al., 2021; Steger & Park, 2012, pp. 172–174). A global meaning system is the composite set of beliefs, goals, and sense of purpose that we operationalize to live our lives. This global meaning system then goes smoothly about its business of assigning good, bad, and neutral meanings to specific situations encountered on the road of life. However, what happens when an extraordinary situation lands in the middle of our nice, safe, justice-for-all, fair-play world and shatters it to the point that our global meaning system overloads and blows a psychological fuse? This fusion of the event and global meaning system can become central to identity, disrupting the individual's entire belief system (Kramer et al., 2020). Neimeyer and Vaughans (2021) discuss a constructivist approach when the trauma involves grief. The traumatic loss provokes a crisis of meaning as individuals try to make sense of conflicting narratives (Niemeyer & Sands, 2011). When this chasm in meaning occurs, loss of control, predictability, or ability to comprehend the world as one once knew it as a reasonable, predictable one goes in the dumpster, and in our attempts to control the emotional and cognitive dysregulation that occurs, PTSD emerges as a major player in our now modified and distorted global belief system.

Meaning making is the attempt to restore the original global meaning system and not let it be driven by the one traumatic event that changed it. Meaning making calls for reviewing and reframing the traumatic event in such a way that an acceptable appraisal of the event can be made. The bottom line is that the event itself can never be undone, but both the negative self and global appraisals of it can (Steger & Park, 2012, pp. 174–175). Billie Mac's tortured narrative is one component of a comprehensive therapeutic endeavor to bring meaning back into his life.

Narrative Exposure Through Journaling. For clients diagnosed with PTSD, speaking of what has happened to them is extremely difficult. Journaling is an excellent method of opening up affect and allowing nonverbal catharsis to occur. By engaging in written narrative exposure, putting down their thoughts in their own words and then hearing them, individuals place the terrible memories at a safe enough psychological distance that they and the human services worker can analyze them (Wei & Chen, 2021).

Journal writing gives the human services worker a catalyst for encouraging the kind of free association necessary to open the crystallized defenses of the individual who might otherwise never explore the traumatic event (Progoff, 1975). One of the veterans who formed the basis of our composite combat therapy group character, Billie Mac, writes a description of one of those endless nights when no sleep will come or, worse, when the terror comes with sleep as the introduction to the group.

Where Did B.M. Go?

What happened to B.M.—the boy from Mississippi—happy-go-lucky, not a care in the world, who loved life, sports, the sunshine, the rain . . . and everything in the used-to-be-beautiful world. Everyone told B.M., "Go to school. Play sports. Go to college." But B.M. decided what he wanted to do for his country. B.M. wanted to go to war and fight to win . . . to serve his country . . . to make everyone proud of him. B.M. went to war. B.M. killed, massacred, mutilated, burnt, hated—a hate that was like a drunk hate—tore his own heart out a little at a time, time after time.

B.M. fought and survived a war that 127 warriors that went with B.M. didn't.

B.M. looked at everyone around him and wondered why the people hated him.

Why they were scared of him . . . why they feared the warrior from Vietnam who went to a fight they were scared to fight.

B.M. wanted to love . . . to be loved. It seemed like the world was completely different from him and didn't have the same ideals about life and love.

B.M. became a drunk. He drank to forget the war, the brave warriors who had given their lives in Vietnam, to forget the people that he was living around. To these people, B.M. was a cold-blooded murdering S.O.B.—a baby-killing M.F.

B.M. had been taught all his life, "Thou shalt not kill, love thine enemy." B.M. lost his morals. B.M. killed his enemies. B.M. cut the heads and ears off some of his enemies. B.M. lost his soul. B.M. is lost to God and can't be forgiven. People can say, "Ask God to forgive you, B.M." But B.M. can't forgive himself and can't ask for forgiveness. B.M. has accepted that feeling like someone took his heart out and stomped it into the ground. There is not a day in his life that he doesn't feel hurt or hurt the ones he loves.

B.M. just wants to be loved . . . to love himself again; to get rid of that hard feeling deep down inside of his heart. B.M. wants to have peace of mind. Is it too much for him to ask, to seek, to search for? Is death what it will take for B.M. to finally find peace within himself?

Why can't B.M. get out of all these depressing moods he stays in . . . and cries about nothing when he is driving down the road?

Sometimes B.M. thinks he is a crazy S.O.B. Maybe the people are right. Why can't B.M. keep a job? Because B.M. was a fuck-up after he got back from Vietnam.

His vengeance and his screwed-up attitude keep him in trouble. B.M. would get so much on his mind and B.M. would keep putting it back inside. The more he put it back, the worse his depression would get until it would erupt in a rage of vengeance, which would always wind up hurting himself or the people he loved.

Even the government deceived B.M. They told B.M., "Don't worry, B.M. You go and fight this war for your country, and if anything happens, we will take care of you." B.M.'s response to this is, "Fine! I will do all I can for my government and my country." But give me my heart and soul back. Make me sleep at night. Make me quit crying. Take this depression away. Help me find a job and help me feel alive again. Give me back what you took from me. B.M. is what you took, and I want myself back.

I wish I could give back the lives I have taken from the world, but I know that I can't. I would if I could, and I am the one that will have to live with that in my heart throughout eternity.

B.M. vividly and dramatically illustrates the anguish of PTSD in his writing—anguish from both an intrapersonal and interpersonal standpoint, of guilt he feels within himself for his moral transgressions and rage at the transgressions visited on him by an impersonal government and an uncaring society; anguish over what he was and is and how he is now attempting to resolve and reintegrate these two vastly different people that were and are B.M. Billie Mac continuously uses his initials, pointing over and over to himself, but in the third person. Only in the last paragraph does his plea change clearly to subjective, first-person owning statements. Even these statements are couched in terms of magical thinking—wish fulfillment. The use of Billie Mac's initials as an identifier of what he really perceives himself to be is not happenstance. The initials "B.M." also stand for "bowel movement." Indeed, Billie Mac's self-assessment is that he is mostly worthless "shit" to himself and others. This is typical of the kind of self-condemnation that an individual who is both victim and victimizer experiences.

This excruciating piece of writing is an initiating step in the long process that moves from self-condemnation to what Lifton (1973) calls **animated guilt**. Animated guilt enables the individual to start taking responsibility for past actions and start to experience new degrees of personal liberation. This rather dramatic example of journal writing was done voluntarily, but when clients in a crisis situation will not talk about their experiences, sometimes suggesting that they write down their feelings can be a way of breaking the impasse (James & Gilliland, 2003). Keeping a journal not only can be an extremely effective way of dealing with unbidden feelings and thoughts as they surface but also can provide the worker and the client with an assessment of how therapy is progressing (Pearsons, 1965). Journaling goes beyond standard Cognitive Processing Theory work of writing down daily monitoring of events, thoughts, and emotions of which one must be trauma-related (Monson & Shnaider, 2014, p. 70). For anyone like Billie Mac, who suffers survivor's guilt or victim/victimizer status, journaling may be a particularly effective way to ventilate feelings the person might otherwise be unable to communicate with the worker but now can because it is on paper and psychologically distanced. Billie Mac's journaling is a very good personal analysis of what went badly wrong in Vietnam.

Billie Mac: I was 18 when the plane set down at Da Nang. The crew chief told us to hit the ground running because Da Nang was under a rocket attack.

I was scared stiff. Well, Da Nang was heaven, rockets and all, compared to what later happened. It got a lot, lot worse than that.

Lack of Goals. No territory was ever "won," so there was no concrete feeling of accomplishment. Combat troops felt betrayed by U.S. politics over a war for which there were no fixed goals for winning and a command structure that was waging a war of attrition, with "body counts" being the primary way of judging whether a mission was successful (Lifton, 1974; MacPherson, 1984, p. 58).

Billie Mac: We swept that one village at least a half dozen times. Sometimes we'd dig in and dare the NVA to hit us, and they did. We lost a half dozen guys in that pesthole. For what? For nothin'. We gave it up, and they moved right back in.

Victim/Victimizer. It further compounded the virulent psychological milieu of Vietnam that veterans, unlike most individuals who experience PTSD, played two roles—victim and victimizer. Because both enemies and allies were Vietnamese, a soldier could not distinguish friend from foe, nor could vigilance be relaxed around women or children because of their potential lethality. Also, because the enemy was Asian and had extremely different cultural values from Americans, it was relatively simple to dehumanize killing or maiming them, particularly when troops saw such things done to their comrades. The nasty way guerrilla war is fought brought out brutality on both sides (Lifton, 1974). Shifts of role from victim to aggressor could occur in seconds (Brende & Parson, 1985, p. 96).

Billie Mac: I couldn't imagine killing a kid or woman. That was true until our medic tried to take care of a kid covered with blood. We all thought he was wounded. When John went over to the dink, he opened up his arms and had a grenade. Blew him and the medic away. Kill them after that? You bet!

Bonding, Debriefing, and Guilt. Research has shown that unit cohesion is an important factor to protect against developing PTSD (Lee et al., 2022). However, the way the armed services filled units during the Vietnam War had much to do with the lack of a support system within the service itself. Personnel replacements were parceled piecemeal into units, which is a bad idea if you are trying to avoid PTSD. Research indicates that unit cohesion is a critical buffer against PTSD (Armistead-Jehle et al., 2011). Although this method put rookies with veterans, it was not the best way to bind a unit together. The rotation system also took its psychological toll. Each person did a 365-day tour. The stress of being "short" caused men to become very self-preservative and immobilized. Units as a whole were never moved out of combat, and a man who entered combat singly returned singly without the benefit of debriefing time. The war was essentially fought in patrol and platoon actions. It was a loner's war, and the soldier who fought alone went home alone (MacPherson, 1984, pp. 64–65). A man might be sweating out an ambush in the jungle one day and two days later be sitting on his front porch back home.

It is no great surprise that returning soldiers who had no transition period from Vietnam to the United States were viewed as "different" and "changed" by their relatives (Brende & Parson, 1985, pp. 48–49). Such rapid transitions out of life-threatening situations left many with survivor's guilt (Spiegel, 1981). They were glad to be out of Vietnam but felt guilty of betrayal for leaving comrades behind, or they took responsibility when they were away from their units and friends were hurt or killed (MacPherson, 1984, p. 237).

Billie Mac: It was inside of a week from jungle to home. My folks thought it was pretty weird because I put my fatigues on and slept in the woods. I just couldn't take being confined in that house. I kept thinking about the guy who took my place as squad leader, Johnson. I knew he was gonna get somebody wasted. I needed to be there, but I sure didn't want to be. I immediately got drunk and stayed that way for a long time.

Civilian Adjustment. Acculturation to civilian life from military life is a recognized problem (Mitchell et al., 2020). Mitchell et al. (2020) state that key factors affecting the transition are combat experience and social support. Veterans stationed in Vietnam likely had extensive combat experience and probably not a lot of social support when returning to the United States. The rapid change from intense alertness to preserve one's life to trying to readjust to a humdrum society made many question where the "real world" was. Furthermore, the returnee's basic belief system would be quickly jarred when, on his arrival home, he was greeted with insensitivity and hostility for having

risked his life for his country (Brende & Parson, 1985, p. 72). Veterans quickly found that for all the ability they had shown in making command decisions of life-or-death importance and the authority they had exercised over expensive equipment in Vietnam, the onus of having been there relegated them to civilian jobs far below their capabilities (MacPherson, 1984, p. 65).

Billie Mac: Any job I could get stunk. They were all menial, and they acted like they were doing me a favor. Hell! I'd made a lot bigger and smarter decisions than anybody I ever had as a boss.

Substance Abuse. The ease with which soldiers could obtain alcohol and drugs to numb themselves and escape mentally from the reality of Vietnam had severe consequences, both in addiction on return and in the public's growing misconception that veterans were all "drug-crazed baby killers," to be shunned as erratic and undependable (Brende & Parson, 1985, p. 72; MacPherson, 1984, pp. 64–65, 221–222). Substance misuse is a major comorbid player in PTSD (Ouimette & Read, 2014), and alcohol is a major self-medication used in attempting to get rid of the torment and terrors in the hellish dream worlds of those individuals who have PTSD as their bedmates.

Billie Mac: Yeah, I drank. Yeah, I shot kids. I drank mainly to try to forget about shooting kids. Anybody who hadn't been there could never understand. I drink now to get some sleep and keep the damned nightmares at bay. I drink after I get fired from a job, I drink when I have fights with the ole lady. I drink when the cops are chasing me at 100 miles an hour. Sounds like I need to be in AA rather than this combat group.

Attitude. The time period during which a vet served in Vietnam seems to be highly correlated with PTSD. Historically the war can be divided into trimesters. Anyone serving in Vietnam during the last two trimesters, from the time of the Tet offensive in 1968 to the U.S. withdrawal in 1973, would have, from a psychological standpoint, a much greater reason to question the purpose of being there than those who had served early on. The prevailing attitude of "Nobody can win, so just concentrate on surviving" cynicism was in direct opposition to the "Save a democracy from the perils of communism" idealism of the first trimester (Laufer et al., 1981).

Antiwar Sentiment. The impact of the antiwar sentiment some people espoused that veterans met on their return home cannot be minimized. It is unique to the Vietnam War and found its focal point in returnees. Veterans were spurned immediately on their arrival in the United States, suffered prejudice on college campuses as they came back to school, were left out of jobs because of antiwar sentiments, and were disenfranchised from government programs through meager GI Bill benefits and government disavowal of physical problems associated with exposure to the chemical defoliant Agent Orange. Perhaps worst of all were the comparisons their fathers made—men who had fought the "honorable" fight of World War II and could not understand the problems their sons suffered in a war that was not black-and-white but a dirty shade of gray (MacPherson, 1984, pp. 54–58). It is interesting to note that Vietnam combat veterans diagnosed with PTSD whose fathers were also combat veterans were likely to have more severe problems than those Vietnam veterans whose fathers had not seen combat (Rosenheck & Fontana, 1998).

Billie Mac: I tried to talk to my old man about it. He'd been in World War II on Okinawa. Hell, he might as well have been in the Revolutionary War for all he could understand about Nam. He finally got so mad that he told me I was nuts and no damn good. He didn't mean that, but I'll never forget it.

All these factors came together in a sort of witch's brew for veterans trying to make meaning out of a situation that was life-threatening and generally considered pointless (Williams, 1983). Emotional support and reintegration with society and family are major tasks for veterans (Whealin et al., 2008), and strong social support is a major antagonist to PTSD (Southwick & Watson, 2015). To survive such a hostile lack of both societal and familial support called for imposing psychological defense mechanisms that made a fertile breeding ground for PTSD. When these psychological defense mechanisms go awry, symptoms are typically seen in the three major PTSD diagnostic categories of intrusive thoughts, avoidance, and increased nervous system arousal.

Intrusive–Repetitive Ideation

Intrusive-repetitive thoughts become so problematic for the individual that these thoughts begin to dominate existence. Intrusive thoughts generally take the form of visual images that are sparked by sights, sounds, smells, or tactile reminders that bring the repressed images to awareness (Donaldson & Gardner, 1985, pp. 371–372).

Billie Mac: That day at the village when Al got it keeps coming back. I don't go fishing in the bayou anymore. It smells and looks like Nam, and every time I'd go I'd start thinking about that village, and I'd get the shakes.

Over time, triggers for intrusive thoughts may become associated with subtle and more generalized stimuli that are seemingly irrelevant to the trauma (van der Kolk & McFarlane, 1996, p. 10). These thoughts occur not only in conscious contact with reality but also in the form of flashbacks and nightmares.

Billie Mac: The reason that got me to the vets center is real simple. I was having these awful nightmares about being in a firefight while on a long-range reconnaissance patrol near Laos. The next thing I know, I'm dug into a bunker watching an enemy truck convoy's headlights come down the Ho Chi Minh Trail with my rifle aimed at them. The only problem was that it was on the banks of the Wolf River in Memphis, Tennessee, and it was headlights on I-40. It was also not 1970 but 1988. I knew if I didn't get help I was going to kill somebody.

Denial/Numbing

Accompanying emotions of guilt, sadness, anger, and rage occur as the thoughts continue to intrude into awareness (Jin et al., 2022). To keep these disturbing thoughts out of awareness, the individual may resort to self-medication in the form of alcohol or drugs. Self-medication may temporarily relieve depressive, hostile, anxious, and fearful mood states (Abram et al., 2021), but what usually occurs is a vicious cycle that alternates between being anesthetized to reality by the narcotic and experiencing elevated intrusion of the trauma with every return to sobriety. The ultimate outcome is increased dependence on the addictive substance as a method of keeping the intrusive thoughts submerged (Luciano et al., 2022).

Billie Mac: The drinkin' is no damn good. I know that, but try going without sleep for a week and knowing every time you nod off, that horrible nightmare's gonna come. Then it starts popping up in the daytime and you drink more to keep it pushed back.

As people attempt to cope with catastrophes, they become passive (immobile and paralyzed) or active (able to cope with the situation). Individual reactions fall into three major groupings: momentary freezing, flight reaction, and denial/numbing. In the prolonged stress of a combat situation, denial/numbing is the most common response and allows the soldier to cope and live with the experience in three ways: by believing he is invulnerable to harm, by becoming fatalistic, or by taking matters into his own hands and becoming extremely aggressive. Any of these proactive stances allow the individual to get through the trauma and cope with it without losing complete control (Figley, 1985, pp. 406–408). Typically, survivors of trauma will let down these defense barriers and will have acute stress disorders immediately after the trauma but will recover. For those who do not, continued emotional numbing and repression can have severe consequences.

Billie Mac: Looking back on it, I can't believe how callous I have become. SOP [standard operating procedure] was "It don't mean nothin', screw it, drive on." This would be right after a B-40 round had blown your buddy's brains all over you. You had to put it behind you to survive. A guy fell off the construction site I was working on last fall and splattered himself all over the pavement. I sat on a steel beam about 30 feet above the guy and just kept eating my lunch. No big deal!

Submerging emotions out of conscious awareness does not mean that they are summarily discarded. The price is that emotional numbing left in place and not relieved can generalize to other aspects of one's life and result in later psychological difficulties (Jin et al., 2022). Shunted into the unconscious for a long time, trigger events in the form of everyday stressors can pile up and cause emotional blowouts when the individual is least prepared for them (Figley, 1985, p. 408).

Increased Nervous Symptom Arousal

Autonomic hyperarousal in people with PTSD causes them to be nondiscriminating to stimuli that may hold no threat to them at all. Acoustic startle response is a cardinal feature of the trauma response (van der Kolk, 1996a, p. 221).

Billie Mac: I can't stand the sound of a chopper. Every time I hear one, I want to run. I get the feeling that every time I hear the 5 o'clock traffic chopper, it's gonna circle in, pick me up, and take me to a hot LZ [landing zone]. One came over the building I was working on. I didn't hear it at first. When I did hear it, I jumped and fell 10 feet and broke my arm.

In the same vein, **hypervigilance**, being on constant guard for threats when there is no immediate threat, is constantly with the person and causes concentration and attention problems. As these problems distort information processing, the resulting inability to decode messages from the central nervous system causes the person to react to the environment in either exaggerated or inhibited ways (van der Kolk & McFarlane, 1996, pp. 14–15).

Billie Mac: This may sound kinda weird, but I don't ever sit with my back to a door. Matter of fact, I really don't like sitting anywhere where my back might be to somebody else! I get real jumpy.

Dissociation

Dissociation symptoms are so potent that the DSM 5-TR (APA, 2022) lists them as a special category of PTSD. Dissociation at the moment of trauma is perhaps the most important long-term predictive variable for PTSD and is invariably connected to "complex" PTSD (Boyd et al., 2020; Kumar et al., 2022). Dissociation can range from numbing or lack of emotional responsiveness to the event to derealization ("this is not real; it isn't happening; it's a bad dream") or depersonalization ("I'm out of my body and looking at this from a grandstand") to complete amnesia of the event.

Dissociation splits off the memory from conscious awareness, but that does not mean the noxious stimulus event is extinguished. To the contrary, dissociation can be a last-resort adaptive way of coping with the trauma while it is going on, but the lack of integration of the traumatic event seems to be a leading cause of PTSD. If dissociation continues, it can severely interfere with daily living and breed disconnectedness and isolation (van der Kolk, 1996b, p. 286). At its penultimate point, dissociation can become dissociative identity disorder (formerly known as multiple personality disorder).

Billie Mac: It's like a lot of times I'm looking at me doing something sorta through a video camera, maybe. Like I'm smaller than real life, and I sorta know it's me, but it's not like I'm really there. The first time I did that was when we were in that village and my buddy Al got it.

What the person needs most is to bring these thoughts and behaviors into conscious awareness and come to grips with them so they can be resolved. Yet, rather than confronting the intrusive and threatening material, the person is more likely to deny its existence and use a variety of avoidance responses to escape from the situation (Horowitz et al., 1980). This issue is particularly problematic in therapy and is why those who experience PTSD may be particularly resistant and noncompliant to approaches that reexpose them to the feared trauma (Bernstein, 1986).

Social Supports

Natural disasters leave so few emotional scars because such disasters often strike intact social support systems simultaneously (Figley, 1988). In natural disasters that affect the whole community, everyone becomes a survivor. As we shall learn in Chapter 16, Disaster Response, community support is critical to the individual returning to a sense of normalcy after a major traumatic event (Halpern & Tramontin, 2007; Harvey et al., 2012). For Billie Mac and his fellow Vietnam veterans, that community support was severely lacking. Family members help each other through the horror of the disaster, and there is no blaming the individual (Figley, 1985, p. 409; Kaniasty & Norris, 1999). One of the keystones for bridging the gap between traumatic events and a return to adequate and wholesome functioning is a strong support system (Perry et al., 2021) that is most generally based within the family (Monson & Shnaider, 2014, pp. 102–103; Southwick & Watson, 2015, p. 24). But when the trauma is intrafamilial and takes the form of child and spouse abuse, those who are most traumatized are most generally the ones who are denied the most social support within the family, and that becomes a major progenitor for PTSD (Courtois & Ford, 2020; Saxe et al., 2007). Those who should provide the most comfort are the ones who are inflicting the most pain (Figley, 1985, p. 411).

Further exacerbating family relationships is the ingrained tendency in trauma victims to "not feel." While the individual would like to be able to demonstrate feelings of caring and love, experience has taught them that exposure of feelings is foolhardy because it invariably makes one vulnerable to further pain. These concepts strike at the very heart of what sustains family life—trust. The response of family members is to feel misunderstood, unloved, fearful, and angry. The response is reciprocal and plunges all members deeper into a vortex of family discordance.

From a family system perspective, if children, parents, or spouses attempt to regulate the continuing warfare in which the individual is engaging, they will be worn down and out by the effort. The individual may also become so dependent on the stabilizing person (usually the spouse) that the individual's needs breed resentment in anyone else who demands time and effort (usually children). The outcome of this spiral is what the individual may fear most from the support system—rejection. Feelings of guilt, numbing, anger, and loss plague the individual, and the spiral continues ever downward into more inappropriate behavior patterns and ultimate disintegration of the family.

Family members who cannot deal with the trauma may paradoxically turn on the victim. Sadly, this is too often the occurrence in the case of mothers who deny their spouses' abuse of the children, finally are confronted with the issue by children and family services, and then blame the children for the trouble they have caused! The same is true for survivors of sexual assault who, if children, may have parents who are psychologically unable to provide support for them and indeed revictimize them for having done something that led to the assault in the first place. If adults, survivors of sexual assault may have a spouse who is unable to respond in supportive ways or who blames the victim for "promiscuous or seductive" behavior that invited the sexual assault or claims the survivor "didn't resist enough" (Notman & Nadelson, 1976).

In attempting to deal with a family member who has suffered a traumatic experience, other members may experience stress to the degree that they may develop similar symptoms (Lenton-Brym et al., 2023). Indeed, if other family members have inadequate coping skills, their own problems may escalate to crisis proportions as the individual's reactions to the trauma create stress within the family. Or, if other members of the family have a hidden agenda of keeping the family in pathological homeostasis, they may engage in enabling the individual's disorder, much as the family of someone with alcohol use disorder may sabotage attempts at recovery. In summary, it should be clear that treating trauma victims also means treating the family (Lenton-Brym et al., 2023).

LO5 A practical way to conceptualize the connection between PTSD and crisis intervention is to view recovery from this mental health disorder as taking place in phases. Brende and Parson (1985, pp. 185–186) compiled the work of Wilson (1980), Figley (1978), and Horowitz (1976) to construct five phases of recovery in the individual with PTSD. These phases directly parallel treatment approaches, with each having its own crisis.

1. **The emergency or outcry phase.** The individual experiences heightened "fight/flight" reactions to the life-threatening situation. This phase lasts as long as the survivor believes the situation to last. Pulse, blood pressure, respiration, and muscle activity are all increased. Concomitant feelings of fear and helplessness predominate. Termination of the event itself is followed by relief and confusion. Questions about why the event happened and what its consequences are dominate the individual's thoughts.

2. **The emotional numbing and denial phase.** The survivor protects psychic well-being by burying the experience in subconscious memory. By avoiding the experience, the individual temporarily reduces anxiety and stress symptoms. Many individuals remain forever at this stage unless they receive professional intervention.

3. **The intrusive-repetitive phase.** The survivor has nightmares, volatile mood swings, intrusive images, and amplified startle responses. Other pathological and antisocial defense mechanisms may be put in place in a futile attempt to rebury the trauma. At this point, the delayed stress becomes so overwhelming that the individual is propelled to seek help or becomes so mired in the pathology of the situation that outside intervention is mandated.

4. **The reflective-transition phase.** The survivor develops a larger personal perspective on the traumatic events and becomes positive and constructive, with a forward- rather than backward-looking perspective. The individual comes to grips with the trauma and confronts the problem.

5. **The integration phase.** The survivor successfully integrates the trauma with all other past experiences and restores a sense of continuity to life. The trauma is successfully placed fully in the past.

Neat and orderly progression for the individual with PTSD through these stages is the exception rather than the rule. More likely is a precipitating crisis far removed in chronological time from the event itself and then a continuing series of crises that escalate until the individual voluntarily seeks help or is forced to seek it. Once intervention occurs, a cyclic pattern of avoidance, recall, recovery, and more avoidance continues until the core issues that gave birth to PTSD are resolved (Figley, 1985, pp. 402–404). The human services worker can expect a series of transcrisis events as this process unfolds.

Maladaptive Patterns Characteristic of PTSD

LO6 Trauma experiences play a major role in the way we perceive ourselves (Keshet et al., 2019). When the trauma results in developing PTSD, five common patterns emerge: death imprint, survivor's guilt, desensitization, estrangement, and emotional enmeshment.

Death Imprint. The traumatic experience provides a clear vision of one's own death in concrete biological terms (Ochberg, 1988, p. 12). Particularly in young individuals, the sense of invulnerability is vanquished and is replaced by rage and anger at one's newfound mortality (Lifton, 1975). For veterans in particular, there is a continuing identity with death. The normal boundary between living and dying is suspended. It is not unusual for veterans to describe themselves as already dead. The only way they have of testing the boundary between life and death is to seek sensation, even if it means danger and physical pain (Brende & Parson, 1985, p. 100). The remodeled criterion E of the DSM 5-TR (APA, 2022) makes pointed reference to reckless and dangerous behavior. Combined with rage reactions, sensation-seeking behaviors put individuals squarely on a collision path with law enforcement agencies, employers, and families.

Billie Mac: After every law officer in Mississippi started chasing me, I ditched the car and ran into a woods. They even had bloodhounds after me. I slipped through them like they were a sieve. It was crazy, but for one of the few times since I've been back, I really felt alive. I'd done that a hundred times on patrol.

Survivor's Guilt. A second pattern is guilt. Guilt comes in a variety of forms: guilt over surviving when others did not, guilt over not preventing the death of another (Stanley & Marx, 2022), guilt over not having somehow been braver under the circumstances, guilt over complaining when others have suffered more, and guilt that the trauma is partly the individual's fault (Frederick, 1980). Most commonly, guilt takes the form of intrusive thoughts such as "I could have done more, and if I had, they'd still be here." or "If I had just done this or that, it (the trauma) wouldn't have happened." Dynamically, the basis of these thoughts may be relief that the other person was the one to die or the individual was lucky to get off so lightly (Egendorf, 1975).

Billie Mac: I was the only one in my outfit to get out of the Tet offensive without a scratch. I wonder why. Why me out of all those people? I've screwed my life up since then. Why did I deserve to get out clean when all those other good men didn't? Going to the wall in D.C. last year tore me to pieces. I cried and cried when I saw the names of my buddies up there. Things really got screwed up after that.

For other types of traumatized individuals, bereavement is closely allied to survivor's guilt. Facilitating grief includes the expression of affect, reconciliation of the loss of a loved one or a missed part of one's life, the ambivalence of not having shared the same fate as others, and moving on to new and meaningful relationships (Ochberg, 1988, p. 10). Because numbing of affect is a major dynamic response to PTSD, it is extremely difficult for survivors to let loose their emotions and grieve.

Desensitization. A third pattern is desensitizing oneself to totally unacceptable events and then trying to return to a semblance of normalcy in a peaceful world. Feelings of guilt and fear may arise over pleasurable responses to physical violence against others. These feelings may become so acute that the individual conceals firearms for protection against imagined enemies but is simultaneously terrified of the guns and what might happen because of the violence that continuously seethes below the individual's own calm outer appearance. These strong bipolar emotional currents that flow back and forth within the individual lead to hostile, defensive, anxious, depressive, and fearful mood states that find little relief (Horowitz & Solomon, 1975).

Billie Mac: I don't hunt anymore. I hate it. Yet this one guy who was my boss didn't know how close he came to getting killed. I was within one inch of taking him out; I was so hot. It would have been a pleasure; the guy was such an ass.

Estrangement. A fourth pattern is the feeling that any future relationships will be counterfeit, that

they mean little or nothing in the great scheme of things. As the person tries to ward off reminders of the experience, severe interpersonal difficulties occur. Because of the vastly different experiences they have undergone, individuals with PTSD become estranged from their peers and truncate social relationships with them because "they don't understand"—and indeed "they" do not. Victimization may also be part of estrangement.

From being victimized in the original trauma to possible secondary victimization by social services, hospitals, and mental health providers, to revictimization by significant others, the survivor is crushed under the weight of dealing with these initial and secondary assaults (Ochberg, 1988). The result is that the person becomes more isolated from social support systems and develops secondary symptoms that range across diagnostic categories of psychopathology (Horowitz & Solomon, 1975).

Billie Mac: I was sitting at my dad's watching TV when Saigon fell. I went nuts and trashed the house. What the hell was it all for? That really cooked it with my old man. I moved out after that and haven't said anything to him since.

Particularly for survivors of sexual abuse, estrangement may take the form of negative intimacy. Invasion of one's personal space and being causes feelings of filthiness and degradation that make reestablishing old relationships or engendering new relationships an extremely difficult ordeal (Ochberg, 1988, pp. 12–13).

Emotional Enmeshment. A fifth pattern is a continuous struggle to move forward following the trauma but with an inability to find any significance in life (Lifton, 1975). Emotional fixation, particularly for veterans, has disastrous effects on family life. Sent to Vietnam as adolescents and exposed to prolonged trauma that the majority of the population will never experience, these individuals cannot bring themselves to engage in equitable relationships with their families and friends, nor can their families begin to understand their aberrant behavior (Brende & Parson, 1985, pp. 116–117). Depression, anger, avoidance, and alcohol misuse are hallmarks of veterans with PTSD, and these show up in mediating family functioning (Evans et al., 2003). It should not be surprising that those angry feelings are reciprocated by family members and create large fractures in a family structure that is already cracked and breaking.

Billie Mac: I can't believe what I've done to my kids. I love them more than anything in the world. At times, I'm the greatest dad in the world, coach the Little League team, take them everywhere. The next minute I'm all over them. I've knocked them around in a rage, and that scares the hell out of me. I'm some kind of Jekyll and Hyde, and my kids are afraid of me. My wife hates my guts for it and said if I didn't shape up *now* she was leaving. My solution to that was to go get drunk. When I came home, she was gone with the kids. They and me would be better off if I was dead.

Now that you have read the foregoing descriptors of PTSD and Vietnam War veterans, think about the most recent combat theaters in Iraq and Afghanistan. Can you identify any similarities? Do you think there will be Billie Macs (or Sally Smiths) coming home from Iraq or Afghanistan?

The Traumatic Wake of Iraq and Afghanistan

LO7 Although U.S. military personnel have withdrawn from Iraq and Afghanistan, the scars of the deployment remain. Most of these personnel have been exposed to the petri dish of death, violence, bloodshed, and destruction in which PTSD grows so well. As in Vietnam, there are no front lines; it's hard to tell friend from foe; vigilance must be maintained 24/7 because a firefight, bombardment, or IED can occur at any moment or any place; no territory is "won"; political goals become cloudy; some people are increasingly unclear about the purpose or goal for being in those places; and termination dates are ill defined.

Further, there is a clear relationship between the duration and intensity of specific types of trauma exposure and the number of symptoms of posttraumatic stress disorder (Baker et al., 2008). In contrast to Vietnam, which was a one-year rotation and back to the "world," many veterans have served two or three tours of duty in the Middle Eastern conflicts, which piles stress not only on them but on their families as well. Many combat units are National Guard or reserve units based in hometowns rather than on military bases. These soldiers are both male and female, and they are older and have families and jobs as opposed to their younger counterparts who come from intact regular army regiments and divisions.

About half of military service personnel are married, and more than 70 percent have children. In real numbers, that means 1.85 million children have one or both parents in the military, and 900,000 of those children have had one or both parents deployed one or more times since 2001 (Chandra et al., 2008). Those deployments cause all kinds of physical, psychological, personal, social, and academic issues with these children (Barnes et al., 2007; Engel et al., 2010; Flake et al., 2009), and that family stress kicks back to soldiers at the front. Combat stress clinics have found the major precipitating factor in homicide/suicide is a stressful relational event that comes from home via e-mail or telephone (Mental Health Advisory Team V, 2008).

Studies so far indicate the PTSD expectancy rate is somewhere between 11 and 12 percent for Middle East war veterans, in contrast to the estimated 30 percent of Vietnam veterans (National Center for PTSD, 2011, 2023). Even if only 10 percent of service personnel wind up with PTSD, the medical corps and Veterans Administration can expect another 250,000 cases to land on their doorsteps. Now consider the families of these service personnel. Even more ominous, perhaps, is the service suicide rate, which has increased enough to get national headlines. The grimness of these figures is reflected in a study by Matthews (2009), who asked seniors at West Point whether they believed they would develop PTSD. Only 22 percent thought they "would not" or "most likely would not."

The Department of Defense and the Veterans Administration have been very proactive in designing interventions that range from frontline, in-theater crisis intervention with combat troops through Post-Deployment Health Assessment and Reassessment programs that are designed to detect physical and psychological problems of returning active-duty soldiers and veterans and immediately start treating them (Brenner et al., 2009). There are now manualized protocols for treating both the symptoms of PTSD (Resick et al., 2008) and readjustment to civilian life and the stressors that come with it (Whealin et al., 2008). Evidence-based strategies that are specifically tailored to the military have been put into operation (Adler et al., 2011). Further, the Veterans Administration has been extremely proactive in providing outreach programs to veterans who cannot easily reach a VA hospital. However, this is a reactive stance, and with the high incidence of mental health issues, the Army has initiated the Comprehensive Soldier Fitness (CSF) program, which is an integrated, proactive approach to developing psychological resilience in soldiers, family members, and the Army's civilian workforce (Casey, 2011).

The Comprehensive Solider Fitness Program

The Comprehensive Solider Fitness (CSF) program consists of four components. The Global Assessment Tool, which is used online by soldiers, is confidential and provides feedback on the following psychological dimensions: positive emotions; negative emotions and depression; optimism; flexible thinking; work engagement; problem-focused coping; character strengths of wisdom, courage, humanity, justice, temperance, and transcendence; social fitness components of trust and friendship; family fitness; and spiritual fitness. This comprehensive psychological fitness exam also comes with self-help modules for each of these areas that soldiers can access independently (Peterson et al., 2011). However, CSF goes far beyond online self-assessment/help. It is also designed to be delivered face to face.

The Master Resilience Trainer course (Reivich et al., 2011) is designed to train sergeants who will then teach soldiers in their units. The course has three components. The first, preparation, includes resilience and mental toughness, identifying character strengths, and strengthening relationships. The second is a sustaining component, which focuses on sustaining resilience across the deployment cycle. The third is an enhancement component that uses a lot of the following sport psychology concepts: mental skills foundations, which involves understanding the nature of performance, the relationship between training and trusting mindsets, and identifying the connection between thoughts, emotions, physiological states, and performance; building confidence, which involves learning effective ways to create energy, optimism, and enthusiasm; attention control, which addresses the concentration demands associated with critical military tasks; energy management, which consists of practical skills used to activate, sustain, and restore optimal levels of energy while minimizing the negative effects of stress; and integrating imagery, which involves ways of creating successful experiences that can enhance aspects of performance. If you start to get the idea of positive psychology at work, you would be right on target.

As we have indicated, support systems are critical in addressing PTSD. For the current military, the problem is that while there may be instantaneous communication with family members via cell phone, WhatsApp, Skype, X, and other internet access, they are physically thousands of miles apart with all the stress that distance brings. The family skills component (Gottman et al., 2011) is designed to educate both service personnel and families on how to alleviate much

of this stress. Frontline troops can take relationship enrichment courses along with their families, who are linked via the internet to access the course materials. Topics include creating and maintaining friendship and intimacy, increasing trust and honesty, managing conflict constructively and gently, de-escalating conflict, practicing cognitive self-soothing, containing cognitive flooding and physical stress responses, soothing and calming one's partner, converting posttraumatic stress to posttraumatic growth through the relationship, building positive relationships and effective discipline with children, and surviving breakups. You don't need a certificate in marriage and family therapy to recognize that this component of the CFS could be a powerful tool in preventing the critical incidents that, according to Mental Health Advisory Team V (2008), turn soldiers' thinking toxic and lethal. In summary, the U.S. Defense Department knows a lot more than it did during the Vietnam War and is now very actively involved in the business of both preventing and alleviating PTSD and its comorbid disorders (Pellerin, 2017).

As of 2015, the Army has issued a series of reports on the effectiveness of the CSF programs and has found them to be generally effective in meeting the designed objective of creating more psychological resilience in soldiers (Harms et al., 2013). However, the program has sustained a great deal of criticism from its inception. Chief among these is the fact that it is a massive research project and has no human protection of its subjects. In addition, the definition of the problem is so ill-defined meaning that results would be global and not conclusive. Generally speaking, the project seeks to promulgate religious values and that war is bad. The result is that, since CFS is designed to help soldiers become "better" warriors, yet war is bad, it is seemingly contradictory. A critical concern is that the basic premises are bad because the research is not based on military personnel but on a civilian population, and outcomes on that original format have not been all that positive, and focus should be on the primary prevention of PTSD rather than building resistance to it through CSF (Dyckman, 2011; Eidelson et al., 2011; Krueger, 2011; Phipps, 2011). Indeed, critics have railed at the lack of objective review and analysis of CSF and have issued calls for independent reviews of it (Smith, 2013; Steenkamp et al., 2013). Each of these criticisms has been vigorously counterpointed (Lester et al., 2013), so it will be interesting to learn how one of the largest psychological experiments ever created will eventually turn out.

Components of Treatment for Adults

Given the constellation of problems that afflict the person with PTSD, treatment is complex, and the human services worker can expect numerous transcrisis events and crisis points to occur during treatment. The treatment of PTSD has three principal components: (1) processing and coming to terms with the horrifying, overwhelming experience; (2) controlling and mastering physiological and biological stress reactions; and (3) reestablishing secure social connections and interpersonal efficacy (van der Kolk et al., 2002). For individuals with complex PTSD, treatment priorities are somewhat different and will be dealt with in Chapter 9, "Sexual Assault." Before the worker tackles any of these components, however, comprehensive assessment needs to occur. Assessment is particularly important in PTSD because it is camouflaged by so many other symptoms and problems.

Assessment

LO8   Assessment of PTSD should consider at least four areas: First, are symptoms of PTSD present? Although their presence may seem to be a given, the length of time from onset may mean that different symptoms are more pronounced at different times. Second, diagnoses of presenting problems such as substance misuse are highly associated with PTSD (Rodriguez & Read, 2020). Unless care is taken to assess for prior trauma when the presenting problem is substance abuse, PTSD might be missed. It is highly probable that people in crisis will present with comorbid problems, and PTSD may not be identified as the undergirding problem unless care is taken in assessing for traumatic incidents. Third, the assessment should consider the ability to control affect (Arditte & Mitchell, 2022). The reason is that the difficulty regulating emotion is strongly associated with PTSD (Seligowski et al., 2015). Fourth, because of contextual differences in terms of physical, temporal, social, and political climate, these variables may have a great deal to do with how the event is interpreted (McGhie et al., 2022).

The following examples indicate just how important contextual variables are in assessment. A Vietnam veteran with PTSD in the 1970s would be perceived as a "crazed baby killer," compared to a Gulf War, Afghanistan, or Iraq veteran in the 2000s, who would be viewed with compassion because of the dramatic change in the political climate and the social view of the people who fought in these wars. Likewise, domestic violence, which was formerly seen as a private matter between spouses, is now viewed as a societal ill to the extent that the label "battered woman syndrome" has been attached to women who have experience this form of violence.

The self-reliant and tightly knit community of Joplin, Missouri, with its extended support system, may react to the devastation of a tornado far differently from the way insular and emotionally distant apartment dwellers in New York City react to being forced out of their apartments by the collapse of the WTC towers. Or, even though large urban areas on the eastern seaboard comparable to the terrorist attack on 9/11 have been targeted by terrorists, the cultural and environmental and situational differences survivors and the communities of the Boston marathon bombing and Charleston, South Carolina, church shooting are much more population specific, closer, and personalized. Thus, in determining the potential to acquire PTSD or manifest it, one should always take into consideration a thorough background assessment that includes gender, race, socioeconomic class, experience, culture, religion, time components, geographic area, number of incidents of prior exposure to trauma, strength of interpersonal relationships, occupational risk, sociopolitical attitudes, and a host of other contextual variables that may have unforeseen impact on the resiliency of the individual to withstand or fall victim to PTSD. In short, just because you go through a traumatic event doesn't mean you automatically get PTSD or are even a "victim" as opposed to a "survivor" (Gist et al., 1999; Kaniasty & Norris, 1999; Kroll, 2003).

Assessment of PTSD falls into two main categories: structured or semistructured interviews and empirically derived measures.

Structured Interview. If time is available, the structured interview probably remains the best diagnostic device for determining whether a person has PTSD. One of the best structured interviews that is considered the gold standard is the Clinician-Administered PTSD Scale (CAPS-5) (U.S. Department of Veterans Affairs, 2023). It assesses all the symptoms outlined in the DSM 5 as well as eight associated symptoms: guilt over acts committed or omitted, survivor's guilt, homicidality, disillusionment with authority, feelings of hopelessness, memory impairment, sadness and depression, and feelings of being overwhelmed.

This structured interview also examines the impact of symptoms on social and occupational functioning, improvement in PTSD symptoms since a previous CAPS-5 assessment, overall response validity, and overall PTSD severity. Current status for all symptoms is assessed first, and if criteria for PTSD are not met, the questions are asked again for a "worst case," 1-month period since traumatic onset. The items also have a QV code, for question validity, when the interviewer has doubts about the truthfulness of the response. The CAPS-5 pays very careful attention to the assessment of lifetime PTSD. Its major drawback is the length of time required for administration. Another clinician interview scale is the PTSD Symptom Scale Interview (PSS-I-5) (Foa et al., 2016). The PSS-I-5 is functional for assessment and diagnosis. This scale consists of 20 symptom-related questions and four additional questions to assess distress and interference in daily life as well as symptom onset and duration revised to correspond with criteria listed in the DSM 5-TR. Questions focus on asking respondents with a known trauma history to identify a single traumatic event that causes the most current distress.

Self-Reports. Self-reports are useful for their efficiency in time, cost, and ease of administration (Moshier et al., 2018). Although several self-report assessment methods are used (Moshier et al., 2018; Rosencrans et al., 2021), the quick pace of crisis intervention means assessment must be done quickly. Given that time is of the essence, a rudimentary assessment Traumagram Questionaire developed by Figley's (1989, 1990) a graphically represented client self-report, is effective. It can be self-constructed on the spot. The questionnaire elicits the number of traumatic events, length of time, circumstances, age of client, persons who may have been involved with the events, and self-reported degrees of stress for all previous traumatic experiences and can be easily incorporated into a standard interview format. Clients are then asked to rate their stress level on a 1 (low) to 5 (high) scale at the time of the event, one year later, and in the present. Next, clients are asked to consider each traumatic experience, what helped them cope, and what helped them adjust or not to the aftermath of the traumatic event.

Figley's traumagram is also a useful tool in determining the causes of transcrisis. In the course of therapy, at times, clients present with symptoms and problems that seem to have no logical basis in reality. They are clearly in crisis. Their symptoms are causing them all kinds of trouble at school, at home, and at work, yet there appears to be nothing in real time that would be causing the problem. This puzzling dilemma

is not uncommon when working with people who have been traumatized and have either dismissed the trauma as ancient history or have submerged it from conscious awareness (Shallcross, 2010). At this point, we start examining two distinct possibilities: delayed onset of PTSD or complicated grieving, which we will examine at length in Chapter 12, "Personal Loss: Bereavement and Grief." To ferret out these issues, we have modified Charles Figley's (1989) traumagram protocol in the following way. We ask clients to consider not only stressful events in their life but also losses they have suffered. Clients are urged to consider not only loss to death, but also financial loss, job termination, death of a pet, romantic breakup, divorce, geographic moves, and the acute onset of a disabling condition either for oneself or a loved one.

By plotting the number of events across the length of time they were acutely felt on an x-axis and then plotting the degree of stress on the y-axis using a scale of 1 (minimum) to 10 (maximum), the interviewer can quickly gain a graphic representation of the total number, type, and duration of traumas and the degree of stress the client has experienced. It gives the interviewer a good picture of what the client feels are the relative power of significant events and also gives the interviewer an opportunity to explore the dimensions of each of these events. It also allows the crisis worker to examine one of the "best bet" indicators for delayed PTSD or the inability to resolve a loss—that is, the repeated exposure of the subject to traumatic events. Its major weakness is the subjective bias of the individual, but its strength is that clients may have "aha" experiences as events and losses they had submerged from awareness are brought into the light of day.

Dr. James's traumagram in Figure 7.1 presents a graphic description of his life history of trauma and loss over several decades. Seven events are depicted, as listed below. The intensity or level of stress and the duration of the stress for each event vary considerably. In this traumagram, the darker the area under each graph line, the more stresses that have accumulated during that time.

Event #1. Intensity level is 10+. Dick is 6 years old on his first overnight camping trip with a summer camp group. After the camp counselor sends the boys off to bed with "Old Man Pollywog," the story of a creature who lives in the nearby swamp abducting small boys and carrying them off, Dick is somehow locked out of the cabin and forced to sleep on the ground, easy prey for the swamp thing. A terrorizing night that indelibly imprints

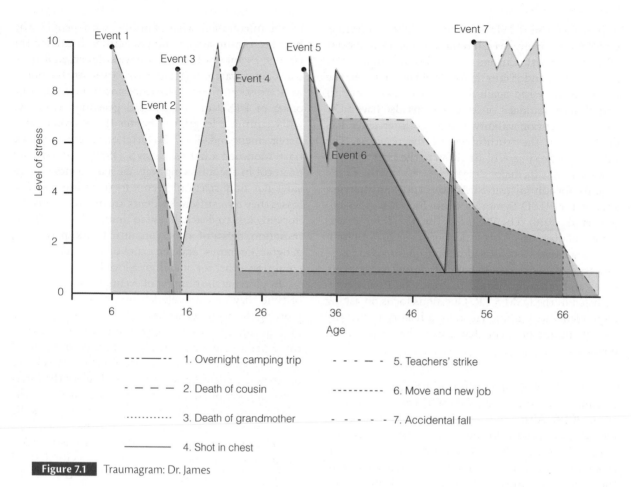

Figure 7.1 Traumagram: Dr. James

young Dickie to the point that he does not camp again until he is 23 years of age and canoeing in the Boundary Waters of Quetico Provincial Park in Ontario. The first night out on this canoeing trip, Dick has an anxiety attack and is in desperate need of support from his mommy. Dick becomes desensitized after 14 days in the wilderness but decides never to camp again if at all possible.

Event #2. Intensity level is 7. Client is 12 years old and is exposed to death for the first time. Traumatic death of 3-year-old cousin due to respiratory paralysis from anesthetic during tonsillectomy. Client is not emotionally close. Onset is acute but quickly resolved over 2-month period.

Event #3. Intensity level is 9. Client is 13 years old. Grandmother dies from cancer. Long-term illness and death expected. Client is emotionally close but reconciled to death. Stress dissipates to zero after 1 month.

Event #4. Intensity level starts at 9, moves to 10+ over a 12-month period. At the age of 21, client is shot in chest while out with girlfriend. Gunshot causes physical problems and what comes to be known 20 years later as PTSD. Client's social relationships plummet. Has anxiety attacks, becomes depressed, socially isolated, and contemplates suicide. After 1 year and 9 months, the bullet is removed. Client seeks counseling. Intensity drops sharply but is residual at a level of 4–5, escalating sharply and acutely for over 3 years in heterosexual relationships until client marries current wife. Intensity level drops to 1 but occasionally spikes during times of severe physical or emotional stress.

Event #5. Intensity level is 9. Client is 32 years old, a married father. Caught in the middle of a teachers' strike. Sees nationally validated program he directed disintegrate. Job loss. Complete job change and geographic change of 300 miles. Depression, anxiety attacks, PTSD symptoms resurface. Seeks counseling, makes commitment to job change out of education. Intensity level goes to 7 due to job change and continues for a year and a half, diminishing to a level of 2–3 with increasing familiarity in new job in petroleum industry.

Event #6. Intensity level is 6. Client is 34 years old, married, and a father. Reenters education with job as university professor. Moves 500 miles. Initial anxiety but mentorship reduces it quickly.

Event #7. Intensity level is 10+. Client is 54, married, and a father of two. Suffers accidental fall with severe external head trauma and edema while repairing roof on daughter's tree house. Severe pain for approximately 2 months from 300+ stitches and 52 staples in skull to reattach scalp. Self-image issues due to facial scarring. Residual injuries and interventions include plastic surgery on head and herniated C-6 disc operation over following 5 years, with spike levels of 10 and residual levels of 1–3.

(There's more, but this is merely an example and not a soap opera of Dr. James's life.)

After completing the traumagram, we query our clients on their affective, behavioral, and cognitive responses to specific traumas, both at the time they occurred and how those incidents are affecting them now. We are looking not just at specific events but at the overall picture of what is occurring. Is the whole greater than the sum of the individual traumas? Does the person show resiliency and stamina with one particular kind of event and not with another? This dialogue is conducted in a user-friendly manner with the admonition, "If some emotions you didn't know were associated with that event pop up, and you get upset and need to take a breather, we'll stop. Just let me know." One of the most critical components of therapy and crisis intervention with a client with PTSD is demonstrating by word and deed that this is a *safe* place to be and that you are a *safe* person to be with (Courtois et al., 2009; Herman, 1992b).

As we query our client, we are searching for recurrent psychodynamic themes that might give us clues to what is driving the current maladaptive behavior. Does the client have continuing anger, regrets, and guilt over past experiences? Is there a common affective, behavioral, or cognitive theme running through traumatic events? Do the events seem as potent now as they were then, with the client suddenly flushed

and angry as he thinks about a physically abusive father who had the unmitigated gall to go and die on him before he could pay the abuser back? If the client has been fired for insubordinate behavior a number of times, can we trace these incidents back to a primary causal agent?

We are also very interested in how the client reports the events. Recently in class, one of our students was going over her traumagram in a very fluid way with even voice tone and a well-modulated voice level—until she came to event 6, which was about her discovery of a longtime close male friend who lied to her about a sexual assault he perpetrated and was later arrested and convicted of it. Her hesitation, loss of words, and trembling voice clearly indicated that this event was profoundly shocking to her and had caused her to deeply question her ability to gauge and assess people she had come to trust. When the professor reflected on her abrupt change in voice, she was taken aback because she had not recognized how deeply it still affected her. In summary, self-reports can sometimes uncover material that normative, empirical scale tests do not.

Empirically Derived Scales. A large variety of empirically derived PTSD instruments have been generated. Of them, the following seem to have reasonable utility in determining if PTSD is present and are reasonably efficient in terms of time and cost to administer. The Mississippi Scale for Combat Related PTSD (Keane et al., 1988) is widely used and has a number of versions for different client populations. The Impact of Events Scale (Horowitz et al., 1979) is one of the most widely used instruments for detecting PTSD and has been employed with a variety of trauma-related populations. The scale assesses only the extent of avoidance/numbing rather than the full scope of PTSD symptoms that are covered by the other tests mentioned here. A revised form of the Impact of Events Scale-Revised (IES-R) (Weiss, 2007) has added five questions to better capture the DSM criteria for PTSD .

The Life Events Checklist is another self-report instrument (Weis et al., 2022). This instrument is designed to gather information about events that have the potential to result in the development of PTSD (Weather et al., 2013). In 2018, Weathers et al. (2023) updated the instrument, which can be accessed at https://www.ptsd.va.gov/professional/assessment/documents/LEC5_Standard_Self-report.PDF. The instrument measures trauma history to predict the possible development of PTSD. Wies et al.'s (2022) research into the scoring instrument provides a reliable method that measures prior trauma history while taking into account individuals' current trauma exposure.

The Keane PK scale of the MMPI/MMPI-2 has been formulated for the specific purpose of diagnosing PTSD (Keane et al., 1984). Because it is embedded in the MMPI/MMPI-2, its score can be compared to the validity scales of the total instrument to determine whether faking or malingering is occurring (Nijdam-Jones et al., 2020). Note that some people, such as insurance claimants, malingerers, or incarcerates, may have less than honorable motives in claiming they have PTSD, and their reports may not be valid.

Overview of Assessment. The responses to questions about social affiliation show a clear distinction between individuals with character disorders and those experiencing PTSD. In general, individuals with PTSD avoid interpersonal relationships, as opposed to the ingratiating gregariousness of a sociopath. Those with PTSD have few close friends, prefer being alone, and discuss few intimate details of their lives. Unexpected contact with other people or stimuli reminiscent of the traumatic event may make these individuals extremely "jumpy" and "edgy" (Keane et al., 1985, p. 270).

The human services worker should never dismiss a report, no matter how trivial it may seem, of involvement in a catastrophic situation or a major loss (Scurfield, 1985, pp. 238–239). Because individuals with PTSD may be very reluctant to talk about the trauma they have been through, human services workers should try to get background information from relatives, coworkers, and any other people who have personal knowledge of the individual. The personal history is particularly important when substance misuse is involved, because if PTSD is not identified, all the efforts of the worker will not ameliorate the substance misuse problem.

Our own and many, many colleagues' clinical experience with clients who are depressed or have a borderline diagnosis has uncovered many who have suffered sexual abuse as children. Often, these individuals also meet the criteria for a diagnosis of PTSD (Kleindienst et al., 2021). Until ruled out, PTSD should be suspected as a causative agent. However, getting at it may prove extremely difficult, particularly given the severe social taboos associated with talking about incestuous and abusive relationships.

Therefore, in an initial assessment, even though the interviewer may have a strong hunch that repression of a traumatic event is causing the problem, the causative agent should never be exposed, interpreted, or even guessed at until a high degree of trust has been built (Scurfield, 1985, pp. 238–239).

Finally, assessment in treatment of PTSD must be ongoing and overarching, particularly during the course of therapy. The changes that occur in the client vacillate dramatically—sometimes daily or even hourly. Because of the intrusive nature of much of the therapy, it is common to see upsurges in symptoms and problem behaviors (Flack et al., 2002).

Assessment of Billie Mac. In the case of Billie Mac, a CAPS-1 interview showed little if any evidence of traumatic experience prior to Vietnam besides the death of a grandfather, to whom he was quite close. In Vietnam, he was in major battle after major battle, interspersed with patrols and sweeps. He was the only man out of his original company to walk away physically unscathed after the Tet offensive.

After Vietnam, the traumatic wake continued. Violent episodes with his father, his wife, and his children; scrapes with the law; drunken binges; barroom brawls; prolonged bouts of depression interspersed with manic acting out; alcohol addiction treatment; job loss due to nonperformance; and suicidal ideation, plus the standard symptoms of PTSD, marked his years since Vietnam with almost continuous crises. There were very few months in the 25 years since his return that he would not rank extremely high on the Triage Assessment Scale. Affectively, he goes far beyond what the situation warrants, with large mood swings that cycle through anger, fear, and sadness. He rarely ranks lower than a 6 on the Affective Severity scale, and his average is a 7.

In the cognitive domain he has suffered physical, psychological, social, and spiritual transgression, threat, and loss. His problem-solving abilities are characterized by self-doubt, confusion, and excessive rumination on Vietnam and his abortive attempts to reacclimatize to the civilian world. His severity rating is consistently an 8 to 9, in the Marked Impairment range.

Billie Mac's behavior invariably makes the situation worse. He either approaches the situation in a hostile-aggressive manner or avoids it for fear of acting out against others. He is immobilized between these two extremes, and significant others report that they feel he is erratic, unpredictable, and dangerous.

A most conservative estimate places him at a minimum of 8 on the Behavioral Severity scale. His total scale score is 24, which places him in the lower range of the Marked Impairment category. Perhaps even more ominously, his individual scale scores frequently hit a 10. As he presents for treatment, he is in serious trouble, and at times of stress, his triage rating scale score spikes into the lethal Severe Impairment range. He has suicidal thoughts, and, at times, his behavior verges on homicidal. His CAPS-1 interview ratings indicate a very high frequency and intensity of PTSD symptoms, and the MMPI-2 PK scale confirms his PTSD surely falls into the more complex variety. If he refuses inpatient treatment, he should have closely supervised outpatient treatment.

Phases of Recovery

LO9 Brende and Parson (1985, pp. 185–186) have compiled the work of Wilson (1980), Figley (1978), and Horowitz (1976) to construct five phases of recovery in the individual with PTSD. These phases directly parallel treatment approaches, and each has its own crisis stage.

1. **The emergency or outcry phase**. The individual experiences heightened "fight/flight" reactions to the life-threatening situation. This phase lasts as long as the survivor believes the situation to last. Pulse, blood pressure, respiration, and muscle activity are all increased. Concomitant feelings of fear and helplessness predominate. Termination of the event itself is followed by relief and confusion. Questions about why the event happened and what its consequences are dominate the individual's thoughts.

2. **The emotional numbing and denial phase**. The survivor protects psychic well-being by burying the experience in subconscious memory. By avoiding the experience, the individual temporarily reduces anxiety and stress symptoms. Many individuals remain forever at this stage unless they receive professional intervention.

3. **The intrusive-repetitive phase**. The survivor has nightmares, volatile mood swings, intrusive images, and amplified startle responses. Other pathological and antisocial defense mechanisms may be put into place in a futile attempt to rebury the trauma. At this point, the delayed stress becomes so overwhelming that the individual is propelled to seek help or becomes so mired in the pathology of the situation that outside intervention is mandated.

4. **The reflective-transition phase**. The survivor develops a larger personal perspective on the traumatic events and becomes positive and constructive, with a forward- rather than backward-looking perspective. The individual comes to grips with the trauma and confronts the problem.

5. **The integration phase**. The survivor successfully integrates the trauma with all other past experiences and restores a sense of continuity to life. The trauma is successfully placed fully in the past.

Neat and orderly progression through these stages for the individual with PTSD is the exception rather than the rule. More likely is a precipitating crisis far removed in chronological time from the event itself and then a continuing series of crises that escalate until the individual voluntarily seeks help or is forced to seek it. Once intervention occurs, a cyclic pattern of avoidance, recall, recovery, and more avoidance continues until the core issues that gave birth to PTSD are resolved (Figley, 1985, pp. 402–404). The human services worker can expect a series of transcrisis events as this process unfolds.

LO10 Initiating Intervention. Generally, survivors of trauma refuse early intervention because they either see the event as too difficult to deal with or believe that people of good character ought to be able to cope with such events on their own without outside intervention. These two faulty assumptions get individuals into the delayed part of the disorder, where most of the treatment population will emerge.

Importance of Acceptance

Given the variety of negative and conflicting emotional baggage the individual brings to the session, it is of paramount importance that the human services worker provide an accepting atmosphere so the individual can start to recount and encounter the trauma. Disclosure of the trauma is difficult for the client with PTSD because recounting what has happened may be horrifying and socially unacceptable. Also, open-minded acceptance of the client's story may be extremely difficult for and repugnant to the human services worker, but if therapeutic progress is to be made, nothing less will do (Brende & Parson, 1985, p. 178).

Billie Mac: (thinking to himself) If I tell about killing that kid, what will the counselor think? A baby killer, that's what! Yet, it's bugging the hell out of me. (Slowly tells the counselor about the incident.)

Human Services Worker (HSW): (stating personal feelings) I can see how hard it was for you to talk about that. A part of me wonders how you or anybody could ever kill a child. However, I understand how scared you were, wondering whether he had a grenade, what a moral quandary that put you in, and the guilt and anguish you feel as you recall the incident.

We currently live in an evidence-based world as far as therapy is concerned as you will soon see in this chapter. However, as in most crisis interventions, initiating and forming a bond with Billie Mac is critical and involves the empathic listening, owning statements, and reflection of feeling demonstrated in this opening dialogue (Lindy, 2012).

Therapy with veterans, either individually or in groups, is ideally conducted with veterans as leaders because of the defensiveness and hostility with which most veterans view professionals who have not undergone the experience of combat. The same is true of the firefighters, police officers, and EMTs you will meet later in the chapter. One could easily extrapolate this notion to group work with other kinds of trauma victims. The problem is that professionals who have also experienced the trauma or the setting within which it occurs are often not readily available. Therefore, the Veterans Center of Memphis published a list of 12 "rules of the road" for establishing the credibility of nonveterans who work therapeutically with veterans (Memphis Vietnam Veterans Center, 1985). These rules should be adapted to any intact group such as police officers, EMTs, nurses, and others whose common bond is more than the incidence of PTSD and where you as the therapist are considered an "outsider" due to your ignorance of their culture, whether it be oil well rigging, farming, or emergency medical responders.

1. The client has the experiential knowledge you don't have; you have the clinical and technical knowledge they don't have. Together, you can forge a working alliance.
2. Make your desire to understand come across so considerable experiential gaps are bridged.
3. Realize clients want you to help them help you understand. In the process, they recreates and reexperiences the sources of the problems, and you, by providing the therapeutic climate, gain an in-depth understanding of the traumatic experience.
4. A different-sex therapist serves as a role model—that is, in the case of a man veteran, a woman who can understand and accept the individual for what he is and has done without prejudging him. The same would be true for a woman veteran with a man as her therapist.
5. Clinical experience and expertise are built over time—as your understanding and technical expertise grow, you will be accepted by the individual or the group despite your lack of direct experience.
6. As a nonmember of the "exclusive" group, you can challenge the defense of exclusivity, that one who wasn't there can't understand, thus serving to break through their feelings of isolation and "contamination."
7. Your technical naiveté often helps individuals explore and express themselves. In their effort to help you understand the technical aspects of combat, emergency medical service, or police tactical procedures, they uncover unknown areas of conflict.
8. At the same time, because of your naiveté, you must guard against becoming too involved in problems and memories, thereby "triggering" situational stress that may need immediate attention and treatment.
9. Realize that moral conflicts will probably be raised for you personally as stories unfold; guard against any display of emotional revulsion to a client who describes atrocities. Be nonjudgmental and objective.
10. Guard against overidentification or hero worship, or you will blunt your problem-solving ability.
11. Expect to need controls and to have to clearly enforce them for your sake and the client's—don't try to do therapy with a client who is drunk or "stoned," refuse to be a party to long tirades on the phone, and bar all weapons and mean it.
12. Heed the signs of burnout: thinking or talking too much about your clients to others, finding yourself having client-specific symptoms such as nightmares, and so on. Step back and evaluate whether you may be too immersed in trying to do too much for too many.

These rules are adaptable to any kind of trauma survivors and the people who work with them *and apply particularly to those who work with adult survivors of childhood sexual abuse or children who have suffered chronic physical and/or sexual abuse.*

One further admonition is necessary for any human services worker who would work with trauma survivors. Frick and Bogart (1982) identified one of the stages that veterans go through as "rage at their counselor." This transference stage (attributing to the human services worker qualities and attributes of significant others in the client's life) is important in coming to terms with the traumatic experience. Human services workers may well become the focal point of all the frustration, grief, fear, lost opportunity, confusion, lack of progress, and attempts at reconciliation with society, family, and friends that mark the trauma survivor's attempt to reintegrate into the social mainstream. Human services workers need to deal with such anger by owning their mistakes in being insensitive to issues, accepting and reflecting the individual's anger while at the same time not being defensive, containing impulsive responses after being attacked, owning their own anger, and not becoming discouraged and giving up.

Risks of Treatment

LO11 The quality of life is affected by anyone diagnosed with PTSD as well as by treatment for this disorder (Fortin et al., 2021). Therefore, human services workers must state clearly the risks inherent in treatment. Making these statements about the prognosis may be difficult, but the individual will probably have pondered many of the same questions. After the initial crisis has passed and the individual is back to a state of at least semi-equilibrium, the human services worker should convey clearly the following risks, as outlined by Brende and Parson (1985, pp. 168–174):

1. There may be only partial recovery; there are no magical cures for this tenacious and pernicious problem.
2. Because of the continuing nature of the crisis, either long bouts with hospitals or weekly trips to the therapist are required that will play havoc with keeping a job.
3. As catharsis of the event occurs, and if exposure therapies are used, it is inevitable that the individual gets worse before getting better. Fear of a psychotic breakdown may occur as the individual learns more about the disorder.
4. As the struggle to find oneself goes forward, personality changes may put heavy burdens on interpersonal relationships as significant others see a very different person emerge from the therapeutic experience.
5. Psychic pain may become almost intolerable as the individual reexperiences disturbing memories

and emotions that, as they are voiced, may cause rejection by friends and professionals alike.

6. Because of the numerous self-constraints placed on volatile emotions, the individual may fear that giving vent to those emotions will lead to uncontrolled anger and result in physical harm to others. Because of the hurt suffered, it will also be very difficult for the individual to give up the idea of revenge on both real and imagined perpetrators of the traumatic event.
7. Because of the compartmentalized and constricted lifestyle that follows the trauma, the individual will safeguard against change and may have extreme difficulty following directions and doing what others may suggest, no matter how reasonable and proper. Giving up such maladaptive self-reliance will put the individual at the mercy of others, a seemingly intolerable situation.
8. A great deal of pain will result from coming to accept the world as it is with all its frailties and injustices. In attempting to gain reentry into such an imperfect world, the individual is in danger of losing patience with it and falling back into the vortex of PTSD.
9. Correlative with accepting the frailties of the world is also the acceptance of one's own set of infirmities; bad memories may return; relationships may not always be excellent; others may obtain better jobs for no legitimate reason.

Acceptance of oneself, including the guilt, sorrow, and regret that go with it, is the sine qua non of getting through PTSD, but it may be an extremely difficult and fearsome task that will call for far more courage than surviving the catastrophe itself.

Multiphasic/Multimodal Treatment

LO12 There is a great deal of support for trauma-focused cognitive-behavioral therapy (TF-CBT) for those who have a wide variety of trauma exposures (Greene et al., 2023; Peters et al., 2021; Pfefferbaum et al., 2019). TF-CBT is a phase-based therapy (Cohen et al., 2017) for children and adolescents (aged 3–18) that has demonstrated flexibility in its application across multiple populations (Goldbeck et al., 2016) and culturally and spiritually diverse settings (Wang et al., 2016). This approach helps children overcome the negative effects of trauma and may also involve parents during treatment and subsequently help them cope with related issues (Greene et al., 2023).

TF-CBT is a short-term component-based intervention. The acronym PRACTICE is used as shorthand to summarize the treatment components. The letters stand for psychoeducation and parenting skills, relaxation skills, affective expression and modulation skills, cognitive coping skills, trauma narration and processing, in vivo mastery of trauma reminders, conjoint youth–parent sessions, and enhancing safety and future development (Cohen et al., 2017). Cohen et al. (2017) operationally divides these components into three treatment phases: Phase 1, stabilization skills (psychoeducation/parenting skills; relaxation, affect modulation, and cognitive coping skills); Phase 2, trauma narration (talking about trauma, sharing trauma narrative with parent [if appropriate], and cognitive processing of the trauma memories); and Phase 3, integration phases (in vivo mastery, conjoint youth–parent sessions, enhancing safety and future development).

Evidence–Based TF-CBT. Several meta-analyses have confirmed that TF-CBTs are the most effective therapies to reduce symptoms (Bisson & Andrews, 2009; Bisson et al., 2007; Bradley et al., 2005; Lenz et al., 2014). Best practices using them have been developed (Forbes et al., 2010) and are now considered the gold standard, first-line treatment modalities by the Veterans Administration (U.S. Department of Veterans Affairs, 2008) and international professional mental health organizations (Australian Center for Posttraumatic Mental Health, 2007; National Institute for Health Care and Excellence, 2005). Indeed, TF-CBT approaches have been the therapeutic modality with the most successful outcome data to date (Bryant et al., 2003; Gradus et al., 2013; Gutner et al., 2013; Iverson et al., 2015; Jeffreys et al., 2014; Reinecke et al., 2014; Voelkel et al., 2015; Wachen et al., 2014; Yoshimura et al., 2014). TF-CBT evidence-based approaches may be divided into three general treatment categories.

Prolonged Exposure (PE). There is a great deal of neurological evidence previously mentioned that indicates trauma rewires the brain and creates the pathological defense mechanisms that are characteristic of PTSD. A good deal of failed therapeutic approaches over the years has taught us that unless the client is returned to conditions that closely approximate the traumatic event, no change will occur (no new rewiring or growth occurs in the brain). Thus, following an in-depth explanation of what this procedure is about and what the unpleasant side effects of it may be, the client is returned to the conditions that closely approximate the traumatic event. This occurs either by imaginal exposure by having clients close their eyes and listen while the therapist recreates the scene or by using computer-generated virtual reality scenarios. Clients may then be given in vivo exposure where they are given gradual but increasing exposure to the feared and threatening stimuli (Bernardy & Friedman, 2015, p. 104).

To do this, a great deal of specific information is collected in regard to the visual, auditory, tactile, and olfactory sensations that existed in the traumatic event so the client is flooded with continuously fear-provoking stimuli from the event. This procedure occurs by continuous and prolonged exposure (PE) until the client becomes desensitized to the previously fear-producing stimuli (Stampfl & Lewis, 1967). Cusack et al. (2016) report this approach is shown to be effective, but client choice for using this approach is important (Shifrin et al., 2022).

Cognitive Processing Therapy (CPT). CPT was developed by Patricia Resick (Resick & Schnicke, 1993) to treat PTSD in sexual assault victims. CPT conceptualizes PTSD as a disorder of nonrecovery in which individuals get "stuck" with distorted beliefs about the traumatic event and can't get out of the psychological ruts their distorted beliefs sunk them into. Evidence with respect to the efficacy of this therapeutic approach is growing (Resick et al., 2017). There are three phases to treatment that involve education about the procedure, trauma processing, and learning how to disrupt the flow of negative feedback individuals generate for themselves. Trauma processing occurs through both written and verbal activities designed to bring the trauma out of the dark and into the light. Homework assignments are given to monitor daily thoughts, feelings, and events, of which at least one must be trauma-related. This procedure is particularly well suited for groups as well as individual sessions. Negative appraisals, attributions, and overgeneralizations about oneself, others, and the world are ferreted out and disputed through worksheets designed to change distorted beliefs into more rational cognitions. Socratic dialogue is used to challenge hot, all-or-none, self-blaming, distorted thinking and create alternative cooler cognitions and more positive self-statements. The overall goal is to create a new narrative about the event that gives the individual hope and a forward-looking positive view of the world and puts the trauma as part of one's history and firmly into the background.

Graziano et al. (2023) report success in decreasing PTSD symptoms using CPT. These researchers collected data over three points during 6 weeks of treatment with two one-hour sessions each week. The data collected involved the connection among symptoms related to PTSD. Graziano et al. (2023) state that even halfway through treatment, individuals reported progress, feeling less startled and cut off from other people. Hyperarousal symptoms also decreased during the treatment. Overall, these findings suggest that progress during treatment may be related to a decline in the centrality of feeling upset at reminders and a reduction of symptoms.

Mindfulness. Therapies using mindfulness are increasingly used for the treatment of PTSD (Nagy et al., 2022; Williston et al., 2021). Mindfulness has been defined as awareness and attention to the present moment without judgment of thoughts, emotions, and sensations as they are experienced (Feldman et al., 2006; Neimeyer & Vaughans, 2021). Williston et al. (2021) liken mindfulness to being open-hearted to the acceptance of experiences and present in the moment. Among the various therapeutic approaches building on this concept are meditation, body scan, yoga, and cognitive behavioral therapies. Not only is this approach showing efficacy in the reduction of psychological symptoms, but promising evidence is also accumulating regarding neurophysiological associations between PTSD and mindfulness (Williston et al. 2021). While more data needs to be collected, this approach holds great promise for treating PTSD.

Stress Inoculation. Stress inoculation was originally developed by Donald Meichenbaum (1985) to deal with anxiety, so it certainly fits well with PTSD, which is chock full of it. It is a three-phase procedure that starts with a good deal of psycho-education about the procedure and an in-depth exploration of where the major physical, behavioral, affective, and cognitive focal points of the anxiety are located in the individual. In the second phase, specific skill acquisition training is done at the anxiety focal points to inoculate the individual. In the third phase, the individual takes the skills learned in therapy and goes out into the real world to test them out and fine-tune them to see how well the inoculation is working.

Tele–Behavioral Health. All of the foregoing TF-CBT techniques can be incorporated into tele-behavioral health components with success. As indicated in Chapter 6, telephone and telehealth have many benefits, such as privacy, convenience, and economy, and most importantly, they seem to work with PTSD (Frueh et al., 2007; Niles et al., 2012; Tuerk et al., 2010). There are now numerous CBT and PTSD apps online and available for download. Chief among them is *PTSD Coach I*, which was constructed by the U.S. Department of Veterans Affairs National Center for PTSD (2014). This application provides reliable information on PTSD and treatments that work, tools for screening and tracking symptoms, techniques to help handle stress symptoms, direct support links, and is operational 365-24-7.

Virtual Reality. Virtual reality (VR) has found a great deal of utility in treating anxiety disorders through prolonged exposure (Goncalves et al., 2012; Nelson, 2013). Abbas and Hoyt's (2014) meta-analysis of VR exposure therapy for TF-CBT found strong treatment effects for its use. VR exposure therapy works on emotional processing and emotional dysregulation of people diagnosed with PTSD by presenting multisensory stimuli targeted to the individual's traumatic memory. In so doing, VR activates their fear response and desensitizes them to it (Reger et al., 2015). A hybrid of imaginal exposure and in vivo exposure, VR therapy typically puts individuals in VR helmets and exposes them to threatening stimuli. An added advantage to this hybrid exposure is that a simulator allows the therapist to increase or decrease exposure of not only sights and sounds but smells and tactile sensations as well.

Ram and associates (2014) used this procedure with veterans from Iraq and Afghanistan against a control condition where exposure was created by watching a television screen with no other stimuli beside the video on the screen. Their results showed significant improvement in experimental conditions against the visual stimuli only group. As measured by the Clinically Administered PTSD Scale (CAPS), these treatment gains held up over time. McLay and associates (2012) used VR with combat service members with PTSD and found that not only did the group achieve gains that held up on PTSD symptoms, but they also had significant reduction on depression and anxiety measures as well.

Brandt (2014) argues that the design of *Virtual Iraq*, a VR system designed to assist clinicians doing prolonged exposure, not only impacts therapeutic practice but also cultural conceptions of therapy as well due to its game-like quality in destigmatizing therapy among young men "digital generation" soldiers. Because of its success, it is now being upgraded into *Virtual Iraq/Afghanistan* with wider applications into medical corpsman, survivors of military sexual assault, and predeployment resiliency training scenarios (Rizzo et al., 2015).

Mindfulness has even found its way into treating PTSD through virtual reality (Mistry et al., 2020). Research conducted by Mistry et al. (2020) found both positive and negative effects of using mindfulness meditation to reduce PTSD symptoms. Positive effects involve a sense of spiritual awe doing meditation using virtual reality. However, individuals with more severe symptoms may experience negative effects such as greater feelings of being ashamed, humiliated, disgraced, embarrassed, and guilt. Attempting to use this treatment method, therefore, should be done with caution and full disclosure to clients.

The Rest of the Evidence-Based TF-CBT Story. While the foregoing approaches generally work well in eradicating the symptoms of PTSD, they are not without controversy. Because they have been extolled as a first-order intervention by the largest single provider of mental health services in the United States, the Veterans Administration's recommendation of these as first-line techniques tends to sway the total treatment field toward blanket approval. However, a number of writers have been critical of the now almost unquestioned approval of these therapies (Holt & Beutler, 2014; Holt et al., 2013; Rothschild, 2010; Steenkamp & Litz, 2014; Wheeler, 2014). Chief among their complaints have been the sometimes disastrous push to remember the trauma in vivid detail, which is one of the reasons that drop out of treatment is high. There are also questions about their validity in the real world as opposed to highly structured randomized controlled studies. Further, while TF-CBT approaches work, the question is do they work well, and do they have lasting effects? Further, are they reliable? Results seem variable. They work well for some and not so well with others, which is actually not too surprising considering how tough and intractable the disorder is to treat.

Wheeler (2014) made a valid argument when she proposed Eye Movement Desensitization and Reprocessing (EMDR) as a valid treatment alternative to TF-CBT. As you will soon read about EMDR, it doesn't involve detailed descriptions of the event, and it doesn't require extended exposure, disputing one's beliefs, or homework involving any of the foregoing. Indeed, the *VA/DOD Clinical Practice Guideline for the Management of Posttraumatic Stress Disorder* (Department of Veterans Affairs & Department of Defense, 2010) recommends EMDR as a first-order treatment, yet Wheeler notes it is not included in the list of disseminated psychotherapies that are evidence-based at the VA.

There are also some tough ethical questions regarding exposure treatment and the individuals who do the treating. These techniques directly target what individuals spend a great deal of psychic energy trying to cover up and submerge from reality. In doing so, they are exposing core beliefs and emotions that are likely to be terrifying and, if not closely monitored and supervised, may put the person in harm's way. As such, these are extremely serious psychotherapeutic techniques and require specific training and supervision in how to use them. Done incorrectly, they can do much harm to clients. In our own practice we have seen some clients become extremely agitated when the uncovering process starts, and it has taken every bit of our years of experience and training to stabilize them. We believe that in-depth psychoeducation, clear informed consent on what will happen, and after-session debriefing are critical to client well-being and safety in these protocols.

As a student, you need to read thoroughly about these potent techniques, ask questions to yourself and your professor, have it modeled, ask more questions of your professor, observe it being done, then ask questions of your clinical supervisor, and then, under close supervision, start to practice it, and then ask more questions of your supervisor. Rothschild (2010, p. 2) states the case admirably when she says that trauma recovery involves more than remembering the trauma because first and foremost it needs to improve one's quality of life, and anything that does that is good for you and anything that doesn't, isn't!

Alternate Approaches. Mindfulness (Rothschild, 2010) and acceptance and commitment therapy (ACT) (Hayes et al., 1999) also target avoidance processes of life problems that surround PTSD but in a much more benign fashion, without strenuous and intrusive exposure protocols. A core component of ACT that is taking root and growing in many therapeutic endeavors is the concept of **acceptance**, being open and aware of unpleasant emotions, thoughts, and experiences and just letting them be without making attempts to alter their frequency or form (Hayes et al., 1999). Finally, by practicing **defusion**, those previously toxic thoughts have much less power than we give them credit for having. Defusion focuses on decreasing the perceived literality (it is absolutely true and fact) of the avoidance language that debilitates and keeps people diagnosed with PTSD stuck in maladaptive value systems. The notion is that clients can be taught to detach from being fused with any idea (Engle & Follette, 2012, pp. 362–365) (including the really bad ones that go with PTSD) by practicing acceptance and mindfulness when negative self and world attributions surface and by continuous practice, they can come to believe that these are "just thoughts" that don't control one's behavior.

Further, because of the idiosyncratic nature of the course of PTSD, various other techniques that employ psychodynamic (Lindy, 1996, pp. 525–536) and humanistic approaches (Turner et al., 1996, pp. 537–558) may also be appropriate. Contextual (Gold, 2009) and contextual behavior therapy (Follette et al., 2009) and eclectic experiential and emotion-focused therapy (Fosha et al., 2009) are newer approaches that specifically target complex traumas. Curran (2013) has published a workbook entitled *101 Trauma-Informed Interventions* that are drawn from tools and techniques from the most effective trauma modalities that are a theoretical smorgasbord. Although this may sound like a haphazard approach, this is not the case. The complexity of this malady calls for some of the very best in integrative/eclectic therapy and treatment planning. Further, an important component of any psychotherapeutic approach in the treatment of PTSD is the use of psychotropic medication.

Psychotropic Medication

LO13 From what is presently known about the biology of PTSD, drugs that regulate neurotransmitters and neuromodulators ought to be helpful in providing at least some palliative relief from the psychophysiological responses that occur with the disorder. Because so many different psychobiological abnormalities may predominate in various PTSD cases, almost every class of psychotropic medication has been prescribed for clients with PTSD (Bernardy & Freidman, 2015; Guidelines Development Panel, 2019; Shifrin et al., 2022). There is as yet no fixed pharmaceutical regimen for PTSD. The effects of medications for PTSD seem to be so narrow for individuals and specific groups that they are often not generalizable to other populations (Davidson & van der Kolk, 1996, p. 511).

As early as 1994, van der Kolk and his associates found that fluoxetine did indeed reduce numbing and arousal responses in a clinical treatment group but *did not* in a group of veterans. Further compounding the problem is that one of the side effects of fluoxetine is that while it may reduce numbing and arousal responses, it can also *increase* startle responses (Davidson & van der Kolk, 1996, p. 512).

Most clinical practice guidelines for drugs now recommend the new anti-depressant selective serotonin reuptake inhibitors (SSRIs) such as sertraline (Zoloft) and escitalopram (Lunestra), and the serotonin-norepinephrine reuptake inhibitors (SNRIs), venlafaxine (Effexor) and duloxetine (Cymbalta) (Guidelines Development Panel, 2019). With the advent of SNRIs such as Effexor and Cymbalta and SSRIs such as Zoloft and Lunestra that additionally have antianxiety properties, the addictive properties of the benzodiazepines are no longer recommended (Bernardy et al., 2015). It appears that these antidepressants alleviate a variety of PTSD symptoms such as irritability, anger, depression, and anxiety along with the intrusion, avoidance, and numbing components of PTSD (Bernardy & Friedman, 2015). If PTSD is in place and comorbid with other disorders such as schizophrenia, then antipsychotics may be used in conjunction with antidepressants (Jeffreys, 2015). These drugs can be considered as generally more effective when they are combined with TF-CBT (Bernardy et al., 2015).

Because presenting symptoms can seriously interfere with treatment, careful prescription and monitoring of psychotropic medication are critical in allowing PTSD therapy to proceed successfully. Medication for PTSD symptoms should be given by someone who has a great deal of medical expertise with the problem and not by a general practitioner. That medical practitioner should also carefully coordinate medication and monitoring with whoever is doing the "talking" part of the therapy.

Individual Intervention Stages
Emergency/Outcry

LO14 In the first phase of recovery, the emergency or outcry phase, the major problem is to get the individual stabilized; this means reducing the anxiety and physical responses associated with the trauma (Meadows & Foa, 1999). Meditation, relaxation, hypnosis, and biofeedback may be used (Evans, 2003; Kolb & Mutalipassi, 1982).

In relaxation training and meditation, the human services worker teaches the client how to relax body muscle groups systematically and to focus calmly on mental images that produce psychic relief of body tensions and stress (Benson, 1976; Wolpe, 1958). Individuals learn how to exercise self-control over many of their stresses and anxieties and dampen debilitating physiological responses.

HSW: OK, Billie Mac. Just imagine that you are lying on the beach with that soft, warm sand, the calm breeze blowing gently over you, the gentle lapping of the cool, crystal-clear water, and just easily focus your attention on that scene. Now just notice the difference in your body too. Notice the difference between how your muscles feel when they are tense and relaxed. Starting with your legs, just tense them up, feel how your muscles tighten up. Now relax them, and just feel that tightness drop away. Notice the difference and the really pleasant feelings that occur when your muscles are just hanging loose and flaccid. Continue to picture the scene on the beach as you work your way up your body, alternating between tensing and relaxing your muscles. Notice as you continue to do this how you can change the way your body feels and what you can focus on in your mind's eye.

The HSW uses relaxation that alone is helpful in alleviating current symptoms and enabling the individual to regain a measure of emotional and behavioral control, and it is also a preliminary step in tackling the cluster of problems characteristic of PTSD. Through deep relaxation or hypnosis, the client may be regressed back to an image of the traumatic event. Regressing the client in this manner is necessary to elevate bad memories of the traumatic event, and the intrusive images that accompany them, to conscious awareness (Brom et al., 1989; Kingsbury, 1988; Spiegel, 1989).

Extinguishing Intrusive Images

Given the previously discussed neuropsychological foundations of PTSD, Ochberg (1988) has concluded that PTSD should be understood first in terms of autonomic nervous system (ANS) arousal, and any treatment should take into consideration the physiological aspects of the disorder. Thus, a standing hypothesis for PTSD treatment has evolved that proposes a return of the client to the original state of elevated psychophysiological arousal in order to affect current maladaptive response sets (Malloy et al., 1983). Once the individual has learned how to relax,

other specific TF-CBT therapeutic strategies such as systematic desensitization, prolonged exposure, flooding, implosion, and Gestalt techniques may be employed to create ANS arousal (Cohen, 2002, 2003; Fairbank & Keane, 1982; Feeny et al., 2003; Foa et al., 2002; Forbes et al., 2003; Hembree et al., 2003; Keane & Kaloupek, 1982; Paunovic, 2002, 2003; Paunovic & Ost, 2001).

The human services worker continues to work slowly through the relaxation exercises and the mental imagery, continuously reinforcing the client for being able to shift to calm, relaxed scenes and away from the intrusive, anxiety-producing images. Practice for the individual in this and the other techniques to be covered in individual therapy is important. We recommend that sessions be audio recorded so the client can practice the procedures at home on a daily basis.

Numbing/Denial

Reexperiencing. Once the individual has learned how to relax, the second phase of intervention occurs, coincident with the individual's emotional numbing and denial phase of recovery. This phase is concerned with bringing to conscious awareness the traumatic event and the hidden facts and emotions about it that the individual denies (Brende & Parson, 1985, pp. 191–192). This is an example of prolonged exposure (PE), and the therapist will audio record it so it can be listened to and processed by the client. In a gentle but forceful way, the human services worker guides the individual, in the here and now of the therapeutic moment, to reexperience in the fullest possible detail what occurred in the traumatic experience so submerged feelings are uncovered and ultimately expunged (Scurfield, 1985, p. 245). While deeply relaxed, the individual is asked to reexperience the terrible events of the trauma, with the injunction that at any time the memories can be switched off and the individual can return to the pleasant image of the beach.

HSW: Now go back to the village and tell me what is happening.

Billie Mac: (lying down, relaxed, eyes closed) The point man all of a sudden comes under fire and gets popped. I see him get hit. He's lying in the open across a ditch about 100 meters from the tree line. It's really getting hot, a lot of fire from concealed bunkers. They're using him as bait. This goes on for about 5 minutes, I guess. All of a sudden, I decide to go and get him. Me and some other guys just get up and run across the open field to the ditch. We're getting all kinds of fire and out of five of us, only me and Al make it to the ditch without getting dinged. The point man is only about 5 meters from me, but I can't get at him. **(Billie Mac breaks into a sweat with slight tremors.)** I finally spot where the concealed bunker is that's making it so hot for us. I've got a LAW [light anti-tank weapon], and I get a bead on the bunker and zap it. At about the same time, there's an explosion right next to me, a B-40 grenade, I guess, and that's all I remember until I wake up on the medevac chopper. **(Breaks into profuse sweating and major tremors.)**

HSW: All right, just shift out of that scene and back to the beach, and just relax. Notice the cool water, the warm sand, the gentle breeze, and just let your muscles relax. **(Billie Mac noticeably relaxes and, with continued directives from the human services worker, returns to a calm, relaxed state.)**

Although the account of the combat situation is fearsome in its intensity, the human services worker suspects that it alone is not responsible for the traumatic reaction. Billie Mac was in many such situations, but this village is the focal point of his nightmares and intrusive thoughts. The human services worker suspects that there is more here than what Billie Mac is revealing and seeks to slowly peel away the psychological walls that defend the trauma from awareness. The human services worker believes that the recounting of the combat situation, despite having psychological value as a defense mechanism, is probably not historically accurate. The individual has left out certain traumatic parts of the story, and the human services worker's job becomes one of trying to fill in the gaps (Horowitz, 1976, pp. 117–118). Having built a very strong rapport and mutual trust with the client (Keane et al., 1985, p. 291), the human services worker probes into the situation and actively seeks to interpret and clarify the content of the client's story with respect to its potentially overwhelming effect (Scurfield, 1985, p. 245).

HSW: Go back to the village and the ditch right before you take out the bunker. What do you see?

Billie Mac: I see the point man. He's alive, but bad off.

HSW: What are you thinking?

Billie Mac: I've got to get him, but I can't. The fire's too heavy.

HSW: What do you feel?

Billie Mac: Scared, I um . . . I can't seem to do anything . . . the rounds are really coming . . .

HSW: What's happening around you?

Billie Mac: Al keeps yelling, "Take the bunker out with the LAW!"

HSW: Then what?

Billie Mac: I . . . can't . . . do it . . . it . . . I'm terrified. **(Starts to shake uncontrollably.)**

HSW: Stay right with that, Billie. I'm right here.

Billie Mac: Al grabs the LAW, stands up and fires it and—Oh, my God! Get down! Oh, Jesus, the B-40 got Al. He's gone. His blood's all over me . . . I killed him. It was my job, and I couldn't do it, and I killed Al. **(Breaks into uncontrollable sobbing and shaking.)**

HSW: It's OK! Just erase that scene from your mind and slide back to that warm, quiet beach. Just put yourself out of the firefight and back to that beach and relax, just focusing that soft sand in your mind.

As the individual breaks through the defenses that have left him numb and shield the actual events from awareness, the full force of the reality of the incident floods over him, along with the overwhelming feelings of fear, guilt, remorse, and terror that accompany the event. As these thoughts come into awareness, they give the human services worker a much clearer picture of the how and why of Billie Mac's phase 2 (denial and numbing) and phase 3 (intrusive-repetitive thoughts). The human services worker, using tolerable doses of reminiscence about the event, seeks to push forward into full awareness of what the true scene at the event was and not what the individual's mind has fantasized it to be.

HSW: Now shift out of the scene at the beach and go back to the village. The B-40 has just gone off and Al is gone. What happens next?

Billie Mac: I can't remember . . . I don't know . . . I passed out.

HSW: **(gently)** Yes, you can. Just think a moment, and picture the scene. It's scary, but you are there now. Go ahead and just let it come and remember. I am here with you and you can get through this.

The worker gently but forcefully urges Billie Mac forward into the core of his trauma and what he fears most. This is a tightwire the worker walks. Coming to grips with the traumatic core is critical if recovery is to occur. Yet pushed too hard, the client may suffer some severe psychological consequences and lose much of the ground they have gained.

Billie Mac: Oh, God! You've got to get the point man now. You've got to go get him. I'm up and running, the fire is terrible, it's only 20 feet to him, but it's like a mile. I'm so damned scared. (**Breath coming in rapid, ragged gasps.**) I've got him and am dragging him back to the ditch. Bullets are kicking up all around me. I'll be cut in two. He weighs a ton. I get to the ditch and roll him and me into it. I turn him over and . . . Oh, Mother of Mary! He's dead. Why, oh why, didn't I get there sooner? I could have saved him. You puke-faced coward. (**Starts uncontrolled sobbing.**)

HSW: (**very calmly**) You are OK. Just shift out of that scene and back to the beach. Just take all the time you need to relax and erase that scene from your mind. Just let the cool breeze blow over you, smell the clean salt air, and enjoy that feeling of being completely relaxed. (**Time passes, and Billie Mac becomes noticeably more relaxed.**) Now I'm going to count up from 1 to 10, and when I reach 10, you'll be fully alert and refreshed.

The human services worker does this and brings Billie Mac back to present time. The worker then processes the events of the imagery session with Billie Mac.

Interpretation. At this point, the worker uses a more psychodynamic approach, actively intervening in the situation by clarifying and interpreting what the client communicates. By dynamically integrating the there and then of the trauma with the client's maladaptive attempts to cope and atone in the here and now of the therapeutic moment, the therapist hopes the client can build a comprehensible picture that will make sense of the memory (Lindy, 1996, p. 534). This interpretation is not typical of TF-CBT and may fly in the face of its structured protocols, but we believe that it is important in that it attempts to empathize with and use words that touch the deeper meaning involved in Billie Mac's anguish (Lindy, 2012, pp. 21–23). With Billie Mac fully awake and the recorder going, the HSW interprets the meaning of the event.

HSW: This is my hunch. See what you think of it and feel free to add, subtract, or tell me I'm full of New Orleans canal water. So it's not just that terrible fight at the village, but more what you didn't do. You feel as if you were a coward there, and that cowardice cost the life of your friend. It's almost as if all these years, you'd been trying to atone for that in the only way you know how—that is, by doing things that would almost guarantee that you die too. The brushes with the law, the uncontrollable rage that winds up in knockdown, drag-out fights, the DWIs, and the suicide attempt.

Billie Mac: I don't know. (**sobbing**) I feel so terrible about it. How could I have frozen? It would have been better if I had got killed rather than live with this.

HSW: Yet you did act. You went after the man, and you couldn't know whether a minute or two would have saved his life. It seems as if that minute or two of indecision has caused 30 years of terrible retribution that you can never pay off. I'd like to suggest that it has been paid with interest, and now the time has come to pay the balance. Are you willing to do that?

Billie Mac: (**shakily**) I guess . . . although I don't know how much more I can take. This stinking shit just blows up in my face and I can't control it. (**Red in the face, shaking, and yelling**) You bitch! How could you do this! This really hurts!

Lindy (2012, pp. 21–25) believes that Billie Mac's heated response contains two important messages. First is the use of what Lindy calls a **trauma metaphor** for clients. "Stinking shit blows up in my face" is an idiosyncratic way of describing and attempting to give symbolic meaning to his current state of being (p. 22). These are metaphors the worker needs to be keenly aware of because they often carry the dysfunctional meaning making message of the survivor. Second, these metaphors are symbolic transference terms that can either speak to the actual event (rocket blowing up in his face) or the therapy blowing up his **emotional dysregulated defense systems** (constant angry attitude with frequent, severe temper outbursts out of proportion to the situation in terms of intensity and duration).

HSW: I understand how rough you feel this is and how callous and uncaring I must seem at times. Now the "shit blowing up" right now I believe is not the "bad shit" of the rocket in the firefight, but if you can believe it, the "good shit" of blowing the cover off and getting it in the open. Remember! We've made it this far. Trust me and yourself. Together we can pull through this.

Even if the human services worker is right on target with her interpretation, getting Billie Mac to integrate the material and also allowing him to reconcile himself to the event are much more difficult. Breaking through the subconscious defenses of the client is not a one-shot deal, and denial is more often the rule than insight and acceptance. Billie Mac's negative reaction to the worker is typical of the client's transference of their ills to the worker as the hurtful effect is brought into awareness. At this point, it is the worker's primary task to remain as empathic as possible to what is going on with the client (Lindy, 1996, p. 536).

Reflection and Transition

Although it can be extremely traumatic for the client, the human services worker will encourage the client to experience the full range of emotional responses they felt at the time of the event as well as the way they try to make sense of it (Donaldson & Gardner, 1985, p. 370). This marks the fourth phase of the crisis, the reflective transition phase (Brende & Parson, 1985, p. 192). The human services worker will help the client by combining behavioral techniques of flooding and thought stopping. The technique of journaling, or having the client write down thoughts as the therapeutic process unfolds, will help the client process the experience.

Flooding/Prolonged Exposure. Flooding or prolonged exposure is one of the most effective, if controversial, techniques for getting rid of the bad memories of PTSD (Feenyet et al., 2003; Keane et al., 1989; Lyons & Keane, 1989). In flooding and exposure (Stampfl & Lewis, 1967), the fear-evoking stimuli are presented continuously. The rationale is that if the individual is literally flooded with anxiety-provoking stimuli, the client will discover that there is no basis for fear. Continuously flooding the client causes the stimuli that are generating the anxiety to diminish; that is, repeating the response without reinforcement diminishes the tendency to perform that response. As the individual reenacts the trauma, the human services worker puts in the missing pieces of the puzzle and ferrets out all conditioned stimuli buried in memory. The result is that no noxious components of memory are left to recondition debilitating responses (Foa et al., 2002; Forbes et al., 2003; Hembree et al., 2003; Keane et al., 1985, p. 265; Paunovic, 2002, 2003; Paunovic & Ost, 2001; S. Taylor, 2003). In Chapter 9, "Sexual Assault," an even more complex variation of

flooding and prolonged exposure combined with cognitive restructuring and guided imagery to extinguish intrusive images will be presented. This technique is a very serious therapeutic endeavor and should not be undertaken by neophytes until they have received supervised training.

Thought Stopping. Thought stopping is a simple but powerful device that enables the individual, with help from the crisis worker, to change debilitating, intrusive thoughts to self-enhancing ones. The crisis worker initially sets the scene and builds the images until the fear-evoking stimuli are at maximum arousal and then shouts "Stop!" and replaces them with positive, self-enhancing thoughts (Williams & Long, 1979, p. 285). The crisis worker tells the individual that at the point when the intrusive scene is most terrifying, the human services worker will slam a book sharply on the table and state in a firm voice, "Stop! Shift back to the beach!" The individual will be passive throughout the procedure, with the human services worker setting and enhancing the scene. A recording of the session is made, and the client is given the assignment of listening to the recording and then using the procedure whenever the intrusive images occur.

HSW: Now erase the beach scene, and come back to the village. You're in the ditch. Smell the stench of that ditch; feel death all around you. You can almost see the grim reaper there. You'd like to run away, but there's nowhere to run. Oh, what a fool you were to ever make the dash out here in no-man's-land! Look back and see your squad members shot up, contorted in pain, with the blood and dirt covering them. Peek over the ditch and see the point man. He's in terrible pain, screaming for help, but there's a blizzard of fire coming from the bunker. It's certain death to stick your head above the dike. Feel the conflict. You want to do something; you know you've got to take the bunker out, but you are paralyzed. You can smell the fear in you, sweating out of your pores. Look at Al. He expects you to do something; you're the squad leader, but you can't. Feel Al's stare. Listen to him yelling, "Take the bunker now, man!" Your fingers are glued to the LAW. Feel Al grab the LAW. Watch him as he stands up in that dreadful hail of death and fires the LAW into the bunker, and in the next instant see the explosion and the dirt fly as the B-40 grenade hits and Al disappears in the flame and smoke. Smell the smoke of cordite and the sheared copper odor of blood. Enhance those images—hear, smell, feel, see, taste that terrible moment. It's all there now as it really was. (**Billie Mac is writhing in the reclining chair.**) NOW STOP! (**Slams book down on desk.**) Shift away.

Billie Mac: (**screaming**) I can't do it!

HSW: (**in a soft but commanding voice**) Yes, you can! Just slide out of that and into that soft, warm sand. Stay with that beach scene. Smell the salt air, the cool breeze, and know that you can do that any time you want. Notice the difference in how your body feels, what goes through your mind. Just enjoy that feeling of knowing you can move into that scene.

This sequence is repeated over and over until the individual is able to switch volitionally from the intrusive image to the relaxing one with ease. The recording can be taken home to diminish the dissociation and permit externalization of the client's inner dialogue about the event and extinguish the fear that goes with it (Tinnin et al., 2002).

Integration

The Gestalt technique of reaching into the individual's past and bringing to conscious awareness what Gestalt practitioners call "unfinished business" (Polster & Polster, 1973) is particularly helpful in draining the pustulant affect that infects the event (Cohen, 2002, 2003; Scurfield, 1985, p. 246). For Billie Mac, this technique will take a different twist and will be the last part of the crisis, that of making atonement, penance, and restitution (Horowitz & Solomon, 1975). A Gestalt technique called the "empty chair" will be used.

HSW: The empty chairs in front of you represent various people. Al, the point man, and other members of your squad that got hit on that day in the village. I want you to tell them what you felt about what you did. I may move to one of the chairs or have you take their place. Right now I want you to imagine Al in that chair over there. What are you going to say to him?

Billie Mac: I'm . . . so sorry. I froze. I shouldn't have done that. I killed you, and I can't ever forget that.

HSW: (**takes Al's chair**) Hey, man, what about that time at Chu Lai, and the A Shau valley? You didn't freeze then. You saved my bacon then. Remember how I froze? You didn't say squat. You think you're perfect?

Billie Mac: You were my best friend, and I let that happen. (**Sobs.**)

HSW: (**as Al**) You think you got a corner on the market? Everybody was scared. I just did it. You gave me back my life a half dozen times. I'll never forget that. You did well by me, buddy. I got no regrets.

Billie Mac: Jesus, I miss you. I loved you so damn much.

HSW: (**as Al**) Then remember the good times we had. That R & R in Bangkok, when we took the town apart. Those are the parts I remember. I love you too, buddy, but it's time we were done with that village. It's time for you to say good-bye to me. (**The HSW gets up and goes over and takes Billie Mac into his arms and hugs him. Billie Mac weeps, releasing a flood of emotion.**)

For each man in the squad, the scene is replayed. Sometimes Billie Mac takes the role of the other man, and sometimes the crisis worker does. Each piece of unfinished business is slowly and patiently worked through until Billie Mac has reconciled accounts with each person who was there on that terrible day. Clearly, Billie Mac goes through a painful but necessary grieving process that must take place if he is to put the event behind him (Brende & Parson, 1985, p. 105). As Billie Mac makes atonement for that day long past and the trauma is expunged, the human services worker seeks to pull him to the present time and help him move forward with his life. Intensive intervention slacks off, and the individual may then go through a series of booster sessions on an "as needed" basis, with a minimum of a booster session once a month for 3 to 4 months (Balson & Dempster, 1980). This point marks the fifth, or integration, phase of the crisis.

Group Treatment

LO15   There are three types of treatment groups for people who have been exposed to trauma. The first type is preventive, short term, and typically used for those suffering acute distress. These are generally known as *debriefing groups* and are composed of members who have just survived a common traumatic experience (Mitchell, 1983). Debriefing for acute traumatic stress is discussed in detail in the last chapter of this book.

The second type of group is a *structured therapy group* that deals in a step-by-step fashion with PTSD symptoms. CPT techniques are well fitted to a group of this type. It typically uses a manualized treatment program and operates as a closed group with a fixed starting and ending point. Homework assignments are provided and worked on from session to session. Typically, groups run about 12 weeks, once a week for 2 hours at a time. Support for this approach is reported by Shnaider et al. (2022) in research with a wide range of trauma experiences including childhood and adult physical and sexual abuse, car accidents, and comorbid diagnoses (e.g., anxiety, mood, substance misuse, obsessive-compulsive disorder, eating disorders). Individuals participating in this research reported improvement in their ability to regulate emotions and a reduction in PTSD symptoms.

The third type is longer term and is typically composed of class-specific members who have been exposed to the same type of trauma but at different times and under different circumstances. It is generally an *open group* that is continuous with different members entering and leaving the group at different times. Commonly called a **support group**, this group deals with a variety of transcrisis issues that have to do with members' attempts to reintegrate themselves into a useful, functioning role in society and is the focal point of this chapter's discussion of group work with clients who experience PTSD.

Support Groups

Rap or support groups were started for veterans in 1970 by Robert Lifton and Chaim Shatan in New York City. Lifton and Shatan were human services professionals who had become disaffected with the Veterans Administration's constant refusal to acknowledge that many Vietnam veterans were suffering from combat-induced psychological problems. The outcome of this dilemma was that professionals finally came to recognize the success of rap groups and to integrate them into more traditional formats (Walker, 1983).

Emotional attachment and social involvement are basic and important ingredients in armor plating the individual against PTSD. For most of those who suffer from PTSD, social isolation and emotional estrangement are the norm. Thus, group work is helpful because of the shared experience, mutual support, sense of community, reduction of stigma, and restoration of self-pride it fosters. The primary task of any group therapy is to help people regain a sense of safety and of mastery because of the shared sense of having gone through the trauma (van der Kolk et al., 1996, p. 433). Further, confrontation by peers

is more acceptable than confrontation by professionals because it is reality oriented (Scurfield, 1985, pp. 247–248).

Groups also serve to educate clients. The terrifying nature of PTSD calls for clearly delineating what is happening and why. Answers to clients' questions—such as "What are common PTSD symptoms?" "Why do people use drugs?" "How long will it take to get better?" "Am I crazy?" "What do I do in this situation?" "Will I ever be as I was before this happened?"—help build a cognitive anchor for the individual (Brewi, 1986).

We now switch our client emphasis to the people who work in police, fire, emergency, and disaster services and who, because of their repeated exposure to trauma, are excellent candidates for PTSD (Bierens de Haan, 1998; Corneil et al., 1999; Dreisbach, 2003; Epstein et al., 1998; Horn, 2002; Tucker et al., 1999; Ursano et al., 1999). We will follow one individual in this group as a generic example of emergency services workers who become at risk for PTSD because of their constant exposure to traumatic events.

The Case of Ryan. Ryan Sanchez is a 35-year-old who has been a patrolman with the police department for 9 years. In that time, he has received numerous commendations and citations for his work. Approximately 1 month ago, he was referred to the police psychologist for a rather dramatic deterioration in job performance. He was caught sleeping on the job, had missed several days of work, and was insubordinate to his field commander when confronted with his inadequate performance at a crime scene. That episode culminated in his being hauled away bodily by other patrol officers after he attempted to punch his field supervisor. He was referred for clinical evaluation by his watch commander. An MMPI-2 administered by the police psychologist indicated a high potential for faking good—presenting a better picture of one's personality than one actually feels about it. The PK scale also indicated a good possibility of PTSD. The police psychologist believed that Ryan's initial interview and his MMPI-2 scores were an attempt by Ryan to present a better picture of his mental health than he was actually experiencing.

The psychologist then conducted a CAPS-1 interview and found a variety of problems that reached into both Ryan's job and family. Prior to Ryan's career with the police department, he served as an EMT for 8 years. He decided to leave EMT work because of its stress but still wanted to work in an "exciting and meaningful" job. He then joined the police department. He has a college degree in biology and a certificate in emergency medical technology. He has been married for 15 years to Mary, a nurse, and has two daughters, Katrina, 12, and Stacey, 8. He has been separated from his wife for 5 months, is currently living with his parents, and sees his daughters on his off-duty days.

He reports that his wife had become progressively more paranoid over other women, accused him of having affairs with them, constantly checked to see if he had perfume or lipstick marks on him after work, and finally attempted to run down, in a mall parking lot, an off-duty female police officer whom she suspected of having an affair with Ryan. That incident resulted in her temporary arrest, but charges were later dropped after she apologized to the female officer.

Ryan reports that at about this time he started suffering a bad case of "nerves." Specifically, he started to experience flashbacks to a series of traumatic events he had experienced as both an EMT and a police officer. He reports a series of instances as an EMT in which he was powerless to save the lives of terminal auto accident victims, a number of them children or adolescents. He reports having become very protective of his daughters as a result and says he wishes "I could put them in a castle with high walls and a moat around it and keep them locked up so nothing could hurt them." His protective view of his children severely strained his relationship with them, and they did not want to go and visit him because of his anger when they were not under his close supervision. He was also an EMT responder to a natural disaster 11 years ago when a propane truck overturned and blew up, killing more than 30 people. They were charred and burned so badly that rigor had set in but were still alive. He was relegated to being the mayor's aide de camp and spent most of his time passing information to the mayor about rescue efforts. He felt completely helpless and out of control and was enraged over his assignment. He very much wanted to be in on the rescue efforts, although he paradoxically reports that it was the most horrific scene he had ever witnessed. He reports having had nightmares about it for a number of months after the event. In the last 6 months, those nightmares have returned with increasing frequency. He also reports that within the last 6 months, he has become severely agitated to the point of a panic attack whenever he is near a propane truck and will go out of his way to avoid them as well

as bulk plants and tank farms where petroleum products are stored.

One other traumatic event is reported as remarkable. This event involved a missing person report while Ryan was a police officer. He and two detectives met the father of a young woman reported missing, at her abandoned apartment. Because they did not have a search warrant, they could not conduct a thorough search of the apartment. Ryan had a hunch that the woman's body was in the apartment buried under a huge mound of bags in a closet, but he was admonished by the detectives that there was nothing they could do. Because it was below freezing in the apartment, there was no foul odor to indicate the presence of a body. Two weeks later, he again met the father at the apartment. The father had come in a rental truck and had begun to haul his daughter's belongings out of the apartment when he noticed a foul odor. On his arrival, Ryan immediately knew the odor was that of a dead body. On entering the apartment, he immediately found the woman under the bags of clothing. He reports an indelible picture of the father sitting in the yellow rental truck with a glazed stare that he cannot get out of his mind. He also reported that his uniform smelled like death and repeated washings would not get rid of it. He finally threw his whole uniform out, but he believes that somehow his new uniforms have soaked up the smell from his leather uniform jacket. He has never undergone formal debriefings for any of these traumatic events and said that although they bothered him some at the time they happened, he moved on past them—or so he thought.

He does not use alcohol, and that fact is confirmed by his watch commander. He reports he has been taking "tranquilizers" and "sleeping medication" since his separation from his wife. He also reports that things are so bad both on the job and at home that he has recently contemplated killing himself, but he has not formulated a plan because he doesn't want his daughters to be labeled because their dad "was another nutso who blew his brains out." He admits to the psychologist that he clearly has lost control of his life and wonders if he indeed does not have PTSD or is suffering a "breakdown" of some kind.

Ryan's symptoms fit a clear diagnosis for PTSD. He has recurrent, intrusive thoughts and dreams about the traumatic events and experiences severe psychological distress to external cues of the events. He now avoids stimuli that remind him of at least two of the events. He has increased arousal symptoms, hypervigilance over his daughters' safety, difficulty concentrating on his job, and problems falling asleep. The psychologist's diagnosis is posttraumatic stress disorder, with delayed onset. Although delayed onset is relatively uncommon (McFarlane & Yehuda, 1996, p. 159), it is not uncommon for a domino effect to occur in emergency medical workers where one event triggers other supposedly long-forgotten ones (van der Kolk & McFarlane, 1996, p. 9). As his social support system has given way at home, Ryan has become increasingly at risk, and the precipitating event of his wife's vehicular assault on a fellow police officer and his subsequent separation from his family has activated the traumatic memories.

Ryan is referred to a behavioral health maintenance organization for individual treatment and is also referred to an independent support group that is cosponsored by the police, fire, and emergency workers unions and the city and county governments. The police psychologist also contacts the human services worker who will be attending Ryan to tell the worker about Ryan's suicidal ideation.

Triage Assessment. Affectively, Ryan is experiencing extended periods of intense negative moods that are markedly stronger than the situation warrants. Although he has no clear intent or plan for dying by suicide, he is agitated and depressed enough to consider it. At times, he perceives his negative mood states as not being very controllable. His affective rating is a 7 to 8. Cognitively, Ryan's thinking is generally equal to the task of moving forward in day-to-day living. However, his ability to control intrusive thoughts and images about the traumatic events is limited, and his perception of events, particularly his obsessiveness about his daughters' safety, differs noticeably from the reality of the situation. His cognitive rating is a 6 to 7. Behaviorally, Ryan's inability to function at work is noticeably affecting his job performance. His behavioral rating is a 6 to 7. Ryan's full-scale triage ranges between 19 and 22. He is in crisis and in need of immediate therapeutic assistance.

Ryan's initial meeting with the human services worker involves obtaining a referral to a psychiatrist to review his medication, explaining what individual therapy will entail, and receiving an invitation to join a support group.

HSW: We've got some men and women that meet on Wednesday night to talk about many of the problems you're trying to deal with now. I think you've got a lot in common with them and believe it might be helpful for you to meet them. They've all been or are in the police, fire, or emergency departments and are trying to come to terms with their experiences there. You don't have to talk if you don't want to; that's up to you. You'll probably feel a lot of different emotions, and some of those aren't going to be too pleasant. However, all of the people you'll meet have been feeling a lot of the same kinds of things, even though they may have different kinds of problems that brought them into the center. From that standpoint, they all know what you're going through, and while it may get tough, they'll support you and not pass judgment. I'd really like to see you come in. You don't have to, but we know that social support is one of the most important ingredients to getting better, and right now it sounds like you could use some of that.

The group meets for an hour and a half each week. The first item is that individuals are asked to introduce themselves by name and unit. This structured event is not just for the purpose of getting into "war stories"; it serves to move people psychologically back in time and place to the starting point of their trauma and to cement the "we-ness" of the group. After introductions, anything on anybody's mind is fair game for conversation. The whole idea is to get you "unstuck" from the rut you're in and get some ideas on how to start moving forward. This will be in addition to the weekly meetings.

The group is composed of "veterans" who have been through many such sessions and "greenhorns" who are at their first meeting. Command officers are separated from rank-and-file members, so there are no possibilities of recriminations by command staff. Everything said in the group is confidential, and members indicate their willingness to abide by that rule by signing a statement to that effect. The groups are run by independent contractors who are not answerable to the city or county government about personnel decisions or any other matters that could put their clients' jobs at risk. Topics range from problems of day-to-day living to the institutions they work for, issues and questions about PTSD and trauma, replays of how and what they did during traumatic events, family and job issues, and how all these problems affect them.

The leaders of the group are a Licensed Professional Counselor and a Licensed Clinical Social Worker who have extensive experience with police, firefighters, and EMTs. Although they have never served in any of those occupations, they have credibility because of their previous work with these groups, and that is critically important. Distrust and suspicion are strong in the early stage of such groups, and human services workers can be expected to be tested over and over again until they have proved themselves to be congruent and trustworthy (Gressard, 1986).

The leaders are not group therapists in the truest sense of the word. They are more like participatory members who have been endowed with the task of keeping the group within loose guidelines concerning time, monopolizing the group, facilitating support and responses from the other members, and, in a few extreme instances, acting as empathic but firm sergeants-at-arms. As leaders, they must be willing to keep a low profile while group members interact. Their leadership role is subtle rather than directive and requires an infinite supply of patience as the group struggles toward resolution of its problems. If therapy in a classical sense of the word is to occur, it happens much later in the game. A clear distinction between the rap/support group and a long-term therapy group is that trauma and the expiation of associated guilt are the main focus, not life adjustment. Life adjustment problems represent another stage in the crisis of this malady and are handled later. The typical support group starts something like this:

HSW: Hi, everybody. We've got some new people here and because they don't know everybody I'd like you all to introduce yourself and your unit. I'm Theo Ewing, a psychologist. I work with the Crisis Intervention Team in the city police department.

Jane: Jane Shore, patrol officer, Delta shift, West Precinct, city. Age 21. (**Rookie on the force, training officer shot in a liquor store holdup. Robbers got away. Feels responsible, nightmares, startle reactions, hypervigilance, some paranoid ideation about abilities.**)

Leann: Leann Sung, EMT, RN, county hospital. Age 50. (**Twenty years' emergency room and ambulance duty, attendant at multiple disasters, catastrophes. Burned out, suicide attempt after caught stealing amphetamines from ER pharmacy, peptic ulcer, numbing of affect.**)

Alonzo: Alonzo Brown, sheriff's deputy, Able shift, north sector, county. Age 42. (**Shot and killed carjacker after carjacker killed hostage by cutting her throat. First shooting, first violent deaths witnessed, nightmares, intrusive images, high blood pressure, alcohol misuse issue.**)

Lamont: Lamont Evans, paramedic, Life Flight. Age 29. (**Life Flight helicopter crashed and burned. He and another paramedic thrown clear. Everybody else died—including two auto accident victims being lifted to hospital. Survivor's guilt, hypervigilance, startle reactions, nightmares, wife has left, phobic reaction to helicopters since accident.**)

Rachelle: Rachelle Johnson, driver, Engine House 47, county fire department. Age 36. (**Saw wall collapse on two members of her engine company during warehouse fire. Helped pull both dead firefighters from rubble. One was her best friend. Nightmares, survivor's guilt, somatic and general anxiety reactions, eating disorder.**)

Ryan: Ryan Sanchez, patrol officer, Charlie shift, Center Precinct, city. (**Personal data previously given.**)

(**Introductions continue around the group, and the group welcomes Ryan.**)

HSW: Has anybody got anything that's hot?

Lamont: Well, two things. I haven't had any more helicopter crashing nightmares since last time; I guess that's something. That prolonged exposure stuff has been tough with Dr. Myer, but I think it's starting to work. I got a prescription for Trazadone which is helping me sleep. And the wife said she might come back.

(**General congratulations from the group.**)

Rachelle: Man! That's something. I wish I could get rid of the damn things. None of those drugs are doing any good. I can't eat. I can't sleep. I don't know how much longer I can take it.

Jane: Ditto that! I can't get by it, and it seems to get worse. I really don't like that flooding stuff. I've heard about EMDR being not so rough, but I don't know who does that.

Lamont: (**gently**) We've all been there and know how tough it is; you knew it'd get worse before it got better; we all told y'all that. It's hell. Y'all been talkin' to your counselors? I'll betcha one of our esteemed facilitators can put you onto somebody who does EMDR (**looks at Dr. James**).

Because of the mutual support and resources within the group, lots of suggestions are given about how Rachelle and Jane can grapple with their emotional turmoil. Survivor's guilt is a common thread that runs through emergency, fire, and police personnel. The expectation is that these people are supposed to lay their lives on the line, and when others die or are injured, there is always second-guessing and fears of being seen as letting their comrades down. Lamont's comments are therapeutic in that they are accepting and understanding of the guilt both women feel.

Rachelle: Yeah, I been talkin' to her. But it just seems like the more stuff comes up, the worse I feel. Why did they die and not me?

HSW: So it still boils down to the survivor's guilt stuff we've talked about. Lamont, Rachelle, and Jane have all talked about the same issues. **(The group leader takes a few minutes to speak to the typical behavioral dynamics of someone who has survived a trauma when others did not, which is typical of the psychoeducational function that is also a part of support groups.)** Any thoughts?

Jane: I've always wanted to be a cop, and I really thought I'd make a good one, but it's tough being a rookie and a woman at that. I've replayed that robbery a thousand times. I don't know what I could have done differently, and Loren, my training officer, told me I did fine. I'm glad he's gonna be all right, but I still think I screwed up somehow. Maybe I'm paranoid, but I'm not so sure the other cops on my shift trust me. Hell! I'm not so sure I trust myself.

Ryan: Well, I'm new here, so I don't know much, but I heard about that, and it sounded OK to me. What did you think you did wrong?

Jane: Well, that's what's driving me nuts. I don't think I did, but I think the others think I did.

Ryan: Well, if it's because you're a woman, lose that thought. I've got a woman for a partner, and she's tops.

HSW: Jane, did you hear what Ryan said?

Jane: Yeah! And thanks. Dr. Myer did give me a phone app that goes with that mindfulness stuff he's also been doin' and that does help some. When I start to feel that negative self-talk overwhelm me, I flip the phone app on. I just let the anxiety come on but then turn it into dandelion seeds and just blow on it and let it float away on the wind and poof! It's gone. **(giggles)** It sounds kinda screwy but it seems to help.

The leader immediately breaks in so two people get reinforcement—the newer member of the group for talking and Jane, who can use the affirmation from a male officer who is a veteran.

Alonzo: So what's happened to cause the change in you, Lamont?

Lamont: I'm not blaming myself as much. I still feel bad about the others that died, but I'm getting reconciled to it. I'm really lucky to be alive, and I've got to start working on putting my life back together. And I'm finally realizing that engine failure had nothing to do with Lamont. My counselor calls it *reframing*, kinda lookin' at it from a different viewpoint. I mean both of you were doing what you were supposed to be doing when those things went down. You can't ask more than that. I been writin' stuff down too, usin' that trauma workbook. Man I haven't had so much homework since college.

Alonzo: I wish I could "reframe" my problems that easy. I mean this crackhead carjacks this woman, practically cuts her head off in front of me. I've got no clear shot until he drops her, then I shoot him. Then the shoot team gives me a clouded report. Should have acted sooner, should have had more patience. How the hell do you do both of those at once? I did it all by the book. What that's all about? Then I get a wrongful death suit laid on me by both the victim and the murderer's families. It's not enough I feel bad about both of them, but now I'm the culprit. I'll never get rid of that image. And no damn support from the department. So now I'm going to 12-step meetings, comin' here with you fine folks and getting stress inoculation training with my shrink. He's doing this imagining stuff about the homicide and he's making noises about getting me ready to go back to the scene and talk it through or something. Man I've been a cop for 19 years, and if I can make it for one more year without having a stroke with this sky-high blood pressure, they can all kiss my ass good-bye. Why shouldn't I drink?

Leann: Yeah well, that's what they do, is use you up. Twenty years at county ER. I've seen it all. When I got caught swiping the speed, I'd been on for four straight shifts through four gun assaults and two knifings, three multiple-injury car accidents, and burn cases of five kids in an apartment fire. I was about to collapse. And I've done that over and over for all these years. And you know what, the ER supervisor who caught me said he could forget it if I could take just the one more shift, said he "knew I needed a pick-me-up." When I said no to that SOB, he turned me in. That's the sum total of my life, no family, a speed freak, a burned-out ER nurse with an ulcer, and a system that uses you up and then dumps you. So tell me why suicide doesn't look like a good career option. (**Starts to weep silently.**)

HSW: Are you still contemplating killing yourself, Leann?

In no uncertain terms, the leader immediately checks out Leann's comment. As she is a past attempter, such comments are never seen as offhand statements.

Leann: No, not really. It just makes me so angry that they'd do that. I told them about that jerk, but they still put me on disciplinary sick leave and didn't do a thing to that blackmailing twerp.

HSW: So it's also the system that you feel betrayed by. It's like after all these years of doing your very best, the system turns its back on you. Not only does it make you madder than hell, but at a deeper level it really hurts to think that somehow an institution that you've given most of your life to would not stick up for you when the chips were down or would even try and blackmail you. (**Leann and Alonzo both nod their heads vigorously in agreement.**)

Although it may appear that the support group has dissolved into a gripe session about uncaring bureaucracies, the stresses put on individuals by notoriously understaffed human services institutions and public safety departments add a great deal to the recipe for posttraumatic stress disorder when emergency situations occur (refer to Chapter 15, "Human Services Workers in Crisis: Burnout, Vicarious Traumatization, and Compassion Fatigue"). Expressing emotion is a potent weapon in the arsenal of opening feelings, which is critical in dealing with PTSD (Tarrier & Humphreys, 2003). The group leader reflects these feelings and gives the members a chance at catharsis but also poses a problem-solving question. Lindy (2012) has been very vocal about neglecting the art of listening to these narratives in favor of manualized cookie-cutter, one-size-fits-all PTSD therapy.

HSW: I wonder what you might do about changing some of that institutional behavior?

Rachelle: I know one thing—if it hadn't been for the union's pushing for this kind of support and now the new debriefing program, we wouldn't be here now. There's got to be more safeguards for people who work in the high-stress jobs we do, and the only way I see that happening is through the

union's collective membership. I think I'll talk to my rep about some of that stuff.

Alonzo: That's right! At least they can get all the certifiables in one place and keep an eye on us. (**Group laughs.**) I know how much that hurts, Leann, 'cause I feel the same way. But you gotta think of all you've done and all the lives you saved and the people you've helped. I'm pretty cynical right now, like you, but I had a person stop me the other day and thank me for something I did a long time ago, that he said kept him out of jail. I couldn't really even remember the incident it's been so long ago, but he sure did. It made me feel good. How many people out there do you suppose you've been involved with who wouldn't be alive now if you hadn't been there?

Alonzo, who has been vitriolic in ventilating his feelings, switches roles and becomes a support person to Leann. In mutual help groups such as this, such role shifts are common, and the need to become a helper rather than a beneficiary is extremely important (Silverman, 1986). Theo, the leader of the group, recognizes this shift and wisely lets Alonzo carry the dialogue.

Alonzo: Eh, ah, Ryan. What's happening with you, man?

Ryan: (**Details his problems.**) I mean, I like you guys and all, but I don't know that this group stuff will help much. I mean you can't fix my marriage, and all this other crazy PTSD stuff. I guess the shrink will sort that out. I just don't know. Dr. James is gonna set up an EMDR session for me so I could let you know how that goes.

Rachelle: I understand, Ryan, I haven't been here that long myself, but I'll tell you this much—these people understand what I'm going through. Maybe we can't save your marriage, but we can sure be here for you, 'cause these other folks have sure been here for me.

Rachelle's comment encapsulates the essence of why it is called a *support group*. As the group session closes, each member is given the floor to speak on what has occurred for them personally during the meeting. No one else is allowed to respond to their comments. Summing statements include both reflections about the impact of the discussion on oneself and reinforcing comments to others. Finally, the group rises, joins hands, and has a silent moment of meditation. The emotionally positive high voltage that flows through the locked hands of some very tough people are both touching and powerful, and it conveys far better than words the caring and support each man and woman feels for their comrades.

Evidence suggests that individuals who have suffered other types of catastrophic intrusion into their lives can profit from support groups. Donaldson and Gardner (1985) report that incest victims quickly gain an intense sense of relief in coming together with others in mutual support groups. A typical comment is "No one else understands, but I can come out of the closet here." Defining these groups at a deeper level is Foulkes's (1948) comment that participants in such support groups can reinforce each other's normal reactions and break down each other's pathological reactions because they collectively constitute the very norm from which the individuals deviate. As such, members of a veterans' rap group one of the authors has worked with have what one member called very good "crap detectors:" "We can smell it immediately when somebody isn't coming clean with us."

The Life Adjustment Group

PTSD may be seen as having a two-generation, or two-phase, treatment approach. In the first generation, treatment focuses on accessing and working through the trauma and its symptoms. Although this will be difficult, the second generation of treatment may be even more so. In the second generation, treatment moves to the client's attempts to readjust to contemporary society, which will generally not be an easy task (Johnson et al., 1994).

As the guilt and horror of the situation are resolved, clients are moved into the life adjustment group, and another crisis ensues. It is not enough to bring to light hidden traumatic experiences. The key is to integrate past experiences, to find meaning and new ways of coping, to make atonement not only for oneself, but also for others, and to find new directions in life (Brende & Parson, 1985, pp. 199–201). The group at this point will diminish and absences will increase. The reason is twofold.

First, threatening material will again be covered. Second, action and behavioral change now become mandatory. Moving from the insight gained about what happened in the past to taking that insight and applying it to the present time is a giant step and one that is guaranteed to be rife with crisis. What is now called for is to get on with the business of living. At this juncture, intervention will take many forms, depending on what the particular problems are that the individual faces. Such problems range from maintaining sobriety to salvaging careers. However, one thread will usually run through the circumstances of all clients at this stage. That thread is of vital importance and must be rewoven into the fabric of their lives. It is their family. Any comprehensive PTSD treatment program should take into consideration the need to reestablish the basic support system of the family, which is of critical importance in helping the survivor move forward in his or her posttraumatic world. Getting family members to open up and express some of their beliefs that influence the client's negative coping behaviors is scary for both the individual and the family; they may believe that discussing their posttraumatic problems would cause so much trouble that the family would disintegrate even though it may presently be in complete chaos (Tarrier & Humphreys, 2003).

Family Treatment

If the trauma is unresolved and chronic, its residue will eventually become enmeshed in the individual's interpersonal network (Figley, 1988, p. 91). As reluctant as the survivor of trauma may be to seek help, often, the family is even more unwilling to participate in the recovery process (Lenton-Brym et al., 2023). Even though family members may be suffering terribly because of the individual's actions toward them and their respondent actions toward the individual and each other, they offer much resistance to changing the status quo, even though they adamantly maintain that change is needed. As strange as it may seem, although families may be stressed to the limit in adapting to the individual with PTSD, they do try to adapt, at times in pathological ways. As the individual changes, the family may be in for a rude awakening and may not be able to make parallel changes. We will learn a great deal of what goes on in families in Chapter 11, "Family Crisis Intervention."

Therefore, one of the crisis worker's major tasks is assessing the family's willingness to engage in treatment. The family's ability to resolve the crisis is a function of the nature of the event, the family's definition of the event, the resources they can bring to bear on it, the buildup of stressors that led to the event, and the effectiveness of their past and current coping skills (Lenton-Brym et al., 2023; Morland et al., 2022).

Treatment objectives are to develop and implement an intervention program to deal with both the stress disorder of the individual and assorted family dysfunctions that were in place prior to the event or that developed after the event. Learning about the disorder, dealing with the boundary distortions of intimacy and separation caused by it, alleviating psychosomatic results of rage and grief, urging recapitulation of the trauma, facilitating resolution of the trauma-inducing family conflicts, clarifying insights and correcting distortions by placing blame and credit more objectively, offering new and more positive and accurate perspectives on the trauma, establishing and maintaining new skills and rules of family communication, and initiating new coping and adapting skills as family dynamics change are some of the many tasks the worker will have to tackle (Lenton-Brym et al., 2023).

The foregoing list of tasks is a major order and is best dealt with by referral to a therapist who specializes in families and conjoint therapy. However, it is practically a must if the family has any hope of survival as a healthy system. The crisis worker should understand that, at an early point in the therapeutic process, the family members need to be apprised of their role in the trauma and urged to become proactive in its solution. Finally, for individuals with PTSD relearning how to be effective members of their families and society calls for the same kind of courage that propelled them into treatment in the first place. However, this time it may be much more difficult, because they will be working with the people they need the most and probably have hurt the most. If outcomes of the family component of the Comprehensive Soldier Fitness program are good, we find no reason why they could not be adapted to other workers in high-risk, high-stress civilian occupations.

Eye Movement Desensitization and Reprocessing (EMDR)

The Controversy over EMDR

LO16 Eye movement desensitization and reprocessing (EMDR) has, to say the least, been a controversial technique. Over the years since the approach was first used, a lot has changed. EMDR has received endorsements from national and international organizations (American Psychological Association, 2017; Department of Veterans Affairs & Department of Defense, 2010; International Society for Traumatic Stress Studies, 2019; National Institute for Clinical Excellence [NICE], (2018). Recent research conducted by Gielkens et al. (2020) found the use of EMDR with older adults diagnosed with PTSD and comorbid psychiatric and somatic disorder had a positive effect on reducing PTSD symptoms to the point of remission. EMDR has also been used in combination with other therapeutic approaches. Negash et al. (2018) found that using EMDR with Emotionally Focused Therapy is effective in helping heal the trauma of infidelity. Used with CBT, EMDR is reported to be effective in reducing negative emotions and avoidance behaviors after a traumatic loss (Lenfering et al., 2020). Although originally met with skepticism, EMDR seems to have emerged with a great deal of support when used properly.

The model uses several stages in the treatment process as listed below. The basic technique of EMDR is to have the person picture the traumatic scene in their mind or think about the thoughts or feelings associated with the trauma while following the therapist's finger with their eyes as it is moved rapidly back and forth in front of the person's face. Newer approaches employ flashing lights that move across the vision field and handheld buzzers that alternate in speed and strength in sending impulses to the client's hands. The procedure is so simplistic and is extolled as so fast and effective in comparison to combinatorial approaches using cognitive behavior and exposure techniques that it has been viewed with skepticism—particularly because PTSD is so intractable that there are as many failures as successes in treating the disorder. However, a number of replicating studies (Jarero & Ureibe, 2012; Lee & Cuijpers, 2013; McGuireet et al., 2014; Urhausen, 2015) do show significant results for EMDR when compared with other treatment modalities. At present, there is no clear scientific explanation of what it does to erase trauma.

However, Bergman (2012) has written extensively on the possible underlying neurobiological mechanisms of EMDR's potential ability to change the functioning of neural circuitry, and it appears that neurobiological effects of EMDR operate differently than the CBT techniques of prolonged exposure, cognitive processing therapy, and stress inoculation (Bergman, 2012; Shapiro, 2014). The hypotheses proposed as to why and how it works mainly revolve around dual processing/focus of attention (if you do two things at once you aren't going to be able to pay attention to both nearly as well as one) or distancing (becoming more detached as you try to process the event while keeping some other activity going on (Bradley et al., 2005; Issacs, 2004; Lee et al., 2006).

So, why use EMDR? There are two major reasons. First, it does seem to work with some people, and not just as a placebo! Your authors have used EMDR with some very cynical, objective, hard-nosed, empirically oriented health service professionals, and they have been absolutely incredulous that the intrusive images have changed and the thoughts and feelings surrounding those traumatic images have diminished. Yet, with some clients we have tried it on, it doesn't work at all! But if it does work, it has been our experience that it works quickly and dramatically.

Second, it is far less intrusive than the cognitive-behavioral therapies that have prolonged exposure as their core treatment element. Bryant and Harvey (2000) warn that exposure therapy should not be used or used with extreme caution when treating clients with anxiety or panic attacks, psychosis, severe depression or suicide risk, substance abuse, borderline personality, marked dissociation, or marked ongoing stressors—which would include most people who have PTSD! At this point, from our experience using it, we agree with Briere and Scott (2006, p. 146) that EMDR appears to be at least as effective in the treatment of simple PTSD as the cognitive-behavioral approaches and is a lot less noxious, but it may run into problems with more complex PTSD.

From the standpoint of client welfare, convenience, ease of use, and cost in time and money, it is at least worth a try as a first-order treatment. Indeed, it has now been used effectively in treating coal miners (Blore, 2014), acute stress disorder (Buydens et al., 2014), dementia (Amano & Toichi, 2014), chronic pain (Tesarz et al., 2014), complex PTSD and dissociation (Knipe, 2015), addiction (Abel & O'Brien, 2015), psychosis (deBont et al., 2013), breast cancer patients with PTSD and depression (Thompson, 2014), massacre aftermath (Jarero & Ureibe, 2012), and children (Diehle et al., 2015). Moving beyond the original protocol in this chapter, EMDR developers have been busy fine-tuning EMDR so there are now protocols being developed for various specific stages and types of PTSD (Shapiro & Laub, 2014).

However, be aware! Like a lot of newcomers into the therapy field, it should become apparent that EMDR has been used metaphorically to attempt to fix everything from the crack of dawn to a broken heart. It is not a panacea. So understand that like every other technique in this business, it has its limits, and nobody knows for sure how or why it works. So, should it indeed be used for serious mental illness like depression, obsessive-compulsive disorder, and psychosis without a lot of controlled research (Logie, 2014)? Given these precautionary statements, here are the basics of EMDR therapy.

EMDR Therapy

Eye movement desensitization (EMD) was developed by Francine Shapiro (1989a, 1989b) at the Mental Research Institute in Palo Alto, California. Shapiro (1991) later added the "R" to the acronym to indicate a reprocessing of information, along with changing to more positive cognitions and desensitization of the traumatic memory. According to Shapiro (1995, pp. 55–73; Shapiro & Maxfield, 2002), there are eight basic treatment components to EMDR: history taking and treatment planning, preparation, assessment, desensitization, installation, body scan, closure, and reevaluation.

History Taking and Treatment Planning. Initially, clients are evaluated for their ability to handle the high levels of disturbance that may occur with treatment. A comprehensive clinical picture of the client is obtained, and a determination is made of the specific targets to be reprocessed; these targets include past events, current stimuli that trigger symptoms, and positive attitudes and behaviors needed for the future (Shapiro, 1995, p. 68; Shapiro & Maxfield, 2002).

HSW: (to Ryan) It appears that at least three events from your past are predominant: the propane truck, the dead body of the missing girl, and the young woman in the auto accident who died in your arms. It also seems that the reemergence of all these traumatic work events occurred closely after your wife, in a fit of jealous rage, attempted to run down the female officer. The constant theme that emerges from all of these events is that you feel powerless, frustrated, and angry, but were and are paralyzed to do much about these events because of a variety of social and job prohibitions and your own moral standards. It appears that at least three triggers set these flashbacks and anxiety attacks off: propane trucks, yellow rental trucks, and verbal battles with your wife—particularly over custody and safety of your daughters.

Preparation. Preparation for therapy entails explaining to the client what is going to happen, the effects that can be expected, and safety procedures. Shapiro also makes a point of discussing secondary gain issues. That is, if the therapy is successful and the pathology is reduced, what will the client have to give up (Shapiro, 1995, p. 69)? Although this may seem strange, a veteran may not want to lose their disability payments or "wounded warrior" status if the PTSD is eradicated.

Assessment. Shapiro (1989a, 1989b, 1995; Shapiro & Maxfield, 2002) proposes that EMDR treats traumatic memory by requiring that the client maintain awareness in one or more of the following: (1) an image of the memory, (2) a negative self-statement or assessment of the trauma, and (3) the physical anxiety response. Once the memory is identified, the client is asked to choose the image that best fits it along with a negative cognition and the chief physical response that goes with it. Although Shapiro (1989a, 1989b, 1995; Shapiro & Maxfield, 2002) proposes that it is optimal when all three conditions are held at the same time, she maintains that the presence of any one is sufficient for desensitization to occur.

Ryan: (**generating images**) I'm standing on the freeway overpass looking down on a scene from Dante's *Inferno*. It looks like a war zone. There are burning wrecks everywhere. I can see blackened bodies. Some are still alive. There are paramedics and firemen and other rescue workers all covered with soot. I can smell burned rubber and flesh. I can hear lots of moans and cries for help and shouting. I can feel the heat coming up out of the freeway on my face and arms. Sometimes when I come upon a propane truck, it all comes back like that. That's why I avoid them if at all possible. (**generating negative self-statements**) I'm powerless. I need to be down there, but I'm not sure I can take it. I've never seen anything like this. I'm a coward. I hate myself for feeling that way. (**generating physical anxiety response**) My skin feels like it's been sandpapered. Every nerve in my body is on fire. I want to run, down there or away, but do something. I can't stand just watching it all.

Anxiety level is assessed by Wolpe's (1982) Subjective Units of Discomfort (SUDs) scale (0 = no anxiety; 10 = highest anxiety possible). Because negative self-cognitions are also part of the disorder, shifts in the client's cognitive view of the traumatic event are also assessed by a Validity of Cognition (VOC) scale that Shapiro (1989a) developed (1 = the cognition is

completely untrue to 7 = the cognition is completely true). Clients are asked to rate themselves on the SUDs and VOC and indicate the physical location of the symptoms (Shapiro, 1989a, 1989b, 1995, p. 70; Shapiro & Maxfield, 2002).

Ryan: The SUDs is way beyond 10. The VOC is 7.

Clients are next asked how they would like to feel and are told to generate a new positive self-statement that reflects the desired feeling (Shapiro, 1989a, 1989b, 1995; Shapiro & Maxfield, 2002).

Ryan: Like I'm in control. I'm not a coward. Not necessarily a hero.

Clients are then asked to judge how true that new statement is (Shapiro, 1989a, 1989b).

Ryan: A generous VOC for that would be 2.

Desensitization. Shapiro (1989b) then gives the client a standard set of instructions designed to diminish performance anxiety and performance demands. She indicates that this step is important because clients may have difficulty accepting the initial changes they feel in themselves. Her instructions are as follows:

> What we will be doing is often a physiology check. I need to know from you exactly what is going on, with as clear feedback as possible. Sometimes things will change and sometimes they won't. I may ask you if the picture changes—sometimes it will and sometimes it won't. I may ask if something else comes up—sometimes it will and sometimes it won't. There are no "supposed to's" in this process. So just give as accurate feedback as you can as to what is happening, without judging whether it should be happening or not. Just let whatever happens, happen. (p. 213)

Clients are then told to generate the scene, the negative statements, and their noxious feelings and visually track the human services worker's finger. The therapist's finger is moved rapidly and rhythmically back and forth, about 1 foot from the client's face, at approximately two back-and-forth movements per second with a sweep of about 12 inches across the client's field of vision. For clients who may have trouble with this approach, Shapiro uses a slightly different format in which the therapist's fingers are to the side of the client's vision field and are alternately moved up and down. The movement is repeated 12 to 24 times for one set. (This is called a *saccade*, which means a sort of pulling or pressing movement.)

After each set of saccades, clients are asked to erase the scene from their minds and take a deep breath. They are then asked to bring up the noxious image again and ascribe a SUDs level to it. If the SUDs level has not changed after two sets of saccades, the client is asked if the picture has changed or if anything new has come into the image. If so, the new image is desensitized before returning to the old image. Periodically, clients are asked to assess the image, cognition, and memory. Their answers are used to determine new insights, perceptions, or alterations.

Ryan: (after two saccades) I dunno. It's not as strong now or something. Maybe an 8. It's like it's moving, or I'm moving. I'm not frozen.

HSW: OK. See yourself moving, and put that "I'm not helpless, I'm moving and taking control" billboard under that picture. Can you think of that?

Ryan: Yeah. It's also like I'm frustrated or angry too now.

HSW: That's OK! New images and thoughts come into this. That's normal. We'll work those through too.

The therapist continues to attack the client's image, but this time has him insert the "I'm a coward" billboard into the scene until it too is diminished and changed to a more positive self-statement. The therapist continues eye movements and processes with Ryan until he reports a SUDs level of 1.

Installation. The idea of the installation phase is to install a new, positive cognition of the event. The installation phase starts once the client's SUDs rating has dropped to a 1 or 0. Ryan has changed his image, and the therapist will continue to pursue this until there are no longer additions to the emotional meaning of the image or there is no longer additional positive input.

Ryan: OK! I'm equal to this. I could handle it down there, but my job is up here coordinating things. I'm where I can do my best.

Note that the cognition is not kept in a negative sense, "I'm not a coward," but is put positively and proactively. While the client focuses on the target image and the new positive cognitions, the eye movements are continued until the client can report a VOC for the new positive thoughts at a level of 6 or 7. If the cognition fails to change after two sets of eye movements, there may be a mismatch between the cognition and the image, or vice versa. In each case, both image and cognition must be congruent with one another. If they are not, then one or the other needs to be replaced (Shapiro, 1989a, 1989b, 1995, p. 71).

Body Scan. After the positive cognition has been fully installed, clients are instructed to think of a physical location of anxiety in their body if the SUDs level remains high. They are asked to concentrate on the body sensation while new saccades are given. When the focal point of physical discomfort subsides, clients are asked to return to the original picture of the trauma and the standard EMDR procedure is resumed (Shapiro, 1989a, 1989b). Shapiro believes there is a physical resonance between the body and dysfunctional material. She believes this phase is important because it can uncover new areas of unprocessed or unthought-of material (Shapiro, 1995, p. 730; Shapiro & Maxfield, 2002).

Ryan: I wish I could jump out of my skin, I'm so anxious. It feels like it's burning from the inside out.

HSW: OK, I want you to focus in on your skin. Feel the burning sensation. (Starts and finishes another saccade.)

Ryan: (after two more saccades) Huh. It's kinda gone now. That's really weird!

Closure. When no new events or negative cognitions are elicited, the EMDR procedure is terminated. The client is never left in a state of emotional disequilibrium, whether reprocessing for the event is done or not. The client is debriefed and reminded that additional intrusive images that may arise after the session are a positive sign of additional processing. Shapiro (1995, p. 73) also recommends that clients keep a journal of their thoughts, situations, dreams, and other information that may come to mind about the memory. This information can be used to target new images at the next session.

Reevaluation. At each new session, an assessment is made of the previous targets. The client is asked to reaccess previously reprocessed targets, and the client's journal is examined for any intrusion of the previously examined material.

Ryan: It's weird. That image of the propane truck explosion is just kinda vague or misty or something. I decided to drive by a bulk plant that I always avoid. It's right on my way to my folks' house. Well, I decided to hell with it, let's see. Usually I'd think I was going to have a panic attack the last couple of months if I went near it. But I drove by it, and it was just a bulk plant. Nothing more! Didn't feel a thing! Fancy that!

In subsequent sessions, the therapist may successively move through images of the propane truck, the body in the closet, the father of the murdered girl in the rental truck, and the scenes with Ryan's estranged wife. However, if the target and the triggers are well worked out, generalization of effect can occur and positive benefits can accrue in other areas of the client's life (Shapiro, 1989a, 1989b, 1995, p. 74; Shapiro & Maxfield, 2002).

Children and PTSD

Diagnostic Criteria for Children

LO17 PTSD is not confined to adults. Children also experience PTSD and manifest symptoms that closely parallel those of adults, with the following notable differences.

The 4th edition of the *Diagnostic and Statistical Manual for Mental Disorders* (DSM-IV) did not have specific criteria for diagnosing PTSD in children, and many of DSM-IV PTSD criteria were not age appropriate for children. As a result, it was difficult (if not impossible) to accurately diagnose PTSD in children. However, the text revised 5th edition of the *Diagnostic and Statistical Manual for Mental Disorders* (APA, 2022) now includes specific guidelines for diagnosing PTSD in children under the age of 6.

The first indicator of PTSD in children age 6 and younger involves exposure to actual violence or the child's perception of threatened death. The violence might be physical injury and/or sexual violence by two of the following; (1) direct exposure, (2) witnessing it happening to someone else, especially a primary caregiver, or (3) just learning that traumatic events happened to a parent or caregiving figure. A key for this indicator is defining who is a primary caregiver. Obviously, for most children, parents are in this group, but it might also include grandparents, siblings, or a babysitter who regularly watches the child. In other words, it is someone with whom the child has a strong emotional attachment.

The second indicator involves intrusion of at least one symptom connected with the traumatic event. These symptoms include recurrent involuntary and intrusive distressing memories of the event. Understand everyone has memories of events, especially of traumatic events, but the crucial issue is the way this affects the typical functioning of the child. Do the memories interfere with usual behavior? Distressing dreams are also a symptom for this indicator. The DSM 5-TR (APA, 2022) cautions that distinguishing the way in which these dreams are or are not connected to the traumatic event may be difficult. Another symptom is that the child may dissociate through experiencing flashbacks and losing awareness of present surroundings. An intense psychological distress when presented with external cues similar to the traumatic event is another symptom. This cue may be almost anything from reading a book in which there is a description of a similar event to someone talking about a comparable trauma, or seeing something on television that brings back the memories. The final symptom of this indicator involves a physiological reaction to reminders of the traumatic event. This reaction can be somatic, such as a headache or stomachache, even to the child becoming petrified.

The third indicator involves persistent avoidance of anything that is a reminder of the traumatic event. The avoidance can involve people, conversations, or interactions that are a reminder of the event. Included in this indicator is that the child may experience changes in cognitions and mood that are negative.

Similar to the indicator for adults, the fourth indicator for children age 6 and younger is hypervigilance. This indicator is observed as overreacting and being startled more than a situation warrants, an inability to concentrate, irritable behavior or angry outbursts, and simply having difficulty sleeping, either going to sleep or staying awake.

The above indicators should last more than one month. During this time, the symptoms should interfere with relationships with parents, siblings, or other caregivers. School behavior may also be disrupted. As in all diagnostic categories in the DSM 5-TR, the problems are not attributed to physiological effects of medications, alcohol, or another medical condition. You might ask: what 6-year-old drinks alcohol? Think about it, the child may accidently drink something, thinking since Dad and Mom drink it, it must be okay.

In summary, children must experience disorganized or agitated behavior. Children usually do not have a sense they are reliving the past but rather relive the trauma through repetitive play. Their nightmares of the traumatic event may change to more generalized nightmares of monsters or of rescuing others. A foreshortened future for a child generally involves a belief that they will never reach adulthood. Children may believe they can see into the future and can forecast ominous events. Physical symptoms may appear that include headaches and stomachaches that were not present before the event (APA, 2022).

For a long time, prevailing wisdom was that young children were not developmentally mature enough to be affected by trauma and as a result couldn't "catch" PTSD (Bosquet, 2004; Osofsky, 1995). If anything, their reaction to disasters would be fleeting. However, with growing research in the field, we now know that is anything but true (An et al., 2022; La Greca et al., 2022). Of the 74 million children in the United States, 30 to 50 percent will experience at least one traumatic event by their 18th birthday and will probably comprise a substantial proportion of the 2.5 billion people who have suffered some kind of disaster in the last decade (Kazdin, 2008). Trauma for children is also homegrown, with about 1 million cases of substantiated child abuse in the United States reported yearly (DeAngelis, 2007).

A survey of a nationally representative sample of over 10,000 adolescents aged 13–18 reported by the National Center for PTSD (2023) estimates that 5 percent of adolescents have met the criteria for PTSD in their lifetime. Prevalence is higher for girls than boys (8.0 percent vs. 2.3 percent), with the differences between the rates increasing as they get older. Overall, the combined rate is 3.9 percent that were surveyed. This report also states that definitive studies on prevalence rates of PTSD in younger children in the general population are not available.

It shouldn't take a PhD in child psychology to figure out that PTSD and its treatment are different in children by the mere fact of their developmental levels (Saxe et al., 2007). There is now accumulating evidence, including age of onset, duration, sequence, and co-occurrence of trauma events, that is providing the groundwork for a developmental model that builds on these variables and begins to plot the trauma pathways that are created as the child moves from middle childhood to adolescent to young adulthood (Peters et al., 2021; Steinberg et al., 2014). Indeed, PTSD manifests itself very differently in children than in adults in terms of symptoms (APA, 2022; DeAngelis, 2007) and in how it affects

the neurodevelopment of children (Saxe et al., 2007, pp. 23–45; Zilberstein, 2014).

Thus, not only because of their age but also because of how children attempt to cognitively handle trauma, even though TF-CBT is seen as a treatment of choice (Chard & Gilman, 2014; Greene et al., 2023; Jensen et al., 2014; Peters et al., 2021), PTSD in children calls for treatment strategies that are very different from those used with adults (Clay, 2010; Cohen et al., 2006; Ford & Courtois, 2020; Malchiodi, 2008; Saxe et al., 2007; Webb, 2007). Reactions to violence and trauma in children vary greatly and are dependent on their temperament and chronological age/developmental stage when the traumatic event occurred. The presence or lack of support systems that are nurturing or toxic is also important in children developing symptoms of PTSD. The ecosystem of the community and the degree and duration of the trauma also play an important role (Fairbank et al., 2014). Together, this means that a one-size-fits-all treatment approach is not effective. Treatment must be tailored to the unique situation given the presence or absence of the above symptoms.

To that end, the National Child Traumatic Stress Network (NCTSN) has been formed (Steinberg et al., 2014) to integrate trauma-informed services and evidence-based practices throughout the United States in clinical and community settings. Practitioners can avail themselves of its services at www.nctsn.org. A wide range of training resources may be downloaded at http://learn.nctsn.org, and NCTSN also has an online knowledge bank developed by network centers at https://www.nctsn.org/.

Support Systems

LO18 By now you should clearly understand that support systems are critical in crisis intervention. Supportive family systems are even more critical for children in their attempts to master a trauma (Bucich et al., 2011; Hambrick et al., 2018; Hicks et al., 2022; Resnick, 2014). Family support systems are important in regard to events both external and internal to the family system (Cimke & Yildririn Gürkan, 2023). Generally, in this chapter, we are speaking of family support in the context of a traumatic event that occurs external to the family, such as a hurricane, 9/11, or a pandemic. We will speak to family support (or lack thereof) when the trauma is generated within the family, as in child abuse, in Chapter 9, "Sexual Assault."

Bowlby's (1982) attachment theory is particularly relevant to traumatized children. In many of the traumas children experience, they are separated from their parents, their homes, and even their communities without warning or preparation. It should come as no surprise that such traumatic separation carries with it a smorgasbord of emotional and personality disturbance. Anxiety disorders, physical maladies, depression, panic attacks, rage reactions, and phobic reactions are common comorbid disorders of childhood PTSD. These are magnified even more when families are rent asunder by a traumatic event and support systems seem to disappear in front of the child's eyes (Hambrick et al., 2018; Hicks et al., 2022) and are even more profound when the young child perceives a threat to the caregiver (Ehrensaft et al., 2017). The final ingredient in this witch's brew of pathology is the unresolved grieving that accompanies the loss of loved ones when children do not yet have the cognitive ability to understand and resolve their loss (Cohen et al., 2006; Gordon et al., 1999; Halpern & Tramontin, 2007; Yule, 1998).

Types of Trauma

LO19 Childhood trauma is important not only for what it does to children but also for the after effects that carry into adulthood (DePierro et al., 2022). Childhood trauma has been compared to being the affective equivalent of rheumatic fever (Terr, 1995, p. 302). Although rheumatic fever is a serious disease of childhood, the damage it causes can later be lethal in adults in a variety of ways. Childhood trauma operates in the same way and can lead to character problems, anxiety disorders, psychotic thinking, dissociation, eating disorders, increased risk of violence by others and by oneself, suicidal ideation and behavior, drug misuse, self-mutilation, and disastrous interpersonal relationships in adulthood (DePierro et al., 2022).

In trying to understand trauma in children, Terr (1995, p. 303) proposes a division of childhood trauma into two categories: Type I, which is one sudden, distinct traumatic experience; and Type II (analogous to complex PTSD), which is long-standing and comes from repeated traumatic ordeals. Lack of full cognitive and moral development causes distinctive differences in how children react to trauma. It appears that even infants have the capacity to remember traumatic experiences (Courtois & Ford, 2020; Hopkins & King, 1994). Children who suffer from Type I traumas appear to exhibit certain symptoms and signs that differentiate their condition from those that result from more complicated Type II traumas. Type I events are characterized by fully detailed, etched-in memories, omens such as retrospective rumination, cognitive reappraisals, reasons, misperceptions, and mistiming of the event (Terr, 1995, p. 309).

In contrast, Type II traumas result in the psyche developing defensive and coping strategies to ward off the repeated assaults on its integrity. Massive denial, psychic numbing, repression, dissociation, self-anesthesia, self-hypnosis, identification with the aggressor, and aggression turned against the self are prominent. Emotions generated from Type II traumas are an absence of feeling and a sense of rage and/or unremitting sadness. These symptoms may be diagnosed in childhood as conduct disorders, attention-span deficit disorders, depressive disorders, or dissociative disorders (Terr, 1995, pp. 311–312). As these children move into adolescence, they have poor grades, drug misuse, and a constellation of other behaviors that get them in trouble (Pynoos et al., 2014). It should come as no surprise that there is a high correlation with youth in the juvenile justice system and multiple traumas in their background (Dierkhising et al., 2014).

Terr's (1983) in-depth, 4-year follow-up on children who were Type I victims of the Chowchilla, California, bus kidnapping is the benchmark study in childhood PTSD. The victims of this trauma were a group of 26 elementary and high school children who were kidnapped together with their school bus driver, were carried about in vans for 11 hours by their kidnappers and were buried alive in a truck trailer for 18 hours before they dug their way out—a horrific Type I trauma.

Etched Memories

Terr (1983) found that the children still had specific feelings of traumatic anxiety over the event after 4 years. When asked to speak about it, children generalized their anxiety from the event to statements like "I'm afraid of the feeling of being afraid." Unlike combat veterans, who might boast about harrowing experiences, the children were profoundly embarrassed by their experience, were unwilling to talk about the event, and shied away from any publicity. They generally voiced feelings of being humiliated and mortified when asked about their experience. Although 8 of 15 children had overcome their fear of vehicles such as vans and buses, they still reported occasional panic attacks triggered by unexpected sudden confrontation with stimuli such as seeing a van parked across the street from their house and vaguely wondering if some of the kidnappers' friends had come back for them.

Eighteen of the children were found to employ suppression or conscious avoidance of the trauma. Parents often aided them in this endeavor, although the two children whose parents encouraged them to talk about the experience were still not spared its residual effects. Their typical response was that they hated the feeling of helplessness they experienced and needed to feel in control of the situation. All the children could remember almost every second and minute of the event. However, they were able to remember few, if any, of the emotions or behaviors they experienced during the ordeal. This remarkable retrieval of full, precise verbal memories of almost all Type I traumas indicates that these memories are indelibly etched into the psyche, no matter how the child tries to suppress them, and are carried forward into adulthood (Terr, 1995, p. 309).

Memory etching may also come from vicariously viewing trauma. Saylor and associates (2003) found that children who saw images of death or injury from the attacks of 9/11 reported more PTSD symptoms than children who did not. Interestingly, the internet had a more profound effect than television or print media. No measurable benefit was reported in seeing positive or heroic images of 9/11.

Developmental Issues

Trauma may have severe repercussions on developmental expectations and acquisition of developmental competencies in children (Ford, 2018). When traumatic events impact a child in the middle of a developmental stage or in transition from one to the next, regressive behaviors occur (Gordon et al., 1999). Eth and Pynoos (1985, p. 44) believe that continuous intrusion of a traumatic event, evolution of a cognitive style of forgetting, and interference with mental processes because of depressed affect very definitely influence school achievement. Children who experience trauma are likely to have problems with "narrative coherence"—the ability to organize material into a beginning, a middle, and an end (Kongshøj & Berntsen, 2023). This inability to organize a linear story has direct repercussions on reading, writing, and communicative ability (Pynoos et al., 1996, p. 342).

Early childhood PTSD is marked by general personality traits that include mood instability, difficulty delaying gratification, withdrawal from or obsessive attention seeking, attention deficit and task completion problems, and oppositional defiance (Manly et al., 2001). Toddlers specifically demonstrate nonverbal attempts to communicate fears and anxiety: continuous crying, screaming tantrums, excessive clinging, immobility with trembling, frightened expressions, and either running toward the adult or aimless motion. Regression to thumb sucking, bed wetting, loss of bowel and bladder control, a variety of fears, night terrors, sleeping with a light on or an adult present, marked sensitivity to loud noises, speech difficulties, and eating problems may occur (Gordon et al., 1999). These symptoms are indicative of the effect survival-threatening stressors can have in rupturing the early attachment bonds that are so critical to development (Ford, 2009, p. 47).

Fears and anxiety continue to predominate in elementary school children, as do the previously mentioned regressive behaviors. School problems also emerge and range from outright refusal to go to school to poor academic performance, fighting, and loss of ability to concentrate (Gordon et al., 1999). Trauma may cause anxious attachment to caretakers and separation anxiety. The child regresses socially, which can result in poor affiliation with peers, social isolation, and avoidance of school. Parents may exacerbate this behavior because of their own unresolved fears of the traumatic event and may become overprotective of the child. Conversely, memories in which the primary caretaker was either unable or unwilling to provide help and succor during the traumatic event do severe harm to the developmental expectation that the caregiver is capable of providing nurturance and security (Kongshøj & Berntsen, 2023). A constellation of behavioral problems may appear, such as depression, panic and anxiety attacks, conduct and impulse control disorders, eating and sleep disorders, and sexual identity issues (Cook et al., 2005).

Adolescents who experience trauma invariably find disruption in their peer relationships and their school life. An et al. (2022) report a contributor to symptoms following a trauma is difficulty sleeping. Peers who were not traumatized may shun them because of their "weird" behavior and not know how to offer support. Any outward physical problems may exacerbate their fragile self-concept and ability to fit into the peer group. Behavioral trouble signs include withdrawal and isolation, antisocial behavior, awareness of their own mortality, suicidal ideation, academic failure, alcohol and drug misuse, sleep disturbance, night terrors, depression, mental confusion, school failure, truancy, problems with the legal system, gang involvement, teen pregnancy, and various physical complaints (Correia-Santos et al., 2023; Ford, 2017; Gušicwt et al., 2018; Kerig & Modrowski, 2018; Lau-Zhu et al., 2019).

Other Responses to Type I Trauma

Sense of a Foreshortened Future. Terr (1983) found that intrusive thoughts did not repeatedly enter the children's conscious thoughts; however, sleep brought very different problems. While a few reported daydreams, more children had nightmares through which ran many repetitive themes of death. The children believed these dreams to be highly predictive of the future and made comments such as "I'm 11 now, but I don't think I'll live very long, maybe 12, 'cause somebody will come along and shoot me." Adolescents in particular are brought face-to-face with their own vulnerability and, in the case of those who have experienced the murder of a parent, report that they will never marry or have children because they fear history will be repeated (Cohen et al., 2006, p. 9; Eth & Pynoos, 1985, p. 48; Terr, 1995, p. 308).

Reenactment. In an attempt to gain mastery over a Type I trauma, children replay the event and develop a reason or purpose for it. Once the reason is found, children often feel intensely guilty about it. "I should have listened to what Mom said and come home right after school!" In Type I traumas, the question is, "How could I have avoided that?" as opposed to the question of Type II traumas, "How will I avoid it the next time?" (Terr, 1995, p. 310).

The play of children with PTSD is very distinctive because of its thematic quality, longevity, dangerousness, intensity, contagiousness for siblings, and unconscious linkage to the traumatic event (Maclean, 1977; Terr, 1981). The clearly prevalent dynamic is a continuing reenactment of the children's plight during the trauma (Eth & Pynoos, 1985, p. 42). This thematic play can be characterized as burdened, constricted, and joyless (Wallerstein & Kelly, 1975). Traumatic play is also problematic because it replaces normal developmental play that is a vital component in childhood maturation (Parker & Gottman, 1989). For adolescents, reenactment may take the form of delinquent behavior (Eth & Pynoos, 1985, p. 47), ranging from truancy, sexual activity, and theft to reckless driving, drug misuse, and obtaining weapons (Newman, 1976).

Physical Responses. Approximately half the children in the Chowchilla kidnapping manifested physical problems that could be construed to be related to the trauma of being held prisoner without food, water, or bathroom access (Terr, 1983). In young children suffering from PTSD, regression may occur, and previously learned skills such as toilet training may have to be retaught (Bloch et al., 1956). Sleep disturbances and severe startle responses can cause a variety of educational and social problems in school (Pynoos et al., 1996, p. 350).

Displacement. In the Chowchilla survivors, a great deal of displacement of affect occurred, with emotions about the event being shifted to a related time, an associated idea, or another person—particularly the interviewing psychiatrist. Prior to the follow-up interviews, children displayed a variety of displaced behaviors, including the belief by one of the children that the psychiatrist had placed notes posing questions about the kidnapping in her school locker (Terr, 1983).

Transposition. Misperceptions, visual hallucinations, and peculiar time distortions often occur in children who have experienced Type I traumas—as opposed to Type II traumas, in which the perpetrators and events have a long history with the children and are rarely misperceived once the events are brought to awareness (Terr, 1995, p. 311). In the Chowchilla survivors, one of the most profound changes occurred in the transposition of events surrounding the trauma. Events that happened after the trauma were remembered as having happened before the trauma (Terr, 1983). Also, there was a general belief that the traumatic events were predictive of what was about to happen to them. Ayalon (1983), in a study of victims of terrorism, found a similar effect in children. Children attempted to resolve their vulnerability and lack of control by saying they should have listened to the omens and "shouldn't have stepped in the bad luck square." In PTSD, such distortions of time become part of the child's developing personality and are attempts to take personal responsibility and even feel guilty for events over which they had no control.

Terr's (1983) study indicates that while children behave differently from adults in their attempt to resolve the traumatic event, they are no more flexible or adaptable than adults after a trauma, and it would be erroneous to assume that they "just grow out of the event." Furthermore, these children did not become toughened by their experience but simply narrowed their sphere of influence in very restrictive ways to control their environment better.

Type II Traumas

Children who have suffered continued physical and sexual abuse and refugee children from war-torn countries are typical victims of Type II traumas. They are poster children for the affective dysregulation that goes with complex PTSD. Massive denial and psychic numbing are primarily associated with Type II traumas. These children avoid talking about themselves, go years without talking about their ordeals, and try to look as normal as they can. If they do tell their stories, they may later deny they did. This aspect is quite different from Type I children, who tell their stories over and over again. Denial may become so complete that Type II children will forget whole spans of their childhood (Terr, 1995, p. 312). Type II children are indifferent to pain, lack empathy, fail to define or acknowledge feelings, and absolutely avoid psychological intimacy. In adulthood, this massive denial cuts across narcissistic, antisocial, borderline, and avoidant personality disorders (Terr, 1995, p. 313). Although self-hypnosis and dissociation in Type II children may take the form of dissociation identity disorders (formerly known as multiple personality disorder) in adulthood, such children most often develop anesthesia to pain and to sex and emotionally distance themselves in the extreme (Terr, 1995, p. 314). That does not mean the rage at what happened to them is not there. Rage includes anger turned inward against the self and outward toward others and can range from self-mutilation to murder. Reenactments of anger occur so frequently in Type II traumas that habitual patterns of aggression are formed, and the seething anger is probably as debilitating as the chronic numbing. Paradoxically, defenses may be formed, whereby the child becomes completely passive or identifies with the aggressor (Terr, 1995, p. 315).

At times, crossover changes from Type I to Type II traumas may occur, as when a single event such as an accident that requires long-term hospitalization and many painful operations turns into a Type II trauma. Children who come out of Type I traumas with permanent physical disabilities such as traumatic brain injury, loss of a limb, long-term pain, or loss of significant others may be forced into adaptational techniques of Type II traumas but still retain clear and vivid memories of the event. Children who are physically injured or have permanent physical change and suffer psychic trauma tend to perpetually mourn their old selves and may employ regression, denial, guilt, shame, and rage over their disabilities (Terr, 1995, p. 316). When traumatic shock interferes with the normal course of bereavement, unresolved grief continues, and the child becomes a candidate for a major depressive disorder (Terr, 1995, pp. 316–317).

A variety of problems that have to do with how a traumatized child looks, acts, feels, and thinks may promote secondary stressors in their social milieu (Pynoos et al., 1996, p. 341). Communicable diseases, altered physical appearance, social distancing, memory impairment, decreased intellectual functioning, guilt, and shame are a few of the problems that can follow in the wake of a trauma. All these problems may present very different before-and-after pictures of the child and alter perceptions by family, peers, and teachers to the detriment of the child. These negative response patterns are then additive to the initial trauma and present additional psychological burdens to adaptation.

A third type of trauma, Type III, is proposed by Kira et al. (2023). These researchers report that continuous trauma has a different effect than a onetime trauma or repeated exposure to trauma. Type III traumas emerge from multiple stressors that are ongoing for an extended period. When these multiple stressors intersect, the trauma is different. Children and adolescents experiencing this intersection of trauma have a different reaction and develop more acute mental health and cognitive conditions. These researchers recommend that this new understanding of types of trauma should be a consideration for treatment.

Intervention Strategies

LO20 The methods of assessment and therapy used with children are different from those used for adults. Early assessment is critical in determining the potential for trauma (Terr, 1979, 1981, 1983) and should happen as soon as possible after the event (Mowbray, 1988, p. 206). Generally, assessment needs to occur in two complementary areas: trauma-specific issues and generic behavioral issues. While we are interested in isolating specific traumatic events and their effects, focusing on them may miss more general issues of depression or behavior problems.

Interviewing. There is some evidence that allowing children to talk about their experience in an interview format also helps in reducing long-term symptoms of PTSD (Nader, 1997, p. 293). However, parent resistance may be severe, and interviewers should carefully explain to both the parents and the child what the purpose of the interview is and how it is going to be done. Interviewing should involve determining the degree and severity of exposure to trauma and assessing the child's response as it relates to the degree of exposure (Pynoos & Nader, 1988).

Pynoos et al. (1996, pp. 336–337) suggest that more precise rather than general features of the traumatic experience be elicited, such as hearing unanswered screams for assistance, smelling bad odors, being close to the threat, being trapped, witnessing atrocities, and remembering the degree of brutality and other specific traumatic conditions. Given the targeting of what will probably be very traumatizing material, the crisis worker needs to proceed in as patient, caring, and empathic a way as possible.

Because children's reports may be affected by fear of disclosure, shame, guilt, and other negative attributions, it is also important to get corroboration from parents or other significant adults about the trauma.

Instruments. Because of the need to systematically measure the response of children to trauma, a number of instruments specifically designed for children have been developed. The Trauma Symptom Checklist for Young Children is a caregiver rating for children ages 3–12. It has validity scales and measures a variety of posttraumatic responses plus sexual concerns, anxiety, depression, dissociation, and anger/aggression (Briere, 2005). The Clinician-Administered PTSD Scale for Children (CAPS-C) (Nader et al., 1994) is a comprehensive children's version of the adult CAPS. It measures standard PTSD symptoms plus symptoms of childhood PTSD. It further determines social and scholastic functioning, along with how well the child is coping with the event. The Diagnostic Interview for Children and Adolescents–Revised (DICA-R; Reich et al., 1991) is a widely used semi-structured interview to assess common psychiatric diagnoses and includes a PTSD subscale. Briere (1996) has also developed a self-report checklist for children, which covers anxiety, depression, anger, posttraumatic stress, sexual concerns, and dissociation. It has an alternate form that leaves out sexual concerns. The Trauma Symptom Inventory (Briere, 1995) is useful for older adolescents who tend to act out their distress. It also has two validity scales that assess under- and over-endorsement in rating items. The Child PTSD Symptom Scale has been developed to assess the severity of PTSD in children exposed to trauma (Foa et al., 2001). The Child Behavior Checklist is a widely used scale that has parents, teacher, and youth self-report forms. This test looks at both external issues such as behavior problems and internal issues such as anxiety and depression, as well as how resilient children are at adapting to stressors (Achenbach, 1991). Finally, the University of California Los Angeles Reaction Index (Steinberg et al., 2004) is particularly noteworthy because it has reliability and validity across age, sex, race/ethnicity, and trauma variety (Steinberg et al., 2013).

Projective Techniques. Because children submerge their affect and parents are loath to deal with the trauma until it causes severe repercussions in their lives, children are rarely brought in for counseling until behavior has reached crisis proportions (Mowbray, 1988, p. 206). Triage assessment at this time may not reveal that trauma is the underlying agent. In that regard, the crisis worker who works with children should have a good knowledge of both projective and question-and-answer personality inventories that will ferret out the trauma. A classic example is the artwork of sexually abused children whose drawings are replete with exaggerated genitalia (Kaufman & Wohl, 1992).

Therapy

Treatment of PTSD directed specifically to children falls into two main categories: cognitive-behavioral therapy and play therapy. EMDR may also be used in combination with or exclusive of cognitive-behavioral or play therapy. Also of critical importance is building a caring and supportive social context pre-trauma and post-trauma (LaGreca et al., 2022).

Cognitive–Behavioral Therapy. There is a great deal of support for cognitive-behavioral therapy as the treatment of choice for children (Cohen et al., 2006; de Arellano et al., 2014; Herpertz-Dahlmann et al., 2005; Neubaueret et al., 2007; Webb et al., 2014). Although Saigh (1987) has reported success using flooding techniques with school-age children, it should be strongly emphasized that this is a *hazardous* procedure for children and may exacerbate symptoms. A more benign and controlled approach is the use of desensitization procedures that alternate between relaxing the child and presenting scenes of the trauma that are progressively enhanced to their full florid detail. This is a stepwise procedure that makes small approximations toward exposing the child to the total traumatic event. The key to this approach is that the child can be immediately removed from the noxious image and transferred to a safe, calm, tranquil scene.

Any cognitive-behavioral therapy should give the child a sense of empowerment and control. A key aspect using this approach is the therapeutic alliance (Ovenstad et al., 2020). Allowing children to generate the material generally promotes a stronger alliance and a more personalized therapeutic experience. Relaxation techniques, cognitive restructuring, stress inoculation, anger management, desensitization, and any other behavioral or cognitive-behavioral techniques should be paced *at the child's speed*. A good deal of discussion with the child and the caretakers about what is going to occur, how the child has the power and control over what will be included, and providing adequate time for processing, debriefing, and follow-up should all be a part of the therapeutic regimen (deArellano et al., 2014).

Play Therapy. Play is the child's work. Being able to play is at the central core of positive child development. However, the ability to do that must invariably have the support of reliable and nontoxic caregiving and parenting for that to occur. When children suffer chronic deprivation, abuse, or neglect with little positive parental support, there is no space, time, or permission to engage in curiosity and discovery through positive play (Tuber et al., 2014). When traumatized children play, it is not about the joy of social relationships or discovery of new and wonderful things but rather a reflection of the toxic trauma they have experienced. We believe, therefore, that play therapy is a primary therapeutic vehicle for removing that toxicity.

Creative arts and play therapy have considerable merit and can be efficacious with PTSD in children (Gordon et al., 1999; Johnson, 2000b; Malchiodi, 2008; Webb, 2007). Play therapy generally falls into two distinct categories: directive, which is collaborative and interactive between the child and the interventionist; and nondirective, which is child centered and interventionist passive. However, nondirective play therapy may be ill advised because **restitutive play** (attempting to reenact the trauma through play and somehow resolve it) becomes increasingly destructive and serves only to increase anxieties that are allowed to go ungoverned (Terr, 1979). We believe a safer approach to reenacting the trauma is to involve the interventionist collaboratively using a variety of play

therapy techniques (Gordon et al., 1999; Landreth, 1987; Malchiodi, 2008) that include artwork (Drucker, 2001; Loumeau-May, 2008), puppets (Carter, 1987; James & Myer, 1987), sand play (Allan & Berry, 1987; Bethel & Oates, 2007; Vinturella & James, 1987; Zarzaur, 2005), dance (Johnson, 2000a), poetry (Gladding, 1987), writing (Brand, 1987), music (Bowman, 1987; Hilliard, 2008), bibliotherapy (Malchiodi & Ginns-Gruenberg, 2008), computer art (Johnson, 1987), storytelling (White, 2005), and drama (Haen, 2008; Irwin, 1987), as well as drawing the traumatic event and telling a story about it (Chapman et al., 2001; Eth & Pynoos, 1985, p. 37; James, 2003; Schreier et al., 2005). Play therapy is also a nonthreatening way to involve parents in the therapeutic intervention with children who have had trauma exposure (Cattanach, 2008; Haen, 2008; Echterling & Stewart, 2008; Steele & Malchiodi, 2008). All these techniques may be controlled and paced by the therapist in consideration of the psychological safety of the child.

The overarching reason for any of the foregoing techniques is to take the global, nebulous, uncontrollable chaos of the crisis event and make it into a concrete, real object that the child can gain a sense of control over. Play therapy would seem efficacious because it enables the therapist to enter the trauma on the child's cognitive terms, reduce the threat of the trauma, establish trust, and determine the child's current means of coping and ways of defending against the trauma (Gumaer, 1984). Play therapy is a safe exposure technique that allows clients (including adults) to integrate their traumatic memories into active consciousness without the fear of reactivating the sensory trauma demons they are so afraid of letting resurface (Steele & Raider, 2001). Furthermore, as thematic trauma-related play subsides and more socially appropriate play reappears, this is an excellent assessment device for determining how well treatment is proceeding. We will examine three very different cases of how play therapy is used with children in Chapter 9, "Sexual Assault"; Chapter 13, "Crises in Schools"; and Chapter 16, "Disaster Response."

EMDR. EMDR seems to be effective with children in symptom reduction of PTSD (Adúriz et al., 2011; Oras et al., 2004; Shapiro & Brown, 2019). Shapiro (1995, pp. 276–281) indicates a number of special considerations for using EMDR, especially with young children. First, the worker must give special consideration to safety concerns. Although Shapiro does not believe parents should attend the session with the child, she does believe parents should brief the worker with the child present. Then, the parent should leave and allow the child to present their version. This two-step sequence allows the parents' authority to be transferred to the worker and also gives the child a sense of being special when the worker's attention is focused exclusively on them.

For children, average EMDR sessions should be no longer than 45 minutes, with eye movements interspersed with other activities. Because children do not have the cognitive ability to conceptualize SUDs units, more concrete representations of the degree of discomfort need to be devised. Holding a hand close to the floor can represent a "little" hurt, while holding a hand at shoulder height can represent a much "bigger" hurt. Because most children are familiar with the workings of a body thermometer, we have used pictorial representations of a thermometer to let children indicate how much discomfort they are feeling.

Because play is such an integral part of a child's world, eye exercises can be accomplished more easily by drawing puppets on the worker's fingers or using finger puppets to perform the saccades. Creativity in helping the child "bring up the picture" is important, so sound effects such as starting an engine or "blowing up the picture" with a loud explosion can involve the children at their experiential level. Installing new, positive cognitions needs to be simplified. "I'm fine" or "I'm safe" may be highly appropriate because of their simplicity and straightforwardness for young children.

Artwork may also be effective in helping to concretize the memory. Having the child draw the event and then hold the picture in their mind while eye exercises are conducted gives the child a concrete way of visualizing the memory. Shapiro (1995) reports that (much as in Gumaer's [1984] method of serial drawing to determine if treatment is effective) when the child is asked to redraw the event after successive eye movements, the intensity of the event as depicted in the drawings is likely to diminish.

Mindfulness. The use of mindfulness as treatment for PTSD and trauma has been gaining acceptance (West et al., 2017). Mindfulness focuses on ways to be and focus on the present (Tran et al. 2022). There are many ways to cultivate mindfulness, including mindfulness-based psychotherapy approaches (e.g., dialectical behavior therapy, acceptance and commitment therapy, mindfulness-based stress reduction, meditation training), all of which can be beneficial in the treatment of trauma. The goal of this approach is to focus on the present in a nonjudgmental manner (McCollum, 2015). Several studies have found this approach helps to reduce stress by creating awareness and nonjudgmental attitudes toward distress, which, in turn, may increase distress tolerance and reduce impulsivity (Somohano et al., 2022). This approach holds great promise for use with children who have experienced trauma (Bauer et al., 2019).

Final Words on the Case of Carlos

Before moving to the final words in this chapter, we want to describe the crisis intervention with Carlos. Carlos is the EMT who came to the local mental health center at the insistence of his wife, who accompanied him. The reason his wife stated for bringing him to get some help was that Carlos was not himself after responding to a horrific car accident in which a drunk driver slammed into a family's vehicle, killing all but one member of the family. After a brief conflict with the receptionist, the receptionist was able to arrange for Carlos to see a therapist immediately. Betty, the therapist, escorted Carlos to her office. Forty-five minutes has gone by since that contact. During that time, Betty used Providing Support and Allowing Catharsis to deescalate Carlos' reactions. At this point in the intervention process, Carlos' affective reaction is a 6, behavioral is a 5, and cognitive is a 6, with the overall rating at 17.

Betty: How are you doing Carlos?

Carlos: (Pause) Better I guess. I still can't get the picture out of my mind. Every time I see my daughters I think about what if they were in that car. Fuckin drunk driver, oh sorry I just get so mad and it is so pointless. Why did I have to be the first one on the scene?

Betty: I hear the anger and fear Carlos. We talked about that. Do you remember?

Carlos: Kind of, you said something about PTSD, but to be honest, I don't remember everything you said.

Betty: (Shakes her head positively) I don't expect you to remember everything. What do you remember?

Carlos: Hmmmmm. Something about why I get pissed off, I mean angry, sorry. And I am so protective. And, well, you want to talk with me some more.

Betty: Good Carlos. You remembered the important stuff. And I do think it would be good for us to meet again. I am here to help you understand everything that you have been thinking and feeling about the car accident.

Carlos: Yeah I guess, I just cannot seem to get it out of my head and all the worry.

Betty: Remember we talked about how that is not unusual. Many people have seen lots of terrible things you have. They go on with their lives, then one day, something snaps and it just is too much.

Carlos: Yea now that you say that I remember.

Betty: Remember I also said having your wife be with us sometimes when we talk will also help.

Carlos: (Smiles a little.) Yeah, she will like that I am sure.

Betty: Okay. Let's go out front and talk with the receptionist Gabriella and make an appointment for next week.

Betty uses the final minutes of the crisis intervention session to follow up and get a commitment from Carlos about continuing to talk with her. Notice that Carlos' emotions and thinking still are focused on the crisis event with only limited control. Carlos also is having difficulty remembering everything he and Betty discussed. That is not unusual for a person in crisis. That is the reason to follow up asking individuals in crisis to recall what was discussed. This follow up is critical in getting a commitment to carry out a plan. Betty accomplishes that very skillfully through reinforcing what Carlos did recall and also gently reminding him of other important aspects of the intervention. Carlos is now ready to move beyond the crisis and start working on making meaning out of what he has seen and his reaction to it.

Moving Beyond the Trauma

LO21 We understand that reading this long introductory chapter into the trench warfare of typical crisis events has been pretty grim and maybe even depressing. Therefore, we want to finish with what we believe is some light at the end of the tunnel. So don't give up! One way survivors move from the tightly wrapped intrapersonal world of agony they have lived in to a more self-actualized and healthy interpersonal focus is to use their experience to help other victims (Lifton, 1973, pp. 99–133). Review the exchange between two Vietnam veterans, one a volunteer and one a professional in the human services field:

Jim: I'm in the group not because of what happened in Nam. I'm pretty much through that. A year's worth of the VA and some excellent help from other people got me over being nuts. I'm here because I owe those folks and maybe, I'm not sure how, to pay some back for what I got.

George: Why did I become a social worker at the vet center? Because I'd been in Nam, hassled with my own stuff, and thought I knew something about it and could help other people. Frankly, I think I've done about all I can here, and I believe I'm ready to start something else professionally. I'm going back to school and would like to concentrate on working with kids.

For both of these men, the ghosts of PTSD have been exorcised. They have integrated all aspects of the traumatic experience, both the positive and the negative. They know pretty clearly who they were before, during, and after the event. They have accepted responsibility for their own actions, as imperfect as those actions may have been at the time, and have made atonement for any guilt they carried (Scurfield, 1985, p. 246). They epitomize the full meaning of the Chinese characters for *crisis* that represent both danger and opportunity. Yet, do these two tough and resilient combat veterans represent what really happens to people with PTSD? Do the Chinese characters really represent what happens to most people, or can they ever climb out of the sump hole of PTSD? Tedeschi and Calhoun (1995) believe so and have formulated the concept of posttraumatic growth to characterize the personal positive changes that can come out of individuals' struggle with trauma.

Their evolving model (Tedeschi & McNally, 2011) has five components: First, trauma survivors need to understand the negative aspects of PTSD, especially one's shaken assumptions about oneself, others, and the future. They should also understand that the physiological and psychological responses are *normal* reactions to traumatic experiences. (We take some exception to the use of the word *normal* as a way of toning down the very nasty responses people have to trauma. To our minds, there is nothing remotely "normal" about it. It is about as abnormal as one can get without becoming psychotic. Therefore, we prefer to use the term *common* to denote that it is anything but pleasant but is about what almost everybody can expect to happen.) However, challenges to one's core beliefs have been shown to strongly predict posttraumatic growth (Lindstrom et al., 2013).

Second, learning to gain emotional regulation over intrusive thoughts and images allows the sympathetic nervous system to calm down and let people start to engage in effective rumination over the trauma rather than brooding over it. Rumination occurs in two ways. **Autonomic/intrusive rumination** is the initial intrusion of unwanted thoughts that assails an individual after the trauma. **Deliberate rumination** is a process that issues out of a reflective state when a thorough reexamination of the traumatic event causes the individual to reframe their view of life and, in fact, grow from the experience (Su & Chen, 2015).

Third is constructive self-disclosure that does not harp on the trauma or its symptoms but, by telling the story to others, unravels the cognitive and emotional tangles that go with the trauma, forms new relationships and bonds, and reconciles the past with the deceased who may have been part of the original trauma. Calhoun and Tedeschi (1998) believe that social support is a critical component in allowing this process to occur.

Fourth is creating a trauma narrative out of self-disclosure that understands the paradoxes of how loss and gain, gaining control and giving up control, and vulnerability and strength are not mutually exclusive. By doing so, individuals begin to build new structures of their personality that are based on personal strength, enhanced relationships with others, spiritual change, appreciation of life, and zest for new opportunities.

Finally, Tedeschi and McNally (2011) propose that the end point (or the beginning, for that matter) is to reframe the trauma as a positive, life-transforming experience that involves becoming more charitable to oneself and others, accepting growth from the traumatic event without guilt, understanding that the experience has transformed oneself in ways others may not be able to comprehend, and becoming a person more in tune and empathic with the human condition and the spiritual aspects that go with it.

Studies are finding that people do indeed grow from traumatic experiences and that positive posttraumatic growth does occur and may even be underestimated (Fraus et al., 2023; Kramer et al., 2020; Wu et al., 2019). For those who have PTSD and for those who treat it, that is heartening research.

Summary

Posttraumatic stress disorder (PTSD) has probably been in existence as long as humankind has been rational enough to personalize the disasters that assail us. However, it was the debacle of the Vietnam War that brought PTSD enough publicity to become a classifiable malady. The psychologically virulent milieu that was the Vietnam War became a breeding ground for trauma, which found its way back to the United States in an estimated 960,000 service personnel who have PTSD or related disorders.

PTSD has multiple symptoms and, for that reason, is often confused with a variety of other disorders. Its basis is maladaptive adjustment to a traumatic event. The disorder is both acute and chronic. In its chronic form, it is insidious and may take months or years to appear. Its symptoms include, but are not limited to, anxiety, depression, substance misuse, hypervigilance, eating disorders, intrusive-repetitive thoughts, sleep disturbances, somatic problems, poor social relationships, suicidal ideation, and denial and affective numbing of the traumatic event. Both natural and human-made disasters may be responsible for PTSD, but it is far more likely to occur in individuals who have been exposed to some human-made disaster that should have been prevented and is beyond accepted moral and societal bounds.

Slow to recognize the disorder, human services professionals did little to ameliorate problems returning Vietnam veterans suffered. Self-help groups were started by veterans when they had no other place to turn. Through lobbying efforts by such men, Vietnam Veterans Centers were set up throughout the United States. Along with other mental health professionals who had been grappling with the problems of veterans and other victims of trauma, staffers at the centers began doing research and developing treatment approaches for PTSD. Those research and treatment approaches have spread out to civilian areas of trauma, and much common ground is being found between war-related and civilian-related traumatic events. Recent research on the psychobiological aspects of PTSD is uncovering a great deal of the intricate interplay between traumatic events and the brain's physiological responses to them. Contemporary treatment includes both group and individual intervention that is multimodal and considers psychological, biological, and social bases as equally important. The United States Army is currently putting in place a comprehensive program that attempts to provide psychological fitness to soldiers to inoculate them against PTSD and other emotional disorders that go with combat.

Children are not immune to PTSD, and they do not just "grow out of it." If PTSD has taught the human services one thing, it is that no traumatic experience should ever be dismissed in a cursory manner and that any initial assessment of a crisis client should investigate the possibility of a traumatic event buried somewhere in the client's past. Assessment and intervention are particularly difficult when the traumatic event is of a familial or sexual nature. A great deal of finesse and skill is necessary to uncover and treat such problems because of clients' reluctance to

talk about socially taboo subjects or the feeling that a person should have the intestinal fortitude to bear up under the trauma. From what we now know, the latter assumption is patently false; under the right circumstances, anyone can fall victim to PTSD.

There are three books we think can be helpful to you if you are going to get into or are already in the PTSD business. They are focused on the military but could surely be adapted for civilian use and are as follows: *Clinician's Guide to Treating Stress After War: Education and Coping Interventions for Veterans* (Whealin et al., 2008), *The Veterans and Active Duty Military Psychotherapy Treatment Planner* (Moore & Jongsma, 2009), and Curran's (2013) *101 Trauma-Informed Interventions*. These books have lots of useful tips and worksheets that can be adapted for use with most anyone who has PTSD.

Crisis of Lethality

8

Learning Objectives

After studying this chapter, you will be able to:

1. Describe the scope of suicide and its ramifications for crisis intervention.
2. Discuss the moral issues surrounding suicide and its impact on interventionist decision making and performance.
3. Explain different theories and models of why people complete suicide.
4. Identify the common characteristics of people who are concurrently suicidal and homicidal and their implications for practice.
5. Recognize the myths that surround suicide and their implications for practice.
6. Recognize warning signs and risk factors for suicide and their implications for practice.
7. Explain suicide intervention strategies and how they might be applied.
8. Describe how crisis management for suicide works and how it may be applied.
9. Recognize the "dos and don'ts" of suicide case management and their importance in practice.
10. Describe what a psychological autopsy is and why it is used.
11. Discuss the reasons for postvention after a completed suicide and why they are important.
12. Describe the crisis worker's own issues after losing a person to suicide and the importance of processing the loss.

Background

In crisis work, the possibility of dealing with suicidal and/or homicidal clients is always present. Thus, in Chapter 3, "The Intervention and Assessment Models," the importance of the crisis worker's continuous awareness and assessment of risk level for all clients in crisis was emphasized. In this chapter, strategies are presented to help crisis workers strengthen their skills in assessing, counseling for, intervening in, and preventing lethal behavior, with the major emphasis on suicide. While this chapter's focus on lethal behavior is mainly concerned with the intent to harm oneself, others may not be exempt from harm. Sometimes, an individual in crisis may be homicidal and target a specific victim or random victims. These homicides are not about the person who murders a shopkeeper in a holdup or the wife who kills her husband for insurance or to be able to marry another person. Those are **instrumental** acts of homicide that occur for some financial or other concrete gain. Rather, a suicidal/homicidal person in this chapter is one who is engaged in an **expressive** act of homicide that is designed to reduce psychological pain. Such suicidal/homicidal people are likely to be emotionally distraught, may feel gravely wronged, depressed, helpless, disempowered, and hopeless, and may attempt to solve their own dilemmas through harm to others and then to themselves.

According to Edwin Shneidman, the founder of suicidology, "Currently in the Western world, suicide is a conscious act of self-induced annihilation, best understood as a multidimensional malaise in a needful individual who defines an issue for which the suicide is perceived as the best solution" (Shneidman, 1999a, p. 155) and who falls into a category of intense and unendurable psychological pain that is caused by unfulfilled psychological needs (Shneidman, 2001, p. 203). To Shneidman's definition we would add "or the murder of significant others."

The Scope of the Suicide Crisis

LO1 As with other topics discussed in this book, suicide has its own exhaustive statistics. We are going to include a lot of demographic statistics to give you an idea of how widespread the issue is and what populations are most vulnerable. However, given all the huge numbers, you can be forgiven if your eyes glaze over. So, before we start, here's a pretty graphic statistic to get your attention. Let's say it takes you about an hour to speed-read through this chapter with snacks and text breaks. In that time, six people in the United States have purposefully died by suicide, which is about one person every eleven minutes. Not only that, but in 2020, 12.2 million people in the United States thought about death by suicide, 3.2 million took the time to plan on doing it, and 1.2 million attempted suicide (American Foundation for Suicide Prevention, 2022; Centers for Disease Control and Prevention [CDC, 2023]).

Ascertaining accurate suicide statistics is very challenging, and, as such, there are often differences between statistics reported by various agencies. Moreover, there are several factors that can lead to inaccurate suicide data. Many suicides are ruled accidental either because of political, religious, and emotional considerations or because medical examiners just can't say for sure what the cause of death was (Granello & Granello, 2007, pp. 3–5). Indeed, most official reports indicate that the real numbers of suicide attempts, as well as injuries caused by suicide attempts, are grossly underreported.

Suicide is a worldwide concern. According to the World Health Organization (WHO, 2021), the global suicide rate in 2019 was 703,000. Further, according to the WHO (2021), there were "more deaths due to suicide than to malaria, HIV/AIDS, breast cancer, or war and homicide" in 2019 (p. 1). For the period of 2000 through 2019, the highest suicide rates were found in Africa, followed by Europe, Southeast Asia, the Americas, the Western Pacific, and the Eastern Mediterranean regions, respectively (WHO, 2021). The suicide rates in Africa, Europe, and Southeast Asia exceed the global average suicide rate. Although the global suicide rate between 2000 and 2019 decreased overall, the Americas were the only region to experience an increase in suicides (WHO, 2021).

Until 2020, suicide ranked as a leading cause of death in the United States, and the rates of suicide had progressively increased in the prior 20 years (Hedegaard et al., 2021). In 2020, with the high rates of death due to COVID-19, suicide dropped from the top 10 leading causes of death nationwide (U.S.) in 2020 (Murphy et al., 2021). However, suicide is a significant public health concern. Each year in the United States, approximately 46,000 people take their own lives (Curtin et al., 2021). This statistic reflects a slight decline from previous years (Curtin et al., 2021). Nonetheless, this translates to approximately 4.9 percent (over 12 million people) of U.S. adults who report serious suicide ideation each year, based on self-report of adults ages 18 and older in 2020 (Substance Abuse and Mental Health Services Administration [SAMHSA], 2021). Drilling down to suicide plans and suicide attempts, one can observe even more distressing statistics. Again, referring to U.S. adults ages 18 and older in 2020, approximately 1.3 percent (over 3 million people) reported having a suicide plan and 0.5 percent (1.2 million people) reported a suicide attempt (SAMHSA, 2021, p. 35). In other words, lots of people think about suicide, some attempt it, and relatively few die by suicide, compared to the rates of suicide ideation and suicide attempts. Yet those "few" numbers are in the hundreds of thousands when taken worldwide, and the traumatic wake they leave for survivors numbers in the millions (McIntosh & Drapeau, 2014). Submerged in those statistics are certain at-risk groups.

Gender differences in suicide seem to trend globally. Worldwide, men tend to take their lives at approximately two to three times the rate of women (12.6 per 100,000 for males and 5.4 per 100,000 for females; WHO, 2021, p. 5). In the United States, men take their lives at approximately four times the rate of women (Curtin et al., 2021). Most data is still reported using binary gender categories and, as such, data is not yet widely available for individuals who do not identify as a male or female. However, some research points to a markedly elevated risk of suicidal thoughts and behaviors in transgender and gender diverse individuals (Cramer et al., 2022; Virupaksha et al., 2016). Moreover, the 2015 Transgender Survey, conducted by the National Center for Transgender Equality, indicated that approximately 40 percent of transgender respondents reported a lifetime suicide attempt (James et al., 2016). This particularly high suicide attempt rate might be attributed, in large part, to the experience of maltreatment across various life domains (e.g., rejection from family and/or faith-based supports, medical mistreatment, harassment and/or violence, unemployment, homelessness and/or housing discrimination, and mistreatment from law enforcement) and associated limited access to support and/or health care (James et al., 2016).

Suicide trends based on age group can vary across time and region. Based on worldwide data collected in 2019, it appears that suicide rates are highest among late adolescents and early adults, tapering down at middle adulthood (WHO, 2021). For the period of 2000 through 2019, the WHO (2021) reports that "suicide was the fourth leading cause of death in young people aged 15–29 years for both sexes, after road injury, tuberculosis and interpersonal violence" (p. 7). In the United States in 2020, 12 percent of adolescents ages 12 to 17 reported having "serious thoughts of suicide," 5.3 percent reported making a suicide plan, and 2.5 percent reported attempting suicide within the past year (SAMHSA, 2021, p. 36). In all age groups from 15 to 64, the suicide rate averages around 15 per 100,000 people, and the highest risk age group for U.S. males tends to be ages 25 to 34 (Curtin et al., 2021). However, suicide rates are also particularly high for adults ages 75 years and older (Centers for Disease Control and Prevention, 2023).

Data on racial and ethnic groups present some important patterns. The highest U.S. suicide rates tend to occur within the non-Hispanic American Indian or Alaska Native population, followed by the non-Hispanic White population (Curtin et al., 2021). Suicide rates among the Black and African American populations are similar to the suicide rates among the Hispanic population, which were approximately half that of the non-Hispanic White population (Curtin et al., 2021). In the United States, the non-Hispanic Asian population has the lowest reported suicide rate (Curtin et al., 2021), but no cultural group is immune to the impact of suicide. Based on the foregoing statistics, suicide is clearly a major public health issue and has resulted in

the birth of 988, the National Suicide and Crisis Lifeline that serves as a connector to local hotlines.

It is important to note, though, that not all individuals who experience suicidality are in crisis. For some individuals who contemplate suicide, the decision is made rationally (e.g., end-of-life planning, response to chronic pain and/or health issues) or the decision is made with deliberation and forethought (e.g., persistent mental illness, unescapable negative life condition).

It's pretty safe to say that no other chapter in this book has more written about it, more research done about it, more models and theories of why it occurs and what it actually is than this chapter on suicide. However, suicide rates continue to generally trend upward, despite various systematic efforts, suicide prevention training programs, and public outreach. In response to the continued struggle with suicide loss in the United States, the American Foundation for Suicide Prevention (AFSP) has introduced Project 2025, which they describe as "A nationwide initiative to reduce the annual rate of suicide in the United States 20 percent by 2025" (n.d.). To achieve this goal, the AFSP (n.d.) has identified four key areas of reform: (1) firearms and suicide prevention (mandating suicide prevention training for firearms ownership and teaching safe storage of firearms), (2) health care systems (working with primary health care providers to more effectively identify the signs of suicide risk and provide appropriate intervention), (3) emergency departments (incorporating suicide screening and appropriate "follow-up services" in EDs), and (4) corrections settings (improving psychoeducation on mental health and suicide prevention monitoring in corrections settings). Nationwide implementation of these initiatives will likely be a multigenerational task.

Suicide and the Moral Dilemma

LO2 Shneidman's (1980) quote from *Moby Dick*'s opening paragraph, a "damp, drizzly November in my soul," captures the essence of what most suicide is: a dreary, wintry storm of endless life-or-death debate. It is at times low, moaning, and incessant, and at other times howling and strident in its demands that consciousness must STOP! It is a titanic and reasoned argument that constantly questions and pleads against the continued struggle in the storm of life. It is into this wind-lashed, flat, frozen, forbidding wasteland of despair that the crisis interventionist enters. It is neither a simple nor a painless place to be.

If you are planning to become a mental health professional, the odds are about one in four that you will work with someone who is considering suicide (Granello & Granello, 2007, p. 1). Indeed, according to a meta-analysis conducted by Stene-Larsen and Renéflot (2019), approximately 31 percent of individuals who take their life were in contact with a mental health professional within the 12 months prior to their death. However, suicide prevention is not only about therapeutic intervention, but suicide prevention also includes psychoeducation about suicide, training suicide gatekeepers within the community, and sending the message that help is available.

In both prevention and intervention work, suicidal ideation and behavior raise complex moral, legal, ethical, and philosophical questions (Allam et al., 2022; Landy & Shah, 2022; Rottman et al., 2014), particularly for crisis interventionists (Fitzpatrick, 2022; Kanel, 2018; Myer et al., 2022), medical personnel (Ford et al., 2021; Pronk et al., 2021), and mental health providers (Calkins & Swetz, 2019; Kious & Battin, 2019). Indeed, cultural mores, religious and spiritual beliefs, and personal experiences of suicide can shape our values and beliefs about suicide. As Boedjarath (2022) states, "cultural practices and experiences are scripted and become tendencies in responsive behavior" (p. 181). Even the most well-intentioned professionals may inadvertently allow personal values and beliefs about suicide to skew their judgment, but self-awareness is the first line of defense for problematic value imposition.

To be sure, our ideas about suicide may not only affect our response to individuals who are suicidal, but they may also play a role when we experience desperation and suicidality. Phillips and Luth (2020) examined the social acceptability of suicide in the United States within the general population and found that the perceived acceptability of suicide was directly correlated to higher rates of suicide. They also found varying acceptance toward suicide based on the circumstances surrounding the suicide (e.g., "incurable disease," "tired of living," "family dishonor," and bankruptcy), the age of the individual who takes their life, and the age and gender of the respondent (Phillips & Luth, 2020, p. 421). Colucci and associates (2013) have examined the reasons why culture is of critical importance in understanding why suicide varies across borders, regions, and ethnicities. Their work pretty much substantiates why Chapter 2, "Culturally Effective Helping," in Crisis is important to know when dealing with suicide.

Now, compare your own philosophical view of death to what Everstine (1998, p. 15) has to say about various kinds of deaths: "Death by murder carries no stigma and is seen as a tragedy" (i.e., It is a criminal act, and somebody must pay). "Accidental death is fully condoned providing the person didn't do something stupid or careless" (i.e., It is a tragedy—unless they were bungee jumping or sky diving, then it was idiotic). "Death by natural causes and resistance to the end allows grieving without animosity" (i.e., It was a tragedy, but they lived a long, good life; or they were too young and heroic to the end). "Less forgivable is natural death by neglect or overindulgence" (i.e., The speeder had it coming; or what did he think drinking would do to his liver?). "The least forgivable death is suicide, for which there is little sympathy and no absolution" (i.e., A sin! A moral flaw! A character deficit! Not up to the task of living).

While in Eastern culture, suicide may be seen as a way of removing dishonor, shame, and humiliation from oneself and one's family (Granello & Granello, 2007, p. 17), that has not been so in the Western world. Historically, suicide has been seen as a sin by almost every major religion. It has been seen by civil authority as an abrogation of the citizen's contract to serve the state and for a long time was called "self-murder." "Self-murder" was often blamed on the instigation of the devil. In the Middle Ages in England, self-murder was an offense against the king and nature, and all of the deceased's lands and goods were forfeit to the crown. Indeed, it was not until 1961 that the common law of felony self-murder was repealed in England. Further, a Christian burial was denied, and people who died by suicide were often buried in the middle of a crossroads with a stake driven through the heart (Williams, 1997, p. 12). (The reason for the middle of the crossroads is rumored to be that horses and ox carts would stop at a crossroad and animals would relieve themselves there).

Euthanasia

Counterpointed against suicide as an act of the devil has been the notion from the Stoic and Epicurean philosophers that suicide could be the right thing to do given terminal illness, unremitting pain, and/or astronomical financial burdens (Williams, 1997, p. 12). Beginning in the latter half of the 20th century, much attention has been paid to **assisted suicide** and **euthanasia** in both the literature and the popular media. The two terms are not synonymous. Stone (1999, pp. 76–89) differentiates between the two by pointing out that in **assisted suicide**, someone else provides the means (lethal agent), but the person who is dying administers it. In **euthanasia**, someone else administers it.

We live in a time characterized by what Stone (1999, p. 77) calls "prolonged dying." Prior to the 20th century, people typically died fairly young and fairly quickly at home. They generally died as a result of infectious diseases or injury. Consider that in comparison to the average lifespan in the United States in 2021, which was 76.4 years (Xu et al., 2022). The lifespan dipped slightly following the onset of the COVID-19 pandemic (Xu et al., 2022). And, not surprisingly, COVID-19 became the third leading cause of death in the United States in 2020 and 2021 behind heart disease and cancer (Xu et al., 2022). Today, a large portion of adults will die in an institution, such as a hospital or nursing home, and probably as a result of a medical condition. Our deaths may be prolonged, painful, and financially draining for ourselves, our families, and society. Do we have a right to refuse medical treatment, to refuse heroic or artificial interventions to keep us alive when there is no hope of getting better or even of survival? Further, should a mental health professional intervene when it is clear that a person wishes to die to end suffering? Every facet of these questions must be examined by our society as we confront the changing human conditions and health care problems in this new millennium (Stone, 1999, pp. 76–82). However, in this chapter, the position is that it is the appropriate role of the crisis worker to intervene and attempt to prevent all suicides and homicides to the degree possible.

The Dynamics of Suicide

Psychological Theories

LO3 There are various ways to conceptualize the pathway toward suicide and suicide crises. Therein lies the problem because suicide cannot be encapsulated into a singular theory or model; indeed, suicidality is a complex phenomenon, and the following theories and models are the field's attempts to come to grips with that complexity. See which ones seems to best fit your thoughts on the matter.

Freudian Inward Aggression. In the Freudian (1916) psychodynamic view, suicide is triggered by an intrapsychic conflict that emerges when a person experiences great psychological stress. Sometimes, such stress emerges either as a regression to a more primitive ego state or as an inhibition of one's hostility toward other people or toward society so that one's aggressive feelings are turned inward toward the self. Freud called this a melancholic state, and it is what we now call depression. In extreme cases, the melancholy becomes so severe that self-destruction or self-punishment is chosen over urges to lash out at others.

Developmental. Developmental psychology views suicide in terms of life stages. Individuals who do not successfully navigate life stages become mistrustful, guilt ridden, isolated, and stagnant (Erikson, 1963) until they are unable to cope any longer and may choose suicide as a way out.

Deficiencies. This model is embedded in the mental illness tradition and proposes that there is some mental deficiency in the suicidal individual compared to the nonsuicidal person. These mental deficiencies then become risk factors that can lead to suicide (Rogers, 2001a). From this perspective, various factors may be conceptualized as "deficiencies," (e.g., pervasive mood disorders and/or anxiety disorders, difficulty coping) although modern practitioners would certainly rebuke such conceptualizations and, instead, view the clients' experiences through the lens of established mental health diagnoses.

Escape. Escapist suicide is one of flight from a situation sensed by the person as intolerable (Baumeister, 1990). This theory has a six-step causal chain. The first step involves individuals' beliefs that they fall short of their own or others' imposed standards. Second, self-blame occurs for falling short, and a heightened state of awareness as to those shortcomings occurs in the third step. Negative affect follows as a fourth step. The result is cognitive disintegration that becomes more narrowly focused on deficits to the exclusion of broader, more integrative, aspects of self until the only option is suicide. Closely allied to escape theory is the concept of perfectionism, where less than perfect behavior becomes less and less tolerable, amplifies hopelessness, psychache, and the risk of suicide (Gordon et al., 2014).

Hopelessness. The hopelessness theory (Abramson et al., 2000) posits that some individuals believe that highly desired outcomes will not occur, or that highly aversive outcomes will occur and that there is nothing they can do to change the situation. Hopelessness represents a key cognitive vulnerability for suicide risk. The only escape is death. Beck's (Beck et al., 1979) cognitive triad of negative thoughts about self, the world, and the future are at the heart of hopelessness.

Psychache. Psychache is a term coined by the founder of suicidology, Edwin Shneidman (1993). Shneidman's (1987) **cubic model** combines psychache, **perturbation** (how disturbed one is and degree of pain), and **press** (stress increased due to more negative factors piling up). When all three are combined, they create the critical mass necessary to activate a suicide. While it's hard to define behaviorally, it's about the most impactful word Shneidman could have thought up to describe what most people with suicidal ideation are going through. **Psychache** refers to the hurt, anguish, soreness, and aching pain of the psyche or mind. It may have to do with guilt, shame, fear of growing old, love lost, or any debilitating cognition or affect. Intolerable psychological pain is the one variable that relates to all suicides. Psychache is tied to frustrated, blocked, and thwarted psychological needs. Suicide thus serves to eliminate the tension related to those blocked needs (Shneidman, 2001). As psychache increases, perturbation increases as well, and the need-press to end it all becomes severe.

Sociological Theory

Durkheim's Social Integration. The most important sociological theory about suicide was originally proposed in 1897 by Emile Durkheim and still holds as the top sociological theory more than a century later. In Durkheim's (1897/1951) approach, societal integration (the degree to which people are bound together in social networks) and social regulation (the degree to which the individual's desires and emotions are regulated by societal norms and customs) are major determinants of suicidal behavior. Durkheim identified four types of suicide: egoistic, anomic, altruistic, and fatalistic (pp. 152–176).

Egoistic, Anomic, Altruistic, and Fatalistic Suicide. Egoistic suicide is related to one's lack of integration or identification with a group. **Anomic** suicide arises from a perceived or real breakdown in the norms of society, such as the financial and economic ruin of the Great Depression. **Altruistic** suicide is related to perceived or real social solidarity, such as the traditional Japanese *hara-kiri* or, to put it in a current context, the suicide attacks by members of Middle Eastern extremist groups. **Fatalistic** suicide occurs when a person sees no way out of an intolerable or oppressive situation, such as being confined in a concentration camp. Although multiple differences exist for incarcerated individuals compared to individuals confined in a concentration camp, the fatalistic perspective may account for some degree of the elevated risk for suicide experienced by incarcerated individuals.

Suicide Trajectory Model. This model considers the total constellation of risk factors: biological (substance misuse, being assigned male at birth, genetic predisposition to depression); psychological (low self-concept, hopelessness, borderline personality disorder); cognitive (rigid, dogmatic, irrational, black-and-white, all-or-none thinking); and environmental (access to firearms, high-stress occupations, loss, family and job stressors). The more these factors are present and pile up, the greater the potential for suicide (Stillion & McDowell, 1996).

Three Element Model. The three elements composing this model are predisposing factors such as drug misuse and mental illness and potentiating factors ranging from family history to romantic and occupational loses to whether one has easy access to weapons. When enough predisposing and potentiating components are mixed together, over time, at some point, a critical mass is created, and a threshold into suicidal ideation and behavior is crossed (Westefeld et al., 2000).

Interpersonal–Psychological Theory. According to Joiner (2007), two interpersonal states, lack of belongingness and the feeling of burdensomeness, are primary motivators in the need to complete suicide. When combined with the acquired capability to act upon one's suicide thoughts, this triad signifies those who are most at risk for suicide. Thwarted belongingness is manifested by loneliness and the absence of positive, reciprocal relationships, and burdensomeness is the perception that one is a burden on significant others who will be better off if the individual is dead. Further, one may overcome the natural fear of pain and acquire a capability toward suicide, or a *fearlessness* of pain or death, through a variety of means, such as previous suicide attempts, non-suicidal self-injury, repetitive fighting, frequent accidents, and high-risk work environments.

Self-injury, in particular, has garnered increasing attention as a possible mechanism through which one may acquire a capability for suicide (Huang et al., 2020; Smith et al., 2010; Willoughby et al., 2015).

According to the International Society for the Study of Self-Injury (n.d.), nonsuicidal self-injury is defined as "the deliberate, self-directed damage of body tissue without suicidal intent and for purposes not socially or culturally sanctioned."

This seemingly simplistic, straightforward statement ties neatly into three central components of interpersonal theory. First and foremost, people acquire suicidal capability by decreasing their innate fear of death by habituating themselves to the fear and pain of self-injury. Second, they perceive burdensomeness to others to the extent that they are so flawed or defective they are beyond repair. They see themselves as such a millstone for themselves, their family, or society that everyone will be better off as a result of their death. Third, failed belongingness means that the person has no perceived attachments or value to any other member of society. The theory proposes that while many people consider completing suicide, and large numbers develop the capability, relatively few actually do so because all three factors must be present concurrently to create the critical mass necessary for the suicide act to occur (Joiner, 2007). Interestingly, an ancillary component of this theory is that those whose job entails exposure to others' pain will, themselves, have higher suicide rates than others because of vicariously experiencing others' pain and, thus, habituating themselves to it. Indeed, there is a fair amount of research that supports this theory (Hill & Pettit, 2014).

Existential–Constructivist Framework. The existentialist side of the framework comes from Yalom's (1980) work on human pathology and involves what he believes are the four corner posts of existence: (1) *death,* which is unavoidable; (2) *existential isolation,* which means that each of us enters existence alone and leaves it alone; (3) *meaninglessness,* our attempt to make sense out of a universe that is beyond knowing; and (4) *freedom,* the absence of external structure, which means that each person is responsible for making choices, taking actions, and enjoying or suffering the consequences of those decisions.

On the other side of the frame, constructivism views death, existential isolation, and meaninglessness as the principal ingredients that provide the motivation for meaning-making activities central to human life (Neimeyer & Mahoney, 1995). As individuals construct their view of self, others, and their relationships, they also construct a worldview where they encounter environmental challenges to which they have to respond.

They essentially have three options in response to these challenges. They can retain their original constructions, alter them to build new constructions, or decide that neither response is viable nor consider suicide as a final construct. This final construct occurs because trigger events that come from suicide trajectory risk factors (Stillion & McDowell, 1996) combine to form the critical mass that allows the individual to construct a worldview that it is a better choice to no longer view the world at all (Rogers, 2001b). A study of suicide notes' motivational components (Rogers et al., 2007) supports the existential-constructivist model of suicide. The researchers found that suicide notes contained relational, spiritual, somatic, and psychological motivators that are the primary motivational components of the existential-constructivist model.

Other Explanations

Accident. Not all people who take their life truly want to die; ambivalence about living and dying may well be implicated in some deaths that may otherwise be considered accidental (Bergmans et al., 2017). Although, by conducting a psychological autopsy, it may be possible to discern accidents from suicide with some measure of accuracy (Freuchen et al., 2012). Problematically, the high rates of death by accident (National Center for Health Statistics & Heron, 2021) leave a lot of room for error in determining the intent behind some deaths by accident. This may be particularly true for impulsive acts, wherein suicide warning signs and/or suicide planning may not have been present. Additionally, in some cases, unintentional severe self-injury may result in death, although the intent may not have been suicidal in nature. According to Muller et al. (2020), unintentional severe self-injury may occur when very high levels of negative affect are present, coupled with a sense of loss of control and the use of unfamiliar self-injurious methods.

Neurochemical or Neurophysiological Malfunction. This theory proposes that neurochemical imbalances or neurophysiological malfunction are primary underlying causes of suicidal behavior (Jackson & Jabbi, 2022). Because some affective responses are shared by common neural pathways and affected by common neurochemistry, it is difficult to separate out distinct emotional reactions that are overtly linked to suicide, such as depression, from other emotions, such as anger. In fact, research suggests that anger/aggression and depression are closely implicated in suicide (Popova et al., 2022; Weniger et al., 2017), and emerging research points to the particularly important role of anger in suicide (Naifeh et al., 2021; Schafer et al., 2022; Wilson et al., 2016; Yarar et al., 2023). Often, though, anger may be a response to various life events, such as trauma (Naifeh et al., 2021; Yarar et al., 2023), or injury, such as traumatic brain injury (Wilks et al., 2019). As such, it can be difficult to discern a neurochemical or neurophysiological foundation as the cause/source of anger versus an environmental response to overwhelming life stressors.

However, Bongard and Sullivan (2013, p. 31) report that, over the last thirty years, research demonstrates that neurochemical changes seem to be highly correlated with attempted and completed suicides. In fact, Liu et al. (2023) found that individuals who have a mental illness and who attempt suicide tend to display abnormal "social decision-making" (p. 11). The researchers also found evidence to suggest that "P2, theta-gamma PAC, and beta-gamma PAC may be neuro-electrophysiological biomarkers associated with decision making" (Liu et al., 2023). There is evidence of the role of 5-HT receptors in aggression, depression, and suicide (Popova et al., 2022), and some research points to the role of cortisol levels in suicidality (Akan et al., 2021). While these biological differences may be correlates and not causes of suicide, evidence continues to mount that they do play a role in suicidality.

Chaos. Chaos theory proposes that, paradoxically, unpredictable behavior can occur within predictable systems. Relatively minor environmental events may lead to suicidal behavior or not within the same individual at different points in time (Rogers, 2001a), while major ecosystem events such as financial depressions can do the same.

Dying With Dignity/Rational Suicide. This type of suicide is typified by a person rationally choosing death in the face of a painful, decimating, and incurable illness or some other major calamity that has no foreseeable positive outcome (Balasubramaniam, 2018; Gramaglia et al., 2019; Pronk et al., 2021). The person has further considered the impact on others and found the action to be more beneficial than harmful. As a result, the person makes a reasoned decision to end their life (Gramaglia et al., 2019).

Ecological/Integrative. In seeking to understand suicide, an ecosystemic/integrative theory takes into account that the painful intrapsychic factors within the individual interact with negative interpersonal and societal issues on multiple systemic levels (Leenaars, 1996, 2004; Potter, 2001). Leenaars (2004) proposes that, while a person may be highly perturbed and suffer a great deal of psychic pain, lethality must be present for the person to complete suicide. An ecological/integrative theory proposes that both perturbation and lethality, and the resultant contemplation of suicide, can only result from a complex interaction of all these environmental variables with the individual (Potter, 2001).

Interactional. Everstine's (1998) interactional view of suicide is in direct contrast to Freud's and Durkheim's. Everstine proposes that suicide is not fomented by anger turned inward or social isolation but by an external rage toward another. It is not at all passive toward the significant other but is highly aggressive and has a "get even" attitude and revenge as its goal. The suicidal person's hatred and desire to punish is so consuming that the aggrieved one's life or a significant other's life is used as a weapon against the hated other person. The hope is that the survivors have the albatross of guilt over the suicide or homicide hung around their own necks forever.

Ludic. Ludic suicides (Baechler, 1979) relate to the desire to experience an ordeal or a way to prove oneself in gamesmanship. Perhaps the ultimate such game of proving oneself is Russian roulette. Any communal rite of passage in which death may be an outcome could be considered a ludic suicide.

Oblative. Oblative suicides (Baechler, 1979) are those that are sacrificial in nature and seen to transfigure one to a higher, transcendental plane. Buddhist monks who set themselves on fire and the LSD user who "wants to meet God personally" and overdoses on a smorgasbord of drugs fall into this category.

Overlap Model. The overlap model includes a lack of social support; a biological propensity to suicide; the presence of psychiatric disorders; personality issues such as impulsivity, hostility, and depression; and a family history of suicide. The more these areas overlap, the greater the potential for suicide (Blumenthal & Kupfer, 1986).

Parasuicide. **Parasuicide** (closely resembling suicide) involves intentional acts which, although not directly lethal, can habituate persons to the pain necessary to kill themselves by inflicting **hesitation wounds** (the idea that it is extremely difficult to kill oneself and people hesitate in their initial attempts to complete the act (Joiner et al., 2009, p. 8). Clients may also engage in self-injurious behavior, such as cutting or burning their bodies to reconnect to reality from a dissociative state. Or, they may indirectly set themselves up to harm themselves by engaging in risky and/or impulsive behavior, such as abusing alcohol, driving too fast, combining the two, or engaging in other risky, daredevil behaviors (Jobes, 2006, p. 90). Any one of these acts may end up with the person dead, injured, disabled, or with other permanent indicators of their distress.

Suicide by Cop. More a method than a theory or model, suicide by cop (as described in Chapter 5) occurs when distraught people get the police to kill them by engaging in a threatening act toward the police or someone else, such as in a hostage situation. It is an **indirect** suicide in which suicidal persons may not have the courage to kill themselves, or they seek to publicize their deaths through the media by "going out in a blaze of glory." Suicide by cop is now so common that many cases get a coroner's verdict of **suicide by legal intervention** (Lindsay & Lester, 2004; Miller, 2006).

So, what do you make of all these models? At various times, each of these models has had its moments of stardom, then, like pop hit tunes and their genres, have faded into "oldies but goodies" with die hard adherents supporting them to the exclusion of any other explanations. Our own belief is that the devil is in the details. That is to say, that each individual follows their own idiosyncratic path to suicide, which might fit well into any of or in combination with the foregoing models.

Characteristics of People Who Complete Suicide

LO4 What is it about a person's inner dynamics that may make suicide or expressive homicide seem sensible? Shneidman formulated 10 common characteristics present in an individual who dies by suicide. His characteristics are grouped under six aspects (1985, pp. 121–149; italics added throughout):

1. **Situational characteristics:** (1) "The common *stimulus* in suicide is unendurable psychological pain" (p. 124); and (2) "The common *stressor* in suicide is frustrated psychological needs" (p. 126).

2. **Motivational characteristics:** (1) "The common *purpose* of suicide is to seek solution" (p. 129); (2) "The common *goal* of suicide is cessation of consciousness" (p. 129).

3. **Affective characteristics:** "The common *emotions* in suicide are hopelessness and helplessness" (p. 131).

4. **Cognitive characteristics:** (1) "The common *cognitive state* in suicide is ambivalence between doing it and wanting to be rescued" (p. 135); (2) "The common *perception* is of constriction such that one's options become very narrow and the world is seen through tunnel vision so that no alternative thoughts can emerge" (p. 138).

5. **Relational characteristics:** (1) "The common *interpersonal act* in suicide is communication of intention" (letting another person know that one's decision makes sense) (p. 143); and (2) "The common *action* in suicide is egression" (the right to exit or go out as one wishes, or the right to autonomously find a way out of one's pain) (p. 144).

6. **Serial characteristic:** "The common *consistency* in suicide is with lifelong coping patterns when deep perturbation, distress, threat, and psychological pain are present" (p. 147).

This list of characteristics points us toward what makes sense to the individual about to embark on suicide. It is not meant to suggest that all suicides are alike. In using the word "common," Shneidman reminds us that suicides, taken together, do reflect similarities. However, he is also careful to note that each suicide is idiosyncratic and that there are no absolutes or universals (1985, pp. 121–122).

Overarching these characteristics and common to all suicides is the individual's sense of perturbation and degree of lethality (Shneidman, 1999a). *Perturbation* is the degree to which the individual is upset. Perturbation by itself does not lead to suicide. Many of us are upset by events, people, and things a great deal of the time, but we get over being upset. However, when perturbation is combined with how oriented the person is toward death, the lethality level rises, and the person becomes more prone to suicide or homicide.

Similarities Between Suicide and Homicide

LO5 Often, the person who is homicidal is often suicidal (Basocak et al., 2021; Capellan et al., 2023; Fridel & Zimmerman, 2019; Lankford et al., 2021). However, there is debate among researchers regarding whether or not other-aggression/homicide (Fridel & Zimmerman, 2019) or self-aggression/suicide

(Lankford et al., 2021) is the primary motivator. As such, there may also be an increased risk for homicide in those who are suicidal (O'Donnell et al., 2015). Furnes et al. (2020) found that approximately 12 percent of their sample of acute psychiatric Norwegian inpatients demonstrated signs of cooccurring suicidality and homicidality. There may be large differences in risk factors between mass shooters (Capellan et al., 2023) and individuals who murder within their family system (Rouchy et al., 2020), although a history of violent behavior (Fridel & Zimmerman, 2019), legal issues (Rouchy et al., 2020), and trauma (Rouchy et al., 2020) tend to be common to both those who are suicidal and those who are homicidal.

There is a thin line between murder and suicide as an expressive act. According to Everstine (1998, p. 103), suicide is often intended to take the place of homicide and brand the intended victim as the person who is really responsible for the suicide. Given the right circumstances, the choice of homicide or suicide or both may tilt in either or both directions. The major problem is predicting when either will happen because lethal behavior is internally generated and highly idiosyncratic. Thus, it is not easy for an external observer to ascertain or predict when the individual's thoughts cross a threshold to action (Pridemore & Water, 2013).

Analyzing Suicide/Homicide Notes

Suicide/homicide notes can provide valuable information, but they do not necessarily provide an open pathway to understanding suicidal/homicidal intention. Contrary to popular opinion, suicide notes are not commonly left. Only approximately 18 percent of individuals who die by suicide leave notes (Cerel et al., 2015). Suicide/homicide notes may generally be characterized by their dichotomous (black-and-white) logic, hostility, and self-blame. Interestingly, there tends to be less evidence of how one is thinking and much more about how one is feeling. Although suicide notes tend to differ by gender, there are some common elements that tend to emerge in suicide notes. Often, writers beg for forgiveness (Mejías-Martín et al., 2023), discuss their unbearable distress (Mejías-Martín et al., 2023) or mental illness (Furqan et al., 2019), address their desire to not be a burden to others (Fernández-Cabana et al., 2015; Mejías-Martín et al., 2023), describe their self-dislike (Synnott et al., 2018), and talk about their lack of belonging or feelings of aloneness (Fernández-Cabana et al., 2015).

Interestingly, Synnott et al. (2018) found that individuals who die by suicide are more likely to mention concepts related to religion (i.e., "God, a Heaven or a Hell, or an afterlife") than individuals who survived a suicide attempt (p. 775). This finding is counter to the common assumption that religiosity might be a protective factor against suicide. It is challenging to generalize the thought processes and emotional experiences that bring someone to suicide. The available information is based on individuals who survive a suicide attempt and those who leave a suicide note, but the decision making for those who die by suicide and do not leave a note remains unclear.

What suicide notes indicate over and over are the idiosyncratic reasons for the suicides and the tunneled, constricted view that there is absolutely no other way out. Paradoxically, while suicide notes are rather barren in themselves, when they are put into context with a detailed life history of the individual, they can tell us a great deal about why the individual took their own life (Shneidman, 1999c). An examination of the following suicide/homicide note graphically illustrates what Shneidman's (1973) research into suicide notes has uncovered.

An Analysis of Seung-hui Cho. Seung-hui Cho, a student at Virginia Polytechnic Institute and State University, killed 32 people, wounded 14 more, and then took his own life on the Virginia Tech campus. His "note," in the form of a videotape he sent to NBC News, certainly gives a description of him that fits well into Shneidman's (1985) typology of the classic suicidal person who crosses through a psychological door into becoming homicidal as well. Here, again, are Shneidman's characteristics, supported by Cho's videotaped statements as excerpted from the *Memphis Commercial Appeal*, April 19, 2007 (Apuzzo, 2007):

1. *Situational characteristics* of unendurable pain: "You have vandalized my heart and raped my soul." His needs are frustrated: "You forced me in a corner."

2. *Motivational characteristics* directed toward ending his emotional problems and becoming a martyr for all the weak and disenfranchised: "You thought it was one weak boy you were extinguishing. Thanks to you, I die like Jesus Christ to inspire generations of the weak and defenseless."

3. *Affective characteristics* of hopelessness, helplessness, and abandonment: "You loved to crucify me. You loved inducing cancer in my head, terror in my heart, and ripping my soul all this time."

4. *Cognitive characteristics* indicated in his previous history of psychotic behavior and by his tunnel vision

of an unjust world, with logic-tight compartments of being persecuted by the rich: "Your Mercedes wasn't enough, you brats. Golden necklaces weren't enough, you snobs." Collectively, such statements mark him as a person with paranoid schizophrenia and extremely dangerous to both himself and others.

5. *Relational characteristics* marked by his communication of intention, stating why his rampage across the campus makes absolute sense: "You had a hundred billion chances, but forced me into a corner and gave me no option."

6. *Serial characteristic* discerned in a long history of difficulty in coping, of being different, and of being bullied (refer to Chapter 13, "Crises in Schools"). The intended victims are those "who had everything and spit on my face and shoved trash down my throat."

The continuing and unendurable *psychache* (Shneidman, 1993) Cho felt and verbalized in the foregoing statements propelled him toward an *egoistic* (Durkheim, 1897/1951) suicidal/homicidal rampage. His alienation, along with a lack of integration into and identification with the group, was both chronic and acute. His isolation and aloneness, manifest in the videotape, were profound, and he brooded over real and imagined injustices he had suffered that caused him "to be humiliated and be impaled upon a cross to bleed to death for your amusement."

At some point, his egoistic suicidal impulses transgress a psychological line to move into Everstine's (1998) *interactional* model of suicide. As with other mass murderers, Cho's depression and pent-up anger turn inside out in a classic Freudian dynamic example of the suicidal and homicidal person (Freud, 1916). At that point, the paranoid rage he feels explodes outward and focuses externally on others who have persecuted him. When that occurs, and blame is externalized, Seung-hui Cho becomes a candidate to commit mass murder on that large, amorphous mass of his tormentors. Why is this so? To the survivors, it makes no sense and is the very essence of *chaos* theory (Rogers, 2001a) at work. To Seung-hui Cho, with malice and coldness aforethought, it makes perfect sense to end his pain and air his narcissistic grievances to the world. Why? His martyr-like rationalization to justify his act is: "If not for me, for my children and my brothers and sisters . . . I did it for them." But finally, the real reason very simply is, "I had to."

Myths About Suicide

LO6 There are a good many commonly held myths about suicide (Berman & Silverman, 2022; Joiner, 2010; Nicholas et al., 2020) that the crisis worker should know and take into account when assessing potentially suicidal clients. Some of the myths are as follows:

1. **Discussing suicide will cause the client to move toward doing it.** The opposite is generally true. Discussing suicide with an empathic person will more likely provide the client with a sense of relief and a desire to buy time to regain control.

2. **Clients who threaten suicide don't do it.** A large percentage of people who kill themselves have previously threatened it or disclosed their intent to others. In fact, many individuals who take their life have recently been seen by a medical professional with complaints associated with the heightened suicide risk (e.g., depression and anxiety and the associated symptomatology; Kammer et al., 2021).

3. **Suicide is an irrational act.** Nearly all suicides and suicide attempts make *perfect sense* when viewed from the perspective of the people doing them. Granted, individuals who are in suicide crisis may not be thinking with the same level of clarity as usual, but the line of reasoning makes sense to them. We sometimes refer to this as "suicide tunnel vision," in which individuals are in pain and so desperately want the pain to end that suicide seems to be the only viable option. From an external lens, others may not see the logic and may attempt to refute the suicidal individual's logic, but the point is that suicide often seems reasonable to the person who is suffering.

4. **People who complete suicide are insane.** There is evidence of a high degree of association between mental illness and suicide, particularly with chronic depression (Cybulski et al., 2022; Ielmini et al., 2022; Li et al., 2020), post-traumatic stress symptoms (Bentley et al., 2016; Saulnier et al., 2023), and substance use (Pereira–Morales et al., 2017; Ramos Silva & Pucci, 2021). There are mixed perspectives on the role of anxiety in suicidality (Bentley et al., 2016; Coryell et al., 2019; Ramos Silva & Pucci, 2021), However, most suicidal people do not necessarily have a prior psychiatric diagnosis, but are acutely depressed, lonely, hopeless, helpless, newly

aggrieved, shocked, deeply disappointed, jilted, or otherwise overcome by some emotionally charged situation.

5. **Suicide runs in families—it is an inherited tendency.** This may or may not be a myth. Sometimes more than one member of a family does complete suicide. Some research points to a hereditable characteristic of suicide, or at least the underlying risk factors that are implicated in suicide (Akan et al., 2021; Jackson & Jabbi, 2022; Ruderfer et al., 2020). In counterpoint to a purely gene pool theory, self-destructive tendencies may be learned, situational, or linked to depression or other hopeless environmental conditions. The very act of completion in one family member may propel other family members to think that suicide is an option during times of heightened distress.

6. **Once suicidal, always suicidal.** Many people contemplate suicide at some time during their lives. Most of them recover from the immediate threat, learn appropriate responses and controls, live long and productive lives free of the threat of self-inflicted harm, and never again consider it.

7. **When a person has attempted suicide and pulls out of it, the danger is over.** Unfortunately, there is an extremely elevated risk for suicide within three months of discharge from psychiatric care, but this elevated risk can continue for years (Chung et al., 2017). Individuals who received inpatient psychiatric care may be inherently at higher risk than the general public due to the presence of psychological disorders that are linked to suicide risk (Chung et al., 2017). However, it is also important to consider individuals who attempt suicide but do not receive inpatient psychiatric care. Those individuals may have learned lessons about what does and does not work to end one's life. And, if their distress is left unaddressed, their suicide risk can continue.

8. **Suicidal individuals who seem to be doing better are out of the woods.** *Contrary to common belief,* one danger signal is a period of euphoria following a depressed or suicidal episode. This often means the person has everything settled and planned, and the person is at peace with the idea of completing suicide. In fact, a notable portion of individuals who attempt suicide will reattempt or complete suicide (Parra-Uribe et al., 2017).

9. **A suicidal person who begins to show generosity and share personal possessions shows signs of renewal and recovery.** Many suicidal people begin to dispose of their most prized possessions once they experience enough upswing in energy to make a definite plan. Such disposal of personal effects is sometimes tantamount to acting out the last will and testament.

10. **Suicide is always an impulsive act.** There are several types of suicide. Some involve impulsive actions; others are very deliberately planned and carried out. Individuals who impulsively take their life tend to be younger and experience lower levels of suicidality than their counterparts who plan suicide (Lim et al., 2016).

11. **Suicide strikes only the rich.** Suicide does not discriminate; it strikes at all levels of society. However, unemployment is implicated in many suicide deaths (Amiri, 2022).

12. **Suicide happens without warning.** The vast majority of people invariably give many signs and symptoms of their suicidal intentions. However, those warning signs and symptoms may be veiled and difficult for others to conceptualize as possible indicators of suicide risk.

13. **Suicide is a painless way to die.** It often is not, and many suicide attempts that go awry, bring terrible suffering in the form of chronic pain and permanent disfigurement.

14. **Few professional people kill themselves.** It is perhaps unsurprising, albeit devastating, to consider the elevated suicide rates in occupations that are characterized by high levels of stress and physical and psychological demand. However, individuals with high educational attainment who work in high stress professions are also subject to elevated risk for suicide. Examples include physicians and other medical professionals (Dutheil et al., 2019) and laborers and agricultural workers (Milner et al., 2013). Moreover, first responders, mental health professionals, and crisis workers are exposed to an inordinate number of suicides and, as a result, experience heightened levels of depression, anxiety, and posttraumatic stress disorder (PTSD) symptoms (Aldrich & Cerel, 2022).

15. **The Christmas season is lethal.** Myths surrounding heightened suicide around the winter holidays are, in fact, only myths. However, individuals who struggle with suicidality may be at an increased risk on or around important personal, relational, or familial anniversaries.

16. **Women don't use guns to kill themselves because of disfigurement.** Women use guns more often than drugs to kill themselves.

17. **More suicides occur during a full moon.** There is no increased number of suicides during a full moon.

18. **Most older adults who complete suicide are terminally ill.** While many older adults who attempt suicide may be depressed, only a portion are terminally ill. However, they may have lost most or all of their loved ones and subsequently feel alone in this world. One might also consider the role of existential loss associated with losing the most important relationships that help to bring meaning to one's life, such as work and recreational activity loss, along with the relationships that go with them.

19. **Suicide is limited to the young.** Suicide rates across the lifespan tend to vary but recent figures suggest a particularly elevated suicide rate around middle age and in older people.

20. **Suicidal thoughts are relatively rare.** A significant portion of individuals consider suicide at some point in their life. A smaller portion ruminate on suicide and seriously consider taking their life. And a smaller portion plan suicide (SAMHSA, 2021). The fact is that thinking about suicide during stressful or painful times is not uncommon, but ruminating and planning are notable warning signs for suicide that should not be ignored.

Assessment

Suicide Clues

LO7 The overarching, cardinal rule for *all* crisis workers is this: Workers who deal with *any type* of crisis client should always assess for the presence of clues and risk factors for lethal behavior. Fortunately for the crisis worker, nearly all suicidal/homicidal people reveal some kind of clues or cries for help. According to Shneidman, Farberow, and associates (1976), no one is 100 percent suicidal. People with the strongest death wishes are invariably ambivalent, confused, and grasping for life (p. 128). Most suicidal clients, feeling high levels of ambivalence or inner conflict, either emit some clues or hints about their serious trouble or call for help in some way (pp. 429–440). The clues may be verbal, behavioral, situational, or syndromatic.

Verbal clues are spoken or written statements, which may be either direct ("I'm going to do it this time—kill myself") or indirect ("I'm of no use to anyone anymore").

Behavioral clues may range from prowling the internet suicide sites to slashing one's wrist as a "practice run" or suicidal gesture.

Situational clues might include concerns over a wide array of conditions such as the death of a spouse, divorce, a painful physical injury or terminal illness, sudden bankruptcy, preoccupation with the anniversary of a loved one's death, or other drastic changes in one's life situation.

Syndromatic clues include such constellations of suicidal symptoms as severe depression, loneliness, hopelessness, dependence, and dissatisfaction with life (Shneidman et al., 1976, pp. 431–434).

All of these clues may be considered cries for help, no matter how subtle or camouflaged they are.

Warning Signs

Warning signs are different from symptoms. While symptoms can only be described, warning signs are observable. Working with the American Association for Suicidology, Rudd et al. (2006) identified nine "proximal" indicators of suicide risk. These include the following: (1) "hopelessness;" (2) "rage, anger, seeking revenge;" (3) "acting reckless or engaging in risky activities, seemingly without thinking;" (4) "feeling trapped—like there's no way out;" (5) "increasing alcohol or drug use;" (6) "withdrawing from friends, family, or society;" (7) "anxiety, agitation, unable to sleep, or sleeping all the time;" (8) "dramatic changes in mood;" and/or (9) "no reason for living; no sense of purpose in life" (Rudd et al., 2006, p. 259). The presence of a constellation of these warning signs indicates the need for intervention to address the underlying causes and, if present, reduce suicide risk.

People often ask if the presence of one warning sign can be enough to indicate suicide risk. The answer is a resounding "yes." However, when seen in isolation, the behavior may be indicative of a different etiology—something other than suicide. Regardless, when in doubt, the best way to help individuals who display these or other suicide warning signs is to check it out immediately. Shyness or embarrassment or fear of asking if they intend to kill themselves is not acceptable and says a lot about the interventionist's professional inadequacy to handle threatening issues. Additionally, some behaviors may be so inherently dangerous that they require an immediate response.

Rudd et al. (2006) also identify indicators that immediate intervention is required to sustain life:

(1) "someone threatening to hurt or kill themselves;" (2) "someone looking for ways to kill themselves: seeking access to pills, weapons, or other means; and/or (3) "someone talking or writing about death, dying, or suicide" (p. 259). As previously mentioned, most people who struggle with suicide display some warning signs. The question is whether or not others are able to identify those warning signs as possible indicators of suicide.

There are a number of acronyms that can be used to identify suicide. The American Association of Suicidology (n.d.) has created one of the more common lists of suicide warning signs with the mnemonic IS PATH WARM:

> I is for ideation.
> S is for substance abuse.
> P is for purposelessness.
> A is for anxiety and agitation.
> T is for feeling trapped.
> H is for hopelessness.
> W is for withdrawal.
> A is for anger.
> R is for recklessness.
> M is for mood fluctuations.

So how many letters do you have to fill before the path to suicide changes from warm to hot? That's a great question. Maybe only one or maybe all of them, depending on your clinical judgment. But regarding due diligence and any future legal problems, it's best to have done as thorough of a risk assessment as you are able to do under the circumstances (Bongard & Sullivan, 2013; Kleespies, 2014). A thorough risk assessment is helpful when providing justification for your level of intervention, whether it is low or high. We previously talked about the ABCs of crisis intervention. Imagine an individual whose warning signs spell out IPAHWAM, and on the Triage Assessment Form, their scores were A=8, B=9, C=10 for a total TAF of 27. Those assessment results provide justification for your efforts to help the client get a night's rest in a secure facility, followed by a thorough assessment administered by the receiving facility.

Risk Factors

Let's suppose you fall into some of the foregoing categories and have decided life isn't worth living, and you are going to kill yourself. How good a candidate are you to take yourself off this planet? Here are some of the high-probability suicide risk categories, so

check them off to determine your level of risk (Amiri, 2022; Berman & Canning, 2022; Farmani et al., 2023; Li et al., 2020; Olfson et al., 2022; Sueki, 2022; X. Xu et al., 2021): You are older than 70 or younger than 20 and a White man. You came out of a troubled home and got in trouble at school for fighting. You still get in trouble for fighting, except now it's in bars. You have a history of alcohol misuse, and you abuse other drugs. You have been diagnosed with (choose one or more): (a) schizophrenia, (b) bipolar disorder, (c) borderline personality disorder, (d) anorexia, or you are just plain (e) depressed. You are single, and you don't have a very good job because you recently lost a really good job. To make up for that, you got drunk, had a hit-and-run accident, were caught, and are now spending your first night in jail. Your spouse has announced their intent to divorce you, and most of your former friends won't speak to you anymore. This isn't the first time you've tried to kill yourself, and you have thought about it quite a bit since that time. You collect guns and know how to use every one of them and know a nice, quiet wooded area where no one ventures at night. It is 5 days after Christmas, and the only cards you got were from a lawyer foreclosing your house and the Internal Revenue Service, who sent you an audit notice. Meanwhile, your rheumatoid arthritis is really bothering you, and the only drug that helped you is now off the market. You've been to an internist twice in the last two months for stomach pains, but you didn't mention anything about being depressed, and the doctor didn't ask. Sadly and ominously, your mother and your mother's father both died by suicide. To top it all off, you originally come from a European country that has a lot of low notes in its national anthem, and you think it's pretty gloomy. If this now sounds like a bad country music song and you fit most of these criteria, do not despair or go step in front of a train (all really good country songs must include a train, so that is the way you are going to kill yourself, but you better not do it in Japan, or the train company will make your estate pay for the damages since so many people do just that in Japan).

The ability to predict suicide and who will attempt or complete it is problematic, to say the least. Here's a really good example of the problem. Research evidence indicates that most people who complete suicide had seen a medical doctor for a health problem in the 90 days prior to killing themselves (Kammer et al., 2021). This variable is so significant that there are efforts underway to implement universal suicide screenings in medical care facilities (American Foundation for

Suicide Prevention, n.d.; Frick et al., 2021; Mancinelli-Hough et al., 2022; Snyder et al., 2020). So okay, how many of you have been to the doctor in the last three months and never thought about killing yourself or someone else? Get the point? While all of the foregoing demographics, personality traits, behaviors, and socioeconomic risk factors can predict incident rates by group and are certainly risk factors, none of them taken singly or collectively predicts very well whether an individual will complete a suicide (Bonner, 2001; Goldney, 2000; Granello & Granello, 2007). So, what a crisis interventionist needs is a fast checklist when face-to-face on a bridge with a jumper and here it is.

Assessment Instruments

A variety of instruments have been used in an attempt to identify suicidal ideation and behavior. They cover personality characteristics, risk factors, and warning signs. The Columbia-Suicide Severity Rating Scale (C-SSRS; Posner et al., 2011), Minnesota Multiphasic Personality Inventory–2RF (Ben-Porath & Tellegen, 2008; Sunhae Kim et al., 2020), Beck Hopelessness Scale (Beck, 1993), and Beck Depression Inventory (Beck et al., 1996) are examples of tests that can be used for suicide risk identification and assessment.

In applying the Interpersonal Psychological Theory of Suicide, there are instruments that can be used to measure the three distinct constructs. The Interpersonal Needs Questionnaire (Van Orden et al., 2012) assesses the critical interpersonal issues of burdensomeness to others and lack of belongingness (Silva et al., 2023). The Acquired Capability for Suicide Scale (Ribeiro et al., 2014) is a brief self-report scale that is intended to measure acquired capability for suicide. And the Painful and Provocative Events Scale Revised (Forrest et al., 2019) is a self-report of how much the client engages in impulsive, dangerous, pathological, and risk-taking activities. These scales can provide a strong estimate of a client's lethality, probably particularly so when utilized in tandem. When assessing acquired capability for suicide, though, it might be most important to examine the client's "fearlessness about death, practical capability, and pain tolerance" (Shahnaz et al., 2020, p. 1230).

A number of other instruments, such as SAD PERSONS (Sex, Age, Depressive Symptoms, Previous Attempts, Ethanol use, Rational thinking loss, Social support lacking, Organized Plan; Patterson et al., 1983), are designed to assess manifestations of clinical suicide ideation and empirical factors that have been previously identified as being related to risk for suicide attempts. These scales accumulate data on relevant demographics, symptoms of suicidal behavior, stress, resources outside of self, personal and social history, and historical and situational variables currently identified in the suicide literature as significant predictors of suicide attempts. However, these devices alone have had a poor track record for prediction (Katz et al., 2017). Best practice in suicide risk assessment requires utilization of a thorough clinical interview and assessment of related treatment issues that may be implicated in heightened suicide risk (e.g., anxiety, trauma, substance misuse).

Clinical Interview. As we have previously discussed, researchers and suicidologists have identified numerous risk factors and warning signs that may help the crisis worker in assessing suicide potential. While there are all kinds of scoring systems for the wide variety of checklists available today, they are rife with the possibility of yielding false positives or, worse yet, false negatives (Sullivan & Bongar, 2006). Here is where science and art commingle, and the crisis workers' interviewing and diagnostic skills come into play. Whenever a person manifests one or five of these risk factors, it should be an immediate signal for the crisis worker to treat the person as high risk in terms of suicide potential.

1. Exhibits the presence of suicidal or homicidal impulses and serious intent
2. Has a family history of suicide, threats of harm, and/or abuse of others
3. Has ongoing substance misuse
4. Has a history of previous attempts
5. Has formulated a specific plan
6. Has experienced the recent loss of a loved one through death, divorce, or separation
7. Is part of a family that is destabilized as a result of loss, personal abuse, violence, and/or because the client has been sexually abused
8. Is preoccupied with the anniversary of a particularly traumatic loss
9. Experiences psychosis (and may have discontinued taking psychotropic medications)
10. Has had recent physical and/or psychological trauma or a history of it as a child
11. Has a history of unsuccessful medical treatment, chronic pain, or terminal illness
12. Is living alone and is cut off from contact with others
13. Is depressed, recovering from depression, or has recently been hospitalized for depression

14. Is giving away prized possessions or putting personal affairs in order

15. Displays radical shifts in characteristic behaviors or moods, such as apathy, withdrawal, isolation, irritability, panic, or anxiety, or changed social, sleeping, eating, study, dress, grooming, or work habits

16. Is experiencing a pervasive feeling of hopelessness and/or helplessness

17. Is preoccupied and troubled by earlier episodes of experienced physical, emotional, or sexual abuse

18. Exhibits a profound degree of one or more intense emotions—such as anger, aggression, loneliness, guilt, hostility, grief, or disappointment—that are uncharacteristic of the individual's normal emotional behavior

19. Faces a threatened financial loss

20. Exhibits ideas of persecution

21. Is experiencing challenges regarding one's sexual orientation and/or is experiencing stigmatization or ostracism based on one's sexual orientation

22. Has an unplanned and unwanted pregnancy

23. Has a history of running away or of incarceration

24. Manifests ideas and themes of depression, death, and suicide in conversation, written essays, reading selections, artwork, or drawings

25. Has black-and-white thinking, all-or-none cognitions, tunnel vision, limited problem-solving ability, difficult self-soothing and resolving guilt. Is perfectionistic

26. Perceives oneself as a burden and doesn't feel belongingness. Makes statements or suggestions that they would not be missed if gone

27. Easy access to firearms, medications, and other fast, lethal means

28. Experiences chronic or acute stressors and perseverates on them

29. Has used the internet or social media to explore suicide methods

30. Has recently been to a medical doctor in the last 3 to 6 months for reasons other than an annual physical check-up

In and of themselves, some of these factors may mean little in regard to suicide. Further, this extensive suicide shopping list of risk factors would suggest that a lot of people are suicidal who do not have the remotest notion of killing themselves (a false positive in statistical terms). The crisis worker must realize that assessing suicidal or homicidal risk is no simple matter. Indeed, some risk factors, such as previous attempts or having a concrete plan, are more lethal than others and must be given more weight or attention. There are no direct "if-then" connections. Suicidal risk factors are much more relevant when identifying groups than individuals (Chiles & Strosahl, 1995, p. 8). Yet as these risk factors pile up, the potential for the individual to engage in a lethal act most certainly increases. Therefore, the clinical interview, and how it is structured and handled, is critical in making on-target assessments of lethality.

CAMS. The Collaborative Assessment and Management of Suicidality (CAMS) is a risk assessment clinical interview framework developed by Jobes et al. (2005). Creation of the therapeutic alliance is critical to this framework, so the emphasis is on collaboration (Jobes et al., 2005, 2018). Section A of the Suicide Status Form is used in this interview to measure "six key constructs: psychological pain, stress, agitation, hopelessness, self-hate, and overall behavioral risk of suicide" (Jobes et al., 2018, p. 244). The client is asked to self-rate across these six constructs and provide qualitative responses to questions pertaining to the first five constructs of "psychological pain, stress, agitation, hopelessness, and self-hate" (Jobes et al., 2018, p. 244). These ratings generate the "SSF Core Assessment" (Jobes et al., 2018, p. 244), and additional questions are asked to help generate a more detailed clinical picture. Section B addresses the client's history related to suicide behavior (Jobes et al., 2018). Section C addresses the treatment plan with special attention toward stabilization and barriers to treatment (Jobes et al., 2018). CAMS is a stepped care model that incorporates a thorough clinical evaluation, treatment planning, and recursive re-evaluations.

CASE. Chronological Assessment of Suicide Events (CASE) is a risk assessment clinical interview framework developed by Shea (2002, 1998). CASE has two primary assumptions: first, that people rarely kill themselves without engaging in concrete planning and making plans to do so; and second, that clients may not voluntarily come forward with information about their suicidal thoughts without a lot of rapport building on the part of the interviewer. The CASE approach involves collecting information from four time frames as it relates to the client's suicidality: "immediate events, presenting events, recent events, and past events" (Shea, 2017, p. 423). Discussing key aspects of these four periods of time allows the interviewer to "sensitively uncover a patient's suicidal ideation, planning, actions, and intent" (Shea, 2017, p. 422).

RFL. The Reasons for Living scale (RFL; Linehan et al., 1983) is a different kind of suicide assessment tool in that it queries a person's reasons for staying alive by posing 48 questions as to why people would *not* kill themselves. It has a six-point Likert scoring system (0-5) for each question, and the items can be categorized into six factors: "survival and coping, responsibility to family, child-related concerns, fear of suicide, fear of social disapproval, and moral objections (Linehan et al., 1983, p. 282). The RFL has been adapted for specific populations, such as military members (Deutsch & Lande, 2017) and older adults (Lutz et al., 2019).

SRADT. The Suicide Risk Assessment Decision Tree (SRADT) is a risk assessment clinical interview framework (Cukrowicz et al., 2004) that moves through a series of yes-or-no questions to come to a decision about how present and pronounced the person's acquired capability of killing themself is. The decision tree framework (Joiner et al., 1999) is utilized to determine the level of relative risk for suicide. Interviewers query three domains: previous suicidal behavior, current suicidal symptoms, and empirically related variables that would exacerbate (hopelessness, impulsivity) or diminish (engaging with social supports, stopping drug abuse) suicidal behavior (Cukrowicz et al., 2004). Completing the decision tree involves obtaining information about the aforementioned areas, inputting the data into the decision tree to determine how high the acquired capability of suicide attempt risk level is, and then using the risk level to determine appropriate intervention.

So, we've given you all these scales, instruments, and assessment acronyms, but they still don't amount to much in the way of a "no miss, on target" suicide prediction device. Further, you may be in a situation where you simply do not have time or access to any of the foregoing instruments. What's to be done in a fast and furious fashion that will give you a best bet predictor? First and foremost, use the TAF. If that score is in the upper twenties, whether suicide or homicide is ever mentioned, you need to get that person secure in a safe place where they can't accomplish either. Second, while some institutions and state legal mandates may call for you to employ certain assessment devices, the simple acronym PIMP (Granello & Granello, 2007) works pretty well when you are backed into a corner

and need to get a fast lethality assessment. The P is for a plan and how lethal it is. I is for intent and how serious and goal oriented it is. M is for method, involving access and availability to means, timeline to attempt, isolation of place, and help. P is for previous attempts, one of the best indicators of commitment to kill oneself.

Using the Triage Assessment Form in Addressing Lethality

Crisis workers intervening with clients in acute crises should *never* omit an assessment for suicide lethality (Jobes et al., 2005; McGlothlin, 2008; Shea, 1998). The worker must not hesitate to ask questions such as "Are you thinking about killing yourself?" ". . . about killing someone else?" "How?" "When?" "Where?" We absolutely agree with McGlothin (2008) that you don't sugarcoat this question for fear of activating suicidal urges in the client or of sounding callous or offensive in broaching such a personal and culturally sensitive topic (p. 39). Mealy mouthed questions such as "Have you . . . considered hurting yourself," "thought about giving up," "felt overwhelmed/really down/strung out/at the end of your rope," along with qualifiers such as "sorta" or "kinda," are not the same as straight questions about "killing yourself" and imply wholly different interpretations that can cause the worker to completely miss lethal ideation.

Asking *the* question about killing oneself or others does not mean doing so in an abrasive, callous manner. As in the CAM and CASE interview formats previously mentioned, collaboration and empathy are key components. Asking *the* question about killing oneself or others is a closed-ended question that seeks a yes-or-no response. However, there are varying degrees of "yesness" that range from "Well, not in a long time!" to "I have the 9 mm cleaned and loaded and am going out to the state park this afternoon" (McGlothin, 2008, pp. 38–39). Therefore, if you get a positive answer, you need to fully explore the dimensions and degree of that lethality by assessing across affective, behavioral, and cognitive dimensions. McGlothin's (2008, pp. 36–37) acronym SIMPLE STEPS provides a step-by-step method to assess lethality and get a good read on the client's affective, behavioral, and cognitive representation of the dilemma.

Suicidal/Homicidal? Are you thinking of killing yourself/someone else?

Ideation: Using a scale of 0-10, how likely are you to kill yourself/somebody else in the next 72 hours?

Method: Do you have a plan for how you will kill yourself/somebody else? Do you have access to the means of executing that plan?

Perturbation: On a scale of 0 to 10, how much psychological pain are you in at the moment? Is there anything you can think of that would make it go higher?

Loss: Have you suffered a loss recently or a significant loss in the past you are not over?

Earlier Attempts: Have you ever tried to kill yourself/somebody else before? What happened such that you are (or the other person is) still alive today? What was your response to discovering that you/the other person lived?

Substance Use: Are you currently drinking alcohol or using drugs? What medications are you taking, and are you taking them as prescribed?

Troubleshooting: How tied up in this are your job, family, and so on? And what might change to stop this? Are you willing not to consider killing yourself/somebody? If a miracle happened and you awakened tomorrow and everything was fine, what would that look like?

Emotions/Diagnosis: Have you ever been diagnosed with a physical or psychological illness? How are you feeling right now (e.g., depression, hopelessness, helplessness, loneliness, anger, agitation, impulsiveness) and have you ever felt this way before? If so, how often? Have you seen, or are you currently seeing, a mental health professional of any kind for this problem?

Protective Factors (Lack of): Who can you depend on when you are having a rough time? What coping skills have you previously found to help you manage when you are struggling? Do you have a medical or mental health provider who has helped you previously and who might be a good resource right now?

Stressors and Life Events: What is going on in your life that leads you to think that suicide/homicide is a viable option or solution to your problems?

The triage assessment of the client in acute crisis provides for immediate revision of the worker's estimate of crisis severity based on the client's responses to these important and necessary questions or on rapidly elevated TAF ratings due to a sudden change in client feeling, behaving, or thinking about suicide or homicide when previously there was no indication of ideation. A client triage profile that may have looked safe before such answers may look quite different a few moments later. If the client is seriously thinking of killing or harming some specific other person, the worker will need to consider the duty to warn and/or duty to protect implications dictated by law developed in the *Tarasoff* case.

Consider the following example. *Before* the lethality questions, the client's presenting problem to a career counselor is job loss due to a plant closing. The counselor identifies the client's depression and frustration over their failure to find a suitable replacement job, but the estimated TAF affect value of 3 or 4, cognition score of 6 or 7, and behavior score of 4 or 5 (total TAF of 13 to 16) yields a "low to moderate" severity summary. Such a total score shows no urgent or immediate concern for the client's severity/lethality status.

Nevertheless, the career counselor senses that something is not quite right. The client's voice reveals a hint of verbal euphoria, while the body language seems to contradict the verbal behavior with a slight hint of hopelessness. The worker further knows that job loss, particularly after a lengthy tenure, and suicide are related (Stack, 2001). As a result of the emerging hints and cues (as an example, the client makes a nonchalant side remark implying that they will not be around much longer), the counselor probes directly into the client's inner world by asking, "What does that mean?" "How?" "When?" and "Where?" and then rethinks and reframes the TAF assessment.

After the lethality questions—the client's responses, which reflect obvious stress and depression, are "For me, there is no future, no life left. I am too old to re-train, and nobody wants me anyway! I might as well curl up and die," and the client answers "Yes" to the question "Are you thinking of killing yourself because things look so hopeless?"—a second TAF assessment of 9 or 10 on affect, 8 or 9 on cognition, and 8 or 9 on behavior (total of 25 to 28), amounts to a dramatic escalation and would trigger an intervention strategy of immediate hospitalization to ensure the client's safety.

This example of using the TAF as a rapid assessment tool shows how quickly the emotional tone may change in a crisis intervention case. It clearly demonstrates that whenever a crisis worker begins to suspect a higher level of severity or lethality than at first revealed, the worker should not hesitate to directly ask the question and probe deeply into the emotionally charged world of the client. A similar rapid increase in the worker's assessment of lethality is also applicable in cases of homicidal intent or any other situation involving threats of harm to self or others.

Level of Risk. The last piece of this complex puzzle is the level of risk. Joiner and associates (1999) and Bryan and Rudd (2006) have put together risk tables that range from nonexistent to extreme. Bryan and Rudd (2006) have established four risk categories and risk levels. Risk categories include "baseline, acute, chronic high risk, and chronic high risk with acute exacerbation" (Bryan & Rudd, 2006, p. 197). The risk level can be explained through the five descriptors of "nonexistent, mild, moderate, severe, and extreme" (Bryan & Rudd, 2006, p. 198). These categorizations can be used to help guide intervention because, as individuals move up the scale to an extreme level, these following things happen. They develop more courage and a sense of competence as they make preparations for and practice run the attempt. Most likely, they have made attempts before that did not result in death, and they have learned from these attempts. They have continuous, intense, and enduring ideation, impaired self-control, severe feelings of hopelessness, multiple other symptoms, and no protective factors. Making determinations about the potential for lethal behavior should not simply involve the calculation of risk based on established instruments but also on information gleaned from a thorough clinical interview (Kleespies, 2014). The **structured professional judgment**, presented by Kleespies (2014, pp. 108–122), combines what professional crisis workers' experience tell them as they use the foregoing verbal and visual assessments along with reliable and valid assessment instruments—if time is available to make decisions on potential lethality.

Intervention Strategies

LO8 This section contains examples of general counseling strategies to use with adults of different ages and different problems who are manifesting potentially lethal thoughts and behaviors. Lethal children will be addressed in Chapter 13, "Crises in Schools." Before you even start reading this section, your question might well be should one even try, with treatment outcomes so equivocal? While there are no absolutes in suicide treatment, there are some promising approaches (Brown et al., 2005; Cukrowicz et al., 2004; Diamond et al., 2021; Jobes et al., 2005, 2018; Linehan et al., 2006), and it is these that will be considered. Suicide intervention strategies involve "interrupting a suicide attempt that is imminent or in the process of occurring" (Fujimura et al., 1985, p. 612). Crisis intervention with suicidal/homicidal clients generally falls into two broad categories, dealing with perturbations and reducing lethality levels.

The Three I's

The major causes of perturbation have to do with the three Is. The person confronts a situation they believe to be **inescapable** (I can't get away from this pain no matter what I do), **intolerable** (I've gone beyond what any human could endure), and **interminable** (If I don't do something about this now, it'll go on forever). The goal of intervention is to change one or more of these Is (Chiles & Strosahl, 1995, p. 74). At the beginning of the interview, the crisis worker must quickly establish a sense of rapport and trust to create a working relationship and provide clients with an anchor to life (Michel, 2011). In that regard, you are running a social locations SAFETY checklist as you attempt to establish a bond when the client is unknown to you. It is also important to begin to reestablish in clients a sense of hope and to diminish their sense of helplessness—to take immediate steps to speak and act on clients' current pain and knowing where their hotspots are on SAFETY will help you do that.

The most effective way to do this is to address not the lethality directly but the perturbation the Is are causing. When the perturbation level of the three Is is lowered and some modicum of control and hope is restored in the person's life, lethality will drop below the explosive level. What this means is not just dealing passively with only the intrapersonal issues but actively confronting the interpersonal and environmental issues that afflict and assail the individual as well (Shneidman, 1999a).

Clients need to be taught to either use existing problem-solving skills or generate new ones so they can shed the inescapability of unsolvable problems. Clients need to develop self-awareness and self-observation strategies to observe natural fluctuations in pain levels and make associations between doing things a bit differently and feeling better. As a result, they can learn that emotional pain will not be constantly intense and interminable. Clients also need to learn that negative feelings can be tolerated by distancing and distraction skills so they are seen as a part of life and not something that is overwhelming and interminable (Chiles & Strosahl, 1995, p. 74). Typically, some form of cognitive-behavioral therapy will be used that employs active support for the person;

teaches cognitive restructuring, emotional regulation, and learning to balance change and acceptance of how things are and will be; and changes destructive and negative behaviors through psychoeducation and problem-solving (Bryan, 2019; Wu et al., 2022). The following cases demonstrate how a crisis interventionist goes about "dotting the Is."

LeAnn, Age 21. LeAnn was a senior at a large university. During her freshman year at a small liberal arts college, she had experienced an emotional and suicidal breakdown as the anniversary date of her older sister's suicide approached. She had left the small college, returned home, and undergone psychiatric treatment. LeAnn had later enrolled in the university in her hometown, where she lived in a residence hall. She went home frequently but managed to succeed fairly well in her studies and social life. LeAnn was referred to the crisis worker by her mother following a weekend mother–daughter discussion during which LeAnn disclosed some recurring suicidal thoughts. The mother expressed concern that the fifth anniversary of her sister's suicide seemed to be looming in LeAnn's mind and asked the crisis worker to call LeAnn in for a conference. During the first interview with LeAnn, the worker established that LeAnn did not have a specific, highly lethal plan, but that she did have a lot of suicidal ruminations.

LeAnn: I think Mother thinks I'm crazy. Sometimes I wonder if she's right. (**Long pause**.) I don't seem to handle stress very well, and this is my last semester with my senior thesis due. . . Sometimes I think I am about to lose it. Do you think I may be going crazy?

CW: No, I certainly don't. What I'm hearing is a lot of confusion and unsettled emotion and a lot of pressure. I'm glad you feel comfortable enough to ask me. I'm wondering what's happening in you to bring up the question. Are you thinking of killing yourself?

LeAnn: Well, I've just been sitting in my room by myself, staring at the wall. I can't get anywhere on that stupid thesis. Not sleeping, not eating, not going out. And I've had this strange sensation of both wanting to run and scream and to just give up. And I've thought about my sister's death constantly. More than at any time since I was a freshman. It's like I'm destined to go the way she went. Sometimes I think I can't stand it any longer.

Then I catch myself and wonder if I *am* nuts. My sister killed herself, and her birthday is coming up. I miss her so much.

CW: Okay, I'm going to ask you a bunch of questions and I've got a couple of forms I want you to fill out. Some of the questions may seem a little intrusive but it's a way of determining where we are going to need to go. When we're done, I'll tell you where I think we need to go.

LeAnn's thoughts and responses are enough to activate the worker to conduct a suicidal assessment process. He first gives her the Suicide Status Form (Jobes et al., 2005). Her scores for psychological pain are 3. She reports missing her sister, particularly on the anniversary of her death. Her stress is a 4–5, but she mainly sees her stressors as completing her thesis. Her agitation is low, with no sense of need to take any action that would lead to suicide. She feels a bit hopeless, but again, this has more to do with her senior thesis completion and resulting graduation. She indicates no self-hatred and gives it no score at all. She rates her overall risk of suicide as extremely low. Her reasons for living are graduation, her parents and friends, and a chance to go on to graduate school. She has no reasons for dying, other than she might see her sister in heaven. Her wish to live is "very much" and her wish to die is "not at all." Her Interpersonal Needs Questionnaire (Van Orden et al., 2012) indicates she does not feel she is a burden and has a very strong sense of belonging to her parents and college sorority sisters. Follow-up questions by the worker using McGlothin's (2008) SIMPLE STEPS indicate few if any of the "hot" cognitions that activate suicidal thinking. The worker relays this information to her in a straightforward, collaborative, and empathic manner.

CW: As you can see, your scale scores are really low, all well within a normal range. I believe that more than anything the anniversary of your sister's death and how much you miss her are contributing to the loneliness and isolation you are feeling. I also think you are pretty normal and reacting pretty normally to school. I wonder if we might talk about those a little and help you make some plans to get out of this rut?

Many people who have suicidal ideation believe they are "going crazy." While some people who experience psychosis or suffer from personality disorders are suicidal, suicide is not the first step on the road to "going crazy." The crisis worker positively affirms that LeAnn is not going "nuts" and seeks to normalize the crisis. The crisis worker focuses on the underlying emotional content of the loss of her sister and the upcoming anniversary as likely a key element in decreasing the client's perturbation.

The same is true of getting a handle on a huge source that would perturb most any student—the dreaded senior project. While her suicidal ideation is not dismissed out of hand, it is put into perspective as one component of her overall response to the loss of her sister and the other normal stressors she is experiencing at school. For many individuals, a suicidal crisis may be a one-time occurrence brought on by acute situational events that, once handled, disappears forever.

Deborah, Age 27. Deborah had been in therapy, on and off, for 11 years—since she was 16. Deborah (1) had a history of suicide attempts, some of them serious, some of them gestures; (2) had used a wide variety of drugs in her college years—in fact, she had dropped out of college after 2 years because of drug use and resulting poor academic performance; (3) had a history of episodes of severe depression, loneliness, hopelessness, and helplessness followed by mood swings to euphoric and deep religious activity and commitment; (4) had been hospitalized numerous times for psychiatric care; (5) had experienced a great sense of loss and grief at the divorce of her parents when she was 16; (6) had recently gone into self-imposed isolation and remorse—cutting herself off from friends, family, and coworkers; and (7) was feeling a new sense of meaninglessness related to her career—she had been seeking something that she really chose to do (as opposed to working for her father). Deborah, in tears, was trembling and in a state of acute anxiety and standing on the railing of a Mississippi River bridge, preparing to jump.

The crisis worker is a Crisis Intervention Team police officer, described in Chapter 5, "Crisis Case Handling." Police and highway patrol officers have stopped all traffic, and people are out of their cars, watching. The scene is tense, and it appears that, at any moment, Deborah will jump. The officer immediately implements Cochran's game plan model of giving their name (play one) and getting the client's name (play two) in order to establish personal contact. The CIT officer's use of "I" owning statements (play three) and reflection and summarization (play 4) (Kirchberg, et al., 2013) are designed to let the client know that the CIT officer is listening and focused in on her alone and, hopefully, to develop a working bond.

CIT Officer: (in a clearly audible but confident, soft, caring, and empathic voice) My name is Sam. Tell me your name.

Deborah: (hesitantly) My name . . . is . . . Deborah. What . . . what do you want?

CIT Officer: I want to help you, if I can, Deborah. I can see that you are under some kind of terrible pressure to make you think about jumping off this bridge. I'd like to talk to you and see if there is any way I can be of help to you.

Deborah: I don't know that anybody can help me. (a little indignantly) Certainly not a cop! Shrinks haven't helped. How can you?

CIT Officer: Deborah, I'm concerned about your safety and about what's bothering you right now. I'm a cop all right, but I am also a Crisis Intervention Team officer. I deal with all kinds of people in crisis, and that's why they called me. For you to consider jumping, there must be a lot of pain that you can't seem to get relief from. If the shrinks haven't worked, how about giving a cop a chance? What's the harm? We have plenty of time.

The CIT officer immediately seeks to establish rapport with the jumper by establishing a first-name basis of communication. Sam validates Deborah's suicidal actions as a way to relieve emotional pain by matter-of-factly stating what Deborah is doing and seeks to elicit what is causing her to do it. Sam uses a validation technique from dialectical behavior therapy (DBT; Linehan, 2014) that sets up what at first might seem the exact opposite of what one would do. Sam promotes the central "dialectic" in DBT, which is that they accept the client exactly as she is in the moment, with her suicide attempt as being her best problem-solving attempt available, but simultaneously pushes the client toward changing the maladaptive behavior patterns that have gotten her onto the bridge (Rizvi, 2011). Sam further acknowledges their role as a CIT officer and what the CIT officer can do, without any false promises. They work very hard to immediately build a trusting, empathic relationship that demonstrates congruence, honesty, and caring (Kirchberg, et al., 2013). While it may seem like we are harping on this subject, building a therapeutic alliance (and this most certainly includes this police officer on the bridge with this client) is absolutely critical. Sam is also empathically seeking to touch and acknowledge the Affect SAFETY social location of her distress. Michel and Jobes's (2011) book spends more than

400 pages on this topic, providing clinicians with an arsenal of theoretical techniques on how to build the relationship. Michel (2011) quotes a woman whom he met in a support group for people with depression who had attempted suicide. She had the chainsaw scars around her neck to prove the gruesome way she had attempted to kill herself. He asked why these people had not sought help. She said, "We could only have talked to another person we knew would not be afraid of listening, without judging. In a suicidal crisis we could never have trusted a person who would want to talk us out of it" (pp. 5–6).

More than other types of crisis workers, though, the CIT officer's job is dealing with the imminent lethality of the situation. The safety of a suicidal/homicidal client (Rudd et al., 2004, p. 152) is the overriding priority, along with the safety of the officer (Memphis Police Department, 2011).

CIT Officer: With the wind blowing and all the commotion around here, I'm having a difficult time hearing you. I need for you to come down off that railing and come over here to the curb and sit down so we can talk. You look like you could use a friendly ear to listen, and I'll take the time to do just that.

Deborah: I'm not sure talking will do any good. Just go away and leave me alone. I don't need you here.

CIT Officer: Deborah, do you remember my name? My name is Sam. Let's take some time to talk. We've got time, plenty of time to just sit down together and talk. You do remember my name, don't you?

The crisis worker makes a point to try to establish a first-name mutual communication with Deborah. Whenever a person such as Deborah is emotionally overwhelmed and immobile, one effective way to break through that immobility is to *personalize* the interaction. A good way to personalize a relationship with a client in crisis is to establish first-name communication as early as possible (Memphis Police Department, 2011). Sam also attempts to slow the emotionally charged situation by repeating that there is time, plenty of time, to find out what is going on. That tells the client that in this moment, the CIT officer is committed to the relationship, as transitory as it may be. "We have plenty of time" is almost a default phrase for us to slow the rapid cognitive and affective cycling that is present in many kinds of crisis down and convey a sense of patience, understanding, interest, and thoroughness that usually

is missing in crisis clients' relationships (Kirchberg et al., 2013). From a social locations SAFETY standpoint, it is an attempt to reduce the **Friction** that has heated the client enough to cause her to choose this radical action to take the psychological heat away.

Deborah: Your name is Sam. So? How do I know I can trust you, Sam? I don't see how you can make my life any better. I've about had it with this life, with this great big lump of hurt deep inside me that won't go away. I'm really tired of this. Anyway, how do I know you won't just put me in jail or that nuthouse they put me in last time?

CIT Officer: (in a calm, low-key, confident, reassuring, caring voice tone) Deborah, what I want to do is to understand what's bothering you, so I can get you some help. What is it that we need to focus on to get you some relief? Right now, all I'm asking you to do for me is just to come over here to the curb, so you and I can take plenty of time to talk, so I can clearly understand just what is upsetting you. I'm certainly *not* here to put you in jail. What I want to do is to try to find out what part of you is hurting inside so that I can get you to some place to get the help that you deserve. I can see you're carrying such a heavy load to think that the only way of unburdening yourself is jumping off this bridge. I don't want to see you get hurt. So, could you at least step off the railing?

Deborah: (Steps down off the railing and takes a few tentative steps toward the CIT officer.) It's just so overwhelming and hopeless. Nothing seems to work. Everything I touch turns to crap, school, love life, job, parents. I am tired of it. So tired.

CIT Officer: Okay, thanks for getting off the railing. (Deborah sits down. Sam slowly moves by her side, sits down, and listens to her story unfold.) Wow! That *is* a load. No wonder you felt like jumping. It takes some courage to step away from ending all that pain and taking a chance on talking to me. I really appreciate that. I want to take you to a guy I know. He's not a shrink. He's a former police resource officer who works on the mobile crisis team. First, I have to take you to the medical center and get you checked out. Is that okay?

Deborah: Will they give me electroshock treatments? I don't want those.

CIT Officer: No, they'll just evaluate you. Look! I want you to ride down there with me. I'll have to put you in handcuffs for the ride there because that's part of the police procedure. That may mean an all-night stay at the medical center, I don't know. But I think I can get them to do the evaluation and then see about getting you out of there pretty quickly to a place and a guy I know about. While they are doing that, I'll call Pete, the guy I told you about. As soon as you are checked out, I'll come back and get you and take you to see Pete—with no handcuffs. You ride up front with me. I think you'd like talking to him. I know sometimes I sure do when I'm in a bind. But let's just sit down here and talk awhile, so I can kinda clue Pete in. Would that be okay?

Deborah: What the heck! I've never had my head shrunk by a cop. It can't get any worse. Okay! (Talks a bit more about what got her here while the CIT officer listens attentively.)

In this case, the crisis worker was able, in a few minutes' time, to validate themself to Deborah and gain her trust by focusing in on what is disturbing her and exploring her issues (Leenaars, 1994). Suicidal clients often cannot concentrate, so the crisis worker repeats himself using the broken record technique and themself seeks to slow things down. Sam also attempts to get Deborah to a place of safety by asking her to move off the railing. Sam immediately reinforces Deborah for getting off the bridge and again for being willing to talk with them. Sam does not make a promise they cannot keep. As an example, Sam promises her no electric shock treatments. They can do that because that procedure has not been done in years in this jurisdiction.

CIT officers like Sam have a great deal of discretion in what they can do with emotionally distressed individuals they take into protective custody. While Sam might be able to get Deborah off the railing by lying to her about not taking her to jail, the next time a police officer was asked to deal with Deborah, she would remember the lie and be much more difficult to work with. Deborah complied with the crisis worker's request and was later taken to the emergency room of a public hospital, where she received medical and psychological evaluations.

The case of Deborah provides a brief example of how some simple verbal techniques, delivered with compassion, caring, and genuineness, can make a dramatic difference in the compliance and survival of many clients who are in acute disequilibrium and actively trying to kill themselves. Deborah's TAF score diminished markedly from an initial score of 30 (A=10, B=10, C=10) to a terminal score of approximately 21(A=8, B=7, C=6). After being checked out, Deborah meets Pete.

CW: I'm Pete, and you must be Deborah. Sam told me about you. I'm glad to meet you. It sounds like you had a heck of a night, and Sam tells me this isn't the first time you've felt so bad you wanted to kill yourself.

Deborah: Sam's right. I don't know why I didn't just go ahead. I was as close as I've ever been. I think next time that will be it.

CW: I'd like to do something a little different from what you are maybe used to. Instead of doing crisis intervention, I kinda do crisis management here with the Midtown mobile crisis unit. Are you interested in learning how to manage some of this stuff?

Deborah: Man, if I just could. That would be something else.

Crisis Management

LO9 Dealing with chronic or episodic suicidal behavior is different from onetime suicide attempts. **Crisis management** refers to the act of planning a response to recurring suicidal behavior in *collaboration* with the client (Bongar & Sullivan, 2013, pp. 157–240; Chiles & Strosahl, 1995, pp. 125–147; Jobes et al., 2005; Kleespies, 2014, pp. 20–24). While we are indeed involved in the treatment of a lethal behavior, there is an important distinction between treatment and management. Treatment implies an end point "cure." Management implies an ongoing problem that needs a continuous collaborative effort between the client and the worker until such time as the client decides that lethality really is no longer a viable option (Jobes, 2006, p. 69). LivingWorks Education explains this as suicide "first aid" in the Applied Suicide Intervention Skills Training (ASIST) framework (Lang et al., 2020). Utilizing the Pathway for Assisting Life (PAL), crisis workers can help clients discuss what brought them to the point of suicide, identify reasons for living or agreeing to "stay safe for now," and develop a plan to increase safety (Lang et al., 2020, p. 2). In this manner, crisis workers are attempting to increase stabilization to a level at which the client can obtain additional support and mental health intervention to help address the underlying causes of the suicidality, as opposed to the goal in crisis intervention, which is not to address the underlying issues but, rather, to promote immediate safety and sufficient stabilization. Little can be done about static (unchanging) risk factors such as race, age, and chronic mental illness, but dynamic factors (modifiable) risk factors such as hopelessness, alcohol misuse, financial crisis, or acute depression can be managed (Kleespies, 2014, p. 21), and those individuals who are operating at a moderate risk level can benefit through outpatient management (Bongard & Sullivan, 2013, pp. 157–200).

The goal is to establish a framework that rewards alternatives to suicidal behavior and minimizes the short-term reinforcements that occur when suicidal ideation and behavior start to develop (Rizvi, 2011; Wenzel et al., 2008, pp. 173–198) and develop a safety plan (Stanley & Brown, 2012). Pete is a member of the mobile crisis team for Midtown Mental Health Unit and a Licensed Professional Counselor. He is a retired police officer and still serves as a resource officer for police officers who are experiencing personal and professional difficulties. He will use a collaborative cognitive-behavioral therapy approach (Brown et al., 2011; Wenzel et al., 2008) with Deborah. To do that, he will need to determine the central cognitive pathway that leads her to consider suicide. He will need answers to the following questions:

1. What about the client's history generates the suicidal behavior?
2. What precipitated this crisis, and is it different from other trigger events?
3. How does the client think about suicide?
4. What does she feel during the crisis?
5. What is she feeling physically?
6. What active or planned suicidal behaviors have occurred or are occurring? (Rudd et al., 2004, p. 67)

He is straightforward, honest, empathic, supportive, a bit cynical, and worldly wise, with little professional psychobabble, one-upmanship, or discounting in his approach. He represents the potential for a perfect match in bonding for a person who has had very few positive attachment figures or trustworthy support persons in her life (Holmes, 2011). Overall, his goals and strategies closely follow Bongard and Sullivan's (2013), Chiles and Strosahl's (1995), Jobes's (2006), Sommers-Flanagan et al.'s (2001), and Joiner and associates' (2009) management plans for continuing treatment of a suicidal client:

1. Destigmatize the suicidal behavior by using an objective, personal (self), scientific approach through teaching self-monitoring and hypothesis testing of behaviors.

2. Objectify the client's suicidal behavior by using reframing and problem solving, validate the emotional pain, move suicidal behavior off center stage, and calmly discuss past, present, and likely future suicidal behavior.
3. Address the likelihood of recurrent suicidal behavior by developing agreements with clients about a behavioral crisis protocol and crisis management plan.
4. Activate problem-solving behavior in the client through teaching problem-solving skills, looking for spontaneous problem solving, reinforcing and enhancing skills, and better understanding of the short- and long-term consequences of behavior.
5. Develop emotional pain tolerance by teaching the distinction between just having and getting rid of a feeling, understanding that suicide is an emotional cop-out; differentiating between emotional involvement and suffering; imparting a contextual approach to negative thoughts and feelings as opposed to a global, pervasive view of negative emotion; and learning how to distance oneself by accepting that negative emotions are merely a part of living and not catastrophic.
6. Develop specific interpersonal problem-solving skills that promote interaction rather than avoidance and isolation. Get the concept of belonging back into her life and the idea that she has something to contribute to the world rather than being a burden on it.
7. Develop intermediate-term life direction through concrete, positive, initial steps that stress the process of goal striving as opposed to the all-or-none, success-or-failure approach to reaching goals.
8. Stay calm while listening with empathy.
9. Instill hope and confidence while establishing a therapeutic alliance.
10. Establish a crisis management plan for living and a backup plan that can be employed at the first sign that suicidal ideation is emerging.
11. Find out what part the specific mini-cultural microsystems (family and community) (Hirsch & Cukrowicz, 2014) play in contributing to suicidal ideation and, conversely, what they can contribute to lethality resistance.
12. Use Hays's **ADDRESSING model** (2001, 2022) to understand and incorporate general cultural components along with Nobbman and colleagues' (2013) specific crisis **SAFETY** social locations into the management plan (See Chapter 2 "Culturally Effective Helping in Crisis" for these acronyms).

CW: Here are some things that I'd like you to think about doing with me. We work together on this, and sometimes other people get involved, but mainly it is you and me. First off, let's just take it as a given that you will probably consider suicide again. That is at present a fact of life. It is not forever, however. What we want to do is take away the reinforcing value of it as a short-term solution and look at the long-term benefits of doing something else. If it happens again, we don't see that as a failure but rather as something to troubleshoot and figure out what we have to do to fine-tune the plan so that it is less and less likely to happen. I also want to look at when you are having thought disorders and mood symptoms. Those are important to know when they start in, so we can do something about them as opposed to just waiting for them to become a tidal wave of emotions and thought that wash over and drown you. The same is true of booze and drugs. If you are using those, we need to do something about that because they go hand in hand with thinking about killing yourself. Are we on the same page thus far?

Deborah: Yeah, I suppose so.

CW: Okay, good. You won't get lectures from me. You choose what it is you want to do about it, and I will support you. If you believe AA or other treatment programs are needed, we can work on that. We need to plan activities that substitute for those times when you might drink or get high. We want to think small, specific, and concrete on this plan and just keep it a few days ahead, so it doesn't get too big and cumbersome and hard to do. We want you to see positive, concrete changes in your life and get control back in it. When that happens, suicide behavior won't happen because you won't see the situation as unchangeable. So, if I were to ask you if you were to do *something* in the next two days, and you could, would you see that as a sign of progress, and would you be able to tell me exactly what that was and why it was a sign of progress? Those are the things we are looking for in this plan. Things like decreasing social isolation, increasing pleasant and healthful activities, engaging in a work or leisure activity with someone you like. Something that is small to start with, but very concrete. Something you can hang your hat on and say, "See, Pete, that is progress!" Does that sound like something you are willing to do?

Deborah: I mean, I guess so. I don't know. This is all overwhelming...and pretty intimidating.

CW: That's okay and totally normal. That's why I am here to help walk you through the process. While this is going to be focused on changing behavior and problem solving, we need to remember that suicidal behavior is supported by emotional pain and the feeling that "I can't escape it, and it is intolerable." To that extent we are going to talk about emotions—journal emotions, tape-record emotions—and take them apart and put them back together again. We are going to listen to those emotions and work through them, so they don't build up and blow up and become all-encompassing and overwhelming.

Now, if suicidal behavior shows up again, we need to plan for it and be in control. We are going to develop what the Army calls a **smart card**; simple rules of the road that keep you straight on task and not off track. You'll have it in your billfold readily accessible when you start to feel things go haywire. Think of it like a diabetic and insulin. Things start to get edgy, haul yourself out of that environment, get a quiet secure place and pull the card and give yourself a shot and review of the instructions so you can de-escalate. We'll write down a crisis protocol smart card, so that you would know exactly what to do. You would be in control of it and not vice versa. On that card, we would put the resources you could use and call on, like telephone numbers, e-mail addresses, hours of operation, and so on. We also want to put two or three cues on the card. Things like "Okay, I am starting to feel anxious. I need to take a deep breath and relax, just relax." Or "Whoa! Wait a second. What am I getting into here? If my hands are sweating, that means I need to step back and take a look at this and see what the behavior is getting me." By having these smart cards, lots of times we can spot trouble and stop it before it gets started. That's a concrete thing we can do together if you are willing.

Deborah: Okay, that sounds doable. I might need some help with it, but the idea is generally okay. Maybe having something like that will help me to remember resources when I feel overwhelmed.

CW: Exactly! That's the point. Also, if it is okay with you, I am going to text you at random to see how you are doing. I may also call you if things get more complex than a text will take care of. This is not going to be "snoopervising." It is going to be concern. The calls won't be long, just brief check-ups of 2 to 3 minutes. You can also text me or call if you want. Just to keep a check on the plan. If things really go to hell in a handcart and you can't get me for some reason, you'll call the local hot-line or the national line. So, there are no cop-outs or excuses on this plan. You always have back-up just like cops call for back-up. Back-up keeps you safe and alive.

Deborah: Ugh, I really don't want to go through this again.

CW: Well, that's why we are also going to talk honestly about when you need to be admitted to a hospital. If that happens, it would be better if you decided to check yourself in for a time-out rather than having me, or somebody like me, involuntarily hospitalize you. I understand that's not really palatable, but it would be you who would be deciding and not somebody else. We are going to do the same thing with medication. What you have been on has not worked very well. I want to look into getting that reevaluated. The whole idea is for you to take more and more control over your decisions. If suicidal behavior should occur, we will see it not as a failure but as an opportunity to troubleshoot what we are doing and change things. The bottom line is that we want to neutralize the reinforcement of suicidal behavior so that it no longer has positive valence, and have other more positive, addicting behaviors and healthful living activities take its place. I will help you manage this, but it is going to be you who will have more and more say in what is to be done. That is a big, long speech. And it sounds like a lot, but we will take it one day and one step at a time. What do you think?

Deborah: It's kinda scary, but kinda thrilling too. I don't know. I kinda feel good for the first time. Maybe like in some control, but that's scary, I've been out of it so long.

The key component in crisis management is normalizing the situation and showing the client that everything comes down to problem solving in a matter-of-fact way. Suicidal behavior will invariably recur in a client like Deborah. To keep her from getting discouraged, we treat suicide as an annoying, inconvenient, but important piece of business that is not catastrophic and does not mean she is an abysmal failure. By focusing on problem solving, developing tolerance to emotional distress, changing disturbing self-images, halting impulsive behaviors, creating anger-management skills, and generating better day-to-day functioning at home and work (Meichenbaum, 2017), we start to build resiliency and emotional toughness in the chronic, suicidal client. This is not an easy task, but it is one that can be done and can be successful.

CW: We are going to work out a treatment plan for living, but first thing is I'm gonna give you my business card with phone and text number and e-mail on it. That is for you to call, no ifs, ands, or buts, if things are really starting to go in the toilet. But the important thing is, it is your crisis card and on the back we are going to brainstorm and come up with five activities that, when things start to go to hell in a handcart, are positive actions that will break that doom-despair thinking and turn off that emotional motor running wild with affective dysregulation, so you don't need to call me but can take control of things yourself. It sounds simplistic, but it works. These are positive activities that will require you to get off your rear end and go do something so you get busy and take your mind off of those inner voices.

Of all the things that don't work in the lethality intervention business, Pete uses a couple of very simple tactics that do work—particularly for those clients who have been hospitalized: follow-up phone calls (Vaiva et al., 2006), text messaging (Berrouiguet et al., 2014) and crisis coping cards (Jobes, 2005, pp. 80–82). The phone calls and texts provide follow-up support that says you belong, and you are not a burden. The protocol card helps clients kick-start their crisis management plan because lots of times, it is difficult for clients to initiate problem-solving skills on their own. A bullet point cue card that is concrete gives them specific, real-time instructions on recognizing warning signs and instituting coping skills (Brown et al., 2011). While there have been online services (Best et al., 2013) and phone apps developed for suicide intervention (Aguirre et al., 2013), they are still so new with little back up research that we are not willing to make any recommendations on them as of yet, although it's fairly clear they'll start to play a larger part in prevention.

Simon, Age 36. Simon was the director of a rape crisis center in a large metropolitan area. He had established a reputation as an effective leader, public relations person, fundraiser, recruiter, and trainer of volunteer workers for the center. He was tireless, dedicated, popular, and widely known as the leader of one of the best organized and most effective crisis agencies in the community.

Now, after six years as director of the center, Simon was approaching burnout. He was also experiencing grief and rage over a broken relationship. Simon was astute enough to finally recognize that he was on the verge of some kind of breakdown and was considering suicide or homicide, so he sought counseling at his agency's employee assistance program (EAP) clinic.

CW: So, Simon, from what I can glean from your intake material and from what you just said, I sense that *you* are fully aware of your vulnerability right now but are keeping up a good front for the troops.

Simon: (in a clinical, detached fashion) That's right. And there's no use in my problems interfering with the work at the center. That's the most important thing. Even so, my issues are affecting me, at least. And, right now, I'm really feeling trapped; no good to them or myself either.

CW: What's the most pressing issue in your entrapment?

Simon: (Starts to tremble and shake with a tremor in his voice.) Well, part of the problem is at home. I've had the rug pulled out from under me . . . literally. (Laughs ironically.) My partner, René, my soul mate for over 6 years, has taken off. It happened right under my nose. (Hits his chest in recrimination.) So stupid! So blind! I didn't see it! She has managed to leave me high and dry with little money and with all the bills. She took most of our furniture, much of which I bought myself. And she took both our dogs, too! That cold-hearted witch! This all happened just when we were getting ready for our one big fundraising event of the year at the center and just as we were preparing for the accreditation site team to visit the center in a few weeks.

I'm feeling so hurt, so humiliated, and so betrayed that I am overwhelmed with anger, disappointment, and depression. I have scarcely slept or eaten for over a week. I thought our relationship was for keeps. I feel like killing her if I could get my hands on the cheating rat, but I still care about her so much! I want the miserable creep back! I'd kill that little blonde witch if I could find out where they took off to. Her, too! I'm feeling so worthless and undesirable and tired of this nightmare that sometimes I just wish I'd sleep forever.

CW: What you've just said worries me. Now I'm concerned about your safety. Are you feeling so depressed and angry that you might consider suicide—or homicide for that matter?

Simon: I don't know how I feel anymore. I guess I wouldn't go that far. Suicide, that is. I want her back more than anything. But I've even thought to myself, "If I can't have her, then nobody can." But I know that's not realistic either.

CW: Simon, does that mean that you might consider doing harm to René or even to her new girlfriend? Have you thought about how you might hurt them if you were going to?

Simon: When it came right down to it, I don't think so. But I'd certainly feel like it sometimes. No, I'm just distraught and mad as hell right now. I'm really harmless, I guess. I don't know what I need. Some space, maybe. Another job, maybe. I don't know. Just some relief and love and rest and to get over this crushing pain.

Simon continues his catharsis about his romantic betrayal and the deep hurt it has caused him for another 30 minutes. The crisis worker listens intently for signs that he may have the means, access, and availability of acting on his stress and perturbation. During that time, he gradually subsides emotionally and regains a good deal of his cognitive ability, to the point the crisis worker rates his affect as 7, behavior as 5, and cognition as 5, for a full-scale score of 17. His Suicide Status Form (Jobes, 2005) is in the average to above range, with 3s and 4s and an overall rating of 3.5. His Interpersonal Needs Questionnaire (Van Orden et al., 2012) indicates some feelings of burdensomeness and a lack of belonging in the middle range "as somewhat true." However, he does give "very true" endorsements of people who care about and support him, which is a major plus. More ominous is his Maslach Burnout Scale (Maslach & Jackson, 1981), which indicates an extremely high score on the Emotional Exhaustion and Depersonalization scale and a low score on the Personal Accomplishment scale, indicating he is well on the road to burnout (refer to Chapter 15, "Human Services Workers in Crisis: Burnout, Vicarious Traumatization, and Compassion Fatigue").

Some safety measures will need to be put in place before he walks out the door.

CW: I believe you, but I need a commitment to treatment from you, written down and signed before you leave here today. Can I trust you to do that?

I also want to institute a treatment plan. Your scores on the two lethality assessments are not in the lethal range, but they are fairly high. The fact that you have considered lethal action is a warning we need to take seriously. You are a smart professional, but even smart professionals don't always know when they are in burnout, and your scores on the burnout scale tell me you are, along with what you self-report.

The case of Simon provides one glimpse of a crisis worker inquiring about both the client's suicidal and homicidal potential. The worker has determined that Simon's possible threat to himself and others is in the low-to-moderate range on all dimensions of the TAF. However, the worker obtains a "Commitment to Treatment" agreement with the client. There is a good deal of divisiveness in regard to "no harm" contracts, but they are generally inadvisable (Bryan & Rudd, 2006; Rudd, Mandrusiak et al., 2006). Notably, "no harm" or "anti-suicide" contracts signed between worker and client have absolutely no legal bearing or support if you get sued, and they absolutely do not substitute for a thorough management and treatment plan (Bongar & Sullivan, 2013, p. 6). Chiles and Strosahl (1995, pp. 131–132) have criticized the no-harm contract because it specifies what a person *should not* do instead of *should* do, and they question its utility if a person starts to feel guilty about not abiding by it and terminates therapy as a result. To that end, the American Psychiatric Association (APA) has stated that no-suicide contracts should not be used with patients who are actively suicidal. Bryan and Rudd (2006) and Rudd, Mandrusiak et al. (2006) discuss the inherent flaws within the no-harm contract and present the Commitment to Treatment Statement (CTS) as a viable alternative. Rudd, Mandrusiak, and colleagues (2006) describe the CTS as an agreement between the patient and clinician in which the patient agrees to make a commitment to the treatment process and living by (1) identifying the roles, obligations, and expectations of both the clinician and the patient in treatment; (2) communicating openly and honestly about all aspects of treatment including suicide; and (3) accessing identified emergency services during periods of crisis that might threaten the patient's ability to honor the agreement (p. 247).

Lamar, Age 51. Lamar was an eminent and successful elementary school principal who had devoted his life to children and the teaching profession. He was exceptionally capable, hardworking, conscientious, and efficient. He was also compulsive and a perfectionist in his work and personal habits. At age 51, Lamar faced some life and career decisions that he regarded as catastrophic: (1) He had recently had bypass heart surgery only to discover he had prostate cancer, and he could not bear to think about his physician's recommendation to accept early retirement and undergo prostate removal surgery. (2) He felt trapped between the two perceived unacceptable choices of continuing to hold the principalship in his debilitating physical condition or becoming the ex-principal who had been forced into early retirement. (3) He was totally unprepared to alter his whole identity, which had included serving the students, faculty, parents, community, school, and the teaching profession. Lamar had no family. He had never married because he had devoted all his energies and talents to education, although he had once been in a long-term relationship with a college roommate. The relationship ended because his partner demanded too much of Lamar's time—time he needed to devote to his students. Lamar came to his longtime friend and colleague, the Jefferson Elementary School counselor, in desperation.

Lamar: (in tears) It is so hopeless. Why me? Why has God forsaken me? I have been a good person. A good teacher. A good principal. What have I done to cause me to come to this? I don't think I can bear it. (Sobs. Pause.) It's so unfair. I have no choice. (Sobs.)

CW: (reaches out and touches Latasha's arm) You're feeling hurt, hopeless, and vulnerable—and you're looking for better answers and choices than you've been able to find so far. Because so far there are none.

Lamar: (still in tears) For the first time in my life, I have no ideas, no options.

CW: I want you to know that I'm glad you have the courage to discuss it. What scares me is the desperation and danger you're feeling. You're feeling that, right now, there are no acceptable choices. That's a really tunnel vision view that's not like you at all.

Lamar: (Still in tears. Nonverbal clues show that he is experiencing acute fear, anxiety, and hopelessness, and has almost given up.) None. None at all. There is no future.

CW: Lamar, it sounds to me like you've considered suicide. I want to know your thinking on this subject.

Lamar: (still in tears) Oh God! I've thought about that a lot. Toyed with it a lot. And I'll have to admit that it becomes more appealing all the time. I have these pain pills for the cancer treatment. I could take them all at once.

CW: Do you have a plan on how to do it?

Lamar: I would put on some Brahms, get a large glass of Chablis, destroy my phone so I wouldn't chicken out. No one would be in the office. It'd be June 9th, the day school is out, about 11:00 in the evening. Everything would be finished up at school, and everybody would be gone. I work late a lot on Friday so security wouldn't bother me. That would give them time to get another principal. I even made some recommendations I have written down. It would be all settled. Actually, I am feeling a little peace with myself as I talk about it. Strange!

Lamar's plan is highly lethal. He has thought carefully about it. He has the means, the method, and the plan is close to irreversible. A fast assessment on the PIMP acronym would affirm high lethal potential. His contemplation that he feels at peace is another highly lethal indication that he has settled his affairs. The fact that his colleague and friend is hearing this makes the decision the school counselor is about to make terribly difficult, but it is one that her training has instilled in her. In such instances, it is critical not to match the client's anxiety level. Moralizing, placating, coercion, lecturing, or other attempts to discount the client will only exacerbate the problem (Chiles & Strosahl, 1995, pp. 113–115). The potential for countertransference to arise in such situations is high. Disregarding cries for help because of their threatening nature, denying the facts because of the personal relationship with the client, feeling a lack of expertise because the person is not an "expert" suicidologist but "merely" a school counselor, and being lulled into a false sense of security by who the client has been as opposed to the state of being the client is now in are serious dangers, and staying in self-control and not becoming vague and tangential are critical to the process of stopping this suicide situation (Leenaars, 1994, pp. 56–57). Duty to protect has just come into play here, and if the school counselor did not assess for suicide and did not take action, she could be held legally accountable as negligent (Granello & Granello, 2007, pp. 266–268).

CW: (Very clearly, empathically, and emphatically makes the following declaratory and exclamatory statements.) What you have just said scares the daylights out of me, Lamar. I cannot and will not let you do that! If you won't go to the superintendent with me right now and tell him you need some help, I will call him myself! If I have to, I will call the school resource police officer to contain you until we can get you to a place of safety. I believe that you have become so constricted you see no options. There are options, and you need to stay alive to find them out! I don't think you would have talked to me if you didn't believe there was something left, and you needed another view. Well, I am giving you that view. So, which do you wish to do? Go with me to the superintendent or have me make the call? You could run right out of here and go swallow all those pills, I suppose, but then we would call an ambulance and they would take you out in front of the kids, which I don't think you would see as really uplifting. So, you see there are some choices left, and the first one is, "Do we go now, or do I call now?"

There are no ifs, ands, or buts about this scenario, and there is no need or time to do any kind of written assessment. The TAF puts Lamar clearly in the high 20s. The school counselor is ethically and legally bound to take action (Chiles & Strosahl, 1995, pp. 17–35; Granello & Granello 2007, pp. 266–268) no matter what the client's protestations about confidentiality, broken friendship, trust, or any other pleas might be. The school counselor, like any other helping services professional, has a duty to disclose life-threatening behavior. That the client is her boss makes no difference. The counselor also lays a guilt trip on the principal to stop any impulsive attempts by reminding him that it would not be good form or model very good behavior to be hauled off in front of the school in an ambulance or police car. This tactic is one used by Everstine (1998, pp. 113–114) to remind clients that there are many more potential victims than their constricted view of things allows them to see. Lamar's love for the children of his school would be a powerful deterrent to doing anything foolish and precipitous.

While hospitalizing a client who is potentially suicidal is no guarantee that the person will not kill themselves, given the clear intent to do harm to himself, at the very least, the crisis worker is removing the principal's immediate access to killing himself. Whether he goes ahead in the future is another matter. At present, putting him in the hospital will bring the psychological perturbation he feels into full view of his oncology team, who can then step in to deal with that aspect of his cancer.

While professional ethics frown on close friends or professional associates counseling one another, we believe that crisis lethality issues override that ethical standard. In the real world, this example of a close relationship between two colleagues is included here because, all too often, this is exactly how the discovery of a potential suicide occurs. Close friends should be aware of what they need to do and do it proactively and without guilt (See Chapter 15, Burnout–the Case of Jane). If the worker is not sure what to do, doesn't feel they have the necessary expertise, or is too close to the client personally, the watchwords are "refer if possible" and "consult"! There is no instance in a helping professional's life when consultation with a peer is more important than when dealing with lethality (Leenaars, 1994).

Older Adults

The number of older adults across the world is growing rapidly. As baby boomers age, this fact, combined with the high suicide rate in older adults, means that a lot more service providers for geriatric populations are going to be needed, and those providers are going to need to get into the suicide prevention/intervention business (Erlangsen et al., 2011). Suicide in older adults is treatable and preventable (Barak et al., 2022; Lapierre et al., 2011), yet comparatively little research addresses this high risk population. Various factors may contribute to the elevated suicide risk among older adults, such as loneliness, isolation, physical illness, grief, depression, and cognitive impairment (Minayo & Cavalcante, 2015). The risk of suicide among older adults tends to increase with age (Lobato dos Santos et al., 2021), which might provide credence to the notion that the aforementioned risk factors exacerbate over time if therapeutic or other supportive intervention does not take place.

The worker's assessment brings to the forefront a special consideration for dealing with older people. That assessment should include ego-weakening factors such as chronic and acute physical and mental illness, senior abuse, alcohol misuse, prolonged stress, failure to respond to medical treatment, and complicated/prolonged grief (for a complete description of this phenomenon, refer to Chapter 12, "Personal Loss: Bereavement and Grief"). A variety of social factors, such as having fewer friends, living alone, being excluded or living on the periphery of social and family events, and being separated from the family

through children leaving, all contribute to the potential for suicide (McGlothin, 2008, p. 124–126). Psychodynamic factors most often include the stress and strain of various losses, such as the loss of a spouse, friends, work roles, and income. Chalking these risk factors up to "just growing old" is inappropriate and minimizes the suffering of older adults.

Roy, Age 68. Roy had been a farmer all his life. At age 65, he went into semiretirement, turning his land, equipment, buildings, and livestock over to his two sons, who also were career farmers. One year after he began his semiretirement, his wife died. About a year later, he was despondent and could find no purpose in life, even though he was in excellent health and had the good fortune of financial independence. He has been somewhat alienated and estranged from his two sons because of disagreements and arguments over their "newfangled" farming practices that he doesn't always agree with. The foreman of the farm, Juan, came upon Roy standing on a tractor in the hall of the barn. Roy held a rope with a hangman's noose in it, and he was attaching the rope to an overhead crossbeam. Roy, thinking he was completely alone, was surprised by Juan's appearance.

Juan: What on earth are you doing there, man?

Roy: (**Almost falls off the tractor he is so startled.**) Where the hell did you come from? What are you doing here?

Juan: I'll tell you what I'm gonna do right now! I'm taking that rope away from you this minute! You're going to get in my pickup truck this minute. I'm driving you straight to the mental health center. That's where we're going. And I'll tell those boys of yours what you've tried to do too! Don't you know that it'd just kill those boys if you finished what you were planning to do? What the hell did you think you were doing, anyway?

Juan's alert and decisive actions clearly show that one does not have to be a trained human services worker to contain and control a situation in which human life is at risk. The crisis worker at the mental health center knew nothing about Roy's problems, but he recognized that a person of Roy's age, gender, life circumstance, style, and sense of private independence would rarely, if ever, present himself for counseling (Chiles & Strosahl, 1995, p. 240). In assessing Roy's responses, the worker quickly concluded that he definitely exhibited six of the lethality characteristics that Fujimura et al. (1985) defined as high-risk factors: (1) the plan was definite and readily accessible, (2) the method was irreversible, (3) there was indication of sleep disruption, (4) support people would not be around, (5) rescue would be improbable, and (6) the most valued possessions had been disposed of. Also, the crisis worker knew that among men Roy's age, there are very few suicide gestures or attempts. Older men are more likely to complete suicide than to attempt it (Shneidman et al., 1976; Stone, 2001). The crisis worker immediately suspected loss as a factor in Roy's decision to kill himself. Shea (2011) proposes that older adults are subject to a series of losses, and, as they suffer these losses, the potential for lethality rises. They include the loss of health, mobility, cognitive functioning, ability for self-care, role with family or society, skills, job or job opportunity, means of self-support, home or cherished possessions, and loved ones, including pets.

CW: Roy, lots of times men who have had lots of responsibility find that as they age, their ability to take on those responsibilities becomes more difficult. They also may not feel like they mean much to anyone because they don't have much importance or lose their capabilities—that, in fact, they are becoming a burden. I'm wondering how you feel about what I just said?

Roy: Well, now there's really nothing else to live for. A man's got to have some purpose. I've got nothing to go to—nothing to get up for in the morning. I just don't know what's gonna happen, and I frankly don't give a tinker's damn. My wife's dead. I can't hardly do anything anymore. The boys don't need me to run the farm, and I damn sure don't need no therapy or no shrink.

CW: (**Thinking to himself: "Wow! He's not fooling! With all this intake information pointing toward suicide lethality, I don't need any more assessment data right now. I'm remembering his age, his male image, his having disposed of all his property, his wife's death—these are potent indicators—and this morning, an aborted self-hanging! It's a wonder he's even here!"**) Roy, what happened this morning is scary, indeed. I'm setting up a complete medical evaluation for you today. I have called your family doctor. I have also called your sons, who are on their way in here right now. To say that they are very concerned is putting it mildly. I know you probably hate it that I called them, but we need to get some support systems in place and straighten some things out between you and your family.

While older clients will see their family doctors for a variety of physical complaints, they will seldom, if ever, speak about psychological duress or even consider it as a possibility! In fact, a number of factors may interfere with help-seeking among older individuals who are contemplating suicide (Rasnayake & Navratil, 2022). These may include "a weak social network, poor understanding of depressive and suicidal signs by family members, negative attitudes relating to old age culture, and a crisis of personal perspectives in help-seeking" (Rasnayake & Navratil, 2022, p. 1). All of Roy's symptoms indicate he has slid, ever so gradually, into being at least demoralized, if not depressed, by life's circumstances. Even though he would appear to have everything to live for, the loss of his wife, when they had grand plans for retirement together, the death of other close friends, and the disintegration of his social network as friends die, go to nursing homes, or move away, all have slowly led Roy to perceive life is no longer worth living. Roy's initial TAF score is approximately 27 (A=8, B=10, C=9).

The benign neglect and estrangement with his sons is another piece of the suicide puzzle that needs to be dealt with. While it might be readily apparent why older adults would complete suicide if they were physically abused or neglected, more often their adult children are guilty of benign neglect or annoyance at dealing with the foibles and frailties of older people. Grown children have their own lives to lead. They may either believe that their parents have little or no need of them, or they may become annoyed by their parents' increasing dependence. As a result, they tend to avoid and exclude their parents not only from activities but from decision making.

Social isolation is further compounded by the loss of friends. As a result, one of the key factors in dealing with older adults is to set up in step-by-step fashion a new set of life supports. Reconnecting with people is paramount. If a person is unable to engage in former leisure or work activities because of a decrease in physical or mental functioning, then new activities that are socially connective and challenging to the client's physical and mental capacity need to be instituted.

While at first glance, these therapeutic goals may seem a long way from suicide intervention, they are, in fact, directly related to it! Disengagement (a progressive withdrawal from the wider world), activity (decreased levels of physical, emotional, and cognitive activity), role exit (social usefulness diminishes as work activity ceases), and social exchange (limited ability to engage in new relationships) theories all play a significant part in whether older persons become suicidal (Granello & Granello, 2007, p, 78).

The other compounding problem is medication and neurotransmitter changes. Wenzel et al., (2009, p. 267) propose that older adults may engage in **chronic or passive suicide** when they decide to quit taking their medication because of side effects, cost, or the notion that stopping taking it will hasten death. In many instances, forgetting to take medication, misdosage, polymedication administered by different doctors, and bad drug interactions contribute to depression. For this reason, it is paramount that primary care providers be contacted, and physical and mental health issues be coordinated (McGlothin, 2008, p. 125). Combined with the effects of alcohol or illicit drugs, the potential for psychological problems becomes exponentially greater in older adults (Chiles & Strosahl, 1995, p. 243). Added to the foregoing is the mounting suspicion that serotonin levels are affected by aging. Thus, the mere fact of getting old may biologically predispose a person to suicide (Granello & Granello, 2007; Kanel et al., 2023).

One of the primary techniques for bringing older adult clients out of suicidal ideation is to remotivate them to live. Chiles and Strosahl (1995) have developed a Reasons for Living Inventory that may be given to clients; it covers survival and coping skills, responsibility to family, child-related concerns, fear of suicide, fear of social disapproval, and moral objections. While clients may naysay many items, there are invariably some they will agree with. The crisis worker may then use these items to combat the suicidal ideation and reinforce the older adult client's desire to live.

CW: (Two days after Roy has been medically evaluated for an antidepressant and has had an emotional but positive family session with his two sons.) So, after talking with your boys and taking the inventory, you have said at least these items would be important: not wanting to be seen as a coward or selfish; my sons might not believe I loved them; I do want to watch my grandchildren grow up; others might think I am weak or selfish; I wouldn't want people to think I didn't have control; I have had a love of life; and there are some experiences I haven't had yet. So those are some reasons for living. I further think that the antidepressant the doctor has prescribed will kick in and you will start to feel like your old self. I want to let you know that there is a group of folks that meet at St. Mark's church that I work with. I understand that might be

pretty repulsive to you, but I asked Jim Joyner if he wouldn't mind talking to you about our group. I believe you know him. In the meantime, I'd just like to make sure that if you start to feel down, you know you can call me before we meet next week. I have also done a little investigating and I believe the agriculture teacher at the high school would be very interested in your expertise in no-till planting, the top-flight soil conservation you are known for, and working with him on the school ag program.

Roy: Hell, I guess it wouldn't kill me to listen to Jim. It's gut wrenching, but I do appreciate what you're trying to do. I particularly appreciate the head-to-head with Leroy and Ronnie. I couldn't have done that myself. I do take a lot of pride in them and the grandkids. I don't know what got into me. Hmm! The ag teacher said that? Hmmmm! Well, maybe.

CW: Roy, I want you to know that I feel good about your progress and, given I have dealt with a lot of people in a situation like yours, the prognosis for you is good. There are a couple of things I want to do, though. First off, we are going to put together a treatment plan. It isn't a forever plan, and I really believe that it's about 4 to 6 weeks' worth of work. That plan is going to involve coordinating your medication with your primary care doctor, some more meetings with your sons that I want our family therapist here at the clinic to do, getting you back socially involved again, and not just letting all that knowledge you have sit out there and ossify on 1300 County Road 1321 East. I also want you to make a contract for living with me. It is essentially a plan we will develop together so you have supports and strategies to help you avoid taking your life while we are working on this. Finally, we're going to distill that plan down to a smart card I'd like you to carry around in your billfold. It'll have just basic prompts in it if things start to get out of hand like when "good, old, traditional" butts heads with "new-fangled." You take a time out and read the card as a reminder of the new you and the plans you've put into action.

Getting Roy involved in a support group with a former friend is a key ingredient in getting a social support group of peers in place. Social support is critical and needs to target the peer groups and pleasurable and stimulating activities with which older adults are involved (Wenzel et al., 2008, p. 278). The crisis worker is very directive and active in instigating these interventions because most people who are depressed are going to have a very difficult time initially acting on their own.

CW: (one week later) You have a couple of what we call "automatic thoughts" linked with some recently developed core beliefs that have helped kick this depression into high gear. Listening to you, they are very different from what you typically have thought and are really typical of the kind of thing that gets a person depressed. For instance, some of your core beliefs are "I am on a downhill slide and there's no upside. I am a burden, and I can't stand that." Some of the automatic thoughts are "It's hopeless and I am helpless to do anything about it. I am a weak old man. I might as well give up. They'd be better off without me." That smart card will have what we call positive counter injunctions on it. For instance, when you are at home sitting alone at night watching TV and, all of a sudden, one of those thoughts pops up, I want you to pull this card out and read it. It will say something like "That's not true! I am engaged and I am putting my knowledge back to work. I am not a hopeless piece of used junk. I have reestablished my relationships with my family and am enjoying the hell out of helping raise my grandkids. Yes! I miss Helen, but I know she'd want me involved in rearing our grandkids. I don't have a terminal case of 'I-can't-stand-it-itis.' I have withstood a lot of things in life as tough as this. It's inconvenient, all these aches and pains, but I can move and think, and I intend to do so and enjoy myself, which is what Helen would want."

These are the positive automatic thoughts I want you to get habituated to. I also have another little program called a Hope Kit I want you to assemble. It consists of a container that holds mementos that will serve as reminders to live and enjoy life. It is not about getting all caught up and getting maudlin about what was, but what symbolizes you and the good life you have lived. I particularly would recommend some photographs or keepsakes of the good times and good memories. But this is definitely not about living in the past; in fact, you just might have some new mementos you want to put in there—like that Future Farmers of America hat you are wearing that I might guess you stole (*both laugh*) from the ag teacher. I want you to use that as a negative thought stopping device, so if you get down in the dumps you can pull it out and start going through it.

As simplistic as it sounds, the Hope Kit (Wenzel et al., 2009) is extremely effective because it is a concrete reminder of all the positive aspects of the person's life (Jobes, 2006). The positive counter injunctions are typical of cognitive-behavioral approaches to stop catastrophic thinking (Beck, 1979). Putting these on a crisis card (Rudd et al., 2004) and placing the Hope Kit in a readily accessible place are easily implemented crisis intervention techniques designed to stop negative cognitions in their tracks.

Roy's situation is not unique to older clients. Roy is fortunate in a sense. He is not faced with debilitating financial or health problems, as many of his peers are. These problems further exacerbate the notion that suicide is a viable option. Finally, a compounding problem is that sometimes, the problems older adults face ripple over to spouses or significant other caretakers, who may also come under lethal threat.

Guidelines for Family, Friends, and Associates

The crisis worker often has to deal with gritty issues that involve family. Getting clients like Roy to come to terms with long-smoldering family issues is not easy. Urging clients to engage in new, resocializing activities is also difficult. However, if they can be done, the quality of life goes up and lethality comes down. Mishara and associates (2005) found that direct intervention with families who called into a suicide prevention line resulted in potentially suicidal people having less suicidal ideation, fewer suicide attempts, and fewer depressive symptoms. Family and friends reported less psychological distress and use of more positive coping mechanisms and reported that their communication with the suicidal person was more helpful (Mishara et al., 2005). The family, friends, and associates of the suicidal/homicidal person can do many things to contribute to prevention, especially in the area of correcting the alienated lifestyle that cuts off the at-risk person's connectedness with others. Indeed, there are parent training programs in suicide prevention such as Parents-CARE (Hooven, 2013) that are effective interventions for suicidal adolescents.

Crisis workers can serve an important educational role by helping families, friends, and associates learn about and become attuned to the risk factors, cues, and cries for help that suicidal/homicidal people generally display in some way (Hipple & Cimbolic, 1979, pp. 76–78). The crisis worker who talked with Roy's sons focused on including Roy back in their lives both as grandfather and as a wise consultant whose knowledge and skill of farming can complement their own. Families can and should be an integral part of treatment and should be fully informed about the positive role (along with the limits) they can play (Rudd et al., 2004, p. 105). Perhaps the most important component of family involvement is helping the whole family system become aware of how the suicidal member's feelings and actions influence the family and how they are reciprocally influenced by the family members' feelings (Softas et al., 1998, p. 227). To that end, dealing with past issues and recriminations is out of bounds. At least until the suicidal events are resolved, bringing up old psychological baggage does little good. The emphasis is on the present and future and developing new behavioral contracts for positive change in the total family constellation (McLean & Taylor, 1994).

Family, friends, and associates who attend to the many cues that have been described in this chapter can help the suicidal/homicidal person by genuinely and assertively confronting the lethal issues. For instance, they can watch for the lethal person's preoccupation with an anniversary date of a significant loss, such as the death of a loved one, or the resulting depression that a job loss or academic failure generates and intervene in a directive manner if needed (McLean & Taylor, 1994). Significant others can help the survivors cope with suicide/ homicide after it happens. On the other hand, if fractures in the family system are severe, discretion may be the better part of valor. Pushing family members together who have long-standing agendas of anger and recrimination is the about the last thing that needs to happen.

When family or other bereaved groups cannot get past the shock of the death and/or exhibit excessive blame or guilt, crisis workers can meet with them and help them deal with their grief (Shneidman, 1975). On a final note, McGlothin (2008, p. 137) believes that all of the family needs to be checked out for suicidal/homicidal ideation because, in many families, suicide/homicide and violence are operational ways to settle problems.

Some "Don'ts" and a Few "Dos."

LO10 A number of authors (Bongar & Sullivan, 2013; Jobes, 2006; Kleespies, 2014; Neimeyer & Mahoney, 1995; Shea, 2011) have identified some "don'ts" and dos" of suicide management that serve to supplement the intervention considerations already listed. Our comments are added to each point in the following list. These "don'ts" and "dos" apply to almost any time you work with a person who manifesting

lethal behavior. It's a long list, and you don't need to memorize it, but you do need to remember where it is and check it out—particularly when you get those big furry moths flapping around in your stomach, making you feel really queasy when you have a potentially lethal client in front of you.

1. Don't forget to use established suicide risk assessment measures in addition to a thorough clinical interview if possible. If not, PIMP it.
2. Don't lecture, blame, give advice, judge, or preach to clients. If that had worked, they wouldn't be with you now.
3. Don't criticize clients or their choices or behaviors. Do remember that as odd or confusing as their behavior seems from an outside perspective, the lethal behavior makes perfect sense to the client.
4. Don't debate the pros and cons of suicide. Philosophy has nothing to do with what is going on in a lethality case.
5. Don't be misled by the client telling you the crisis is past. Never just take the client's word that things are "settled" and "okay now." Do keep checking!
6. Don't deny the client's suicidal ideas. Ideation leads to action. If a person says they have lethal intent, even in a joking or offhand way, check it out.
7. Don't try to challenge for shock effects. This is not "Scared Straight" therapy. Challenges may be acted on to show you the client means business.
8. Don't leave the client isolated, unobserved, and disconnected. Provision needs to be made for keeping the client safe and secure, and that means somebody needs to monitor them.
9. Don't diagnose and analyze behavior or confront the client with interpretations during the acute phase. Psychodynamic interpretations involving "why" are unimportant at this point.
10. Don't be passive. Suicides are high on the triage scale. You must become active and directive.
11. Don't overreact. Suicidal/homicidal behavior is scary, but it is behavior that can be handled. Do stay calm and keep your voice well-modulated. That's what this book and chapter are about. You don't have to be a superhero to do this stuff. Just keep calm and practice what you have learned!
12. Don't keep the client's suicidal risk a secret (be trapped in the confidentiality issue) or worry about "snitching" on the client. Whether you are a bosom friend or a professional, this is life-threatening behavior. You do need to tell someone in authority who can keep the client safe.

13. Don't get sidetracked on extraneous or external issues or persons. Forget about all the other real and imagined ills and issues. Do deal with the lethality in a straightforward, business-like manner. The other stuff can and should be acknowledged as important to the person, but that's it.

14. Don't glamorize, martyrize, glorify, heroize, or deify suicidal behavior in others, past or present. If you want somebody to kill themselves or copycat a friend or idol, this is an excellent way to have that happen.

15. Don't become defensive or avoid strong feelings. The possibility for transference is great in lethal behavior. While lethal feelings are scary, they are exactly what need to be discussed and uncovered.

16. Don't hide behind pseudo-professionalism and clinical objectivity as a way of distancing yourself psychologically from painful and scary material. What you are actually trying to do is insulate yourself from the brutal reality of what is going on, and that is not helpful. You must get into the game and build the relationship.

17. Don't fail to identify the precipitating event. Find what specifically caused the client to decide to become lethal. Global reasons are not helpful. Do identify the reason the client got here today, so action plans can be generated to deal with it.

18. Don't forget to follow up (you may get sued if you don't). Do keep track of lethal people until the crisis has passed.

19. Don't forget to document and report (you may get sued if you don't). Do keep good records of your assessment of the client and when and what you did with your recommendations.

20. Don't be so embarrassed or vain that you don't consult (you may get sued if you don't). Substantiation by another professional in a difficult case makes good therapeutic and legal sense.

21. Don't fail to make yourself available and accessible (you may get sued if you don't). If you come in contact with a suicidal/homicidal client, you must stay the course, be available, and have backup support.

22. Do take your time. Don't be hurried. Things may be frantic in the immediate environment, but you are the rock in the middle of the maelstrom. You have time!

23. Do watch for countertransference. Shea (2002, p. 122) poses two questions to keep you grounded. "What am I feeling right now?" "Is there any part of me that doesn't want to hear the truth right now?" Those are caution lights and reality checks on your potential loss of objectivity and treatment goals. Do get supervision.

24. Don't be blackmailed into caving into client demands. Do set limits and keep them. Clients with borderline personality disorder are especially adept at treatment blackmail. For example, keeping one's guns isn't an option with a highly suicidal client. Refusal to comply with treatment is not an option, nor is maintaining the right to kill oneself during treatment. Refusal to treat this client is not abandonment, but good clinical judgment.

25. Don't fail to take adequate protective measures if you are working with an outpatient client who owns guns. Do get them in safe keeping. (You may get sued if you don't). If you are working in an inpatient setting with a suicidal person, follow the institution's protocol to the t crossed and i dotted. The institution may still get sued, but you likely won't.

The Psychological Autopsy

LO11 Shneidman (1987) developed the psychological autopsy technique for the purpose of compiling detailed postmortem mental histories following suicides or deaths that were equivocal (not sure of cause). Psychological autopsies involve examination of personal demographics such as work, criminal, school, and medical records along with in-depth interviews of friends, relatives, coworkers, and health care professionals to attempt to ascertain the suicidal person's intent. They also attempt to determine what the trigger events were that might have contributed to the suicide. For instance, normative data from psychological autopsies indicate that an average of 40 percent of people who die by suicide had a medical illness and that HIV/AIDS and cancer are two particular illnesses that increase suicidal risk (Kleepies et al., 2009). Psychological autopsies also attempt to determine what, if any, psychopathology was present in completed suicides. For example, it appears that between 30 and 40 percent of people who die by suicide may meet criteria for personality disorders. Psychological autopsies have determined that besides the big five psychiatric diagnoses of major depressive, bipolar, anorexia nervosa, schizophrenia, and borderline personality disorder that are precursors to suicide (Joiner et al., 2009), schizoid and antisocial personality disorder also have strong associations with suicidal behavior (Duberstein & Witte, 2009). The autopsy was initially conceived by Shneidman to help clinicians become more cognizant of the warning signs of suicide in cases where intent, reason, and motivation are muddled and unclear.

The following questions seek to flesh out the psychological profile of the decedent's death—indeed, to determine first and foremost whether it was a suicide (Shneidman, 1999d). These questions are posed in an empathic manner to the survivors: Why did the person do it? How did he/she do it? When? That is, why at that particular time? What is the most probable mode of death? Besides details of the death itself, the autopsy seeks to determine the person's personality and lifestyle, typical patterns of reactions to stress, emotional upsets, and periods of disequilibrium, particularly in the recent past. What role did alcohol and/or drugs play in the person's life? What was the nature of his/her interpersonal relationships? What were the person's fantasies, dreams, thoughts, premonitions, or fears relating to death, accident, or suicide? What changes, if any, occurred in the person's habits, hobbies, eating, sexual relations, and other life routines? Information is garnered regarding the person's lifestyle, such as mood up- or downswings, successes, and plans for the future. Not only can these questions help determine whether the death was a suicide, they can also help determine how staff who may have been involved with the client can better prevent suicides (Shneidman, 1999d).

As with many important discoveries, Shneidman (1971) found a serendipitous function of the psychological autopsy. By being empathic and supportive to the survivors in order to elicit more information, the autopsy was therapeutic for the survivors. Thus, the psychological autopsy (Shneidman, 1987) may not only provide information that helps prevent future suicides but may also represent a postvention method of helping survivors either gain a better understanding of why it happened or feel less guilt and responsibility for the deceased's demise. Indeed, what the psychological autopsy spawned was a variety of postvention strategies to help survivors of suicide.

Postvention

LO12 **Emotional Toll.** Suicide can have devastating effects on the family and social units (Cerel et al., 2008; Dutra et al., 2018). Osterweis et al. (1984) report that survivors of the death of a loved one by suicide are thought to be more vulnerable to physical and mental health problems than are grievers from other causes of death (p. 87). The average suicide leaves 6 to 10 survivors who experience extreme grief (Mitchell et al., 2004). Shneidman (2001, p. 154) puts it eloquently when he says that the person who completes suicide puts his psychological skeleton in the survivors' emotional closet. If that is true, then in the United States alone, with about 4 million survivors, the closet is chock-full of skeletons. Survivors are faced with guilt, shock, trauma from body discovery, police interrogation, legal issues, shame, sleep difficulties, concentration problems, denial, family relationship problems, and complicated, long-term grief (Granello & Granello, 2007, pp. 281–282). Survivors may also feel double binds of guilt and anger—guilty that they didn't do enough to stop the suicide and angry that now they are left behind having to raise children alone, struggle with debts, and so on, while the suicidal person is no longer present to assist with those tasks/responsibilities (Shea, 2002, p. 95).

Survivors of suicidal people may encounter more **stigmatization** than other bereaved individuals and experience significant complications to the grieving process (Dutra et al., 2018). Most of us have lost loved ones and been to funerals; we know the routine. Suicide survivors have no such formal guidelines. Survivors frequently sense that they are the objects of gossip and criticism, and they may be right. Bereaved loved ones often blame themselves for the suicide, and more than in any other form of loss, they tend to perceive that they are being neglected by others. Therefore, the loss of a loved one by suicide is doubly stressful. Grieving loved ones left behind by a suicide may refer to themselves as victims because, in addition to the emotional stress of the death itself, the survivors must also deal with burdens such as social stigma, guilt, blame, a search for the cause or meaning, unfinished business, and perceived rejection wrought by the suicide (Rando, 1984, pp. 151–152).

Child Survivors

The potential for children whose parents have completed suicide to suffer severe mental illness is extremely high (Burke et al., 2010; Mittendorfer-Rutz et al., 2008). Psychosomatic disorder, learning disabilities, obesity, running away, tics, delinquency, sleepwalking, fire setting, and encopresis, along with social adjustment problems, depression, and PTSD symptoms fly out of a Pandora's box of adverse outcomes of a parental suicide. Intervention is particularly important in dealing with children coping with a parent's suicide, who may exhibit shame, denial, and concealment and experience ostracism by their peers. If intervention does not occur, these children may experience a host of feelings that lead them to believe they are bound to suffer the same fate as their parent. Feelings of guilt in the child and distortion in communication between adults and children are constant companions. To neglect such children and assume they'll get over it is an extreme therapeutic error. School counselors, school social workers, and school psychologists are particularly critical in understanding what the suicide of a parent may mean to a child and need to be able to intervene with them and their peers. This kind of traumatic event can cause complicated traumatic grief in children and is absolutely within the purview of crisis workers who operate in school buildings (Cohen & Mannarino, 2011).

Parent Survivors

Parents whose children attempt or complete suicide are also likely to suffer severe psychological repercussions as they attempt to come to terms with their loss. There is mixed research, though, regarding the health and mortality risk for parents who have lost a child to suicide (Hendrickson, 2009). Lester (2004) found that the immediate parental response to a child's suicide tends to be hostility toward others, denial of the suicide, and rationalization of the death as accidental. Guilt and depression soon follow, and the likelihood of severe and continuing dysfunction with the surviving family members grows. Getting both children and parents into support groups and keeping them from becoming more isolated with their negative feelings are critical.

Support Groups

Crisis workers need to be aware of local services that provide such group support. Many organizations, school systems, and communities fail to develop postvention plans for suicide/homicide loss, with the result that survivors have psychological issues that affect those systems (Berkowitz et al., 2011). Baton Rouge, Louisiana, has a model comprehensive program that provides immediate referrals for all survivors of suicides from the local coroner. It utilizes an Active Postvention Model that provides trained crisis workers who specialize in the immediate aftermath of a suicide to provide support services to survivors. It provides group support and 24-hour access to

services (Campbell, 2011). Communities could not do better than to adopt this model.

Or, in the contemporary world of behavioral telehealth that delivers services to isolated rural populations, follow the example of the Southern Illinois University College of Medicine's Farm Family Resource Initiative (FFRI) (See Chapter 1, "Introduction" and Chapter 6, "Behavioral Telehealth") which once a month offers a free online educational and support program for people with agricultural ties who are survivors of a significant other's suicide. Bonnie Landwher, LCSW, is the leader of the program. She states it's not just a "Kumbaya feeling of telling our sad stories," but rather its purpose is posing questions and seeking answers to such perplexing questions as, "What can we do about it? "Why is this happening?' and "Why am I feeling this way?" in a supportive group format where people who are often socially isolated given their agricultural geographical area are unable to obtain or easily access a support group. The only criterion for admittance is that a person must be connected with agriculture to preserve the occupational and cultural commonality of the group (Sloup, 2023).

The following model is fairly representative of what these support groups look like. Hatton and Valente (1984) conducted a supportive group therapy experience for parents who sought relief from painful grief after the suicide of a child. They held 10 meetings with parents who felt shame, guilt, self-doubt, confusion, and isolation. The first three meetings were spent sharing and ventilating feelings. Four reactions surfaced. First, there was a prohibition of mourning by the parents' social network. The outside world was seen as hostile and incapable of understanding their grief. Second, former coping mechanisms for dealing with grief were useless. Attempting to share the pain even with spouses was impeded by the fear of burdening or depressing the person even further. Third, extreme isolation was felt both from friends and from family. Fourth, parents developed an identity crisis and questioned their ability to parent and maintain self-control.

The next five meetings were spent doing grief work. Sessions focused on giving support and reassurance, looking at adaptive and maladaptive coping mechanisms, gaining a new perspective on the loss, considering the effect of the suicide on their other children, and dealing with the anger they felt at society and the bureaucratic bumbling of authorities. The last 2 weeks were spent reminiscing about the good times, becoming more future oriented, letting go of anger, and sadness at termination of the group.

Transcrisis Postvention

Resnik (1969) proposes that crisis intervention of a completed suicide should occur in three phases. First is **resuscitation**. Within 24 hours, the crisis worker needs to make a supportive visit to assist the survivors in dealing with their initial shock, grief, anger, and most likely self-recrimination, guilt, and blame. This phase may last for several weeks. Survivors should be encouraged to talk about the suicide and experience the full range of feelings associated with it, without feeling ashamed or embarrassed to do so, and tell the story as many times as it needs to be told (Granello & Granello, 2007, p. 283). Phase two involves **resynthesis**. The crisis worker helps the survivors learn new ways of coping with their loss and prevents the development of pathological family responding. Finding a therapist who is experienced with grief work or a self-help group is critical during this time, and this most assuredly holds for children. This second phase may last for several months. The third phase is **Renewal**. The crisis worker helps the family reformulate itself in a context of growth and movement beyond the suicide. This process may occur up to a year after the suicide and is usually terminated on the first anniversary of the suicide. What Resnick proposes in these chronological phases is a vivid example of dealing with transcrisis states.

The Case of Leah. Leah Nichols, the 54-year-old manager of a branch bank, returned home from work Friday evening and discovered her 24-year-old son, Ronnie, dead from a gunshot wound. Ronnie had left a suicide note where he had apparently killed himself in his bedroom. Leah's husband, a college professor, had been dead (of heart failure) for about a year, and she and Ronnie lived in the family home. Ronnie's siblings, Brenda, age 31, Richard, age 27, and Larry, age 22, were married and living in cities scattered about the region. Ronnie was a warm, friendly, loving, and lovable person who had never married or dated much. He was very sensitive and was given to mood swings from deep depression to euphoria. He had expressed suicidal ideation since his primary school years and had been under psychiatric care since his adolescent years. But in recent months, he had appeared to be gaining in maturity and had gotten off his medication.

Leah's grief had moved progressively toward becoming complicated (see Chapter 12, "Personal Loss: Bereavement and Grief," for a complete description of this problem), but she felt she should set a controlled and circumspect image for the three siblings and other friends and relatives. After being admitted to the emergency room and spending three days in the hospital for nervous exhaustion, she was referred to the crisis worker.

The following intervention strategy was provided for Leah during the days and weeks immediately following Ronnie's suicide and represents one component of Resnik's (1969) resynthesis phase. The individual follow-up grief work dealt with many issues that are common in suicide work: denial, guilt, bargaining, and depression. The issue of Leah's martyrdom came out during an individual session approximately three weeks after Ronnie's funeral.

Leah: My kids think I'm holding back. They say I'm too stoic, too unaffected, or too aloof. They think my lack of showing emotions is not normal—not healthy.

CW: What do you think?

Leah: I don't know. I guess I believe somebody has to keep the lid on—keep a steady head during all this. I haven't wanted to trouble any of them with my problems. Their daddy's death, then Ronnie's. They've had enough without me dumping my grief on them.

CW: What are you saying, at a deep level, below the surface, right now?

Leah: I guess I am saying I'm hurting like hell. I guess my actions have looked pretty cold and strange to them. I guess I've been trying to protect them—to keep them from hurting.

CW: What will it do for you to keep them from hurting?

Leah: Make me a martyr, I guess. I don't know what else it could be.

CW: I wonder if it could keep you from the hurt and anger you have pushed back?

Leah: **(Starts sobbing.)** I . . . I . . . guess . . . I feel so helpless and always have had that feeling for that poor little boy I could not help despite everything I did. **(Weeps while the crisis worker moves over and holds and comforts her.)**

The crisis worker does not attempt to steer Leah to any particular conclusion. Rather, the questioning strategy—a combination of techniques from reality therapy, rational-emotive behavior therapy, and Gestalt therapy—is used to help Leah gain conscious contact with her own inner world. This crisis intervention technique would be ineffective if the worker were trying to analyze or identify pathology in Leah's behavior. Diagnosing, prescribing a cure, and managing Leah's recovery for her would have also been inappropriate. Leah needs to move forward at her own speed and pace to Resnik's (1969) Renewal phase.

The Case of Handley. Adults who have been traumatized by the suicide of a close associate, coworker, or friend can profit as well. A brief example of one type of group intervention/psychological autopsy illustrates this point.

Handley, age 27, killed himself by carbon monoxide poisoning. He had had a chaotic and turbulent life, punctuated by a destabilized family, drug and alcohol misuse disorder, and numerous suicide attempts. Despite all his problems, he was a friendly, energetic, charismatic person who worked in a restaurant supply business. He left behind several friends and coworkers who admired him and were surprised at his suicide, even though some of them were aware of his dilemmas and his occasional suicidal ideations.

Several days after Handley's funeral, his coworkers were still in acute grief. Some were emotionally stuck, asking themselves and each other, "Why?" Some were feeling guilty because they did not pick up on the cues and do something to save Handley. The following description is a modified psychological autopsy/group processing that we have developed to aid coworkers affected by a colleague's suicide. It is a variation of a grief debriefing procedure (Mitchell & Wesner, 2011) that is designed to help people share feelings, thoughts, and behaviors both of the deceased's actions and their own responses.

Handley's modified psychological autopsy was convened by a crisis interventionist who met with the group of bereaved coworkers and led them through the following steps:

1. **Introduction.** The worker made a brief introduction, outlining the purposes and structure of the meeting.
2. **Constructing the "why."** The crisis worker helped the group piece together the cues, clues, and signs (pooled from the knowledge contained within the group) that made Handley's suicide more understandable (from Handley's point of view).
3. **Commemorating the positive traits and accomplishments.** The group made a list of Handley's attributes and achievements that they particularly wanted to highlight and remember.

4. **Saying good-bye.** During the second round, each coworker was given an opportunity to take care of unfinished business with Handley and to verbally say goodbye using the "empty chair" strategy. Some members expressed anger as well as love. This was a very emotional and cathartic experience for everyone.
5. **Turning loose.** The crisis worker summarized the material from the preceding three steps and led the group in brainstorming and making another list, gleaned from Handley's case, to help them learn how to detect and prevent future suicides. Further, it allowed the group to turn loose the idea that they might have been in any way responsible or negligent in Handley's death.
6. **Absolving guilt.** The crisis worker obtained a commitment from a member of the group to edit and distribute the psychological autopsy lists to every member of the group. Last, the crisis worker made a statement that essentially (a) expressed appreciation for the group's participation, (b) assured the members that they were not responsible for Handley's death, and (c) gave the group permission to end the acute grieving phase and enter the long-term period of grief.

The crisis worker tapped into the power and cohesiveness of the group to provide stability and equilibrium for individual members. A variation of this group technique would be appropriate with a family, a fraternal group, the employees in a workplace, a school group, or a church group (any group dealing with a loss-related crisis).

Comans and associates (2013) report on a community intervention program in Australia for people who are bereaved and suffering grief from a suicide. Called the Stand By service, they found that, through direct bereavement and grief intervention, health outcomes, quality adjusted additional life years of living, time off of work, and medical costs were all positively affected by this community service (Comans et al., 2013).

Finally, where specialized support groups are not available, the Samaritans are available 24/7. The Samaritans originated in England but now operate in the United States and Australia. While specifically focused on suicide and grieving, they are an eclectic crisis line manned by highly trained volunteers. People feeling lonely and hopeless are their stock-in-trade (Jordan & McIntosh, 2011). You can reach them by telephone, chat, or text. Besides their

24/7 help line that is tied in to 988 national suicide line, (Just search "Samaritans crisis line" to get one near you), the Samaritans also offer grief support services and community education events. Anecdotally, there are some pretty interesting, informative and uplifting comments on their internet blog site worth reading *Samaritanshope.org* (Samaritans, 2023).

If you or someone you know is in a bind and you or they can't get through on your local hotline and can't get help with feelings of lethality, the national suicide hotline is open 24/7 at 988. Across the world, the Samaritans in England answer e-mails pretty quickly at jo@samaritans.org (Samaritans, 2023). To find help in a language other than English, e-mail *www.befrienders.org* (Befrienders Worldwide, 2023).

Losing a Client to Suicide

LO13   Crisis intervention does not always work. Client incidence of suicide among psychologists, social workers, and counselors ranges from 22 to 33 percent (Kleespies & Ponce, 2009). Sometimes, even the most skilled professionals and crisis workers cannot succeed. We must remember that if people really intend to kill themselves, despite our best efforts to intervene, they can manage to accomplish the task. The following suggestions have been provided to help workers cope with the loss of clients (Farberow, 2001; Sommers-Flanagan, et al., 2001).

Guided debriefings by experts are necessary for workers who have lost a client. Having a client complete suicide or homicide is one of the most stressful events that can occur in the experience of a crisis worker. The guilt, recrimination, rumination, and perseveration may lead to constant second-guessing. The "what ifs," "shoulds," "oughts," and "might have beens" all lead to feelings of owning responsibility. If a client completes a suicide or homicide, a psychological autopsy, or debriefing (see the section on critical incident stress debriefing in Chapter 16, Disaster Response), and supervision should be mandatory for the worker.

Indeed, the impact of losing a client to suicide, or a victim of the client, can be overwhelming and can cause the crisis worker to experience what is called *vicarious traumatization* (see the section on vicarious traumatization in Chapter 15, "Human Service Workers in Crisis: Burnout, Vicarious Traumatization, and Compassion Fatigue"). Such cases call for the utmost of professional expertise to provide intentional and intensive debriefing of the traumatized workers. It is absolutely essential that such workers realistically examine (under the guidance of outside consultants) what happened, learn from the event, and absolve themselves from guilt and responsibility for the regrettable loss. From our experience doing supervision and debriefing of crisis workers who have dealt with client fatalities, it is one of the toughest supervision jobs there is and goes far beyond vicarious trauma in its psychological impact—both in regard to the crisis worker and the supervisor.

Summary

The phenomenon of suicide is democratic in that it affects every segment of society, and it is everybody's business. Suicide and homicide as expressive problem-solving acts have many similarities and parallels in terms of motive, risk, and assessment of lethality. Suicide is a serious problem that is on the rise among all groups, especially youth. Researchers find few common denominators in their quest to identify suicide/homicide risk types and to predict and prevent suicide/homicide. The two oldest and most prevalent theories of suicide are Freud's notion that suicidal behavior is rage at others turned inward and Durkheim's concept that suicide is tied closely to social pressures and influences. Other theories that have emerged more recently see the basis or cause of suicide as largely accidental, a method of escape, a pervasive sense of hopelessness, interactional and revenge driven, biochemically induced, chaotic, interpersonal, or completely rational in the face of unendurable pain or suffering.

The dynamics of suicide are important because crisis workers who deal with suicidal clients need to know that there are several different types and characteristics of suicide. There are many reasons why people kill or attempt to kill themselves, and there are differing moral and cultural points of view about suicide among various social, ethnic, and age groups. Among the many myths of suicide are two that are particularly salient in impeding crisis work: (1) discussing suicide will cause a person to think about doing it or to act upon it, and (2) people who threaten suicide don't do it. Crisis workers are advised to directly question clients who display any suicidal or homicidal ideation.

Many risk factors have been identified that serve as danger signals and help to determine levels of lethality. Some of the highest risks are the presence of serious intent, a history of prior attempts, and evidence of a specific and lethal plan. These risk factors are important criteria for both assessing and acting in the realm of suicide intervention. Workers who are sensitized to the dynamics find that suicidal people often send out subtle but definite clues and/or cries for help.

Intervention strategies show how crisis workers can be appropriately assertive, directive, and forceful. In working with suicidal clients, workers should not be passive. In suicide intervention, workers must consider many environmental and social factors in addition to attending to client safety (e.g., age, gender, social status, availability of supports from family and friends, and community attitudes surrounding the person at risk). Counseling around the issue of suicide/homicide also involves facilitating the grief and healing of clients who are survivors as well as the care and debriefing of crisis workers who experience the loss of clients to suicide or homicide. Finally, the psychological autopsy is a primary way of both learning how to prevent suicides and alleviating the guilt and shame of survivors.

Sexual Assault

9

Learning Objectives

After studying this chapter, you should be able to:

1. Discuss and critique the variability in the wide range of statistics reported for various types of sexual assault.
2. Identify the different definitions of rape/sexual assault and understand the reasons for the intensity of the traumatic wake of a sexual assault.
3. Explain the dynamics of rape.
4. Examine the myths about rape and describe their fallacies.
5. Describe the dynamics of date and acquaintance rape.
6. Identify intervention strategies for rape.
7. Describe how secondary victimization is prevented.
8. Describe and be able to discriminate the variety of responses sexual assault survivors have.
9. Describe the dynamics and symptoms of posttraumatic sexual assault behavior.
10. Discuss how to treat sexual assault survivors who have posttraumatic stress disorder (PTSD).
11. Explain and describe the coping dynamics of adult survivors of childhood sexual abuse.
12. Explain the "false memories" controversy.
13. Discuss treatment strategies for adult survivors with PTSD and how they are applied.
14. Explain the need for support groups for adult survivors of childhood sexual abuse.
15. Explain and describe the dynamics of childhood sexual abuse.
16. Explain and describe the dynamics of family systems in childhood sexual abuse.
17. Explain and describe the phases of child sexual abuse.
18. Explain and describe how intervention strategies with sexually abused children occur.
19. Describe the steps in how a child sexual perpetrator is successfully prosecuted.
20. Describe the traumatic aftermath of child sexual abuse and how it is treated.

The Scope of the Problem

LO1　Before we discuss key statistics to help frame the gravity of sexual assault and its traumatic wake for survivors, we need to begin by establishing some key terms for this crisis. The National Intimate Partner and Sexual Violence Survey, administered by the Centers for Disease Control and Prevention (CDC), Division of Violence Prevention (DVP), utilizes the term "contact sexual violence" to encapsulate four forms of sexual violence which are: "rape, being made to penetrate someone else, sexual coercion, and/or unwanted sexual contact" (Basile et al., 2022, p. 1). In this chapter, we speak primarily of rape, although much of this chapter can pertain to other forms of sexual violence as well. We often use the terms rape and sexual assault synonymously, and we will provide more descriptive definitions for rape and sexual violence later in this chapter. However, other scholars may differentiate between rape and sexual assault, in that sexual assault may include sexual violence that does not involve penetration. The same can be true for individual states, each of which has a specific definition to describe these terms. It is not possible for us to use the terms with fidelity to each state's respective laws. As such, we hope you will read this chapter with the understanding that our primary focus herein is rape, although any form of sexual violence perpetrated against someone can certainly precipitate a crisis. With that in mind, let's turn to some relevant statistics.

Be forewarned that the statistics in this chapter are some of the most controversial and error prone reported in this book! Given the emotional volatility and cultural artifacts that undergird sexual assault, after reading this chapter, we hope you will understand why these statistics may be so prone to error.

The benchmark National Violence Against Women Survey (National Institute of Justice and Centers for Disease Control and Prevention, 1998) conducted in 1997 in the United States found that 1 in 6 U.S. women and 1 in 33 U.S. men had experienced an attempted or completed rape as a child and/or as an adult, using a definition of rape that includes forced vaginal, oral, and anal sex. Although each study yields slightly different results regarding the actual number of sexual assaults occurring annually, they seem to paint a common picture, which is an ever-increasing rate of sexual violence. The *National Intimate Partner and Sexual Violence Survey: 2016/2017 Report on Sexual Violence* indicates that 1 in 4 women and 1 in 26 men report having experienced completed or attempted sexual assault (Basile et al., 2022). This is a notable increase from the aforementioned statistics from 1997. The Bureau of Justice Statistics also found an increase in their study of criminal victimization (Morgan & Oudekerk, 2019). Their results indicate that the rate of sexual assault increased drastically between the years of 2015 to 2018, from 1.6 people ages 12 and older per 1,000 to 2.7 people per 1,000 (Morgan & Oudekerk, 2019). Even more disturbing, nearly half of those who have experienced completed sexual assault were raped when they were minors (Basile et al., 2022).

Sexual assault (Borumandnia et al., 2020) and child sexual abuse (Stoltenborgh et al., 2011) are global problems. In addition, consider the extensive sexual assault experienced by Congolese refugees in South Africa (Alfaro-Velcamp et al., 2019), the "corrective rape" of lesbian women in South Africa (Koraan & Geduld, 2015), the sexual violence committed against Ukrainian women by Russian soldiers (Zechenter, 2023), the elevated rates of sexual assault committed against migrants and refugees in European countries (De Schrijver et al., 2018), and the extensive sex-trafficking within U.S. borders (Haney et al., 2020). These are just a few examples of the heart wrenching and troubling statistics that frame this chapter.

Although sexual assault occurs within all cultures and all groups of people, certain subgroups tend to be disproportionately at higher risk. Examples of high risk groups in the United States include American Indian/Alaskan Native and Multiracial women (Basile et al., 2022); LGBTQIA+ military service members (Schuyler et al., 2020); female military service members (Nichter et al., 2022); individuals with disabilities (Campbell et al., 2021; McGilloway et al., 2020); and members of sexual minority groups (Messinger & Koon-Magnin, 2019).

Contrary to popular myth, these acts were not all committed by strangers and sexual assailants lurking in big-city dark alleys and vacant parking lots. In fact, only a small portion of sexual assault is committed by strangers. In Basile and colleagues' (2022) study based on sexual assaults that took place in 2016 and 2017, in more than half of sexual assault cases, the perpetrator was an acquaintance. For women, 39 percent of perpetrators were intimate partners, 16 percent were family members, and 12 percent were strangers (Basile et al., 2022). For men, 39 percent of perpetrators were acquaintances, 16 percent were family members, and 13 percent were strangers (Basile et al., 2022). It should not be surprising, then, that rape, sexual assault, and child sexual abuse demographics tend to mimic domestic violence statistics. What research is starting to find out regarding intimate sexual assault is not just the severity and duration of the sexual abuse as the root cause of the trauma but the profound sense of betrayal by someone who should have never, ever done something as anathematic as a caregiver (O'Rinn et al., 2013).

Overwhelmingly, the research on sexual assault focuses on men as perpetrators and women or children as their victims. As such, a majority of this chapter is written from the perspective of women and child survivors of sexual assault perpetrated by men. However, no one should labor under the delusion that adult men are not raped (Basile et al., 2022; Reed et al., 2020), although men are less likely than women to conceptualize the assault as rape (Reed et al., 2020). Moreover, it would be absolutely false to believe that women are not capable of some of the most heinous sexual acts, such as raping children (Wijkman & Da Silva, 2021); raping with co-offenders (Wijkman & Da Silva, 2021; Ybarra & Mitchell, 2013) or an intimate partner (Wijkman & Da Silva, 2021); and sexually abusing children (Gölge et al., 2021; McLeod, 2015). Indeed, although still largely under-researched and arguably minimized by society (e.g., consider public reactions to female teachers "having sex with" underage male students), growing evidence demonstrates the disturbing role of female perpetrators of sexual violence.

Underreporting

One reason for debate regarding the actual rates of sexual violence is that sexual assault is drastically underreported to law enforcement officials. Morgan and Oudekerk (2019) found that, in 2018, only approximately 25 percent of sexual assaults were reported to law enforcement. Underreporting could be due to a number of factors, such as survivors' difficulty comprehending procedures (Spencer et al., 2017) or written protocols for reports of sexual assault on college campuses (Taylor, 2018), the perpetuation of rape myths and military culture biases that inhibit disclosure for military personnel who are assaulted (O'Brien et al., 2015), having a prior relationship with the perpetrator (Jones et al., 2009), using substances around the time of the assault (Jones et al., 2009), fear (Spencer et al., 2017), fear of judgment or being blamed for the assault (Spencer et al., 2017), and shame (Spencer et al., 2017).

What's more is that the vast majority of crime survey reports do not report sexual abuse of children under the age of 12. However, the available data based on adult self-report of prior abuse paints a grim picture regarding the prevalence of childhood sexual abuse. In their 2016–2017 survey, Basile et al. (2022) found that 49 percent of women rape victims reported that they were first raped before the age of 18, of which nearly 35 percent were first raped between the ages of 11 and 17, and 14 percent were first assaulted at age 10 or younger. Similarly, nearly 57 percent of men rape victims reported that they were first raped before the age of 18. Of those men, approximately 30 percent reported rape between the ages of 11 and 17 and almost 27 percent reported being the victim of sexual assault at age 10 or younger (Basile et al., 2022).

In addition to various intense, sometimes debilitating, short-term effects of sexual assault (e.g., injury,

fearfulness, sexually transmitted infections, and pregnancy; Basile et al., 2022), abundant evidence suggests that crises resulting from sexual abuse are linked to serious adverse long-term outcomes (Perilloux et al., 2012). Examples of the long-term effects of sexual assault include an increased risk for the development of PTSD symptomatology (Bell, 2016; deMello et al., 2023); higher risk of suicide (DeCou & Lynch, 2019), particularly among sexual minority men (Scheer et al., 2021); disordered eating (Malet-Karas et al., 2022; Oshodi et al., 2020); problematic alcohol consumption (Oshodi et al., 2020); sexual dysfunction (Turchik & Hassija, 2014); and various health issues (Potter et al., 2018). Individuals who experience sexual assault also carry a large financial burden. Peterson et al. (2017) found that the lifetime cost of rape is $122,461 per victim, which equates to over $3 trillion for all victims, combined. The lifetime cost includes expenses related to medical costs, involvement in criminal justice procedures, lost work productivity, and other related expenses (Peterson et al., 2017).

Defining Rape: The Unique Situation of Sexual Abuse/Rape Survivors

LO2 There are many definitions of rape. Some are based on legal constructs; some are derived from other sources. Brownmiller (1975) distinguishes between most legal definitions and what she refers to as a woman's definition of rape. She sees the legal definition of rape as "the forcible perpetration of an act of sexual intercourse on the body of a woman not one's wife" (p. 380) as much too narrow and protective of male supremacy. Brownmiller's preferred definition from a woman's perspective is that rape is "a sexual invasion of the body by force, an incursion into the private, personal inner space without consent—in short, an internal assault from one of several avenues and by one of several methods [that] constitutes a deliberate violation of emotional, physical, and rational integrity and is a hostile, degrading act of violence" (p. 376). That definition appears to encompass the whole scope of rape, as well as other forms of sexual abuse/harassment. Although this definition was originally focused on the woman's perspective, this definition might be more widely applied across gender and sexual identities. For the purposes of this chapter, your authors will use Koss and Achilles' (2008) definition of **rape** as an unwanted act of oral, vaginal, or anal penetration committed through the use of force, threat of force, or when incapacitated; **sexual assault** refers to a broader range of sexual criminal offenses such as sexual battery and sexual coercion, up to and including rape (U.S. Department of Education, 2011).

The Dynamics of Rape

LO3 The etiology of rape has roots deeply embedded in the psychosocial and cultural fabric of the particular society in which it occurs (Brownmiller, 1975; Donat & D'Emilio, 1998; Eisler, 1987–1995; Ullman, 1996a, 1996b). According to Brownmiller (1975) and Eisler (1987–1995), the cultural mechanism of male dominance constitutes the driving force in rape in all cultures. Psychosocial, cultural, and perso-nal attitudes and responses are important dynamics in considering the phenomenon of rape (Benedict, 1985; Williams & Holmes, 1981).

Lussier and Cale (2016) examined the origins of rape and provide a framework through which to understand the evolution of rape theory. They explain three primary models through which to understand sexual aggression perpetrated by men onto women, which have pervaded research and literature over the past forty years. The first model is based on a "propensity for sexual aggression" (p. 72), wherein perpetrators experience some type of propensity for sexual aggression based on various intrapersonal factors, such as the presence of psychopathology and disruptions in their sexual development process (Lussier & Cale, 2016). The second model is based on a propensity for criminal behavior, wherein perpetrators act upon their criminal impulses through sexual aggression, just as they might in the commission of non-sexually aggressive crimes (Lussier & Cale, 2016). Lussier and Cale note that the second model does not hold up robustly to critique. The third model incorporates the two aforementioned models (propensity for sexual aggression and propensity for criminal behavior) to conceptualize the interplay of unique intrapersonal and environmental factors (Lussier & Cale, 2016) that collide to develop a sexual perpetrator. Lussier and Cale further state that emerging research from a "developmental life course" perspective may shed additional light on primary motivators for sexual aggression (p. 74). Indeed, varied factors may contribute to the development of sexual aggression, and identifying these factors may help in the development of evidence-based prevention programming. To truly understand the origins of rape, though, we must also consider sociocultural factors.

Social/Cultural Factors

Baron and Straus (1989) characterize rape as a social phenomenon and theorize four different causes: gender inequality, pornography, social disorganization, and legitimization of violence. **Gender inequality** refers to the economic, political, and legal status of women in comparison to men. Some types of **pornography** can reduce women to sex objects, promote male dominance, and encourage or condone sexual violence against women. **Social disorganization** erodes social control and constraints and undermines freedom of individual behavior and self-determination. **Legitimization of violence** is the support the culture gives to violence, as portrayed in the mass media (such as television programming), violent sports, military exploits, and video games. **Social norms theory** proposes that male peer aggression and female submission are part of the norm and justification for violent sexual interaction (Dardis et al., 2015).

The notion of male supremacy has its roots deep in our cultural history, which has always equated the property rights of men with access to and control over the bodies of women, children, and others who are perceived as dependents (Brownmiller, 1975). Indeed, Eisler (1987–1995, pp. 153–154) describes rape and sexual assault as one of several threats widely used to ensure the continued domination and control of women. Historically, the crime of rape has been understood not as a crime against the woman but as a crime against her father or her husband (Donat & D'Emilio, 1998).

Brownmiller (1975) and others have documented a part of the history of rape as a psychosocial means by which the victors in wars reward themselves and humiliate their vanquished foes. The wholesale rape and killing of helpless women and children represents the ultimate vulnerability and defeat of a people. It likewise represents the ultimate humiliation and subjugation of a person. Whether it is inflicted on thousands, as reported in war, or on one person, the purpose is quite similar—the use of unrestrained power to force the vanquished into total submission.

Personal and Psychological Factors

Personal and psychological factors unique to men who perpetrate sexual abuse affect both their decision to assault and the way the assault is carried out

(Beech et al., 2006; Groth & Birnbaum, 1979; Lisek & Miller, 2002; Lisek & Roth, 1988; Williams & Holmes, 1981). The following may describe the male offender:

1. Acts in a hostile, aggressive, angry, condescending, and domineering manner and believes he is strong, courageous, and manly even though he often feels weak, anxious, inadequate, threatened, and dependent and believes women are inherently dangerous.
2. Lacks the interpersonal skills to make his point in society and particularly with women.
3. May need to exercise *power* to prove to himself and to the victim that he is powerful, omnipotent, and in total control.
4. May show *sadistic* patterns—the sadistic rapist frequently uses extreme violence and often mutilates or murders the victim in order to attain a feeling of total triumph over the victim.
5. Sees women as primarily sexual objects and has sexual urges that he perceives as uncontrollable and all consuming.
6. Holds stereotypical and rigid views of gender roles with hypermasculine self-views that validate he is a "real man."
7. Harbors chronic feelings of anger, hostility, and fear toward women and seeks to control them by his sexual "conquests."

Feminists, with good historical reason, have attempted to define rape as basically an exercise in power and control. On that basis, most rapists have been cast into one of four categories: **anger** (mad at women), **power exploitative** (show they have power over women), **power reassurance** (continuously need to feel that they are powerful over women), and **sadistic** (take joy in hurting women). McCabe and Wauchope (2005) found evidence to support these typologies in two studies, one of men who had only been charged with sexual assault and the other of men who were eventually convicted of sexual assault, but they also found confounding outliers who did not fit any of the four categories well. A number of researchers (Lisek & Miller, 2002; Lisek & Roth, 1988; Scully & Marolla, 1998; Sussman & Bordwell, 1981) have interviewed convicted rapists and have vividly demonstrated that each rapist's reasons for assault are individual. For example:

1. Some men use rape to punish or exact revenge because a specific woman has "done them wrong." They see all women collectively as responsible for one woman's supposed transgressions. Some

negative precipitating event with an intimate partner causes them to "take it out" on and "get even" with some woman who is a total stranger to them. It doesn't make any difference who the person is as long as the intended victim is a woman—a generic symbol of their lost power, virility, and masculinity that they desperately want back.
2. Criminals who commit rape in the perpetration of a crime often see rape as an added bonus. It's there for the taking, so why not?
3. For some men, rape is attaining the unattainable woman, the woman they would never otherwise have a chance with. In this instance, sex is the motivating factor.
4. For some men, rape is an impersonal experience and preferred over any demonstrated caring or mutual affection. There is no obligation, and the power, control, and sexual tension release are gratifying.
5. Finally, in its most heinous form, gang rapists see rape as recreation, adventure, and proving they are "macho." These individuals belong to sexually violent subcultures that reflect both the rapist's views of women and the notion that sexual conquest of as many women as possible is a critical measure of manhood. A gang rape is seen as male bonding at its height. While numerous interviewees stated they regretted their actions and were now sorry for them, the immediate impact on them postrape in regard to what they had done was slight. Ominously, if they felt anything, they generally felt good about what they did.

Yet, the vast majority of rapes have to do with the power relationships between men and women (Sussman & Bordwell, 1981, p. 12). Somehow, the contemporary sociocultural milieu produces some men who feel such an absence of power and control in their lives that they develop a need to "take it" (control). These men come to believe that it is their "right" (p. 5) and proceed to rationalize and justify their behavior, even though they have invaded and taken by force another person's life and body.

Myths About Rape

LO4 One of the most difficult obstacles that human services workers face in dealing with all forms and aspects of rape and sexual abuse is the abundance of debilitating myths in society (Benedict, 1985; Burt, 1998; Ganas et al., 1999; Matsakis, 2003; (Yapp & Quayle, 2018). There are a number of myths that pervade society and affect the rate of sexual assault transgressions: victim blaming (Romero-Sánchez et al., 2018), reporting of sexual assault (Heath et al., 2013; Reed et al., 2020), law enforcement response (Garza & Franklin, 2021); criminal persecution (Ussery, 2022), and the survivor's coping in the aftermath of rape (Bhuptani & Messman-Moore, 2019; Frazier et al., 2017). A few of these myths include the following:

1. **Rape is just rough sex.** The notion that rape equals sex is perhaps the most destructive myth of all. If we believe that rape is sex, then it follows that rape doesn't hurt (physically or psychologically) any more than sex does. We can even believe that the survivor enjoys and is erotically stimulated by its roughness. Rape is violence, torture, and a life-threatening event. It is utterly dehumanizing, and enjoyment of "rough sex" has nothing to do with it. However, research indicates that certain types of rapists are aroused by the use of force and violence against victims, and such arousal may be heightened by aggressive resistance of victims (Drieschner & Lange, 1999; Knight, 1999). Social norms theory supports this myth. Dardis and associates (2015) found that college men's *beliefs* about what their peers thought about sexually aggressive behaviors correlated highly with what their *perception* of the average college men's beliefs were, although in actuality they were not correlated with their friends' *actual* beliefs. However, perpetrators of sexual assault were *highly significant* in their belief in *overestimating* friends' involvement in sexually aggressive behavior.

2. **People "cry rape" to gain revenge.** Ganas and associates (1999) hypothesize that this myth permeates our society because such myths (a) provide comfort for our social structure (people don't want to believe that rape really occurred), (b) serve to focus the blame for sexual violence on victims rather than perpetrators, and (c) are easier to believe than the reality of knowing that rape can happen to anyone. As such, it is one of the most heated and controversial issues in sexual assault. "Revenge" reports are sometimes heard, and at times, the cry of "rape" has been used for secondary gain, such as getting back at a jilted lover, blackmail, job security, or covering up an unwanted pregnancy. A 2 percent rule has been used by the Federal Bureau of Investigation (FBI) in its training as the percentage of false accusations.

Lisek and his associates (2010) found about a 6 percent false accusation rate in their investigation of rape allegations. Ferguson and Malouff (2016) found a similar rate of false reports of sexual assault, 5 percent, in their meta-analytic study. They further note that although there is some evidence that sex crimes are more frequently falsely reported than other types of crimes, there are too many complicating factors to accurately compare false report rates for sex crimes to other types of crimes (Ferguson & Malouff, 2016). To be sure, there is much controversy regarding how false reports are defined (Saunders, 2012) but, as we previously discussed, we know with certainty that sexual assault is under-reported. For that reason, we generally advise to "start with believing."

3. **Rape is motivated by lust.** Eisler (1995) and Scully and Marolla (1998) believe that the motivation for rape is most likely to be domination, power, anger, revenge, control, frustration, or sadism. Benedict (1985, p. 8) and Eisler (1995, pp. 237–239) report that some men may come to associate sex with violence, thus viewing women not as human beings but as objects of prey and/or domination and viewing sex as an act of power, control, and triumph. However, one counterpoint view, based on studies of the evolutionary theories of rape by Thornhill and Palmer (2000), suggests that the rapists' motives are primarily sexual, with the exercise of power mostly a means to an end. This idea is supported at least in part by Scully and Marolla (1998), who found that some of the rapists they interviewed saw it as the only way to get sexual access to women who were unwilling or "out of their league."

4. **Rapists are weird, psychotic loners.** No such contention can be supported by the research. Rapists come from every walk of life. People who rape and commit other forms of sexual abuse have been identified in every stratum of society (Benedict, 1985, pp. 9–10; Burt, 1998). The idea that rapists were mentally ill held sway for a long time (Groth, 1971) and was seen by feminists as a particularly odious way of rationalizing the male-dominated societal power and subjugation motives that undergirded and upheld a repressive, patriarchal society. The sheer number of rapes make it statistically impossible that the typical rapist is "mentally ill," given the small number of psychopathic men in the population (Scully & Marolla, 1998).

5. **Victims or survivors of rape provoked the rape or wanted to be raped, so no harm was done.** This myth is based on the idea that, by acting sexy, wearing sexy clothes or lots of makeup, being at a bar and "coming on" to a man, walking along a road alone at night, or doing laundry or grocery shopping late in the evening, somehow or other a person does something that clearly says, "Come rape me!" The bottom line is that through a series of weak inferences and rationalizations, the rapist is able to condone his sexual assault. The rapist is no longer responsible for the way he acted because the woman, by her actions, brought it on herself (Burt, 1998). Although most rapists deny that they are rapists, rationalize that women provoke or want it, or deny that their sexual assaults are rape, there are virtually no documented cases in which women have lured men into raping them. Ganas and associates (1999) and Sussman and Bordwell (1981) have clearly shown that what the survivor does before the rape has little,"if anything", to do with the rapist's decision to assault.

6. **Only bad women are raped.** This myth is one of the most blatant examples of a "blame the victim" attitude (Brownmiller, 1975). This myth is taken to mean that if the woman has a "bad" reputation, the rape is justified. The stereotypical "damaged goods" notion means that a woman who has said "Yes" once can no longer legitimately say "No." For many, the extension of this myth means that sex workers are so devalued that they have no worth and, therefore, cannot be raped (Silbert, 1988). Regardless of a person's occupation, no one deserves to be assaulted, and everyone is entitled to equal protection and treatment..

7. **Real rapes happen only in bad parts of town, at night, in abandoned buildings or lonely fields by strangers who have knives or guns and who engage in brutally beating the victims when they resist heroically—even unto death.** That's pretty much rubbish! While there are rapes that happen that way, remember that half or more of the perpetrators are someone who knows the victim (Basile et al., 2022). Moreover, approximately one third of rape victims sustain injuries during the assault (Basile et al., 2022).

8. **If the woman doesn't resist, she must have wanted it.** The old stereotypical notion, which has had some coinage in the courts, is that the woman needs to resist unto death or be so physically drained or hurt that she can't resist any longer. Resisting may get a woman killed, particularly if the assailant is armed and is more physically powerful. Furthermore, there are psychological obstacles in the way of resisting, such as tonic immobility, which is "a state of involuntary, temporary motor inhibition" (Möller et al., 2017, p. 932). Ominously, Kassing and Prietio (2003) found that counselors-in-training thought that male rape victims should fight back. There is no conclusive evidence that fighting back or not fighting back is better for the victim (Matsakis, 2003).

It is not easy or simple to eradicate or even to refute the preceding myths in society at large (Ganas et al., 1999). Feminists argue that it is to the advantage of the entire patriarchal society to believe such myths, and it is certainly to the advantage of the rapists (Burt, 1998).

Myths about rape and sexual assault are not the sole domain of women. Here are some of the more prevalent myths about men and sexual assault (Male Survivor, 2011).

1. **Boys and men can't be victims.** Let's suppose that a 350-pound NFL noseguard decides to have his way with you. What do you think will happen? Boys and adult men are often physically weaker than their male attackers or are threatened with weapons. In fact, Basile et al. (2022) found that nearly half of male rape victims were concerned for their safety during the attempt. It is also important to consider that the perpetrator may have power and control over the victim through position, influence, knowledge, and prestige. But it would be downright wrong to assume that only men assault men. In fact, most perpetrators of sexual assault against men are women (DiMarco et al., 2022).

2. **Gay men are usually the perpetrators of sexual abuse of boys.** Pedophiles are pedophiles, regardless of the child's gender. Their sexual orientation is inconsequential. However, there is some evidence that the vast number of offenders of childhood sexual abuse are other juveniles, and this is particularly true for boys (Gewirtz-Meydan & Finkelhor, 2020).

3. **Boys are less traumatized than girls.** Admittedly, there is less research on the childhood sexual abuse of boys than of girls. However, the available research tells a daunting story, in which male survivors of childhood sexual abuse experience similar levels of psychological distress, although there may be some gender-based differences in

symptom presentation (Foster, 2017; Gallo et al., 2018; Payne et al., 2014). To think that boys do not struggle with the effects of sexual abuse would perpetuate false and damaging narratives about male masculinity.

4. **Boys abused by men will later become gay.** The development of adult sexual orientation is complex but sexual assault perpetration by another man does not make one gay. In fact, with men, our own experience is that a number of those who have been victimized by men become homophobic or overcompensate by attempting to prove their manhood by having sex with as many women as possible.

5. **Vampire/zombie syndrome.** The notion is that people who experience childhood sexual abuse will grow up to become perpetrators. The research does not support this assumption (Widom & Massey, 2015). This is an especially dangerous myth because it can stereotype victims as perpetrators, when the victims desperately need help rather than punishment, ridicule, isolation, and abandonment.

6. **If a minor experiences sexual arousal or orgasm from abuse, this means they enjoyed it.** We are hardwired for sex. Physical stimulation is likely to happen during sex. That does not mean the child wanted the experience, fully participated in it, or "got off" or "wanted it" as many perpetrators try to rationalize. The same can be said for adult rape survivors.

7. **If the perpetrator is a women, the survivor just got lucky.** This is a widely held belief and a very, very dangerous stereotype. Some of the most disturbed clients we have seen have been children and adolescent boys abused by women in authority positions and consanguine relationships. The conflict, confusion, rage, and other extremely volatile emotions and thinking they display toward women as adults mark them as threats for harm to women. Above all, these children should receive treatment immediately after discovery of the assault.

For men, these myths have profound effects. One of the major ones is the shame, embarrassment, and guilt they feel that militates against coming forward, and there is still considerable stigma attached to be a male who has been raped (Easton, et al., 2014). The problem is that, even among "educated" people, these myths have remarkable staying power. What's more is that rape myth acceptance may have something to do with pervasive isms, such as sexism, racism, classism, and ageism (Suarez & Gadalla, 2010). To tackle rape myths, Suarez and Gadalla (2010) state that we need to first start with those current isms that skew perception, such as sexism, racism, and classism.

Date and Acquaintance Rape

LO5 Much of the research reported on date and acquaintance rape deals with sexual assaults on college campuses. Little is known about date rape as it applies to high school students. Rape is the most common violent crime at U.S. universities (National Center for Education Statistics, 2022). In 2019, a total of 11,800 "forcible sex offenses" were reported under the *Clery Act*, which accounted for 43 percent of the total reported criminal incidents (National Center for Education Statistics, 2022). Women may decline to report rape for a number of reasons, including the aforementioned erroneous rape myths. Commonly, women decline to report due to fear, perceived shame, self-blame, or not wanting to get the perpetrator in trouble (Spencer et al., 2017). Indeed, in our experience, it is unfortunately all too common for friends and family to blame the victim. Ninety percent of the college women who are raped know their assailants, and most rapes occur in a social situation, such as partying or studying together in a dorm room (Cole, 2006).

Because most of you reading this book are sitting in a college classroom, be advised that nearly 25 percent of first-year women students will be victims of attempted or actual assault through either incapacitated rape (15 percent) or forcible rape (9 percent) (Carey et al., 2015). When looking across the college population, rates are even higher. In 2015, just over 33 percent of women reported rape or attempted rape, and nearly 13 percent of men reported sexual perpetration (Koss et al., 2022). Given the low frequency of reporting of sexual assault, you can assume that any statistic you encounter is probably a pretty conservative estimate of what is really happening (Kariane et al., 2005; Weiss, 2010).

Mills and Granoff (1992) found that 28 percent of college women surveyed acknowledged that they had been victims of rape or attempted rape. In a national survey of college men and women, Koss (1998) found that 8.3 percent of the women felt they had been forced to engage in unwanted sex. Conversely, only 3.4 percent of the men felt they had forced a partner to engage in unwanted sex. Few told anyone about the encounters, although those reporting attempted rape were more likely to tell someone than were those who had actually been raped. A number of male respondents admitted to committing what is legally defined as rape and admitted to continuing to make sexual advances even when their dates had told them "No!" Sexual violence is an ongoing concern for everyone, but particularly for college students.

One of the bigger myths of rape is: *Date rape isn't really rape.* The girl went out with him, didn't she? He probably spent a good deal of money on her. What if she kissed him back and engaged in heavy petting? Then she turned him off? She deserved it and probably even wanted it even though she said "no." Even if it was a boyfriend of long standing, and whatever else may have happened before the rape in terms of sexual foreplay, and no matter how much money was spent, "No!" is "No!" and no one has the right or justification to rape anyone else, including their romantic partner. And, yes, that includes marital partners (Singh & Sharma, 2022).

Candy Is Dandy, but Liquor Is Quicker— and More Violent

Alcohol, partying, sex, and college students. This combination of those factors, alongside a newfound emancipation from parental governance, can make sexual aggression shockingly high among male college students (Shorey et al., 2015). Indeed, barroom groping, kissing, and touching are pervasive and seen as part of the course of partying (Becker & Tinkler, 2015). And, although victims' substance use does not make them responsible for the assault, alcohol consumption (Ray et al., 2021; Turchik & Hassija, 2014) and drug use have been established as risk factors for rape (Sabina et al., 2017; Turchik & Hassija, 2014). In fact, alcohol is the most commonly used date rape drug (Anderson et al., 2017). However, other common date rape drugs include ethanol, benzodiazepines, ketamine, and gamma-hydroxybutyrate (Costa et al., 2020). What's more is that, in one study, 90 percent of male perpetrators of rape stated that they were intoxicated at the time of the assault (Koss et al., 2022). Indeed, although intoxication is certainly not an excuse for sexual perpetration, research indicates that alcohol use can skew one's experience related to consent to engage in sexual activity. Jozkowski and Wiersma (2015) found, in a large sample of students across the United States, that alcohol consumption prior to sexual activity was associated with both external consent (verbal and behavioral cues) and internal consent (feelings associated with giving consent). Although their study does not address rape, it is evident that alcohol consumption plays a role in sexual disinhibition.

Rape victimization while incapacitated Versus rape victimization by force can result in some differences in the survivor's healing from the rape trauma. Fields and colleagues (2022) conducted a study of 74 adults who received outpatient treatment for sexual assault at a mental health clinic. They compared symptomatology and treatment outcomes for individuals who experienced voluntary, involuntary, and no drug or alcohol consumption prior to the rape (Fields et al., 2022). Among the three groups, there was a noticeable difference between those who were raped while intoxicated (either involuntary or voluntary consumption) and those who were not intoxicated during the assault; those who were intoxicated and had impaired trauma memory reported fewer symptoms of post-trauma, such as hyperarousal and hypervigilance, and less anhedonia. However, all rape survivors reported relatively equivalent rates of re-experiencing symptoms.

Ominously, childhood sexual abuse increases the risk for alcohol misuse and that, in turn, increases the chances of engaging in sexually risky behavior (Walsh et al., 2014). Further, engaging in sexually risky behavior has been linked to a higher risk of sexual assault (Ray et al., 2021; Turchik & Hassija, 2014). Again, this does not suggest that victims are responsible for the sexual assault inflicted upon them.

Preventing Date, Acquaintance, and Other Forms of Rape

Sexual assault prevention is a complex task. However, prior to talking about sexual assault prevention programming, we wish to issue a reminder. We are, by no means, suggesting that sexual assault survivors are to blame for the heinous victimization they experience. Rather, there are some evidence-based approaches to prevention programs that include ways to help individuals reduce the likelihood of victimization. Regardless of someone's actions (e.g., drinking or drug use, engaging in sexually risky behaviors, attending a party solo, etc.), there is absolutely no excuse for another person committing a sex crime against them. With that said, let's address a few key components of prevention programming.

Because most research regarding sexual assault prevention comes from the college population and college campus setting, the majority of what we will discuss here addresses college campus sexual assault prevention programs. Sexual assault prevention tends to be compromised of three main domains: "risk reduction, resistance education, and empowerment-based self-defense approaches" (Orchowski et al., 2020, p. 823). Although these three components are individually and collectively needed in prevention programming, there is not yet a comprehensive prevention model established for replication on college campuses (Orchowski et al., 2020). What is known, though, is that one-off (single-incident) prevention yields little in the way of long-term results. Instead, "integrated and sequenced comprehensive programming" is needed to combat the incidence of sexual assault on college campuses (Orchowski et al., 2020, p. 823).

As Suarez and Gadalla (2010) discuss, prevention starts with addressing oppressive beliefs and the various isms that underlie sexual assault. Programming to mitigate the effects of sexism, classism, racism, and oppressive rape myths is a good starting point (Suarez & Gadalla, 2010). Undergirding some of those isms is the perpetuation of sexual violence through abundant access to pornography that conveys skewed and problematic messages about sex (McVey et al., 2021). These oppressive beliefs and isms are largely implicated in the establishment and perpetuation of rape myths. As such, programming that targets rape myth identification and correction can play an important role in sexual assault prevention (Jozkowski, n.d.).

Prevention should not just be a matter of helping potential victims mitigate risk. Rather, prevention should also address the offenders (or potential offenders) and the role of bystanders. Programs that promote awareness among men regarding factors that increase the risk for perpetrating sexual violence can be useful as a prevention strategy (Orchowski et al., 2018). Relatedly, bystander intervention plays a large role in rape prevention. As such, programming that addresses indications of imminent assault, intervention strategies, and empathy for the victim (Cares et al., 2015; Zapp et al., 2021) are important aspects of holistic prevention programming.

Programming for risk reduction among women tends to include risk identification, assertiveness skills, and self-defense. Sexual refusal assertiveness and sexual abstinence can reduce the chances of experiencing sexual assault (Wigderson & Katz, 2015), and learning assertiveness techniques seems to be a key ingredient in any education program for women. Assertiveness skills seem critical and reduced rape

and attempted rapes between experimental and control groups (Senn et al., 2015). Even where there were no differences in sexual assaults between controls and experimentals, women who utilized assertiveness and self-defense skills experienced less self-blame than controls (Gidycz et al., 2015).

Despite our focus here on college-level prevention, awareness programming for sexual assault prevention should begin at an early age to reduce the likelihood of childhood sexual abuse. Safe@Last, developed in 1997 by the Rape and Sexual Abuse Center in Nashville, Tennessee, is one such example. According to Morris et al. (2017), Safe@Last teaches children "(1) to distinguish safe from unsafe people, (2) to differentiate between safe and unsafe situations, (3) problem-solving skills, (4) assertiveness skills, and (5) clear disclosure methods" (p. 296). Safe@Last has demonstrated effectiveness in raising children's knowledge of indicators of sexual threat (Fuqua, 2008; Morris et al., 2017).

Hillenbrand-Gunn and associates (2010) conducted a program for high school students that focused on social norms theory (Perkins & Berkowitz, 1986), which is based on what one thinks one's peers do and believe rather than what the peers actually do and believe. Their program was based on a men as allies philosophy and combined with social norms theory as their theoretical framework. Group psycho-educational/discussion sessions were administered to both male and female high school students through a variety of formats that challenged sexist, coercive, and abusive behavior that is a precursor to thinking that sexual assault is acceptable. Pre- to post-program results indicated that attitudes changed in the experimental group and not in the control group. The results of this methodologically sound experiment held at a 4-week follow-up for both men and women suggest that it holds promise as a creative approach focusing on peers, a formidable force for this age group (Hillenbrand-Gunn et al., 2010).

Similarly, Rowe et al. (2015) used a MY Voice, MY Choice assertive resistance training program that used a virtual immersion program emphasizing assertiveness skills and found at 3-month follow-up that the adolescent girls reported less sexual victimization than a wait list group. They also found that psychological victimization and psychological distress were reduced for those girls who had greater prior victimization at baseline.

Daigneault and her associates (2015) conducted sexual assault awareness workshops for 15- to 17-year-old high school students and were effective in improving general knowledge regarding sexual assault and awareness of resources in the event of experiencing sexual assault. They also found improved attitudes regarding sexual assault, along with their ability to recognize sexual assault in a dating context and diminish responses that deny or minimize assault. Indeed, prevention is an ongoing process, and early prevention efforts may be a key in helping individuals to recognize threats, exercise self-protective behaviors, and override societal messages that perpetuate victimization.

Intervention Strategies for Rape and Battery: The Case of Melody

LO6   Melody Swanson is a 50-year-old teacher. She has been living alone in a small house since the younger of her two children went away to college two months ago. Melody was divorced seven years ago. She had a long weekend off from school and decided to go away to a casino for a minivacation. When she returned home from her trip at 9:30 yesterday evening and emerged from her car in her driveway, she was met by a gunman in his middle 20s.

She dropped a small bag of groceries and some items from her purse as she was abducted at gunpoint and forced into the gunman's car, which was parked on the street. Melody was beaten, driven away to an isolated area several miles from her home, raped, beaten again, robbed, and abandoned, bleeding and bruised, with her clothing in shreds. She was weak and dazed but managed to find her way to the nearest house in the early hours of the morning, where she called for help. It is now 8:30 a.m., and Melody is at the trauma center of a hospital in a large metropolitan city, where she has just been taken by the police. Melody is experiencing physical and emotional trauma. She personifies a traumatized person. She is in shock, shaking, and trembling, has both eyes black, numerous contusions, abrasions, and cuts and is still in the muddy clothes she was abducted in. She is about to meet what will become a very important person in her life—a crisis worker from the local sexual assault and domestic violence center who specializes in rape cases.

Immediate Aftermath

In most situations, the most helpful and appropriate immediate response from a crisis worker is empathy and assurance that the survivor is still alive.

Nowhere in crisis intervention is it more important to provide the core facilitative conditions of building trust, displaying unconditional positive regard, using empathic listening and responding, providing concreteness and clarity, and demonstrating patience. The crisis task is predispositioning the client in regard to what they are going to go through, from vaginal or rectal examinations to law enforcement questioning to the acute stress symptoms that are likely to follow the initial onslaught of emotions they are now experiencing. The worker is going to quickly build what in the psychotherapy trade is called a **working alliance** (a cooperative and trusting working relationship). Melody's rape is a case in point of how this operates in the immediate aftermath of a trauma. Cloitre and her associates (2004) report that building this alliance is as critical as, if not more important than, mastery of any intervention techniques.

The **impact stage** (Matsakis, 2003, pp. 82–90) occurs during the assault and for approximately two weeks following it. During this time, a kaleidoscope of emotions, thoughts, and behaviors may occur, or conversely, the client may be in a state of shock and dissociation, with both physical pain associated with the sexual assault and dissociation, somatic reactions, hypervigilance, nightmares, and startle responses that are symptomatic of the acute stress disorder that often follows. Stability both from a physical and psychological standpoint are critical at this time (Briere & Scott, 2006, p. 273). It is the crisis worker's job to do a number of things as soon as the client comes into the hospital or the crisis center.

Some sense of control needs to be restored so the client can go through the physical exam and, if they so choose, file a report with local law enforcement. Paramount is restoring a sense of safety and security to a person whose world has just been turned upside down. To do this, the crisis worker must accurately assess the client's state of mobility and equilibrium and gently but also with assuredness and confidence enter into this upside-down world. The worker needs to gather information while walking a therapeutic tightrope between sensitivity and the need to ask specific behavioral closed-ended questions. Maximum sensitivity means using empathic prefacing statements followed by gathering behavioral information on the assault. To ask for information without voicing sincere concern for the person's trauma is not only callous and insensitive but likely will also terminate intervention before it starts (McCart et al., 2009). To that end, it is critical that the crisis worker immediately start the predisposition task of our crisis intervention model. Courtois and Ford (2009) propose the following capstone statement in regard to treating survivors of prolonged complex trauma, but we believe it also fits well here. Your job at this point is to provide relational conditions that encourage the safety of the attachment between the client and the worker (p. 190), and this may be anything but easy for you or the client.

CW: (talking slowly while she, with permission, gently picks up Melody's hand in an examining room in the ER) Hi, Melody, I'm Jolee Mabry. I am a counselor from the Metro Sexual Assault Unit. You have been through a terrible experience, that no one should ever go through, but you survived it. I can't begin to know what it feels like to experience all the feelings and thoughts you are having right now, but I do understand as traumatic as this is you have survived and I am going to be with you while you go through this, if you would like.

Melody: (looking fearful and struggling for words) I don't . . . I don't know . . . what to think, do, . . . what will happen? Where is he? Who was he? Why me? Can he get in here? So many things . . . I . . . I am so cold, and it feels like my heart is about to pound through my chest. Is this a nightmare? But I know it's real . . . I think. Where . . . am . . . I? I'm so sorry. I . . . I . . . I don't remember your name. Who are you?

CW: (Picks up a blanket and, with permission, gently pulls it around Melody.) I'm Jolee Mabry. I am a nurse and a counselor at the sexual assault center here. You are safe here. You were brought here by the paramedics and the police. You are in the Trauma Unit. I'm Jolee Mabry, a counselor here in the trauma unit. You were beaten physically by the man who assaulted you and the paramedics brought you here. You were raped and assaulted, that is very real. That's why you are here to get taken care of, and we do a very good job of taking care of people who have been sexually assaulted. That is my job, to take care of you, steer you through this experience and act as your advocate and just take care of things for you. Do you understand what I just said and know where you are?

Melody: Yes. What's going to happen to me? (Starts to shake.)

CW: I can't say it will be pleasant, but the medical staff and police officers who deal with sexual assault

here know their business. The nurse who will do the rape kit exam is a specially trained Sexual Assault Nurse Examiner (SANE). She will make it as painless as possible. You will be asked by the police to describe what happened, and there will be a number of medical procedures. As I said, I'll be with you every step of the way, and when they are done, I'll be with you to make arrangements to see that you stay safe and do what's necessary to get some stability and control back in your life.

Melody: Absolutely, please stay. (Grabs Jolee's hand and grips it.) It was horrible—the rape. I don't know how I came out alive and without any broken bones. He intended to kill me. Part of the time I was in a daze. I don't know what came over me. I must have blacked out. He may have thought I was dead. I don't know how long I lay out there alone after he left me. I certainly didn't fight back or protest. Look at me, I am so dirty. (Recoils in disgust.)

CW: Melody, I'm so proud of you for the way you handled it. You did whatever it took to stay alive. You saved yourself, and that took courage. Whatever you did, whether it was blacking out or offering no protests, was right, because it preserved your life, and that's the important thing right now. We are going to get those clothes off of you and get you cleaned up, but we need to get some pictures and take some samples first, so hang in there a bit longer.

Melody: I feel so damn stupid. Always watchful and just let my guard down. So damn angry at me. I'd kill that bastard if I had a chance. Shoot his nuts off! Lord! Did I just say that? I don't say things like that, but that scurrilous low-life SOB . . . degrading . . . How can I go back to face my students . . . I feel like I'm in a sort of twilight zone. Maybe part of me did die. I'm feeling so alone and vulnerable. It's like this whole damn thing isn't real. It couldn't be happening to me, but I know it is. I know I keep going back to that and all this whirling going on in my head . . . I don't know if I can hold it together.

There is no universal response to rape. Melody represents a few of the conflicting emotions that rampage through someone who has been sexually violated. Dissociative responses are a common defense mechanism to try to bring some stability back into the survivor's life as a whirlwind of emotions blow through the survivor's mind. The laundry list of responses that follows this dialogue represents a good deal of, but not all of, the dirty emotions the client is trying to wash out of their mind. The crisis worker's job is to continuously provide support, safety, and practical assistance. While it may seem to be minimizing and discounting the gravity of the situation to call it **psychological first aid** (National Child Traumatic Stress Network and National Center for PTSD, 2006; National Institute of Mental Health, 2002), that is exactly what the worker is doing. Psychological first aid comprises three primary tasks of our intervention model: predispositioning/bonding, exploration/assessment, and safety. However, how this usually gets done is anything but stepwise. Crisis workers who ply their trade in the field of sexual assault are indeed engaging in a stand-up act where they have to be quick in changing strategies and responses to meet the kaleidoscope of emotions that may range from catatonic-like shock to unbridled rage.

CW: It's really scary, the thought of losing control with all those thoughts and emotions racing around in your head, Melody, but that is common for sexual assault survivors. It may be hard to imagine, but your mind and body are attempting to get order back into what for the past few hours has been complete chaos. It's your mind and body's normal defensive response to a completely abnormal situation. It will pass, and to help move that process along, we are going to take this piece by piece, one step at a time, until you get control back.

Melody: I don't know. I guess, but . . . (**Pause, with an apprehensive look.**) I'm a teacher; I maintain control, but I just can't seem to get a handle on this . . . (**Starts to break down again with muffled sobs.**) I'm so sorry, I'm such a mess, and can't get a grip.

CW: You don't have to be sorry about anything. You are not a mess. Grief is also part of this. You have lost a lot tonight. (**Sits patiently while Melody holds on and sobs quietly with her arm around her.**)

The crisis worker acknowledges her grief, which is a common response to the many losses the client has suffered (Matsakis, 2003, pp. 111–127). She also starts to slowly give her information about the psychological processes occurring within her as a start to developing coping skills and regaining emotional and cognitive control. It is important to start providing basic psychoeducation to clients who are experiencing extreme psychological stress (McCart et al., 2009). Melody is suffering from what we call **peritraumatic**

stress symptoms. Those are traumalike symptoms that almost all persons would suffer given similar circumstances. Whether these symptoms turn into acute traumatic stress disorder, which we discuss in other parts of the book, or turns into PTSD will depend a lot on what happens in the next few hours and days. The worker has to be judicious in how much information on psychological coping mechanisms she gives out to avoid cognitive overload. Indeed, engaging in any formal therapeutic intervention or formal assessment in the next few days is *not* recommended. What is recommended is planning thoroughly for the next few hours and days to keep the client safe, supported, and stabilized. Healing from a rape requires concentration, effort, thought, and time and cannot be rushed (Matsakis, 2003, p. 14).

CW: This whole procedure is going to take about 3 to 4 hours to complete. We want you thoroughly checked out in regard to not only your sexual assault but the physical assault as well. The police will interview you. Lt. Lenise Balay is going to do the interview. She and I work together a lot on these cases, and I trust her completely. She is one of the most empathic police officers I know. She will ask you some pretty pointed questions, but understand she wants to get this just right so we can catch who did this to you. You are also going to get a pelvic exam and a rape kit done. Andrea Little is a SANE nurse who specializes in doing this. It won't be pleasant, but again, she is a specialist in this business and will be very thorough and gentle. I'll be with you every step of the way. OK?

This is a brief synopsis of the practical medical and legal information the worker gives the survivor. In rape cases, thoroughly explaining what is going to happen is critical to not secondarily revictimizing the survivor. The sensitivity that needs to be manifested in doing a rape exam is best demonstrated in Bennett's (2015) article on getting a bra drive going for raped women who did not want the embarrassment of going braless by having to turn their bras over for evidence. The Riverside county multidisciplinary Sexual Assault Response Team conducted a very successful bra collection drive so the SANE nurse could replace the survivor's evidence bra. Sexual Assault Response Teams (SARTs) are growing multidisciplinary teams that provide a variety of support and coordination services for sexual assault survivors throughout the country (Moylan, et al., 2015).

CW: (after the police lieutenant and SANE nurse are done) Excellent! Dr. Zanzar has gone over all your tests and has okayed your release. You got through that well. Where would you like to go, and who would you like to be there with you, someone you really trust?

Melody: Well, my brother, Tom. I'd want him there with me. He's an ex-Marine. Although I don't know how he'd feel about all this and his stupid sister who he's always yapping at to be more vigilant and careful. God! I just feel so ashamed to let him know this happened. But I don't know if I can go back in my driveway or not. That's ridiculous but it still scares me, just the thought of it . . .

CW: I understand how you could feel that way, and the last thing you want to do is tell him about this. Would you like me to call him and get him down here and talk with him? I have done this before, and I think I can help you out with that.

Using Support Systems and Stopping Secondary Victimization

LO7   In the immediate aftermath of the rape, getting support and safety measures in place is a high priority, as is educating the significant others in the survivor's life about the foregoing dynamics. A critical component is steering the person through the medical and police procedures that can have a high potential for secondary victimization (Howell, 1999; Ochberg, 1988; Pauwels, 2003). Secondary victim crisis intervention may also be necessary if there are persons in the support system who might either become homicidal or turn on the survivor and blame them (Pauwels, 2003). Particularly family members and loved ones may need very firm, clear instructions on how they are going to meet the survivor in their first encounter. The difficulty of this initial encounter after the rape cannot be overemphasized. Both from the survivor's and significant others' standpoint, it may be very easy to affix blame as a way of trying to make sense out of what happened. Secondary victimization must not be allowed to occur, so the crisis worker's job will be to educate significant others on how they can best support the client.

Therefore, it is extremely important that a counselor from a rape crisis or sexual assault unit be contacted immediately, as in the preceding example. A nationwide nursing service called the Sexual Assault Nurse Examiner (SANE) program provides specially

trained nurses for first response medical care and crisis intervention. The SANE program provides comprehensive and consistent postrape medical care, such as emergency contraception and sexually transmitted disease prophylaxis, documents forensic evidence accurately, provides expert testimony, promotes psychological recovery, and coordinates multiple service providers to provide comprehensive care for rape survivors (Campbell et al., 2005).

CW: (Meets brother Tom at the center reception desk.)

Tom: (excited, agitated, and loud) What's this all about? What's going on with my sister? What's she doing at the Rape Crisis Center? Is she in trouble? Did she get raped? WHAT THE HELL IS HAPPENING AND WHERE IS MY SISTER?

CW: Your sister has been beaten and sexually assaulted and . . .

Tom: What the . . . where did it happen?

CW: In her driveway, about 9:30 last night. She was just coming back from the casino.

Tom: Casino! What the hell was she doing at the casino? Jesus Christ, when I get hold of her . . .

CW: (Becoming assertive and using a well-modulated but commanding voice, immediately interrupts his ranting.) I understand that you were in the Marines, so tell me this. Is it the Marine Corps creed if a guy gets wounded to go yell at him and tell him how stupid he has been?

Tom: Well no I . . . um . . . but this is different.

CW: Tell me how so. You took care of your wounded buddies, didn't you? What was your rank anyway?

Tom: Well, uh . . . Master Sergeant. But, uh . . . I don't see what that's got to do with it.

CW: (well-modulated but clearly assertive) I'll tell you what, Tom. I didn't get a chance to introduce myself. I am Jolee Mabry, a counselor and nurse with the sexual assault center. I was a nurse in the Gulf War, wore the Eagle, Anchor, and Globe (Marine Corps insignia) myself. First Lieutenant Mabry, USMC retired, at your service. I served in Saudi Arabia and Iraq with mobile surgical units there. If you are as good a marine as I think you are, you retrieved your wounded and did everything possible to keep them alive and safe, did you not? Is that correct, Master Sergeant Swanson?

Tom: (sort of snaps to attention and in a rather tentative voice) Yes, ma'am. That is . . . uh . . . affirmative, ma'am.

CW: Good, so you have a wounded sister. You know about PTSD, right? We don't want her going out on a date with that now, do we? What she needs is all the care and support you can give her, don't we now? No blame, no fault finding, don't you agree? No going out hunting the bad guy because your job is taking care of your troop, and your sister is surely that and more, is she not? A lot of care and understanding, compassion and empathy, for the terrible combat experience she has been through, and make no mistake, it is indeed that. So, Master Sergeant Swanson, can you take this mission on, or do I get somebody else?

Tom: Yes, Lieuten . . . uh, er, ma'am. I can certainly do that.

CW: Semper Fi. Now go in there and take care of your sister. Hold her and tell her how much you love her and take her home. Also tell her how brave she was and how smart she was to survive this. You cannot give her too many "way to go's"! Got it? I'll be in touch with both you and her. Here's my card. If you need help, call me. Marines look out for one another. I'll be back with you two after you spend some time together.

Tom: (sheepishly, wringing his baseball cap in his hands) I am sorry for my initial behavior, ma'am. I was pretty wound up. I am squared away now. Thank you for straightening me out. I won't mess this up.

Secondary victimization of a rape victim is always close at hand. It is certainly not uncommon for relatives to become angry and blaming of the victim when they are confronted with news of a rape as they seek to get control over what they perceive as an uncontrollable situation. The crisis worker changes her approach as soon as she detects the brother's negative attitude and becomes very directive with lots of "I" assertion statements to get the brother's attention. She lays something of a guilt trip on him to get his attention and change his cognitive sets about what needs to happen. She uses a technique that we would generally be critical of but works well here. That is, she uses a number of negative interrogative statements ("Don't you think/agree?") that ask for agreement with her point of view. By doing so, she shifts focus to positive rather than negative support for this wounded survivor.

Although you are probably not a Marine nor usually would by chance meet a survivor's brother who was, the crisis worker manifests the best of creative and adaptive thinking to create a bond and reframe this in terms he can understand. Although he is not now an active Master Sergeant, she knows that once a Marine, always a Marine, and that's why her responses aren't to "Tom" but "Master Sergeant Swanson." That's an all-star performance which goes to the heart of the adaptability that great crisis workers have.

CW: (Reenters the room with Melody and Tom.) You're going to have a lot of different reactions to this. They are not the same for every person, so don't be alarmed if you have some and not others. We will talk about all of this when things have settled down. People have lots of different ways of coping with this. The main thing is for you to feel as safe and secure as you can. I am going to give you a number that is on call 24 hours a day. Do not feel guilty about calling. I am going to be your main contact from the Center, so don't be afraid to call me. I will be doing some checking in with you, if that is OK.

The crisis worker's intuition is right when she guesses that the place of safety and comfort for Melody would be her own home but that the frightening part would be getting past the place in her driveway where she was abducted. The crisis worker is also correct in reassuring Melody for her actions, which brought her out alive. Clients will immediately begin second-guessing themselves as to what they should have done, and negative emotions of guilt, shame, and embarrassment will start building (Courtois & Ford, 2009, p. 188; Matsakis, 2003, pp.118–119; Weiss, 2010). The crisis worker dispels this notion by clearly and empathically stating that what she did was just right because it got her through the ordeal and out the other side alive. If she is able, the crisis worker immediately starts education in gentle and small doses. Primary education concerns getting the client through the next 24 hours, which are indeed going to be unreal for her. Her brother is a critical support and will need to be given some primary education about rape dynamics.

An important issue for rape survivors is control. Whatever will allow Melody to bring some control back in her life is important to do and is a major goal for the crisis worker. That may or may not be attempting to remember details of the assault. They may want to take a long, hot shower, or just sleep. Melody has experienced an emotionally draining loss of control to the attacker, and she needs to be reassured that her loss of control is neither total nor permanent. She did what she had to do to survive, and that took courage. It is important to her for others to recognize her and give her credit. There is no wrong way to survive a rape (Howell, 1999)! Nonjudgmentalism and support are critical so the client immediately starts moving from victim to survivor status (Ganas et al., 1998).

Responses

LO8 Although the cited authors (Benedict, 1985; Matsakis, 2003, pp. 81–98; Williams & Holmes, 1981) assert the following array of responses to rape from a primarily women's perspective, we believe these hold true for all survivors of sexual assault. The person who is assaulted:

1. May respond by exhibiting no emotions—appearing unaffected.
2. May feel humiliated, demeaned, and degraded.
3. May suffer immediate physical and psychological injury as well as long-term trauma.
4. May experience impaired sexual functioning.
5. May blame themself and feel guilty.
6. May experience difficulty relating to and trusting others—especially others from of the same gender as their perpetrator.
7. May experience fantasies, daydreams, and nightmares—vividly reliving the assault or additional encounters with the assailant—or may have mental images of scenes of revenge.
8. Will never be the same, even though most survivors, over time, develop ways to recover, cope, and go on with their lives.
9. May be fearful of reporting the assault to law enforcement or a rape crisis center.
10. May be reluctant to discuss the assault with members of their family, friends, and others because of the risk of rejection and embarrassment.
11. May become severely depressed and suicidal.
12. May be extremely angry and revenge-seeking to the point of becoming lethal.

The Following Three Months

LO9 Rape has high potential for PTSD, depression, suicide, panic attacks, generalized anxiety disorder, social adjustment disorders, sexual dysfunction, eating disorders, dissociation, and more negative worldviews and cognitive distortions. The crisis worker must not let the client regress and retreat into the past. Blaming external factors, self-blaming, and perseverating on why the rape happened are not helpful, along with the guilt of "what if-ing?" oneself to death about where one was, what type of clothing one wore, not paying attention to surroundings, and on and on (Frazier et al., 2001; Matsakis, 2003, pp. 81–98; Weiss, 2010).

Follow-up, proactive, and continuous supportive therapy is essential and may include any of the following topics (Ganas et al., 1998, 1999; Howell, 1999; Matsakis, 2003; Pauwels, 2003).

Critical Needs. During the three months following a sexual assault, a survivor such as Melody:

1. May need continuing medical consultation, advice, or treatment; they may experience soreness, pain, itching, nausea, sleeplessness, loss of appetite, and other physical and somatic symptoms.
2. May have difficulty resuming work; the added stress of the sexual assault may create too much stress in the workplace.
3. Needs to have people reach out to them, listen to them, and verbally assure them—not shun them or fear continuing to relate to them.
4. Needs the acceptance and support of family and friends.
5. May have difficulty resuming sexual relations and needs understanding without pressure.
6. May exhibit unusual mood swings and emotional outbursts, which others will need to understand and allow.
7. May experience nightmares, flashbacks, phobias, denial, disbelief, and other unusual effects.
8. May go into depression, which may be accompanied by suicidal ideation or acute traumatic stress disorder.

PTSD

LO10 As previously indicated, rape ranks second only to combat in the potential for PTSD. Because it is a less noxious approach, your authors would first use EMDR as a therapeutic intervention. It is far less intrusive than the cognitive-behavioral approaches generally recommended. If EMDR didn't work, then we would use a combination of the three recommended cognitive-behavioral treatments (Briere & Scott, 2006; Cloitre & Rosenberg, 2006; Courtois et al., 2009; Ford, & Cloitre, 2009; Foa & Rauch, 2004; Frazier et al., 2001):

1. Exposure treatment, which calls for repeated emotional recounting of the traumatic memory;

2. Affect regulation, which focuses on teaching clients skills to reduce painful internal emotional states; and

3. Cognitive therapy, to replace dysfunctional cognitions with new, more adaptive thoughts.

These procedures will be demonstrated shortly in this chapter in the case of heath, an adult survivor of childhood sexual abuse. Two supplementary therapy issues that are specific to rape need to be mentioned. First, there is the fact of opening up the old wound of the rape. Confronting the rape may be painful, but it is absolutely necessary, and the client needs to clearly understand what is going to happen. However, opening this wound, whether it be the recent rape of Melody or the old ones of Heath's adolescent abuse, needs to be done in a carefully gauged manner. To start exposure therapy means pushing away defenses that are in place to keep the client stabilized, although that stability may be anything but healthy (Courtois et al., 2009). However, because these defense systems are being rent asunder, sexual assault survivors have a tendency to go rather blindly in harm's way. While therapy is occurring, they are almost a sure bet to experience transcrisis points as they form new defensive systems and coping mechanisms. As a result, it is not just the psychological safety but the client's physical safety with which the worker needs to be concerned.

Critical Supports

Support people can be of great help during this phase of recovery. In fact, one of the most important things a crisis counselor can do is to get support systems in place and coordinate them. The recovery of survivors of sexual assault is enhanced by the empathic help and understanding of the people close to them. Whether the survivor's support people are family, friends, associates, medical or legal personnel, crisis workers, or long-term therapists, the important ingredients in the helping relationship are acceptance, genuineness, empathy, caring, and nonjudgmental understanding (Baker, 1995; Benedict, 1985; Howell, 1999; Remer & Ferguson, 1995). These support people can help survivors of sexual assault by:

1. Understanding and accepting the survivor's changed moods, mood swings, and so on, and allowing them the freedom to act them out.

2. Supporting and being available—but not intruding—while encouraging them to regain control and to recover their life.

3. Ensuring that they doesn't have to go home alone (without overprotecting them).

4. Realizing that recovery takes a long time and lots of hard work.

5. Allowing them to make their own decisions about reporting the rape and prosecuting the assailant.

6. Leaving it up to them to decide whether they want to change jobs or place of residence.

7. Responding to them in positive ways, so they do not sense that the support person blames them for "letting it happen" or feels they are not capable of taking care of themself.

8. Allowing them to talk about the assault to whomever they wish, whenever they wish, but not disclosing the assault to anyone without their prior consent.

9. Showing empathy, concern, and understanding without dominating them.

10. Recognizing that they will likely suffer from low self-esteem and finding ways to show them that they are genuinely valued and respected.

11. Recognizing that their hurt will not end when the physical scratches and bruises are gone—that their emotional healing will take a long time.

12. Finding ways to help them trust again—assisting others (friends, coworkers, siblings, parents) to show tolerance, understanding, and confidence.

13. Encouraging coworkers, friends, siblings, and parents to believe in them and not avoid them or avoid talking with them openly about the rape.

14. Including their children, if they have any, in many of the considerations concerning help toward emotional recovery.

15. Referring them to sexual assault support groups for survivors and family members.

16. Recognizing that their spouse, partner, or lover may develop symptoms similar to those of the survivor (nightmares, phobias, rage, guilt, self-blame, self-hate, and such) and may need help similar to that needed by the survivor.

17. Encouraging their spouse or partner to give them time to recover, free from pressure, before resuming sexual activity and to let them know they are still interested in their mate, still desire them, but that former patterns of sex life will be resumed at the survivor's own pace. It is important for a spouse or partner to talk this out openly with the survivor, to clear the air for both parties.

The foregoing is not a grocery list to just be handed to support persons. It is something the interventionist needs to do as part of a psychoeducation program that lets people know what to expect and works with them as they struggle through what will be a period of transcrisis events and points.

Adult Survivors of Childhood Sexual Abuse

LO11 There is ample evidence that the sexual abuse of children wreaks lasting damage in their lives that continues into adulthood (Briere & Runtz, 1987, 1993; Briere & Scott, 2006; Browne & Finkelhor, 2000; Courtois & Ford, 2009; Kessler & Bieschke, 1999; Lamoureaux et al., 2012; Maschi et al., 2013; Mitchell & Morse, 1998; Oshodi et al., 2020; Payne et al., 2014; Rosencrans, 1997). If survivors are left untreated, they may experience recurring episodes of revictimization and exhibit debilitating symptoms (transcrisis points) for many years (Briere & Runtz, 1993; Cloitre & Rosenberg, 2006; Davis et al., 2002; Kessler & Bieschke, 1999; Noll et al., 2003; Van Bruggen et al., 2006).

Psychological Trauma and Sequelae

Effects on adult survivors. The histories of adult survivors of childhood sexual abuse show a higher incidence of (1) depression, anxiety, shame, and humiliation (Briere & Conte, 1993; Briere & Runtz, 1988; Browne & Finkelhor, 2000; Oshodi et al., 2020); (2) borderline personality disorder, dissociative disorder, and posttraumatic stress disorder (Briere & Runtz, 1993; McLean & Gallop, 2003; Mitchell & Morse, 1998; Oshodi et al., 2020); (3) social stigmatization, alienation, inhibitions, introversion, and interpersonal hypersensitivity (Browne & Finkelhor, 2000; Lundberg-Love et al., 1992); (4) more contacts with medical doctors for somatic complaints including chronic pain problems, such as fibromyalgia and irritable bowel syndrome and long-term serious physical health deficits such as pulmonary, heart, and liver disease, unintended pregnancy, and obesity (Hertel & Johnson, 2013; Kendall-Tackett, 2008; Moeller et al., 1993; Bachmann, & Moeller, 1993; Stevenson, 1999); (5) negative self-image (Courtois, 1988; Herman, 1981); (6) poor interpersonal relationships and poor parenting skills (Browne & Finkelhor, 2000); (7) suicide (Tripodi & Pettus-Davis, 2013; Ullman & Brecklin, 2002); (8) substance misuse (Bender et al., 2015); (9) incarceration in prison (Tripodi & Pettus-Davis, 2013); and (10) sexual revictimization (Aakvaag et al., 2017; Waldron et al., 2015; Zlotnik, 2014). Yet, these are not all of the contents of the Pandora's box of childhood sexual assault. Hertel and Johnson (2013) found in their examination of over 17,000 respondents to the Adverse Childhood Experiences study that the higher the number of adverse experiences children suffered, the worse the effects became. Those pernicious effects ranged across physical health problems such as obesity, heart and liver disease, sexually transmitted diseases, unintended pregnancies, partner violence, illicit drug use, suicide attempts, and other mental health and emotional issues.

A long list of studies have found that a significant number of female clients (institutionalized, outpatient, psychiatric patients, and clients in clinics) were sexually abused as children (Briere & Runtz, 1987; Hertel & Johnson, 2013; Kessler & Bieschke, 1999; Maschi et al., 2013; Salter, 1995). Adult female survivors consistently demonstrate symptoms similar to those of combat veterans in addition to compulsive sexual behavior, sadomasochistic sexual fantasy, sexual identity issues, and loss of sexual interest (Briere & Runtz, 1987; Courtois, 1988; Finkelhor, 1979; Herman, 1981; Mitchell & Morse, 1998). And, like combat veterans, child sexual abuse survivors are prone to use alcohol and drugs to submerge bad memories from awareness and to engage in suicidal ideation and attempts (Duncan, 2004; Hien et al., 2009; Rew, 1989; Smith et al., 2014; Ullman & Brecklin, 2003).

Male survivors who were abused by adult men fare no better and report essentially the same symptoms, with concomitant sexual orientation ambiguity, mistrust of adult males, homophobia, hypersexuality, poor physical and mental health, lower emotional and social support, post-trauma symptomatology, social isolation, anxiety, and body image disturbances (Choudhary et al., 2010; Gartner, 2005; Lew, 2004; Myers, 1986; Payne et al., 2014; Rowan, 2006). Perhaps more importantly, Monk-Turner and Light's (2010) study of men who had been sexually assaulted and raped found that if actual penetration of a male's body occurred, it was the major variable in *not* seeking treatment.

Revictimization. Many of the foregoing symptoms appear to be even more profound and multiple if survivors suffered multiple types of childhood abuse, including childhood sexual abuse (Aakvaag et al., 2017; Cloitre & Rosenberg, 2006). Just like their women counterparts, men who were sexually assaulted in childhood are more likely to be assaulted as adults (Aosyed et al., 2011). Early assault is additive, and it appears that the higher the incident rate and the more profound it is, the higher the potential for later problems. If the abuse continues into adolescence, the potential for adult sexual assault also increases (Van Bruggen et al., 2006). Further, if both sexual and physical abuse occur in childhood and adolescence, the chance for revictimization again increases (Ullman & Brecklin, 2003). Survivors of childhood sexual abuse do not usually experience repetition of their victimization on the conscious level; that is, they do not intentionally precipitate abuse. It may be that revictimization or repetition of the sexual abuse tends to recur through the survivor's reenactment of the physical, sexual, or emotional abuse that was experienced during childhood (Schetky, 1990).

Our own feeling from treating such clients is that they have received very few of the typical parental warnings and admonitions that would naturally have been taught to them if they had had a typical childhood. As a result, they tend not to be aware of or reactive to warning signs and cues that would say to most people, "This is not a safe place to be or a safe thing to do or a safe person to be with." They also may respond very much as our combat veterans do by engaging in risky behaviors to achieve adrenaline highs that let them know they are "still alive and kicking." Because of this, the crisis worker needs to provide psychoeducation on warning signs and cues that may stop survivors from blithely going into dangerous settings and engaging with people who will do them harm.

Child Abuse as a Predictor of PTSD. Child sexual abuse has been shown to predict the development of PTSD in later life (Darves-Bornoz et al., 1998; Hannan et al., 2017; Kessler & Bieschke, 1999; Pfefferbaum, 1997; Regehr et al., 1999). In a comparison of the prevalence of PTSD and other diagnoses in abused children, Ackerman and associates (1998) studied three groups: sexual abuse (SA) only, physical abuse (PA) only, and both (BOTH). Children in the BOTH group had more diagnoses overall. PTSD was significantly comorbid (disorder or trauma caused by two variables) with most affective disorders. A younger age of onset of SA and coercion to maintain secrecy predicted a higher number of total diagnoses. Also, children had more diagnoses when PA had come from men rather than from women. The research of Darves-Bornoz and associates (1998) indicated that adding physical assault during the rape of children was predictive of chronic PTSD. However, to suppose that PTSD is the only or major pathological outcome of child sexual abuse is to severely underestimate the negative consequences that accrue. Developmental processes associated with affect regulation and interpersonal relational skills may be severely disrupted and pave the way for future assaults (Cloitre & Rosenberg, 2006).

False Memories

LO12   The "false memory" concept, applied to work with both adults who were abused as children and perpetrators of abuse, has raised concern and controversy among human services workers and scholars (Otgaar et al., 2021; Patihis et al., 2014; Rubin, 1996). This debate raged in the 1990s, although it has garnered less attention in recent years, you should understand that it still plays a role in the criminal defense of accused abusers (Otgaar et al., 2021). Regardless of whether a memory is factually real or false, the belief in a memory's legitimacy creates significant emotional responses in individuals (Laney & Loftus, 2008) and can have lasting, detrimental effects.

The False Memory Syndrome Foundation was created in 1992 by Pamela and Peter Freyd, who had been accused by their daughter of sexual abuse. They propose that false memories occur for three reasons. First is countertransference, in which mental health professionals who have been abused themselves plant the memories to exact revenge and satisfy their own power needs. Second, angry adolescents who are seeking emancipation lash out at their parents by making accusations of sexual abuse. Third is the child who projects her own strong sexual feelings onto the father as his own toward her (Freyd, 1993).

Elizabeth Loftus, an expert in memory, has been part of this debate since the 1970s. Her work on false memories and the fallibility of memory has been critical in the evolution of our understanding of repressed memories. Loftus (1997) states, "it is one thing to change a detail or two in an otherwise intact memory but quite another to plant a false memory of an event that never happened" (p. 7). In her landmark study with Pickrell, Loftus utilized information obtained from participants' family members to construct a "lost-in-the-mall scenario." In this study, participants were provided a pamphlet that contained stories about real events that had transpired during their childhood (information provided by family members) and a made-up story of being lost in the mall at age 5. Twenty-nine percent of participants claimed to remember being lost in the mall at age 5, which never happened, and 25 percent adamantly claimed the event really transpired, even after being told it was a planted memory (Loftus, 1997). In light of these intriguing findings, Loftus notes that "external suggestion can lead to the construction of false childhood memories" (Loftus, 1997), a finding that has major implications of mental health professions.

The debate behind the legitimacy of false (implanted) memories as opposed to recovered memories has been a major part of the ongoing debate. According to Laney and Loftus (2013), there are two primary arguments in this discussion. First, Laney and Loftus (2013) state that there has been debate over whether or not false memories were actually false or if they might be based on actual repressed memories. Determining whether or not something actually happened can be challenging but, as Laney and Loftus describe, some researchers have been able to limit extraneous variables and still demonstrate that memories can be implanted. Second, Laney and Loftus discuss the criticism that participants in false memory studies might have identified the purpose of the study and were playing along to satisfy the researchers. However, researchers have conducted studies in which participants were misled to believe the study addresses something other than memory, and a significant portion of participants still generated false memories based on implantation techniques (Laney & Loftus, 2013). What's more is that it is nearly impossible to differentiate between real and false memories (Laney & Loftus, 2013).

When considering the equivalent emotionality demonstrated by individuals who adopt false memories and those with real memories, the idea of "uncovering repressed memories" that may not be overtly true presents noteworthy challenges for trauma professionals. Feigon and de Rivera (1998) conducted a "recovered memory" survey of 154 psychiatrists, and they concluded that the numbers of false accusations of childhood sexual abuse appearing to emerge from the psychotherapy of adults constitute a real problem. Their study indicates that the specific content of false memories extracted from client interviews depends on the particular interviewer, the way questions are asked, the context in which the interview takes place, and the interviewee's emotional state. Indeed, research continues to demonstrate that emotion has a powerful impact on memory (Kaplan et al., 2016) and that the development of false memories can

be triggered through multiple mechanisms, such as by making general suggestive statements, through dream interpretation or hypnosis, or through making personalized suggestive statements (Muschalla & Schönborn, 2021).

The debate notwithstanding, psychotherapy with and advocacy of survivors should be done by workers who are highly trained and skilled in dealing with the trauma, the repressed and dissociated memory issues, the risks, and the needs of survivors of child sexual abuse. Similarly, professionals who deal with perpetrators' memories should have a thorough understanding of the complex forms of abuser memory and forgetting that are frequently encountered. The discrepancies, emotions, dissociations, memory blackouts, and discomfort with traumatic memories may affect the way both survivors and perpetrators perceive the past abusive events (Rubin, 1996). To that end, anyone who does this work *absolutely must not* bring their own parental or abuse agendas into therapy. We have witnessed such a happening, and it was extremely destructive for clients and the therapist. Clinicians must strive to neither suggest nor suppress reports of remembered or suspected abuse and trauma. Instead, they must practice from a stance of supportive neutrality (Courtois, 2001).

Intervention Strategies for Adult Survivors: The Case of Heath

LO13 Heath was sexually abused by his stepfather regularly from ages 8 through 15. For 20 years, he suppressed most memories and emotions related to the sexual abuse, which had included fondling, digital penetration, and anal intercourse. He has vivid memories of the physical abuse he suffered at both his stepfather's and his mother's hands. It is somewhat ironic that his stepfather was employed as a psychologist at a major university. Now, at age 35, he has regained his memory of the sexual abuse and is experiencing severe symptoms of delayed rape trauma syndrome.

His marriage is ending; his career is in shambles; his communications and relationship with his three children are adversely affected by his personal turmoil; and his rage toward his stepfather and his anger toward his mother have robbed him of his self-respect and his affection toward his parents, who live across the state from him. His only daughter, the middle child, recently had her eighth birthday, and Heath is deeply obsessed with his daughter's safety. Heath feels a great deal of guilt, shame, remorse, and loss of self-esteem. For several years, he has been experiencing some suicidal ideation, and since the recovery of his memory of the sexual abuse, this ideation has seriously intensified.

Interventions with Heath included both individual counseling and support group work, in which he willingly participated. In support group meetings, Heath received the encouragement, validation, and information he needed to absolve himself from guilt, shame, and remorse. He also acquired essential advice from support group members on implementing safety measures he could take to ensure that his 8-year-old daughter would not fall prey to the kinds of sexual abuse he had suffered. That advice allayed his fears and concerns about his daughter's vulnerability. Often, the affirmation and informational resources obtained in support groups are key elements in the emotional healing, fear reduction, enhancement of self-esteem, and rehabilitation of adult survivors of child sexual abuse. It was certainly so with Heath (Mitchell & Morse, 1998, pp. 231–238).

Assessment

Particularly among older individuals, such as Heath, who suffered childhood sexual abuse under severe societal and family strictures of secrecy and denial, the abuse will be disguised and repressed. Often, such clients will have been under the care of mental health professionals and been diagnosed with a variety of psychological disorders, ranging from schizophrenia to depression to borderline personality.

Presenting problems are typically depression, anxiety, dissociation, and compulsive disorders (Courtois, 1988). Although the client may present as competent, responsible, mature, and otherwise capable, these characteristics are a facade for underlying emotional problems. Affectively, behaviorally, and cognitively, abuse victims may present themselves in a labile, quickly vacillating manner, rigidly adhering to one end or the other of the continuum—"I'm great" or "I'm terrible"—or rapidly oscillating between the two (Courtois, 1988). In fact, there is growing acceptance for the conceptualization of borderline personality disorder as a manifestation of complex trauma symptomatology (Luyten et al., 2020).

Triage assessment of these people can be problematic, to say the least. At one moment, they present as affectively calm and controlled, perhaps to the point of rigidity. At the next moment, because of some real or imagined slight, particularly in interpersonal relationships, they may become extremely labile (emotionally unstable) with angry tirades or uncontrolled crying and then offer profuse, guilt-ridden apologies for their behavior. It should come as little surprise that many individuals with a diagnosis of borderline personality disorder have suffered from childhood trauma (Ball & Links, 2009).

Cognitively, they may present themselves as competent and perceptive thinkers and then, when faced with a stimulus that causes a flashback or intrusive image, completely dissociate themselves from present reality and respond in a confused, disjointed manner. Behaviorally, such individuals may run the gamut of Diagnostic and Statistical Manual of Mental Disorders, Fifth Edition, Text Revision (DSM-5-TR) (American Psychiatric Association, (APA, 2022) diagnostic categories—and then appear perfectly appropriate! If there is any key to making an accurate assessment of adult survivors of childhood sexual abuse, it is their consistent inconsistency across triage dimensions. The astute crisis worker who is struggling to make an assessment in which such inconsistency is displayed should consider childhood sexual abuse as a working hypothesis.

A crisis invariably initiates therapy; as in other forms of delayed PTSD, the crisis may seem unrelated to a past traumatic event. During the intake interview, if some of the common symptoms of PTSD are revealed, then childhood sexual abuse should be suspected as a causative agent and further assessment should target it as a possibility. Construction of a traumagram (Figley, 1985) will often provide clues to the origin of the precipitating event. The crisis worker who suspects PTSD in an adult due to childhood sexual abuse should immediately make plans to refer the client for a comprehensive psychiatric assessment after the initiating crisis is contained.

The Case of Heath. Heath is a 35-year-old cisgender man who initially presented at a community mental health center with suicidal thoughts and actions. He had overdosed on sleeping pills, was discovered comatose by a friend, and had been taken to the emergency room, where his stomach was pumped. At intake, he showed the counselor cuts he had inflicted on himself with a box cutter. He was dissociative and saw himself "out of his body" as he drew the knife up and down his arms (Note: Self-injury is typically conceptualized as a coping skill, most commonly as a means of regulating intense emotion). He had also cut off his parakeet's head (a much more ominous suicidal sign of taking out a prized possession), although he was extremely remorseful about its death and could not imagine why he would have done such a terrible thing. He was currently depressed and saw no reason for living.

The counselor rated him overall on the Triage Assessment Form at 27, set up a suicide safety plan with him, and referred him to a psychiatrist for evaluation and medication for depression. After several false starts and stops at counseling, Heath finally admitted the real issue: He had been abused sexually and physically as a child by his stepfather from age 8 to 15, and his mother had denied the abuse. Both parents had engaged in physical abuse of Heath during the same period of time. At age 16, he went to live with his father, who had severe alcohol misuse disorder. Those arrangements were chaotic, but no further physical or sexual abuse occurred. That lasted until he moved away to college.

He reports that the behavior that got him to the ER and into counseling has been getting progressively worse, and he can no longer keep thoughts of the abuse submerged. He is experiencing severe social estrangement and has very few social relationships—none of which are with other men. He wears numerous layers of clothing that hide his figure, even in very hot weather. He is a talented artist and is employed part-time at a graphic design business.

Treatment of Adults. A major component of therapy is to use a posttraumatic stress treatment model that uses some combination of prolonged exposure and cognitive processing or cognitive restructuring (Cloitre & Rosenberg, 2006; Foa & Rauch, 2004; Nishith et al., 2005) along with techniques to deal with the severe affective dysregulation (inability to monitor and control one's emotions) that accompanies this form of trauma (Briere & Scott, 2006, pp. 76–77; Courtois et al. 2009). A meta-analysis by Ehring and associates (2014) that dealt exclusively with PTSD with child sexual abuse as a causative agent in adult survivors examined standard cognitive behavioral therapy (CBT) treatment, trauma-focused CBT treatments, and EMDR. Overall Parcesepe and her associates' (2015) comprehensive review of treatment results found that all three interventions—behavioral, exposure therapy, and EMDR—were more effective in alleviating symptoms than no treatment. However, they did not find significant differences in treatment effectiveness between the three. They found that trauma-focused CBT was the most effective, and treatment including individual sessions fared better than group treatment alone. However, Finkelhor (1987) proposes that the trauma of childhood

sexual abuse goes beyond other causal agents of PTSD because of the unique dynamics of traumatic sexualization, social stigmatization, betrayal of trust by loved ones, and the powerlessness of children, so trust-building and affirmation activities are particularly critical.

Discovery and Admission. For survivors of childhood sexual abuse, particular problems arise in the therapeutic process that are absent with victims of other traumatic experiences. If the client is otherwise in crisis and childhood sexual abuse is suspected, do not explore incest material immediately because of the likelihood of compounding the present crisis through decompensation, regression, or dissociation. Client safety is paramount and should always be a primary or conjoint consideration with exploration of the incest (Courtois, 1988, p. 173). At the time the client chooses to own the trauma of incest, the potential for crisis rises exponentially. Stige et al. (2013) report that when attempts to self-manage the trauma finally give way, a high level of distress is reported prior to help seeking. Sensitivity in respecting and exploring the individual's process of seeking help when offering trauma treatment to survivors cannot be over emphasized. This is a huge undertaking that typically has a mountain of stigma attached to it and is positively related to trauma symptom severity (Deitz et al., 2015). The worker needs to be very sensitive to the client's admission, gently encouraging the client to disclose the abuse and directly and positively affirming the client for doing so. Trust here is critical. Not only have these clients learned that adult caretakers are untrustworthy (Elliot, 1994), but it is more than likely that others in the helping professions have victimized them as well (Ochberg, 1988).

Heath: (apprehensively) I don't know what you'll think about this. But I guess I can trust you. I just can't live with this anymore. (Pauses.)

CW: (suspecting from previous indicators what is coming) Whatever it is, I can see how deeply troubling it is and how difficult it must be. I am here to listen and try to understand. Whatever it is, I want you to know that you will still be the same Heath, and that person is not going to be any different in my eyes. I hope what I've just said makes it easier for you to get it out.

Heath: (starts sobbing) This is really bad.

CW: Heath, I am going to reach over and hold your arm, is that OK? (Heath nods. With permission, the counselor softly touches Heath's arm and speaks gently.) I'm guessing this is about something that somebody did to you or that happened to you, and it's OK, really OK, to talk about it.

Heath: I had sex with my stepfather. (**Relates a long history of sexual and physical torment by his step-father and mother, with the counselor listening and empathically responding.**)

Heath: (gently weeping) I know you're a counselor and all, but you must think I'm horrible.

CW: I can appreciate how terribly difficult that was. I also want you to know that I believe what you said. I don't think you're horrible at all. What I think is that you were a victim and that you are a survivor of those terrible things that shouldn't have happened and did. I want to correct one thing you said. You did not have sex with your stepfather. You were eight years old and had no choice. He forced sex on you. That's a big difference. Now I want to give you an idea of what is happening to you, why these bad memories keep coming back, and what they do to disrupt your life.

The crisis worker uses affirming and supportive statements throughout this opening scene. She touches the client only after being given permission because touching can sometimes be construed as anything but supportive by the client.

There are three general phases to this treatment. The first is safety; the second is processing, remembering, and mourning; and the third is reconnecting and reintegration (Courtois et al., 2009; Mitchell & Morse, 1998, pp. 184–195). The first order of business is keeping the client safe and in full knowledge of what is going to occur. There have been far too many secrets in these clients' lives. There are no secrets here.

Psychoeducation. Psychoeducation about the role that PTSD plays in incest trauma is important at this point because it can help allay clients' fears that they are "different," "dirty," or "mentally ill," and it assures them that PTSD is responsive to treatment. Education about PTSD also removes the mystique, confusion, and "craziness," anchoring present maladaptive behavior as purposive and reasonable given the survivor's traumatic history. It also allows the client to believe that something can be done through treatment (Courtois, 1988, p. 173).

CW: (after an explanation and showing Heath the DSM5-TR PTSD classification) So you are not "nuts." Those are the reasons these things are currently happening. We can treat this. It is a long road, and at times it is going to seem as if things are getting worse instead of better. We will have to go back and dig into those memories, and they are going to be painful. I want you to think about this because it is not an easy task. It is something you will need to choose. If you choose to do so, I want you to know that we'll go through this together. (**The counselor then explains what the treatment procedures will be and answers questions the client has about different components of the treatment.**)

Grounding. Grounding refocuses clients' attention onto the immediate therapeutic environment or, when over the phone or internet, on the physical surroundings they are presently inhabiting as opposed to flashbacks, intrusive thoughts, and dissociative states that are beginning to overwhelm them (Briere & Scott, 2006, pp. 96–97; Sanderson, 2013, pp. 167–174). They propose the following five steps:

1. Attempt to focus the client's attention on the therapist and the therapy. "I am right here. We're together in this room and we are doing exposure therapy. You are not back in the bedroom 20 years ago" are typical verbal responses to a client "going into the wind." At times, gentle touching may also be appropriate but should be used with caution due to the possible retriggering effect for many survivors of interpersonal trauma.

2. Ask the client to describe the internal experience they are presently having. "Describe what's going on right now." If the client has difficulty or appears frightened or otherwise unequal to the task, then move to step 3.

3. Orient the client to the immediate environment that they are in—the room with the worker, where it is, how it looks, what's in it, and how safe it is, and that it is not in the bedroom 20 years in the past.

4. If the client is still indicating stress, start deep breathing, relaxation, and/or grounding techniques (which we recommend teaching to these clients).

5. Repeat step 2 and assess the client's ability to return to therapy.

Grounding is a critical component of this therapy, in which clients are taught to literally put their feet on the ground, get physically and psychologically anchored, and stop the fragmentary thought processes and heightened affect that lead to depersonalization, flashbacks, and overpowering emotions (Matsakis, 2003, pp. 57–58; Mitchell & Morse, 1998, p. 198). Sutherland (1993, p. 23) proposes that focusing on gravity in relation to the body starts to make the client aware of the numbness and disowning of various body parts that she uses to dissociate from the trauma. The client is asked to find and identify a "spot of safety" where they can practice grounding. That spot of safety is a place the client can go and feel absolutely safe. One anchor that grounds clients is carrying a talisman with them, something that can literally be touched to connect them with reality. Coins, charms, key chains, totems, worry stones, and so on can all serve this purpose.

Your authors use this technique with abused and neglected foster children a lot and have used it with adults as well. Matsakis (2003, p. 58) proposes physical grounding, such as holding a familiar or safe item like a teddy bear; emotional grounding by writing oneself an e-mail or leaving a message on one's answering machine and then reading or listening to it; or mental grounding by describing aloud the room one is in, singing, or reading out loud from a magazine.

CW: So, the safest place in the house is the bathroom, with you sitting on the commode. Fine! When some of these cues that we've talked about start happening and you start to feel things sliding away, I want you to go into the bathroom, put your feet flat on the floor, and with the toilet lid down, have a seat, pick up a copy of *Car and Driver* (or any other magazine), and say to yourself, "It is 9:15 p.m., Tuesday evening, January 25, 2016. I am sitting on the toilet in my home, reading *Car and Driver*, and I feel a little silly sitting on the toilet lid, but I am quite safe." So just relax and enjoy that. Just notice your eyes scanning over the articles and looking at the pictures.

At times, when the client is in crisis and away from the worker, grounding the client over the telephone is critical. This can be done by reassuring the client that they are safe and asking them to describe what they see and hear around them. Ask them if they can feel their feet on the floor and if not, press down with their feet and grip something with their hands. Finally, they should keep a list of people they can call and go through the grounding exercise with (Mitchell & Morse, 1998, p. 199).

Mindfulness. A variation on stabilizing a person who is dissociating and derealizing is using mindfulness exercises. Mindfulness is the art of relating to one's experience in the present moment with full awareness and acceptance of whatever comes to mind (Brown et al., 2013). Using mindfulness techniques can significantly reduce distress (Sass et al., 2013) by opening attention to one's experience and keeping an open mind to whatever one encounters (Bishop et al., 2004). This is not a "just do it" exercise but takes practice and should not be done until an individual receives a good deal of psychoeducation (Williams et al., 2007), practice, and tryout with the technique. The major idea is that thoughts are just thoughts—not fixed and immutable facts that can't be changed (Greason, 2015). However, due to the risk of interoceptive reexperiencing, it is very important to prepare clients for mindfulness, remain attuned to indications that they are having reexperiencing symptoms (e.g., rapidly shaking leg, clenching fists, rocking back and forth, crying, shaking), and be prepared to help them ground in the present moment if they begin reexperiencing the trauma in physically debilitating ways.

CW: So, sit on the toilet and focus your attention on the lavatory and just tell me what you see on the countertop as you see it.

Heath: All my hand lotions and pills and stuff and shit! My frickin' razor!

CW: OK, the razor's there, but for the moment focus on something else.

Heath: It's that new oatmeal soap I got at the health food store.

CW: Tell me what's going through your mind as you look at it.

Heath: Well, erh, ah. It's supposed to really clear your complexion up; deep scrubbing gets the oil out and that. I could sure use that after the day I've had and . . . oh man! I am starting to lose it again.

CW: That happens, but now remember the exercise of watching those thoughts we did and how we moved them. You can just watch them float away.

Heath: Ha! I did! By golly I did it! Ha! They just sorta went down the shower drain.

CW: Good! Now let's try something. Get a washcloth and soap up and wash your face. Can you do that?

Heath: (Gets up, wets washcloth, and goes back on the stool and starts soaping his face.) OK I'm washing my face. I did it with cold water. It's rough but it feels kinda good. Cool and like scrubbing you know. Like maybe I could just take a shower and feel clean.

CW: So, you have that in your mind, what your face feels like and can start to imagine how that would feel like if you did take a shower and could just feel that sensation of cleanliness.

Heath: I umh, yeah, I think I could. I am back together pretty much. Thanks Dr. J.

CW: OK! Are we good to go?

Heath: Yes!

The crisis worker uses the "watching" technique to shift the client's attention when he starts heading back down old ineffective trauma-filled paths to give him a sense of control and power over his thoughts (Greason, 2015). The face wash utilizes a different type of mindfulness technique called **body scanning** (Kabat-Zinn, 2013, pp. 75–97). In body scanning, the individual monitors physical sensations throughout the body and gently allows themself to feel, experience, and accept the physical sensations that emanate from various body parts. The crisis worker doesn't panic or attempt to get Heath to stop when he starts to regain control. Rather, he acknowledges that in a matter-of-fact way but gently guides Heath back to ground. If you have ever been camping and got up on a frosty morning and washed your face in a cold mountain stream, you surely understand how quickly you are grounded in that moment with all that cold freshwater on your face and very much aware of the world around you!

Validation. As the client starts through the process of therapy, numerous transcrisis points will occur as long-buried trauma is brought back to awareness. In an active, directive, continuous, and reinforcing manner, the human services worker (Courtois, 1988, pp. 167–170; Longdon, 1994; Mitchell & Morse, 1998, pp. 90–91, 184–188):

1. Validates that the incest did happen, despite the denial of this fact by significant others; the client is not to blame, it is safe to talk about it, and the worker does not loathe the client for having been a participant.
2. Acts as an advocate who is openly and warmly interested in what happened to the survivor as a child and makes owning statements to that effect but still maintains neutrality and neither advocates for nor dismisses legal action. The worker also understands there is a high potential for transference/countertransference and is clear and consistent in maintaining boundaries.

3. Reinforces the resourcefulness of the victim to become a survivor.
4. Provides a mentor/reparenting role model to help with childhood developmental tasks that were missed.

Extinguishing Trauma. Extinguishing trauma means effecting a psychological extinction—that is, facilitating the reduction or loss of a conditioned response as a result of the absence or withdrawal of reinforcement. In practical terms, this means the reduction or loss of both Heath's negative beliefs about himself and his debilitating behaviors that were responses to his childhood sexual abuse. It also means getting rid of the perpetrator.

When the survivor is in therapy, there are always at least three people there—in Heath's case, there are four (Mitchell & Morse, 1998, p. 198): the worker, Heath, and the perpetrators—his mother and stepfather. The crisis worker sought to extinguish Heath's negative beliefs and behaviors by systematically leading Heath to mentally refute his erroneous perceptions that he was responsible, culpable, or guilty and had him reframe his previous beliefs to help him gain a new insight that he was an innocent victim and can now view himself more realistically as a guilt-free survivor.

When working through traumatic events, the client will experience a dramatic increase in affective and autonomic arousal (Ochberg, 1988). The human services worker must be very careful to provide palatable doses of the traumatic material that do not exceed the client's coping abilities (Courtois, 1988, p. 174) and prompt a crisis within the therapy session. Careful processing with the client before and after each session of extinguishing and reframing traumatic memories is important in preventing such crises.

CW: Let's take a look at what we did today.

Heath: I'm pretty scared. I didn't remember a lot of that stuff until we dug that memory up.

CW: That's pretty typical. Any reasonable person would bury that stuff. If you really start to feel like you're losing it, I want you to call me.

Heath: (later that evening, calling) I really hate to disturb you, but I've really got this urge to start cutting myself. I'm also having thoughts about killing my other pet bird. They're starting to get pretty real.

CW: (very directively) Do you feel like you're losing it enough that you need to be hospitalized?

Heath: I don't know. Maybe if I just talk this through.

CW: OK. Go get on the toilet seat, put your feet on the ground, and let's talk. (**Heath does so.**) OK, you there? Feet on the ground? OK! Remember what I said about this being rough. What you went through today brought back a lot of old memories and some ugly fresh ones. That's normal. It's nasty, but it is normal. Now I want you to think of how we changed that scene, how you told yourself all those negative things about yourself being dirty and no good, and what the reality of that scene is. (**A dialogue ensues that recaps the day's events. Heath is able to regain control, and after a 20-minute dialogue is able to feel secure enough to relax and go to bed.**)

The worker should be aware that extinguishing one traumatic event does not lessen the fear and trepidation of moving on to other events. This is particularly true in the case of adult survivors of childhood sexual abuse, who may experience increased intrusive behavioral symptoms and regress to former maladaptive behaviors even though they are making good progress in erasing bad memories (Cogdal & James, 1991). Clients may appear to be getting worse instead of better—which is threatening and scary for both client and worker.

The worker should be prepared for this contingency, tell the client of its likelihood, and affirm that it is totally acceptable for the client to check in with the worker if these symptoms and behaviors reemerge between sessions. The worker's role when this happens is to be understanding, affirming, and calming. Constant validation is important because many clients will be discouraged at the length of treatment, afraid and angry over revictimization and extension of the traumatic experience's "life," and flee from therapy (Courtois, 1988, p. 177). The second phase of therapy involves reclaiming the self. It is a painful business to watch, and there is every urge to rescue the client. This must not happen! The work must be done by the survivor, and dependence cannot be allowed to occur (Mitchell & Morse, 1998, p. 190).

Prolonged Exposure/Cognitive Restructuring. Reframing the client's negative and distorted beliefs about themselves is critical in allowing the client to separate the fact and fiction of an abusive childhood (Courtois, 1988, p. 181). While imaginally flooding the most abusive childhood scene the client can tolerate, clients paste mental billboards under the scene (Cogdal & James, 1991). These billboards typically deliver all the myths and distorted messages that the abuser gave in addition to the client's own childhood negative self-talk. The image of the assault scene is enhanced through prolonged exposure or flooding by loading all the sights, sounds, smells, and noises as if it were happening in real time to the most distressing level the client can tolerate. The idea is to build the noxious stimuli to such an extent that it finally loses its malignant power over the client and becomes benign.

CW: (**with the client deeply relaxed, eyes closed**) Picture that videotape, the bedroom, the "game," him making you get on him and suck his "peter," almost strangling as you do so. Feel the pain and the disgust. But he makes you keep doing it until he gets off, and the semen is running all over, sticky and wet. Notice the messages underneath that scene. "This is what fathers do to their children." "You aren't a good son if you disobey your stepfather." "I'll kill you if you don't keep our secret." Feel the confusion, the fear, and the repulsion as you do this. Put those messages in big block letters underneath that scene. Do you see them?

Heath: (**eyes closed and body twisting**) Yes!

CW: Freeze that scene and the billboards. Take a snapshot of it. Let it develop. Hold it in your hands.

The client is then asked to destroy the image along with the negative parental injunctions and his own negative self-injunctions (Cogdal & James, 1991).

CW: Now, I want you to get rid of that scene. It is in your past, and it is gone, so now get rid of it from your memory also. Do that now, and tell me what is happening.

Heath: I set a match to it. It is burning. It's a huge fire now with yellow, sick-smelling smoke.

CW: Let it burn.

Heath: It's just a crisp cinder now, all gone.

CW: All gone? Is there anything else you want to do with it?

Heath: CRUSH IT!

CW: Do it! What's happening?

Heath: I'm grinding it up with my boot heel. It's nothing; he's nothing.

CW: Fine. Now relax and slip back into that soft, cool mountain glade. Just relax and feel the tranquility, calmness, and peacefulness.

The client then replays the scene, but this time substitutes positive, self-enhancing counter injunctions based on the facts and not on the fictional messages of the event. The worker guides the image and reframes the stepfather in a truer psychological image (Cogdal & James, 1991).

CW: Go back to the bedroom with him now. Picture the scene but change it. See him as small, very small, weak. He is a small, selfish, pouting boy, dressed up in a man's pajamas. He looks ridiculous. Put these billboards under the scene. "The only people he has power over are little kids." "It is his fault this is happening." "It is WRONG!" "It is criminal!" "I should have felt confused, fearful. I had the right to feel that way!" "I also have the right to be *angry* about it." "*Nobody* has the right to do that. Nobody!" Now freeze that picture and snapshot it. Let it develop. Look at it. What are you feeling and thinking?

Heath: (yelling) You asshole! You bastard! You are gone from my life, you puke! You lied to me, you scared me to death, and kept at it. You used me because you were afraid of everybody else. I was the only one you could use, you scumbag. You've got no power over me now, you pissant, or my memories. You are history!

CW: I want you to save that picture. Put it someplace else, safe in your memory, and every time that image starts to come back, pull out the picture and look at it. See that scene for what it really is, and see those billboards, flashing. Have you got it?

Heath: Yes. I've got it.

CW: How do you feel?

Heath: Better, relaxed, relieved maybe.

As the client works through a series of traumatic events, each one is set up as it happened with all of the negative distortions and self-talk that accompanied it. These negative self-attributions carry over into the present time and form maladaptive operating schemas for how the client lives. By rooting out these distortions and modifying them into more positive, self-enhancing, and enabling counter injunctions, clients are able to compare "old" and "new" schemas and not only modify and rid themselves of the debilitating memories but also begin to incorporate those new schemas into their present-day lives (Cloitre & Rosenberg, 2006).

Relearning Feelings. Like combat veterans, survivors of childhood sexual abuse have developed excellent coping skills to deny and numb feelings. But this is even more problematic for survivors of childhood sexual abuse because learning to differentiate feelings is a skill that develops in childhood. For most of these survivors, their childhood environments were anything but nurturing, and their caretakers may have suffered from severe affective dysregulation, alternating between a flood of feelings and none at all. As a result, a condition called **alexithymia** develops in many survivors of childhood sexual abuse. Alexithymia is the inability to recognize and label feelings. Recognizing and labeling feelings is of utmost importance in helping clients give voice to shunted emotions and warded-off feelings. Heath's bitter and angry emotions are not unlike those of combat veterans as they relive and extinguish bad memories.

Developmentally, clients have to literally relearn and identify their emotional states. Cloitre and Rosenberg (2006) use part of their group format on skills training in affect and interpersonal regulation (STAIR) to teach clients to recognize feelings, monitor emotional intensity levels, learn emotional triggers, and formulate coping/reaction responses. Many of the students in survivor groups have absolutely no idea what the visual cues are that others give them.

For example, a professor who gives one of these survivors a quizzical look after asking a question might well be described as angry or mad by the survivor. In working with survivors, one of your authors commonly uses an elementary school classroom guidance technique to train students to recognize feelings. Each student in his survivor groups gets a handout showing emoticons and feeling words attached to them to help the students relabel feelings and discriminate emotional cues from others. Far from seeing this exercise as childish, clients report that they pull out and use these sheets on a daily basis to validate their present emotional state.

Grief Resolution. Beginning to recognize past, buried feelings is to start on the road to acknowledging feelings of anger and rage, as Heath does in the preceding dialogue (Courtois et al., 2009, pp. 93–94). These feelings will ultimately end in sadness and grieving for the loss of a happy childhood, his loss of who he might have been without the trauma, and the loss of a psychologically healthy family instead of the malevolent one he grew up in (Courtois, 1988, p. 181). It is likely to be one of the most painful stages as the client comes to grips with the reality that there is no retrieving the past or changing it and that attempts to do so are fruitless. Only the future holds promise for him, and he can control only that (Hays, 1985). Grieving and resolution, particularly with perpetrators of the abuse, are other transcrisis points in therapy. At this time, the crisis worker will have to move into a grieving and loss mode (see Chapter 12, "Personal Loss: Bereavement and Grief").

Heath: I had a call from my mother last night. I wanted to be assertive with her and tell her how I felt, like I had worked out in group. But when it came down to it, I just couldn't. I haven't got the guts. (**Starts crying.**) I'll never get rid of this. Why couldn't she have been different? Why does she still try that stuff of browbeating me? Wasn't what she did enough?

CW: You have every right to feel sad that she wasn't or still isn't what you'd hope a mother might be. I wish she could change, but I have my doubts. So, if she won't, what will you do?

Heath: I guess she won't. I guess I'll just kiss her off.

CW: You survived with her battering you, and you've survived for 10 years without her. Perhaps it's time you did say goodbye. (**Patiently lets Heath silently weep.**)

Confrontation. The tremendous push-pull between the love and hatred survivors feel for their perpetrators is a difficult issue to resolve. Role-playing with the empty chair technique, writing letters, drawing, and journaling may be ways of mourning the loss. Whether the survivor will ever actually confront the abuser is a question only the survivor can answer. There are a number of reasons it may be good for the survivor to confront the perpetrator, such as empowerment, closure, "setting the record straight," anger, grief, and forgiveness (Cameron, 1994). However, *this must be the survivor's decision*, and the crisis worker must remain scrupulously neutral in this debate. Confronting the abuser is not mandatory for healing (Mitchell & Morse, 1998, p. 162). Further, to believe that the perpetrator will "confess" to the abuse may be very wishful thinking indeed.

The following questions generated by Bass and Davis (1992, p. 134), or some variation of them, need to be asked and processed with the survivor before the decision to confront is made.

1. What is motivating you to do this, and are you prepared to do this?

2. What will you possibly gain, and what will you possibly lose?
3. Could you live with being excluded from family functions and risk losing contact with family members who did not abuse you?
4. Will you be able to handle it if you are labeled "crazy"?
5. Can you handle getting no reaction or denial?

Changing Behavior Through Skill Building and Reconnecting. Although coming to terms with past trauma and stopping maladaptive present behavior are critical to the adult survivor, changing behavior to more self-determining choices is the major end goal of therapy. The vacuum left by the removal of bad memories and the psychic energy previously expended to maintain control of those memories is not easily filled. Some survivors describe living with trauma and then letting go of that trauma as a shift in their identity—learning to discover themselves and thrive, rather than merely surviving in the shadow of intense trauma. Pearson (1994) and Mitchell and Morse (1998) recommend using several categories of techniques for skill building, listed earlier in this chapter.

Reeducation is necessary for survivor skill building, and the worker may assume a teaching role in transmitting basic life skills such as communication, decision making, conflict resolution, cognitive restructuring, and boundary setting (Courtois, 1988, pp. 181–182). Herman (1981) likens the survivor to an immigrant who must literally rebuild her life in a culture that is absolutely foreign to what she experienced as a child. From that standpoint, the crisis worker should not be unsettled by the emergence of some rather unusual and personal questions.

Heath: Er, ah, I was just wondering, Dr. James, how you treat your kids. I mean, if they act up do you ground them, or what? What do you talk about at dinner? And do you and your wife ever argue?

Although such questions may be construed as intruding on the private life of the worker or attempts by the client to shift focus from his problems or create dependency, it is important to answer these questions as honestly and succinctly as possible, without shifting the focus away from the client's personal concerns. The client is testing his perceptions against the most valid and stable validity check he currently has—his therapist. For that reason, it is important to urge survivors to join therapy or support groups so that new behaviors can be tested out and discussed with peers. Because many families of survivors such as Heath's are so completely dysfunctional, clients need education on what a functional family is and how it operates. Duncan (2004) has defined the characteristics of a functioning family (not the Hollywood ideal one), and we believe they are well worth spending time on in a support group.

As these survivors reconstruct their lives and start to become interested in developing meaningful relationships, Sheehan (1994) proposes five basic fears that they will have to deal with: abandonment, exposure, merger, attack, and their own destructive behavior. Fear of abandonment comes because there were never protectors in their young lives. Thus, they avoid emotional encounters because they vow never to be hurt in the same way again and constantly test whether significant others are really committed to them. Fear of merger means fear of losing control and of losing one's selfhood. Survivors have to learn what personal boundaries are because parent/child boundaries were merged into sexual ones. Fear of attack has to do with real or imagined assault, something quite common in most survivors' backgrounds. The anger and rage that accompany the traumatic wake can make survivors wonder whether they can control their own destructive impulses and rage toward themselves or others. These are all topics that involve group work and support and can occasion many transcrisis moments for these people.

Support Groups for Adult Survivors.

LO14 For victims, groups provide a number of potential positive outcomes and help them move from victim to survivor. Victims may be reluctant to participate, but they should be encouraged to do so, although not all survivors of sexual trauma may be ready or immediately able to participate in groups. Education as to what the group is about, who the members are, confidentiality issues, what kinds of problems members are working on, and the safety and support of the group format is a critical component in assessing, selecting, motivating, and committing survivors to group work (Courtois, 1988, pp. 253–262).

Courtois (1988, pp. 245–249) lists the following benefits of group treatment for survivors of childhood sexual abuse:

1. The individual's sense of shame, stigmatization, and negative self-image are reduced by meeting other survivors who appear "normal."

2. Commonality of experience raises members' consciousness about incest, so the experience becomes more normalized and may be seen from an interpersonal and sociocultural perspective rather than an "only me" perspective.

3. The group serves as a new "surrogate" family where new behaviors and methods of communicating, interacting, and problem solving can be practiced in a safe, accepting, and nurturing environment.

4. The group allows for the safe exploration and ventilation of feelings and beliefs that have been denied and submerged from awareness.

5. Childhood messages and rules that were generated within the abusive environment can be challenged and dissected to determine how they still influence the survivor's maladaptive behavior patterns.

In summary, the case of Heath should make it very clear that dealing with an adult survivor of childhood sexual abuse is a complex, tedious, meticulous, and stressful process that is filled with many crisis events. It should come as no surprise that one of the toughest customers a worker will face, the person with borderline personality disorder, runs rampant in this population. It takes a great deal of expertise, patience, empathy, and personal resiliency to work with such cases. The case of Heath should vividly illustrate why compassion fatigue, vicarious traumatization, and burnout are high probabilities in this kind of work.

Religiosity and Spirituality

In a just world where a benevolent and caring God is ever present, rape and childhood sexual assault never happen. Yet, they do happen quite regularly. So, what happens to a person who has a belief that there is a just God out there somewhere who has abandoned them? To examine the role religiosity plays in trauma, ter Kuile and Ehring (2014) queried 293 trauma survivors on their changes in religious beliefs as a result of their trauma. Nearly half reported changes, and as the researchers predicted, shattered assumptions about a just world and a fair God caused a decline in their religious beliefs and increased their chances of "catching" PTSD (ter Kuile & Ehring, 2014). Those who experienced increases in religious activities used them as a positive coping mechanism, and that finding has been supported by other studies as well (Baty, 2013; Glenn, 2014). This issue is covered extensively in Chapter 12, "Personal Loss: Bereavement and Grief," and in Chapter 11, "Family Crisis

Intervention," but suffice it to say that, if at all possible, it appears that for many people, finding meaning in a higher power is a critical ingredient in getting through a sexual trauma.

Helping individuals who have been traumatized after traumatic events to find meaning in what has happened to them is probably the second most important thing after getting them stabilized (Altmaier & Prieto, 2012). Probably above all other traumas, finding forgiveness and resolution is tremendously difficult, particularly when the offender is a family member. However, for some survivors, working through the trauma can trigger the development of personal growth that changes the survivor in profoundly positive ways. Calhoun and Tedeschi (2014) refer to this as posttraumatic growth (PTG). And, although the experience of PTG can be profound, PTG does not invalidate or nullify the suffering incurred as a product of the trauma (Calhoun & Tedeschi, 2014). Understanding the central role of spirituality or religion in the healing process and the development of PTG for many people, the crisis worker must work with each client to assess the sexual abuse's impact and what part spirituality and religion can (or can't) play in helping the client move forward in a posttraumatic growth mode. To that end, the crisis worker should attempt to determine whether the spiritual distress comes from God for not being there when the abuse happened or not giving the person the strength to get through it. This is a slippery slope, particularly when the person has been strong in their faith. At such times, referral to a pastoral counselor with expertise in the area is highly recommended (Young, 2015).

Sexual Abuse in Childhood

The fact is that child sexual abuse has always been with us (DeMause, 1974; McCauley et al., 2001), but a variety of political, social, and cultural factors have kept child abuse—and most particularly, child sexual abuse—behind closed doors in the United States (Costin et al., 1996) and throughout the world (Schwartz-Kenney et al., 2001). By the time one of your authors was a school counselor in 1966, mandatory reporting laws for physical abuse had been enacted in all 50 states (McCauley et al., 2001)—although there was considerable comment at that time on just how exactly one was to report such abuse and the still unclear question of whether one could get sued or fired for doing so no matter what

the law said! (Indeed, no matter what the law says today, you should be aware that when the subject of child physical or sexual abuse rears its ugly head in a school building, there can be, and often are, repercussions when abusing parents are confronted.) Oftentimes, legal, ethical, moral, and political issues collide when child physical and/or sexual abuse is involved. (For that reason, you should know exactly what you need to do and how to substantiate it when making a report. We believe it is absolutely mandatory to consult with another professional and have that professional bear witness when doing so.)

However, it wasn't until the rise of the women's movement and child advocates in the 1970s and their lobbying efforts to open up the blinds that had been closed on this topic that the public really started to become aware of the extent of the problem. In 1974, the Child Abuse Prevention and Treatment Act was passed in the United States, and its definition of what might be covered under the law included sexual abuse. Just as Leontine Young's book *Wednesday's Children* (1964) raised consciousness levels about the physical abuse of children, David Finkelhor's book *Sexually Victimized Children* (1979) did the same for awareness about child sexual abuse.

The Numbers

As we discussed earlier, childhood sexual abuse numbers are staggering. Finkelhor et al. (2014) utilized data collected in 2003, 2008, and 2011 to estimate rates of sexual abuse or rape occurring by age 17 in the United States. Participants were ages 15 through 17 years at the time of data collection. The researchers found that over 26 percent of women and 5 percent of men reported childhood sexual abuse or rape. Of those, just over 11 percent of women and nearly 2 percent of men reported that they were assaulted by an adult (Finkelhor et al., 2014). Basile et al. (2022) conducted a study in 2016-2017 with adults who reported sexual assault and abuse histories. They found that approximately 49 percent of women were first raped prior to age 18. Further, of that 49 percent of women who experienced childhood sexual abuse, 35 percent of them were first raped between ages 11 and 17, and 14 percent were first assaulted at age 10 or younger (Basile et al., 2022). The numbers for men are similar. Almost 57 percent of men who experienced sexual assault reported that they were first raped prior to age 18. Of those men, approximately 30 percent reported rape between ages 11 and 17, and almost 27 percent reported being the victim of sexual assault at age

10 or younger (Basile et al., 2022). What's more is that an estimated 325,000 children are at risk of becoming victims of commercial sexual exploitation each year (Adams et al., 2010). Michael Salter's (2013) book, *Organised Sexual Abuse,* provides a chilling look into all of the different groups that organize to sexually abuse children. It goes without saying that the prevention and early identification of childhood sexual abuse remains a significant challenge and concern for both mental health professionals and communities at large.

Dynamics of Sexual Abuse in Childhood

LO15 Manifestations of PTSD do not just spring forth full-blown in adulthood (McLeer et al., 1992). In fact, Kisiel et al. (2014) used data collected through the National Child Traumatic Stress Network Core Data Set to examine symptoms and functional impairments in children who experienced trauma and sexual trauma. They found that children who experienced sexual trauma had high rates of PTSD, symptoms of depression, suicidal ideation, and sexualized behaviors (Kisiel et al., 2014). Likewise, Amado et al. (2015) conducted a meta-analysis of studies that examine the effects of childhood and/or adolescent sexual abuse, and they found significant rates of symptom presentation. Specifically, children and adolescents who experience sexual abuse are highly likely (approximately 70 percent chance) to develop symptoms of depression, anxiety, and general emotional suffering (Amado et al., 2015). Casanovas et al. (2022) found similar results in their study of adolescent women who experienced sexual assault. They found that adolescent sexual assault survivors experienced high rates of somatic symptoms, depression, and anxiety (Casanovas et al., 2022). Even when considering clustering of other types of childhood traumatic caregiver events such as physical abuse, neglect, domestic abuse, emotional abuse, and noncaregivers' trauma such as natural disasters or severe medical problems, when sexual abuse was factored in, child sexual abuse had a potent and additive effect on the duration and degree of trauma experienced (Kisiel et al., 2014). Probably the most ominous finding of this rogue's gallery of behavioral outcomes was a study that Fox and associates (2015) did on over 22,000 delinquent juveniles in Florida. They found that each additional adverse traumatic event the child suffered on the Adverse Childhood Experiences Index increased their movement toward becoming serious violent and chronic offenders. It is abundantly evident that childhood sexual trauma affects children's mental health and, as we discussed earlier, childhood trauma can have lasting effects into adulthood.

Even when rape and sexual assault on children and adolescents do not later result in full-blown PTSD, the emotional and behavioral fallout is far reaching and destructive. In addition, these children have a wide variety of other problems that include concentration difficulties, poor grades, aggressive behavior, social withdrawing, somatic complaints, overcompliance, depression, antisocial tendencies, behavioral regression, poor body image/self-esteem, eating and sleep disturbances, encopresis and enuresis (loss of bowel and bladder control), hyperactivity, suicidal ideation, and extreme, generalized fears (Conte & Schuerman, 1988; Knauer, 2000; Miller-Perrin, 2001; Sgroi et al., 1982).

Although the foregoing symptoms may be indicative of many disorders of childhood, the following are not and are rarely ever found with any stressor other than sexual abuse (Goodwin, 1988; Knauer, 2000, pp. 3–30; McLeer et al., 1992; Miller-Perrin, 2001; Salter, 1988, pp. 230–235). Sexually abused children come to school early, stay late, and are rarely or never absent. They barricade themselves in their rooms or otherwise hide and attempt to seal themselves off from their assailants. They may be "perfect" children to the world and to their teachers.

To the contrary, they may engage in inappropriate and persistent sexual play with peers. They may have a sexually transmitted disease. They will have a detailed and age-inappropriate understanding of sexual behavior. They may have physical and somatic symptoms with overlying sexual content such as vaginal or anal bleeding and odors. Sexual drawings, stories, or dreams are common occurrences. They may suddenly have money or gifts that can't be explained. They may display blatant sexually suggestive poses such as wide-open legs, rubbing of genital areas, and provocative dress. They may engage in excessive, compulsive, and even public masturbation, and may even approach other adults sexually. Small children may act out sexually with real or stuffed animals. Teenagers may run away and engage in sex work. They may engage in self-injury by, for example, cutting or burning themselves. They may have a sudden dislike for someone or demonstrate inordinate clinging behavior. These behaviors provide a template with which varying patterns of psychopathology seen in adult survivors are drawn.

A particular subset of childhood PTSD is the effects of parental abuse and neglect that often occur in the course of childhood sexual assault. The differences between how PTSD manifests in abused children with PTSD versus adults with PTSD have become profound enough that a team from the National Child Traumatic Stress Network has designated a new disorder called developmental trauma disorder (DTD; DeAngelis, 2007). DTD is characterized by exposure to one or more developmentally adverse interpersonal traumas such as abandonment, betrayal, physical or sexual abuse, and emotional abuse. Emotional outcomes range across rage, fear, betrayal, resignation, defeat, and shame. A major marker of DTD is dysregulated development that affects physical health, behavior, cognition, relationships, and self-attribution. Negative expectations about caregivers develop because of their abusive history. As a result, these children stop expecting protection from others and believe future victimization is inevitable (van der Kolk, 2005).

Dynamics of Sexual Abuse in Families

LO16 The incestuous family may operate much like an alcoholic or battered family does in developing a series of messages or rules that pivot around denial, duplicity, deceit, role confusion, violence, and social isolation (Courtois, 1988, p. 45). Children receive messages such as:

1. Do not show feelings, especially anger.
2. Be in control at all times; do not ask for help.
3. Deny what is happening, and do not believe your own senses/perceptions.
4. No one is trustworthy.
5. Keep the secret because no one will believe you anyway.
6. Be ashamed of yourself; you are to blame for everything.

Intergenerational Transmission of Sexual Abuse. Typically, there is high potential for intergenerational transmission of sexual abuse in these families. This is not to say that all, or even most, individuals who are sexually abused as children will grow to be sexually abusive toward others. However, research seems to bear out that perpetrators of childhood sexual abuse have extensive histories of abuse during their own childhood (Cutajar et al., 2011). It is difficult to pinpoint the reasons for this cycle of abuse. Parents who themselves have been abused often seem to have blind

spots for what is occurring in front of them. Further, Knauer (2000, pp. 18–19) proposes that the original attraction to the abuser is because of the familiar traits that the person sees in the abuser that ring true within her own abusive family of origin. Others propose that early attachment is severely disrupted when childhood sexual abuse occurs, and those disrupted attachment patterns can manifest in harmful adult patterns in which the person perpetuates the abuse they experienced at a young age (Grady et al., 2017).

Incestuous fathers display inordinate amounts of jealousy and paranoia over their daughters' dating and relationships with other men and attempt to rigidly control behavior through threats and intimidation, and the same may happen with mothers who abuse their sons (Knauer, 2000, pp. 49–61; Rosencrans, 1997, pp. 69–83; Salter, 1988, p. 237). Abusive fathers are controlling tyrants who erect a facade of respectability in the community and often try to isolate their children and spouses or partners by forbidding them to socialize outside the home and refusing to let them have close friends. However, because of their sensitivity to power, they become meek and contrite when confronted with their abuse (Herman, 1981, p. 178).

Children born to mothers who have experienced sexual abuse are at an increased risk of experiencing childhood sexual abuse (Hornor, 2010). Mothers of children who are being sexually abused are often oppressed and economically dependent, abused by their mates, and products of incestuous families themselves (Courtois, 1988, pp. 54–55; Herman, 1981, pp. 178–179). Mothers may be physically or mentally disabled, causing the eldest daughter to take on the role of "little mother," which extends to fulfilling the father's sexual demands (Herman, 1981, p. 179). Knott and Fabre (2014) describe common reactions by mothers in response to their child's report of sexual abuse. They discuss the interplay of the mother's own childhood sexual abuse history and the mother's relationship with the abuser as major determinants of the mother's response (Knott & Fabre, 2014). Citing multiple prior studies, they also talk about the role of domestic violence in the mother's willingness to believe the report or ability to respond to the report, and the role of the mother's substance use and how addiction can affect her responsiveness (Knott & Fabre, 2014). Knott and Fabre (2014) also discuss the child's age as a major factor in whether the mother believes the allegations of sexual abuse, wherein mothers tend to believe younger children more than older children. Although some mothers may confront the abuse once they discover it, many others engage in denial and helplessness, and when confronted with the reality of the situation, may revictimize the child by physical or verbal abuse (Salter, 1988, p. 209). In those situations, the child becomes the scapegoat for the family's problems (Knauer, 2000, p. 18).

Female Abusers. Females who are abusers are not as much of an anomaly as one might think and are more than likely underreported as sexual abusers. Using data collected in 1998 from a Canadian sample, Peter (2009) found nearly a 11 percent prevalence rate for female-perpetrated sexual abuse. Allen (1991) believes there are about 1.5 million victims in the United States, and Elliot (1994, p. 220) reports a figure of about 500,000 in Canada who have been abused by women. While these numbers may seem outrageously high, they also may not be. A study of Latino and European American adolescents who had been sexually abused found that among male high school students, 52.8 percent reported that they had been abused by women (Newcomb, et al., 2009).

A few studies have reported on female sexual abusers and the outcomes for their victims (Allen, 1991; Elliot, 1994; Fehrenbach & Monastersky, 1988; Knopp & Lackey, 1987; Mathews et al., 1989; McCarty, 1986; Nathan & Ward, 2001; Rosencrans, 1997). More often, they are discovered as coabusers (Elliot, 1994; Rosencrans, 1997; Wijkman & Da Silva, 2021), but women are known to sexually abuse children, particularly their own relatives (Gölge et al., 2021; McLeod, 2015). The traumatic wake they leave is generally even more devastating because they are seen as the primary caregivers and the persons in whom most trust and nurturing are placed.

In particular, it is important to disabuse the myth that boys are not troubled by such sexual behavior and "gain experience from older women." Rosencrans' research (1997, pp. 245–253) indicates quite the opposite. The young man who has (or is forced or coerced to have) sex with an older woman, even if the young man believes the sexual encounter to have been consensual, is placed in a double bind. If any part of the experience felt good, the victim may believe it wasn't abusive. If it didn't feel good, then he may have all kinds of recriminations, and the experience may trigger a crisis of sexuality (Lew, 2004, p. 61). Lew (2004, p. 61) believes that this causes male survivors to repress memories of abuse by women far more than they do abuse by men. And when those memories do

return with a vengeance, they are far more devastating. That outcome is exponentially true when the perpetrator is the victim's mother.

"Motherfucker" is one of the most pejorative, vulgar, and demeaning terms in the English language and has all kinds of negative connotations for boys who might engage in such deviant behavior. That term presupposes the son is the instigator of such illicit sexual contact (Gartner, 2005, pp. 29–30). Research indicates that is anything but true. The Freudian notion of an Oedipal complex wherein the son lusts after the mother has little validity. The social myths and cultural artifacts that mask the true malevolence of female perpetrators on male children minimize this problem in much the same way as the issue of male perpetrators was minimized in the past (Speigel, 2003, p. 15). If we turn that term around as "son fucker," does that reframe your thinking on the matter and shed light on who the true aggressor is?

The sexual identity problem that boys face when they have been abused by female caretakers, and particularly mothers, is a psychological abattoir (Elliot, 1994; Mitchell & Morse, 1998; Rosencrans, 1997). Gartner (2005, pp. 106–120) proposes that it can be cataclysmic for the victim to acknowledge he is in an incestuous relationship with his mother. While the erotic excitement he feels is disturbing, it can also lead to a sense of sexual prowess that can plant the seeds of some very deviant and pathological beliefs about women. This is not a movie plot in which a young man becomes a mature and skillful lover at the hands of an experienced, beautiful, and competent woman. It is sexual abuse at the hands of a woman who seeks to satisfy her own needs and wishes at any expense to the children she abuses. Indeed, out of the bad seeds of these relationships may grow some very poisonous adult relationships for these boys. The bottom line is that adult female abuse of boys is extremely serious and can lead to ominous outcomes (Deering & Mellor, 2011).

As an example, two adult men one of your authors has encountered in his own practice who were sexually abused by their mothers were potentially the most dangerous to women he has ever seen. They had wildly vacillating "Madonna–whore" complexes about women they had targeted for their affection that could turn these women from the purest virgin to the "sluttiest streetwalker" in a moment, all because of some imagined travesty the women had committed. The really scary part of their delusions was that the women had no idea any of this was going on! Rosencrans's (1997, p. 252) informal interview with law enforcement officers tends to confirm that these abused men have a high potential for sexually related crimes.

Our overall knowledge of female sexual abusers probably compares to what we knew about male child abusers 50 years ago. Therefore, the astute crisis worker may ask the following when doing an intake interview with men who experienced sexual abuse.

CW: We have talked about the perpetrator. Did anybody else sexually abuse you? I am wondering if there were any women who ever did those sorts of things to you?

Because of the high incidence of sexual abuse perpetrated on boys and their reluctance to talk about being sexually abused as children, tactful questions should be asked of any age man, even when this is not the presenting problem. The plain and simple fact is that we still tend to dismiss sexual acts and the harmful aspects they present in males (Alaggia & Millington, 2008; O'Leary, 2009). A case in point is the filing of criminal charges against abusers of male children. While the cases filed against perpetrators when the child is female are woefully small in relation to the number committed, a study conducted by Edelson and Joa (2010) found that charges are even less likely to be filed against perpetrators when the victim is a male child.

Phases of Child Sexual Abuse

LO17 Childhood sexual abuse, whether it takes place online through the production and/or consumption of child pornography or scheduling of virtual abuse sessions (Ali et al., 2023) or in-person, occurs at disturbingly high rates. Greene-Colozzi et al. (2020) surveyed undergraduate college students at two U.S. universities. Approximately one quarter of the students they surveyed reported a history of communicating with an adult online as a minor. Of those, 65 percent stated that they were sexually propositioned during their online communication with an adult. Further, 23 percent of their sample reported a history of online sexual grooming by an adult (Ali et al., 2023). Of the participants who met their predator in-person, a substantial percentage reported being raped by the predator. So, how do vulnerable children fall prey to child molesters? Sgroi (1982) found that the abuser's behavior can be traced

through five phases: (1) engagement, (2) sexual interaction, (3) secrecy, (4) disclosure, and (5) suppression. These phases apply to both intra- and extrafamilial abuse. The focus of our discussion here is on sexual predators.

Engagement Phase. The abuser's objective in the engagement phase is to get the child involved in sexual activity with the abuser. Both access to the child and opportunity (privacy) are needed if the abuser is to be successful. Therefore, if one were looking for possible instances of unreported abuse, one would identify times and situations when the potential abuser and the child were alone together. One must also consider the different strategies that two different types of abusers (child molesters and child rapists) may employ.

Called **grooming,** molesters enter a seduction phase during which they successively approximate a child to accept that the sexual abuse is okay, appropriate, educational, acceptable, and even a duty. This seduction phase is prior to actual sexual abuse and is not well defined, and there is a lack of consensus on what it actually entails (Bennett & Odonohue, 2014). However, molesters tend to use enticement and entrapment to get the child engaged in sexual activity. **Enticement** may include deceit, trickery, rewards, flattery, or the use of adult authority to tell the child in a matter-of-fact way that the child is expected to participate. **Entrapment** is used to manipulate the child into feeling obligated to participate through traps, blackmail, and so forth. Molesters may make pornographic pictures or videotapes and convince the child that there is no choice other than going along with the secret activity and may also seek to impose guilt by making the child feel responsible for the abuse.

In modern society, grooming often takes place within the online realm. The adage your grandparents told your parents, "Never talk to strangers!" really, really applies here, except you don't talk to them on the internet either. Whittle and associates (2013) examined both familial factors such as close parental supervision of internet use when integrated with contextual and environmental risk factors (low income, poor schools, decaying neighborhoods) and found a heightened risk for potential contact with potential molesters. If you've seen any police sting operations on television, you know how prominent this is and continues to be even with the stings! It is indeed illegal to proposition a child on the internet for sexual interaction, even if that "child" is a 22-year-old police officer.

Factually, though, and stings aside, not a lot is yet known about how molesters operate. One reason for the dearth of literature on online predators is that molesters often get tied in with child exploitative material, and that muddles the picture. Online offenders may engage in only internet action or become **solicitation/traveling offenders**. Those are offenders who will attempt to entice a child to meet with them to have sex or encourage them to run away with together (Seto , 2013).

Child rapists use persuasion, threats (particularly the threat of harm), or the imposition of superior physical *force* to engage the child in the abusive activity. Typically, the rapist will threaten to kill or injure the child or someone dear to the child or destroy something the child holds dear, like a pet, or threaten suicide himself, convincing the child that they will be blamed for the rapist's death if the child resists or reports the rape. In using superior force, the rapist may simply overpower the child, restrain the child, give the child drugs or alcohol, or physically brutalize the child into submission.

In an online environment, predators may use coercion, pressure, and threats to ensure compliance. Often, this is done under the guise of someone else, likely of the victims' approximate age. Seymour-Smith and Kloess (2021) conducted a discourse analysis of actual chat room interaction between one convicted child molester and five of his young male victims. They found that the predator used highly sexualized content, aggressive communication, and explicit threats to secure compliance (Seymour-Smith & Kloess, 2021). Interestingly, Seymour-Smith and Kloess (2021) found a theme of parity that ran throughout the communication, wherein the predator used various excuses to make the victim perceive that the predator had not been treated fairly by the victim. However, when faced with potential noncompliance by the victim, the molester made threats to publish sexualized images of the child online, which triggered an exchange of "deal-making." (Seymour-Smith & Kloess, 2021). This practice has been termed "sextortion," which is defined as "the act of coercing people into sending explicit images of themselves and subsequently blackmailing victims with the public release of said images" (Hong et al., 2020, p. 192). According to Hong et al. (2020), sextortion is a common, growing practice among online child predators.

The vast majority (about 80 percent) of abusers use the first two strategies—enticement and entrapment. Abusers tend to repeat their engagement patterns and show little tendency to move from nonviolent to violent strategies. Molesters are apt to consistently entice or trap children, while child rapists tend to use threat or force almost exclusively. The strategy used by the abuser is an important issue in treatment because survivors typically wonder throughout their lives why they "permitted" the abuse to occur. In actuality, no child is able to provide consent, and the full responsibility for the abuse lies with the perpetrator. Helping survivors, regardless of age, to understand that they were not responsible for the abuse is a monumental task.

Sexual Interaction Phase. Types of abuse may include (blatant or surreptitious) masturbation (the abuser may masturbate prior to making physical contact with the child), fondling, digital penetration, oral or anal penetration, dry intercourse, intercourse, forcing or coercing the child into touching the abuser's genitals, forced prostitution, and exploitative material. Children may be coaxed into cooperating, though not consenting, because abusers—as adult authority figures—often command, engage, or enlist cooperation from the child. Children lack the maturity, experience, and age to be able to consent, but they may cooperate because of their subservient status.

Secrecy Phase. Abusers communicate to children that others must not discover the sexual activity. The objective of abusers is to continue the abuse. This necessitates avoiding detection and maintaining access to the child while continuing the abuse. The techniques for maintaining the secrecy may involve incorporating "rules" or "games," implicating the child in the activity, and setting the child up to be responsible for keeping the secret.

Disclosure Phase. Sometimes, the abuser is discovered accidentally. Other times, the abuse is disclosed intentionally by the child or someone else. Intentional disclosure is usually made by the child. Intentional disclosure often enormously complicates the discovery and existence of sexual abuse because parents and others refuse to face it or believe it. Accidental discovery may occur as a result of such consequences as pregnancy, STDs, sexual acting out, promiscuity, and physical trauma. The way the abuse is disclosed can affect the child's self-esteem and reaction to treatment. For instance, disbelieving adults some-times respond by blaming and punishing the child—and allow the sexual abuse to continue.

Suppression Phase. The suppression phase may begin as soon as disclosure takes place. Suppression may be attempted by the abuser, the child, the parents, other family members, professionals, the community, or an institution. There are many reasons for suppression: fear of publicity; fear of reprisal; to protect the reputation of a family, an abuser, or an institution; to avoid prosecution; to avoid responsibility; to protect the child; to avoid embarrassment; to avoid the kinds of confrontation and intervention required to deal effectively with the difficult and sensitive situation; and fear of getting involved.

Survival Phase. On the basis of our own experiences and the reports of other writers (Besharov, 1990; Kendrick, 1991), we have added another phase, the survival phase. During this phase, it is important to implement strategies for helping the child and the family respond to and recover from the abuse as much as possible. This phase includes stopping the abuse, providing needed medical and psychological treatment for the child, and helping the significant others close to the child overcome the trauma, fear, anger, betrayal, and despair caused by the abuse (Benedict, 1985). It also involves preventing further abuse (Bass & Thornton, 1983) and prosecuting and/or getting counseling for the abuser (Benedict, 1985).

Intervention Strategies with Children

LO18 **Assessment.** Assessment includes thorough documentation of the abusive events for possible legal use. Using anatomically correct dolls helps confirm what actually occurred in the abuse. No specific measures currently exist for measuring the effects of psychological abuse in young children, although a complete psychological evaluation may be useful in gauging the child's overall level of functioning (McLeer et al., 1992; Wheeler & Berliner, 1988, p. 235). The previously mentioned behavioral indicators of childhood sexual abuse and PTSD criteria for children are currently the best indicators that sexual abuse has occurred.

Peterson and Hardin (1997) have developed a guide for screening children's art for sexual abuse.

The child is asked not to verbally disclose but rather illustrate different subjects and situations. Different indicators of sexual abuse may appear as the child illustrates the requested subject matter—such as a picture of people doing something at home. Assessment includes an analysis of style, treatment of figures, and actions with negative aspects. Point values are awarded for a variety of criteria commonly found in abused children's drawings. Once the point value reaches a certain level, child abuse should be suspected (Peterson & Zamboni, 1998). However, it doesn't take a doctorate in projective techniques to see how different the drawings of children who have been abused are (Kaufman & Wohl, 1992). We would propose that most children do not draw families that are joined by penises and vaginas or have clubs growing out of their arms that are raining blows down on other family members—but sexually and physically abused children do because that's the way their families interact.

Therapeutic Options

Because of the complex nature of child abuse, interventions should comprise multiple components targeting a variety of problem areas (Miller-Perrin, 2001). We group these into three categories: play therapy, Trauma-Focused CBT (TF-CBT), and trauma-informed care. Although there are various forms of evidence-based practice for treating children who experience sexual trauma, we believe these three components have the most support and tend to be the most efficacious.

The first component is play therapy (Gumaer, 1984; Malchiodi, 2008; Webb, 2007; White & Allers, 1994). There are various forms and models of play therapy, ranging from unstructured child-centered (Landreth, 2012) to prescriptive play therapy (Gil & Shaw, 2009). Although we focus on play therapy in this chapter, it should be noted that multiple expressive modalities (Malchiodi, 2003) and sandtray therapy (Homeyer & Sweeney, 2022) are also highly useful approaches for working with child sexual trauma survivors. Regardless of the specific modality, it is common understanding that play is the means through which children communicate. Talking about sexual trauma is challenging for adults, and assuming that children, particularly young children, have the words or emotional intelligence to be able to express their internal experience would be a catastrophic mistake. As such, utilizing play therapy to address sexual trauma in children allows a pathway for children to make sense of and express their internal experience without the use of words or cognitive understanding of complex emotions.

Play is natural for children, and mental health professionals can build rapport with children and help them resolve trauma through effective application of play therapy. However, utilizing play in therapy is not just about letting children play with toys while the therapists observes; there is a lot of theory and technique involved in effective application of play therapy. The TEEL model by Draper and colleagues (2009) summarizes some of the key features of play therapy. TEEL stands for "tracking (T), empathy (E), encouragement (E), and limit setting (L)" (Draper et al., 2009, p. 229). Tracking refers to the therapist's nonintrusive and nonjudgmental observation of the child's behavior and stating that behavior back to the child, such as "You are looking at all of the puppets and trying to figure out which one to use" or "You are stacking the blocks, one by one." Tracking helps the child know that the therapist is paying attention, similar to minimal encouragers. Empathy is demonstrated through reflections of feeling, which helps children to put words to their internal experience. Encouragement is used through reflecting the child's intent or effort; encouragement is not praise (Draper et al., 2009). Examples of encouragement might include "You are working very hard on that building" or "You are searching through all of the colors, trying to pick the one that is just right." Finally, limit setting is about helping the child to understand limits or boundaries and make choices regarding their actions and the consequences of those actions. Limit setting is typically phrased as "_____ is not for _____. If you choose to _____, then you choose to _____." For example, "The walls are not for writing on. If you choose to write on the walls, you choose not to play with the crayons any more today." Because the child has a choice to make, limit setting helps to promote autonomy and accountability through decision making. There are many more techniques and strategies for play therapy. Authors such as Eliana Gil (Gil, 2016), Garry Landreth (Landreth, 2012), and Terry Kottman (Kottman, 2014) offer extensive descriptions of the therapeutic application of play. Perhaps the most widely recognized literature on using play therapy with sexually traumatized children comes from Eliana Gil (Gil, 2016).

The second component is CBT that is trauma focused (Cohen et al., 2006; Neubauer et al., 2007). Trauma-Focused CBT (TF-CBT) has a strong research base (Cohen & Mannarino, 2015; Konanur et al., 2015; Lenz & Hollenbaugh, 2015; Lindebø Knutsen et al., 2020; McGuire et al., 2021) and is recognized by the National Child Traumatic Stress Network (NCTSN) as an evidence-based therapy for children and adolescents, ages three to 21, who experience trauma, including sexual trauma (National Child Traumatic Stress Network, 2017). TF-CBT is typically implemented in 8 to 25 sessions, and it combines both individual work with the child/adolescent and conjoint sessions with the caregiver (Trauma-Focused Cognitive Behavioral Therapy & National Therapist Certification Program, 2021). Active caregiver participation plays a significant role in TF-CBT and can markedly increase treatment efficacy (Cohen & Mannarino, 2015). TF-CBT is designed to target multiple symptoms that may manifest, such as "Posttraumatic Stress Disorder (PTSD), depression, anxiety, externalizing behavior problems, relationship and attachment problems, school problems and cognitive problems" (National Child Traumatic Stress Network, 2017, p. 1). Major components of TF-CBT include parent skills training, psychoeducation about trauma, affect regulation and relaxation skills, cognitive coping skills, narrative restorying of the trauma, and grief processing (National Child Traumatic Stress Network, 2017). TF-CBT has been adapted for use in various contexts, including group therapy (Deblinger et al., 2016), unaccompanied minor refugee children (Unterhitzenberger et al., 2015), and via telebehavioral health implementation (Stewart et al., 2017).

The third component is a trauma systems approach (Saxe et al., 2007). The NCTSN (2018) defines trauma-informed systems as those in which "all parties involved recognize and respond to the impact of traumatic stress on those who have contact with the system including children, caregivers, and service providers" (p. 1). The NCTSN delineates the following aspects of trauma-informed systems: (1) routine screening for trauma and trauma-related symptoms; (2) using evidence-based and culturally appropriate assessment and treatments; (3) disseminating psychoeducational information on trauma and its related symptomatology; (4) strengthening protective factors and resilience among those affected by trauma and their family systems; (5) addressing the impact of trauma on parents/caregivers and the family unit; (6) interprofessional collaboration to enhance holistic treatment and continuity of care; and (7) supporting staff wellness and creating a work environment that minimizes the likelihood of employees developing empathy-based stress reactions (The National Child Traumatic Stress Network, 2018).

Incorporating an ecosystemic approach that involves not only children and parents but also community systems such as social services agencies, mental health facilities, and schools increases the chances of stopping emotional and behavioral dysregulation across the entire system where the trauma operates. Saxe and his associates (2007) propose that two major components are operating with a traumatized child. First, a traumatized child has difficulty regulating emotional and behavioral states. Second, the social environment and system of care are not able to help the child regulate these emotions and behaviors.

You will soon meet crisis workers from the Carl Perkins Child Abuse Center, who operate out of Jackson, Tennessee and cover much of rural west Tennessee. They operationalize all of the following 10 principles, and then some! Saxe and associates (2007, pp. 95–108) propose 10 principles of treatment if the system is to be changed. Additions from the Carl Perkins Center case manager, Chase Sanders, are included as in-the-field support (Sanders, 2023).

1. Fix a broken system, not just the identified client. Relentlessly attack the whole trauma system. Working with parents or other supports of the child is as critical as working with the child. In many cases, parents, who themselves received little love and lots of abuse, need to be reeducated along with their child's therapy (Sanders, 2023).

2. Put safety first. Nothing takes precedence over safety. That view of safety includes the trauma of court appearances or having to say over and over again what happened to them. Particularly in the case of young children, efforts to minimize the trauma of "telling the story" are made by video recording as admissible evidence. For physical safety, removing the child from the harmful environment is paramount. If school or agency personnel become aware of a child's potential abuse, in Tennessee, they are required to immediately call DCS and have a worker interviewing the child within two hours of the initial call. If abuse is determined, the child is then transported to a safe environment and a child advocate from the Center is assigned for safekeeping and support until adjudication occurs (Sanders, 2023).

3. Create clear, focused plans that are based on facts and target specific components of the child's emotional dysregulation and the level of instability in the child's environment and system of care. The Carl Perkins Center uses an evidence-based approach that is built on a cognitive behavioral and trauma-informed protocol, which follows the state Department of Human Services treatment requirements. They typically have a 12-session limit on therapy. However, if needed, the Center may extend the number of therapy sessions. Play therapy techniques may be used to enhance bonding and trust when some children have generalized trust issues and are scared to talk to the therapist. Depending on the support systems available, the Center may work independently with supports or conjointly with them. The Center may also use Eye Movement Desensitization and Reprocessing (EMDR) with older children. The total approach is that, while standard therapy protocols are employed, intervention is not cookie-cutter mass production but is tailored to the idiosyncratic nature of the abuse and is continuously monitored in regard to outcomes through case staffing (Sanders, 2023).

4. Don't "Go" before being "Ready." Build an alliance with the family, understand logistical problems such as childcare and transportation, and create an understanding of what treatment will involve and who will be included. Before even a forensic interview is made, the child and support persons will be thoroughly oriented as to the therapeutic and legal processes by an advocate assigned by the Center. That advocate will stay with the child until the complaint is adjudicated and trouble shoot any issues that arise (Sanders, 2023).

5. Use resources to gain maximum benefit. Carefully plan and coordinate the tactics and strategy with the system's players for the best possible outcome. Time and money are scarce in the treatment world. Plan carefully so neither gets wasted. Carl Perkins Center executives are very good at obtaining money from a variety of sources to provide intensive and extensive service. However, case management balances on a fine line of providing quality service and moving client back into a nontherapeutic world (Saunders, 2023).

6. Accountability is critical. Accountability has two parts. First is the worker's ability to put words into action and evaluate how well those actions are working and change them if they aren't. Second,

and more daunting, is requiring that children, parents, and others in the social ecosystem be accountable as well. Case staffings have built in accountability. If things are not going forward, the staff assume a stance of what needs to be changed as opposed to a "business as usual" approach (Sanders, 2023).

7. Deal with the reality of the situation. If resources aren't there, if family systems are compromised, if children are developmentally delayed, then understand the reality of the situation and adjust goals and expectations to it. If we have a child client with autism spectrum disorder (ASD), we work out an acceptable and doable intervention that utilizes communication strategies appropriate to the child's needs. It isn't always perfect, but we continuously try to improve (Sanders, 2023).

8. Take care of yourself and the treatment team. All the king's horses and all the king's men do not put Humpty-Dumpty back together again if the horses and men are broken themselves. There's a chapter ahead of you in this book on burnout. Guess what one specific area of crisis intervention has high burnout rates? That chapter is the real deal if you are going into this business, so read it carefully. The Carl Perkins center has and still does about the best job of preventing burnout we know of (Bottoms, 1999; Sanders, 2023, East et al., 2001).

9. Look for the strengths in the system. The trauma system of the child is rife with pathology and failure. It is easy to find things wrong. Yet, there is resiliency and strength within this system. It is your job to keep a positive view of it and make lemonade out of the lemons. We work from a positive, strength-based, resiliency format. There is no "can't" here at Carl Perkins (Sanders, 2023).

10. Leave a better system. As with all crisis intervention, you are not an adoption agency taking on children and families to raise forever. Teaching families how to take care of themselves is the end goal. Our standard is a twelve-session limit imposed by the state Department of Human Services. We might go longer if need be and we have if the occasion warrants, but not too long and not too often. We have a parent support group parents can attend but long-term therapy is not our business. (Sanders, 2023).

When the entire ecosystem of the child is brought into play, involving all of the players in the treatment

using combinations of trauma-based cognitive-behavioral therapy (Cohen & Mannarino, 2000b; Deblinger et al., 2015) overlaid with play therapy techniques (Everstein & Everstein, 2019; Geraci, 2022; Knell, 1995; Moffatt, 2013), outcomes for parents include better parenting practices, improvement in depressive symptoms, reduction in abuse-specific emotional distress, and greater support for the child. Children have less externalization of problems, fewer depressive symptoms, reduced behavior problems at home and school, and feel less shame, guilt, depression, and anger due to the abuse. Perhaps even more important, social services, schools, law enforcement, judiciaries, and mental health services all play well together (Cohen & Mannarino, 1996, 1998, 2000a, 2000b; Everstein & Everstein, 2019; Lanktree & Brier, 1995; Trask et al., 2011). When this happens, the sum is indeed greater than its parts.

Need for Affirmation and Safety. Initial intervention techniques call for intentionally and positively managing the crisis of disclosure and the resulting fear and anxiety. Affirmation and validation are crucial in regard to what has happened, what is happening, and what will happen to the child, the offender, and significant others. The admonition in the PTSD chapter on *not* using flooding techniques with children holds even more firmly with sexual abuse. If prolonged exposure techniques are to be used, they should be done with gradual and graded exposure to the aversive stimulus, with plenty of time for processing between exposures. Children should also be taught progressive relaxation techniques so they can learn how to remove themselves from the feared stimuli. Because small children are not fully developed cognitively, most instrumental and operant behavioral techniques that may be used with adult survivors are also not efficacious. Yet anxiety about and fear of the abusive events and the abuser need to be reduced, and this calls for reexposure to the trauma.

Regaining a Sense of Control. Anger and grief are emotional by-products for children of sexual abuse. Venting of these feelings should be encouraged, particularly because most adults are not comfortable with them and may attempt to repress such feelings when children exhibit them (Wheeler & Berliner, 1988, p. 237). Drawing, painting, modeling clay, sand play, writing, and learning to communicate emotions are all therapeutic vehicles to ventilate angry feelings and loss. Play techniques can also give the child a renewed sense of empowerment by allowing play figures to be acted on, thus reducing long-standing feelings of helplessness (James, 2003; Malchiodi, 2008; Sadowski & Loesch, 1993; Webb, 2007). Punching out a Bobo doll or picking up a play telephone and calling the police can give children a sense of control in a situation in which they have little (Salter, 1988, p. 215). Along with relaxation and other stress reduction measures, play techniques such as sand tray therapy can be used to teach the child to control anger when the child constantly acts out with peers or significant others.

Education. Education about adult sex offenders and sex itself is important for children because they will have little if any knowledge of why or what has happened to them. Shame is a predominant feature of the child's response to abuse (Knauer, 2000, pp. 74–82). Children need to know that it is the adult and not the child who made the mistake. Children who have been physically injured need to have these injuries explained and be told that their bodies will be okay. Many children believe that others will be able to tell what happened by looking at them. Children need to know that although they may feel different, sexual abuse does not make them look different.

Understanding developmental stages is critical in what kind of education is provided and how therapy is delivered (Saxe et al., 2008, pp. 7–12). Cognitively, young children usually have little understanding of sexual functions. Typically, they will not initiate questions about sex, but when workers initiate education about sex through slides or books, children will respond with their own questions. Every child who has been sexually assaulted needs some type of sex education and information on what the assault means (Baker, 1995; McLeer et al., 1992; Oates et al., 1994; Salter, 1988, pp. 217–218). In addition to the play therapy techniques (such as drawing, painting, modeling, and sand play) mentioned earlier, a highly effective means of teaching important social and survival lessons to children is through outreach services into schools, religious institutions, and community centers with professionally developed puppetry programs.

Assertiveness Training. Assertiveness training may be seen as more of a preventive measure to keep children out of harm's way than a remedial measure for sexually abused children. Yet, sexually abused children have learned, as a self-protective measure, to be compliant to deviant requests and need to learn that it is okay to protect themselves and to "Just say NO!" (Salter, 1988, p. 219). Because abused children are at greater risk for revictimization (Walker et al., 2019), teaching them cues and warning signs and appropriate assertion responses is important so that they can learn self-protective measures that may limit their exposure to future abuse (Castro et al., 2019; Miller-Perrin, 2001; Wheeler & Berliner, 1988, p. 242).

Intervention Strategies for Child Sexual Abuse: The Case of Elizabeth

Elizabeth, age 8, is the middle child in the family. She, her 11-year-old brother, and a 5-year-old sister live with her mother and stepfather, whom her mother married nearly 2 years ago. Elizabeth's mother, Mona, and father divorced when the youngest child was about 1 year old. Elizabeth's stepfather started off by fondling her. This went on for several weeks. Although Elizabeth was bewildered, scared, and intimidated, no one else knew about the abusive activity. Recently, while everyone else was out of the house, her stepfather raped her. He threatened to kill Elizabeth, Mona, and her sister if she told anyone. The following morning Elizabeth confided in her brother, who, in turn, told Mona what had happened.

Incredulous over this discovery and paralyzed as to what to do, Mona called the child abuse hotline that she remembered seeing advertised on TV and in the local newspaper.

The following simulated dialogue was generated by Delaine Bottoms (1999) vice president for operations of Carl Perkins Child Abuse Center with new supporting protocols contributed by Case Sanders, current case manager at Carl Perkins. It should be noted that the procedures detailed follow Tennessee law and may not be generally applicable to all states, territories, provinces, and countries.

Disclosure.

Mona: (calling the child advocacy hotline; angry, crying uncontrollably, barely in control) Hello. Hello! I want to report a (choke, sob) rape. He . . . that bastard . . . he raped my baby. That piece of trash raped my daughter. Oh, how could I have not seen . . . How could I have let this happen? (Continues crying and screaming uncontrollably, beseeching the hotline worker for help and railing at her husband.)

CW: OK, I understand you're extremely upset and have every right to be, but I need for you to be in control right now. My name's Delaine. I need to know your name, where you live, and whether you're safe from who did this to your daughter.

Mona: (Regaining a bit of control, gives her name and address.) It was my . . . It was . . . my husband . . . Leon. Her asshole stepfather . . . I found her underwear. It was all bloody . . . Oh my God! My baby . . . My poor baby. He's gone in his truck . . . He's headed for Chicago on a run . . . I'll kill him . . . I will kill him if it's the last thing I ever do!

CW: So you are safe, and he's not in the house. How badly hurt is your daughter? Does she need an ambulance and medical attention?

Mona: I don't know. She's kinda in a daze. Just walking around holding on to her teddy bear. Oh, that bastard! I'll castrate that bastard before I kill him!

CW: Mona, I hear how angry and shocked you are, but I need for you to follow me very closely. This is extremely important. I want you not to do anything with Elizabeth. Don't wash her up or change her clothes. I want you to take her to Madison County General Hospital and bring her underwear with you in a paper bag. Do you have a way to get to the hospital? Are you okay enough to get to the hospital? (Gets acknowledgment from the mother that she can get to the hospital.) There are going to be people at the hospital who are going to want to talk to you and Elizabeth, and we're going to need to do a medical exam of her. This is not going to be easy, but we know how to do this. You did the right thing. I'll meet you at the hospital, and I'll help you get through this. We will get through this! Do you understand? Now tell me what you're going to do and when you'll get to the hospital. (Mona restates what the crisis worker has told her and assures the worker she can do those things.)

The initial shock that accompanies discovery and disclosure is invariably highly dramatic and volatile for parents who have been blind to the perpetrator's intent. Because rape is a violent crime, the primary consideration of the crisis worker is to determine if people are now safe from the perpetrator and if they need medical attention. The initiating crisis is multifold. The crisis worker needs to make sure that there is no physical injury to the child and that the out-of-control parent is sufficiently functional to take care of the child and do the things necessary to preserve evidence. She will also need to restore the mother to equilibrium. Exacting revenge by assaulting the perpetrator would put both mother and daughter in jeopardy. The scene at the hospital can be extremely threatening, and the crisis worker does all she can to indicate that the mother has done the right thing and that, as difficult as it may be, the crisis worker will be there with her to the conclusion. The crisis worker's initial job will be to do crisis intervention with the mother by making sure everyone is safe and helping her get back in control of her emotions and actions (Bottoms, 1999; Knauer, 2000, pp. 31–47).

Immediate Aftermath. In cases where there is physical injury, the survivor will need immediate medical evaluation and care. The crisis worker, after determining that the mother can get herself and her daughter to the hospital, immediately makes other phone calls to the Department of Human Services and law enforcement. She also calls the hospital and informs them that a child sexual assault victim is on her way and that a sexual assault team needs to be assembled. After making these phone calls, she immediately leaves for the hospital.

Mona: (at the hospital, in a room with the crisis worker) All I can think about is that no-good lying creep. He's lucky he's on the road, or he'd be dead now. I'd shoot his balls right off of him. I've got a .38 Special, and by God . . . as God is my witness . . . I will do it. What's happening to my daughter? They took her away. Is she going to be all right? I've read some stuff on this. It's not just him raping her now, but she'll be scarred for life! How could it happen? How could I be so stupid? What in the hell is wrong with me? He was so nice to her, to all of us! How, oh how could I have been so stupid? (Starts uncontrolled sobbing and pacing, slamming her purse down again and again.)

CW: You've certainly been through a lot in the last few hours. And you've done a remarkable job of taking care of Elizabeth. Your concerns about her physical injuries now and her psychological injuries later are certainly justified. I'm not going to sugarcoat this. You're obviously a very good mother who has suddenly been thrust into this—nothing you or Elizabeth did caused it. It was perpetrated on her and you. We are here to assist you in any way we can. We want to provide someone to be with you and Elizabeth during these critical hours, as well as providing aftercare and follow-up counseling.

But right now, even though your husband is away, I'm concerned about your anger. It's certainly justifiable, but what Elizabeth needs is for you to be the best mother you can be right now. If you shoot your husband, how will you be able to support your daughter when she needs you most? You won't! You will be in jail. That's where your husband deserves to be, not you. Let law enforcement handle your husband. What we need to do is handle this and care for Elizabeth. Can you do this? That's really what you want, isn't it, to help your daughter get through this?

Mona: I . . . I . . . I guess so. I appreciate it. Everything happened so fast! I don't know how I managed without falling apart. It's like a wild, awful dream—an ugly nightmare. I don't know how I'll handle it when the dust settles. I'm so mad— I could kill him! I feel like I've been raped too. There's so much on me right now. I don't know if I'm capable of bearing up under all that's got to be done. Damn, damn, damn that man! Excuse me, I shouldn't blow up like that.

CW: That's all right. You have a perfect right to be angry and to say it. It's good that you care enough to be upset, and it's good to see you direct your anger at him—the real cause of Elizabeth's hurt and your anger. Both of you deserve better treatment than he gave you, and no child should ever experience sexual assault.

Mona: That's right. I trusted him! And he took advantage of her. She was helpless—a helpless child. I've got to show her where I stand on this. First, I'm going to take good care of her, and then I'm going to send that rotten louse to jail for good!

CW: Mona, I know things are really crazy right now, and you don't know what's happening. I want to take care of that by telling you what's going to happen and how things are going to be done, so you know what's going on and don't feel so out of control. I'll go through each step of what is going to happen today and what we can do to ensure that Elizabeth gets through this in good shape. I'm going to explain what will happen very carefully to you. If you have any questions, stop me. There are no stupid questions about this. I want you to fully understand what's happening, so you can start to get back in control. Mona, the important thing is

that you gain control. Right now, I'm being very directive, and will be doing so until you get past this emergency and back on top of things. You have choices, and if, at any time, you feel like making any of the choices yourself, please feel free to do so. You can stop me at any time, and that will be OK. **(The crisis worker patiently goes through all the details of what is going to happen, stopping whenever Mona has questions, and checking to see that she understands what she's being told.)**

The crisis worker permits her to express her anger, isn't threatened by Mona's outburst, encourages her to keep owning and expressing her feelings, and lets her know that neither she nor Elizabeth was to blame for the assault. That strategy is important in letting Mona know that she can be in control and that the worker believes in her without the worker jumping in and expressing the anger for her. This is no place for the human services worker who is not calm, cool, and detached in their professional demeanor. The worker must be solid during a crisis, acting as the client's rock. There is probably nothing more heart wrenching and sickening than the aftermath of a severe sexual or physical assault on a child. Intervention here clearly calls for a strong constitution. But, more importantly, if the worker manifests their own anger directly at the parent or the perpetrator, that anger may be misinterpreted as being directed toward the victim (Bottoms, 1999).

At times, when the perpetrator is still an immediate threat, the worker must take on the trappings of a crisis worker who deals with survivors of intimate partner violence. The family may need to be moved to a safe place until the perpetrator is apprehended. The crisis worker continuously reinforces the mother for doing the right thing and for caring about her daughter. This is an extremely important strategy because adult caregivers may engage in severe guilt and recrimination because they believe they should have been more vigilant (Sanders, 2023). The crisis worker also must make sure that the mother will not exact revenge on the perpetrator and put herself in jeopardy with the law (Knauer, 2000, p. 46). It will indeed do Elizabeth little good if her mother is facing a charge of assault with intent to commit murder. Finally, the crisis worker patiently educates the parent on what is going to happen. Education about the aftermath of a child assault is critical in giving parents back the sense of control they feel they have lost.

Two components of education are important. First, detailing what the legal proceedings are and what the mother and child need to prepare for allows them to know what is ahead of them and not be blindsided by all the legal, social, and psychological ramifications of a child sexual assault. Second, giving the parent information on how to deal with the child in the immediate aftermath of the discovery is critical in ensuring that the child is not revictimized and that the parent does not feel guilty for doing or saying the wrong thing (Bottoms, 1999). An even more shocking revelation may occur during the initial disclosure and interview. That is, it is not uncommon for the parent to disclose that she was also sexually abused as a child and swore this would never happen to any of her own children (Bottoms, 1999).

Mona: (head in her hands, slumped over) It's my fault. I let this happen. God knows I should have known. Uncle Ralph did the same thing to me when I was 14. I tried to tell Mom, but she just blew it off 'cause Uncle Ralph helped us out when Mom went through her divorce. And now my own daughter . . . I couldn't even protect her. I'm no better than my mother.

CW: (reacting coolly, letting Mona talk through her own sexual assault) There's a big difference. As I hear you say it, your mother didn't follow up because she was afraid and dependent on your uncle. You weren't afraid, and when you found out you took immediate action. See the difference? A big difference! Right now, you are being the best mother possible. Do you see that difference?

The worker, although taken aback, immediately discriminates between what Mona's mother didn't do and what Mona did do. She underscores and reinforces Mona for taking action and reaffirms her as a fit parent.

Prosecuting the Perpetrator

LO19 **Interviewing the Child.** Whenever a child is sexually assaulted, there are two primary concerns. The first is taking care of the child and seeing that the child is safe. The second is obtaining evidence to prosecute the perpetrator. If the child has not been injured or if the discovery is made a good while after the assault, then an interview needs to be conducted that will allow the necessary evidence to be obtained. In the past, report of a child assault would entail numerous interviews with medical staff, law enforcement, and social services. The intimidating circumstances and the necessity to repeat the story over and over have a high potential for making the child feel terrorized, guilty, confused, and unequal to the task of meeting the demands of a variety of strange and threatening adults. The potential for revictimizing the child and the parent while going through this procedure is extremely high if not handled appropriately (Bottoms, 1999).

To stop this from happening, the Carl Perkins Center uses an interview procedure that many other child advocacy agencies employ. This approach is a good model for dealing with cases of sexual or severe physical assault on children and is now starting to be instituted across the country. One *trained* forensic interviewer with a listening device in their ear conducts the interview and is video recorded, and the video is sent to a viewing center where other social service and law enforcement officials can view and listen to the interview (Sanders, 2023). The child's psychological well-being is critical in the aftermath of disclosure, and a typical law enforcement interrogation would likely put the child under severe duress. Therefore, whoever conducts the interview should be skillful not only in obtaining evidence but also in making the child feel safe while the interview occurs. At the Carl Perkins Center, the interview is conducted in a pleasant, child-friendly room by a very caring child-centered forensic worker at the center, not in the stark confines of a police interrogation room (Bottoms, 1999). The child is shown the cameras and microphones, where they go to, who will be listening, and what and how the interview is going to proceed, so nothing is hidden as to what is going to occur (Sanders, 2023). The worker may also use "good touch–bad touch" with a doll or a figure drawing to have the child indicate where on their body (e.g., genitals, mouth) the assault took place. (Note: *Mouth* is included here because oral sex is a common occurrence in child sexual abuse [Knauer, 2000, pp. 5–6].)

Note how the emphasis in the above description was on *trained* interviewers. Because this is a criminal matter, the worker needs to be able to obtain information without biasing the child's testimony. In other words, the typical mental health worker will not have the expertise to do this. For that reason, crisis workers do not typically interview children to obtain information for prosecution; rather, forensic interviewers are utilized to collect information that may be used for prosecution without further traumatizing the child or biasing the child's disclosures (O'Donohue & Fanetti, 2016). Those who conduct child forensic interviews following sexual trauma should be skillful not only in obtaining evidence, but also in making the child feel safe while the interview occurs. The Carl Perkins center training staff take great pains in training school personnel to NOT try and conduct an interview regarding what happened. Doing so can be problematic when trying to secure a conviction. The bottom line is to report the suspected abuse immediately and then let the experts take over. Conversely, when there is no prior knowledge of abuse and the child discloses an assault in a spontaneous manner, the crisis worker needs to be cool-headed, listen to the child, and be prepared to make an immediate referral.

After the examination, the crisis worker needs to affirm to children that they are okay physically, that some part of their body is not "broken," that they will not die, and in the case of victims who are able to become pregnant, reassuring them that they are not pregnant (Bottoms, 1999).

CW: (Very empathic, sits down beside Elizabeth and takes her hand.) Elizabeth, I'm Delaine from the Center for Children. I'm guessing some pretty scary things have happened, and you're probably having some pretty scary feelings right now. I want to talk to you about some of those scary things. It's okay to be scared, because it was a scary thing that happened. But you're safe now, and your mom and I are going to make sure you stay safe. So, if you'd like, I'll try to answer any questions you have about what happened and what's going to happen.

Elizabeth: (after the examination and the initial interview by a forensic expert) When Leon did this to me and he stuck his peter in me, it really hurt. Am I gonna die, 'cause I started bleeding? Will I get pregnant?

CW: No, you're not going to die. It's normal to feel sore after all that and to bleed some. But the doctors said you were okay, and Dr. Ann will be back to see you and tell you you're okay. I checked with the doctor, and you're not old enough to get pregnant yet. Dr. Ann will tell you about all this, so don't worry about that.

It is extremely important for young children who have little information about how their body functions to immediately allay fears of what may happen to their body as a result of the assault. Children should also be prepared for the medical evaluation. It is advisable to have a sexual assault nurse examiner (SANE) to conduct an evaluation of the child. Doing so not only allows the child to receive proper medical care, but Golding et al. (2015) note that the testimony of a SANE tends to increase the jury's likelihood of rendering a guilty verdict in a court of law. As such, a proper sexual assault evaluation can be an important part of helping the child obtain legal justice for the incomprehensible acts completed against them.

Preparing the Child for Testimony. Interviewing children about their potential sexual abuse is a tricky business, and it should absolutely be done by qualified and practiced forensic examiners. There is no set protocol free of trial ramifications, so the goal is to elicit reliable and complete information without tainting it (Saywitz & Dorodo, 2013). The last thing that needs to happen is raising the specter of "false memories." Sexual assault is a criminal matter, and at some point, the child will probably have to testify in a courtroom. That appearance may be terrifying to a small child who will have to give testimony against a caretaker who may have either been very nice to the child or made threats against the child and their family. Depending on the child's age, the Carl Perkins Center uses puppets, books, and videos to educate the child on what testimony in a courtroom entails. Immediately before the child's appearance in court, an advocate from the center will take the child to the courtroom to acclimate the child to what may be perceived as a frightening experience. The staff explains everybody's role and how things will happen. The staff member will role-play traffic court, so the child gets an idea of how courts operate. Children can explore the courtroom, ask questions, and sit in the judge's and witness chairs, so they become familiarized with a courtroom and are not terror stricken when they are asked to engage in the real situation (Sanders, 2023).

Another problematic area is the time of the court appearance. Courts are notorious for not starting on time. Sitting all day on a bench outside a court waiting for it to convene while the perpetrator is seated on an adjacent bench is clearly not conducive to the child's or the family's good mental health. As a result, the Carl Perkins staff keeps the child and the family at the center until a call is received from the courthouse that the court is about to convene. Only then are the child and family transported to the courthouse. After the court appearance, the child is brought back to the center and debriefed. Questions such as "How did that feel?" and "What was that like for you?" are posed to alleviate the residual fears of having confronted the perpetrator at close range (Bottoms, 1999; Sanders, 2023).

The span of time from disclosure and discovery of the assault to the court appearance may be up to a year, and there will be lots of transcrisis points as time seems to drag on interminably. It is important that each of these crisis points be met head-on by crisis workers. Thus, the Carl Perkins Center staff immediately swings into action in dealing with the child and the family and stays with them in support and therapeutic roles for up to a year after the initial contact is made (Bottoms, 1999; Sanders, 2023).

Aftermath

LO20 It should be a given from all you have read in this chapter that any child who has been sexually abused needs counseling (Knauer, 2000, p. 46). Discovery of an incestuous relationship throws the entire family into crisis. Parents face loss of what has become an addictive behavior, possible criminal sanctions, loss of their family, and social stigmatization. The nonoffending parent finds themself torn between their partner and the assaulted child. The child may find themself discredited, shamed, punished, and still unprotected (Herman, 1981, p. 183). The worker will also face a crisis in deciding what to do and whether or not to believe the child's story. However, discovery of child sexual abuse is no different from discovery of any other physical abuse, and state laws mandate that it must be reported (Sandberg et al., 1988). It is a criminal activity and should be dealt with in that manner.

Conversely, it is not uncommon for children to retract their complaints under pressure from the family (Weiss & Alexander, 2013). Therefore, until clearly proved otherwise, the child's allegations should be accepted as valid, and the worker's primary consideration should be reporting the abuse to Child Protective Services and obtaining safety for the child (Sandberg et al., 1988).

Because the behavior is both criminal and addictive, treating the problem via family therapy is fruitless. What is called for is immediately referring the problem to and cooperating with family services and law enforcement agencies that do not subscribe to a family reunification policy (Sandberg et al., 1988). It then becomes much more possible to remove the offender from the home through a court order. Removing the child from the home has negative ramifications because it may be construed as banishment and may also serve to strengthen parent bonds

against the child. The child needs assurance that they are not to blame for the incest; they should be praised for their courage and clearly told that they are helping, not hurting, their family and will not be abandoned even if they retract their story (Herman, 1981, pp. 184–185).

Counseling

Aftercare is critically important to prevent a host of maladies from appearing in later childhood and carrying on into adulthood. Universal characteristics such as lying, stealing, fighting, verbal and behavioral oppositional defiance, and promiscuity are typical aftermath behaviors that will assail children who have been sexually victimized. Boys may perpetrate sexual assaults on other children, bully other kids, vandalize property, and generally direct their anger outward. Girls typically turn their anger inward and engage in alcohol and drug misuse, eating disorders, and promiscuity. Reducing problem behavior is important along with dealing with the trauma (Miller-Perrin, 2001). These issues should be addressed before they become major behavioral problems. The aforementioned use of play therapy, Trauma-Focused CBT, and trauma-informed care systems is critical in supporting children who experience sexual trauma.

Group Support Work with Nonoffending Parents

For nonoffending parents, the notion of entering counseling or a support/therapy group may be very threatening. However, it is quite possibly the only way they will be able to get their families back together. Nonoffending parents are secondary victims of child sexual assault (Cyr et al., 2018; Fuller, 2016). Nonoffending parents play a key role in their child's treatment, and they also have very specific needs related to their own healing and to parenting a child survivor of sexual trauma (Deblinger et al., 2015; Sanders, 2023). Support groups for spouses of abusers can be a helpful recovery tool (Vilvens et al., 2021), enabling members to come to regain a sense of control and empowerment in themselves and their families, reduce blame and guilt in themselves, and restore family bonds (Brittain & Merriam, 1988; Salter, 1988, p. 211; Sanders, 2023).

Preventing Parental Dependence. Perhaps most tragic of all the issues that assail a family is the nonoffending parent's overreliance on the child. Often, a role reversal occurs whereby the child not only is the sexual object of the perpetrating parent but also becomes the chief confidant and comfort provider for the nonoffending parent. The nonoffender parent becomes emotionally overdependent on the child as a source of support (Alexander et al., 2000). Therefore, crisis workers spend a good deal of time with nonoffending parents, teaching them to reassume the role as head of household and to stand their ground when the child attempts to reassume their pseudo-adult role. Finally, time is spent on talking about the nonoffending parent not falling into another relationship that has the same outcome as the parent may be highly likely to do (Bottoms, 1999).

Crisis Session. Trauma therapy is an evolving field, and researchers continue to uncover elements of best practice in working with sexually traumatized children. Although trauma therapy occurs after the immediate aftermath of the assault or disclosure/discovery, in trauma therapy with children who have experienced sexual assault, the fact is that there are transcrises aplenty with which to reckon. We return to the case illustration of Elizabeth, who has been building a world in her sandtray, for an example of transcrisis in therapy.

Elizabeth: (Tears up the carefully made new family she has been building in the sand tray and breaks down in tears.) This won't ever come true! Some kids at school said Leon's gonna get out just like their daddies did and will be right back at home. I HATE THIS STUPID SAND TRAY! THIS IS HOPELESS. WE'LL NEVER BE SAFE, AND I HATE THERAPY, AND YOU TOO, MISS DELAINE, so you can just kiss my ass goodbye! (Stands defiantly as an 8-year-old can, tearfully regarding Delaine with as evil a look as she can muster.)

CW: (Says nothing but picks up some modeling clay and popsicle sticks and starts constructing something.)

Elizabeth: (Sits over in the corner, staring balefully at the worker. Slowly comes over to the worker.) Whatcha doing with that clay and those stupid popsicle sticks?

CW: I am going to build something I think might help when things are really down. I guess you are so hopeless and helpless right now you couldn't help me, but is it okay if I make a change to your sand tray?

Elizabeth: I didn't say that. What is it? I guess you can change it.

CW: (Sweeps the sand away in the sand tray and parts it to reveal a broad swath of blue board.) It is a bridge. I am building a bridge over troubled waters. But it has to be a strong bridge with good foundations, strong girders, and support wire because it has to stay solid and mustn't fall in. It carries very important people on it . . . like your mom and you.

Your stepfather may get out some day, but you will be a grown woman by then. But there are going to be other troubles that will get you down and things that will appear just as hopeless, maybe things you do, or your mom does, or maybe what other people say or do. So, it's got to be a strong bridge. I'd like to put this family on the other side with palm trees and beach chairs and sunshine, not on this side with the swamp and all the nasty swamp things that live in it. But I can't build this alone. It is your bridge.

Elizabeth: (Grudgingly starts to help mold pillars for the bridge.) I guess so.

CW: (after bridge is done) How do you feel? You see, you have a real way to get out of the swamp. I am going to take a picture of this, and I want you to put it in the book. This is very important because it shows that you can get to the other side, and you can make your own bridge to get you there. So remember where you have come from. You have indeed crossed over that bridge with all the work we have done. There is no going back; you are across, but every once in a while, when things get tough, it's good to remember that this bridge we just built really is your bridge, Elizabeth. It is something you now own and can use forever. Now stand over there by the bridge and give me a big cheesy smile!

Drawing or constructing a bridge lets clients concretely fill in gaps when they see little way across "troubled waters." Bridging exercises are mainly used for assessment to determine where people have been and where they are going (Martin, 2008). Here, we use bridging as a therapeutic vehicle to get Elizabeth mobilized again and show her where she has been, whence she has come, and where she is going. Here, the crisis worker takes action and very actively and directly gets into the game, but as soon as Elizabeth mobilizes herself, the crisis worker assumes a collaborative mode and then becomes nondirective as Elizabeth regains control.

Summary

The sexual assault research consistently finds that the incidence of sexual assault is greatly underreported. The majority of reported rapists and other sexual abusers are males, and they come from all walks of life. Most abusers appear to perceive those they attack as objects of prey rather than as people. They usually assault not out of lust or desire for sexual gratification but out of a perceived need to control, exert power over, punish, vanquish, defeat, hurt, destroy, degrade, or humiliate others. Typically, abusers deny, minimize, and/or rationalize their behavior to the extent that they themselves rarely define their attacks as abuse. Instead, they usually claim that the survivor asked for, deserved, seduced, wanted, or needed the experience in order to grow up or somehow caused the abusive activity to occur.

Rape is a complex phenomenon that encompasses and affects the psychosocial, cultural, and personal aspects of society. There are no cause-and-effect formulas that explain why one person sexually assaults another. Consequently, many erroneous assumptions, beliefs, and myths about rape are held by different people, and gender influences perceptions about rape.

Date and acquaintance rape, especially on college campuses, has become a pressing problem. The problem is exacerbated by the use of drugs and/or alcohol that are usually found to be associated with date rape. One impediment to preventing date and acquaintance rape is the endorsement of rape myths, which perpetuate erroneous and dangerous ideas about sex and rape.

Recently, the human services professions have directed a great deal of attention to rape and sexual assault on children. Substantive work has been done in the areas of crisis work, counseling, legal, social, and psychological interventions to help children and to prevent child sexual abuse. Such intervention and prevention have been made even more urgent in light of recent findings that child sexual abuse extends debilitating traumas far into the adulthood of survivors. An enormous amount of research has shown that adult survivors of child sexual abuse often suffer a wide diversity of emotional, physical, psychological, and social pathologies that manifest themselves in various degrees of transcrisis and PTSD symptoms later in adulthood. These findings have produced greater urgency than ever before to help victims of sexual abuse and to stop offenders from assaulting.

Crisis intervention and other human services work in the area of rape and sexual assault of children requires unique and specialized knowledge and strategies. Children are vulnerable to many kinds of pressures, and perpetrators of child sexual abuse know all the angles needed to ensnare child victims. The legal, medical, social, mental health, law enforcement, and human services professions, as well as the court system, are becoming increasingly integrated in attempting to stop the abuse and to work with abused children and their families. There is ominous research on sexual predators' use of the internet for the dissemination and consumption of child exploitative material and for predatorial interaction with minors.

In recent years, the public, too, has become increasingly aware of the phenomenon of rape and other forms of sexual abuse, and that new awareness appears to have ushered in a greater sensitivity to and advocacy for the rights and needs of survivors. However, much remains to be done. Society still needs to overcome a number of long-standing myths about rape and other forms of sexual abuse. And survivors' families, friends, and coworkers need to be willing and able to respond to survivors with openness, genuineness, acceptance, understanding, and respect, all of which are key attitudes or conditions for nurturing recovery from the debilitating trauma and effects of sexual assault. Given the high incidence of sexual assault and its underreporting, it is highly likely that a number of you may have experienced this crisis. As a result of reading this chapter, you may experience or be experiencing some of the repercussions this chapter speaks of in people who have been sexually assaulted and abused. We urge you to not be ashamed, embarrassed, or guilty but to understand that this crisis is common to a whole lot of people and to get help! If you don't feel there is help in your community or you are too embarrassed to ask, call the National Office on Violence Against Women's hotlines: the Rape, Abuse, and Incest National Network Hotline at 1-800-656-HOPE (4673) or the National Teen Dating Abuse Helpline at 1-800-799-7233 (SAFE). If you are attempting to recover on your own from a sexual assault, get Aphrodite Matsakis's *The Rape Recovery Handbook* (2003). It is a step-by-step help program for survivors of sexual assault. It's user friendly, talks straight to you, and has really helpful exercises in it.

Partner Violence

10

Learning Objectives

After studying this chapter, you should be able to:

1. Describe the pervasiveness of partner violence that cuts across all cultures and socioeconomic classes.
2. Explain how approaches to partner violence are changing.
3. Summarize the dynamics of partner violence.
4. Explicate the psychological factors that contribute to partner violence.
5. Identify the stressors that lead to partner violence.
6. Critique the myths that surround partner violence.
7. Classify the different types of perpetrators of partner violence.
8. Explain the cycle of abuse.
9. Describe the factors that contribute to abused individuals staying in violent relationships.
10. Identify assessment strategies for battering relationships.
11. Summarize the intervention components for intimate partner violence.
12. Describe the dynamics of living in a shelter.
13. Describe what occurs in follow-up after leaving the shelter.
14. Explain how to intervene with children who live in an abusive environment.
15. Describe the dynamics of dating violence.
16. Describe the dynamics of stalking.
17. Explain how treatment for perpetrators of abuse occurs.
18. Delineate how a typical domestic violence reduction group operates.

Introduction

LO1 In this chapter, we address intimate partner violence (IPV), which is often used interchangeably with the term *domestic violence* (DV) (Burelomova et al., 2018). The World Health Organization (WHO, 2022) defines IPV as "behaviour within an intimate relationship that causes physical, sexual or psychological harm, including acts of physical aggression, sexual coercion, psychological abuse and controlling behaviours. This definition covers violence by both current and former spouses and partners" (para. 1). According to the Centers for Disease Control and Prevention (CDC), Violence Prevention Injury Center (2023), IPV may include physical violence, sexual violence, stalking, and psychological aggression.

The pervasiveness of IPV is so great that it cuts across social, economic, religious, ethnic, cultural, racial, and geographical boundaries (Atteraya et al., 2015; Bott et al., 2019; Chuemchit et al., 2018; Cools & Kotsadam, 2017; Domenech Del Rio & Sirvent Garcia Del Valle, 2017; Fidan & Bui, 2016; Gebrezgi et al., 2017; Ghafournia, 2017; Katiti et al., 2016; Lacey et al., 2015; Lövestad et al., 2017; Lysova et al., 2019;

Martín-Fernández et al., 2019; Moffitt et al., 2022; Peterman et al., 2017; Sanz-Barbero et al., 2018; Sardinha et al., 2022; Stöckl & Penhale, 2015). Indeed, a review of the American Psychological Association's abstracts reveals that almost every country the *National Geographic* covers has had a study done on IPV. Culture plays a large part in what is defined as IPV or if it even exists. Further, if we define culture in terms of the social locations that Laura Brown (2008) speaks so eloquently to, we need to examine other diversity factors, such as being transgender (Peitzmeier et al., 2020), pregnant (Chisholm et al., 2017; Suglia et al., 2010), disabled (Ballan et al., 2014), homeless (Yeater et al., 2011), low income (Ahmadabadi et al., 2020; Okuda et al., 2015), HIV positive or a sex worker (Ulibarri et al., 2010), and neighborhood of residence (Beyer et al., 2015) as some of the many social locations that lead to violence between intimate partners.

Certainly, abuse in domestic situations is not limited to spousal relationships; IPV occurs within all intimate relationships and across gender identities and sexual orientations (Chen et al., 2020; Kolbe & Büttner, 2020; Laskey et al., 2019; Oliffe et al., 2014). Although women are statistically more likely than men to have partner violence perpetrated against them (Breiding, 2014), men also experience violence perpetrated by their intimate partners (Chen et al., 2020; Hines et al., 2007; Kolbe & Büttner, 2020), and men may be involved in same-sex relationships in which both partners perpetrate IPV against the other (Walsh & Stephenson, 2023). Moreover, research on IPV within the LGBTQIA+ community suggests significantly elevated rates (Chen et al., 2020; Peitzmeier et al., 2020). Therefore, it should be clearly understood that the concepts discussed in this chapter apply to *all* partners or people involved in any established current or former cohabiting or intimate relationship. However, because women form the major target group of severe partner violence and the bulk of available research is on women survivors of male perpetrated violence, this chapter focuses mainly on crisis intervention with women who experience partner violence and the men who hurt them.

The Incidence of Partner Violence

The history of IPV in Western society goes as far back as the patriarchal system does. While an assault on or rape of another man's wife caused and still causes immediate and severe legal punishment and moral outrage, abuse by a man of his own wife is quite

another story (Pleck, 1987). Common law in the United States early acknowledged the right of a man to chastise his wife for misbehavior without being prosecuted for doing so (*Bradley v. State of Mississippi,* 1824). Indeed, the law's attitude toward the abuse of one's spouse to the current day is aptly summarized in the case of the *State of North Carolina v. Oliver* in 1874. The court ruled that "if no permanent injury has been inflicted, it is better to draw the curtains, shut out the public eye, and leave the parties to forgive and forget." The implications of such "blind" justice are ominous.

There is no more anxiety-provoking call for a law enforcement officer (LEO) than a domestic disturbance call. In fact, responding to domestic disturbances is one of the most dangerous emergencies to which LEOs respond, following other high-violence calls such as serving warrants, transporting prisoners, and bar fights (Johnson, 2017). Between 1980 and 2006, there were nearly 4,200 assaults on LEOs annually when responding to domestic violence calls (Johnson, 2017). And between 2011 and 2020, over 8 percent of LEO deaths were attributed to domestic violence (Tucker, 2022). Moreover, research has demonstrated that when women are the primary criminal offenders (not solely in domestic violence situations), they are likely to be perpetrators of violence against LEOs (Covington et al., 2014).

In the United States between 2009 and 2015, LEOs responded to approximately 1.3 million nonfatal domestic violence calls annually (Reaves, 2017). And, during the COVID-19 pandemic, 911 calls for domestic violence in the United States increased (Richards et al., 2021). Globally, approximately 27 percent of "ever partnered" women have experienced physical or sexual IPV at some point in their life (Sardinha et al., 2022, p. 807). However, Gracia (2004) talks about the iceberg of IPV reporting, wherein the available data likely only reflects a small portion of those who actually experience IPV. Indeed, IPV is underreported for a variety of reasons, such as lack of anonymity in research-based reporting (Cullen, 2023); gender bias, as it applies to male victims of female IPV perpetration (Erickson et al., 2017); victim blaming attitudes (Gracia, 2004, 2014; Prochuk, 2018); dependence on the perpetrator, including financial dependence (Gracia, 2004); fear of retaliation or reprisal (Gracia, 2004); shame, embarrassment, or perceived guilt (Gracia, 2004; Prochuk, 2018); lack of access to resources (Gurm et al., 2020); and social imbalances that disempower women (Gracia, 2004), to name a few.

To improve identification and intervention for individuals who experience IPV, several measures have been taken in recent years. If you have been to a medical provider recently, you probably noticed that the intake form included at least one item pertaining to relationship violence and/or direct questions asked about IPV by your medical provider. This is particularly true for physicians who specialize in reproductive and sexual health. However, many primary care physicians and emergency receiving departments also utilize this practice. When looking across multiple studies, it appears that data from these screenings indicates an approximately lifetime IPV prevalence rate of 38 percent of clients in primary care settings and 40 percent in emergency settings (Sprague et al., 2014).

Although the intent behind these medical setting screening measures is commendable, the actual implementation and data collection may be complicated by a number of factors. Let's first examine screening for IPV perpetrators. Limited rapport between the patient and medical provider can lead to patients' hesitancy to disclose IPV perpetration (Portnoy et al., 2020), particularly when patients are concerned about judgment from the medical provider related to perpetration of IPV (Portnoy et al., 2020). Moreover, patients who perpetrate IPV may be hesitant to acknowledge their trespasses for fear of legal consequences (Portnoy et al., 2020). For IPV survivors, in addition to the above cited reasons for not disclosing IPV, some reason for survivors not disclosing IPV specifically to their medical provider might include feeling like the medical provider does not actually care for them or that they are not taken seriously (Pratt-Eriksson et al., 2014), being asked about IPV when others are present (Correa et al., 2020), and not being asked clear and direct questions about IPV (Correa et al., 2020). Naturally, the reasons patients may not disclose IPV to their medical provider abound, but some of these reasons could be rooted in the medical provider's willingness (or unwillingness) to broach the topic. When considering providers' perspectives, some limitations may include limited time during which to properly conduct the screening (Aluko et al., 2015), concerns about offending clients (Aluko et al., 2015), limited training on IPV for medical staff (Clark et al., 2020), and limited psychoeducational and referral resources for individuals experiencing IPV (Clark et al., 2020). It might be that screening conducted by medical assistants is more likely to result in IPV disclosures than screenings performed by physicians (Sharples et al., 2018),

which might be the result of factors such as increased relatability to a medical assistant and/or more time spent with the patient during which to build rapport.

When considering risk factors for experiencing IPV, the research abounds. Common risk factors may include living in a culture that justifies "wife beating" and upholds laws that disadvantage women (Heise & Kotsadam, 2015, p. 338); experiencing childhood maltreatment (Kolbe & Büttner, 2020; Li et al., 2019) or witnessing abuse of one's mother during childhood (Stöckl & Penhale, 2015); being sexually victimized early in life (Stöckl & Penhale, 2015); being of lower socioeconomic status (Ahmadabadi et al., 2020; Reichel, 2017); having children (Sanz-Barbero et al., 2018); being of immigrant status (Sanz-Barbero et al., 2018); having a romantic partner who misuses alcohol (Cunradi, 2007; Kraanen et al., 2014; Stöckl & Penhale, 2015) and substance misuse by the victim (Kraanen et al., 2014); belonging to the LGBTQIA+ community, particularly for those who are transgender (Langenderfer-Magrud et al., 2016); and, for women, having lower levels of power within the relationship (Diamond-Smith et al., n.d.).

In terms of risk factors for perpetrating IPV, being a survivor of family or partner violence is one of the strongest predictors (Okuda et al., 2015). However, other factors that may contribute to the risk for becoming an IPV perpetrator include the following: the presence of a personality disorder and/or alcohol use disorder, being lower income earning status, having limited social support, and being young (Okuda et al., 2015). Denial and rationalization among IPV perpetrators are common. Perpetrators often victim blame to justify their abusive actions (Russell & Hamel, 2022). However, when they acknowledge their trespasses, it may be that IPV perpetrators are more likely to report some types of IPV that are less socially admonished (e.g., emotional abuse) and deny types of IPV that are met with high amounts of social disapproval (e.g., physical abuse, sexual abuse; Walsh & Stephenson, 2023). Even in cases in which individuals have previously acknowledged their abusive behavior, they may deny their IPV perpetration when faced with social and/or legal consequences (Walsh & Stephenson, 2023).

The aforementioned risk factors for IPV only capture a limited number of the aspects that contribute to the increased risk of violence within romantic relationships. One can observe that some of the same risk factors for experiencing IPV are also risk factors for perpetrating IPV, such as experiencing violence within the home as a child and current substance misuse. This does not suggest, though, that all, or even most, individuals who are reared in an abusive home will grow up to either perpetrate or experience partner violence. Indeed, the constellation of factors that lead to IPV are unique for each individual and couple, and there are far more individuals than not who survive childhood maltreatment and go on to live highly productive lives with emotionally rich and supportive relationships. Regrettably, those are not the types of relationships that are the focus of this chapter, though.

Emerging Approaches to Partner Violence

LO2 Despite the long history of partner abuse, only since 1974 has there been a consistent and planned systematic approach to the problem. Erin Pizzey's book *Scream Quietly or the Neighbors Will Hear* (1974) was responsible for the start of the first women's shelter in England. Subsequently, in the United States, the National Organization for Women, along with grassroots organizations such as the Massachusetts Coalition Against Sexual Assault and Domestic Violence, has come to the forefront in developing funding sources, shelters, support groups, organizing and training manuals, and legislation for those who experience IPV. Such increased public awareness and the efforts of feminist and other citizens' groups resulted in the formation of the National Coalition Against Domestic Violence to promote a national power base for abused individuals and families (Capps, 1982). This group has exerted a good deal of social and legislative pressure to combat the problem of IPV. The Domestic Abuse Intervention Project in Duluth, Minnesota, has become internationally known as the Duluth model for its integrated approach to the problem (Pence & Shepard, 1999). The Duluth model has become internationally known because of its massive and sustained effort to get every agency that comes in contact with an IPV incident—from 911 dispatch that receives the first call to the last judge, probation officer, or therapist who signs off on the IPV perpetrator as finished with intervention—involved in a systematic and integrated manner so that no abused person or IPV perpetrator falls through the cracks (Home of the Duluth Model, 2011).

Thus, over the last four decades, the country's approach to IPV has changed dramatically. First,

there has been a shift in law enforcement departments, increased prosecution of partner violence, and enhanced legal protection through tougher protective orders and warrantless arrests. In many cities and states, a LEO call to a domestic dispute in which violence is involved now results in a mandatory arrest; and if convicted, the perpetrator is mandated by the court to either participate in counseling and a Batterer Intervention Program (BIP; now often referred to as Domestic Violence Perpetrator Programs) or go to jail (Goodman & Epstein, 2011; Pence & Shepard, 1999; Shupe et al., 1987). Second, as a result of lobbying efforts by activists, state legislatures have enacted protection laws with teeth in them that allow judges to tailor-make orders of protections suited to individual cases (Goodman & Epstein, 2011). Third, countywide coordinated community responses on the order of the Duluth model have been formed (Goodman & Epstein, 2011). Fourth, domestic violence units have been formed in law enforcement departments, probation and parole offices, states attorneys' offices, and domestic violence courts, which all coordinate efforts to reduce partner violence (Chalk & King, 1998, p. 172; Pence & Shepard, 1999).

A growing number of academicians have focused research on family violence, gender roles, and male dominance. Their scholarship has resulted in social activism that has debunked the "safe haven" notion of the family (Jasinski & Williams, 1998, pp. vi–vii), and brought partner and family violence into public view. The Violence Against Women Act of 1994 provided $1.2 billion for the improvement of services and community support for domestic violence victims, the criminal justice system's response to violent crimes against women, safety for women in public transit and public parks, assistance to victims of sexual assault, and support for a variety of educational, health, and database services. This bill was reauthorized in 2000 with an increase of $3.3 billion over 5 years to community services to aid survivors of domestic violence, sexual assault, and stalking. It was reauthorized again in 2005, 2013, and 2022 and has received continuous funding. An overview of its many activities can be found at the website of the Department of Justice's Office of Violence Against Women (https://nnedv.org).

Media attention about the severity of the problem has raised public consciousness. Television documentaries, newspaper articles, media coverage, and social media posts have attracted attention, changed public perspectives, and removed some of the cloak of secrecy from IPV. Stories such as those of Francine Hughes (subject of the movie *The Burning Bed*), who suffered prolonged and severe beatings by her husband and who finally killed him by pouring kerosene around his bed and setting it on fire, have had an impact on the courts by challenging legal precedents and assumptions about homicide and self-defense (Edwards, 1989). Indeed, psychologist Lenore Walker's (1989) book *Terrifying Love* is a chilling and eye-opening account of her experiences as an expert witness in murder trials of battering victims who have killed their assailants. The result has been the recognition of a history of abuse called the **battered wife syndrome** (posttraumatic stress disorder [PTSD]-like symptoms due to battering) (Walker, 2000, pp. 160–161), which is now known as **battered women syndrome**, as a valid part of a legal defense for abused women who kill their husbands (Chalk & King, 1998, pp. 171–172).

Once arrested, IPV perpetrators are required to go through a variety of different educational programs to teach them not to abuse (Geffner & Rosenbaum, 2002; Mederos, 1999; Rosenbaum & Kunkel, 2009; Sonkin & Dutton, 2003). Treating perpetrators has become a big-time business. For example, in 2006, there were 450 registered BIPs, serving more than 25,000 perpetrators in California alone (California State Auditor, 2006). There is no way of knowing how many BIPs operate in the United States as a whole, but as of 2017, 47 states employed standards or guidelines pertaining to BIPs (Ferraro, 2017). However, the effectiveness of BIPs is controversial, and some authors argue that revisions are needed to align BIPs more closely with the evidence base (Babcock et al., 2016). Programs for female offenders are fewer, and the evidence for program effectiveness is also lacking (Clearinghouse for Military Family Readiness, 2017). However, all states now have laws on the books that make IPV a crime, and domestic violence courts may mandate sentences ranging from jail time to BIPs (Rosenbaum & Kunkel, 2009).

Dynamics of Partner Violence

Psychosocial and Cultural Dynamics

LO3 The overarching dynamic that has held sway over violence directed toward women is the belief in male supremacy. This belief is the result of a long-term sexist, paternalistic social order that rewards aggressive behavior in men but expects women to be passive and submissive (Benjamin & Walz, 1983, p. 65; Pence & Shepard, 1999). This stereotypical and dated view has produced a volatile mix of personality dynamics between the "traditional" man and woman. The flash point of such a mix occurs when the man who lives the traditional male image of chief breadwinner and director of the family perceives himself as losing power in the conjugal relationship.

The question of power is the fuse that ignites this explosive mixture. In this view, the woman's position is to obey, conciliate, perform traditional domestic duties, and, in general, be subservient. Any attempt to establish herself in her own right is likely to be met with punishment for overstepping her bounds (Benjamin & Walz, 1983, pp. 74–77; Pence & Shepard, 1999). Violence, though, is not something that develops only in families. It involves a complex interplay of social, cultural, and psychological factors, and to say that a patriarchal system alone is responsible for partner and family violence would seem to fall far short of the mark (Dutton, 1995, pp. 27–62).

The fact is that a great many men who have patriarchal attitudes go through their entire partnered lives without assaulting their spouse, and abusers' sociopolitical beliefs don't discriminate them from nonabusers (Hotaling & Sugarman, 1986; Straus & Gelles, 1986). So, is there one true theory of the abusive/assaultive personality that leads to partner violence? The answer to that question is a resounding "No!"—although most of the following theories have their fervent supporters who would vehemently disagree with that statement. The following theories encapsulate past and present thinking about the causes of IPV. Most of these theories were originally proposed from the perspective of women survivors and male offenders of IPV. However, many of the underlying assumptions could be extended to transgender, gender nonbinary individuals, and men who experience IPV.

Attachment/traumatic Bonding Theory. Attachment theory is one means through which to conceptualize the origins of IPV (Dutton & White, 2012; Katafiasz, 2020). Disruptions of attachment in early life arouse intense anger, grief, sorrow, and anxiety in the child and diminish the child's ability to form mutual and trusting relationships as an adult (Bowlby, 1988). Although various forms of insecure adult attachment do not typically lead to violent relational patterns, some evidence points to the role of disrupted attachment patterns in the development of IPV during adulthood (Doumas et al., 2008; Velotti et al., 2022).

For example, Doumas and colleagues (2008) found higher rates of male and female perpetrated IPV when the male partners demonstrated avoidant attachment (i.e., emotionally detached, untrusting) and the female partners demonstrated anxious attachment (i.e., fear abandonment, seek validation and intense closeness). And Velotti and colleagues (2022) found that anxious attachment patterns were related to all forms of IPV. Take, for example, a child whose parents were unreliable, abusive, needy, or otherwise unequal to the task of child rearing. As an adult, that person may be very sensitive to fears of abandonment and enmeshment. The partner may contribute to these fears through their own fears of abandonment. Each partner creates ways to control the other to avoid being abandoned. One of those ways is through violence. Traumatic bonding may explain why some people stay with or return to their abusive partners (Dutton & Painter, 1993). However, some scholar suggest that attachment-based therapy may be a suitable approach to treating IPV (Gibby & Whiting, 2023).

Coercive Control. Morgan (1982) used the term **conjugal or intimate terrorism** to describe a tactic akin to brainwashing and political terrorism in which violence or the threat of violence is used to break the victim's resistance and bend them to the terrorist's (abuser's) will. Typical brainwashing and terrorist tools such as social and physical isolation, torture, sleep deprivation, malnourishment, dictating the use of the victim's time, bondage, false confessions, and denouncing and belittling the victim to significant others are all standard operating procedures of abusers to enhance the victim's dependency on them. Johnson (1995) identifies this type of offender as indeed a terrorist, representative of the type that people who seek out protective shelters describe. People who are abused by these offenders have more injuries, take more painkillers, have more PTSD symptoms, are attacked more frequently, and are less likely to have the violence stop (Johnson & Leone, 2005). This pathological offender is very different from the general population of situational abusers and is extremely dangerous.

Cultural Reinforcement. Sociological theories cover a wide gamut of specific theories that are psychosocially and culturally bound. These theories find the roots of violence in institutions ranging from the culture at large down to the family unit. Societal attitudes about the legitimate use of violence to achieve personal ends have their roots in a tradition of perceived "national interest." As a nation, we promote and glorify the controlled use of aggression for protection, law and order, self-defense, and national interest (Benjamin & Walz, 1983, pp. 64–66). Force is a major resource in maintaining the existing social structure and projecting national presence. This notion has been extended to the family by at least implicit permission of the state. For the state, the family is the basic disciplinary agent—family over individual, man over woman, adult over child. Control is direct, continuous, personalized, and an efficient way of keeping intact the past social order of the state (Capps, 1982).

Exchange Theory. Exchange theory (Gelles & Cornell, 1985) is a variant of a learning theory approach. It proposes that perpetrators of abuse hit people because they can (Carden, 1994). As long as the costs for being violent do not outweigh the rewards, violence will invariably be used as a method of control (Hampton et al., 1999). Particularly when social control agents such as law enforcement, criminal charges, imprisonment, loss of status, and loss of income are not used as negative sanctions that increase the cost of the behavior, perpetrators will continue to engage in abusive behavior. Gender inequality in physical size, financial resources, and social status allows abusers to become violent without fear of retribution. Although there may be loss of status in the larger society for being a perpetrator of abuse, there are certain subcultures in which aggressive and violent behaviors are proof of being strong. Finally, exacting "costs" from a partner to pay for their supposed "sins and transgressions" is itself satisfying to the perpetrator (Gelles & Cornell, 1985, pp. 120–125).

Feminist Theory. For generations, patriarchal structures of society have enforced or permitted various crimes against women, such as IPV, rape, incest, sexual mutilation, nonconsensual sex work, and a host of other sexist restrictions to keep women in servile positions. Early feminist theory conceptualized IPV as the product of patriarchal systems (George & Stith, 2014) and is credited with being a driving force in shifting social conceptualizations surrounding men's marital right to abuse women (Cannon, 2020). However, modern feminism is largely characterized by a social justice focus that acts in opposition to oppressive systems for all minoritized groups (George & Stith, 2014). From this view, IPV is not singularly and causally connected to patriarchal social systems. Rather, modern feminist theorists conceptualize IPV as the result of a complex intersection of oppression related to multiple aspects of one's identity, such as race, ethnicity, religion, gender, educational achievement, ability status, and socioeconomic status (Cardenas, 2023; George & Stith, 2014). Furthermore, modern application of feminist theory to IPV has sought to examine the dynamics of female perpetration of IPV and "deconstruct gender and power binaries" for all couples, including couples within the LGBTQIA+ community (Cannon et al., 2015, p. 681).

Intraindividual Theory. There is evidence that psychopathology and neurophysiological disorders may play a greater part in some perpetrators of IPV than was previously thought. Personality disorders, such as antisocial personality disorder and borderline personality disorder, may be related particularly to IPV perpetration but potentially also to IPV victimization (Collison & Lynam, 2021). Additionally, the presence of PTSD was found to be related to the perpetration of IPV by both men and women in a South African sample (Breet et al., 2019). And correlations were found between IPV, depression, alcohol misuse, and other mental health disorders among both active duty and veteran military personnel (Sparrow et al., 2017). We spoke earlier about the role of alcohol misuse in the incidence of IPV, but there is also research to support cocaine use as a factor in the perpetration of IPV for both men and women (Crane et al., 2014). These studies illustrate the point that a wide variety of mental health conditions play a significant role in IPV perpetration and victimization.

Learned Helplessness/Battered Woman Syndrome. Learning theory approaches operate on the principle that both perpetration and acceptance of physical and psychological abuse are conditioned and learned behaviors. A great deal of research examines the relationship between being abused by parents and/or witnessing interparental violence as a child and being violent toward a partner as an adult (Godbout et al., 2019; Li et al., 2020; Sijtsema et al., 2020). Foremost among these theories is Lenore Walker's (1984, 1989, 2000) theory of learned helplessness, which she adapted from animal studies conducted on random, noncontingent punishment (Seligman, 1972). Applied to IPV in particular, the theory proposes that abused individuals stay in abusive relationships because they have been conditioned to believe they cannot predict their own safety and that nothing they or anyone

else does will alter their terrible circumstances. Over time, through continuous conditioning, the person loses hope and feels completely incapable of leaving. Walker's (2017) book, *Battered Women Syndrome* provides a rich description of the cycle of abuse and characterization of PTSD-like symptomatology of battered women syndrome.

Walker (1984, 1989, 2000) proposed a number of factors in childhood and adulthood that are building blocks for learned helplessness. Childhood factors include witnessing or experiencing physical abuse, sexual abuse or molestation, health problems or chronic illness, stereotypical sex roles, and rigid tradition. Such experiences teach the child that external, autocratic, and often whimsical forces dictate outcomes. In adulthood, factors that are instigated by the abuser include an emergent pattern of violence; sexual abuse; jealousy; overpossessiveness; intrusiveness and isolation; threat of harm; observed violence toward other people, animals, or things; and alcohol or drug abuse misuse. Given these conditions, the victim cannot escape the noncontingent punishment and, thus, loses any effectiveness in being able to control what happens to them (Walker, 2000, pp. 10–12).

The term **helplessness** has caused a great deal of furor from feminists because they see this pejorative term as casting women in a victim role with few resources or little empowerment. However, according to Walker (1989), women are not helpless in the standard sense of the term. What **learned helplessness** means is that battered women choose behavioral responses that have the highest predictability of causing them the least harm in the known situation (pp. 50–52) or what Gondolf and Fisher (1988) call the survivor hypothesis, in which women become very active and resourceful in protecting themselves and their children (Browne, 1997). Because of the extreme and often lethal violence that occurs when these women attempt to leave and the lack of social support for making any attempt, it is understandable that a "Better the devil I know!" philosophy predominates for many abused women.

Masochism. Psychoanalytic theory, which has held masochism to be the primary motivating factor in abusive relationships, is now mostly obsolete in the therapeutic community. There is no empirical research to substantiate the notion that erotic enjoyment of pain through battering is a trait found in abused women (Okun, 1986; Stark & Flitcraft, 1988). From a feminist point of view, this theory held sway for a long time because the male-dominated field of psychiatry found it a convenient pigeonhole for a troublesome problem. Until interest in the problem was generated in the 1970s, little research was presented to refute the idea.

Nested Ecological Theory. Because no single factor theory has effectively explained the IPV phenomenon, an integrated, multifactor approach may be the best way to understand the complexities of IPV (Brewster, 2002). Dutton (1985, 1995) proposed an ecological theory that integrates many of the foregoing theories. Four layers of variables operate within the ecosystem. First is a core of individual experience composed of intrapersonal psychological factors such as shame, denial, and hostility. Second is a family system layer, in which the individual experiences such negative actions as abandonment, neglect, and abuse. Third is a community/peer layer, which inculcates fundamental religious training, alcohol and drug use, and rigid gender role socialization. Finally, in a larger societal context, the individual is exposed to sociopolitical gender inequities, media portrayal of subjugation and violence against women, and racial/ethnic prejudices. As a result, it is not just one but many factors that operate within the individual, in interpersonal relationships, and throughout the larger social environment that are communicated and synthesized to rationalize IPV as a viable option (Hampton et al., 1999), despite the objective wrongness of such actions.

Psychological Entrapment. Psychological entrapment proposes that individuals experiencing IPV do not leave the relationship because they feel as though they have too much time, energy, and emotion invested in the relationship (Brewster, 2002), or they would feel shame if their terrible secret were found out (Buchbinder & Eisikovits, 2003). They engage in wishful thinking that some miracle will occur or that they can somehow change the significant other, and a nonviolent, intimate, and loving relationship will emerge. For some people, the shame of their abuse and the failed relationship is so great that they will do anything to keep it from public view. This shame-based reaction is based on the assumption that the person experiencing the abuse is somehow responsible for the abuse. Although we factually realize that is not true, perpetrators of IPV are highly skilled in making their victims feel responsible for the abusive actions perpetrated against them.

Stockholm Syndrome. This intriguing psychological reaction to abduction has its origins in 1973 during a bank heist in Stockholm, Sweden, in which individuals held captive developed an affectionate relationship with their captors (Klein, 2019). After 130 hours trapped in a bank vault with the captors, hostages felt a special affection for the captors, even going so far as to defend and protect the captors (Klein, 2019). Perhaps this was in response to perceived kindness from the captors and the belief that the captors spared the hostages' lives (Klein, 2019). Despite ongoing debate regarding the clinical utility of Stockholm Syndrome (Namnyak et al., 2008), the concept continues to be used in lay vernacular to describe situations in which abused or captive individuals develop attachment toward their perpetrator(s). Applied to IPV, it might be that the individual who experiences IPV becomes so completely isolated and subjugated by their abuser that any form of perceived kindness (no matter how small) is conceptualized by the victim as sincere care from the perpetrator. There is some continued query into the application of Stockholm Syndrome to IPV (Ahmad et al., n.d.; Chattoraj, 2022; Hertlein & Teichert, 2023), although this remains a debated topic. Stockholm Syndrome may be better conceptualized as an appeasement strategy used for survival (Bailey et al., 2023).

Psychological Factors

LO4 Psychologically, both parties to an abusive relationship may have certain identifiable characteristics. You should clearly understand that these are not just separate and individual ingredients but complex forces that interrelate with one another and, thus, increase the odds of IPV. To that point, it can also be helpful to understand that IPV is not always unidirectional (only one partner engaging in abusive behavior) but may be bidirectional (both parties engaging in abusive behavior) in a reciprocal manner (Plouffe et al., 2022). For exemplative purposes, let's examine some common characteristics of violent partners.

To be sure, IPV occurs within transgender and gender-nonconforming couples, likely at higher rates than in cisgender couples (Valentine et al., 2017). However, most research on psychological factors that may contribute to IPV is based on gender binary samples. Robertson and colleagues (2020) conducted a meta-analysis of 43 studies from 10 countries that addressed the presence of psychopathy among individuals who perpetrate IPV, among both men and women. They found evidence to suggest that the presence of psychopathy is related to IPV perpetration. However, they were unable to identify distinct patterns in the type of psychopathy and the perpetration of IPV (Robertson et al., 2020). Beyond psychopathy in particular, other studies address the presence of specific personality traits and behaviors that may be implicated in IPV perpetration. Some common characteristics of men who perpetrate IPV include the following: higher than average patterns of anger (Eckhardt et al., 2008; Norlander & Eckhardt, 2005) and hostility (Norlander & Eckhardt, 2005), difficulties related to alcohol and/or substance misuse (Amegbor & Pascoe, 2021; Eckhardt et al., 2008; Singh et al., 2014), patterns of impulsivity (Caetano et al., 2008), feelings of powerlessness (Caetano et al., 2008), low self-esteem (Dowgwillo et al., 2016), and patterns of emotion dysregulation (Ross, 2011). Interestingly, Ross (2011) found that men tend to endorse retaliation as their primary reason for engaging in abusive behavior. However, Ross was unable to identify situational or relational factors against which the participants were retaliating. Instead, due to their high endorsement of Borderline Personality Disorder (BPD) symptoms, Ross hypothesizes that retaliation among men perpetrators of IPV might be more reflective of personality traits than of situational factors that may trigger retaliatory responses. Maneta et al. (2013) found similar patterns in their examination of BPD traits and IPV perpetration and victimization among men and women. Specifically, they found that BPD traits were associated in men with both IPV perpetration and IPV victimization, while BPD traits were only associated with IPV victimization in women (Maneta et al., 2013). Further, in our experience, we have found that many men who use violence in their intimate relationships tend to have rigid ideas regarding relationships and expectations for their partner, are often prone to jealousy, may lack in empathy, and can appear very charming to others outside of the relationship. The latter descriptors often pertain to characteristics of Antisocial Personality Disorder, which aligns with research conducted by Dowgwillo and colleagues (2016). Deciphering the factors leading to IPV is not an exact science, though, and it is impossible to develop a character sketch for those who will perpetrate violence against their partners and those who will not. Further, it should go without saying that this list is not exhaustive, but it helps to demonstrate that there are some common characteristics of men who tend to perpetrate violence against

their partners. And knowing these characteristics can aid in screening for IPV.

The research on women who perpetrate violence against their intimate partners is fairly limited (Laskey, 2016), but make no mistake that women can also commit violence against their partners with devastating effects (Morgan & Wells, 2016; White & Dutton, 2013). Available studies suggest some commonalities in women partners who are violent: patterns of impulsivity (Caetano et al., 2008), feelings of powerlessness (Caetano et al., 2008), difficulties with emotion regulation (Ross, 2011), disagreeableness (Dowgwillo et al., 2016), difficulty with emotional closeness (Dowgwillo et al., 2016), and presence of one or more personality disorders (Spidel et al., 2013). To the latter point, Spidel and colleagues (2013) found that Antisocial Personality Disorder (APD), Borderline Personality Disorder (BPD), and Narcissistic Personality Disorder (NPD) were highly implicated in women who perpetrate violence in their relationships. In fact, they found that women who met the diagnostic threshold for BPD tended to be physically violent, women who demonstrated traits of NPD tended to engage in higher rates of verbal violence, and women who displayed traits of ASP tended to engage in both physical and verbal abuse (Spidel et al., 2013). Interestingly, they also found that nearly three quarters of their sample met criteria for PTSD, suggesting a trauma-informed conceptualization of personality disorder traits (Spidel et al., 2013). Although not related to personality characteristics, Caetano and colleagues (2008) found that women who are employed are more likely to perpetrate IPV than women who are unemployed. (Caetano et al., 2008). However, it is important to note that some violence perpetrated by women may be reactionary to violence perpetrated by their opposite gender partner (Herrera et al., 2008; Plouffe et al., 2022; Ross, 2011) or as retaliation against real or perceived hostile dynamics and/or high levels of control within the relationship (Ross, 2011). Research does not abound on the converse (i.e., men defending themselves against women perpetrators), but it is certainly the case that some men engage in hostile defensive behavior as a self-protective measure.

IPV emerges in response to complex and intense interpersonal and intrapersonal factors. Although there tend to be commonalities among individuals who exercise violence within their relationships, it should be noted that the above-mentioned characteristics address correlations rather than causations.

Put another way, just because individuals may possess some of the aforementioned characteristics does not mean they will become abusive in their relationships.

Stressors. If power is the fuse, then stress is the match that lights the fuse. As the idealized image of the relationship breaks down and environmental stresses build up, couples can become engaged in an ever-increasing spiral of violent interaction (Barnett et al., 1980). Although they are not generic to all partner violence, a list of factors that seem to appear over and over in IPV follows (Ahmadabadi et al., 2020; Barnett et al., 1980, pp. 7–9; Benjamin & Walz, 1983; Bograd, 2005; Brown et al., 2010; Cunradi, 2007; Finkelhor et al., 1983; Gelles & Cornell, 1985; Halbsgut, 2011; Jasinski & Williams, 1998; Koverola & Panchanadeswaran, 2004; Okun, 1986; Parker et al., 1993; Schwab-Reese et al., 2016; Stuart et al., 2006; Walker, 1984, p. 51; Williams et al., 2008). These factors may be introduced by the abuser to control the situation, may occur as a product of the relationship itself, or may be environmentally introduced from outside the relationship.

1. **Geographic isolation.** Because of geographic location, the victim has no friends nearby who can provide a support system. A person living in a remote area who cannot drive is an example of the worst case—literally being marooned and held captive by an abusive partner.
2. **Social isolation.** Because of extreme emotional dependence, the abused individual expects all needs to be met by their partner and has no significant others to turn to when they are assaulted.
3. **Economic stress.** When a partner is unemployed or underemployed, has inadequate housing, is pressured by creditors, and cannot feed and clothe their children by themself, they become financially dependent on the abusive partner.
4. **Medical conditions.** Long-term, chronic medical conditions for either spouse or children exact tremendous financial and emotional costs.
5. **Conflict over parenting.** A lack of knowledge of effective parenting skills and/or conflict over parental roles can lead to situations that start as minor disciplinary problems and escalate into violence in the family.
6. **Pregnancy.** Abusive acts might include interfering with the childbearing partner's use of birth control, pressuring them to give birth to an unwanted child, creating anxiety over providing for the new baby, or arousing jealousy over attention given to a newborn. Regardless of the specific manifestation of the event, pregnancy is an especially acute crisis point for potential abuse.
7. **Family dysfunction.** A veritable kaleidoscope of problems causes dysfunction in the family. Some of these problems are related to age and number of children, presence of stepchildren, loyalty conflicts, death, desertion, and career change.
8. **Alcohol and drug misuse.** Chemical dependence serious enough to cause economic chaos and severe emotional disturbance characterizes addictive families and has spin-offs that commonly include IPV. The insidious problem with alcohol and drugs is that they are often used as an excuse for abusive behavior that is normally prohibited by societal norms and standards.
9. **Educational and/or vocational disparity.** When one partner in a relationship has higher educational attainment or higher vocational status than the other, this may raise questions of adequacy and responsibility with both parties. This may be particularly problematic when the individual whose social constructs enforce a sense of gender-based responsibility and/or superiority is unable to provide for their family.
10. **Age.** One of the most consistent risk factors for IPV perpetration is age. Research seems to consistently demonstrate that individuals at younger ages are more likely to engage in abuse within their relationships.
11. **Disenfranchisement.** Seeking help from the authorities for IPV may be very aversive to racial and ethnic monitories, members of the LGBTQIA+ community, individuals of immigrant status, and other marginalized groups because of their previous negative experiences with or fear of retribution from the system.
12. **Rejection.** The abuser's perception of rejection is an antecedent to abuse. Particularly for men, having a family of origin in which rejection frequently occurred tends to yield adults who are extremely sensitive to any behavior construed as rejection. Their response is likely to be aggressive.
13. **Threat to masculinity.** Some men who perceive themselves as less masculine see their use of threat and/or violence as affirming their masculinity in comparison to men who have good self-concepts who do not perpetrate abuse.

Myths About IPV

LO6 The following myths encapsulate numerous arguments used by those who would submerge, camouflage, and diminish IPV (Gelles & Cornell, 1985; Hampton et al., 1999; Massachusetts Coalition of Battered Women Service Groups, 1981; Okun, 1986; Roberts, 2002; Rollero & De Piccoli, 2020; Stark & Flitcraft, 1988; Straus et al., 1980; Weitzman, 2000).

1. **"Abused individuals overstate the case."** Any person who has contusions, lacerations, and broken bones is not overstating anything. In any other instance, such outcomes are referred to as *assault and battery*.

2. **"Abused individuals provoke the abuse."** Minor perceived infractions can serve as justification for perpetrators to abuse their romantic partners, thereby perpetuating a scenario in which the abused party begins to internalize feelings of responsibility for the abuse. Even in cases in which the abused person engages in antagonizing behavior, there is no excuse for perpetrating violence against one's partner.

3. **"Abuse is a private, family matter."** When abused individuals are disenfranchised from their homes and the children of abusive relationships learn the pathological roles of IPV perpetuated by their parent(s), IPV transcends the home and becomes society's problem. All 50 states now have warrantless arrest policies for IPV. Abuse is anything but private.

4. **"Alcohol misuse is the prime reason for IPV."** Although alcohol plays a part in many cases of abuse and is present and used by both men and women who engage in violent relationships, it may be only an excuse for, and not the cause of, violent behavior. There are many violent relationships in which alcohol is not present.

5. **"IPV occurs only in problem families."** The dynamic representation of stress factors that assail families shows that any family, at any given point, may be classified as "problem;" there is no such thing as a perfect family.

6. **"Only low-income and working-class families experience violence."** Although members of those socioeconomic classes often come to the attention of law enforcement agencies at a much greater frequency than middle- or upper-class members, statistics from shelters, 911 calls, and crisis line calls indicate that IPV has no class boundaries.

7. **"The abuse cannot be that bad or the abused would not stay."** The host of personal factors that tie an abused person to the relationship militate heavily against simply picking up and leaving.

8. **"A husband has patriarchal rights."** What a man does in his own family is not his own business when the emotional overflow of what he does spills over into the community. No amount or kind of justification can excuse IPV.

9. **"The abused individual exaggerates the problem to exact revenge."** Reporting IPV—whether committed by a total stranger or one's spouse—is no exaggeration. If revenge were the motive, there would be a host of ways of going about revenge that would be far less traumatic than calling or showing up at an abuse shelter.

10. **"Women are too sensitive, especially when they are pregnant."** If a person is too sensitive because she objects to being beaten, thrown down a flight of stairs, or hit in the face with a lamp, then we would suppose that everyone is overly sensitive.

11. **"IPV is rare."** The statistics reported in this chapter clearly indicate otherwise. Partner and family violence is endemic in society.

12. **"IPV is confined to mentally disturbed or 'sick' people."** Although there may be a correlation between IPV and certain psychological disorders, there is no definitive connection between any given psychiatric diagnosis and perpetration of IPV. And countless other individuals who meet diagnostic criteria for those same disorders do not engage in IPV. Remember that correlation is not causation.

13. **"Violence and love cannot coexist."** Strange as it may seem, members of violent families may still love one another. This paradoxical aspect is most problematic because children in such families may grow up believing that people hit those they love. Although they may learn otherwise in adulthood, those early disruptions to attachment and social modeling can present challenges pertaining to their intimate relationships.

14. **"Elder abuse between intimates is neither prevalent nor dangerous."** Because of the debilitating factors that come with aging, the potential for physical abuse becomes greater and more lethal as partners can become more frustrated, angry, and depressed over the declining physical and mental capabilities of both themselves and their partners.

Profiling the IPV Perpetrator

LO7   Researchers have examined multiple personality and behavioral typologies of abusers/ batterers. Dutton (1995), Fowler and Western (2011), Gondolf (1985), Hastings and Hamberger (1988), Holtzworth-Munroe and Stuart (1994), Holzworth-Munroe and associates (1999, 2003), and Saunders (1992) have all developed typologies of abusers based on clusters of demographic, personality, and abuse variables. Holtzworth-Munroe and Stuart (1994) and Holtzworth-Munroe and associates (1999, 2003) have compiled three major groupings—family only, dysphoric (anxious)/borderline, and generally violent/ antisocial—and a fourth subgroup, low-level antisocial. Characteristics of the **family only abuser** include high dependency, impulsivity, poor communication skills, and family-of-origin violence. The **dysphoric/ borderline abuser** has a history of parental rejection and child abuse, delinquent acts, poor communication and social skills, violence-as-a-solution ideation, extreme fears of abandonment, and low remorse. The **low-level antisocial abuser** has antisocial behavior and moderate levels of domestic and general violence. Fowler and Western's (2011) typologies conform closely to the foregoing types with psychopathic, hostile/controlling, and borderline/dependent. The **generally violent/antisocial abuser** has all the foregoing characteristics but to a much more profound degree and probably falls into what Jasinski and Williams (1998, p. 1) call the **terroristic abuser.** Such people are extremely aggressive and impulsive and view violence as appropriate to any provocation inside or outside the home.

The family only abusers are the largest group, and their behavior is consistent with Walker's (1979) cycle of violence. Its members are likely to be contrite and apologetic after IPV incidents. Approximately half of abusers fall within this category (Petersson & Strand, 2020). The dysphoric/borderline and antisocial types are typical of how women who flee to shelters describe their abusers. They are the most dangerous types of abusers. Differences in these groups in regard to their level of violence appear to remain somewhat stable over time, and they do not appear to move from one group to the other (Cavanaugh & Gelles, 2005). Thankfully, not all partner violence escalates, nor does it evolve into more dangerous personality types (Holtzworth-Munroe et al., 2003).

There is a good deal of debate over the use of profiling because of the diversity of typologies in IPV populations. However, Gibbons et al. (2011) used the Millon Clinical Multiaxial Inventory with a sample of 177 batterers and found that 54 percent fell into a personality disorder category and 37 percent could be characterized as having severe pathology. Taking the foregoing typologies together with an assessment device like the Millon, consider that Eke and associates (2011) found that of their sample of men who had murdered or attempted to murder an intimate partner, 42 percent had previously committed crimes, 18 percent had a psychiatric history, and 15 percent had both. These individuals were given the Ontario Domestic Assault Risk Assessment. Their mean score was in the 80th percentile of "at risk" for domestic violence. The researchers concluded that the use of validated risk assessment data for abusers and indicators of pathology and/or criminal behavior would increase the ability to predict who would violently assault an intimate partner and hopefully aid in intervention and the prevention of homicidal acts toward intimate partners. Loinaz (2014) used the Brief Spousal Assault Form for the Evaluation of Risk (B-SAFER) to classify offenders and predict recidivism. His study on incarcerated abusers in Spain found high predictive validity with both the nonpathological group and the antisocial/pathological group. He further found that the antisocial pathological group had about a 2 to 1 recidivism rate. We believe some fine-tuning of these instruments, applied to all abusers, would be of some worth in determining their degree of potential lethality and guiding judicial disposition as to what kind of intervention they should receive. Combined with an improved understanding of demographic factors, cooccurring mental health issues, and the assailant's readiness to change, understanding typology can be an important aspect of tailoring treatment for IPV (Butters et al., 2021).

The Cycle of Violence

LO8   Barnett and associates (1980) schematically represented the phases leading to the explosion of violence in the family. Walker's (1984) cycle theory of violence—(1) tension building, (2) battering and abuse, (3) contrition and loving respite—closely parallels these phases, and her research supports the theory (p. 95).

> **Phase I. Tranquility prevails.** The relationship mainly have been characterized as calm to this point, with no previous violent incidents, or a period of calm may follow an earlier violent episode.

Phase II. Tension starts to build. A variety of stressors impinge on the relationship. They may come in combination or singly from the common group already mentioned. However, there is no reduction of tension, and the situation grows more strained.

Phase III. A violent episode occurs. The episode may range from harsh words to a severe beating. At this phase, communication has broken down, and the situation is out of control.

Phase IV. The relationship takes on crisis proportions. A variety of options becomes available.

a. The abuser becomes remorseful and asks forgiveness. Sooner or later, the victim forgives the abuser, and calm is restored.

b. The abuser is not remorseful and feels their control over the situation has been established. The victim gives in and relinquishes control, and calm is restored.

c. The victim takes new action. Within this option are two possibilities: the abuser negotiates the situation, and, given that the negotiation is agreeable to the victim, calm is restored; or the abuser rejects the new action, and a crisis state continues.

It is at this last point, in which no possibility of resolution exists, that the victim is most likely to seek help by contacting an abuse center. Walker found that as the abuse continues, the loving contrition phase diminishes, and abuse becomes more prevalent (2000, p. 128). If effective assessment and intervention do not occur when the violence emerges (Phase III), the likelihood that the violence will recur and will be of greater intensity is dramatically increased (Barnett et al., 1980, p. 34). Dutton (1995, pp. 126–139) has demonstrated that this cycle closely fits that of the Borderline Personality Disorder (BPD) type of abuser.

Not all IPV relationships fit the cycle of violence. Abuse between partners may be a once-in-a-lifetime affair. But many women have reported being constantly terrorized and assaulted with no intermittent periods of relief (Dutton & Starzomski, 1993). These are most probably the victims of the antisocial, psychopathic type of abuser, who sees little need for contrition or remorse in dealing with a partner—or anybody else, for that matter.

Realities for Abused Individuals

LO9 Why, then, do individuals stay in an abusive relationship? For those who have no experience with violence in a relationship, it is an easy thing to say, "Leave the loser!" or "I wouldn't tolerate that. I'd call the cops and have them arrested!" or "Forget you, nobody does that to me, I'm leaving!" In actuality, most people who are in abusive relationships do leave, and this in itself is a courageous act because it is one of the most dangerous things they can do. The abuser tends to do poorly on their own and would often rather kill or die than be separated from their partner because they are more terrified of abandonment than violence or punishment (Walker, 1989, p. 65). It is remarkable that a number of people do leave, given their clear understanding that lives hang in the balance—their own, those of their children, and even the abuser's.

The same question could be asked of people who perpetrate IPV. Why do they stay? Henning and Connor-Smith (2011) examined more than 1,000 men who had been adjudicated for abusing their partners. More than half said they were planning on staying in the relationship. Their reasons included being older, caring about their children, attributing less blame to the woman for the alleged offenses and their arrest, and coming from a family where they saw the same thing as children and regretted modeling their parents' assaultive behavior. Ominously, the researchers also found that some men who were continuing the relationship had low relationship satisfaction predictors: having children, expressing hostile attitudes toward women, being jealous, blaming the victim for the arrest, and describing the victim as being aggressive.

Most women leave an abusive relationship an average of seven times but do so with varying degrees of permanency (Women Against Abuse, n.d.). The following reasons for staying in the relationship have been gleaned from a number of researchers (Benjamin & Walz, 1983; Bograd, 2005; Koverola & Panchanadeswaran, 2004; Okun, 1986; Pagelow, 1981; Storer et al., 2021; Walker, 1979, 1984, 1989, 2000), and these realities have nothing to do with the myths listed previously.

1. The abused person has a fear of reprisal or of aggravating the attacks even more.
2. Even though the situation may be intolerable for the victim, the children have their basic physical needs met.
3. The abused person will suffer shame, embarrassment, humiliation, and even ridicule if their secret gets out.
4. The abused person's self-concept is so strongly dependent on the relationship and perceived social

approval that leaving would be very destructive to them.

5. Early affection and prior love in the relationship persist, and by staying, the abused person hopes to salvage them.

6. If financially well off, the abused person is unable to forgo a reduction in their financial freedom.

7. In the cyclic nature of abuse, the mate may not be terrible 24 hours a day, 7 days a week. The abused person may tend to forget the abuse and remember only the good times.

8. Early role models of an abusive parent may lead the abused person to believe that relationships exist in no other way.

9. The abused person may hold religious values that strongly militate against separation, divorce, or anything less than filial subjugation to their partner's wishes.

10. The abused person may be undereducated, have small children to raise, and have limited or no job skills.

11. The abused person may be kept so socially, physically, geographically, and financially isolated that they have no resources of any kind to help them get out.

12. The abused person may be so badly injured that they are unable physically to leave.

13. The abused person may believe their partner's promise to reform.

14. The abused person may be concerned for children who are still at home.

15. Love or sorrow at the mate's professed inability to exist without them may impel them to stay.

16. Because of previous negative experiences with the authorities, the abused person may believe they have no options.

17. Due to language barriers or immigration status, the abused person may be unable to communicate the abuse, or they may be afraid to seek help.

18. The abused person may fear enforcing racial stereotypes by making their abuse known to others.

Secondary victimization may result by labeling abused women as hysterical, emotional, dramatic, untrustworthy, irresponsible, unlovable, or a bad parent, for example. Such labeling may provide professionals with "reasons" to do things to abused women, ranging from overmedication with psychotropic medications to sending them to jail and removing their children from the home. Any one of the revictimizations by well-meaning or not-so-well-meaning

institutions undermines assertiveness and reinforces submissiveness and compliance, which, in turn, increases vulnerability to abuse (Stark & Flitcraft, 1988; Walker, 1989). It is little wonder that a woman making her first call to an abuse center may be taking only an initial step in a series that sometimes goes on for years before she can make a complete break from the abusive relationship.

Intervention Strategies

In the past half decade, the raising of consciousness that IPV is endemic and that it exacts tremendous financial and emotional costs on society has caused an exponential rise in attempts at intervention. To that end, intervention strategies for IPV are different from other types of crises because they target both the abused and the abuser.

Assessment

LO10 Assessment of IPV is complex, is subject to controversy, and there are many unanswered questions in regard to its precursors, onset, and outcomes for both the abused and the abuser. Assessment is also problematic because of the transcrisis nature of IPV. Both perpetrators and those whom they abuse do not present themselves in a "steady state" that is amenable to stable and consistent measurement. Nonetheless, screening for IPV is a critically important process that should be part of both medical (Rabin et al., 2009) and clinical intake procedures.

Assessing the Risk of IPV. Graham et al. (2021) conducted a systematic review of available instruments that are intended to detect both IPV and the risk of partner homicide. They examined the reliability and validity of various instruments, such as the Brief Spousal Assault Form for the Evaluation of Risk (Kropp & Hart, 2004), the Danger Assessment (Campbell et al., 2009), the Spouse Violence Risk Assessment Inventory (Dayan et al., 2013), and multiple other instruments. In total, they synthesized 43 studies from the available research base to review reliability and validity for 18 different instruments used in varying settings and administered by different types of professionals, such as mental health workers, medical workers, and first responders (Graham et al., 2021). They found that many of the 18 instruments did not have a robust psychometric basis, although some instruments were supported by an adequate research base. Further, their analysis provided evidence of limited psychometric analyses pertaining to the application of these instruments with gender-diverse and same-sex couples (Graham et al., 2021). Graham et al. (2021) call attention to the need for enhanced analysis of IPV and partner homicide risk assessment instruments.

Personality Measures. Take a moment to imagine, if you have not personally experienced it, living in a home in which you are abused daily, whether it be emotionally, physically, sexually, financially, or a combination of them. Imagine that you feel stuck and hopeless that you will ever be free from your perpetrator's wrath. To be sure, individuals who live daily in IPV experience shifts in the way they perceive and interact with the world and the way they perceive themselves. To think that IPV does not dramatically affect survivors is to invalidate the gravity of the situation. However, the specific mechanisms by which IPV affects individuals are not uniform.

Assessment of survivors of IPV by personality measures is somewhat confounding and contradictory to what one might logically expect. One never really knows whether the personality factors found in IPV survivors were present before they were abused or are the result of the victimization (Abd El Moez et al., 2014). Indeed, the assessment of "psychological injury" is challenging, at best, and presents concerning implications for legal proceedings (Fariña Rivera et al., 2014). However, some authors suggest that reliable and valid assessment tools, such as the Minnesota Multiphasic Personality Inventory (MMPI), can be used as part of a holistic assessment process to help build the victim's credibility and identify key mental health markers that are highly related to trauma (Akl et al., 2023; Butcher et al., 2015). However, other authors suggest that there is not a single psychological profile of IPV survivors, and, as such, assessments such as the MMPI do not yield reliable results (Allen, 2020). Research demonstrates key aspects of survivors' mental health functioning, though, that are likely indicative of IPV victimization, such as depression, obsessive-compulsive behavior, anxiety and phobic anxiety, sensitivity in interpersonal interactions, paranoid thought processes, somatization, hostility (Vilariño et al., 2018), problems with intimacy, distorted cognition, suspiciousness, and emotional restriction (Torres et al., 2013), to name a few. To that end, the Battered Woman Syndrome Questionnaire (Millen et al., 2019) is used to help identify

women who display characteristic symptoms of IPV. Overall, women who experienced IPV may present many of the symptoms of posttraumatic stress disorder and can be placed for diagnostic purposes within the PTSD category of the DSM 5-TR (American Psychiatric Association, 2022).

Clinical Interview. Probably the best assessment device for partner abuse is a clinical interview. Any family history obtained during a clinical interview should include questions about hitting, threats, controlling, destruction of property or pets, forced sex, alcohol and drug use, and the partner's hyper-vigilance and paranoia about the client's actions (Jasinski & Williams, 1998, p. 37). Walker (1984, p. 122) also has one major rule of assessment that supersedes all others and to which your authors strongly subscribe: *When a person reports experiencing IPV, believe them and start intervention immediately.* It is a safe bet that whenever an IPV survivor seeks help, they are not carrying out the act as some means by which to get back at their partner; IPV survivors tend to only ask for help after the abuse has reached a critical point and become exceedingly serious.

Walker (1984, p. 26) found that only 14 percent of battered women surveyed would seek help after a first incident, 22 percent would seek help after a second incident, and 49 percent would seek help only after a series of incidents had taken place. Walker's data is dated, but current research suggests a continued trend toward limited help seeking, particularly through formal supports (Satyen et al., 2019). Given the length of time that passes and the degree of severity of the crisis that is typically reached before help is sought, triage assessment of the IPV survivor should first and foremost examine the survivor's safety and the safety of significant others, such as children. We can assume that an IPV survivor making an initial call to a crisis line will be at the extremely high end of the assessment scale. The survivor may be behaviorally out of control because of physical abuse that has just occurred. The survivor may be affectively out of control because of the trauma and the threat of more to come. Cognitively, the survivor may be just holding things together and may not be far from dissociating from the terrible reality of the situation.

Sadly, many people in the helping professions still confuse the effects of IPV with symptoms of other diagnoses. It is extremely important to be aware of the symptoms that may mask the underlying IPV. For example, compared to women who are not abused, women who experience IPV are at an elevated risk for suicide (Cavanaugh et al., 2011; MacIsaac et al., 2017), substance misuse (Stone & Rothman, 2019), and various medical conditions (Black, 2011). As we have already mentioned, there are a myriad of ways that individuals may respond to IPV, and the symptomatology for IPV is too diverse to pinpoint. However, helping professionals should remain attuned to possible indicators of trauma (e.g., magnified startle response, reexperiencing, anxiety, emotional lability), harmful attempts to cope with the trauma (e.g., substance misuse, self-injury, disordered eating), and physical indicators of abuse.

Crisis workers typically encounter IPV victims in the following four settings: in hospital emergency rooms and other medical care settings, on telephone crisis lines, in law enforcement follow-up operations on domestic violence calls at crisis centers, and at shelters (discussed later in this chapter). The operational strategy in all of these settings should be twofold. First and foremost, ask! Ask if the person has been abused, even if the presenting problem appears to have little to do with IPV. Chang and associates (2005) advise that workers give a reason for why they are asking about IPV to reduce the client's suspicions and minimize stigma and that they provide information, support, safety, and access to resources whether or not the client discloses IPV. By doing so, crisis workers are not seen as trying to diagnose a pathological condition but to communicate compassion, provide valuable information, and open the door for clients to self-disclose IPV and consider seeking services.

That show of concern creates increased levels of trust when questions about IPV are asked in an empathic manner, confidentiality is discussed, and nonjudgmental and supportive responses and concern for the person's safety are made with offers to provide help, even if IPV is not the basic issue that brings the client into counseling (Battaglia et al., 2003). The smorgasbord of symptoms presented in this chapter all come out of IPV. While there may be other reasons, one of the biggest mistakes a crisis worker can make is to not empathically query a person about IPV and validate their experiences (Day, 2009; Spangaro et al., 2011). When a client is validated by an external source who reaffirms that IPV is unacceptable, that act is a major contributor to the client taking action to remove themself from the abusive relationship (Day, 2009). Congruent with validation is the client's sense of support from community resources in providing them with information and supporting them

in making the countless decisions that range from career and geographic moves to religious and moral qualms they have over leaving the abusive relationship (McLeod et al., 2010).

Crisis Lines

Of all the dilemmas a crisis telephone worker faces, IPV is one of the worst. IPV survivors may present emotions that range from icily detached to hysterical to white-hot anger. No matter what the client's emotional response, the crisis worker's job is to try to help the client cope with the immediate situation (Roberts & Roberts, 2002). That immediate situation may include the perpetrator being present while the client makes the call. The client may call a crisis line instead of law enforcement in hopes that law enforcement will not have to become involved, but the notification of the abuse to an outside agency will make the abuser stop.

At times, the client may ask the crisis worker to talk to the abuser. In almost all cases, that is not a wise choice. The client should be asked if they are in danger and need law enforcement assistance. The focus is on the caller and the caller's safety, not attempting to defuse the abuser. If the abuser truly wants to be defused, then they may call the crisis line separately. Although the threat of further injury or death to the client may be extremely high, unless the crisis worker feels danger is imminent and can get the client to give their name and address so a 911 call can be made, the best the crisis worker can do is to offer short-term assistance to help ease physical pain and calm the client emotionally. The duty to warn certainly takes precedence over confidentiality, but deciding whether the danger is sufficiently imminent and lethal to necessitate a call to law enforcement is tricky and has future ramifications. Even then, the crisis worker may have raging internal debates about what to do. If the client is helped to get to a safe place, will that only enrage the abuser even more? Is the client really ready to make such a move? What assets does the client have to enable them to leave the relationship? What does the client need to enable them to be able to leave the abusive relationship? That is why the worker should carefully go over each area, making sure that all pertinent information and all possibilities of available action have been carefully considered. No other type of crisis presents as critical a need for comprehensive yet fast assessment than does IPV.

It is also worth remembering that if the crisis worker calls back a week later, the client may be going through a "honeymoon phase" and may seem not to have a care in the world, only to turn around later at the next abuse incident and beseech the crisis worker's help again. These situations, oscillating from extreme need one day to little, if any, need the next, can make crisis workers cynical and uncaring if they do not carefully manage their stress levels. Yet, such ambivalence is more typical than not as clients slowly come to grips with the risks and realities of leaving the situation or, quite possibly, facing death from their abuser.

Components of Intervention

LO11 Although modern crisis services tend to offer support through phone, live chat, and text, let's use the example of a hotline phone call to explore Juanita's situation. Imagine that a call comes into the crisis call center/hotline, and the crisis worker picks up the phone. The assessment process begins with active listening. The crisis worker immediately has to be concerned with a variety of roles. The worker must be not only a good listener but also supportive, facilitative, and concerned with the caller's safety and must act as an advocate (Barnett et al., 1980, p. 44). Indeed, the crisis worker should demonstrate effective use of client-centered/survivor-centered communication skills and practice (Grossmann et al., 2019).

Listening. Empathy and facilitative listening are crucial to assisting the crisis hotline caller (Kalafat et al., 2007). The client must know that the crisis worker has some understanding of and accepts their present situation in a nonjudgmental, non-value-laden manner. Only then will the IPV client be able to open up and openly share their feelings about their predicament (Heppner, 1978). The crisis worker also immediately reflects that they understand the difficulty and urgency of the situation by positively reinforcing the client for calling and taking a first step toward resolving the problem. Let's turn to a case involving Juanita, who is in an abusive relationship and has called a crisis line. The case picks up after initial introductions have been made.

CW: You did the right thing by calling. No matter how bad it seems and what terrible things have happened, you've made a big step on the road to straightening it out. We're here to help, and we'll stick with it as long as it takes.

Juanita: I . . . I . . . don't know. It's gone on so long. I feel so ashamed. I don't know what to do! It's so confusing.

CW: I appreciate how difficult it was to make this call. The hurt, the fear, the uncertainty of it all. So, start anywhere you want. We won't do anything unless *you* decide it's best for you. Right now, I want to listen to what you have to say. I'll listen for as long as it takes, so take your time and tell me what's happened.

Supporting. The caller/client is given both explicit and implicit permission to ventilate. Allowing clients to talk openly about their situation in a nonjudgmental context is a key component of effective response for crisis line workers (Kalafat et al., 2007). The free flow of the client's anger, hurt, fear, guilt, and other debilitating feelings may take minutes, hours, and even months to reconcile. In crisis work, we wish to create a safe place in which clients can express their raw emotions, but we also try to help clients avoid getting caught in the spiral of emotions that can move them from action to emotional paralysis. So, emotional discharge/catharsis is facilitated with care. Supportiveness means empathizing but not sympathizing with the client. A sense of lack of social support is one of the major factors for IPV survivors, and this lack of support may be particularly severe for individuals who do not have a family, group of loved ones, or other form of support network. It may be that the client has become isolated from their support network by the abuser or that they did not have a support network prior to entering the relationship with the abuser (e.g., individuals who immigrated from other countries or who are refugees, individuals whose family members are deceased or out of the picture). Many IPV victims are only partially mobile, and any action steps they take may be months away from happening. Thus, supporting an IPV victim often requires multiple interventions. In situations in which follow-up with clients is feasible, the crisis worker may have to exert an excruciating amount of patience over a long period of time as the client slowly moves toward making a decision and/or preparations to take action. In situations in which follow-up is not feasible, callers may reach out multiple times to the hotline for support over a period of time. No matter how bad the client's situation looks to the crisis worker, only the client can decide when they are ready or able to take action to leave the traumatic circumstances (Dagastino, 1984).

CW: OK! I understand it's a hard decision to make—getting out. Your marriage has had some good times, and you'd really like to hang onto that part of it, even though the abuse is happening more often. You say you want some time to think about it. That's OK! It's your decision, and we'll help whenever you need us.

Breaking away from an abusive relationship is a slow process. The crisis worker cannot move the client any faster than they are willing to go. The worker must be acutely aware of becoming overly sympathetic to the client's needs to the point of accepting responsibility for the client and attempting to "fix" things for the client. Many times, the IPV survivor will project anger onto law enforcement, spiritual or religious leaders, or other significant persons. Often, this anger or frustration with authority figures may signify what Heppner (1978) calls the *wishing and hoping syndrome.* The survivor wishes the situation would change, that the relationship would return to the way it used to be, and hopes the crisis worker can make the abusive partner change. However, cessation of abusive behavior by the perpetrator rarely happens without legal or therapeutic intervention (Dagastino, 1984). Under no circumstances should the crisis worker attempt to rescue the IPV survivor by talking to the abuser. It is dangerous and takes responsibility and autonomy away from the survivor. Instead, the conversation should be redirected away from what can be done to "fix" the abuser and toward how the survivor can be empowered to leave the abusive relationship.

CW: Although I hear you wanting me to come and straighten your partner out and make things the way they were, I can't do that. I wish I could, but I'm not able to change people or make them do the right thing. If you think marriage counseling would work, I can give you some names of people who do that. What I can do is help you make some decisions about what you want to do right now.

Perhaps out of fear, feelings of helplessness, and sheer frustration, a typical response to the crisis worker's refusal to fix the problem is anger.

Juanita: You're no damn help at all. You're just as bad as the rest. You're a horrible counselor. I'm gonna have to go back to him, and he'll kill me, just because you wouldn't do anything.

Because crisis workers do not want to lose clients, such ploys often rub a raw nerve in the workers and propel them to do something they may later regret. The crisis worker should realize that when the client doubts the crisis worker's ability, she is also doubting her own ability. She is probably looking for a

way to resume the relationship and may be displacing her own current inability (due to any of multiple factors, such as financial restrictions, learned helplessness, fear of retaliation, and isolation) to make changes by blaming the worker (Dagastino, 1984). The best response the crisis worker can make is not to be confrontive but to be empathic, realizing that right now, the client is in an overwhelming situation that is characterized by complex and confusing emotions. Often, despite logic, the IPV survivor often talks themselves out of leaving the relationship and, instead, tries to find a way to repair the relationship and return to their partner. It is important to remember the cycle of abuse and the myriad ways that IPV shifts the survivor's perception such that the survivor feels entirely dependent on the abuser. There should be no judgment of the client for "wanting" to return to their abuser because this "want" is perceived more as a need, and the client may have absolutely no idea of how to get their needs met if they leave the relationship.

CW: I'm sorry you're angry with me because I won't talk to your partner. I can imagine the frustration you feel. Yet I'm also not like the others who'll tell you how to act and what to do. I am here to support you and help you figure out a plan that works for you. I will not rush you, and I will not shame you. You are in control here.

The excerpt typifies the response of a crisis worker who is being supportive yet not taking over for the survivor. Usually, abuse survivors have not been able to be independent for quite some time, and they can quickly fall back into a dependent state. If the crisis worker keeps foremost in mind that the client is ultimately going to have to be their own defender and protector, the crisis worker is not likely to fall into a sympathy trap. The crisis worker who becomes angry or engages in denouncing or criticizing the abuser is making a fundamental mistake. The crisis worker may provoke the survivor to defend the IPV perpetrator and to verbally attack the crisis worker (Dagastino, 1984). This is a common reaction, in part, because IPV is characterized by a complex web of love and fear.

Facilitating. To facilitate the client's movement toward action takes a great deal of tenacity and patience. Helping callers think more clearly and explore options for responding to the situation are key aspects of crisis line work (Kalafat et al., 2007). Typically, the crisis worker will need to manage the client's feelings of dependency, ambivalence, and depression, which are all clear-cut signs of the client's immobility due to the chronic abuse. Overarching these immobilizing feelings is the learned helplessness referred to earlier. To generate movement in the client, the crisis worker strongly reinforces the client's attempts at rational decision-making, self-control, and statements of personal power (Heppner, 1978).

CW: You said that you couldn't do anything, but that's not true. You called here, didn't you? When you first started talking, you were crying uncontrollably, and now you're speaking in a level, controlled voice. I also notice a lot of "I" statements, which say to me you're starting to feel some sense of independence. Maybe you don't know it, but those are all signs that you're starting to feel some personal power for the first time in a long while, and I think that's great!

Ambivalence about the situation is predominant in most IPV survivors. Ambivalence is particularly strong with regard to the IPV perpetrator who may be quite tender at times, showing remorse and asking for forgiveness for their violent behavior (Scheffer et al., 2008). The perpetrator may even shower their abused partner with gifts and tells their partner what they want to hear (Conroy, 1982). Because of the complexity of emotions involved in IPV, some authors suggest that the process of leaving an abusive relationship is best viewed through Stages of Change model (Cluss et al., 2006; Khaw & Hardesty, 2007). To manage ambivalence, the crisis worker cycles between asking open-ended questions and reflecting and clarifying the client's feelings as an effective means of helping the client begin to examine previously denied feelings and thoughts. In so doing, crisis workers may help to enhance psychological readiness for change.

CW: What were you thinking and feeling while he was beating you?

Juanita: It was like I was standing off to the side watching a movie of this. It was like this can't really be happening, especially to me.

CW: So that's how you cope with it. Kind of separating yourself from the beating, as if it's happening to someone else.

Juanita: Yes, I guess I've done it that way for a long time. I'd lose my mind otherwise.

CW: What is your understanding of why he is abusing you?

Juanita: I don't know. I guess I'm just not a good wife.

CW: *It seems to you that* you're not living up to his expectations. How about your own expectations?

Juanita: I'm not sure. I mean, I've never thought of that. It's always been what he wants.

CW: How do you cope with the abuse other than just kind of separating yourself from the situation when it happens?

Juanita: I try to do what he wants, but when it starts to build—the tension—I just try to stay out of his way and be nice, although I know sooner or later, I'm gonna get his wrath. I dread the waiting. Actually, sometimes I push the issue just to get it over with. I know he'll always apologize afterward and treat me nice, at least for a while.

CW: So you do what he wishes even though you know the bottom line is a beating. Yet because of the anxiety, you may even push things to get it over with. Seems like you're willing to pay a steep price to get his love back.

Juanita: When you say that, I can't believe I'm letting this happen to me. What a fool . . . a stupid fool!

CW: You are not a fool. People who abuse are really skilled at making their victims feel that way, though. Tell me, what's keeping you in the relationship?

Juanita: God! I don't know. Love! Honor! Obey! The kids. The good times. Martyrdom. I don't have a job, and I'm pregnant again. I've got to get out. He'll wind up killing me, and maybe even this baby. I have to protect my kids and my baby.

Using open-ended questions, restatement, and reflection, the crisis worker relentlessly hammers at the survivor's faulty and illogical cognitive perception of the abusive situation. Only by placing themselves in the survivor's position can the crisis worker form an accurate perception of what steps to take and how the crisis worker will operate on the nondirective-to-directive continuum of intervention. People who have been abused also have in common the feeling of depression. Invariably, once a survivor has related the details of the assault, their affect becomes flat. Depression has taken over. Beneath the depression is a volcano of residual anger that is trying to find an outlet. The crisis worker's job is to help move the survivor out of the depressed state and let the angry feelings out (Dagastino, 1984) without letting the anger become destructive. This is the first step toward taking action.

CW: As you relate the details, it sounds like you're reporting it but not living it. I wonder if that's a typical way you hold it in . . . control it.

Juanita: I guess . . . if I really thought about it, I'd kill the bastard. How could he do this to me?

CW: How does it feel to let some of those angry feelings out?

Juanita: Scary! I'm really scared I would kill him if I got the chance.

CW: That is a legitimate feeling after what you've been through, but that won't get you where you want to go. Let's take a look at some of the alternatives between killing and being killed.

In summarizing the facilitation of the survivor's movement from an immobile to a mobile state, the Massachusetts Coalition of Battered Women Service Groups (1981, pp. 25, 67) has made the following recommendations for crisis workers.

1. **Be real.** Don't hide behind a role. You are what you are. To pretend to be something else makes the crisis worker false and discredited in the survivor's eyes.

2. **Set limits.** The crisis worker is not a superhero. Owning feelings of puzzlement, anger, stupidity, tiredness, and so forth allows the crisis worker to stay on top of the situation. If the crisis worker is tired, is taking on a lot of anger, and cannot work it through with the client, the crisis worker should own those feelings, ask for a time-out, and get out of the situation (hand the client off to another crisis worker who can assist) until the problem can be gone over with a fellow professional and a fresh start can be attempted.

3. **Give the survivor space and time to experience their raw emotions.** Remember that the survivor is experiencing a flood of emotions that have been building over a long period of time. Knowing that anger is one step on the way to finding their identity and independence again can be reassuring and empowering to the survivor. Give them time to ventilate before settling down to a plan of action.

4. **Allow the survivor to go through the pain but stay with them.** Your first response may be to become a psychological crutch because the survivor is so fragile at this point. The crisis worker who remembers that the survivor has been down a long road of abuse and is just now beginning to experience that pain (because they have had to push the pain away for so long to function in the abusive relationship), will realize that it is immensely hard to leave an abusive relationship. Belief in the survivor's ability to escape from the abuse is of overriding importance.

5. **Stay present and observe nonverbal communication.** The client's nonverbal and verbal responses are both very important; they tell the crisis worker whether what the survivor is saying is congruent with what the client is doing. Reading nonverbal responses may be difficult over the phone, but the worker needs to be aware of intonations, pauses, and sighs. How something is said may be as important as what is said. Also, what is not said may be as important as what is said.

6. **Be respectful and nonjudgmental.** The survivor's actions must be carefully separated from the survivor themself. What the survivor does may seem illogical when viewed through the lens of logic. But that logical lens is corrupted for IPV survivors, who are subject to all sorts of psychological manipulation and physical harm from their abuser. The client may reference religious and moral issues about leaving the relationship, with which the crisis worker may not agree. judgment time for debates or judgment. Clients should feel free to express their conflicting thoughts and feelings without being shut down by their crisis worker.

7. **Restate and reflect the survivor's thoughts and feelings.** As simple as this sounds, it is often extremely difficult. There is no greater therapeutic help than manifesting these skills.

8. **Set priorities together.** Two heads are better than one. This is why the crisis worker is there. If the client could manage the problem alone, they would. Likewise, the crisis worker is not in business of running clients' lives for them. The process must be collaborative.

9. **Examine options.** Brainstorming can uncover a variety of previously hidden ideas, options, and actions.

10. **Stay away from "whys."** Asking *why* a person does something like staying in an abusive relationship often leads the client, rightly or wrongly, to assume they are being judged. When a client feels they are being judged, they are apt to respond in defensive ways that do little to help them in their situation. Imagine if someone queried you about why you made some of the decisions you have made in your relationships. Add IPV to the equation, and there simply are no clear-cut answers.

11. **Give the survivor time to experience catharsis, but do not let them get stuck in self-pity.** The client needs to accomplish movement, and the crisis worker needs to move gently from nurturing emotional release to helping the client start to make plans, however small, concerning their predicament.

12. **Get back to the survivor.** Even if the client says, "I guess I can make it now," get the client's phone number and, if possible, call a few days later to make sure they are getting along all right. Many abused people experience so much embarrassment and shame that they cannot bring themselves to make another call for help. (Note: It is important to determine whether the call can be made without compromising the client's safety. Consider, for example, when the perpetrator is likely to be home and if the call can be tracked. If the exchange is happening over the internet or through mobile applications, data privacy settings and history tracking are important considerations (Havron et al., 2019) because the abuser may have access to and control over the client's internet-based accounts and devices.

13. **Peer supervision and feedback are essential for IPV crisis workers.** The intensity of partner abuse is such that few, if any, crisis workers can remain totally objective all the time. Cross-supervision by trusted co-professionals keeps the crisis worker on track, reduces personal stress, and helps avoid burnout.

Ensuring Safety. The crisis worker's first job is to determine how critical the situation is (Roberts & Roberts, 2002; Walker, 1984, p. 122). Is this a crisis call where danger is imminent, or does the client just need a chance to cathart? All the listening and responding skills known to humanity are of little use if the client has multiple bone fractures or if their significant other has threatened to come back and kill them. The crisis worker calmly and cautiously makes an assessment of how bad the situation is. Does the survivor need and want medical attention, shelter, a place to send their children, or a way out of the house if the abuser returns?

All these questions are posed in a measured, deliberate manner to avoid adding to the panic the client already feels. Although the situation may be critical and the best alternative may be for the client to go directly to the shelter, the crisis worker has

to remember that the client cannot be forced into making that choice. This does not mean, however, that the worker cannot make such a recommendation.

CW: From what you've said, it sounds like the situation is bad. Bad enough that you might consider leaving and going to a shelter for individuals who are experiencing partner violence. I need to ask a few questions to help me get a better idea of the current level of risk you and your children are in. Do you feel as if you or your children are in danger now? Is he there now? Do you want me to call the police? Do you need medical attention?

Because of a fear of the unknown, the client may balk at this alternative (Dagastino, 1984). Patiently, the crisis worker explains the role and function of the shelter, answers any questions the survivor has, and tries to allay the client's fears. If, after all this, the client is still unwilling or unable to make a decision, the crisis worker does not push the issue. In initially reporting the abuse, survivors often appear to feel that it is an isolated incident rather than abuse. They cannot see the insidious nature of IPV described by Scheffer Lindgren and Renck (2008). They delude themselves with the belief that "My partner really does love me, and if I'm a better person, it'll never happen again." As the crisis worker intervenes, the crisis worker should be aware that such incidents are not isolated. Indeed, there is a consistent pattern leading up to the climax of abuse (Walker, 1984, p. 24). The crisis worker endeavors to lay that pattern out so the client recognizes it not as isolated but as continuous and predictable. Recognizing the pattern is particularly important when the client is not sure whether to leave or stay. Walker proposes that instead of speaking about the cycle of violence, the crisis worker should lay out the escalating behavior in a graphical form. Having the client draw a graph of the ever-escalating violence and the shorter periods of tranquility can be an eye-opening event that allows the client to decide to get out (Walker, 2000, pp. 136–137).

CW: As you tell me about it, I hear a sort of pattern. For about a week, he gets surly, starts criticizing the way the house looks, the way you look, the food you cook, and your control over the kids. Those criticisms start out mild but become more severe until you finally have had enough and say something to the effect that he ought to take more responsibility if he doesn't like things. That winds up with your getting beat up. I wonder if you can look back and see how the situation has repeated itself. Just take a pencil and piece of paper and make a graph back for the past couple of months. Put down the length of time when there has been peace and tranquility. Then, put down how many hours or days the tension builds and he gets psychologically abusive, then put down when the fights start and how long they go on before he comes back and says he's sorry.

Juanita: Well, I don't know. I really think it was different this time. I mean, this was the first time I needed emergency treatment. He was really sorry afterward. **(draws out graph)** Well, maybe it is getting worse. He seems to be getting madder faster.

CW: OK. So, you see! What's different is that the pattern seems to be repeating itself more frequently, and it's getting more intense.

Juanita: Dang! I do see! I just don't know, though.

Often the client may be psychologically immobile and may not even hear the question, so the worker may need to pose it again (Dagastino, 1984).

CW: When did he say he'd be back, and what'd he say he'd do?

Juanita: I just don't know whether to take it anymore. I love him, but I'm really scared.

CW: OK, I understand you are afraid, but I need to know how much time we've got and what threats he made.

By gently guiding the client back to immediate and pressing issues, the crisis worker keeps the session on track but does not deny the emotional hurt and confusion the survivor is experiencing.

By the time the abused person becomes desperate enough to make the call for help, they do not have time to be analyzed. What the person needs is some behavioral action-oriented techniques they can use on a short-term basis (Walker, 1979, pp. 75–77). Just having a plan allows the client to regain some composure and feel they have obtained some control over the situation. The whole focus of the conversation is to prepare the client to get through that one day. At this time, the crisis worker does not worry about tomorrow or any other time. If follow up is an option, the crisis worker may call the client and talk about the next day. If the crisis worker attempts to deal with future events that extend beyond a week, the client often gets lost in the details (Dagastino, 1984).

Because of the flood of critical needs on behalf of the client, the worker must realistically judge which needs may require immediate action and which ones can be deferred. To help make sense of the heavy flow of information, the crisis worker documents what the client says so that the crisis worker can quickly identify and set priorities on the very practical and pressing concerns. Use of a structured set of questions and information ensure that crisis line workers cover critical needs and provide clients with consistent information (Dagastino, 1984; Roberts & Roberts, 2005). Immediate actions and follow-up actions need to be covered and checked. Issues such as getting enough money for the children's lunch the next day may be just as important as taking care of a broken nose, and the crisis worker will need to remember this. By calmly, clearly, and concisely feeding back to the survivor their written summary, the crisis worker takes the survivor step-by-step through a review of their most critical needs. By dissecting the crisis in this manner, the worker assures the survivor that their problems can be broken down into manageable chunks (Dagastino, 1984).

CW: Here are all the things I hear happening to you right now. No wonder you're feeling paralyzed; anyone in that situation would feel the same. You've said you have no job, the children don't want to leave, and that he might kill you. You also indicated that it was against your faith to get a divorce, and particularly coming from Colombia, there are some really strong cultural prohibitions. That's a lot. Let's take them one at a time and sort through each problem and put them back together.

A careful examination of the client's fears about these problems, what priorities need to be set on them, and the options she has in dealing with them is extremely important. Until the abused person can confront such fears openly, they cannot begin developing strategies to deal with her problems (Heppner, 1978).

CW: You're afraid to leave because you feel sure he will come after you when he comes back, and you're not sure what he might do, so that causes tension to build. Yet I really believe if we make a plan right now, you'll feel better, even if you don't have to use it.

If the client states that they do not know what to do, the crisis worker immediately looks at the two basic alternatives—staying and leaving. What has the client done before? How is this time different, if at all, from the times before? If so, what different action needs to be taken now? A key ingredient is determining the level of danger at home. Is the abuser really going to act out, or is the fear of the abuser acting out propelling the client into making the call? To learn what has happened before, the crisis worker asks questions such as "When your partner has gone out and gotten drunk before, what has your partner done?" "What have you done?" From these answers, the crisis worker gains a realistic assessment of the danger level of the situation. If the client is unwilling or unable to leave the house, the crisis worker could work with the client to brainstorm what the situation might be once their abuser returns home. The crisis worker goes through, in a systematic way, each situation of potential confrontation and then discusses the potential positive and negative outcomes of the client's attempt to handle the confrontation (Dagastino, 1984).

CW: Imagine that your partner comes home very late at night and starts trying to pick a verbal altercation with you over something, anything. Let's say he starts fussing about your son's math grade. Maybe he says something like "Where is Jonathan? I want to see his report card right now! He is a worthless little rat, and I'm going to teach him a lesson about responsibility!"

Juanita: Ugh, I can't stand being around him when he's drunk. I would probably say something like "There you go again with your drunken rage, trying to prove yourself." But he would get even more angry at that point. I cannot stand it when he tries to pull our kids into his rages, though.

CW: Let's be clear, you have every right to say something like that. You and your kids have been through far too much in this relationship, and, of course, you are exhausted and just fed up with the way you are treated. That being said, you mentioned that you would say something snarky, and he would get even more upset. I wonder what would happen if you were to have a different response, maybe one that is direct but not snarky. Maybe something like "You have been drinking, and now is not the time to talk with him about his grades. It's time for me to go to bed. Goodnight." How do you think he might respond to that?

Juanita: He's hard to predict, but that is probably less likely to get him further riled up.

CW: It's one option. Again, please do not think that I am saying that you do anything to cause or excuse his behavior. Quite the opposite. It is never okay for someone to intentionally hurt their partner or children. However, when you are trying to figure out a way out of the relationship, it might be helpful to use strategies that reduce the likelihood of a major blow up. It's all about keeping you and the kids safe, and your baby, too.

Juanita: I see your point. I mean, it's worth a try. I have had that type of reaction in the past, and I don't think he got quite as angry. So, I can probably try that again.

By looking at options and posing alternative ways of behaving, the crisis worker attempts to provide coping and/or communication techniques that may help to defuse the crisis. By the time the crisis worker is done, the client is feeding back a plan, point by point, either for staying in the home or for moving out. Having an escape plan is critical (Walker, 1984, p. 122).

CW: All right! You've figured out how to get out of the house. You'll keep the back door open. You've given the kids a note to go over to the neighbors. You've got our number, and you know you can get to your car, parked out back, and get to a safe place before calling us.

As indicated in Chapter 6, "Telephone and Online Crisis Counseling," computers and electronic technology play a huge role in our lives. And for individuals living within violent relationships, virtual support options and mobile applications are an integral part of promoting safety, providing treatment or intervention, and promoting psychoeducation about IPV (Anderson et al., 2021; Baird et al., 2022). For instance, the National Domestic Violence Helpline offers 24/7 access via phone (1-800-799-SAFE), live chat (www.thehotline.org), and text (text "START" to 88788). Various states also offer state-level help lines for their residents. There are countless IPV apps, but perhaps one of the most widely known is Aspire News, which has versions available for iOS and Android. Not all apps are created equal, though, and there are a number of IPV apps that are of questionable quality (Moret et al., 2022). As such, if crisis workers wish to recommend apps to their clients, it is imperative that crisis workers verify the quality, function, and utility of those apps prior to making such recommendations.

In summary, both short- and long-term safety depends on helping abused individuals take action steps rather than remaining psychologically immobilized. For many IPV survivors, taking first, tentative steps toward action is likely to be extremely frightening, confusing, and full of trepidation. The following points seem worthwhile for crisis workers to know and understand in helping individuals experiencing IPV to make such decisions and take action (Massachusetts Coalition of Battered Women Service Groups, 1981, pp. 25, 67).

1. Help survivors think and act on their situation by providing legitimate reinforcement for their efforts.
2. Help survivors figure out what they want by providing a sounding board for examining ideas and alternatives.
3. Help survivors identify feelings that prevent them from making decisions.
4. Be honest. The crisis worker cannot tell a person what to do, but the crisis worker can clearly state from their own life how the situation would affect them.
5. Help survivors to do things for themselves, making sure to not foster dependency on the crisis worker.
6. Know and offer resources from which IPV survivors can get specific kinds of assistance: Spell out *who, what, where, when,* and *how.*
7. Help survivors gain a sense of self-confidence and the ability to take care of themselves.
8. Be challenging. Support survivors, but do not be afraid to coax them toward a decision-making point.
9. Be open to choices. Each IPV survivor has control over their life; the crisis worker must not attempt to assume control for clients.
10. Hear and understand what survivors have to say, particularly if it does not run parallel to the crisis worker's own beliefs, attitudes, and outlooks.
11. Build on the commonalities that survivors share, but recognize the worth of the individual differences of each person.
12. Assess lethality. "I'm fed up with all of this" may really mean "I'm ready to take my life."

The following crisis worker's response to a woman experiencing IPV, who, after two hours of talking on the telephone, could not decide what to do, aptly illustrates the application of the 12 points just made.

CW: I understand your mixed feelings of wanting to stay and wanting to leave, also the constant fear you live with while waiting for the next time, maybe even wishing it would happen quickly so the tension will ease off. But my guess is that tension reduction only occurs for a short period and then starts to build all over again. I also understand that you feel like you're locked into this, but there are some alternatives, which we have gone over. I want you to pick at least one of those, whichever seems best for you, and do it. This is important. Do something that will make you feel better right now. I think it would be safer for you to go to the shelter right now, but if you don't really feel you can do that, I understand. However, if you feel the tension start to rise and you feel like you just can't take it anymore, I want you to promise to call back here. If you think it's safe for me to do so, I want to call you tomorrow afternoon to see how things are going. Do you think that will be okay?

Advocacy. Because IPV survivors have been isolated for long periods of time, they generally have little knowledge of alternatives available to them. This is especially true with respect to their rights and options with both legal and social service systems. Providing court advocates who understand the laws and how to weave through bureaucratic obstacles and how to cut through the red tape that often interferes with someone seeking help from the system is of paramount importance. Weaving one's way through the state employment and social service system to obtain financial aid and job training requires support and advocacy. The crisis worker needs to have an excellent networking system to tap into and get immediate help for a variety of problems IPV survivors will face.

Transcrisis Perspective. All the preceding intervention procedures cannot be accomplished in a 20-minute intervention. Even minor crises may require two or three calls to get the client stabilized, in touch with their feelings, and into some semblance of preabuse equilibrium. The crisis worker is not providing a short-term elixir that merely calms the survivor and then blithely sends the survivor on their way. What is being provided is a blend that not only deals with the immediate crisis but also has a long-term application. Because of the profound effects of the abuse, particularly in terms of the IPV survivor's sense of self, IPV survivors often find that they need to go through a complete rediscovery process about who they are and what they can do. This process should not be hurried.

Indeed, the transcrisis of the abused individual does not end when the client gets off the phone and decides to get out of the relationship. The initiating interview or hotline call is only the first part of the crisis resolution. Other crises will continue to emerge. Ibrahim and Herr's (1987) work with abused women who were involved in a group counseling format that concentrated on vocational exploration and economic independence is an excellent example of a transcrisis point. When these women reached the stage of vocational implementation, ready actually to go out into the world of work and test their skills, they experienced all kinds of threatening and anxious feelings and became immobile and paralyzed. The women needed 15 two-hour sessions of intensive support from the group leaders to work through this stage. Although much has changed in the nearly four decades since Ibrahim and Herr's study, the fact that IPV survivors often question their self-efficacy and competency remains an ongoing reality; IPV perpetrators are keenly skilled in their ability to eat away at their victims' confidence, independence, autonomy, and general belief that the victim can do anything in the absence of their abuser.

Shelters

LO12 While a hotline deals with short-term, remote crisis intervention and/or counseling through phone, text, and/or chat, a shelter is a longer-term facility where survivors and their families can seek refuge for short or extended periods of time. Both the hotline and shelter tend to be staffed around the clock with 24-hour access, although 24-hour intakes at some rural shelters may not be feasible.

Not only do shelters provide a place of residence that is often safeguarded by security systems, they also often include related supports, such as childcare, support groups, individual counseling, legal advocacy, medical assistance, and resources regarding employment and government/social support options (Macy et al., 2013; Rogers, 2019). Typically staffed by both professionals and volunteers, shelters provide a safe place for clients to stabilize and begin rebuilding their lives after escaping IPV.

According to Sullivan (2018), domestic violence shelter staff work with clients in the following capacities:

1. providing information about adult and child survivors' rights, options and experiences; (2) safety planning; (3) building skills; (4) offering encouragement, empathy, and respect; (5) supportive counseling; (6) increasing access to community resources and opportunities; (7) increasing social support and community connections; and (8) community change and systems change work (p. 126).

As such, domestic violence shelters work toward the overarching goals of increasing self-efficacy for residents and their children, instilling hope for the future, and increasing access to various sources of supports (Sullivan, 2018).

Although, as we have previously discussed, IPV is not exclusive to cisgender heterosexual couples, and IPV perpetrators can be of any gender, the majority of IPV perpetrators are men who are in relationships with women. As such, the vast majority of IPV shelters are for women, regardless of their sexual orientation, although gender inclusive shelters are growing in number. It should be noted, though, that shelters designed to support women rarely, if ever, accept men as clients. You might imagine the challenges of having men as clients in shelters where most residents are women who have fled violent relationships with men. Particularly in rural areas, men and transmen are hard-pressed to find support in the form of IPV shelters. That is an unfortunate reality, and perhaps by the time the 10th edition of this book is published, more progress will be made in that area. For now, though, we turn to discussing the experience of women in shelters with the understanding that much of this content could be applicable to other shelter residents.

Individuals who enter shelters often have conflicted feelings regarding the termination of the relationship with their abusive partner (Fisher & Stylianou, 2019). If the person has children, the children may not understand the reasons for leaving and may long for their other parent, which can be compelling toward reunification. Scheffer et al. (2008) interviewed women who had left abusive relationships. A central theme was the emotional pull the women experienced between leaving and staying in the relationship, often fluctuating between both ends of the emotional continuum of hate and love within short periods of time (Scheffer et al., 2008). When working with women who have not yet reached the pivotal "releasing turning point" that Scheffer and associates (2008) describe, it is important for the crisis worker at the shelter to maintain consistent contact and reinforce these survivors for having the courage to come to the shelter.

CW: I'm glad you made it. I know it took a lot of courage.

CW: (a few minutes later) Getting settled in? Come on with me. There are some other women I would like you to meet.

CW: (2 hours later) How are things going? Got the kids settled in? They seem like great kids. Want to have a cup of coffee and talk?

Vacillation between going back and staying is common for newcomers to the shelter, not only because of conflicting feelings regarding their relationship with their abuser. Residents may also leave for reasons such as wanting to find permanent housing, separation from loved ones and/or children, conflict with other residents, issues with shelter staff, restrictive shelter policies, being displaced from their community, and subpar shelter facilities/conditions (Fisher & Stylianou, 2019). Restrictive rules are a common point of contention for shelter residents (Gregory et al., 2021), leading some experts to propose rule reduction strategies for shelters (Kulkarni et al., 2019). However, the longer residents stay at the shelter, the greater the probability is that they will not return to their mates. Until residents can recover their self-esteem and come to understand that they are not the cause of the abuse, they are at risk of leaving and going back to their abusive partner (Schutte et al., 1986). The crisis worker does not try to force residents to stay at the shelter but does try to get them to take some psychological "time-out" to review their situation in a more objective way (Dagastino, 1984).

Juanita: I'm all mixed up. I don't know if I'm wrong or not. I'm Catholic, and I'm Colombian. Women in my family just don't walk out of a marriage. The church and my family both say we just need to work things out, but I really think he'll kill me.

CW: Let's assume you're taking a 1-day vacation, so you can get some rest before you go back and deal with it. It's fine if you want to go back home, but do this much for me—just take it easy for a while. I can see that you're physically all right and not hurt, and I'm relieved about that. This is a great time to talk about what you can do if you do or don't go back.

The crisis worker checks repeatedly with Juanita and reinforces her decision to come. She conveys her concern for Juanita and, with the help of other women in the shelter, sees that the survivor and her family are settled. The focus is on the here and now. During the first few hours of the survivor's separation from her abuser, the crisis worker will probably have to be very directive. By merit of the abuse they have endured, few women at this time have the ego strength to stand on their own, and most need an abundance of support and help. The objective is to keep the survivor moving, thinking, and acting so she is preoccupied and does not have time to let fear, guilt, or any other debilitating and anxiety-ridden emotions overcome her. The crisis worker should be carefully attuned to the survivor's needs. Some may find help by sitting, talking, or crying with a worker or a group of other women. Others may be so exhausted that they need to go to bed and sleep. Whatever the survivor needs, the worker should be adaptable to those needs and flexible enough to change as circumstances demand (Dagastino, 1984).

Shelter Dynamics

A variety of positive dynamics occur at shelters. There is substantial support from other residents who have experienced similar trauma. This support enables survivors to begin regaining the courage to face people, recover their lost self-esteem, and learn that the abuse is not their fault (Schechter, 1982, pp. 55–60).

Domestic violence/emergency shelters are not vacation spas where one's every whim is catered to. Although an abundance of peer support occurs, life in a shelter is challenging and requires major adjustment. Privacy is limited, conflicts occur between residents, facilities may be uncomfortable, and rules and curfews can feel overbearing. Add to that the possibility of being uprooted from familiar sources of support and loved ones, having limited personal belongings, and feeling a nagging sense of unsettledness associated with wondering if the perpetrator will find them, shelter residents experience a swift and marked transition upon entry into emergency shelters. Coping with those changes can be a major stressor in and of itself.

Shelter resident: Getting used to a shelter is overwhelming. You like it, but you don't want to be there, 'cause it isn't home. You've got to put together all your psychological know-how in getting along with different types of people. Wondering if you're going to make it, especially when you see all the pain and confusion and don't know whether it's yours or theirs or what, and hoping nobody finds out you're here. Trying to be understood and feeling like you are a blabbermouth here when you couldn't talk at home. Trying to look forward and all the time wanting to forget . . . wanting to forget . . . wanting to forget (Schechter, 1982, pp. 59–60).

At a shelter, everything is not always as it seems. Some residents who come to the shelter are extremely dependent and exceptionally adept at intentionally or unintentionally manipulating the workers there (Walker, 1984, p. 126). They have been taught by their abuser that they cannot and should not try to function independently. Those abusive messages and the learned helplessness that accompanies them can take root within the survivor's mind and interfere with recovery. A statement like "You really understand—you've made my whole life better" is reinforcing to the worker but may actually be manipulation. Emergency shelters are intended to be temporary solutions, although many residents may need to reside at the shelter for months at a time. When residents become dependent on the shelter and its staff, and they are not making progress toward independence, shelter workers often have to change tactics to encourage those residents to take initiative.

CW: I appreciate what you said, and I appreciate your wanting to cook my dinner and all the other things you want to do for me. It has been a pleasure getting to know you, but I am hoping you may start making progress toward reclaiming your independence. A more effective use of your time and mine could be working on getting you set up in an apartment and looking for a job.

Grief. Besides being dependent, many abused individuals go through a grief process. Sorrow and depression, guilt and self-blame, and decision-making difficulty are all hallmarks of the grieving process. What would be viewed as normal in a person who suffered the death of an intimate partner may be viewed as pathological in an abused individual. However, these responses are just as legitimate for an abused individual who is trying to come to terms with the loss of a significant relationship, shared parental responsibilities, and a clearly defined role as a partner (Campbell, 1989).

There are a lot of *yes, buts* as workers start to confront survivors with building a new future. As survivors shift from a depersonalized view of their situation to depression over it, the process can be uncomfortable to a shelter worker who does not conceptualize the relationship loss within a grief framework. The survivor's grief often puzzles others who objectively look at the abusive relationship and think that the survivor should be relieved rather than grieving. Many human services workers may be threatened by these feelings and deny the survivor's need to mourn by concentrating on dealing with concrete aspects of the survivor's dilemma.

The survivor's grief can be understood, however, if one asks the question "For what are they mourning?" In most cases, the survivor has defined themselves in terms of their relationship with the abuser, and if that relationship ends, the survivor feels as if they have lost everything—including their sense of self (Turner & Shapiro, 1986). Survivors cling quite tightly to the dreams they once had or may still have for the relationship. When the relationship ends, survivors must come to terms with the fact that those dreams will never materialize. Therefore, survivors are not grieving so much for what was, but for what they hoped could have been (Spanno, 1990). A crisis worker can and should validate that the survivor's loss is very real and that the survivor has a legitimate right to mourn and experience feelings of loss (Russell & Uhlemann, 1994). At this point, the counseling process is little different from grief due to the death of a loved one (refer to Chapter 12, "Personal Loss: Bereavement and Grief").

Juanita: I wanted this to work so much. We could have had it so good, but I couldn't take him abusing me and the kids, too. What went wrong with that good-looking, happy couple in this picture? He was so handsome and so good to me in the beginning. Then it just slowly went to hell, and now this. **(Weeps while slowly turning over in her hands a wedding picture that she brought with her to the shelter.)**

CW: It's really hard to say goodbye to all those things that were and might have been. It must hurt even more than the abuse to know that all those hopes and dreams won't come to pass.

Juanita: It tears my heart out, but I know I did the right thing. Sooner or later, he would have killed me or the kids in one of his rages. It's so weird! I still love him, but I also hate him.

CW: The grief you're feeling is as real as if a close friend or a relative had died. Perhaps even more tragic because when this relationship died, a part of you died with it, Juanita. The part of you who struggled out of a single-parent home, went to college, got an education, made a success of herself, married the perfect man, and then had all those expectations dashed because of the way he treated you and the children.

Juanita: I can't let that stop me. Nothing else did. I made the right decision coming here. I also made the right decision getting a temporary protective order against him. Maybe that last act of love will get him the help he needs or the jolt he needs to wake him up so he doesn't do it to somebody else. But I can't worry about him anymore. I have to focus on me and my kids, and my baby.

CW: As you say that, I see so much determination coming through the tears. I also see a new, different, stronger person as you say those farewells, as tough as they are.

A person who has been involved in an abusive relationship needs to grieve and to have that grief validated. The crisis worker does this while reinforcing that although there is now an altered future, it has the potential to be a good future. It is through this process that the survivor can come to see the relationship for what it really was—abusive. The crisis worker will make a very bad therapeutic mistake if they expect the survivor to rejoice. If the survivor is expected to be happy for leaving and is discouraged from feeling a sense of loss and expressing it, the survivor may never confront the truth about the relationship. The end result may well be a return to the partner or someone else just like the perpetrator (Spanno, 1990).

Depression. Depression comes in many guises. Many survivors who come into the shelter sleep much of the time. On first appearance, they may seem to be lazy. Actually, they may be going through a stage of trying to regroup their psychic energy. The crisis worker's task becomes one of trying to help them move past their inactivity, but not by pressuring them or taking them on a guilt trip (Massachusetts Coalition of Battered Women Service Groups, 1981, p. 27).

CW: I've noticed you pretty much sticking to your room and sleeping a lot. I was a little concerned and was wondering how you were feeling. I wonder if you've had a chance to talk to anyone about how you feel since you got here.

Juanita: I feel so guilty. It seems like I have slept ever since I've gotten here, and the other women have been so good to take care of the kids. I'm not really like this. I just don't seem to have any get-up-and-go. I'm really sorry to be so much trouble.

CW: What you are doing is exactly what you should be doing, getting your energy back. You burned up a tremendous amount of it making the decision to get out and get here. The other women have felt the same way, so they understand. In a few days, you'll do the same for somebody else. If you want to talk, we're here. If you want to rest, that's just fine too. The main thing is you're safe, and that's what's important right now.

Terror. For many survivors, a stress-related syndrome similar to agoraphobia arises after they have been in the shelter for a while (Massachusetts Coalition of Battered Women Service Groups, 1981, p. 27). They may have extreme and unexplainable attacks of terror that are touched off by seemingly innocuous incidents. These incidents greatly restrict their activities and new freedom. Fear of their abusive partner, fear of their predicament, fear of their separation from a definable past, and fear of an undefinable future can all cause the onset of terror. Under no circumstances should the shelter worker allow terror to continue. Survivors must be encouraged and helped step-by-step to pull themselves away from the security blanket of the shelter and get themselves out into the real world, albeit at a reasonable pace.

Such progress may take place in very small, slow steps, but the steps must be taken. As survivors take these steps, they receive very specific, positive reinforcement for what they have accomplished, enabling them not to fall back into learned helplessness but instead to take responsibility for their future (Weincourt, 1985). Invariably, survivors will not be able to see that they have done much of anything, or they tend to diminish their successes. For survivors who are faced with leaving a relationship with no means of support, structural change in their economic environment is imperative. Independent housing, job training and opportunities, affordable childcare, and social support services are critical. Programs such as the Job Readiness program that is run in a number of Kentucky shelters provide job training to make survivors employable (Websdale & Johnson, 2005). However, such preparation may bring on its own developmental crises as these survivors venture into new, unfamiliar territory.

CW: I know you're still scared to death to go down and talk to them at FedEx about that job. It's a big step, but a week ago you couldn't walk down to the grocery store, and now you're doing that fine.

So, let's take it one step at a time. Look at what you have overcome already. We can plan for the job interview, slow and steady, talk about what might happen in the interview, and give you a chance to really become confident about going down there.

Those Who Have Decided to Leave. There are some survivors who have definitely made their choice about leaving their abusive partner. They come to the shelter for immediate assistance and quickly begin working on the next steps toward their independence. The crisis worker deals with immediate specifics, such as finding a place to live, financial aid, and childcare. Emotional support has a low priority because these survivors are so busy that all they want and need is very practical advice and support. They are very different from those experiencing acute crisis because they are highly motivated to change their lives. They are much easier to work with because they have made a decision to escape their domestic pressure cooker (Dagastino, 1984).

Follow-Up

LO13 Once survivors leave the shelter, they should be provided with follow-up care (Tutty & Rothery, 2002). As immediate demands are relieved, the emotional impact of their decision to escape the abusive relationship should be dealt with over the long term. Survivors are encouraged to pursue counseling because IPV is typically, by its very nature, psychologically damaging. It is not uncommon for survivors to be so busy putting their lives back together that their emotional reactions are delayed. Survivors may be out on their own, well-established, and seemingly doing quite well when they experience a sudden onslaught of emotions in response to the IPV. The crisis worker apprises the survivor of what to expect in the way of emotional aftershocks.

CW: Even though you feel like you've made the break from your husband, don't be surprised if, later on, you get depressed and really feel like you need and miss him. Or maybe it just all hits you at once, seemingly out of the blue. That's to be expected with this type of trauma. We know that, and we're here to help then, too!

Indeed, in the worst of scenarios, survivors may become lonely, forget about the terrible abuse they suffered in the past, invite their ex-partner over for dinner, and find themselves again experiencing violence from the person they thought they might be able to forgive. Or, because of urging from children and/or their ex-partner, survivors may feel pressured into reuniting (Tutty & Rothery, 2002). Therefore, in following up with the survivor, the crisis worker should understand that there may be relapses and that the survivor may fall into old ways of feeling or behaving. The crisis worker should not shame the survivor for those relapses, which are part of the separation and healing process for many survivors.

CW: Hello, Juanita. Just called to see if you've been able to make that appointment for counseling at the Human Services Clinic. I know it's hard to get in there at times and thought if you hadn't, I could call the clinic to help you get started.

The crisis worker continues to be a support system until the survivor is well connected to a long-term support source (McLeod et al., 2010), and only then does the crisis worker fade from the survivor's life. Long-term support is particularly critical for IPV survivors. Support and advocacy are critical during this time frame. Those who have a support group and advocates who help them access services do significantly better in reaching their goals than survivors who lack such services (Sullivan et al., 1994). Support services also build self-esteem, increase locus of control, reduce stress, and enhance feelings of belongingness and support (Tutty et al., 1993). Follow-up and support are particularly important for survivors who have little education, few job skills, and minimal financial support (Webersinn et al., 1991).

Intervention with Children

LO14 Children are sometimes the forgotten victims in IPV. Even when the abuse is not perpetrated directly against the child, the IPV is highly damaging to children, so much so that witnessing IPV is considered a form of child abuse (Dodaj, 2020). Living in homes in which IPV occurs not only puts children at risk for direct abuse but also can make them feel responsible for abuse perpetrated by the adult(s) (Pingley, 2017). Further, as Pingley (2017) states, exposure to IPV "can lead to physical health, mental health, challenges in the development of social skills, and changes in cognitive processing" (p. 26). As such, crisis workers need to be as concerned for children as they are for the parents who experience abusive relationships.

Of primary concern is the safety of the children, so a lethality assessment should be conducted to determine where the children should reside and who will supervise them during visitation and other occasions where the perpetrator may be present. For children who are old enough to take action on their own, a safety plan should entail how to determine whether the situation is becoming lethal, how to get away from the perpetrator, and where they can go to be safe. If they are in a shelter, they need to know how to keep the location a secret, not only from the perpetrator, but also from other relatives and acquaintances. If there is evidence of abuse toward the children, which is highly likely in partner violence, the crisis worker is mandated to report the abuse to the respective child protection agency. Laws on mandated reporting differ by state and country of residence. As such, crisis workers should be keenly aware of the relevant child abuse mandated reporting laws for the location in which they practice.

Children who have witnessed partner violence or have just fled or been removed from a home can benefit from immediate short-term intervention to reduce the longer-term effects of the abuse (Arroyo et al., 2017) that can follow them into adulthood (Anderson et al., 2011). (Refer to the sections on children in Chapter 7, "Posttraumatic Stress Disorder", and Chapter 9, "Sexual Assault", for more detailed assessment and intervention strategies.) Research demonstrates that cognitive-behavioral approaches that are tailored to the client tend to be the most efficacious, although many types of interventions seem to have some level of therapeutic quality (Arroyo et al., 2017). Perhaps the act of having someone address the emotional impact of IPV is, in and of itself, therapeutic. Knowing that someone cares and being able to emotionally cathart, cognitively process the events, enhance coping skills, and address maladaptive cognition are common components of short-term interventions. But first and foremost, a trained crisis worker should perform a safety assessment to ensure that the child is not in immediate danger. Then, children may wish to process the events and their reaction to the events verbally or through play. The crisis worker will also work to correct negative misattributions about self-blame. Specific problem-solving strategies need to be developed in which the child's affect is normalized, and the child learns how to anticipate and deal with uncomfortable emotions (Lehmann & Rabenstein, 2002). Crisis workers should not engage in forensic interviews for child sexual assault survivors, though, unless specifically trained and authorized to do so. Forensic interviewing for childhood sexual assault survivors is a highly specialized field of practice, which is discussed in Chapter 9, "Sexual Assault."

Longer-term therapeutic intervention is particularly effective in reducing the long-term impact of IPV for children (Arroyo et al., 2017). Work done conjointly with caregivers is critical. Trauma-Focused Cognitive Behavioral Therapy (TF-CBT) (Cohen et al., 2003) is perhaps the most widely utilized trauma-informed approach for treating children. TF-CBT has been specifically adapted for multiple groups, such as child victims of Commercial Sexual Exploitation, children of military families, LGBTQIA+ youth, children in foster care, and children from minoritized groups (Trauma-Focused Cognitive Behavioral Therapy & National Therapist Certification Program, 2021b). TF-CBT is typically implemented in 8 to 25 sessions, and it combines both individual work with the child/adolescent and conjoint sessions with the caregiver (Trauma-Focused Cognitive Behavioral Therapy & National Therapist Certification Program, 2021a). Active caregiver participation plays a significant role in TF-CBT and can markedly increase treatment efficacy (Cohen & Mannarino, 2015). Major components of TF-CBT include parent skills training, psychoeducation about trauma, affect regulation and relaxation skills, cognitive coping skills, narrative restorying of the trauma, and grief processing (National Child Traumatic Stress Network, 2017). Although TF-CBT has strong support in the research, expressive and play therapy techniques have also demonstrated efficacy for traumatized children.

Malchiodi (2008, p. 254) recommends art and play therapy as a primary therapeutic mode because many children may not be able to verbally process the violence they have witnessed. Advocates of play therapy describe play as the child's natural way of communicating. Particularly for young children, but also applicable to older children and adolescents, expressive and play therapy allows for the expression of the child's innermost experience without the barrier of finding the right words or even having to cognitively understand the complex flow of thoughts and emotions. Treatment goals for children and the victimized parent include (Malchiodi, 2008; Weinreb & Groves, 2007):

1. Creating an alliance with the parent to help the child heal.
2. Providing psychoeducation to both parent and child about the trauma and therapy.
3. Restoring the parent's self-esteem and confidence to parent.
4. Establishing a safe therapeutic environment for the child to express thoughts and feelings.

5. Relieving the child's symptoms, including difficulty with living transitions, sleeping, nightmares, and other trauma symptoms.

6. Reestablishing the child's previous level of cognitive functioning and strong attachment with the nonoffending caregiver.

7. Reassurance that what has happened is not the child's fault and the child is not guilty of anything.

8. Helping the child express thoughts and feelings and regain cognitive and emotional regulation.

9. Providing stress reduction strategies to aid in stopping emotional dysregulation.

Weinreb and Groves (2007) provide an excellent example of why using play therapy is effective with children coming out of IPV situations. In this instance, a 7-year-old girl had witnessed severe beatings of her mother by her father. She was introduced to therapy by being brought into a play therapy room and invited to play. She used drawing and playing with figurines that represented her violent environment to work through a constellation of conflicted feelings about the traumatic events and separation of her family. She expressed that she was afraid of, yet missed, her father, which are all too common ambivalent feelings about the offending parent. Trying to verbalize these ambivalent, conflicted feelings and integrate them is extremely difficult for an elementary school-age child. Working them out through play and anchoring them with drawings, models, and other concrete representations is far more appropriate to the child's emotional and cognitive development than trying to use talk therapy.

Many times, group work (Malchiodi, 2008, pp. 252–263) may be used with children; benefits include decreasing isolation, bonding with other survivors, and seeing others moving forward from the trauma of the IPV they experienced. Malchiodi (2008, pp. 258–261) has adapted Herman's (1992) three-phase trauma recovery model to her groups, which generally meet for 90 minutes for up to 12 sessions. Phase 1 is about establishing safety rules, confidentiality, personal space, and boundaries, which may be put on a colorful poster and signed by the children as part of their behavioral contract. The group engages in activities such as making feeling thermometers; reading about Brave Bart, the traumatized cat who gets into a group of other traumatized cats; creating safety hands with "safe" adult names and phone numbers on it; learning relaxation and yoga activities; and free drawing and play time. Phase 2 is about

telling the trauma story and includes activities such as creating collages of being powerless and powerful, making "how hands can hurt" posters, drawing a picture of "your family," reading therapeutic storybooks, engaging in relaxation and stress reduction activities, practicing scaling techniques with feeling thermometers, learning simple cognitive-behavioral techniques to reduce negative thinking, and free play and art time. The final phase has to do with returning to the community and reconnecting with significant adults in the child's life who are central to their emotional recovery. These caregivers are asked to participate in the final two sessions. Children can share their artwork and have parents engage in reconstructing artwork, cooperatively creating or adding to safety hands to reinforce the child's sense of security and creating past, present, and future collages to show where they have been, where they are now, and the hopeful future they are moving toward.

Outcomes for the children should include the following (Malchiodi, 2008, p. 261):

1. Increased knowledge of the emotional and physical effects of family violence

2. Understanding that violence in the family is not okay, and it is not their fault

3. A reduction in stress-related or PTSD symptoms; increased ability to self-regulate emotions

4. Decreased negative self-talk

5. Improved ability to identify feelings and the ability to communicate those to peers and adults

6. Increased sense of social support

7. Stronger connection with the nonabusive parent

8. Resilience to cope with future crises

Finally, many children are still involved with both parents, and long-term monitoring and intervention are needed. The Duluth Family Visitation Center ("Duluth Family Visitation Center," n.d.) is based on the Duluth Model and provides "supervised exchanges, visits, and communication, where we focus on building safe and positive relationships" (para. 1). Centers like the Duluth Family Visitation Center operate on the premise that some level of reunification with the offending parent is likely to occur and that parent training is critical for both parents so children will not be used as messengers, negotiators, or witnesses to further verbal or physical abuse. As such, staff members in this type of center attempt to remain neutral and to act as advocates for the children with both parents by providing a safe place to exchange children, helping parents develop good parenting relationships with their children, and providing valid information to courts regarding custody and visitation rights (McMahon et al., 1999).

Teen Dating Violence

LO15 IPV is certainly not restricted to marital and cohabiting relationships. In fact, teen dating violence (TDV) occurs often and is a critical issue for adolescents. According to the National Intimate Partner and Sexual Violence Survey: 2016/2017 Report on Intimate Partner Violence (Leemis et al., 2022), approximately 25 percent of women and 20 percent of men who have experienced IPV state that their first incident with partner violence occurred prior to age 18. And in one study, nearly 65 percent of women and nearly 62 percent of men reported TDV victimization between the ages of 13 and 19 (Bonomi et al., 2012). TDV comes in many forms, not just physical abuse. TDV may also involve problematic behavior, such as verbal aggression, sexual aggression, extreme jealousy, monitoring behavior (e.g., monitoring internet and social media use), and excessive possessiveness. We have already said this generally about IPV, but it is worth saying again. It is not only men who perpetrate TDV; women are often TDV perpetrators as well (Duval et al., 2020).

There are a number of risk factors for TDV. It might not come as a surprise that substance misuse is often associated with TDV (Duval et al., 2020; Maldonado et al., 2015). To varying degrees, personal factors such as mood and level of self-control may be related to TDV (Duval et al., 2020). And, perhaps most unsurprisingly, teens who experience violence within their homes or childhood maltreatment are at an increased risk of perpetrating and/or experiencing TDV (Duval et al., 2020; Maldonado et al., 2015; Wolfe et al., 2009). For many individuals who are perpetrators or victims of TDV, one must consider whether or not the teens have a realistic idea of what constitutes a healthy relationship. For that reason, researchers suggest that psychoeducation on relationships plays a critical role in addressing TDV (Bonomi et al., 2012; Duval et al., 2020). Loveisrespect.org provides a wealth of resources for teens regarding healthy relationships, safety, how to support others who experience TDV, and how to get help. They also offer a crisis line, live chat, and texting options to support teens who experience TDV.

In that regard, the best directive your authors can offer to anyone who is physically assaulted even once in a dating relationship is, no matter how great the love, how great the good times, how great the attraction, how many flowers, apologies, and promises to change are given after an initial assault, *get out of the relationship now!* No abused person we have met set out with the intention to partner with someone who would beat them. However, by rationalizing those red flags early in the relationship, many people inadvertently get caught up in the dizzying cycle of abuse.

And if *you* have assaulted someone in a dating relationship, *get help now!* "Assaulted" doesn't necessarily mean that you put the person in the hospital. It may have been a series of hard shakes, a shove or two, or a slap in the heat of an argument or a moment of jealousy. Although you can easily rationalize this behavior away, the chances are good that this behavior will increase in the future. Besides the harm you do to someone you profess to love, the changes in the law and increased judicial sensitivity to partner violence mean that you will probably spend some time incarcerated if you are convicted of an assault on your romantic partner.

Stalking

LO16 Although, like any type of interpersonal violence, it is challenging to pinpoint a precise prevalence rate for stalking, some research suggests that approximately 4.5 percent of adults in the United States have experienced stalking (Basile et al., 2006), with the National Intimate Partner and Sexual Violence Survey pegging the stalking rate at 15.2 percent for women and 5.7 percent for men (Breiding, 2015). That percentage is most likely a lot worse on college campuses. Shorey et al. (2015) found that in their study, 38 percent of men and women in a current dating relationship had been stalked in the previous 6 months. But those cases often go unreported because of fear of violence, gender norms, and shame (Cass & Mallicoat, 2015). So, for those who are victims of a stalker, the official definition of stalking is "the willful or intentional commission of a series of acts that would cause a reasonable person to fear death or serious bodily injury and that, in fact, does place the victim in fear of death or serious bodily injury" (Office for Victims of Crime, 2002, p. 1). Stalking is real, and it is frightening.

Stalking is generally defined as repeated harassment, following, and/or threats that are committed with the intent of causing the victim emotional distress, fear of bodily harm, and/or actual bodily harm. Racine and Billick (2014) provide an overview of the common typology systems for stalkers, including the following: (1) "Zona's stalker–victim types" of (i) simple obsessional (based on some type of previous relationship through which the stalker developed an obsession), (ii) love obsessional (not based on a prior relationship; the stalker is likely entirely unknown to the victim), and (iii) erotomanic (based on a delusion that the victim is in love with the stalker); (2) "Mullen's Stalker Typology" of (i) rejected (based on a prior relationship for which the stalker seeks revenge or reconciliation), (ii) intimacy seeking (based in delusion or infatuation, in which the stalker seeks an intimate relationship with the victim), (iii) incompetent (based on the stalker's sense of "entitlement" to possess the victim without recognition that the victim does not reciprocate), (iv) resentful (based on a sense of being "wronged" by the victim and is often characterized by threats toward the victim), and (v) predatory (based on willful intent to sexually violate the victim); and (3) the "RECON Typology of Stalking" with Type I ("intimate and acquaintance" stalkers) and Type II ("public figure and private stranger stalkers") (pp. 251–252). They note that the RECON system allows for identification based on identifiable risk factors (Racine & Billick, 2014).

Public figure/celebrity stalkers who typically target movie stars may send out hundreds of e-mails, letters, or phone calls. Most of these stalkers are not targeting their victims for violence or murder; in fact, many public figure stalkers are women who stalk men and display psychotic features (Racine & Billick, 2014). One of your authors once worked with a woman who was diagnosed with schizophrenia. She believed the singer Meatloaf was in love with her. Although she did not stalk Meatloaf, this erotomanic delusion exemplifies the type of delusion that may precipitate public figure stalking. Private stranger stalkers direct their predatory behavior toward individuals who are not public figures but are not directly known to the stalker (Racine & Billick, 2014). These stalkers have a tendency to escalate to violence (Racine & Billick, 2014). Intimate stalkers are the most common and perhaps the most dangerous; these are stalkers who were previously in a relationship with their victim (Racine & Billick, 2014). Finally, acquaintance stalkers know their victim but have not been in a romantic relationship with their victim (Racine & Billick, 2014).

They may be prone to violence, but much less so than intimate stalkers (Racine & Billick, 2014). However, Tjaden and Thoennes (2000) reported that injury rates were four times higher among women stalked by acquaintances as opposed to strangers.

It may interest you to know that the first state stalking law in California didn't come into existence until 1990, although all 50 states in the United States now have stalking laws (Lawson, 2013). However, stalking is not just a problem in the United States; stalking occurs worldwide (Maran et al., 2014; McKeon et al., 2015; Pengpid & Peltzer, 2014). For example, in a Finnish sample of university students, over 22 percent reported that they had been a victim of stalking once, and over 26 percent reported being stalked two or more times (Björklund et al., 2010). And in a Portuguese community sample, the lifetime prevalence of stalking was nearly 20 percent (Matos et al., 2019). Concerningly, McKeon and associates (2015) found that, in their Australian sample, males tend to minimize the problem by believing stalking isn't really serious, that it's romantic, and that victims are to blame when it happens. Indeed, it is better you are stalked by a stranger from that standpoint because Scott and associates (2014) found that the victim was perceived as more responsible when the stalker was known to her as opposed to a lurking stranger. Clearly, there is no excuse for stalking, and we never hold victims accountable for being stalked. The point is that individuals who perpetrate others can expertly twist their rationale to fit their preferred narrative.

Cyberstalking

There is probably no more terrifying experience than being stalked, and cyberstalking adds a whole new level of access to stalkers. Cyberstalking allows the stalker to collect information about their victim and then, when communicating with the victim, reveal those personal facts. With the ever-increasing global reliance on the internet and the substantial use of social media, it is no surprise that the internet is a cyberstalker's best friend. Indeed, for those with the know-how and utter disregard for others' privacy, most anything about anyone can be found online.

What's more is that many people freely post candid details about their lives on social media for anyone to consume at any time. With little effort, cyberstalkers can learn about their victims' daily routine, favorite places to eat, pets' names, vacation schedule, and countless other personal details. Stop for a moment to think about common security questions on your online accounts, such as your mother's maiden name, your childhood street address, your pets' names, the location at which you first met your romantic partner, and even your birthdate. Now, reflect on how much of that information you have posted online. If you have not posted much of that information, either purposefully or inadvertently, good job! But if you feel a knot in your stomach thinking about everything you have posted, perhaps now is the time to set this book aside and do a little personal data clean-up on your accounts. Regardless of the measures we take to be cautious, though, anyone who has a digital trail is subject to cyberstalking.

Research on cyberstalking can be difficult to interpret due to researchers using varying definitions and criteria to determine a threshold for cyberstalking (Wilson et al., 2022), making prevalence difficult to ascertain (Kaur et al., 2021). Moreover, there is debate regarding relevant classification systems for cyberstalking or if cyberstalking should be considered as an extension of general stalking behavior (Kaur et al., 2021). Indeed, increased consensus among researchers is needed to generate a valid framework for understanding and evaluating cyberstalking. However, the available research paints a concerning picture.

Cavezza and McEwan (2014) found that while cyberstalkers were more likely to be ex-intimate partners and less likely to approach their victims, the majority still combined off-line stalking as well, and this behavior was also affirmed by Strawhun and associates (2013). We have mentioned numerous times that women perpetrate IPV quite often, and the same is true for cyberstalking. In fact, there is some evidence to suggest that women may engage in more cyberstalking than men (Alexy et al., 2005; Kalaitzaki, 2020; Strawhun et al., 2013).

Stalking victims have many of the same PTSD-like symptoms that IPV survivors do and resort to the same kinds of strategies when the stalking becomes intolerable, such as changing one's address, moving away, quitting one's job, changing one's name and appearance, and going underground (Knox & Roberts, 2005). Stalking victims often experience profound psychological reactions, such as intense anxiety and symptoms of posttraumatic stress disorder (Short et al., 2015). Moreover, Short and colleagues (2015) talk about the pervasiveness of cyberstalking, wherein perpetrators can access their victims at all hours of the day and in all contexts, thereby creating a situation in which victims feel like they have

no reprieve. In fact, many victims of cyberstalking report issues related to their relationships, work, and finances (Short et al., 2015).

Stopping stalking can be highly frustrating because the authorities likely cannot intervene unless the individual has some proof that they are being stalked (Brewster, 2002). Persons who are being stalked need to keep a recorded log of sightings, phone calls, copies of e-mails and letters, and any witnesses to the stalking. If you are being stalked, we encourage you to call law enforcement now! There are victims' advocacy groups that know how to deal with this problem, and many of them will help their clients navigate the process of reporting their stalking to the authorities. Federal anti-stalking legislation was implemented as part of the Violence Against Women Act in 1996, and all 50 states now have laws regarding stalking (Knox & Roberts, 2005). While many jurisdictions have paid little heed to stalking problems in the past, increased awareness has caused the instigation of counterstalking programs like the Nashville Metropolitan Police Department's Counterstalking Plan, which uses a wide array of technology to trap and prosecute stalkers (Roberts & Kurst-Swanger, 2002). Michele Path (2002) has written an excellent survival manual for stalking victims.

Treating IPV Perpetrators

The treatment of individuals who perpetrate IPV is challenging, complicated, and subject to high rates of recidivism. What's more is that the vast majority of treatment programs for IPV perpetrators are directed toward men who are perpetrators, even though it is well established that women and gender nonbinary individuals also perpetrate IPV at significant rates. For that reason, modern approaches to IPV treatment are often individualized to address the client's unique needs (Butters et al., 2021; Crane & Easton, 2017). Common treatment issues include, but are certainly not limited to, the following:

1. Assessment of IPV and related treatment issues. We spoke earlier regarding assessments that can be used to help gauge the likelihood of IPV and/or partner homicide. We also spoke about the presence of alcohol and/or substance misuse in many cases of IPV as well as related treatment issues. Accordingly, alcohol and substance misuse assessments should always be administered. Common examples include the Alcohol Use Disorders

Identification Test, Substance Abuse Subtle Screening Inventory, and Drug Abuse Screening Test. In addition to the role alcohol and drug use play in IPV perpetration, any individual who is under the influence of a mind-altering substance cannot actively participate in treatment. So, as you might imagine, alcohol and drug screening, assessment, and treatment are very important in the treatment of IPV perpetrators (Butters et al., 2021; Karakurt et al., 2019). When measuring related personality constructs such as anger and psychopathy, common tools include the Millon Clinical Multiaxial Inventory and the Minnesota Multiphasic Personality Inventory.

2. Whether or not to use a conjoint/couples counseling approach. There are some important arguments behind this recommendation, one of which is the assumption that perpetrators are involved in heterosexual relationships (Armenti & Babcock, 2016) and that bidirectional/reciprocal IPV is not occurring. Conjoint counseling is probably most suitable for couples who experience situational violence and problematic communication (Armenti & Babcock, 2016).

3. Managing anger, power, and control. For some IPV perpetrators, stopping their abusive behavior can feel akin to managing a substance addiction (Arvidsson & Caman, 2022); managing their anger and behavior takes thoughtful and consistent effort and is not as simple as turning off a faucet. For that reason, learning anger identification and management skills can be particularly helpful for IPV perpetrators (Morrison et al., 2018).

4. Managing previous trauma. Because of the established link between trauma and IPV perpetration (Gil-Gonzalez et al., 2008; Maldonado & Murphy, 2021; Okuda et al., 2015), trauma treatment is an important part of a holistic treatment program for IPV perpetrators (Karakurt et al., 2019).

5. Increasing motivation. Seeking professional support for violent interpersonal behavior is no small feat. And, although some clients may describe an ultimatum as a turning point (Arvidsson & Caman, 2022), motivation remains a key obstacle to treatment for many clients. As such, Motivational Interviewing (Miller & Rollnick, 2013) can be a powerful tool in the treatment of IPV perpetrators (Butters et al., 2021; Pinto e Silva et al., 2022).

6. Psychoeducation on IPV. Helping clients understand IPV and what constitutes healthy and unhealthy relationships is a significant aspect of treatment (Morrison et al., 2018). This may be quite challenging for individuals who have never experienced or seen a healthy relationship modeled. Reconceptualizing what constitutes a healthy relationship might be particularly challenging for individuals who have very strict ideas of gender roles or expectations of their partner. For that reason, addressing flawed cognition can be helpful as a means of teaching IPV perpetrators to examine the origin of their concepts/beliefs regarding relationships and how their thoughts influence their behaviors. However, relatedly, clients should learn to take accountability for their actions (Morrison et al., 2018).

7. Teaching healthy communication and conflict resolution skills. Although assertive, rather than aggressive, communication may seemingly come natural for many of you who are reading this book, assertive communication is a learned skill. Teaching IPV perpetrators how to express themselves effectively is a key aspect of treatment (Morrison et al., 2018). This may be particularly challenging for IPV perpetrators who are used to exercising their dominance to get their wishes and needs immediately met without compromise. And this might also be difficult for clients because of flawed gender roles that prevent expression of the full range of human emotion. But learning to communicate assertively and manage conflict in a manner that does not intentionally hurt others is critical to establishing and maintaining healthy relationships.

There are various approaches to *treating* IPV perpetrators, but the most widely known IPV *intervention* model is called the Duluth Model.

The Duluth Model

LO17 During the early 1980s, the Coalition for Justice for Battered Women in San Francisco was instrumental in getting law enforcement to redefine how they handle domestic disputes and how the district attorney prosecutes IPV cases (Sonkin et al., 1985, p. 25). Law enforcement do not mediate but arrest, and district attorneys do not dismiss but prosecute. In short, IPV perpetrators need to realize that partner violence is a punishable crime (Sonkin et al., 1985, p. 41), and in more and more cities and states, it is becoming exactly that.

Although arrest may deter violence while the perpetrator is incarcerated (Gondolf, 1984; Sherman & Berk, 1984), that same perpetrator will come back to their family, or at least be in close proximity to their family or inevitably form a relationship with another partner. While many believe that "throwing them in jail" is justified because of the abuse, incarceration will not have changed the perpetrator's attitudes and behavior in any way, and the perpetrator will continue to be a threat (Bent-Goodley et al., 2011).

Many communities and most states have adopted some form of diversion program modeled along the lines of the program the Coalition for Justice for Battered Women in San Francisco and the Domestic Abuse Intervention Program intervention model developed in Duluth, Minnesota (the Duluth model). These are *intervention* models as opposed to *treatment* models. Note the distinction between *intervention* and *treatment*. As with many systemic crises, there are philosophical issues between grassroots activists who organized and lobbied for aggressive intervention with IPV perpetrators and mental health professionals, who came after them, who focus on the perpetrator's underlying pathology and seek to provide treatment to change the personality structures that cause the battering (Rosenbaum & Kunkel, 2009).

The Duluth model is based on a Coordinated Community Response model ("What Is The Duluth Model?," n.d.) and requires a tremendous amount of commitment and integration of community agencies, mental health facilities and institutions, law enforcement, and the judiciary to provide services for abused individuals. As you might well imagine, getting all these agencies and institutions working on the same page is equivalent to herding cats. Lindsay and Brady (2002) acknowledge and discuss some of these issues when such massive integration of services is undertaken. The treatment aspect of the model contains a cognitive-behavioral component to it. However, it also examines the historic separation of roles and power for men and women and seeks to knock down those stereotypes. But this process requires adherence to traditional gender roles, and binary gender roles are not applicable to a large group of IPV perpetrators and victims. The program's aim is to give IPV perpetrators insight into their mistaken beliefs and goals based on these age-old stereotypes about marital roles and functions and to change their belief systems in regard to marriage, relationships, women, masculinity, and the use of aggression to solve problems (Aymer, 2008; Miller, 2010; Pence & McDonnell, 2000).

Most other models have a cognitive-behavioral basis that focuses on cognitive restructuring of IPV perpetrators' irrational thinking (Rosenbaum & Kunkle, 2009). Models that emphasize the perpetrators' strengths rather than deficits are being tried (Lehmann & Simmons, 2009). Other models provide skill building through self-empowerment strategies. This model works off the notion that targeting self-empowerment can revise and regulate feelings of powerlessness and worthlessness, which are hypothesized as core values that lead to the abuse. In this model, then, abuse is seen as a problem not of the abused partner but rather of the abuser's own feelings of inadequacy and failure to develop compassion for loved ones (Stosny, 1995).

From a therapeutic treatment viewpoint, cognitive-behavioral treatments are seen as the preferred mode of operation. Treatment professionals take umbrage at the notion that this is "anger management training" because they see the issues that IPV perpetrators are attempting to overcome as far more complex than that. Thus, it will probably come as a surprise to you that most programs and many states prohibit "anger management" as a primary treatment because they see it as an excuse to rationalize a controlled behavior (Rosenbaum & Kunkel, 2009). The fact is that in many instances, the Duluth model has been combined with cognitive-behavioral therapy for IPV perpetrators, so there is a great deal of variance between programs that claim to follow the Duluth model (Bennett & Vincent, 2001; Healy et al., 1998).

Summary

IPV has deep roots in the psychological, sociological, and cultural makeup of the United States and many other countries that extend back to the beginnings of their patriarchal systems. IPV is pervasive through all socioeconomic levels of society and knows no ethnic, racial, religious, gender, or sexual orientation boundaries. Dynamically, IPV may be seen as having much to do with the concept of power. A number of stressors that insinuate themselves into a relationship can escalate relational problems to violence.

A variety of theories have been proposed to explain why IPV occurs. However, it is still unclear what propels people into using violence in their relationships and what will keep them from being abusive again. IPV is sequential, developmental, and dynamic. The situation of the abused client is unlike that of many others in crisis in that it is almost always transcrisis in nature; that is, it is cyclic, reaching many peak levels over extended periods of time. For a variety of reasons, it is rare that a person leaves a violent relationship for good after the first episode of abuse. Continued and increased violence over a period of years is the typical pattern of abusive relationships.

Crisis lines, emergency shelters, and programs for IPV survivors and their children continue to grow across the United States. Courts and law enforcement agencies have become much more proactive in protecting the rights of these IPV victims, particularly women. However, the number of IPV survivors still far exceeds the capacity of human services to comprehensively and effectively provide care. One of the most frustrating components of intervention with clients who are IPV survivors is the intense difficulty they have in escaping from their partner's grasp.

Providing counseling in such trying circumstances calls for a great deal of empathic understanding. The crisis worker's job is to help keep the client as safe as possible, provide options, and work patiently with the survivor, help them explore alternatives and choose a plan of action. Recently, the focus on IPV has shifted to include comprehensive and integrated intervention and treatment programs that involve social services agencies, law enforcement, and the judicial system. These programs operate throughout the country. Typically sent to such groups by court order, IPV perpetrators learn to understand the factors that lead them to violence, learn to recognize and communicate their feelings, and learn to avoid or stop confrontations that lead them to act out their feelings in violent ways. If you are being abused and don't know what to do, and there don't seem to be resources in your community, call the National Domestic Violence Hotline at 1-800-799-SAFE(7233) or 1-800-787-3224 (TTY). You can also text (send START to 88788) or live chat with someone who can help. If you are a teen experiencing dating abuse, call the LoveIsRespect Helpline at 1-866-331-9474 or 1-866-331-8453 (TTY). You can also text (send "LOVEIS" to 22522) or live chat with someone who can help.

Family Crisis Intervention

Introduction

Everyone probably knows a family that seems to be in a constant state of chaos. For these families, as soon as one chaotic situation is resolved or averted, another pops up to take its place. A family member loses a job, another family member is diagnosed with a chronic medical condition, and that is followed by someone being in a car accident. Topping it all off, another family member is arrested for some alleged illegal activity, and the family continues to spiral out of control. One frenzied situation after another produces an unremitting sense of pandemonium, and in these families, dull moments are few and far between. You very likely shake your head, wondering what is needed to assist this family. The thought crosses your mind that a reality television series or daytime soap opera could feature this family.

A few families are like this, but the vast majority are not. Most families live in a stable, predictable manner, following the same routine day in and day out. However, even for stable families, crises are a fact of life. No family is immune (Hoffet et al., 2009; Rolland, 2012). All families bump or maybe crash into something that taxes them and disrupts routines. In the early months of 2020 and those following, even the most stable families likely experienced one form or another of a crisis because of the pandemic (Gurwitch et al., 2020).

Some family crises come suddenly and unexpectedly, disrupting day-to-day life. Other crises are the result of fatigue that develops from a series of events that have worn down a family's resilience (Golan, 1987; Walsh, 2012a). Still other crises are insidious, creeping up on families, and suddenly they find themselves besieged with decisions they are not prepared to make. These families may not even realize they are in crisis until things start crumbling around them. Regardless of the type of crisis, the usual way of coping no longer works, and families scramble simply to survive.

Even if your practice is exclusively with individuals, individual crises always entangle family members (Rosenfeldet et al., 2005; Walsh, 2012a). In fact, understanding the effect of a crisis from a family perspective may just be the way to ease the pressure and facilitate the ability to restore an individual's coping mechanisms. Using an intervention model designed for family crisis situations is critical (Walsh, 2012a). Just as personal theories and intervention models fall short in individual crisis intervention, family therapy models also may not be effective in crisis situations.

In this chapter, you will meet the Medina family, who are experiencing a crisis because of a tragedy that seems to take place almost on a daily basis, a mass shooting. These shootings have occurred in almost every setting you can think of, including retail outlets, faith-based organizations, public and private schools, universities, workplaces, and even in back yards. Given the sheer number of mass shootings, odds are that you may be asked to provide crisis intervention services at some point in your career.

Eva, the mother in the Medina family, worked as a cashier at a large box store and was recently severely injured during a mass shooting. Although not life threatening, the injury required hospitalization for five weeks plus physical rehabilitation. One employee was pronounced dead at the scene. Six customers shopping at the store also did not survive. Another three employees and four customers received various levels of injuries from minor to serious. The case presented is not representative of any specific mass shooting. The case is simply used to represent a family in crisis.

This chapter begins by presenting information that forms the foundation for working with families in crises. We begin by defining family crisis and transcrisis. The next section provides historical context for family crisis intervention by summarizing research on family crises, followed by a discussion of various models for understanding families in distress. The models discussed in this section trace the development of family crisis intervention since World War II. As you will read, the models have evolved over time and now emphasize resiliency. The next section discusses the types of crises families encounter, followed by an introduction to the Medina family. The remainder of the chapter uses the Medina family to illustrate "hands on" practical information for helping families in crisis.

Definition of Family Crisis

LO1 The effect of crises on families is mentioned in many chapters in this book. Chapter 18 (online) on addictions talks about "family rules and addictions" and "children in families who abuse alcohol." The next chapter on partner violence obviously involves a family crisis. Chapter 9, "Sexual Assault"; Chapter 10, "Partner Violence"; Chapter 12, Personal Loss: Bereavement and Grief; and Chapter 16, "Disaster Response" each discuss family issues related to those crises. In each of these chapters, the focus is on understanding and helping the individual having the crisis. The chapter on partner violence focuses on Juanita and helping her as she navigates and moves beyond her situation of domestic violence. The crisis intervention with Heather in the chapter on sexual assault addresses her working through feelings about being assaulted by her stepfather. While the Benefield family are the targeted characters in the disaster chapter, the focus is still on how each one of those members copes with the trauma they have been through rather than looking at the total family system as they struggle to regain pre-disaster homeostasis. Yet, all of these crises affecting individuals also have the capacity to significantly change the family system. And understanding the effect of crises on families begins by defining a family crisis.

Chapter 1, "Approaching Crisis Intervention," introduced our definition for a crisis as individuals being overwhelmed and unable to marshal the resources needed at that moment to attend to what has happened. Included in the discussion was a brief description of systemic crises that applies to families, organizations, and communities. That discussion is an excellent foundation for shaping a definition of family crises. However, coming up with a definitive definition of a family crisis is like trying to grasp a handful of mud. The more you squeeze the mud, the more it slips through your fingers. You might ask why a definition for family crisis is so slippery. First, the different starting points and intensity levels for a family crisis make it difficult to pin down an all-encompassing, perfect definition. No matter the starting and ending points, something always seems to be missed. Second, attempting to understand family crises from the reactions of individual family members' reactions is an exercise in futility (Etcherling et al., 2005). A systems understanding is needed because the whole is greater than the sum of the parts. Understanding individual reactions is essential, but when working with families, a broader, more comprehensive view is needed to be effective.

As suggested in Chapter 1, "Approaching Crisis Intervention," some family crises start with one family member experiencing a personal crisis that ripples through the family, causing a larger crisis (Walsh, 2012a). These metastasizing crises leach into the family, pulling in all members one at a time. An individual crisis generally takes the path of least resistance in families, seeping into the most vulnerable places. Take, for example, the crisis of a family member losing a job. While only one family member lost a job, the crisis has the potential to affect the family in many ways, such as changing spending patterns, causing others to get jobs to make ends meet, or disrupting relationships in the family. Other family crises begin outside the family and come without warning, affecting family members simultaneously, such as a sudden accidental death in the family (Hoff et al., 2009). This type of crisis hits the family all at once. Like a head-on collision, all family members feel the brunt of the crisis instantaneously. In general, natural and technological disasters fall into this category and are a major cause of family crises, causing relocations, injuries, major financial issues, and so on (Everstine & Everstine, 2006).

The intensity with which a family experiences crises must also be considered. For some family members, the crisis might be quite intense, while for others, the situation might be more of a disruption (Myer & Moore, 2006). Members of a family in which someone has sustained a debilitating injury causing extended rehabilitation and physical therapy might experience different levels of intensity. Some members of the family might have their entire schedule disrupted, taking care of the person, taking them to appointments, and caring for them in the home. Others in the family might only experience minor inconveniences, having to alter their lives occasionally to help and support the injured person. Taking this a step further, a complicating factor for family crisis occurs when some members of a family believe a crisis is occurring and other family members do not even acknowledge a crisis exists (Al et al., 2011). When family members are not on the same page with respect to the crisis, intensity is difficult to gauge. Many times, this situation involves making a decision of some kind, such as placing an older family member in a nursing home or similar care facility. Some family members may get caught up struggling with ways to address the crisis,

while others may ignore it or discount that there is even a problem. The latter simply want to make a decision and move on. Working with these families calls for crisis workers to use patience to help family members find a common ground to address the crisis.

We found several definitions that shed light on just exactly what a family crisis is. These definitions are like a diamond with many facets. Each facet offers a different perspective on family crises.

1. Family crisis occurs when a disaster or trauma damages the bonds that connect people and destroys the basic tissues of social life and the prevailing sense of community (Rosenfeld et al., 2010).
2. A crisis results when a stress comes to bear upon the system and requires change outside the system's usual repertoire, causing nonspecific changes in the system (Pittman, 1987).
3. A crisis results from families feeling dismemberment (loss of family member), accession (unexpected addition of a member), demoralization (loss of morale and family unit), or a combination of the three (Hill, 1965).
4. A crisis occurs depending on how a family defines an event that disrupts the social networks of a family, thereby changing its configuration (Hoff et al., 2009).
5. A crisis takes place when traumatic events wreck a family's homeostatic balance and render the system nonfunctional (Everstine & Everstine, 2006).
6. A crisis is an unexpected, negative event that does not allow the family to continue functioning in their usual manner; further, most families are unprepared for the crisis and find addressing such circumstances both challenging and stressful (Webb & Dickson, 2012).

Just as with the definitions for individuals in crisis, clearly different perspectives are used to define family crisis. These definitions focus on various aspects, including structural changes in relationships, lack or deactivation of coping mechanisms, a sense of loss within the family, family communication, inability to function in the usual manner, and balance within the system. Integrating components of the definitions above with the one in Chapter 1 "Approaching Crisis Intervention," for individual crisis shapes our characterization for family crisis. Our definition of a **family crisis** is: *A crisis occurs when perceptions or experiencing of an event bears on the family as a whole, testing the family's structural integrity, because the usual repertoire of problem-solving skills and communication styles are not* *adequate or have been exhausted. Unless relief is obtained, the crisis jeopardizes family homeostasis and has the potential to strip family resilience.*

Transcrisis

LO2   Transcrisis (Ford, 2021; Gilliand & James, 1988) is a concept recognizing that crises may at times not be fully resolved and what van der Kolk and McFarlane (1996) identify as the black hole of trauma. If not fully resolved, the feelings, behaviors, and cognitions may become submerged and out of awareness. These feelings, behaviors, and cognitions can lay dormant for extended periods of time and have no effect on day-to-day living. However, when new stressors occur, the feelings, behaviors, and cognitions surface, resulting in a reaction similar to the original crisis. Unlike post-traumatic stress disorder, **family transcrisis** is not a diagnosable Diagnostic and Statistical Manual of Mental Disorders, Fifth Edition, Text Revision (*DSM-5-TR*) disorder. Rather, transcrisis is present as more of a low-level, lurking, residual state that surfaces when the situation activates the suppressed feelings, behaviors, and cognitions associated with the original crisis.

The way a family addresses and attempts to resolve a crisis has a significant impact on the development of issues that lead to longer effects and possibly to a transcrisis state (Vos et al., 2021). Families can stifle a crisis, hoping it simply will evaporate, ignore it thinking it will go away, or hide from it hoping the storm will blow over. Regardless, in the end, the issues related to the crisis fade, receding to a point where they are below conscious awareness and not affecting day-to-day functioning. The issues are an undercurrent swirling just below the surface, seemingly waiting for the opportunity to erupt when a new stressor is encountered. Just as with individuals, the eruptions into a transcrisis state are not predictable and may not occur for weeks, months, or even years after the original crisis. Between the flare-ups, families attain homeostasis, behaving as if nothing is wrong. Interactions of family members between the outbursts are typically filled with usual, everyday, customary activities. Family members understand the expectations and function in a consistent, routine manner. However, the experience of a novel stressor can catapult families into a transcrisis state and reopen old wounds. Issues not resolved from the original crisis rocket to the forefront, leaving families wondering what is happening. Families might experience an empty, sinking feeling that nothing has changed from the original crisis event, and they are just experiencing another setback in a long line of aftershocks, which they attempt to survive while waiting for the next aftershock because the original issue has never been resolved.

Interactions among family members often provide a window into identifying a transcrisis state in families. These interactions can be obvious or subtle but almost always refer to previous experiences when families were not able to satisfactorily resolve a crisis. Obvious transcrisis statements are relatively easy to detect. A family member might say something like "Here we go again, just like before." Other typical statements include "This is just like before, you did not listen to me then and you are not listening now," "You keep saying the same thing, over and over and over, you never change," or "We just cannot get this right." Each of these statements refers back to previous experiences that are clues for considering if families are in a transcrisis state. Many times, less obvious subtle indicators are seen in the form of nonverbal behaviors. Family members may shake their heads as if saying "Here we go again," or roll their eyes communicating "Not the same thing we did before." Recognition of the transcrisis state means crisis intervention strategies are needed to facilitate families' satisfactory resolution of the original crisis.

Research on Family Crisis

LO3   The framework of crisis intervention for working with families is somewhat unclear (Al et al., 2011). A possible reason for the ambiguity is that much of the research in this area has concentrated on identifying specific factors associated with families in crisis such as economic factors, individual family member history, race or ethnicity, spirituality and beliefs, stage of the family life cycle, parental behaviors, education level, recovery, and so on (Gil-Rivas et al., 2010; Price et al., 2010; Rosenfeld et al., 2010; Yorgason, 2010). Research has also focused on specific situations that tax the ability of families to respond (Price et al., 2010). The results of this research provide a model for identifying risk factors and issues related to families in crisis. Keep in mind that this research is just the framework, not a complete grasp of the nuances of the unique ways individual families react to and cope with crises. Like using the same blueprint to build two houses, the basic frame of the houses is the same, yet the insides are very different. One house might have smooth walls, while the other might have textured or paneled walls. Soft pastel colors might be the color scheme for one house, while the other house has bright, bold colors for the walls. The two houses have the same floor plan, yet each is very different. Similarly, two families might have the same or similar risk factors and have experienced the exact same crisis situation, but their reactions are very different. The research findings allow crisis workers to sort through relevant and not relevant issues, but do not address the intervention process.

Medical Crises

Probably the most extensive research with families in crisis situations involves the disruption of family life because of medical issues (Gonzalez, 2013; Lutz et al., 2011; Metha et al., 2009; Tunick et al., 2013). A catalyst for much of this research has been advances in health care that extend life beyond what was previously possible even a few years ago (Rolland, 2012). This emphasis is not surprising since the question is not if families will face a medical crisis, but when and what type of medical crisis. Sooner or later, all families face decisions about medical treatment, such as end-of-life care, management of chronic illnesses, choices regarding critical care, and/or supporting family members who are not able to care for themselves. Research on decision making has examined family processes regarding end-of-life issues (Gonzalez, 2013; Haley et al., 2002; Metha et al., 2009), elderly care (Buhr et al., 2006; Ducharme et al., 2012), choices involving critical care (Tunick et al., 2013; White et al., 2012), treatment of chronic illness (Hickman & Douglas, 2010; Yorgason, 2010), and aftercare (Lutz et al., 2011).

The COVID-19 pandemic adds an entirely new layer to medical issues. Families had to cope with disrupted attachment crises (Gurwitch et al., 2020). Maybe someone had to drop a family member at a hospital emergency room and was not able to wait with them to see a doctor. That situation occurred regardless of the medical issue but was even worse if the family member had COVID symptoms early in the pandemic, not knowing if they would ever see their family member alive again. You probably saw news media reporting on this situation, often showing family members outside the hospital window or using video conferencing to see and talk with the family member. A complication of this crisis involves not being able to access other social support. As you think back on that time, you may have had limited contact with extended family and other support systems such as faith-based communities. This all took place when the support was most needed. Even worse, if the family member did not survive, a funeral was probably delayed until a time when the COVID-19 pandemic was not at a high level. Children were especially affected when a parent, grandparent, and/or sibling did not survive (Gurwitch et al., 2020).

Medical crises such as these can cause family members to struggle and sometimes battle over limited choices, none of which are optimal. Reactions range from cooperative coordination of efforts to chaotic and even mean-spirited attempts at taking advantage of the disorder surrounding the situation. Emotions bubble up, maybe even exploding into full-blown politically incorrect name calling. Behavioral reactions might be smooth and well-coordinated or restrained to the point of being paralyzed, with no one willing to do anything. Behavioral reactions also can erupt into something less than appropriate to the point of physical altercations at times. Family members might scheme and/or conspire to deliberately manipulate the situation to cause other family members' feelings of guilt or to take responsibility for all the ills ever experienced by the family. They may attempt to sabotage efforts to address the crisis to punish or finagle an advantage for themselves. Forewarned is forearmed so you are not blindsided as families grapple with medical crises. Simply stated, the variety of reactions is limitless.

Disaster Recovery

Risk factors, resilience, and recovery from disaster are other areas that have been the focus of crisis intervention with families (Gurwitch et al., 2020; Knowles et al., 2010, Whitmand & Mattord, 2021). Research in this area typically takes place in the aftermath of disasters such as the Three Mile Island nuclear accident (Handford et al., 1986), the terrorist bombing in Oklahoma City (Sitterle & Gurwitch, 1999), the terrorist attacks of 9/11 (Devoe et al., 2011), Hurricane Katrina (Gil-Rivas et al., 2010; Knowles et al., 2010; Shanhinfar et al., 2010) and most recently, the COVID pandemic (Gurwitch et al., 2020; Pfefferbaum, 2021). These situations can shatter the day-to-day activities of families in an instant, resulting in considerable change (Everstine & Everstine, 2006). The result is that families are thrust into a novel and stressful situation that is often chaotic, without forewarning and/or experience to manage all that needs to be accomplished. Many times, resources are scarce, and families have difficulty accessing these in a timely manner (Rosenfeld et al., 2010; Webb, 2005).

Much of the attention in the research on families in disaster recovery addresses the role of parents and caregivers in family members' reactions, specifically children and adolescents (Gil-Rivas et al., 2010). This research found that caregivers significantly influence children's and adolescents' adjustment positively or negatively following a disaster (Devoe et al., 2011; Felix et al., 2015; Polusny et al., 2011). As would be expected, negative reactions to a disaster such as increased anxiety or chronic unwanted thoughts in caregivers had high transference to youth in their care. On the other hand, caregivers who demonstrated resilience and growth after a disaster had high transference value to children and adolescents in their care as well. Researchers have also discovered that a critical factor following a disaster involves the capacity of communities to meet the ongoing needs of families following a disaster (Kilmer & Gil-Rivas, 2010). Kilmer and Gil-Rivas believe that communities must go beyond traditional mental health intervention and develop comprehensive disaster response services that address families' needs in the longer term.

Family Crisis Models

LO4   Theoretical explanations of families in crisis have been in existence since 1949 (Hill). These models describe families' reactions to distress or stress depending on the developer's experience with and observations of families experiencing hardship. For example, the ABC-X model was developed to explain families' experience of absences due to military deployment and the reunion of families (Price et al., 2010), while the family distress model builds on the developers' experience in family medicine and was created to explain families who need but are reluctant to seek external support (Weber, 2011). The models offer different vantage points to view families' crises, with each one presenting valuable insight into understanding the experience of crises as they impact families.

ABC-X and Double ABC-X Model. The first and one of the better-known family crisis models is the ABC-X formula (Boss, 2002). The ABC-X model can be broken down into four key components: (1) the stressor event, (2) the family's resources, (3) the family's perception of the stressor, and (4) the crisis (Price et al., 2021; Weber, 2011). These four components happen sequentially, with each contributing to families experiencing a crisis.

The catalyst for the development of this model was the return of soldiers following World War II (Price et al., 2010). Since the model's inception in 1949 (Hill) and initial reconsideration in 1958, many researchers in the field have adjusted and adapted the model for a wide variety of crises (Boss, 2002). The most significant change in the model was made by McCubbin and Paterson (1983), who expanded the model to include risk and protective variables that influence the crisis following the event to explain ways families adapt. The expanded model, known as the double ABC-X model, is used to explain families' reactions to and recovery from events ranging from internal and external disruptions to family functioning.

The elegance of the ABC-X and double ABC-X model is its simplicity. The model starts by focusing on precrisis, with the "A" being the precipitating event and/or stressor (Weber, 2011). These events are ones for which families have little to no prior experience. As a result, families experience hardships they are not able to manage because of the lack of competence and/or resources (Rosenfeld et al., 2010). "B" represents the resources available to families to cope with the event (Price et al., 2010). If adequate resources are available, families avert falling into a crisis. If resources are not accessible, a crisis may occur depending on the interpretation of the event. This brings us to the "C" in the model that stands for families' interpretation of the event (Weber, 2011). When families interpret the event as a crisis producing problems that exceed their physical and psychological resources, a crisis "X" is experienced, requiring potential changes in structure and interactions to restore stability (Rosenfeld et al., 2010).

Double aA. The double "aA" refers to the immediate stressor plus the demands and shifts that occur in families and individual family members, resulting in a stacking of stresses one on top of the other (Boss, 2002; Rosino, 2016). As the stresses continue to stack up, families feel even more squeezed, thus increasing the severity of the crisis. The "bB" in the equation concerns activating existing resources as well as seeking additional resources from outside the family (Price et al., 2021; Rosino, 2016). The double "cC" of the model involves families' perceptions about the way to restore balance (Rosenfeld et al., 2010; Rosino, 2016). For example, if the primary breadwinner loses the job, a family might decide that other members of the family need to secure jobs to offset the loss of income. The family might also cancel planned vacations to cut costs, change eating habits such as dining out, and so on. All these measures are perceived methods to restore balance to the family. "xX' refers to families' adaptation process to crises (Price et al., 2021). Successful adaptation is termed **bonadaptation**, and the lack of balance is called **maladaptation** (Rosenfeld et al., 2010). Bonadaptation is considered to be good, useful, and healthy, whereas maladaptation is negative, ineffective, and unhealthy. Understand that what is bonadaptation for one family may not be the same for other families. The same is true for maladaptation. Also, bonadaptation in one situation is not necessarily true for another, and the same holds true for maladaptation.

Contextual Model. The **contextual model** of family stress builds on the ABC-X model (Weber, 2011). Introduced by Boss (2002), this model recognizes that families are unique and that events, the same or similar, will be experienced in distinctive ways. As a result, this model considers families' internal and external context as major factors in shaping reactions to stress and crisis situations. Internal context refers to things families can control and are divided into structural, psychological, and philosophical context (Boss, 2002). The structural context of families includes issues around boundaries and communication patterns that can be manipulated by families. Issues related to families' psychological context concern affective and cognitive perceptions of the stressor or crisis (Weber, 2011). Philosophical contextual issues concern values and belief systems held by families (Boss, 2002). Boss believes that because internal contextual issues are regulated by families, these should be addressed in the intervention process.

However, many external contextual issues are beyond the control of families. Issues such as history, macroeconomic human development, heredity, and culture fall into this category (Boss, 2002). Families cannot control historical events, nor can they control global finances, for example, whether a recession takes place. These issues are global and are a result of a multitude of interacting factors. Aging is another external factor over which families have no control, although some try through cosmetic surgery or anti-aging products. The biological and genetic makeup of families is an external factor (Boss, 2002). Boss contends that we are born into families not by choice and that some families' genetic makeup is more resilient than others. The final external factor concerns culture and the way it interprets events (Boss, 2002).

Research supports this concept by examining cultures and studying the way some cultures react to traumatic situations (deVries, 1996). External contextual factors should be recognized as contributing to family reactions and used as a framework for understanding families' experiences (Boss, 2002).

Family Distress Model. The **family distress model (FDM)** was first introduced by Cornille and Boroto (1992) and later was enhanced by the **family outreach model (FOM)** (Cornille et al., 2008). The purpose for the model is to identify families' patterns of coping to develop interventions designed to support attempts at managing the situation (Weber, 2011). FDM states that when in distress, families use strategies that are different from their daily predictable patterns (Cornille et al., 2008). If the changes in routine are not successful in reducing the stress, crises arise. FDM was broadened by the formation of FOM, which added a practical intervention component. FOM goes beyond traditional family intervention models based on conceptualizations of pathology that must be diagnosed or dysfunctional families that require expert assessment (Cornille et al., 2008). This assessment leads to making intentional choices about intervention approaches, both collaborative and directive styles, to support and help families during the crisis. The intervention style used is determined by what best fits with what specific families want and need (Cornille et al., 2008). According to the developers, FOM can be used to identify families' needs and direct the intervention process from collaborative to directive approaches.

FDM consists of five phases that move from the initial encounter with a stressful event to the tools for assisting families. Phase 1 of FDM assumes families have predictable patterns that are typical and desirable and include routines, rituals, and rules used for decision making (Weber, 2011). Decisions can be conscious or automatic, occurring with little to no thought, such as when dinner is served, who is responsible for cleaning bathrooms, who drives the family car, and so on. However, internal or external situations arise that disrupt day-to-day patterns resulting in families moving to Phase 2 of FDM (Weber, 2011). Tried and true strategies to correct the disturbance are attempted in this phase. These strategies have been successfully used to manage previous disturbances and are designed to reduce stress, therefore returning families to typical functioning. If these methods are not successful, a family crisis occurs.

Phases 3 to 5 involve families organizing around the crisis, seeking resources to manage the situation, and finally reorganizing to create a new pattern of stability (Cornille et al., 2008). In these phases, families become preoccupied with the crisis and a great deal of collective energy is used to control the disruptions (Weber, 2011). Weber states that unless families are able to access support to manage the crisis, patterns either beneficial or maladaptive will adjust to accommodate the crisis state. If, however, support is found, families will regain stability through activating old patterns or developing new patterns.

Family Communication Model. The **family communication model** depicts an approach for families to cope with and prevail during crises using internal and external verbal interactions. The model makes the assumption that the root of family crises is communication (Webb & Dickson, 2012). According to this model, communication patterns change to discuss challenging topics that are not typically discussed. Examples of topics challenging to discuss are a family member's terminal illness and the effect on everyone in the family or the excessive consumption of alcohol or use of illegal substances by one or more members in the family. Generally, issues such as these are not the average topic for day-to-day conversations; rather, they are discussed as needed and in extraordinary circumstances. The authors add that communication can be internal discussion with family members only and/or external communication with others. Webb and Dickson stress that these difficult conversations are the key element for coping with crises. The goal of this communication is the co-construction of a rational explanation that makes meaning of the experience to create a positive view of the ultimate outcome for crises. Webb and Dickson caution that any change in communication patterns be strategic rather than unregulated disclosure. According to them, discussion should be tailored for individual family members with respect to the amount of information given and to whom it is shared and how it can be handled.

Webb and Dickson (2012) further state that effective family coping with crises involves two types of communication. The first type of communication is instrumental and concerns the exchange of information. Instrumental communication involves discussions that are unique to crises and are deliberate in nature. For example, in the case of weather-related crises such as hurricanes, floods, or tornadoes, families would discuss issues such as evacuation plans and locations to meet in case members are separated. Instrumental communication is based on a "need-to-know" basis, with not everyone being given the same information. The second type of communication is emotion based. These discussions can involve sharing feelings previously not disclosed that relate to the crisis. According to Dickson and Webb, communication of emotions is vital in helping family members develop healthy coping mechanisms.

Resiliency Model. The **resiliency model** represents a current focus of family crisis intervention and views families not as damaged but rather challenged by adversities (Walsh, 2012b). This model concentrates on the potential for recovery and restoration of functioning rather than pathologizing families' reactions while experiencing adversity (Walsh, 2021). Through activating families' belief systems, organizational patterns, and communication processes, families have potential for personal and interaction transformation and growth (Walsh, 2012b). According to Walsh (2021), when adversity strikes families, a dynamic process occurs that sets a trajectory for families' reactions to the situation. Belief systems involve families' ability to make meaning of the crisis, develop a positive outlook, and include spiritual traditions. These elements create a perspective families employ to approach crises. Organizational patterns include the capacity of families to be flexible, feel a sense of connectedness, and the ability to access social and economic resources. These elements must be clarified and marshaled in light of modern families' structures and resources. Walsh (2012b) states there is no common configuration and, therefore, organizing crises will be unique for families. Finally, communication involves problem solving and includes clear messages, open emotional expression, and collaboration. Walsh recognizes culture is important and significantly influences the communication process. This influence includes the way emotions are shared along with what feelings are acceptable to communicate.

Although other models for family crises can be found, the ones presented in this chapter are representative and practical in planning and coping with a family wide crisis. Each model provides a different perspective in working with families in crisis, and specific use is dependent on context, time, and socioeconomic and cultural environment.

Types of Crisis Families Encounter

LO5 Family crises come in all shapes, sizes, and forms, with each having idiosyncratic qualities. Generally, the types of crises families experience mirror the types described in Chapter 1, "Approaching Crisis Intervention," such as developmental, situational, and so on. Just as with individuals, some crises come from seemingly nowhere, shattering a family's homeostasis, while others creep up insidiously on families and before they know it, full-blown chaos reigns (Walsh, 2021). With families, however, several special types of crises can occur. These crises develop because as a system, stressors placed on families have an effect on the collective whole, as well as individual family members (Myer & Moore, 2006).

Knowledge of the types of crises experienced by families is critical for identifying possible issues that may be causing problems and is important for understanding effective approaches for helping them climb out of the crisis. Recognize that although the types of crises families experience will be discussed as separate types, crises are not usually that distinct. Some issues and problems are common to all types of family crises. The most distinguishing aspect of family crises is their origin. Also, you need to appreciate that families may present a crisis situation in such a way that makes it difficult to identify the type. The watch words here are "be flexible" and willing to adjust as you find out more about what is happening.

Developmental Crises. As families develop and mature, crises are inevitable (Pittman, 1987) because the transitions brought on by development strain family coping and resilience, creating the potential for stressors to accumulate and disrupting their ability to function (Bonnefil & Jacobson, 1979; Peterson et al., 2010). Crises falling into this category in many ways are governed by families' culture. In fact, the concept of family is greatly influenced by culture (McGoldrick & Ashton, 2010). For example, in many cultures, family refers to the nuclear family, while in others, family has a multigenerational connotation. For some traditional families living in Eastern countries, a crisis might occur if members of the family eschew a collective identity and strike out on their own, leaving customs behind. In contrast, a family in a Western culture might have a crisis because of the "failure to launch" that happens when young adults do not separate from parents and do not leave home. More will be said about culture later in the chapter.

Most **developmental crises** can be anticipated and therefore planned, while others cannot (McGoldrick & Shisbusawa, 2010; Pittman, 1987). Getting married, having children, children beginning school, midlife transitions, retirement, and so on are all examples of predictable situations that may cause developmental crises (Cowan & Cowan, 2012). These situations have the potential to shift a family's day-to-day functioning (Peterson et al., 2010), straining its coping abilities and resources. If stretched far enough, a crisis occurs.

Off-time developmental crises occur when transitions are out of sequence, not happening in the expected order (McGoldrick & Ashton, 2012). By nature, these situations are particularly troublesome as they can be extremely disruptive to families' resilience and capacity to cope (Peterson et al., 2010). Examples of off-time developmental situations are the untimely death of a parent, unplanned pregnancies, forced retirement, disability due to chronic illness, and so on. Families may not be prepared to mobilize the resources needed to manage the demands and could spiral into crises (Cowan & Cowan, 2012).

Bolts From the Blue. Bolts from the blue family crises (Pittman, 1987) are akin to individual situational crises in that these are unexpected, resulting in families feeling as if they have smashed into a brick wall at full speed. No matter how prepared families might be, these crises fracture the family homeostasis, disrupting the day-to-day functioning of a family. This category of crises includes, but is not limited to, off-time developmental crises. Most of the crises falling into this category are largely universal in nature, crossing cultural boundaries. These crises are generated both internally and externally to families (Weber, 2011). Examples of internally generated crises of this nature include infidelity, mental illness, a parent abandoning the family, desertion, chronic gambling, and diagnosis with a chronic illness. Externally generated crises include loss of job, disasters, sexual assault, victim of a crime, and lawsuits.

Pile Up Crises. Pile up crises for families take place when stressors accumulate to the point that they derail families' ability to function (Walsh, 2012b). The idiom "the straw that broke the camel's back" captures the essence of pile up crises. Pile up crises occur when families experience a series of internal and/or external stressors over a short period of time (Patterson, 2002). Initially, families cope well, but as the stressors accumulate, the capacity to cope falters and breaks down, plunging families into a crisis. Families may not be aware they are experiencing a pile up crisis. Instead, they may perceive the situations as isolated events that unfortunately have come all at once. Families may ask for assistance with just the latest of the series of events. Yet the persistent challenges eventually drain the available resources and coping mechanisms. The refrigerator stops working one day, which may not have been a major surprise. However, the same day the family car has a flat and you discover while getting the flat fixed a new set of tires is needed, not to mention the brake pads are too thin to drive safely and both must be replaced immediately. The financial strain is great but manageable with effort. Later in the day, the family discovers that an extended family member with whom they have been close has been diagnosed with a potentially fatal medical problem. Following this comes a revelation that one of the children in the family is not doing well in school and, in fact, is close to flunking. One situation after another ensues, none of which on its own is insurmountable, but combined eventually overwhelms families' capacity to bounce back. The breakdown of coping mechanisms and the rapid depletion of resources send the family into a nosedive and a pile up crisis is the result.

Exhaustion Crises. Exhaustion crises are similar to pile up crises but instead occur over a more prolonged period. These crises occur when families experience stressors over an extended period of time. Unlike pile up crises that involve multiple stressors, crises of this type may be due to one stressor that has unrelentingly beleaguered families over an extended period of time. Take, for example, a situation where a child has a medical condition that requires repeated attention. The medical condition is not life threatening but requires numerous visits to a physician and periodic stays in the hospital. Initially, families may find this situation manageable, but after a few months, fatigue begins to take its toll on the family, disrupting its day-to-day function. As resilience wears down and exhaustion sets in, a crisis of some type surfaces (Patterson, 2002; Walsh, 2012b).

An example of an exhaustion crisis is the continued stress experienced by a family when one member, maybe even two, misuse medications, street drugs, or alcohol. If you or a loved one are struggling with crisis fatigue, contact the Substance Abuse and Mental Health Services Administration (SAMHSA) National Helpline at 1-800-662-4357 for information

on support and treatment facilities in your area. For more mental health resources, refer to the National Helpline Database.

Perpetual Crises. Some families roll from one crisis to the next with virtually no time between the crises (Kagan & Schlosberg, 1989). This is a kind of hybrid transcrisis with no one particular stimulus but a constant refrain of the "If it weren't for bad luck, I'd have no luck at all" song. Crises for these families are a way of life as they are unable to cope on a day-to-day basis because the threshold for tolerating even minimal stressors is so low almost every situation evokes a crisis response. Families in perpetual crises specialize in getting others involved, including welfare offices, schools, child protective services, and so on (Kagan & Scholsberg, 1989). Families in this category may have structural problems that constantly intentionally or unintentionally cause crises (Pittman, 1987). Examples of structural issues that cause continuous crises in families include members who abuse alcohol and disrupt family functioning or family members in persistent trouble with the law, resulting in families living in a constant state of uncertainty, not knowing if the sheriff will be knocking on the door. These families live as if they are not at the edge of the cliff but have already taken a step off that cliff.

Crises for these families are different from metastasizing crises discussed in Chapter 1, "Approaching Crisis Intervention." Metastasizing crises can be traced back to an isolated catalyst that spreads into other areas of families' day-to-day life. That is, you can trace a starting point to the series of crises that are linked together. However, there seems to be no starting point for families in perpetual crises. These families act out themes repeatedly, caught in a loop that never stops (Ford, 2021; Kagan & Scholsberg, 1989). The situations causing the crises are separate and unrelated, yet the same modus operandi is used regardless of its appropriateness. The families may be able to acknowledge the futility of the situation but lack the energy, knowledge, or will to do anything different. Instead, they rely on others to rescue them from crises.

Ambiguous Loss. Ambiguous loss is a special type of family crisis worth mentioning (Boss, 2006). Families having an ambiguous crisis experience the incongruity between physical and psychological presence and absence of family members (Price et al., 2010). A clear example of an ambiguous loss would be families with a member who is a soldier listed as missing in action.

Another example is the families of passengers of the Malaysian flight 370 that crashed, and no wreckage or bodies were found. Yet family crises of this nature also involve times when someone may be physically present but not psychologically or emotionally, such as family members with dementia or possibly a chronic mental illness (Price et al., 2010). According to Price et al., these crises unsettle the functioning of families because of the lack of clarity in the situation. The lack of clarity prevents families from reorganizing the relationship with absent family members and completing social rituals that enable adjustment to the loss (Weber, 2011).

Dynamics of Family Intervention

LO6   **LO7**   Families create systematic patterns of relating to one another and the world around them in order to maintain equilibrium as they live together (McWhirter et al., 2013). These patterns establish the instrumental and expressive dynamics within the family that ease daily life so families function effectively (Knowles et al., 2010). Instrumental dynamics include the roles family members assume to meet the functional needs of day-to-day living (Cochran & Niego, 2002). Think about your family; everyone has a pretty good idea of who is responsible for what and when tasks need to be completed. You do not have to consult about who takes out the trash; you know who has that responsibility. You also know the rules about whose turn it is to set or clear the table. Your family might take turns, but it may be that the person who cooks does not have to help clean up after dinner. Boundaries are also part of instrumental dynamics and manage the interactions within and outside the family (McLendon & Petr, 2005). In your family, what can you say, and who can you say that to? Are you supposed to talk with your friends about the argument that happened the previous evening? Can you tell a parent or others in the family about problems you are having with school, relationships, or other issues? These are examples of the boundaries for your family.

On the other hand, expressive dynamics of families involve the ways family members interact with one another (Pierce et al., 1996), how conflicts are negotiated (Knowles et al., 2010), as well as values and goals held by families (Myer et al., 2014). In your family, you know the person best able to provide emotional support and comfort. You probably have a good idea about how differences of opinion or conflicts are resolved in your family. Some families might get quite loud when clashing with one another, while other families might know that discussing differences is forbidden or limited to certain times of the day. You also know that ignoring family values will cause trouble, possibly resulting in punishment of some type. However, when families face a crisis, these dynamics, instrumental and expressive, are turned upside down and become confusing (Ectherling et al., 2005; Peterson et al., 2010). The usual way of doing things no longer works, and families are forced into making adjustments (Rosenfeld et al., 2010). This discontinuity can be a turning point for families (Patterson, 2002). Understanding these dynamics is critical to work with families who are in a crisis (Myer et al., 2014).

Based on the family crisis intervention models discussed previously, six dynamics are particularly sensitive to the break of family dynamics (Myer et al., 2014). Crises seem to weave their way through these dynamics, causing distractions, disturbances, and interruptions as families work to overcome the situation. However, resolving a family crisis is not easy and, in fact, is very complicated. Often, the changes in dynamics hamper, stall, and otherwise thwart the resolution process as families struggle to right themselves. In fact, the modifications to dynamics may cause other crises to surface. Therefore, a critical aspect of the crisis intervention process is recognizing the shift in routine functioning to help families bring this shift into focus.

Roles. Probably the most visible dynamic altered by a crisis is the roles family members play. Customary roles are no longer performed, leaving gaps in families' capacity to function (Price et al., 2010). A wide range of alterations in roles can take place, but they generally fall into two categories. First, suppose a family member develops a chronic illness or an accident occurs, and they are no longer able to fulfill a role because of not being able to go up and down stairs. Someone else in the family must assume the roles the debilitated family member fulfilled. Or the family's primary "breadwinner" is fired or furloughed, leaving finances uncertain. Other family members must pick up the slack, and adolescent family members potentially must find jobs to make up for the loss of income. The second way roles change in the wake of crises involves the creation of new roles. For example, new roles are created when crises incapacitate members, resulting in the need for a caretaker. Both of these changes occur because families are trying to maintain homeostasis while coping with crises.

A **role** is defined as a practical function taken on by someone within the family (Goldenberg & Goldenberg, 2013). Roles within the family may be assigned because of the status of individuals within the family such as "mother," "father," "oldest," and "youngest." However, roles may also be assigned because of an individual's abilities or availability to perform certain tasks. For example, someone who is very good at organization may be assigned to manage paying the bills. An individual who has a talent for cooking, regardless of traditional gender roles, may take the role of planning and preparing meals. Families learn to expect that the roles assigned to specific members will be carried out (Gladding, 2010). In the face of a crisis, roles within families become blurred or performed inconsistently (McLendon & Petr, 2005; Price et al., 2010). The absence of one or more family members due to the crisis may result in another member assuming the absent member's role (Price et al., 2010). At times, a shift in roles is in some ways socially sanctioned—for example, in the case where a parent leaves the family either through divorce or death and the oldest same-gender child is expected to assume the departed parent's roles. For example, in some families, the well-intentioned statement "Now that your father has gone, you are the man of the family" signifies a shift in roles for the adolescent male who hears this statement. Shifts in the roles can be viewed as a family system's attempt to survive and adapt to the crisis (Gillespie & Campbell, 2011). The number of role shifts and the degree of those shifts in roles compared to prior role functioning can be used as one measure of a family's reaction to a crisis. Generally speaking, the greater the number and the more pronounced the shifts in roles, the more severe the crisis. Thus, assessment of the nature of the changes to roles within the family is critical for effective crisis intervention as it offers an understanding into one aspect of the chaos and conflict that may be observed in a family system during a crisis.

Assignment of roles during a crisis can be negotiated and agreed on by families, or they can be presumptuous, with specific family members being aggressive and forcing their way into certain roles or imposing roles onto others. Roles may also be assigned with a family member taking control and dictating the roles family members should fulfill. Often, conflicts will arise regarding who in the family takes various roles. These conflicts limit a family's ability to adapt and adjust to a crisis (Rosenfeld et al., 2010). Navigating through these conflicts can be treacherous as family members vie for their preferred roles. Sorting through these situations must be carefully done and caution exercised not to take sides. Even though family members may not agree on their roles, interference can result in an immediate attack if this is from someone outside the family.

Boundaries. Family boundaries are used to manage internal and external interactions (McLendon & Petr, 2005). Boundaries help create order as families manage daily activities by setting up subsystems and coalitions, controlling relationships and contact with others. According to Brown and Manning (2009), boundaries can be physical and psychological. Physical boundaries shape interactions within the family as well as outside the family. These can restrict or encourage interactions. An example of a typical physical boundary is that between parents and children. Another example of a traditional physical boundary is between the men and women in families. Psychological boundaries serve as an injunction/expectation for when and how family members interact with others (Brown & Manning, 2009).

In crisis situations, families find themselves in unfamiliar territory as they face forces pushing families and individual family members in many directions (Ford, 2021; Price et al., 2010). Families' status quo with respect to organizational patterns is tested in ways never before encountered. The result is that new organizational patterns may be formed to meet the needs of the current situation (Myer et al., 2014). In crises, boundary shifts can become more permeable or rigid depending on families' perceptions (Carroll et al., 2007). Families might find these shifts in organizational patterns necessary and advantageous as they adapt. However, some families and possibly individual family members may resist modifications and be either unable or unwilling to make changes.

A key issue for families in crisis is flexibility in organizational patterns (Walsh, 2012b). Families that are able to adjust boundaries in the wake of crisis situations fare better than those whose organizational patterns become more rigid. Families with rigid boundaries can lose their sense of connectedness as they work to overcome the challenges presented by crises (Walsh, 2012b). This connectedness permits mutual support and collaboration and respects individual family members' needs and differences.

Communication. Communication is another dynamic often altered as families struggle to cope with crises (Ford, 2021; Webb & Dickson, 2012). These authors state that changes occur because families are challenged to make sense of crises, resulting in disruptions of communication patterns. These changes can be disruptive or beneficial depending on the families. Disruptive communication in families is commonly experienced because of uncertainties embedded in crises (Tjersland et al., 2006), disagreement about what actions are needed (Sofka, 2004), and the desire to regain a sense of control (Hoff et al., 2009). Troublesome communication following crises can become either truncated or expanded (Ratnarajah & Schofield, 2008). Truncated communication is generally to the point without embellishment, including only facts, whereas expanded communication can involve enhancing stories with great bravado, including emotional details and minute details. While neither of these two patterns is inherently negative, these can lead to misunderstanding and annoy other family members. Often, these are a gauge to families' reactions to crisis situations. The more severe the reaction, the more difficult it will be for families to work through and adapt to the new situation.

On the other hand, good communication has the potential to facilitate positive outcomes in the resolution of families' crises (Yorgason, 2010). Open communication seems to be a key factor in facilitating families working through crises (Webb & Dickson, 2012). Clear, consistent messages and clarity of information is indispensable for families weathering crises (Walsh, 2012b). In addition, open emotional expression and collaborative problem-solving help families adjust as they live through the demands placed on them by crises (Knowles et al., 2010; Walsh, 2012b).

Rules. Rules govern families' day-to-day behaviors and are negotiated in the formation of families (Imber-Black, 2012). Rules fall into two categories: (1) procedural and (2) ritualistic. **Procedural rules** set the basis for family structure and provide consistency. When followed, procedural rules result in families maintaining a state of equilibrium. These rules/processes determine internal and external interactions of family members as well as set the standard for topics for conversation (Murray et al., 2010). Breaking procedural rules has the potential to destabilize by undermining the foundation on which a family is built. The behavior of family members is not predictable, and families must try to reestablish stability. The second type of rule involves expectations involving rituals within families. Rules around rituals are ever present in families' lives and create meaning as they remember special times in their lives (Imber-Black, 2012). **Ritualistic rules** can be as mundane as kissing your partner as you leave for work or tucking in children at bedtime. Celebrations on birthdays, anniversaries, and holidays also are covered by ritualistic rules. For example, on Memorial Day, the extended family gathers for a backyard barbeque or at Christmas, breakfast always entails baking homemade pecan caramel rolls. Hannukah is another example of a holiday in which families observe ritual rules. Abiding by ritualistic rules symbolizes families' connectedness with the past, gratitude for the present, and hope for the future (Imber-Black, 2012).

Crises can result in changes for both procedural and ritualistic rules. Families become sidetracked and embroiled in addressing the immediacy of crises and might neglect, forget, or otherwise ignore family rules (Myer et al., 2014). Procedural rules may no longer be effective given the demands of crisis situations. Generally speaking, the more severe the crisis, the more likely procedural rules will be broken. For example, even though a procedural rule is not to talk about family matters with someone not in the family, this rule may be ignored as family members seek support. At times, crises force a change in procedural rules. Some family members might perceive these as beneficial, while others in the family might have a very different perception. Other times, families choose to alter these rules by making deliberate decisions to change them.

Ritualistic rules are also at the mercy of family crises. Birthdays might be forgotten, or celebrations of holidays could be postponed. Emotions can run high if celebrations such as these are forgotten or missed, even though families are struggling through a crisis. Cognitions can also run hot because expectations were not met regarding rules around rituals. However, ritualistic rules can be an important anchor for families in certain types of crises. The reason is that many of these rules revolve around faith-based functions and beliefs (Rosenfeld et al., 2010). These can help families ground themselves and give security as they work through crises (Imber-Black, 2012). Ritualistic rules support family members' efforts at coming to terms and finding meaning in crises.

Values. Arising out of families' belief systems, **values** are those things deemed important for morale (Greenstone & Leviton, 2011), and they drive families' perceptions. As such, values play an important role in crises (Boss, 2002), influencing families' reactions as they attempt to make sense of the situation (Walsh, 2012b). Two different aspects of values are involved in families making sense of crises. First, values play a critical role in the way families interpret crises. Families use causal or explanatory attributions based on their values to assign meaning to crises. Cultural heritage, faith-based beliefs, beliefs held because of ethnic background, and political beliefs, along with others (Boss, 2002; Humphrey, 2009; Robert & Kelly, 2015; Rosenfeld et al., 2010; Walsh, 2012b) all contribute to families' perceptions of crisis situations. Some families might attribute crises to being "God's will," while others might explain the situation as an "act of nature." Still other families might attribute crises to simply having bad luck. It is important to remember that families are unique with respect to the way and the degree that belief systems influence their values (Boss, 2002). Second, families use values to determine their ability to handle the situation. Values help to create a sense of coherence that allows families to tackle crises together (Hansson & Cederblad, 2004). Families whose values lead them to be optimistic and positive tend to have greater success in facing crises (Walsh, 2012b), while a fatalistic perspective can be a barrier to coping with these situations (Boss, 2002). Some families rely on their faith to see them through crises. Other families might trust their political beliefs or their feelings the government will come to their rescue.

Crises often challenge and even alter families' values (Schmidt & Welsh, 2010). The challenge comes when values are unable to provide guidance on how to make sense of crises. Families may feel as if they are trying to fit a square peg into a round hole or a round peg into a square hole. No matter what, there will be gaps. Families struggling to make sense of crises will try to fill in the gaps in order to maintain allegiance to their values. If these efforts fail, families will look for ways to rationalize the experience. In these situations, some values may take precedence over others. Values can also change because of crises. Values prized by families may no longer be practical or functional because of crises. Values such as education, leisure, political involvement, religious affiliation, and community service may be reconsidered as families grapple with the consequences of crises.

Goals. Goals motivate families in their desire to attain or achieve something (Rosenfeld et al., 2010). Obviously, some goals involve physical objects, such as having the biggest house or new vehicles every year. Other goals may not be so large, such as having the nicest yard in their community or having pretty flowering plants on the porch. Other goals are less tangible and might include contributing to retirement funds or being a member of a prestigious country club. Not all family goals are expressed—some may be unspoken. Expressed family goals might include stable employment that provides income or becoming a home owner. Unspoken family goals can help children become independent or maintain a healthy lifestyle and live a long, happy life. Regardless of the type of goal, crises bring into focus the uncertainty of the future (Galvin et al., 2012). Families might reconsider the goal of living to a ripe old age when medical crises arise. Disasters might cause families to learn to appreciate health rather than focus on obtaining material possessions (Rosenfeld et al., 2010). Faced with changes brought on by a new reality, families are compelled to reexamine goals, making changes as required (Myer & Moore, 2006).

In crisis situations, families' goals may undergo dramatic and unexpected changes (Rosenfeld et al., 2010) and interrupt families' abilities to reach goals (Weber, 2011). Collective and individual ambitions are at stake as families struggle to weather and resolve crises. Goals are put on hold or abandoned altogether as crises send shock waves through families. Shock waves have the potential to stir up issues that can either be beneficial or detrimental to working through crises. More often than not, family members initially rally around each other for support. Differences are put aside, and families work together to get through the crisis. Yet as the crisis wears on, those differences have the tendency to resurface. Families with positive stable, lasting supportive interactions will fare much better (Boss, 2002). In fact, these families have the tendency to get stronger. Unfortunately, the same happens with families who have a history of uncooperative dealings. These families often experience an upsurge of these types of interactions as crises cause friction among family members.

Although these dynamics are discussed as distinct and separate, in reality, these are interrelated. Changes in one of the dynamics listed above generally cause changes in one or usually more of the others. Later in this chapter, we will introduce a modification of the Triage Assessment Form that can be used with families. The form for families was developed based on the dynamics listed above and can be used much in the same way as the original.

Case Vignette

Meet the Medina family: a typical middle-class family, in which the parents have been married only to each other. The family lives in a two-story house on a nice street in a middle-class neighborhood in a suburb of a major metropolitan area. The three children in the family all attend public school and are active in extra-curricular activities. The Medina family is used throughout the remainder of the chapter to illustrate crisis intervention with families. The case will be discussed at various points in the family's journey after Eva, the mother and wife, survives a mass shooting at her work. Below is a brief history of the Medina family as well as the mass shooting that catapults the family into a full-blown crisis.

Daniel, the husband, is 43 and a foreman in a local electric motor factory. He has been employed there for 15 years and is well liked by all. Eva, the mother, works part-time as a cashier in a local big box store. She started working after all the children started school. Dominic, the eldest child in the family, is in his last year of high school. He is active in sports and participates in whatever sport is in season. Emily, the Medinas' second child, is 16 and participates in extra school activities plus is socially active on social media. She is a good student but spends a lot of time on social media, even though her parents discourage her from this as much as possible. The youngest child was a surprise for the Medinas. Eloise is 10 and still in primary school. She likes to spend her time reading and being with friends.

Hearing about the mass shooting, Daniel, the father, immediately called his wife. After several tries with no answer, Daniel left work and rushed in a panic to the store where Eva worked. During the trip, he contacted Dominic and told him to collect his sisters and go home. Confused, Dominic asked why, and Daniel responded "Just do it!" Upon arriving at the scene, Daniel searched frantically to find his wife. He finally was able to talk with local law enforcement, who said several people were transported to the city hospital. Not knowing if Eva was alive or dead, he jumped into his car and sped down to the hospital.

Hybrid Model Applied to Families

LO8 Chapter 3, "The Intervention and Assessment Models," introduced the hybrid model for crisis intervention. The flexibility of this model makes it extremely useful for working with families in crisis. The seven tasks imbedded in the model can guide the process of helping families in crisis. Three tasks: (1) safety, (2) assessment, and (3) support are continuously worked on throughout the intervention (Myer et al., 2013). The other four tasks: (4) making contact/predispositioning, (5) examining the problem, (6) reestablishing control, and (7) follow-up are incorporated into crisis intervention as needed (Myer et al., 2013). Once these tasks are completed, crisis workers can move to another one. However, the chaotic, fluid nature of crises may cause crisis workers to return to these tasks several times during the intervention.

In this chapter, the focus is primarily on the tasks rooted in the model, not the model itself. Although the application is very similar to the one with individuals, differences arise when working with families. These differences are analogous to the application of basic counseling techniques with individuals and families or groups. The techniques and strategies are the same but adapted for use with families.

Making Contact/Predispositioning. **Making contact/predispositioning** is a task with families in crisis that involves placing yourself in a position of being helpful (Ford, 2021). Kanel (2011) views making contact as the foundation for being able to assist families in crisis. Ectherling et al. (2005) echoed this sentiment, stating that making contact is a fundamental connection that demonstrates a genuine commitment by the counselor's willingness to stand by the client. This process of making contact/predispositioning is very different than traditional rapport building (Myer et al., 2013). Rapport develops over time, often taking several weeks, whereas making contact/predispositioning is established in the first few moments of the crisis intervention process. The goal of this task is to quickly connect and bond with families in a way that makes them receptive and cooperative to the intervention process.

As with individuals, making contact/predispositioning begins before the first contact. The crisis worker should position themself as someone who has the family's best interest at heart and acts as an advocate. This mind set is particularly important when the family runs head on into the bureaucracy of a large institution like a regional trauma unit hospital as the Medinas are about to do. They are going to be confronted with every one of the hybrid model's tasks, and they are now going to be doing it on what may be considered alien territory. As such, if the crisis worker is seen as a representative of a bureaucratic system, this can derail at worst, or set back at best, the entire intervention. Instead, you must communicate being knowledgeable yet not subservient to the system. As stated in Chapter 3, "The Intervention and Assessment Models," the way in which introductions are made is critical. Long-winded introductions listing your degrees, licenses, and certifications only serve to make you seem important and do not necessarily help families. If requested, by all means provide these. However, in the initial contact, tell families your name, your profession, and that you are sorry for what is happening. You will also want to allow them to introduce themselves to you and if possible, greet family members individually. This process helps to connect with everyone as well as the families as a whole. Clarify your intentions by telling families the purpose of you being with them, and then start employing the basic listening and responding skills detailed to you in Chapter 4, "The Tools of the Trade."

Although the task begins with the initial contact, making contact/predispositioning may need to be repeated periodically. One reason for repeating this task is that family members may arrive at different times. As family members arrive, you will need to recycle back to this task and introduce yourself and allow them to do the same. Take time to listen to the new arrivals' concerns and bring them up to date with the discussion to that point. This process validates their participation and incorporates them into the discussion. Another reason for returning to this task is the fluid, chaotic nature of crises. As crises evolve, families or individual family members may question the relevance of the presence of crisis workers. Their perception may change and cause them to question the purpose of a crisis worker's presence. Care must be taken not to overreact or become defensive. When this situation occurs, crisis workers must make contact for a second, third, and fourth time and predisposition themselves with families. Revisiting this task is also needed as families move through the recovery stages. Crisis workers must redefine, that is, predisposition, themselves as families move through the recovery process. The need for revisiting/predispositioning is the changing role and function of crisis workers as families move through recovery. As families begin to adapt and stabilize, the role of crisis workers shifts from being the "go to" person to more of a "guide," steering them on an as-needed basis. The stages of recovery for families will be discussed in the next section of this chapter.

The following exchange takes place in the first few minutes after Daniel arrives at the hospital. Daniel had first tried to locate his wife at the store but discovered she had been taken to the hospital.

The information he had was that Eva had been shot and taken to the hospital, nothing about the seriousness of her condition. After arriving at the Emergency Room, the receptionist and a nurse guided him to a private room. Both the receptionist and nurse assured him someone would be coming to talk with him as quickly as possible. A couple of minutes passed, and the social worker named Christine knocked on the door and entered the room.

Christine: (opens the door slowly) May I come in?

Daniel: Are you the doctor? Where is my wife? I need to see her right now!

Christine: No sir, I am a social worker who works in the ER. My name is Christine (holds out her identification card hanging on her neck)

Daniel: I need to see her now! Make it happen!

Christine: I know you are scared and angry. Your name is Daniel, right? And Eva your wife?

Daniel: F...king right I need to see her now. (He gets up from the chair and starts for the door.) Christine, I want to see her. (takes a deep breath). I just need to know she is alive. They could not tell me at the store.

Christine: Again Daniel my name is Christine, I am not the doctor, but I work in the ER with families when someone is brought here.

Daniel: Fine CHRISTINE, now let me see my wife.

Christine: (Talks quietly) Daniel, the EMTs brought in several people from the shooting, if you can sit down for a minute I will find out where your wife is. The nurse told me her name is Eva, is that right?

Daniel: Yea and be quick......please.

A few minutes pass and Christine returns.

Daniel: Did you find her? Is she alright? Did you talk to her? Can I see her?

Christine: Daniel, I know you are scared and worried out of your mind. I would be if I were you. I talked to the head nurse, and he said Eva is in surgery.

Daniel: Surgery, why is she in surgery, is she going to be okay, is she going to die? (Starts to breathe heavily)

Christine: (Talks quietly) Eva is in surgery to remove a bullet and repair the damage it did. (pauses) Daniel, listen to me. (pauses) Eva was seriously injured but will live. The doctors told me she will not die, and I believe them. I need you to believe that too.

Daniel: Are they sure? How do they know? Where was she shot?

Christine: (**Looks him in the eye**). She was shot in the leg. There are no "sures" when somebody gets shot Daniel, but the report is Eva's doing well in surgery. The doctor who's operating will see you when they're done. I do understand that's your concern and anxiety, and knowing how your wife is doing is your number one priority, and it's mine as well. Do you understand what I am saying? If so, I want to hear it back so we're on the same page.

Daniel: (**A bit calmer, regaining composure**). She got shot in the leg, serious, but good chances of surviving.

Christine: That's right. Now I'm gonna check with some other people who've come to see about other survivors. I'll be back and give you updates as I get them. I need to know if there's anybody who needs to be called or contacted.

Daniel: No, I've called the rest of the family. They're on their way.

As soon as Christine arrives, she begins working on the task of making contact/predispositioning. Note that as soon as Christine walks into the room, she introduces herself and confirms that she is talking to Daniel and that Eva is his wife. Throughout the short conversation, Christine uses Daniel's and Eva's names repeatedly as a way to make contact. Christine also several times repeats her name. Why would she do that? Many times, a person in crisis has difficulty tracking a conversation, and information needs to be repeated several times. Christine also repeats what the doctor said about Eva's condition several times. This was purposeful because Daniel's reaction to the crisis is high. Christine's report is empathic but objective. No false promises or guarantees are given. Daniel's affective reaction is pushing 7, if not 8, and his behavioral reaction is in the range of 6. Cognitively, Daniel's reaction is probably an 8, as evidenced by him asking two, three, and four questions at a time. As Christine talks, she uses a quiet voice in an attempt to lower Daniel's affective reaction. She asks him to wait to lower the behavioral reaction. She mostly tries to lower his cognitive reaction by speaking in clear, simple statements, saying Eva is injured severely but has a good chance of surviving. She repeats this information several times in order to get Daniel to hear it. She also affirms that she is going to be his go-to support person and, although busy with others, will stick with him until Eva is out of surgery and he can see her. She further checks to see that other support persons will be accessible before she attends to others seeking information on other survivors.

Safety. **Safety** is a default task and is particularly important when working with families in crisis (Rosenfeld et al., 2010). You may automatically think client safety (for this chapter, that means families) is essential and the first item of business in crisis intervention. As we stated in Chapter 3, "The Intervention and Assessment Models," this task includes *your* safety, not just the family's safety. The first consideration is your safety when working with families in crisis. There are very valid reasons why responding to a domestic violence call is one of the most dangerous that police officers make. You are no exception when dealing with distraught, upset, angry families that have thrown rationality right out of their psychological windows when a crisis turns into a behavioral emergency. You must first and foremost consider your safety as the priority. Do not place yourself in a situation that compromises your safety. It goes without saying, right? Not so! Why, you might ask? First, your training will almost assuredly not prepare you for those situations. Second, crisis intervention is not a video game that gives you multiple lives to keep playing so you don't push boundaries in the heat of the moment. Third, although you mean well and are a caring, sharing, wonderfully empathic human being, families in the chaos of crises can suddenly, without clear provocation, lash out at anyone perceived as a threat, whether that is accurate or not. For example, you might be called to a home to work with a family in crisis. Even though you are there to help, individual family members may not appreciate your presence. Family members might think you are sticking your nose where it does not belong. Some individuals could look for chances to sabotage your attempts to help. Something that is said could be interpreted negatively, taken as an affront to the family or individual members. A comment might be construed as derogatory and questioning the family's integrity or their intelligence. In an instant, families as a whole or individual members can lash out at you unexpectedly. Therefore, safety for crisis intervention means being mindful of your well-being at all times, and this is particularly true in the present situation where highly distraught family members and supporters are coming into a hospital after a traumatic injury has occurred. Paradoxical as it may sound, in a behavioral emergency (Kleespies, 2014), strengthening the tenuous relationship by communicating empathic and nonjudgmental understanding and forging a bond as a supportive team member, as the social worker does with Daniel, can defuse and de-escalate a potentially volatile situation. (Ford, 2021, p. 27).

Prevention and preparation are key aspects for safety. A guideline is to have two crisis intervention workers present when working with families if possible. Having two crisis workers allows one to take the lead in the intervention while the other is watching and alert for changes in milieu and interactions in the family. Understandably, having two crisis workers is not always possible, but when possible, it is recommended. Being aware of your surroundings is also essential when working with families in crisis. Awareness of your surroundings is especially important if you are asked to make home visits. Gather information and know the nearby area if working with families on their home turf so to speak. Where is the closest place to get help if needed? Is there a fire station nearby? Is a police substation close by? What other places could you get to quickly if needed? Being able to communicate with the office is important. Let someone know not just where you will be but also when you expect to return. Set check-in times so if you are unable to, someone will contact you. Also, have a signal so if you call and use a word or phrase, they are alerted that you need assistance immediately. While seemingly common sense, prevention and preparation create a measure of safety for you as well as families.

Throughout the intervention process, vigilance is needed to guard your and the family's safety. This means being constantly mindful of the environment through observing the verbal and nonverbal behaviors of all family members. What are family members communicating? Is anyone making threats, directly or indirectly? Has someone said something that might be considered a veiled threat? **Veiled threats** are circuitous statements that do not express a direct warning but contain a menacing message beyond the words (Braverman, 1999). Are any intimidating statements pointed at individuals or groups of family members? Being mindful of nonverbal communication is also vital. Threatening moves such as shaking a fist at someone or making a slight lunge are moves that might put safety at risk. Have family members communicated by raising their voices, speaking louder or more rapidly or otherwise communicating anger or distress? Anger or fear can be a catalyst for threatening behavior that jeopardizes safety. Relentless and continual watchfulness is central to providing safety for yourself and families as well as allowing you to gather the information needed to help.

The following exchange takes place approximately 45 minutes after Daniel arrived at the hospital. Christine has been with him much of the time, only leaving periodically to check if the doctors have sent any information from the surgery. Daniel's reactions were initially severe but seem to have lowered some. He vacillates between sitting and pacing the floor. Dominic arrives with his two sisters, Emily and Eloise. They were shown to the room by hospital security. The door is open, and they walk into the room. The two girls immediately go to their father, giving him a hug. However, Dominic hangs back a little.

Dominic: Dad, what is going on? Who is this? (Pointing to Christine)

Daniel: **(Takes a breath)** Are you guys okay, did you get here safe?

Emily: Yea, Dad, we are okay, but where is Mom?

Christine: You must be Dominic (**pointing to him**) and let's see, you are Emily, and you have to be Eloise. I have been here with your Dad since he got here.

Daniel: Oh yea this is umm..... Christine. She is a social worker or something.

Eloise: **(staying close to her Dad and holding his hand)** Do you work here?

Christine: Yes, I work here. My name is Christine; I work in the ER and talk to families when they are here.

Daniel: Oh sorry, yes she talks with families. She has been helping me. Can you guys sit down? We have something to tell you.

Emily: What? We heard about the shooting on the radio coming here. They said a lot of people died. (**She starts to cry**). Is....Is....Mom dead?

Daniel: No sweetie. Mom is not dead, but she got shot and hurt pretty bad. (**He looks over at Christine for support**)

Christine: Your mom is alive. I realize this is really scary hearing your mother was shot, and you are frantic with worry, so please take a seat and let me explain.

The three children take a breath of relief.
Everyone sits down, the girls on a couch with their Dad and Dominic in another chair. Christine sits across from them.

Dominic: She will be okay won't she?

Christine: (**says quietly but with assertion**) I need for you to hear me carefully. I need you to sit down and listen to what I have to say. I want to help you see her as soon as possible, but I need for you to cooperate with me now. Okay?

Daniel: (**Looks at each child and motions to be quiet**) She knows what is going on. Listen, okay?

All three children nod yes.

Christine: Your Mom was shot in the leg during the shooting and hurt... well pretty bad. The doctors are doing surgery. I was told she was bleeding a lot, so you understand the surgery unit is off limits, right? The risk of infection and all. As soon as she wakes up you can see her. (Pauses.) I am told she will go to the ICU and be there for a couple of days. You can see when she gets there, but she will still be asleep from the surgery. She won't be able to talk to you. (Pauses) Do you understand that she will not be able to see you or talk to you? Do you understand?

Emily: What do you mean, will she ever be able to talk to us?

Christine: Emily ...she will be able to talk probably tomorrow, but she will just be asleep from the surgery. (**pauses**) I'll be your conduit of information until the surgeon is done and then she'll talk to you. She is in good hands with Dr. Melton. She is an excellent surgeon. I'd want her working on my own mother if it came to it. Stay here for right now. I know you need to be together. I will get you all something to drink and a little snack. I'll give you a few moments alone. I'll be back. And see you through this until she comes out of surgery, then I'll also follow up with you tomorrow. .

Dominic: (**still standing and pacing back and forth agitated**) Wait......Are you sure she is not going to die or something? (**said in a demanding voice**)

Eloise: Mom is dying? (**cries more but sits down**)

Christine: No one said that . . . it was just a question. Your Mom is not dying. The doctors will tell me if that would happen.

Daniel: Mom is not going to die. Stop thinking that way.

Christine: Stay here. I do need for all of you to sit. I understand you are scared out of your mind; I will be back with something to drink and a snack in five minutes. I'll also see if the doctor has given any updates.

Throughout the exchange, safety is the first and foremost concern. Christine continues to use a soft calming voice to ease the Medinas' anxiety. Reduction of their anxiety is essential to maintain everyone's safety. Several times, she uses owning statements to express her compassion and concern to make a connection with the Medinas. The owning statements are straight out of Chapter 4, "The Tools of the Trade." These statements are used to express understanding and engender trust (Ford, 2021, pp. 26–27). The goal is that if trust is built, the Medinas will find a way to compose themselves; not doing anything that would endanger their well-being. In making contact with the children, Christine uses their names and also predispositions them on what to expect when their Mother is out of surgery. She also uses "I understand" statements to acknowledge their affective state.

All of the family are individually high-moderate to high on the individual triage scale, and she cannot let them remain there for their safety as well as the safety of others in the hospital. At this time, the triage rating for the family is difficult to determine. A good estimate would also be in the high-moderate range, meaning Christine should partner with the family and use a "we" intervention approach. Why do you think that Christine says she is getting them something to drink and eat? This tactic can be used to create a stronger connection with the family and to divert their attention for a moment using the strategy of Providing Protection and Guidance.

Assessment.   When working with families in crisis, you will have to sort through an overwhelming amount of data (Bonnefil & Jacobson, 1979). The ability to shift through this information quickly and efficiently is critical. This assessment should focus on gathering the information needed to assist families as they work their way through crises. This means having criteria or a model to use to organize the information (Bonnefil & Jacobson, 1979). The model should be flexible enough to use with various crises and should also be adaptable to use with families that have different structural configurations. The assessment process should also provide real-time information that can immediately be used in the intervention process.

Family assessment has come a long way since the early days of family therapy (Lebow & Stroud, 2012). Among the more established methods are self-report instruments such as the Family Environment Scale, F-COPES, FACES IV (Family Adaptability and Cohesion Evaluation Scale IV), and Sources of Stress Scale (Lebow & Stroud, 2012). A few more recently developed scales include The Support Seeking Scale (Marshal et al., 2023) and the Parent Report on Externalization Symptom Scale (Rivers et al., 2022). These instruments provide an insider's perspective on the way families are functioning and seem relevant in crises. Yet, self-report instruments have limitations when being used in family crisis situations. Can you imagine the challenge of completing self-report instruments when families are in the midst of crises? The emotional or cognitive disruptions from crises can make completing any assessment instruments problematic. The question of reliability also surfaces since it is not known if individuals are responding based on only their perception or based on the collective functioning of their family (Lebow & Stroud, 2012). In addition, measures of functioning from these types of instruments are partial and are not able to examine all aspects of families in crisis (Lebow & Stroud, 2012). Another problem is that these instruments must be scored and the data deciphered into information useful for the intervention process. While useful, these instruments may not be the best choice for crises. So, the default option is the triage scale (Figure 11.1), which Christine uses to make her determination whether it is safe to leave the Medinas for a while.

We have adapted the Triage Assessment Form: Crisis Intervention (TAF:CI) described in Chapter 2, "Culturally Effective Helping in Crisis," for use with families. The Triage Assessment Form: Family Therapist (TAF:FT) uses a similar format as the TAF:CI and is based on crisis workers' observations and interactions with families. Just as with the original form, the severity of families' reactions to crises are rated in affective, behavior, and cognitive scales. Anchors for ratings were developed using the six dynamics described earlier (i.e., roles, boundaries, communication, rules, values, goals). Figure 11.1 is the TAF:FT. As with the original form, a rule out method is best for rating the severity of families' reactions. Assume all families in crisis are a 10 on each of the scales. Does a family fit any of the anchors for a rating of 10? If not, move to the 8/9 anchors of marked impairment. Do any of those anchors describe your observations? Again, if not, move to 6/7 and keep moving down the scale until at least one of the anchors matches your observations. If families match half or more, the higher number in the category is most likely correct; if less than half, the lower number is probably accurate. Scores on individual scales suggest the reaction needing attention the most with the highest being the reaction needing attention at

that moment. The composite or total score indicates the directedness of the intervention, whether that be a nondirect, collaborative, or direct. The higher the total score, the more direct the intervention should be.

Assessment can be confusing when working with families. The confusion involves assessing family members individually and the families as a whole. What happens if one family member seems rather calm and collected, while another person in the family is reacting just the opposite and is particularly distressed to the point of being extremely emotional? What and how do you assess these situations? The original TAF:CI can be used to assess individual family members and the family as a whole using the TAF:FT. Crises causing a wide range of reactions among individual family members means that you should attend to individual family members with extreme reactions while simultaneously helping families address the hardships caused by the crisis. These situations call on crisis workers to do a juggling act, moving between addressing individual needs and helping families deal with crises as a unit. A general guideline is to attend to individuals' reactions if these are interfering with helping families as a whole.

The following excerpt shows Christine switching between helping the Medina family and concentrating on the reactions of individual family members. In this excerpt, Christine has returned from talking with the Head Nurse about the progress of Eva's surgery. During the exchange, Daniel becomes overwhelmed cognitively as he confronts the reality of Eva's injuries. He becomes caught in a loop of thinking that does not let him or other family members address the pressing issues caused by the crisis. The severity of his reactions on the TAF:CI is 6 to 7 for the affective and behavioral scales, while the cognitive scale is an 8. Christine must take steps to help Daniel stop his merry-go-round thinking patterns before she can address family issues. Eloise, the youngest in the family, seems to be feeling and mirroring the reaction of her sister being crushed by the emotional weight, with her affective reaction reaching an 8 or even 9. Christine understands that Eloise is feeling abandoned and needs support from her father. Dominic is sitting quietly but fidgeting while Emily appears to be holding back tears and taking quick short breaths. Christine weaves in and out of focusing on the individual family members while also addressing family dynamics within this session.

Crisis Date: _____   Office Visit Date: _____

Family Members: Name, Age, and Role (present and not present) _____

_____

_____

Crisis Description _____

_____

Attempt/s at Resolution: _____

_____

Observations and Reported Behaviors (Check as many that apply**)**

___ inability to provide daily needs (___food
___clothing ___shelter ___ utilities)***

___ self-medication by one or more members

___ major health concerns reported *

___ family violence ***

___ neglect of children (emotional, physical)***

___ verbal threats to self or others

___ suicidal/homicidal thinking/verbalizing *

___ suicidal/homicidal gestures/behaviors *

___ suicidal/homicidal plan clear *

___ disagreements within family

___ family members disengaged

___ lack of energy within family

___ isolation from social support systems

___ approval seeking by family members

___ refusal to communicate with other family members

___ demanding special attention by family members

___ tension among family members

___ denial by family members

___ family members nonresponsive

___ family members responses guarded

Notes: _____

_____

***** *Referral to Social Service Recommended *Referral for Specialized Support***

TRIAGE ASSESSMENT

Feelings	**Behavioral**	**Thinking**
___ Anger ___ Fear ___ Sadness	___ Approach ___ Avoidance ___ Immobile	___ Transgression ___ Threat ___ Loss
1 2 3 4 5 6 7 8 9 10	1 2 3 4 5 6 7 8 9 10	1 2 3 4 5 6 7 8 9 10

Total Score: ___

Figure 11.1   Triage Assessment Form: Family Therapist

SEVERITY SCALES

	1 No Impairment	2/3 Minimal Impairment	4/5 Low Impairment	6/7 Moderate Impairment	8/9 Marked Impairment	10 Severe Impairment
A F F E C T I V E	○ Stable mood, control of feelings suggesting family resiliency.	○ Brief periods of elevated negative mood with little effect on family resiliency.	○ Evidence of negative mood noticeable causing family resiliency to fluctuate.	○ Mood primarily negative causing family resiliency to be ineffectual.	○ Mood is negative causing family resiliency to fail.	○ Mood is shutting down ability to respond to the crisis causing family resiliency to disappear.
	○ Affect is appropriate with no effect on boundaries.	○ Affect elevated but generally appropriate with little effect on boundaries.	○ Affect intensity is longer than situation warrants causing boundary disruptions.	○ Affect control is difficult and not always successful causing changes in boundaries.	○ Affected not controlled with significant boundary shifts.	○ Affect control absent causing danger to family or others and boundaries to be ignored.
	○ Emotions are under control with no impact on family values.	○ Emotions are substantially under control with no effect on family values.	○ Emotions are controlled but influenced by crisis with minimal effect on family values.	○ Emotions not under control and focused on crisis and influencing family values.	○ Emotions generalize from crisis event to other situations and changing family values.	○ Emotions of the crisis are generalized to situations substantially changing family values.
	○ Responses to questions/ requests are calm and composed.	○ Responses to questions/ requests are emotional but composed.	○ Responses to questions/ requests vary from rapid and agitated to slow and subdued.	○ Responses to questions/ requests are emotionally volatile.	○ Responses to questions/ requests noncompliant due to interference of emotions.	○ Cannot respond to questions/requests because of interference of emotions.
B E H A V I O R A L	○ Behaviors are socially appropriate.	○ Behaviors mostly effective, outbursts if present are inconsequential.	○ Behaviors are ineffective, yet not dangerous.	○ Behaviors are maladaptive but not immediately destructive.	○ Behaviors are likely to intensify crisis situation.	○ Behaviors are ineffective and accelerate the crisis.
	○ Family rules unaffected.	○ Family rules mostly followed.	○ Family rules recognized but adjusted.	○ Family rules altered.	○ Family rules suspended	○ Family rules abandoned.
	○ Daily routine unimpeded.	○ Daily routine mostly followed with minimal effort.	○ Daily routine experiencing periodic disruptions.	○ Daily routine noticeably compromised.	○ Daily routine experiencing significant disruptions.	○ Daily functioning not preformed.
	○ Behaviors are not a threat or danger nonexistent.	○ Behaviors demonstrates frustration, but is nonthreatening.	○ Behaviors minimal threat to family or others.	○ Behaviors are a potential threat to family or others.	○ Behaviors are impulsive and harmful to family or others.	○ Behaviors are highly destructive possibly to cause injury/death to family or others.
	○ Roles are stable.	○ Roles mostly stable but still functional for daily living.	○ Roles fluctuating but still functional for daily living.	○ Roles fluctuating and not functional for daily living.	○ Role overlap interrupts functioning for daily living.	○ Role breakdown prevents functioning for daily living.

Figure 11.1   (continued)

SEVERITY SCALES *(continued)*

	1 No Impairment	2/3 Minimal Impairment	4/5 Low Impairment	6/7 Moderate Impairment	8/9 Marked Impairment	10 Severe Impairment
C O G N I T I V E	○ Decisions are considerate of family members.	○ Decisions are not consistently considerate of family members.	○ Decisions are inconsiderate of family members.	○ Decisions are arbitrary and antagonistic of family members.	○ Decisions are random with a potential to be harmful to family members.	○ Decisions are a clear and present danger to family members.
	○ Decisions are logical and reasonable.	○ Decisions are indecisive but only with respect to crisis.	○ Decisions are inconsistent and sometimes unreasonable.	○ Decisions are erratic and reality and interfering with daily functioning.	○ Decisions are illogical, have little basis in and generalized beyond crisis.	○ Decision making frenetic or frozen and not based in reality and shuts down daily functioning.
	○ Discussion of crisis event substantially matches reality with communication being normal within the family.	○ Discussion influenced by crisis, but communication not effected.	○ Discussion focused on crisis but with prompting still able to consider other issues within family.	○ Discussion is limited to crisis situation disrupting communication within family.	○ Discussion about crisis intrusive to communication within family.	○ Discussion is chaotic shutting down communication within the family.
	○ Accept views of others in family.	○ Acknowledge views of others in family.	○ Acknowledging views of others in family difficult.	○ Disagreement with views of others in family.	○ Antagonistic of views of others in family.	○ Aggressively confronting views of others.
	○ Problem solving strategy agreed on.	○ Problem solving agreed on with minimal dissent.	○ Problem solving inconsistency within family.	○ Problem solving disputed with no agreement.	○ Problem solving argued with no consensus.	○ Problem solving not observable with no ability to focus.

CIP-Solutions, March, 2009

Figure 11.1   (continued)

Christine: (**Knocks and enters the room. Immediately, all attention is given to her,**) I am sorry; that took longer than I thought. How are you?

Daniel: Well not so good. What did they say? Is Eva out of surgery? How is she?

All three children kind of sit back, with Eloise grabbing Daniel's arm and pulling close to him.

Dominic: Yeah what is going on?

Christine: I have good news. (**Takes a deep breath in an attempt to calm the family's reaction then smiles**). Eva, your mother is out of surgery. She did great.

Daniel: Can we see her? Can I talk to her? What did the doctors say?

Christine: Let's slow down just a bit. (**Looks at Eloise**). How are you Eloise?

Eloise: *(**Looks at dad in a quavering voice**)* I just want to see my mom.

Christine: I would too, and you will. (**Looks at Dominic**) Dominic you seem really anxious.

Dominic: You're fucking right.

Daniel: Son there is no need for that kind of language.

Dominic: (**Whispers.**) Sorry, just what is taking so long?

Christine: I know waiting is the hardest part. You will see your mother soon.

Daniel: How soon? I just want to talk to her. When will she be able to come home?

Christine: You will see her as soon as she gets to a room in the ICU. Now Emily what is going on with you?

Emily: (**Says nothing and bursts into tears.**)

Christine: (**Takes a deep breath and while doing so looks at each family member.**) I can see you all are scared and love your mother, wife a great deal. Like I said, I have good news. Your wife, mother, did great in surgery and will completely recover.

Daniel: (Audible sigh of relief.)

Christine: (Smiles.) But I need you to listen now. Can you do that?

Everyone nods but Dominic.

Christine: Your wife, mother, will completely recover, but the doctors said that will take time.

Daniel: How much time?

Christine: The doctors cannot pinpoint an exact amount of time. But probably a few months. She will need to go to rehabilitation after leaving the hospital and then to physical therapy.

Dominic: What do you mean? You said she will be okay?

Christine: Dominic, she will, but it will take time. Okay, (**takes a deep breath again trying to settle down the family.**) Eva, your wife and mother, will need time to get back to herself physically and probably emotionally. She has gone through a lot and will need lots and lots of support from each of you.

Daniel: What kind of support? What do you mean?

Christine: Eloise, I can see your mother is very important to you; Emily, I am sure that is true for you as well. And Dominic, your reaction tells me you too love her. Daniel I also see you love her because you came here immediately after hearing about the shooting. You all are going to have to work together to help Eva recover. She is not going to be the same person when she first comes home. You will need to be patient with her.

In this brief exchange, Christine recognizes that the Medinas' reactions are in the moderate to marked category. Using this knowledge, she addresses each family member as an individual and uses broken record, positive reinforcement, and owning statements with each family member to hammer home not only to each individual but also to the total family their love for their mother and the need to support her. This response may seem overly redundant, but it is not because her individual and universal statements about loving Eva are designed to glue the family together because in the months ahead, there will be many opportunities for them to come unglued. During this time, she is using her knowledge of the way families react while in crisis to begin assessing the family system's reaction on the TAF:FT. Using the strategies of Providing Guidance and Support, Christine eases the Medinas into what to expect during the recovery short and long term for Eva. From Daniel's rebut of Dominic for using colorful language, Christine assumes he is the disciplinarian in the family. Eloise grabbing onto her father shows they have a strong bond. Christine sees Emily sitting close to her father but guesses she may be closer to her mother. The overall family's affective reaction vacillates between being scared to anger with a rating of a 6 and maybe a 7 on the TAF:FT. The behavioral reaction appears to be approached by their desire to immediately see Eva, with a rating again of 6 to 7. Christine acknowledges their desire but works to shift the reaction to being immobile, asking them to be patient. Cognitively the reaction is equally that of transgression and threat and a rating of 7 on the TAF:TF. Christine needs to slow down their worrying about the worst and focus on reality.

After a few minutes, a nurse knocks on the door and says the family can see their mother. Everyone jumps up, including Christine. The nurse tells the family that Eva is in ICU, and they will only be able to see her through a window. The nurse adds that before seeing her, the doctor needs to talk with them. At that moment, the doctor enters the room. She says Eva did wonderfully in the surgery, and there were no complications. She adds she will completely recover, but it will take time. She addresses everyone in the room and answers their questions. After that, Christine and the nurse accompany the family to the ICU and stay with them while they look through the window at Eva. After about 15 minutes, Christine says Eva will be asleep the rest of the day and may be asleep or groggy tomorrow. The doctor said she will be sedated for a few days so her body can start healing itself. Christine suggests they all go home and get some rest and eat something. She also says when they come back to stop by her office.

The overall severity ratings for the TAF:FT appear to have lowered to the moderate range in the middle teens from 15 to 17. The affective ratings are probably around a 5, and the Medinas' family communication, boundaries, and rules are undoubtably going to be disturbed as they cope. Although the Medinas do not know this yet, Christine anticipates these changes. The family's daily routine will be in flux as they attend to Eva's recovery. The Medinas' behavioral reactions are in the moderate range at this time as the family copes with the consequences of Eva's injuries. Family rules will likely be ignored or completely dismissed, causing significant changes in the way they interact with each other. Dynamics associated with cognitive reactions are in the moderate range as communications have changed since they cannot communicate with Eva and decisions about family goals may be challenged.

Support.   Plain and simple—families in crisis need **support**. As discussed in Chapter 3, "The Intervention and Assessment Models," crisis workers must be able to communicate a sense of caring to help clients in crisis. The same holds true for families. In fact, the crisis intervention process may be the best opportunity for families to find the needed support. Often, families believe they are alone, marginalized, and otherwise not deserving of support when faced with crises. The pioneer mindset of self-sufficiency might emerge, with families believing no support is needed, that they can do it themselves, and that they are self-sufficient. While this attitude is admirable and often allows families to weather crises, sometimes this belief is not enough. Everyone, including families, needs someone to lean on from time to time.

Support can be considered the cornerstone of crisis intervention. Support provides a foundation on which families can rebuild their lives following crises. This means listening to families as a group talk about their experience (Ectherling et al., 2005). As individual family members share their experiences, group understanding or "knowing" will evolve. "*Knowing*" refers to the family forming a meaning of crises as a collective apart from individual family members (Boss, 2002). The support that is needed comes in four different forms: (1) psychological, (2) logistical, (3) social, and/or (4) informational. Each of these types of support is important in the intervention process. Families almost always need more than one of these supports to face the adversities brought on by crises. Psychological support for families involves crisis workers joining the struggle of families as they search for ways to overcome the hardships brought on by crises. Joining with the family conveys you are connected with the family, and you will be with them through crises (Peterson et al., 2010). The connection ranges from being a sounding board for mild crises to taking a direct role in decision making with families with more severe reactions.

Logistical support comes in the form of helping families access resources (Myers & Wee, 2005). Resources may range from referring families to appropriate agencies that give assistance to actually contacting and possibly arranging transportation for families to access the resource. For example, families may need logistical support following a fire that destroyed their home and most of their belongings. Crisis workers can help these families locate resources for clothing, shelter, and so on. If they do not have transportation, you might have to arrange for that as well. Social support concerns connecting families with others with a shoulder to lean on. This may be with families having similar experiences or organizations (e.g., church, community centers) that can provide ongoing, longer-term support. Social support has been shown to be very important for families experiencing crises, creating a network of families to talk with about their experiences (Cohen, 2004; Myers & Wee, 2005). Helping families recognize they are not alone by connecting them with others having similar experiences is a powerful tool to facilitate recovery. Informational support involves facilitating families in gathering the data needed to make decisions. Because crises are not planned, families more often than not do not have the experience or knowledge base to face the effects of crises. Educating families through informational support gives families the knowledge needed to work toward a positive resolution to crises.

The next day, the Medinas return to the hospital and immediately go to the ICU. They are allowed to look at Eva through the window again, and the nurses assure them that Eva had a quiet night and is doing very well. A nurse calls Christine to let her know the Medinas are there. Christine comes up to the ICU and greets the family. Daniel apologizes for not coming to her office, saying he forgot but just needed to see his wife and the children to see their mother. Christine says not to worry but asks them to come down to her office. The family agrees and accompanies Christine to her office. When they arrive, the two girls, Emily and Eloise, again sit with their father on a couch while Dominic sits by himself.

Christine: I am glad you came down. (**Scans the room looking at each family member.**) How are you doing?

Daniel: I guess okay under the circumstances.

Christine: I can only imagine how tough last night was. Did you get any sleep?

Daniel: Not so much, but I think the girls slept, and I am not sure about Dominic.

Dominic: (**Shrugs**) Some, I guess. Mostly I am pissed off about all this. Why did it happen?

Daniel: (**Glares at Dominic.**) Language, we talked about that.

Dominic: Sorry Dad, but it is so unfair.

Christine: (**Interrupts.**) Yes, Dominic, it is not fair; no family deserves to go through this. How about this morning? What was that like?

Eloise: I miss my Mom. I wanted her to make pancakes, that makes me feel better.

Daniel: We went to the breakfast place, and you got pancakes.

Eloise: They were not the way Mom makes them.

Emily: I will make them tomorrow. I know how mom makes them; she has been teaching me.

Eloise: (**Smiles.**) Okay.

Daniel: NO, you won't... You have to go to school. There is not enough time.

Emily: Dadddddd........

Christine: That is what I want to talk with you about. Anything else different about this morning?

Daniel: I guess pretty much everything. I called off work and they understood. And I could not make the kids go to school. And they never miss.

In this brief exchange, the crisis is resulting in several family characteristics that have been affected by the crisis. As you read through the exchange, which characteristics can you identify? Christine recognizes the communications affected by noticing which family members are talking to each other. Rules are also being suspended and boundaries as well. The value of never missing school or calling off work is also suspended. Another characteristic is roles. Emily offered to step in for her mother and start making breakfast for Eloise. Immediately, her father tries to squash that change, probably in an attempt to keep things the way they were. Communication is also altered by what the family is discussing. Christine observes this change and anticipates even more changes. She shows support for the family, and near the end of the exchange, she shifts from Providing Support to Providing Guidance, suggesting that more changes are likely as a result of Eva being a victim of a mass shooting. The TAF:FT overall rating is likely in the mid-teens and possibly a little lower, with the affective rating around 4 to 5 and the behavioral and cognitive ratings about the same.

Reestablish Control. Reestablishing control is an essential, recurring task as families search, sometimes desperately, for ways to regain stable, predictable functioning. This is essential because reestablishing control is the basis for climbing back to a sense of normality because of the unpredictable nature of crises that cause setbacks as families labor to regain equilibrium. The immediate goal is to stop families' downward spiral because familiar methods of functioning become increasingly ineffective when in a crisis situation. Once the downhill slide is halted, the objective becomes one of rebuilding families' capacity to maintain the restored stability and begin a steady climb back to functioning, as much as possible, in a routine manner. Setting short-term, concrete goals is generally the most effective way to help families reestablish control. These goals might be set for the next few minutes, hours, or possibly for a day or two. The time frame greatly depends on the severity of families' reactions to crises. Typically, the more severely families react, the shorter the time frame for goals. Accomplishing the goals helps families regain control and create a foundation on which to restore day-to-day functioning.

Reestablishing control often means helping families simply slow down and calm themselves. Families in crisis may find themselves going at full throttle as they scramble to maintain order and manage the after effects of the situation. The frenetic pace may be thought of as the only way to survive and manage the chaos. Often, families might believe that with just a little more effort, normality will reemerge. Yet from the outside, the frenzied pace suggests families are in disarray with limited to no ability to manage the fallout from crises. Slowing down families creates a situation that will allow them to take one thing at a time rather than trying to untangle a jumbled mess all at once. Taking things one at a time is central to reestablishing control. Helping families prioritize the list of daily tasks lets them address the situation in manageable chunks, little by little.

Reestablishing control also helps families sort through the chaos to discover and create a new foundation to regulate the effect of crises. Generating a new base allows them to start the climb to a reliable, routine day-to-day functioning that may not be the same as before experiencing the crisis. An aspect of reestablishing contol in between reestablishing and can involve a psychoeducational component. Information is a powerful tool to allay fears that they are dysfunctional in some way or another. Providing information on typical reactions, what to expect, the potential for setbacks, and so on all eases the anxiety of not knowing what is happening. This newly established level of functioning can be the basis for new ways of coping and developing resilience (Boss, 2002).

Christine has set the stage for the Medinas to understand that changes in the way the family operates will come. She understands that communication is a key element as the family faces the changes in the way they function during the next few weeks and possibly longer. The changes that will mostly affect the Medinas are roles and rules. These will be affected in the short term, while other family characteristics will experience an impact later in Eva's recovery. The following exchange takes place in Christine's office after Daniel was allowed to sit with and talk briefly with his wife.

Christine: (Looking at Daniel.) How was the visit?

Daniel: (Looks at each of the children, then Christine, and talks in a slow, quiet voice.) I guess as good as it could be. I told her all the kids are here and everyone is praying for her........she kind of smiled but really could not talk. I told her I loved her, and the doctors said she did really good. She smiled when I said that. (Tears form in his eyes, and the two girls, one on each side, lean in to hold him.)

Christine: I can see that really meant a lot to you. Were you able to talk with the doctor?

Daniel: Yea, she said Eva did really good but had a long road ahead of her. Oh yeah, and she might need a wheelchair and a walker for a while.

Emily: Dad, what do you mean, she can't walk? Will she be in a wheelchair forever?

Daniel: No sweetie, not forever but maybe a few months.

Dominic: But what does that mean? A few months?

Christine: That is what I want to talk with you about. You all probably know Eva, your mother, is going to need a lot of support and help. (Looks at each family member then focuses in on Daniel.) That will cause some changes in how you do things.

Daniel: Yea, I guess. (Shrugs his shoulders.)

Dominic: Will she be able to cook and things like that?

Eloise: Daddy who is going to take me to school?

Christine: Great questions. Let's talk about that. Okay?

This exchange demonstrates Christine's support for Daniel after his visit with Eva. She then uses the information the doctor gave him as a springboard to enter into a discussion about probable changes that will occur during Eva's recovery period. The purpose of the discussion is to help the Medinas understand the changes and begin to plan for those. Take a moment and imagine how the conversation might go, what the topics might be, and ways to ensure the Medinas maintain good lines of communication as the family adjusts to a new way of functioning on a day-to-day basis. As stated earlier, the most immediate and noticeable family characteristics affected are roles and rules. Family boundaries will also be modified inside as well as outside the family. The characteristic of communication is key to maintaining family functioning and problem solving. The other family characteristics of values and goals are also affected by the crisis but will be felt later. Take a moment and list ways you might anticipate changes in these characteristics around the Medinas ability to function.

Problem Exploration. Problem exploration is critical with families because of the inclination to compartmentalize the effect of crises (Myer & Moore, 2006). The tendency is to define and understand crises on an individual basis, not the families as a collective unit. The impact of crises on families as a system is an afterthought and sometimes disregarded. Attention is concentrated on helping individual family members, while intervening with families as a unit is neglected (Myer et al., 2013). Consequently, family dynamics and issues are not addressed. Not addressing these issues can be the seed of problems emerging in the future.

Problem exploration involves listening to all family members. All family members are affected, although the impact may be experienced in a different way (Myer & Moore, 2006). Every family member should have a voice in this task. Care must be exercised not to allow a single family member to dominate and arbitrarily assign meaning to crises or to demarcate the boundaries of the resolution process.

Problem exploration means focusing on the immediate effect of crises on families' ability to function. Digging up skeletons of past problems or dissecting the causes and undercurrents of families' misfortunes is not the goal of crisis intervention. Although these issues influence families' reactions, attention should remain on identifying and addressing the issues surfacing because of the current crisis. Problem exploration should be directed at recognizing the dynamics being affected, identifying potential actions leading to a positive resolution, and channeling families' energies in that direction. How have families' dynamics changed in the aftermath of crises? Are the changes beneficial or detracting from families' ability to work through crises? These questions help in appreciating the effect of crises on families.

What are some actions families can take to manage the current circumstances? How do these actions affect and/or influence family dynamics? Brainstorming can be helpful to facilitate families' movement in identifying possible actions to take in the midst of crises. Another technique is "priming the pump." In times past, priming the pump was needed if you could not get water out of a pump. No matter how hard you pumped the handle, no water would come up. However, by pouring a little water into the pump and then pumping the water, it created suction, making the pump work. In crisis intervention, this method means crisis workers offer a few suggestions, priming the pump in a manner of speaking, which will hopefully kick-start families to begin coming up with their own solutions. Helping families channel energies into constructive solutions and actions is also part of problem exploration. At times, this means crisis workers taking the lead, while at other times, this involves pointing families in the most practical and beneficial direction.

Eva was released from the ICU two days after the shooting. Christine met with the family most times they visited the hospital. Twice, she set specific meetings to see how the plan they developed was working. A few adjustments were needed, but overall, the plan they developed worked. As the family discussed the changes and problem solved, Christine used the strategies of Providing Guidance, Encouraging Mobilization, and Providing Support. The other nine strategies discussed in Chapter 4, "The Tools of the Trade," could also be used. In what ways would these be useful? The overall TAF:FT started in the high teens to lower twenties. That rating meant Christine partnered with the family in a fairly directive way. After a week or so, the TAF:FT ratings dropped to the lower teens, and Christine's role shifted to being a consultant.

Follow-up. Follow-up as a task occurs periodically during the intervention, not just at the end or after a few days. Crisis workers should periodically check with clients in crisis to ensure they are aware of what is happening. Attending to this task can feel boring and almost tedious. However, remember that families' awareness of immediate circumstances is often compromised, and as a group or individual, family members are preoccupied with thinking about the crisis (Myer et al., 2013). Families may seem to be paying attention, yet the focus on the crisis impairs their ability to respond to questions and follow simple instructions. Periodically "checking in" allows crisis workers to monitor families' attentiveness to the current situation and ability to take action on plans to resolve the crisis.

A second type of follow-up is short-term follow-up (Greenstone & Leviton, 2011), and it may be either formal or informal (Roberts, 2005). Short term does not mean weeks or months but rather hours and days. Depending on the situation, accomplishing this task ranges from easy to impossible. Christine can easily follow up with the Medinas by meeting them when Eva is in the rehabilitation unit of the hospital. She can also possibly check in while Eva is in physical therapy. Not all family members will be present, but by making this effort, she shows support and continued interest in seeing that they are doing well and continuing to function on a day-to-day basis. In other situations, short-term follow-up is more difficult because families are not easily accessible. These situations might require setting a meeting time for families to come to an office or visiting them in their homes. Phone contact might also be useful to check in with families.

Long-term follow-up is a third type that is useful with families. Long-term follow-up involves monitoring families for mental health issues that could emerge a few months or longer after disasters. These problems may arise because families fail to adjust to life after a crisis. The result is continued strife in the family as they strive to reconcile the changes in their dynamics. Long-term follow-up also allows crisis workers to check for symptoms related to a diagnosis with a mental health disorder (Myer, 2014). If these surface, referral for personal counseling is recommended (Kolski et al., 2012).

Crisis intervention with families involves working on these tasks. Sometimes the process moves very quickly, while at other times, moving through the tasks takes more time. Safety, assessment, and support are continuously worked on through the intervention process, while the tasks of making contact/predispositioning, reestablishing control, problem exploration, and follow-up are addressed as needed. Periodically during the intervention, these later four tasks may need to be worked on when families are sidetracked.

Stages of Family Resolution of Crises

LO9 Historically, crises were typically considered to be resolved in 6 to 8 weeks. However, over the past decade, it has been recognized that the impact of crises can be longer (Myer & Moore, 2006). Depending on the specific crisis, families' recovery may range from months to years. This section continues to follow the Medina family as they struggle with the consequences of Eva being a victim of a mass shooting. Up to now, only Christine has been involved in helping the Medinas in the few days following the shooting. However, Eva's discharge is imminent, which means the Medinas will be confronted with a new set of hardships. Christine may be able to continue to work with the family based on hospital policy and procedures but also may need to refer them to another service provider.

Families go through a predictable series of stages as they work to resolve crises. What is not as predictable is the time frame through these stages. The number of stages families experience following a crisis varies among the assorted models (Weber, 2011). Movement through these involves restoring the family's functional, historical, interpersonal, and spiritual continuity (Rosenfeld et al., 2010). A condensed three-stage model seems most practical for working with families experiencing crises. The stages are survival, adjustment, and adaptation (Myer, 2014). Each of the phases presents a unique set of issues and challenges for helping families (Walsh, 2012b). As a result, crisis intervention strategies fluctuate depending on the phase of recovery. Some families race through the stages, barely missing a beat or experiencing much disruption. Other families seem to move through the stages as if their feet are stuck in molasses while going uphill with weights dragging them back. They epitomize a transcrisis state, which can become a way of life and has the potential to redefine the family in terms of the crisis as permanent and unsolvable (Ford, 2021, p. 28). Both internal and external factors have a significant role as families work to recapture their ability to move on and function on a day-to-day basis (Boss, 2002). Among these factors are their experiences with similar situations (Boss, 2002), the amount of change resulting from crises (Myer & Moore, 2006), family cohesion (Olson, 2000), resilience (Rosenfeld et al., 2010), and their reliance on their faith and spirituality (Robert & Kelly, 2015; Walker et al., 2015). It is important to recognize the family's stage in order to match the intervention process accordingly.

Survival Stage. The survival stage of recovery occurs from the first few hours through possibly 3 to 4 weeks following crises and restoring functional continuity (Rosenfeld et al., 2010). Initially, the focus of this stage is to meet the physical needs of families if needed (Snider et al., 2010). For example, families in crisis following a disaster might need assistance locating shelter, food, and clothing. If physical issues such as shelter, food, or injuries are not a concern, the survival stage involves helping families recognize and acknowledge a new reality brought on by the crisis. While this is easily said, in some situations, it is not so easily done. Families may cling to and long for familiar ways, ignoring and resisting change to ward off uncomfortable thoughts and feelings (Walsh, 2012b). A family may long to walk the dog around the block like they did almost every evening. They may seek "comfort" food such as mom's meatloaf and mashed potatoes smothered in gravy or Dad's smoked pork loin with grilled vegetables. Families will want to find anything familiar that reminds them of fond memories of better times.

Many families will also seek guidance and comfort through connections in their spiritual tradition (Walker et al., 2015; Walsh, 2012b) in the survival stage. Crises can be a catalyst for families to find the strength in their spirituality to withstand the hardships resulting from crises (Boss, 2002; Richards et al., 2015; Walsh, 2009). However, some families might not find solace in their spiritual tradition or culture. Instead, crises may cause them to have reservations about their spirituality and cultural traditions (Public Broadcasting Service, 2002). Addressing these issues in crisis intervention depends on the setting and should be done with care. The setting plays a major role in the way spirituality is discussed. For example, Christine may refer the Medinas to someone who has expertise in career development and occupational therapy if the family needs this support.

Patience is critical as you listen to families as a group talk about their experiences (Ectherling et al., 2005). They may need to tell their story not just once but multiple times as they attempt to make meaning of the crisis. As individual family members share their experiences as a group, understanding or "knowing" will evolve (Boss, 2002). Allowing families to tell their story is very important in this stage (Rosenfeld et al., 2010) as new feelings and thoughts are uncovered with each telling of the story as they try to make meaning from all that happened (Echterling et al., 2005; Williams, 2004). As this attempt to make meaning unfolds, watch for a hierarchy of suffering that alienates family members (Myer et al., 2003). Family members might try to play one-upmanship on others in the family either directly or indirectly. Family members may say something like, "I was more scared than you [another survivor] because I saw this or heard that." Or "You can't be as stressed as me ... you weren't even around when the disaster happened; you were out of town." Indirectly, they may say, "No one knows how much I suffered; I don't even know yet." Defusing interactions that create hierarchies of suffering involves carefully listening and facilitating respect for everyone's experience. A second word of caution concerns family relationships and interactions. Initially, families will typically "circle the wagons" and let bygones be bygones. However, after the initial coming together, the relationships that existed prior to the disaster will most likely be exaggerated. Families with healthy relationships and interactions will tend to become healthier. At the same time, families with destructive or unhealthy relationships and interactions will move more in that direction. Of course, this situation does not occur 100 percent of the time; exceptions do exist.

As Christine meets with the Medinas during Eva's recovery, she quietly monitors the family's interactions, internal and external. This is accomplished by observing which family members sit together and who talks to whom. Early in the exchanges, Christine notices Dominic always sits by himself, while the girls sit with their father. This information may be a clue to family boundaries and possible conflict between Daniel and Dominic. Christine can also take note of which family members regularly come to the hospital. Any conclusions from this information depend on the unique circumstances of the family. Maybe Dominic cannot be present because of school functions, or he may have a part-time job. The girls also may be pulled in different directions because of friends or outside activities. Yet, the information is important as Christine works to support the family during the survival stage. As Christine talks with the family, she learns that extended family members have stepped up to help the Medinas function on a day-to-day basis. Family friends have also pitched in. Meals are brought to the family, and offers to transport the children to school and other activities abound. Daniel says all this support helped relieve the stress and trauma of the crisis; he is so grateful so many people have lent a helping hand.

Another aspect of crisis intervention in this stage involves preparing families for postcrisis experiences (Rosenfeld et al., 2010). Using a psychoeducational approach helps prevent discouragement and frustration from setting in (Kolski et al., 2012). Knowing what to expect strengthens families' resilience in the wake of setbacks. Guidance and ordering are both useful strategies for organizing families' thoughts about life after the crisis. Some families might simply need a gentle push, while others will need their hands held during the survival stage. A special case occurs when the death of a family member is involved. Families that have lost a loved one might need to be prepared to identify the body at a morgue (Rosenfeld et al., 2010).

Adaptation Stage. The adaptation stage typically starts a few days up to 3 weeks after the crisis and spreads over several months and, in some situations, longer. In this stage, families will assess their ability to carry on and search for explanations (Weber, 2011) and recognize that recovery may be a daunting task that will not happen overnight (Price et al., 2010). A stark realization floods into consciousness as people see their world has been turned upside down, and righting it will take hard work. Victories and defeats will be weathered as families work through this stage. Although the experience of families in this stage is idiosyncratic, several general types can be described. Some families rise to the challenge, not being afraid to take the first step on the long road of recovery (Echterling et al., 2005). Families reacting in this manner generally view the crisis as a shared problem and may only need guidance and a little support (Walsh, 2012b). Other families will react as if they hit a brick wall, giving up and deciding the work is too much. These families become immobile and will need support and inspiration as they work to overcome the challenges brought on by crises. Still other families are slowly worn down as they seemingly trudge through adjusting to the hardship that beset them (Rosenfeld et al., 2010). These families will need encouragement and caring to sustain their efforts at resolving the crisis.

Be on alert for families in which the crisis has reignited past unresolved crises in their lives. As we said earlier, families may have "unfinished business" about a crisis submerged below their awareness that can be triggered by a current crisis. The new crisis causes unresolved issues to emerge, resulting in a roller-coaster-type experience. This situation is very possible during the adjustment stage as families are faced with numerous challenges as they put their lives back together.

Although all the strategies are useful during the adaptation phase of recovery, a few merit special attention. **Mobilization** is one of those strategies. According to Myer and James (2005), mobilization involves helping survivors activate internal strengths and trigger dormant coping mechanisms. The amount of involvement depends on the severity of families' reactions. The more severe the survivors' reactions, the more direct you will be as a disaster counselor. You may find yourself being a cheerleader when using this strategy. From a Solution Focused Brief Therapy (SFBT) (De Shazer, 1994) standpoint, the worker will be encouraging and cheering families along as they struggle to regain a daily routine (Sklare, 1997, p. 49; Walter & Peller, 1992). Indeed, the Medina family will continue to experience difficulties as Eva recovers. Setbacks will likely occur. These setbacks will possibly build and become "pile-up" crises linked to the original crisis. The crisis of "exhaustion" is also possible during this phase of recovery. Maintaining contact with the family in long-term follow-up can help the Medinas as related but new crises emerge. Individual family members may also have personal setbacks. Given the crisis being caused by a mass shooting, additional mental health issues may surface, including but not limited to posttraumatic stress disorder, attachment disorder, major depression, and so on. The emergence of these problems suggests the need for more trauma-informed counseling on a longer-term basis.

Families who seem adrift and scattered, not able to concentrate on what needs to be done in this stage, will benefit from focusing (Myer & James, 2005). Families may be collapsing under the weight of the tasks being heaped on them in the recovery process. They might think all is lost and feel a sense of helplessness. **Focusing** helps families sort through what seems like a junk pile of responsibilities in order to focus on the most important ones at that moment. A direct approach may be indicated for survivors who are floundering and not able to even know what needs to be done. A less direct approach is required for families who may have a list of things that need to be done but simply cannot decide where to start. Leading these families involves helping them make that decision by listening patiently and getting them to focus on the most important issues. Setting and meeting short-term goals builds confidence for these families.

The flip side of the coin from focusing is expansion (Myer & James, 2005). **Expansion** allows families to see alternative perspectives to understand and recover from their experience. Families with a restricted, narrow perspective may need to have their view expanded to see other approaches to recovery. Expansion is effective with families who find themselves in a "velvet rut." A velvet rut involves being comfortable trying the same thing time after time even though no change occurs. In other words, thinking only one way will work to help them dig out from the aftermath of crises. The family might say something to the effect we have always done things this way, why should we change, it has worked in the past. Although comfortable, the rut hinders recovery because it is inefficient at best and counterproductive at worst. Helping families entertain other viewpoints lets them reframe their experience and consider additional paths to recovery.

A final strategy useful in this stage is **creating order**. This strategy is used to help survivors rank order a list of what needs to be done and in what order these things should be worked on (Myer & James, 2005). Some families may be stuck, not knowing where to start. Other families may know what needs to be done but be confused about what needs to be done first. An important part of using this strategy with families is to help them understand that the most important things needing attention are not always what need to be done first. Many long-term goals fall into the category of important tasks. For example, recovery for some survivors involves rebuilding a house or returning to work to have a paycheck. Arguably these are tremendously important; however, they may not be the first thing that needs to be done. Helping families rank order the issues enables them to break these into manageable portions so they can move forward and reestablish a routine in their lives.

A little over two months after Eva was released from the hospital, Christine set up a family meeting to follow-up with the Medinas. Eva was still going to rehabilitation four days a week. Rehabilitation was going well, but she still had limited mobility and needed assistance going to rehab and around the house.

Christine: Please come in and sit down.

(The Medinas enter her office and sit down. Daniel helps Eva sit down and then sits by her. Dominic sits in a separate chair slouched over, eyes on the ceiling, while Emily sits next to her mother tapping her foot rapidly with a sullen look on her face.)

Christine: Thanks for coming. Is Eloise here?

Dominic: Ummmm....no. She wouldn't come today the little snot.

Eva: Well, that is not exactly right. We thought that we needed to talk without her today.

Dominic: (Sarcastic). Miss Goody too good to pitch in and pull her load ain't comin' cause she's pissed off, the little shit. She's threatening to run away and I'd pitch in for the bus ticket!

Daniel: (Threatening look directed at Dominic). I won't tell you about that foul language again. You mind your mouth young man.

Emily: (Sneeringly). Look at whose talkin' Mr. All Dominic America who's too busy with sports to do other than a spit and a lick at keeping his room cleaned, clothes washed, and forget about housework that's women's work. So watch where you're throwing gripes cause they bounce off us like rubber and stick like glue and land on you.

Dominic: (Sarcastic). Yeah and I see killing us all with your cooking is part of your master plan for fixing this family. So just blow it out your nose short pants. See no foul language okay Dad?

Daniel: (Yells). SHUT UP! I'm sick of this arguing that's all I hear and now you bring it here.

Eva: (Starts crying).

Daniel: (Caustic, glaring at Dominic and Emily) Now look what you ungrateful, selfish brats have done making your mom cry. I'm getting pretty sick of you frankly.

Christine: Whoa! What am I missing?

Daniel: (Sighs.) Sorry. Well you know things have gotten hard.

Christine: What do you mean hard?

Daniel: (Lets out a slow breath.) Well maybe not hard, I mean all the kids want to help but.....well things just are happening.

Eva: (Rubs her husband's arm. Still sniffling, wipes tears away) Sweetheart can I explain.

Daniel: (Nods yes.)

Eva: Dominic and Emily are both in high school and Eloise is still small. They have lots of extra stuff to do and want to be with their friends, and then stuff seems to land on Eloise to do. (Tears again form in her eyes.) And I need so much help and am such a burden. Daniel has to work extra hours because of the medical bills so a lot of stuff falls on them to get things done. I don't want them to miss out on anything and it's not fair to Eloise and it's such a mess (breaks down).

Dominic: (Shrugs) Mom it is just hard to do everything.

Daniel: At first everyone was great. Eva's sister would come over and clean the house, the neighbors brought food almost every day. My sister volunteered to take Eva to rehab. My work even gave me a little time off. But now.....

Eva: Now it feels like we are on our own. I can't do it, and Daniel has to work so a lot of responsibility has fallen on Dominic and Emily and all we ever do is wind up getting angry and arguing like just now. It's awful.

Christine: (Gently, but firmly in a well-modulated voice). TIME OUT. I need to explain something to you. What just happened here can be pretty typical when a crisis hits and things go topsy turvy as far as family roles are concerned. It's anything but pleasant, but it can be expected and there are ways of maybe not solving everything, but making reasonable adaptations and saying for now it's good enough until things get back on an even keel. I'm gonna model what I call a Family Planning Meeting. I am going to recommend you have one of these every week for a while. Maybe on Sunday night when you can eat a pizza and just relax, talk, and plan and trouble shoot things. Here's the deal. There are just two rules. I'll be the referee here to show you how this works, but I think Eva, you need to be the referee for meetings at home. I'll call time if these rules are violated.

Two simple rules: First when you talk, everything has got to start with "I." No "yous" or "theys" allowed. You need to say what you want or need, not what others might or should do. Once you finish what you need to say, the next person has to restate what you said and get acknowledgement that what was restated is correct. Then, you can start out with "I." These two communication rules will cause some good things to happen. First and foremost, you have to own your own thoughts and feelings and not project them onto others. Second, it will slow things down and cause you all to listen more closely to one another. Third, you'll have to think about what they said before you respond, and that will cause you to consider your response more carefully. If you follow those rules, I believe you'll find conversations will be a lot more civil and productive. Your meeting time should be done when things are calmer and you're refreshed, and problem hurdles are low and fewer.

Example: It's Friday night, payday, groceries are in, but the car battery dies. It's inconvenient, but not a catastrophe, so the hurdles the family has to get over to solve the problem are low. On the contrary, Monday morning mom needs to go to rehab, Dominic needs to cut practice early and drive her, it's the end of the month and bills are due, money is scarce, and the battery dies. Are things a little different, hurdles higher? Might tempers and stress get stretched a little more on Monday? So plan a time for the meeting when everyone can chill out and yes, attendance is required by all.

A Family Planning Meeting is limited to talking about problems and solving them, not talking about the failings of family members. The only time we talk about people is in regard to who solved it with a "WAY TO GO." It is about a CAN DO not a CAN'T DO family, and we are going to think that way as the only option. Finally mom, I'd like you to keep a chart that'll look like this:

Unacceptable Undesirable Trivial Tolerable Acceptable Desirable

Problem name start:_____

Unacceptable Undesirable Trivial Tolerable Acceptable Desirable

Problem name finish:_____

When you discuss a problem, I'd like you to mark where it is when you start to tackle it. I think you'll find that a lot of problems can really be put into the trivial category and may not be worth spending much time on. But after you've worked on it for a week, go back and rate it again. What are you willing to settle for? It doesn't have to be **Desirable** although that would nice. Maybe **Tolerable** is good enough.

Now, I want to start that right now, and I'd like to hear what each thinks needs to be the one thing to work on for next week, get some consensus and go at it. Okay?

Dominic: Like do we all have to agree? I mean there's lots of problems since mom still uses a wheelchair.

Christine: You may generate a priority list and agree on how and what you'll work on, but right now, I'd like for us to practice and get the hang of a Family Planning Meeting and settle on one thing and give it a try. Then we'll meet next week and debrief it and see how it goes.

As you can readily observe, the Medinas are in the midst of adapting to the new reality of the aftermath from Eva's injuries and are moving toward a behavioral emergency (Kleespies, 2014). Eloise's threat to run away cannot be taken as idle and will need to be investigated by the crisis worker. The Medinas are in disarray as family roles are in flux and communication has broken down. The family goals and values are also being confronted and ruptured as they adjust to the new reality of Eva's physical restrictions. The historical and interpersonal continuity is in disorder as the family works through the new reality of Eva's rehabilitation. Christine determines problem solving is stuck at best or totally absent. She rates the family in the high teens to low twenties on the family version of the TAF. Given that rating, she will become much more directive in attempting to change the negative system dynamics that have emerged.

She uses techniques from James' (1970) Parent Effectiveness Training (PET) to implement order, stop the chaos, shift to positive planning, and support and mobilize the family. From her experience, Christine knows that this will take time and probably involve meeting with them at least once or twice to fine tune their ability to reorient themselves to the new reality they are facing and start to make progress out of the emotional dysphoria in which they are currently mired.

Adjustment Phase. As families adapt to the changes brought on by a crisis, the adjustment stage begins. This stage involves the integration of changes resulting from crises into their day-to-day functioning, although they may have periodic setbacks, especially at anniversaries or holidays. The historical, interpersonal, and spiritual continuity is reestablished as families integrate the crisis as part of their life. Typically, adjustment begins in the first few months following a crisis, but the time frame for this stage to begin depends on individual families. Some families move into this stage quickly, while others take time to adjust (Price et al., 2010). A key element in the amount of time needed to adjust is the amount of change experienced by survivors (Myer & Moore, 2006). Crises causing significant shifts in families' priorities generally result in this stage being prolonged. The more severe the crisis, the more likely families will need extra time to fully adjust to the new realities brought on by crises.

An important aspect of the adjustment stage is watching for the emergence of symptoms related to mental health disorders. Yet, care must be exercised not to over diagnose, even though survivors seem to be experiencing symptoms consistent with a diagnostic label (Violanti, 2000). Myer et al. (2003) caution that a diagnostic model is not always the most beneficial for understanding reactions to crises. Etcherling et al. (2005) concur, saying that reactions to crises cannot be viewed only as mental health concerns. The most important consideration is what will help you understand and provide interventions that will facilitate families' process of recovery (Myer et al., 2003). A strength-based rather than symptom-based approach may be more therapeutic in this stage (Stuhlmiller & Dunning, 2000), and that is exactly what Christine is doing.

Being open to creative approaches that are based on research and innovation is valuable in the adjustment phase of recovery. In that regard, James (1974) developed the Parent Effectiveness Training program, which was a 10 session, 3-hour program that taught parent groups behavior management and communications skills to help them with underachieving, socially and emotionally maladjusted junior high school students who grappled with academic, behavioral, social, and emotional adjustment problems in school. Parents could be identified as being in frustrated transcrisis states in attempting to deal with the long-standing chronic school problems their children were having. Pre-post academic achievement scores, behavioral baselines, and social adjustment scales of students were compared with a parent group who underwent training, a motivated parent group waiting for training, and a control group whose parents rejected training. Significant pre-post gains on achievement scores, decreases in disruptive classroom behavior, increases in proactive classroom behavior, and gains on social and personal adjustment scales were found for the students whose parents underwent the training protocol (James, 1974). As an anecdotal note, the groups generated social support systems and would provide personal telephone crisis calls with one another when things were not going well.

Key dates. During this stage of recovery, anniversaries and holidays are important (Myer & Moore, 2006). At these times, families will remember and reminisce about the way life was before the crisis. Some families may express regrets about lost opportunities with respect to what they wish they had done or said (Eliason et al., 2008). Listening and validating these expressions is important for families as they move forward. At these times, families will reexperience the same feelings, behaviors, and cognitions suffered at the time of the crisis. Reminiscing at these points is a way for families to integrate the new reality and make meaning of the hardships faced during the crisis. Take care not to allow families to become too melancholy and sink into a pit of self-pity as they reflect at these times. If this situation occurs, families will slip back into a crisis requiring a new round of crisis intervention services.

Spirituality. Pervasive throughout traumatic events that slam into and wreak havoc with most family systems is that, for some families, their belief in a higher power is questioned. The degree of the higher power's involvement in the traumatic event itself and the traumatic wake of the event's aftermath result in questions with which many families struggle. Denied by, unsure of, and embarrassed by it, many therapists deflect or attempt to ignore it as a topic to be included in therapy (Walker et al., 2004). Walker et al. (2015, p. 5) report that the gap between the validity of spirituality as an integral part of therapy and the validity the general public places in it is huge. This gap is further exacerbated by the fact that only a few psychotherapy training programs address spirituality or religion. There is good reason that spirituality appears in the Triage Assessment Form under the cognitive domain. For most people, when they come to grips with a trauma and try to make meaning from it, spirituality, religion, and how one communicates with a higher power are critical in finding peace and resolution toward traumatic events (Humphrey, 2009; Slattery & Park, 2015; Van Deusen & Courtois, 2015). A **spiritual crisis** occurs when a previously held religious or spiritual belief is called into question or completely abandoned (Richards et al., 2015, p. 85).

In the aftermath of the mass shooting, the Medina family's faith may be tested. Unless Christine has specific training in this area, she should work with the family and refer them to someone who is qualified. We would recommend a person with training in counseling and also a degree in theology. Many programs include courses, and some programs have specialty areas of training on spirituality and faith. Individuals graduating from these programs have specific training and supervision for helping people in this area.

Cultural Issues

Up to now, issues related to families' culture and ethnicity have only been touched upon, yet these play an important role in crisis intervention. Chapter 2, "Culturally Effective Helping in Crisis," discusses in detail the importance of culturally effective helping, especially with respect to the concept of social locations (Brown, 2008). Just as with individuals, families have social locations (McGoldrick & Ashton, 2012). Social location for families uses a multidimensional perspective that helps to avoid the stereotyping that often occurs when using a one-dimensional viewpoint. Instead of using just ethnic background or racial origins, the concept of social location incorporates many aspects of families' lives. In addition to typical things such as race and ethnicity, social location for families can also include such things as education levels, spirituality, socioeconomic status, generational status, geographical location, family structure (e.g., blended, divorced), and so on, as ways to understand families.

A useful way to understand families is to begin at home by looking at the dynamics in your family. What did your family value? What were your family's goals? What roles did family members fill? How were rules viewed and enforced? What boundaries did your family use, and how did your family communicate? This knowledge gives you a foundation for how families in crisis are similar or different from yours. The awareness and insight gained from looking at how your family functions will be invaluable in understanding families in crisis.

In crisis intervention, situations may occur when doggedly sticking with cultural values and beliefs can hinder or even prevent families' recovery. In these situations, crisis workers may need to help families look beyond and possibly suspend devotion to their cultural values and beliefs to help them find the support needed to recover. A judgment will need to be made whether or not families' culture is preventing or just slowing progress toward recovery. This situation is especially true when families' safety and/or immediate well-being is jeopardized. Some medical crises might also fit the category with cultural values and beliefs that impede families' recovery. Take, for example, a family member with dementia who has become a danger to self and others. Although cultural values and beliefs maintain that families should care for this family member, the family member would be safer and better served in a setting with people trained to work with those who have this condition.

Summary

Working with families in crisis can be both challenging and rewarding. The challenge centers on trying to understand and then help families stabilize their lives. Families have been thrown into disarray by a tragic event and are unable to manage what is happening around them. Regardless of the severity of families' reactions, helping them weather, overcome, and grow from the experience involves understanding not just the effect on individual members but on the system as well. The information in this chapter furnishes a strong foundation for understanding the changes that occur when the typical ways of coping are ineffective. These changes generally occur around the six dynamics (i.e., roles, boundaries, communication, rules, values, and goals) discussed earlier.

When combined, these dynamics interact, making each family's reaction unique. The Triage Assessment Form: Family Therapist introduced in this chapter gives crisis workers the ability to assess these dynamics quickly and effectively so interventions can address families' reactions needing attention. Spirituality is often a key component in dealing with a crisis and should never be arbitrarily dismissed as unimportant or not within the purview of crisis intervention.

The reward comes when you observe families overcome the hardships and establish a new routine. The tasks imbedded in the hybrid model can guide the intervention as you work with families to survive, adapt, and ultimately adjust to the new reality they are facing. Patience and time are generally key elements of helping families work toward the goal of resuming a day-to-day routine. While the pace of recovery for families varies, eventually, families are able to function hopefully for the better.

Personal Loss Bereavement and Grief

Learning Objectives

After studying this chapter, you should be able to:

1. Appreciate that loss is universal and that you will have to deal with it in its many manifestations if you go into the human services business.
2. List the terms necessary to speak the language of loss.
3. Describe the cultural dynamics that influence how people deal with loss.
4. Understand the role of spirituality and religion in loss.
5. List the different models of loss.
6. Recognize the different types of grief assessment tools.
7. Recognize the different types of loss.
8. Understand the principles of treatment for loss in different subgroups.
9. Identify the criteria for complicated grief.
10. Know the treatment techniques for complicated grief.

Introduction

One of your authors is about to fill his gas tank at a self-serve when he notices an older woman struggling to fill her tank. It becomes apparent to your knight-in-shining-armor that he needs to render assistance to this clearly distraught and frustrated woman. He does so and immediately gets into a grief counseling session as the woman has an emotional come apart at the gas pump. Her husband, you see, took care of all the "mechanical" issues in their lives, including filling the car with gas, for 50 years of marriage. After he dropped dead from a heart attack 2 months ago, this woman's world turned from a very secure, knowable, and predictable life into a fairly good working analysis of what we describe in Chapter 1, "Approaching Crisis Intervention," as chaos theory. An hour and a half later, your caring and kindly, somewhat disheveled author, now late for a meeting with the dean, who, while sitting in

a car in a strip mall parking lot, has experienced a range of emotions from his unintended client that range from hysterical grief to rage against her husband's chauvinism that has left her helpless with things "mechanical," gets her somewhat stabilized after a cell phone call to a friend of the woman to come and take her home and a commitment from this bereaved and grief-stricken woman to go to a church in town that has workshops and counseling for the newly widowed.

Dr. James is not a good one-trial learner. A number of years ago, when he was a junior high school counselor who had become a self-styled expert in parent training (subject of his doctoral dissertation), he decided to really show how astute he was at ferreting out parenting issues after he invited a school psychologist buddy over to see how his revolutionary communications/behavior management parenting class (it was 1971) worked. A mother was talking about her seventh-grade daughter who was acting rebellious and oppositional defiant since her father passed away more than a year ago. It was about 8:30 P.M. with another half hour to go in the meeting. Dr. Freud (aka Dick James) decided to make an astute interpretation of the mother's complaints and reflected to her that it appeared it was not just the daughter but also she who had not gotten over the death of her husband. That keen insight started a delayed grieving process that was not the highlight of the evening for the other parents, who would have rather been almost anywhere than the teacher's lounge of Jefferson Junior High School at that point in time. The ending of this story occurred at about 10:30 P.M., when your now thoroughly ego-deflated and wrung-out author drove the parent back to her home in a small rural community 15 miles from school and had to listen to his school psychologist friend, who had to follow him out to her farm, needling him about his therapeutic insight on the ride back to town. This is a trilogy, as most tales of wisdom are, so there is one anecdote more to go.

At one point in his life, your Dr. James was thoroughly burned out with education and counseling and decided to get into the oil business. He ran a bulk petroleum products plant in Manitowoc/Two Rivers, Wisconsin. In that capacity, he served a number of dairy farmers by making home deliveries of gas and diesel fuel in his tank delivery truck. One farmer in particular was a jovial if somewhat rowdy individual who had a reputation for wrecking bars when he got a little too much beer in his system. As a result, this robust young dairy farmer had a good deal of respect and some bit of fear from his neighbors. One spring day, he was gearing up to cultivate for spring planting. His 5-year-old son was badgering him to ride on the tractor, but dad thought it too dangerous, so he was sent back into the yard to play. Somehow, the 5-year-old was able to get over the locked gate into the feed lot. There, he turned on the automatic feeding system, got caught on an auger and was dismembered. This was a horribly traumatic death with a closed casket. Empty words or no words of condolence could be said to the devastated parents. Your author had a Ph.D. in counseling psychology but had little experience in grief work, as the previous anecdote would indicate. No one knew what to say, or indeed was afraid to say anything to attempt to assuage his grief and self-blame for his son's death. Finally, after watching this desolated and isolated young man for a month after the funeral, your author sucked up his courage, made plans to finish his route early, walked into the milking parlor, and told the aggrieved farmer

that in another life, he had been a counselor and was willing to talk and listen to him about his son's death and the circumstances surrounding it. That conversation went on for 2 hours. It was one of the toughest counseling sessions your author ever had. It was also a turning point, because it convinced him that he didn't want to be a millionaire oil baron but needed to get back into the business of counseling. So the point of this long-winded opening is . . .

LO1 To be human in the world as we know it is to experience loss. Although universal, the experience of loss is individual. Not everyone reacts to loss and grieves in the same way, not even within families. One family member might be angry and feel loss, another feels scared and has a sense of transgression, while a third feels deep sadness and cannot marshal energy to do almost anything. The interruption in past, present and anticipated relationships probably causes most of these reactions. In addition, factors unrelated to the loss also affect the way individuals grieve. What is going on and has happened in grieving individuals' lives, such as their experience with loss, proximity to the loss (i.e., physical and psychological), and the amount of change resulting from the loss combined, affects the way individuals react. Appreciating these factors for you is different than anyone you talk with and key to helping grieving individuals.

Almost every chapter in this book has statistics about the chapter's topic. This chapter doesn't, because sooner or later, you are all going to experience at least one loss—your own! Besides that ultimate loss, you will also experience loss in two other ways. First, you will lose something near and dear to you. The loss could be almost anything; a job, a family heirloom, the dream of a career, your first car, your health. Second, and just as important, if you go into the human services business, you are also going to experience dealing with clients who have experienced loss. In fact, you are going to deal with it a lot more than you think because it's not just death you are dealing with, but almost any other kind of loss you can think of having. Therefore, this chapter on loss is indeed about you and perhaps your denial and fear of it.

Of all the tough issues that crisis workers face, probably none is more difficult than working with individuals who have experienced a traumatic loss. People who are assailed by a violent loss have significantly higher symptom levels of prolonged grief disorder, posttraumatic stress disorder (PTSD), and depression compared to persons bereaved by nonviolent losses (Boelen et al., 2015). Boelen and his associates found in their study of 496 bereaved individuals that indices of unrealness, negative cognitions about self and the future along with catastrophic misinterpretations about the world and depressive avoidance of the traumatic loss were all significant mediators of prolonged grief, PTSD, and depression. The Dyregrovs (2008) captured the essence of this finding in a father's response to the traumatic death of his child: "We are taught to handle most situations, but whenever sudden, traumatic death occurs, we are completely helpless both in terms of handling it personally and giving others support" (p. 47).

As you read and discuss this chapter you may experience some potent feelings regarding loss that you thought were pretty much buried. That is not uncommon. As we indicated in Chapter 7, "Posttraumatic Stress Disorder," when we use Charles Figley's (1985) traumagram, we always ask people to graph their losses as well as their traumas. At times, when we are absolutely perplexed about the reasons people are manifesting puzzling problems and symptoms that defy a primary cause, the reason generally lies with an unreconciled loss. Understand that what you read in this chapter may well cause some of the same feelings to surface. For that reason, our course syllabus in crisis intervention specifically states that if you have suffered a recent or unreconciled loss, taking the course at another time may be advisable. That being said, if you are experiencing discomfort in reading this chapter, we urge you to talk to your professor or supervisor to find a grief counselor and talk though your loss.

Recovery from major **primary losses**, such as the death of a friend, child, parent, or spouse requires time, possibly several years, and the traumatic event may have a profoundly lasting effect on the remainder of an individual's life (Costa & Holliday, 1994; Finkbeiner, 1998; Lenferink et al., 2022; Lerner, 2000; McCown & Davies, 1995; Morse, 2000; Pearlman et al., 2010). Although generally not as catastrophic as death, other loss events—e.g., job loss, bankruptcy, physical paralysis, disability, a forced move to a different residence, chronic illness (both physical and mental), geographic and school changes, limb amputation, divorce, or loss of one's home or possessions from flood or fire—can have many or all of the same ramifications (Colgrove et al., 1991, p. 2; Farina, 2000; Lerner, 2000; McCown & Davies, 1995; Michaels, 2009; Morse, 2000; Schliebner & Peregoy, 1994).

In probably no other area of crisis does belief (or lack of it) in a religion and/or a higher power come into play in attempts to make sense of loss, specifically death, and derive meaning from it (Van Tongeren, 2021). To that end, the questions that spirituality and religion bring to the table tend to cause most crisis workers indigestion and heartburn as they struggle to deal with it—both for the individual and themselves. To that end, besides what else we have to say on the subject in this chapter, it is well worth memorizing the list that Aten and associates (2015) propose crisis workers use when dealing with religion (found in Chapter 16, "Disaster Response").

Terms Critical to Understanding Loss

LO2 The objective of this chapter is to provide a general survey of ways in which crisis workers may help clients understand and cope with losses without attempting to deal with the infinite ways in which losses occur and clients attempt to resolve them. To that end, it is important to understand a number of terms that coexist with crisis intervention involving loss.

Bereavement is a period of sorrow following the death of someone significant to you (Humphrey, 2009, p. 6) and is a common life transition rather than a clinical disorder (Neimeyer & Kosminsky, 2014). It is an objective state or condition of deprivation that is especially caused by death and is then followed or accompanied by grief (Pine, 1996). In Rubin's (1999) two-track model of bereavement, the first track is the individual's own adjustment (or lack thereof) in overall biopsychosocial functioning—affective, behavioral, cognitive, social, somatic, and meaning-making systems. The second track involves the individual's affective-cognitive relationship to the deceased and how that is reconciled over time.

Uncomplicated bereavement is the process that occurs as the bereaved individual works through a variety of tasks to integrate the reality of moving forward in life without the person who died (Cohen et al., 2002, p. 309). Those tasks include: (1) moving from an interactive, living relationship to memories that establish continuing bonds with the deceased; (2) coming to terms with the reality of death; (3) experiencing and working though the painful, negative emotions associated with the loss; (4) finding meaning in the loved one's death; (5) adjusting to life without the loved one and forming new relationships with other peers; and (6) becoming open to the possibility of changing negative attitudes such as fear, sadness, anger, and bitterness about life and one's loss into joy and happiness as new opportunities, relationships, and transformations evolve and develop (Cohen et al., 2004; Van Praagh, 2000; Worden, 1991). For most individuals, bereavement is transitory, and, with resilience, they return to former levels of functioning over the course of several months (Neimeyer & Kosminsky, 2014).

Grief is a state or condition of mental anguish or emotional suffering and is a result of or in anticipation of the bereavement (Pine, 1996). Grief is highly unique and multidimensional; a person's affective, behavioral, and cognitive makeup are affected. In addition, contextual and ecosystemic influences affect grief, shaping the experience. Grief and grieving may apply to both primary and secondary losses. Although grief is a universal experience, there is no universal agreement on what it is, and considerable controversy exists over its "normal" duration (Howarth, 2011). *Prolonged Grief Disorder* (PGD), or as it has been referred to as Complicated Grief, is now an official disorder in the Diagnostic and Statistical Manual of Mental Disorders, Fifth Edition, Text Revision (DSM-5-TR) (American Psychiatric Association, 2022).

The majority of people who experience loss and grief do not manifest PGD (Bellet et al., 2020). While grief itself is not a sign of mental illness, prolonged grief is now considered a mental health issue and is designated as such in the DSM 5-TR. Persons experiencing PGD are preoccupied with the deceased and may have recurrent, intrusive images or thoughts of the death. Common symptoms include shock, disbelief and anger about the death, loneliness and isolation, a feeling that a part of the self has died along with the deceased, and a feeling that the future holds little worth (Neimeyer & Kosminsky, 2014). People with complicated grief experience prolonged grieving that causes distress and impairment that can affect both physical and mental health (Shear & Mulhare, 2008).

Traumatic grief is generally subsumed under complicated or prolonged grief, with the additional requirement that the person witnessed or was in close proximity to the violent, sudden, unexpected, horrifying death of a loved one (Lenferink et al., 2022). Lenferink et al. (2022) also state that anger is common when death occurs due to violence and unnatural causes. These authors add that an angry reaction is a typical response in cases where another person is responsible for the death, such as homicide, but it can also be observed when the death occurs by chance, such as in a fatal traffic accident. Often, survivors will also experience symptoms consistent with or even develop PTSD.

Disenfranchised grief occurs when a person has experienced a deep and meaningful attachment, experienced loss, and cannot openly acknowledge or grieve the loss or have it validated by others (Doka, 1989; Stroebe et al., 2008). It might be erroneously thought that disenfranchised grief occurs only in clandestine relationships involving affairs outside of marriage. However, cultural and societal norms may also forbid—or at least not sanction—displays of grief between coworkers, men, various types of professionals such as medical doctors, and other people who should "keep it together" or "not care all that much."

Further, individuals may feel ashamed about the relationship, be afraid that an overt display of emotion could hurt them professionally, or just experience emotions that inhibit the grieving process (Doka, 1989). Many people would believe it "silly and overemotional" to grieve over a pet. They may keep their feelings of grief closely to themselves unless they feel they are absolutely safe in sharing them. Yet to act as if the death means nothing for the sake of "having a stiff upper lip" can be a harmful variation of disenfranchised grief—particularly for children and older adults (Doka, 1994).

Loss is a universal human phenomenon, but people respond to it with varying degrees of grief and mourning (Howarth, 2011). Any loss is some form of death. Death of a loved one, death of a relationship through the breakup of a marriage or a friendship, leaving a job, putting down a pet, repossession of a home, moving geographically away from friends and family, and even the loss of precious keepsakes can constitute a loss that becomes a crisis. All losses produce some degree of grieving (Giunta & Giunta, 2002, p. 4).

Primary loss is a significant event such as a death. **Secondary loss** is a consequence of a primary loss. Death of a spouse may cause loss of status, social contacts, financial security, and sexual intimacy, which are secondary losses. Primary loss of a job may cause financial insecurity, reduced self-esteem as a family provider, and a lack of self-confidence in vocational ability, which are secondary losses (Humphrey, 2009, p. 20).

Ambiguous loss is of two types. The first is when a person is physically absent but psychologically present, as in the case of a missing person. A prime example of this type of loss is a parent who is incarcerated (Arditti, 2016). In this situation, a parent or other loved one is convicted and imprisoned in a location that families or loved ones cannot visit. The second is when a person is physically present but psychologically absent, as in the case of dementia or schizophrenia (Boss, 2006). Imagine visiting your parent or other loved one, and you are remembered as a 10-year-old even though you are 45 years old.

New meaning to ambiguous loss came about because of the COVID-19 pandemic (Govermale et al., 2023; Kokou-Koklou et al., 2020). Loss during the height of the pandemic, especially in the early months, generally meant that funeral services were either postponed or simply did not happen. Family members, friends, or other significant persons were trapped with ambiguous loss until closure could be achieved (LeRoy et al., 2020). This situation was especially true when family members or other loved ones were scattered across a large geographical region and travel was restricted or not advised. Video conferencing may have been used to remember the person who died. However, video conferencing is not the same as being physically present at a service. Honoring the person who died may have also been delayed until travel was considered "safe" and a memorial service was held. Although the memorial service created closure the bereavement process was prolonged. Research related to ambiguous loss and the pandemic is needed to understand the full impact on grief and bereavement.

Nonfinite loss. Nonfinite losses are those loss experiences that are enduring in nature, usually precipitated by a negative life event or episode that retains a physical and/or psychological presence in an ongoing manner (Bruce & Schultz, 2002). The anxiety, guilt, stress, and trepidation of adult caregivers in deciding to move a parent into a nursing facility is an example of a nonfinite loss. Such losses are closely related to ambiguous loss in that the person is still alive, but the major ties that characterized the prior relationship are dramatically changed and largely absent. Harris (2020) describes nonfinite losses as internal in nature and taking on a sense of uncertainty, vulnerability, and helplessness in continuing to foster the relationships and they can lead to chronic guilt and sorrow in the caregiver.

Preloss grief, also referred to as anticipatory grief, is the reaction that occurs when an individual is diagnosed with an illness that will likely end in death (Singer et al., 2020). Not only must family members

and loved ones struggle to come to terms with the potential loss of a loved one but also the changes that result as the loved one's health declines (Nielsen et al., 2016). Family members' and loved ones' reactions span a wide range of responses. These might include emotional distress and confusion about individuals' role in life. Reactions also may result in everyone, including the individual diagnosed with the illness, being surprised and shocked as they search to understand the meaning of the diagnosis (Singer et al., 2020). They are forced to weather the shock of a loved one's likely death. Singer et al. (2020) state that, as with bereavement, most family members ultimately adapt and tap into their resilience as the journey plays out. Some individuals are able to adjust after a short time, while others may exhibit more intense reactions. These reactions have the ability to cause significant impairment that persists even after their loved one has died.

Mourning is a social or cultural state or condition expressing grief or feeling because of bereavement (Pine, 1996). Mourning is a communal rather than an individual reaction to loss, generally prescribed by cultural protocol and the time frame in which it occurs (Bedikian, 2008; Humphrey, 2009, p. 5; Morgan & Laungani, 2002; Stroebe et al., 2008). The public appearances one makes, the clothing one wears, the music one listens to, the religious rituals one performs, and even the food one eats are many of the artifacts prescribed for mourning. Mourning can apply to both death and nondeath losses (Humphrey, 2009, p. 10).

Thus, when dealing with the crisis of personal loss, crisis workers are likely to encounter a variety of issues. First are the individuals enduring the loss, which may range from a terminal illness to the breakup of a teenage romance to the loss of a job to the loss of a pet—all of which may be perceived as intolerable and catastrophic. Second are their caregivers, who must provide help and succor not only for those experiencing the loss but also for themselves (Allen et al., 2006; Okun & Nowinski, 2011). Third are survivors who may be experiencing problems that range from shame, sorrow, guilt, and anger to prolonged grief, depression, substance abuse, serious physical illness, and suicidal behavior (Boelen & Prigerson, 2007; Giunta & Giunta, 2002; Parkes & Prigerson, 2010; Rosenblatt, 2010; Wakefield et al., 2011). Further complicating the issues that confront workers who are dealing with grieving individuals are the cultural contexts within which their clients operate.

Dynamics of Bereavement

Cultural Dynamics

LO3 No area of crisis intervention is quite so culturally sensitive as mourning and bereavement after a loss. While grief responses are largely biological and common across all societies, mourning and bereavement are culturally based and vary greatly from society to society (Morgan & Laugani, 2002, 2003, 2004a, 2004b; Morgan et al., 2009; Stroebe et al., 2008; Weiss, 1998). Humphrey (2009, pp. 8–9) exhorts us to recognize that loss and grief occur in the multiple and fluid context of personal, familial, social, cultural, and historical influences. Humphrey proposes that an individual's grieving is a continuous negotiation process among a wide array of sociocultural influences specific to the person and the environment in which they live. These influences range from beliefs and values about meaning to rules and conduct for behaving, to support networks to religious practices and healers, to an individual or collectivist society, to traditions and rituals, to communication style, to levels of acculturation and assimilation, and to ethnicity (Humphrey, 2008, p. 8). Suffice it to say that Brown's (2008) social locations you read about in Chapter 2, "Culturally Effective Helping in Crisis," play a huge role and act in infinite ways to form the individual's response to loss.

Consider the term *culture* in the broadest possible context. Race, religion, gender, geographic region, sexual orientation, disabling condition, socioeconomic class, and temporal context all factor in multiple ways into the loss experience (Doka & Davidson, 1998). The manner in which humans grieve differs from culture to culture and from time to time. As Bedikian (2008) suggests, the ecosystem within which we operate has a great deal to do with how we mourn and grieve. The prolonged grief that Queen Victoria felt for Prince Albert in late-nineteenth-century Great Britain translated into rigid rules of mourning for women that included heavy black costumes and black crepe veils for up to 4 years after the dearly beloved's demise to show their grief. The advent of World War I brought that practice to a screeching halt because women went to work in factories and formal mourning etiquette gave way to the necessity of showing up for work in work clothes. That somber and extended approach to mourning has given way to wearing a dark dress or suit to a visitation or memorial service of a half hour and going back to work that afternoon.

Thus, each culture develops its own beliefs, mores, norms, standards, and attitudes toward death, and these can change over time to meet changing conditions (Dutro, 1994). Further, groups from differing backgrounds within a particular culture may have vastly divergent attitudes and perceptions about death (Dutro, 1994), and individuals within that group may further differ dramatically in how they construct and make meaning from the loss (Neimeyer, 2001).

Rando (1984) stated that "for all societies there seem to be three general patterns of response: **death accepting**, **death defying**, or **death denying**" (p. 51, bold added). Joffrion and Douglas (1994) characterize modern Western society as a death-defying culture. Kübler-Ross (1975) writes that, in our culture, "death has become a dreaded and unspeakable issue to be avoided by every means possible," noting "that death reminds us of our human vulnerability in spite of our technological advances" (p. 5). Do you suppose that is why there are drive-by funeral homes in California where you can view the body from your car without ever having to get out? Ramshaw (2010) proposes that while postmodern Euro-American Protestant funerals have become highly impersonal, there still exists a desire and a need to personalize rituals as a celebration of the person's life.

Contrast that drive-by visitation to being in the second line at a New Orleans funeral procession (the mourners following the funeral band) as the body is carried to the cemetery. Do you believe you would see a very different view of how death is dealt with in Louisiana and how emotionally involved you were in it? Let's suppose you were the main object of attention. Would you prefer the drive-by visitation (barely in sight, quickly out of mind) or a Black family's 2-hour funeral ritual in Kentucky that was full of reverence, respect, open grief, and spiritualism for the departed plus a lot of singing, music, and dinner on the church grounds (Collins & Doolittle, 2006)?

For example, Muslim suicide terrorists may be viewed as martyrs absolutely merged with God and God's will in their willingness to sacrifice themselves. Indeed, for Muslims in general, prolonged public mourning and expressions of grief are discouraged because of the great value placed on the acceptance of God's will with restraint and understanding. While Muslims may cherish memories of the departed and grieve mightily in private, their return to public functioning after a loss is strongly encouraged (Rubin & Yasien-Esmael, 2004).

Contrast that notion again with Mexican American families as they handle traumatic grief. Perhaps because of the mingling of historical indigenous and Catholic beliefs about death as a way into a new life and beginning along with the strong family bonding that predominates in the Mexican culture, death plays a prominent role. Besides the well-known Día de los Muertos (i.e., Day of the Dead), when parades and festivities honor deceased family members, living family members honor and maintain a strong bond to the deceased through storytelling, dreams, keepsakes, ongoing faith-based altars at home, and rituals through church (Doran & Hansen, 2006).

Finally, consider the way two very different cultures half a world apart process grief. Bonanno and his associates (2005) measured grief processing and deliberate grief avoidance in the United States and the People's Republic of China. These researchers report that the way people in both cultures grieved initially predicted how they would process their grief later on. However, contrary to the way people in the United States fared, continued grief processing or avoidance did not predict negative psychological consequences for the Chinese.

What needs to happen as far as grieving is concerned and what the culture expects to happen often butt heads. When expatriates move into foreign countries and suffer loss, particularly if it is traumatic in nature such as in hurricanes or floods, they may experience what Smid and Boelen (2021) refer to as *cultural incongruity*. This situation arises when the beliefs between the host nation and the new arrivals differ for handling, physically and emotionally, the death of loved ones. Van der Heijden and Swartz (2010) investigated a peer-led HIV/AIDS prevention strategy in South Africa for vulnerable children who had lost parents to the disease. The intervention ran into trouble because attempts to talk about death and elicit memories of loved ones ran counter to the cultural practice of maintaining silence about the deceased and protecting children from unpleasantness. What all of the foregoing boils down to is that loss and its reconciliation constitute one of the most culturally sensitive areas into which a crisis interventionist ventures. To say that one must tread lightly here and be very observant when dealing with cross-cultural loss is one of the bigger understatements made in this book!

Sociocultural Mores

Schoenberg (1980) describes how societal mores and attitudes toward life, death, and dying in the United States have changed over the years. As the country has shifted from a rural to an urban orientation and lifestyle, there has been a shift from a death-defying culture to a death-denying culture (pp. 51–56). While farm families usually came in contact with the birth, life, and death of animals as well as people, city dwellers rarely encountered dead animals or dead people. People in rural communities cared for their own dying relatives and friends. They prepared the corpses for burial and dug the graves by hand. They laid out the bodies of the dead in the parlor and commemorated the lives of the departed; then, they buried them in the family or community cemetery. That's quite a contrast to the way dying, death, grieving in public, and funerals are carried out in most communities in the United States today. Death in modern Western societies has been sanitized and generally removed from the context of everyday life (Crase, 1994; Joffrion & Douglas, 1994; Morgan & Laungani, 2003; Schoenberg, 1980), although the COVID-19 pandemic brought death to everyone's front door either by the disease itself or graphic videos on television of refrigerated trailer trucks full of the dead from overflowing hospital morgues.

The social organization of bereavement and the social reaction to the loss of loved ones have changed partly because of shifts in age-specific mortality patterns (Osterweis et al., 1984). In former times, adult life expectancy was short, and infant mortality was high. Epidemics and famines frequently wiped out large numbers of people. Communities were small and close-knit. Death was taken personally by everyone in the community, and mourning rituals were community-wide events (pp. 199–200). People saw death every day, and fiery sermons about hell, death, and eternal damnation made people acutely aware that they were always one step away from the grave. Changes in families, geographic mobility, urbanization, information technology, aging patterns, the job market, birth control and child-rearing practices, medical and nutritional improvements and advances, and information dissemination and processing have greatly affected the way society views and deals with death, loss, and grief (Green, 2008; Morgan & Laungani, 2003, 2004a).

In modern times, the bereavement process has tended to become standardized by laws, regulations, and the development of specialists who carry out these laws and regulations. Death usually occurs in a hospital or nursing home. Frequently, the deceased are older people who have been out of the mainstream of community activity for a number of years; as a result, they are not as widely known as they were in their younger years. Mourning has tended to move out of the home and into funeral parlors and hospital chapels. Laws affecting the role of funeral directors and the policies of employers have influenced the ways society mourns. Workplaces have established rules governing the time employees can take off from work following the death of a close family member or loved one. Many institutional constraints on behavior have tended to impose social uniformity on the previously diverse patterns of grief and bereavement (Green, 2008; Morgan & Laungani, 2003, 2004a).

Grief that follows a death has become much more institutionalized (Osterweiset et al., 1984, pp. 201–202), but such institutionalization is not necessarily negative. For example, some funeral homes offer professional grief counseling programs for their clientele and communities (Riordan & Allen, 1989). Thus, the sociocultural changes that occurred between 1900 and 2000 brought about important changes in reliance on such helpers as physicians, nurses, psychologists, social workers, counselors, rehabilitation specialists, hospice workers, and caregivers for survivors of loss (Dershimer, 1990, pp. 14–36; Huber, 1993; Schneider, 1984, p. ix). Indeed, Morgan and Laungani's (2002, 2003, 2004a, 2004b) multivolume set on a global perspective of death and bereavement looks like a Dictionary of Occupational Titles search in regard to the wide array of occupations that are represented in the contributing authors.

Spirituality and Religion

LO4 One of the major reasons religions exist is to make meaning of and understand death (Slattery & Park, 2015; Van Tongeren et al., 2021). Whether you believe in Zeus, Odin, God, Buddha, Isis, Allah, the Great Spirit, or Charlie Brown's Great Pumpkin, the human quest for meaning in life and death has looked to some deity to provide the answers. Whether you believe in Valhalla, Heaven, Nirvana, paradise, reincarnation, or anything else that means a secure, happy, peaceful place in the hereafter, humans have continuously attempted to cheat the finality of death by creating an afterlife and making sense of why bad things happen to good people and why the good die young (Drescher & Foy, 2010; Giunta & Giunta, 2002; Green, 2008; Walsh, 2009). Faith, beliefs, and religious practices are often the foundation stones for dealing with life's end and the loss of loved ones (Aten et al., 2019; Morris Trainor, 2019). Each of these offers comfort, hope, support, and connection when one feels hopeless, unsupported, and

disconnected (Aten et al., 2019). Spiritual resources provide guidance to family members and friends on how to honor the deceased and mourn their loss across the world and through the millennia (Walsh, 2009). To that end, Kaut (2006) proposes that any end-of-life assessment and counseling should include a bio-psycho-social-spiritual network.

However, religion, spirituality, and supreme beings are double-edged swords. What they bequeath as far as hope is concerned, they can also snatch away. The COVID-19 pandemic brought this issue to the forefront, with people struggling to understand not just the death of a loved one but the millions around the world who also died (Zhang et al., 2021). According to Zhang et al. (2021), these struggles involve wanting a divine intervention to heal the dying loved one, strength to endure the outcome, and simply make everything all better. Questioning faith when loss occurs as a result of a disaster is also an issue (Aten et al., 2019). For people, longstanding beliefs are called into question in the wake of a disaster. The Frontline video titled Faith and Doubt at Ground Zero, first aired in September 2002, brings to life the struggles experienced by survivors of the terrorist attack. This video can be viewed on youtube.com. The loss resulting from disaster sometimes not only involves the death of a loved one but can also involve the loss of a home, heirlooms, family photos, and so on. Each of these losses takes a toll, many times resulting in some people questioning their faith.

One of the biggest problems people encounter when faced with loss is making meaning structures that work and help them move through the grief. That's fairly easy in a just and equitable world, but in the world of crisis intervention, as you should know by now, it is very often anything but fair and equitable. Because not everything is fair, people may question their particular deity of choice when their beliefs, attitudes, assumptions, values, and everything else they hold dear to make sense of the world become ruptured, disjointed, and chaotic (LeRoy et al., 2020). If the Great Pumpkin continues to dash Charlie Brown's hopes for a meeting, it may challenge one of his deepest held beliefs and then lead him to question whether this whole "spiritual" thing is just one giant house of cards, and he needs to find another vegetable deity or just go worship Lucy!

So, it should become clear that attempting to make sense and meaning of a loss can challenge one's most deeply held religious and spiritual beliefs (Humphrey, 2009, p. 26), and that is especially true when the loss is traumatic, interpersonally caused, chronic, or occurs over time during significant developmental stages of a person's life (Walker et al., 2015). On the other edge of this spiritual sword, the Giuntas (2002) are among a multitude of authors who spend a great many pages of print hooking all of the many facets of grief up with why God has not left the building with Elvis and is still a shoulder to lean on. The process of making sense or meaning out of loss, then, involves examining those constructs that help make sense out of life up to the point of the loss and then renewing, redefining, or revising them to restore homeostasis and equilibrium (Humphrey, 2009, p. 26).

In that regard, in the areas of death and major losses, a significant proportion of people (in all societies, including ours), perhaps a majority, find faith to be their most important resource for coping, recovery, and growth. Crisis workers must be comfortable in allowing grieving clients to find healing in their faith and spirituality (Culliford, 2002). This stand does not, of course, mean that crisis workers should inject or impose their own religious beliefs on their grieving clients.

Conceptual Approaches to Bereavement

LO5   There are a variety of models, ranging from psychodynamic to constructivist to cognitive-behavioral approaches, that seek to deal with loss (Bowlby, 1969, 1973, 1980; Cohen et al., 2006; Gillies & Neimeyer, 2006; Neimeyer & Levitt, 2000; Osterweis et al., 1984; Neimeyer & Vaughns, 2022; Powers & Griffith, 1987; Raphael, 1983; Wass & Neimeyer, 2018). Historically, stage/phase models (Bowlby, 1969, 1973, 1980; Kübler-Ross, 1969; Kübler-Ross & Kessler, 2005) have achieved a great deal of fame and notoriety.

Stage/Phase Models

Kübler–Ross's Stages. Probably the loss model best known to the general public is that of Elisabeth Kübler-Ross (1969), which views loss as a series of five stages—denial, anger, bargaining, depression, and acceptance—that people go through as they come to grips with their own imminent death. She later used these five stages to describe grief and the grieving process (Kübler-Ross & Kessler, 2005). While never intended as a strictly linear, stepwise model, it has come to be perceived as such.

As popular and valid as this model has become in the general public's mind, there is little research to substantiate its validity (Konigsberg, 2011). Thus, while its simplicity gives it a lot of curb appeal to the public, there is little empirical evidence to substantiate its use, and it causes problems when people stubbornly refuse to move through its stages as Kübler-Ross proposed. No matter how much people want a neat ribbon-wrapped package that sets out simple rules and stages for grief, there are simply no stages of grief that fit all persons (Friedman & James, 2009). As a result, Kübler-Ross's and most other stage models have been pretty much consigned to history's dustbin.

Bowlby's Attachment Theory. Attachment theory is one of the better known theories in the therapy field that was generated from studies of separation and reunion of young children with their parents (Bowlby, 1969, 1973, 1980). Attachment theory is a linear phase model that focuses on the nature of the griever's relationship to the deceased. The breaking of affective bonds and the disruption caused by the loss require grieving. Failure to grieve intensely is seen as problematic in not coming to terms with the loss of the object. The need to emotionally turn loose or "detach" from the person or object is the end goal of the grief process. This phase model also has its share of controversy and criticism. Grief may not follow a prescribed set of stages the way Bowlby proposes. Moreover, failing to grieve intensely may be a sign of resilience rather than a pathologically avoidant suppression of feelings. Finally, detachment may not necessarily be preferable to continuing to keep bonds and memories of the lost object (Shaver & Fraley, 2008).

Schneider's Growth Model. We feel that one of the better stage/phase models is Schneider's (1984) eight-stage process model of loss. It is a holistic, growth-promoting model designed to nurture as much personal growth as possible within a context of stress, loss, and grief and has attracted a great deal of attention in the study of the potential positive aspects for growth in the wake of a trauma (Cann et al., 2011a, 2011b; Triplett et al., 2011).

The model includes the following stages (Schneider, 1984, pp. 104–226): (1) initial awareness of a loss, which is generally a significant stressor; (2) attempts to limit awareness of the loss, holding on by means of concentrating one's thoughts and emotional energy for a period of time on whatever positive aspects of the loss one can recognize and making use of whatever inner resources one has to immediately stave off immobility and disequilibrium; (3) attempts at limiting awareness by letting go, which involves recognizing one's personal limits with regard to the loss and letting go of unrealistic goals, unwarranted assumptions, and unnecessary illusions; (4) awareness of the extent of the loss, recognizable as mourning—the most painful, lonely, helpless, and hopeless phase through which the loss sufferer goes; (5) gaining perspective on the loss, reaching a point of accepting that what is done is done and providing time to make peace with the past; (6) resolving the loss, which occurs when the bereaved can see and pursue activities unconnected with the loss without it being a reaction against (letting go) or identifying with (holding on) the lost person or object; (7) reformulating loss in a context of growth, which involves discovering potential rather than limits, seeing problems as challenges, being curious again, and seeking a balance between the different aspects of self; and (8) transforming loss into new levels of attainment, which involves an integration of the physical, emotional, cognitive, behavioral, and spiritual aspects of the person and is an integral part of the process of reformulation to higher levels of understanding and acceptance of the loss.

A Counterpoint to Traditional Models

Dutro (1994) has described how our concepts of grief and loss have become more dynamic, moving from the medical or pathology theories to more interactive models. Dutro's comprehensive and dynamic model views grief and loss from the perspective that each individual experiences loss according to psychophysiological, affective, and cognitive-behavioral factors, such as the mode of death, relationship of the deceased, prior losses experienced, and dominant subcultural norms. These factors figure into a dynamic structural model of grief that, according to Dutro, is in sync with sociocultural life in the 21st century. His and others' dynamic, individualistic grief models (Dyregrov & Dyregrov, 2008; Humphrey, 2009; Konigsberg, 2011; Neimeyer, 2000; Worden, 2002) refute many ideas about grief that have been associated with older stage theories:

1. The common assumptions concerning "stages" of grief are not supported.
2. Placing time limitations on grief is inappropriate.

3. The withholding or suppression of sadness in response to bereavement is not necessarily pathological.
4. Insistence on severing ties or detaching oneself from lost objects denies lifelong bonding and usefulness of positive memories.
5. One-size-fits-all models don't work because each individual griever's experience is unique. Grief is not a unitary phenomenon but rather a multidimensional, interactive, individual experience for every bereaved person, based on a complex set of interwoven variables.
6. There are no fixed beginning and ending points in grieving.
7. While grief does not end, it does change.

From that standpoint, the dual process model (Neimeyer 2018; Neimeyer & Vaughns, 2022; Stroebe & Schut, 2001; Stroebe et al., 2008) and the adaptive grieving model (Martin & Doka, 2000), seem to best represent current thinking (Doughty, 2009; Humphrey, 2009) on the fluid, idiosyncratic nature of grief and grieving and how the crisis worker should consider approaching them.

The Dual Process Model. The dual process model may be characterized as an approach-avoidance model that has two components: loss orientation and restoration orientation. **Loss orientation** stressors are associated with the loss itself, which may be experienced in ruminating about it and having behavioral, emotional, and cognitive reactions to it that oscillate between avoiding and confronting the disrupted bond with the object of the loss (Stroebe & Schut, 2001; Stroebe et al., 2008). Stroebe and Schut see this process as a normal and natural process of loss adaptation. For instance, a college student may feel sadness and anger over the loss of a girlfriend (confronting the stressors) but begin working out and increase their study time (avoiding the stressors) in efforts to put lost love out of their mind. As the loss recedes in time, and in line with how processing models are supposed to operate, a restoration orientation begins. So, both avoidance and confrontation are to be seen as a normal and natural process of loss adaptation (Humphrey, 2009, p. 47).

Restoration orientation occurs when grievers start to come to grips with the consequences of the loss and begin to form new roles and identities, develop new relationships, make life changes, and engage in new activities that distract from their grief. The newly aggrieved widow we met at the gas pump at the beginning of this chapter may start to engage in restoration orientation by alternately avoiding her confrontation with loneliness by sitting in front of the TV for hours on end and deciding to confront it by joining a church renewal group that her newly met crisis counselor and pump jockey told her about. The primary task of restoration orientation is attending to rather than avoiding life changes, doing new things, seeking distraction from grief, and dealing with new roles, identities, and relationships (Humphrey, 2009, p. 48). One of the major advantages of this model is that it recognizes that grief is not static but is a series of waves with crests and troughs that ebb and flow at their own pace but gradually move into more quiet, placid, and calm affective, behavioral, and cognitive waters that nourish growth. However—and this is a big "however"—these researchers propose that the griever can get into hot water and move into prolonged grief if this ebb and flow does not occur (Stroebe et al., 2008). Neimeyer (2018) proposes that moving back and forth between denial of an unrequited grieving state and attempting to adjust to the new reality of the missing person and then a turnabout into abject grieving and denial of the new reality are a normal reaction. So, the crisis worker who uses this model should understand that it will make absolute sense when the griever seems to randomly bounce back and forth between a loss and a restoration orientation that operates on a sometimes rapid approach-avoidance continuum. If you understand this model, then, it is not upsetting but rather understandable that people are not static or stable as they grieve but move back and forth as they attempt to bring equilibrium and homeostasis back into their lives and will require the worker to be elastic and flexible when these switches occur.

The Adaptive Model. Martin and Doka (2000) identify grieving as three basic styles that operate along a continuum, with *intuitive* grieving on one end, *instrumental* grieving on the other, and an infinite number of variations between the two. Intuitive grievers respond to loss mainly in terms of emotion, while instrumental grievers think through their grief and/or act on it. Most people, Martin and Doka believe, operate somewhere in the middle and have a blended style. The other component of the adaptive model targets the preferred affective, behavioral, cognitive, and spiritual strategies that grievers use to adapt to the loss. Martin and Doka place a heavy emphasis on spiritual components because of the model's strong

theoretical basis in Jungian psychology and the fact that many people place a great deal of emphasis on the spiritual aspects of adaptive grieving.

It is important to note that adaptive strategies are a good deal more than, and different from, coping strategies. Coping implies "getting along" or "bearing up," while adaptation means engaging in behavior that will result in change. Interestingly, the same adaptive strategies may be used by persons at both ends of the intuitive-instrumental continuum but for entirely different reasons. For example, the common practice of going through a photo album of the deceased and reminiscing about happier times may be used by both intuitive and instrumental grievers. For intuitive grievers, it is a cathartic release of emotions as memories flood conscious awareness and are relived. For the instrumental grievers, the photo album may be a way of remembering, organizing, and planning activities. So, for the intuitive griever, pictures of riding horses on the family farm bring back memories of Sunday afternoon rides, picnics by the river, the smell of horses and harness leather, and grandfather's wide-brimmed Stetson cowboy hat bobbing along in front on his horse Whiplash. For instrumental grievers, the same photos may remind them that the upcoming sale of the farm equipment needs to be inventoried and favorite items parceled out according to requests from brothers and sisters.

It should be clearly understood that adaptive styles do not necessarily mean a rose-covered remembrance path down memory lane. Adaptive styles that are useful in the short term may be counterproductive in the long term. Emotional catharsis verging on hysteria may be fine at the funeral, but level-headed business sense is called for when the family farm is put on the auction block. Also, if primary grievers have different grieving styles, they may butt heads. An instrumental griever who throws herself back into her work may be confounded by a husband who continues to emote at any small remembrance of a daughter who has died in an auto accident. Likewise, he may be appalled that she is so callous and cold as to start packing their beloved daughter's clothing to give to Goodwill six months after the funeral. While they are both using adaptive strategies that serve them well, the interpersonal divisiveness that may occur is something else to behold and, in this example, may wind up in divorce court with little idea that their grieving styles are the friction point that got them there.

People get into trouble with the adaptive model by employing **dissonant response** modes that are consistent with the opposite grieving style. This sets up a discrepancy between people's inner experience and their outward expression of grief, so persons with intuitive grieving styles tend to act like people with a more instrumental style. A "stiff upper lip" worn to meet peer social expectations of "moving on, getting back to normal," finally cracks from the emotional turmoil raging in the person to be let out. When that happens, the person has taken a large step toward complicated grief (Humphrey, 2009, p. 42).

The Constructivist Model The emergent model of how a majority of grief work is being done today is based on George Kelly's (1955) constructivist model of psychotherapy. Robert Neimeyer (1993, 1996, 2004, 2009, 2018; Neimeyer & Vaughns, 2022) has been the leading proponent of this approach. Simply put, a constructivist approach emphasizes humankind's need to impose meaning on their lives. That meaning making results in a stable self-narrative which allows them to get up every morning with a view of a positive future (Neimeyer, 2009). From a constructivist standpoint, loss, especially sudden, traumatic loss, can wreck core beliefs and rend asunder how one lives life and makes meaning of it through their self-narrative (Neimeyer et al., 2009). In constructivist terms, there are two ways of handling this loss, either by *assimilating* it or *accommodating* it (Janoff-Bulman, 1992). The bereaved can reassimilate into their pre-loss beliefs and self-narratives by reconstructing this new world without the significant other by staying ensconced with unchanged old beliefs and operating systems (Janoff-Bulman, 1992). A pathological example of assimilation is the unchanged bedroom décor of a teenager 10 years after she died in an auto accident. Or, an alternative is to accommodate the loss by reorganizing, expanding, and engaging in an in-depth examination of who they are and what their self-narrative will now be given the dramatic change the loss has caused (Janoff-Bulman, 1992). A pathological outcome by overdone accommodation is denial of the impact of the loss by plunging into bad, knee-jerk romantic, financial, and other negative decisions without regard to a stable, prior to the loss, self-narrative.

From a positive standpoint, either assimilation or accommodation is acceptable to a constructivist therapist if it can re-establish a coherent self-narrative that is actualizing, forward-looking, and has resolved the incongruence between the sense of loss and a renewed sense of meaning (Neimeyer et al., 2009).

It should come as no surprise that a constructivist approach to therapy involves an eclectic therapeutic smorgasbord of narrating activities that range from writing to dancing to ferret out new meaning making (Neimeyer & Vaughans, 2021).

It should become readily apparent to you as the crisis worker that being able to ferret out and understand these styles and the models that go with them can be critical in helping grieving individuals move through grief and, even more importantly, in helping significant others understand that the bereaved's grief is not some weird, aberrant pathology but a highly functional, idiosyncratic adaptive measure that works for them.

Assessment Tools

LO6 **The Texas Revised Inventory of Grief (TRIG).**
The TRIG (Faschingbauer et al., 1987) is probably the most widely used inventory to measure grief. It has two scales, Current Grief and Past Disruption. Because of their temporal nature, the two scales allow the worker to determine what kind of progress in grief resolution has been made. The inventory asks respondents to rate themselves on a Likert scale (1 = completely false to 5 = completely true) in response to 8 questions about past behavior at the time the person died (I felt a need to do things the deceased had wanted to do; I was angry at the person; I found it hard to sleep) and 13 questions about how the respondent presently feels about the person's death (still cry when I think of the person who died; I cannot accept this person's death; I hide my tears when I think of the person who died). It has few validity studies, and some of the items ("crying") are replicated, while other well-known concepts, such as guilt, are left out. Yet, it has been used with a wide variety of groups, providing good cross-comparisons and a wealth of normative data.

Grief Experience Inventory (GEI). The GEI (Sanders et al., 1985) assesses the longitudinal course of grief. Self-descriptive items that are answered true/false comprise the inventory. Nine clinical scales cover Despair, Anger/Hostility, Guilt, Social Isolation, Loss of Control, Rumination, Depersonalization, Somatization, and Death Anxiety; six research scales include Sleep Disturbance, Appetite, Loss of Vigor, Physical Symptoms, Optimism–Despair, and Dependency; and three validity scales cover Denial, Atypical Response, and Social Desirability.

Hogan Grief Reaction Checklist (HGRC). The HGRC (Hogan et al., 2001) is designed to discriminate grief reactions from depression or anxiety. Its 61 items target categories of Despair, Panic, Blame/Anger, Disorganization, Detachment, and Personal Growth. It can discriminate variability in the grieving process as a function of the cause of death and time elapsed since the death.

Inventory of Complicated Grief (ICG). The ICG (Prigerson et al., 1995) specifically targets symptoms of grief that are distinct from bereavement-related depression and anxiety and predicts long-term functional impairments. Its items are rated on a Likert scale from "never" to "always." Items target long-term grief, such as not accepting the death, feeling anger or disbelief, avoidance, and auditory and visual hallucinations of the person.

The Persistent Complex Bereavement Inventory (PCBI). The PCBI (Lee, 2015) was developed to assess for persistent complex bereavement disorder (complicated grief). It is a 16-item self-report that rates items on a five-point scale from 0 (none) to 4 (severe–nearly every day). The items are grouped into three subscales of *core grief* (i.e., preoccupation with the deceased), *reactive distress* (i.e., difficulty accepting the death), and *social identity disrupting* (i.e., the desire to die). To achieve a diagnosis of prolonged complex grief, each of the subscales has to have ratings of at least 3 to 4 and have persisted for at least 12 months for adults and six months for children (Lee & Milman, 2021).

The Social Meaning in Life Events Scale (SMILE). The SMILE (Bellet et al., 2018) is a 26-item self-report instrument that measures the degree to which social interactions help or inhibit an individual's ability to make meaning of a life event. Respondents rate themselves 1 (strongly disagree) to 5 (strongly agree) on the Social Validation scale (i.e., talking to other people about the event). Higher scores indicate better efforts at making meaning of the event. The Social Invalidation scale measures the extent to which the mourner's social environment frustrates or casts aspersion on the deceased (i.e., I feel more distant from others when I talk to them about this event). Higher scores indicate thwarted efforts to make sense of the event. The clinical use of the SMILE is for understanding the potential roadblocks with the individual's interpersonal environment in making sense of the loss (Bellet, 2021).

Quality of Relationships Inventory Bereavement Version QRI-B). The QRI-B (Bottomley et al., 2017) is a 13-item self-report instrument that assesses predeath relationship quality between the departed and the survivor. A 4-point Likert scale from 1 (not at all) to 4 (very much) measures the frequency and magnitude of items on a *Closeness* subscale, which focuses on the warmth, support, and trust prior to death (i.e., How positive a role did the person play in your life?). The *Conflict* subscale measures the degree to which predeath relationships were marked by discord and distress (i.e., How upset did this person make you feel?). The clinical application of this scale can be used to assess the impact of the relationship with the deceased and also be used to look at possible ways to intervene into a disrupted bereavement process (Bottomley & Neimeyer, 2021).

Types of Loss

LO7 People may encounter many different types of loss that produce stress, trauma, and/or grief. Following are several types of loss that crisis workers may encounter. It is not the purpose of this text to provide crisis intervention techniques for dealing with every specific type of loss. What is shown here is that loss covers a broad scope and that certain fundamental helping skills and strategies apply in a generic way to helping individuals who are suffering from loss.

Death of a Spouse

An unimaginable, indescribable loss has taken place, and the numbness and excruciating pain is so deep because someone you love has died, and it is unmatched for its emptiness and profound sadness (Kübler-Ross & Kessler, 2005, p. 29; Parkes & Prigerson, 2010). The death of a spouse is one of the most emotionally stressful and disruptive events in life (Cramer et al., 1990; Daggett, 2002; Leahy, 1993). Camelley and associates (2006) studied the long-term effects of widowhood. They found that the widows continued to talk, think, and feel emotions about their lost spouses decades later. Twenty years post loss, they would still reminisce about their spouse every week or two and had a conversation about their spouse once a month on average. Twelve and a half years post loss, they reported still feeling upset between "sometimes" and "rarely" when thinking about their dead spouse.

Based on this research, does it surprise you when, at the end of a year, the surviving spouse is not "over it"? Losing a mate is, in a way, as if part of yourself has died. You are now alone when you need your significant other the most, and you are stricken to think that what you have built over your entire life is now pretty meaningless (Van Praagh, 2000, p. 96). As James Van Praagh states, "On the day my mother died my father was not the man I had known all my life" (p. 97). That simple statement is as well put as we can find and pretty much encapsulates what is going to take place as the widowed spouse attempts to put life back together. Van Praagh's statement makes two points. First is clearly what will happen with dad and how he will come to grips with his loss. The other component is not only how the family will handle their grief over the loss of their mom but also how they will handle their dad. This issue becomes even more critical if their dad is now responsible for raising young children alone (Glazer et al., 2010).

There are more women survivors (widows) than men (widowers), and the bereaved spouse typically faces a number of problems and stages of bereavement alone (Kübler-Ross, 1969; Kübler-Ross & Kessler, 2005). In addition to the immediate shock and stress, many survivors face serious personal, physical, emotional, economic, social, career, family, and community problems (Buckley et al., 2010; Johnson, 1977; Khosravan et al., 2010; Osterweis et al., 1984, pp. 71–75; Pizzetti & Manfredini, 2008; Rando, 1984, pp. 144–149; Vahtera et al., 2006). More ominously for older adults, the death of a spouse increases the mortality rate for the surviving spouse (Elwert & Christakis, 2008; Hart et al., 2007).

It appears that other variables intrude into mortality rates of surviving spouses as well. Elwert and Christakis (2006) found that race played a significant role in mortality rates of surviving spouses, with White spouses suffering a large and enduring effect of mortality, while Black people did not suffer a detectable effect. Religion may also affect how long people live after a spouse dies. Abei and Kruger (2009) found that Catholic men lived 2.2 years longer than Jewish men after a wife died, and Catholic women lived 1.5 years longer after their husbands died than Jewish women.

So should you be calmed if you are a Black Catholic and anxious if you are Jewish? Not necessarily, but you should understand as a crisis worker that a multitude of variables go into survivorship and realize that some common mundane demographics go into

what you need to be observant of when dealing with grief and bereavement. Further, while some may argue that bereavement and grief should not be classified as mental illness, an abundance of research indicates that there is a Pandora's box of evil hornets that can sting some survivors in multiple ways, and if some of those survivors do not have good immune systems, it can hasten their deaths. Therefore, it would appear important that crisis workers and medical health care workers in particular be aware of the part bereavement and grief play in physical health issues.

Loss Due to Caregiving

The stress of caregiving has become so widely recognized as a potential mental illness that it has been classified in the International Classification of Diseases, *Tenth Revision, Clinical Modification (ICD-10-CM)* (2023) under *"Other specific problems related to primary family support group."* It is also suspected as the underlying cause for physical ailments in caretakers as well (Amankwaa, 2017).

Caregiving is a major issue for spouses and parents. Long-term care causes radical changes not only in attitudes toward the receiver but in the provider as well. You might stereotypically think in terms of someone in this category as providing heroic years-on-end efforts in caring for a bedridden individual with some terminal disease or chronic disability. Think also about the parents of a 28-year-old son with schizophrenia who has delusions of persecution to the extent that he is on a first name basis with the local CIT, goes off his medication, and becomes dangerous to the extent that his parents sleep in watches and have a heavy-duty reinforced deadbolt on their steel bedroom door. In other words, there are many brands of caretakers, there are a lot of them, and there are going to be even more as the baby boomer generation ages and continuing advances in medical science prolong more lives, saving those who otherwise might have died but are cognitively and physically disabled.

Grief and bereavement over lost relationships are compounded by frustration over any ambiguity of the loss. The receiver of care is alive but not there for the caregiver either mentally, physically, or both, so former behavioral duties (e.g., who takes care of the taxes, bills, car, kids' lunches), affective relationships (emotional support, sexual activity), and cognitive abilities (figuring out job moves, college decisions, buying a house) are no longer functional (Betz & Thorngren, 2006). Caregivers often report a sense of loss of their identity (Dickson et al., 2010)—for example, from former spouse and lover to caregiver and nurse—as they move farther and deeper into caretaker roles.

Bad things happen to good caretakers who take care of individuals with spinal cord injuries, internal head trauma, multiple sclerosis, end-stage cancer, renal disease, Alzheimer's disease, dementia, the cognitively and physically challenged, people with mental illness, and others who are so incapacitated by their maladies that they require constant care and or vigilance. Those who wound up having complicated grief reported that there were more intense end-of-life family conflicts and problems dealing with other family members who refused to accept the illness or manner of care (Kramer et al., 2010).

Caregivers reported a kaleidoscope of problems. They experience depression, sadness, anger, guilt, worry, isolation, resentment, financial difficulties, frustration, relational deprivation, loss of employability, worry about the future of the person they care for if they are older, and have their own physical health problems that are often exacerbated by the constant physical and psychological stress of caregiving (Adams, 2006; Morgan, 2009; Ott et al., 2007; Office on Women's Health, 2023; Taylor et al., 2008). The length of time in dying also has an effect on the surviving caregiver. Keene and Prokos (2008) found that, compared to spouses who were noncaregivers or short-term caregivers, long-term caregivers reported more relief and less depressive symptoms than their counterparts. As coldhearted as it may seem, relief from long-term care of the terminally ill seems to allow caregivers to cope with their loss better.

It is a safe bet that the caregiver population is going to grow in the United States as the baby boomer population ages into degenerative disease territory. Other countries provide supportive services at the national level; how well these programs are working is still an open question. In the United States, this population is underserved and depends on charitable organizations such as the National Alliance for the Mentally Ill, the Alzheimer's Association, and other malady-specific support groups. Most caregivers constantly live in subtranscrisis or transcrisis states due to the ever-present threat of medical or financial crises for the disabled person and their own continual stress in caring for them.

These caregivers and the people they care for often come to the attention of first responders such as CIT officers. Helping these individuals find support groups, get relief through time off/out programs, plan for future events, obtain psychological first aid or supportive psychotherapy, normalize negative feelings, find outside help, obtain financial, medical, and legal advice, acquire psychoeducation about caregiver issues, and develop meaningful narratives about their losses are all program components that crisis workers might well provide (Adams, 2006; Dillenburger & McKerr, 2009; Haley et al., 2008; Morgan, 2009; Office on Women's Health, 2023). *Envisioning Transitions* (Neimeyer & Vaughans, 2021) is a technique that can be helpful when making a final decision for caretakers to move individuals into extended care facilities and can forestall grappling with nonfinite losses. The National Eldercare Locator, a service of the U.S. Administration on Aging, can help you find caregiving services in your area. You also can contact your local area Agency on Aging.

Death by Euthanasia

Since the turn of the century and more so within the past decade, euthanasia and physician-assisted suicide are becoming more prevalent and legal (Andriessen et al., 2020). Several countries, including the Netherlands, Belgium, Canada, Luxembourg, and Colombia, allow euthanasia or physician-assisted suicide (Dyer et al., 2015). In 2015, Quebec was the first Canadian province to legalize a form of euthanasia termed *medical assistance in dying* (MAiD), and it was legalized across the country in 2016 (McKinnon et al., 2021). In the United States, the "good death," as it is sometimes referred to, is allowed in at least eight states, including California, Colorado, the District of Columbia, Hawaii, Montana, Oregon, Vermont, and Washington (Andriessen et al., 2020). Andriessen et al. (2020) found losing a loved one in this manner comes with a host of issues, some of which are positive, while others have more a negative valance. The positive issues include being able to finish business with the loved one, having honored the loved one's last wishes, and having set the time and place for death. Ethical and moral issues top the list for more negative issues. Loved ones may feel guilt and responsibility for allowing the death to occur. Issues with authorities can also complicate bereavement when death occurs in this way. Finally, loved ones may have to respond to questions from the community and friends that can muddle the grieving process. The consequence is that loved ones may be cautious about sharing the cause of death with anyone outside a very small circle of people.

A major ethical dilemma can occur for crisis workers who adhere to their professional organization's ethical standards, particularly in states, provinces, and countries where euthanasia is legal. In Canada, counseling someone to choose death by suicide or aiding a suicide without medical assistance are criminal offenses that carry prison sentences. The same is generally true in the United States.

However, providing information on MAiD is entirely legal for Canadian human service workers. Simply said, that is not a simple solution. In legal terms, a rational assisted suicide precludes having severe emotional distress. If a therapist is approached by a client who proposes euthanasia as a solution to chronic depression, the reporting law of imminent harm supersedes simple referral or agreement of MAiD as a viable solution (McKinnon et al., 2021).

Therein lies the typical conundrum faced by crisis interventionists. Does the autonomy of the client override nonmaleficence where euthanasia is legal and the therapist acts as a sort of paradoxical gatekeeper? McKinnon and associates (2021, p. 58) put it really well when they state that therapists are tasked with creating options for clients, but when they are working with a death option, that removes all other options. From our own standpoint, being cast in the role of a decision maker in regard to another person's life, even if on a legally sanctioned treatment team, is fraught with peril. Whatever your own personal moral beliefs about the good or evil of euthanasia, it behooves you to be absolutely cognizant of your state, province, or country's law on the matter. The best advice we can offer is, when in doubt, refer back to our crisis ethics LASER protocol in Chapter 3, "The Intervention and Assessment Models," and pay particular attention to the **Legal** component.

Death of a Child

Regardless of the ages of the parents or children, the death of a child is always a major loss (Dias et al., 2021; Edelstein, 1984; Finkbeiner, 1998; Kübler-Ross, 1983; Rando, 1986; Romanoff, 1993; Silverman, 2000). The death of a child is perhaps the ultimate loss for a person to endure (Dias et al., 2021). Parents are left to deal with the incomprehensible fact that their child died before they did and often feel enormous guilt that they should have done something differently to have prevented it (Van Praagh, 2000, pp. 154–155). The death of a child is another type of loss that survivors don't "get over" quickly. In a review of the literature, Dias et al. (2021) found that parents who have lost a child develop psychological, cognitive, and social health outcomes that differ from the general population. Their research states that bereaved parents have lower levels of physical functioning, higher levels of anxiety, and more sleep disturbance than parents who have not experienced the loss of a child.

Every parent is unique in terms of needs, history, personality, coping style, relationships to others, social concerns, family situation, and sense of meaning regarding the death of a child (Braun & Berg, 1994; Finkbeiner, 1998; Romanoff, 1993). Therefore, every parent suffers the loss of a child somewhat differently. The death of a child is traumatic for parents, whether it occurs as a stillbirth or sudden infant death syndrome (SIDS) or follows accident or illness in adolescence or young adulthood (Osterweis et al., 1984, pp. 75–79). It is equally traumatic for aged parents to lose their children who may be middle aged or older.

Frei-Landau et al. (2020) report that for many people, attachment to God plays an important role in mediating the loss of a child. These researchers state that attachment to God evolves out of the early experiences in relationships that are internalized into mental representations that later guide individuals' information processing later in life. Individuals who experience secure relationships view God as comforting, making a strong attachment to God. Individuals with a strong attachment to God can find solace in making meaning of the loss.

Ann Finkbeiner (1998, pp. xxi, 37, 44, 54), after several years of grief and healing, shared her deep personal meanings regarding the loss of her only child, an 18-year-old son who was killed in a train accident. Her comments cut to the core of what it means to lose a child:

> I learned two things about the long-term effects of losing a child. One is that a child's death is disorienting. The human mind is wired to find patterns and attach meanings, to associate things that are alike, to generalize from one example to another, in short, to make sense of things. Your mind could no more consciously stop this than your heart could consciously stop beating. But children's deaths make no sense, have no precedents, are part of no pattern; their deaths are unnatural and wrong. So parents fight against their wiring, change their perspectives, and adjust to a reality that makes little sense.
>
> The other thing I learned is that letting go of a child is impossible. One of my earliest and most persistent reactions to T.C.'s death was surprise. I had no idea whatsoever how much he had meant to

me. All I knew was that I hadn't wanted to think about it. Our children are in our blood; the bond with them doesn't seem to break, and the parents find subtle and apparently unconscious ways of preserving that bond.

Bereavement in Childhood

Children who experience the death of a parent or sibling may show overt signs of bereavement, but sometimes, their grief may be covert, leading caregivers to assume that the children are not affected by the loss (Burns et al., 2020). However, Salinas (2021) has documented the fact that *young children do grieve*. While most children that experience the loss of a loved one go through mourning as a normal process and do not necessarily end up with pathological responses (Glazer, 2010), they may be at a higher risk of developing both mental health and behavioral health problems (Clow et al., 2023) that develop into complicated/prolonged grief (Cohen & Mannarino, 2011; Cohen et al., 2006, pp. 199–203; Cowan, 2010; Crenshaw & Lee, 2010; Howarth, 2011), Because the majority of the time that children and adolescents spend outside of the home is at school, it necessarily follows that strengthening school support systems that can deal with traumatic grief in childhood is important (Cohen & Mannarino, 2011; Heath & Hudnall, 2011; go to Chapter 13, "Crises in Schools"), particularly in supporting caregivers who may be having their own difficulties resolving grief issues.

Studies by Gudas (1990) suggest that signs and symptoms of behavioral and psychological difficulty occur differently between bereaved preschool and school-age children. Older children, with concepts of the permanence of death and personalization of their own mortality, experience more anxiety, depression, and somatic symptoms than younger children. Depending on the age and cognitive development of the child, their understanding of death may be very different and unsettling. From a Piagetian standpoint, the preoperational child's egocentric view of death may be laced with magical thinking and fantasy with no clear view about death's finality (Brown, 1988, pp. 70–74). Children at the concrete operational stage may understand the "why" of death as a specific cause-and-effect event, while children at the formal operational stage can understand the finality and irreversibility of death and have all kinds of questions concerning the "whys" (Brown, 1988, pp. 7–81; Matter & Matter, 1982).

Toddlers. Toddlers ages 18 months to 3 years do not understand how death differs from going away. Because they live in an egocentric world, they may well assume that they caused the death to occur. While death does not have meaning as such for them, they do understand when something is lost, and that loss may be very distressing. They may exhibit high levels of anxiety, seen in agitated/restless behavior, excessive crying, thumb sucking, biting, and tantrums. While it is unlikely they will retain a strong memory of the traumatic event of the person's passing, they may have some physical memoirs (Giunta & Giunta, 2002, p. 244).

Preschoolers. Children ages 3 to 5 also experience profound reactions to loss and may display feelings of sadness, anger, crying spells, feelings of remorse and guilt, somatization, and separation anxiety (Gudas, 1990). At about age 4, children have a limited and unclear understanding of death. Because they are still ego centered, they may believe they caused the death. They are not yet able, for the most part, to understand the permanency of death (Webb, 2007). While they are much clearer about who died and the sense of loss in their lives, they are usually quite literal about their interpretation of what it means to go to heaven, perhaps wondering "Does Bobbie get to have pizza and birthday cake and other little angels over to his house on his birthday?" Because of their egocentric stage of development, they also may feel that they caused the death (Webb, 2011), for example: "Bobby gets everything, mommy and daddy love him most, and I wish he was dead."

At this age, children will start to play the event out, often to the dismay of parents who, horrified and distressed from their own grief, forbid children to do so. There is likely to be severe separation anxiety from caretakers, including excessive clinging and crying on separation, needing to be held, and not wanting to sleep alone. Children this age may see a change in daily routine as a threat and feel angry and rejected for no apparent reason. They may become mute and withdrawn, with extended periods of sadness. There may be noticeable regression in physical independence, such as the inability to dress themselves, tie shoes, go to the bathroom, or eat with utensils. Bed-wetting and night terrors may occur (Giunta & Giunta, 2002, p. 245). Because their vocabulary is still very limited, when preschoolers hear words such as "passed," "lost," "gone over," and other euphemisms for death, these words will be taken quite literally (Webb, 2011), so if dad is "lost," it is the family's or police's duty to go find him.

Primary School Age. At about age 6 or 7, most children understand the universality and irreversibility of death. Death is now more specific, precise, and factual. Elementary school-age children generally operate in the concrete stage of development. As such, they may report matter-of-factly the gory details of a pet getting run over and thus be seen by adults as cold and uncaring (Gudas, 1990.) Conversely, because of their sensitivity to pain, they may become quite agitated if they hear the gory details about how mutilated the body was and will attempt to avoid such conversations (Webb, 2011). They may also be able to run a balance sheet and see that while their sister's death is a sad thing, their parents will now be able to spend more time and money on them.

Play is used extensively to attempt to work through the trauma. If play becomes both extensive and intensive and is focused on the trauma, it has now moved into traumatic childhood grief (Terr, 1981; found in Chapter 7, "Posttraumatic Stress Disorder"). At this point, there will be difficulty concentrating in school, with commensurate behavior and/or academic problems. Numerous somatic complaints may arise (headaches, stomachaches, dizziness, unspecified malaise with numerous school absences). Primary school-age children may have increased difficulty controlling their own behavior and may exhibit radical changes from quiet and shy to verbally aggressive and acting out or vice versa (Cohen & Mannarino, 2011; Giunta & Giunta, 2002, p. 245).

Intermediate/Middle School Age. While children at this age will generally understand the permanence of death, they may exhibit a good deal of anger and rage at the unfairness of it. They may develop a sense of foreboding and doom about a foreshortened future and see their existence as now pretty meaningless. They may alternately feel euphoria and excitement at having survived, then feel guilty for having survived when others didn't. Such mood swings may occur often and dramatically as they attempt to cope with emotional dysregulation. They may become highly judgmental about their own and others' behavior, particularly in regard to the deceased or the handling of events surrounding the trauma (Cohen & Mannirino, 2011; Giunta & Giunta, 2002, p. 246; Webb, 2011).

However, to suppose that a child's concept of death progresses in an orderly chronological manner is to suppose wrongly. Life experiences have much to do with a child's perspective and understanding of

what death is (Silverman, 2000, pp. 47–53). One can only imagine the difference in perspective and view of death between the average 6-year-old in Baghdad, Iraq, and an average 6-year-old in Des Moines, Iowa.

Intervention and Treatment

LO8   **Intervention and Treatment.** Children's affective, behavioral, and cognitive responses must be approached not in terms of adult perspectives but in terms of each child's understanding and developmental stage (Rando, 1984, pp. 157–162). Children are especially vulnerable during periods of major loss because their inexperience and their undeveloped personalities can easily lead to confusion and a misinterpretation of events and a lack of grieving (Schoenberg, 1980, p. 200). Because children's personalities are growing and absorbing social stimuli at a very rapid and concentrated rate, care must be taken to provide reassurance and support during family bereavement (Schonfeld, 1989). They may ask the same questions over and over about the loss, not so much for the factual information but for reassurance that the adult view is consistent, that the story has not changed, and that the grieving adults and children are safe. Children need to hear, over and over again, the simple, truthful, reassuring words of adults who are relatively secure and who show genuine concern for the children's feelings (Osterweis et al., 1984, p. 100).

Some people believe that children should be shielded and protected from exposure to death and loss. Sugar-coating death, such as daddy having gone away, should not happen. While death is indeed a dirty word for some people in contemporary society, it is one that needs to be used to honestly convey what has happened. The research suggests very strongly that bereaved children will make healthier adjustments to loss if they are informed about the loss truthfully and permitted to participate actively in mourning (Osterweis et al., 1984, pp. 99–127; Rando, 1984, p. 155; Schoenberg, 1980, pp. 151–154). Even though children may exhibit behavioral responses during the bereavement process that adults may interpret as "not caring" or "not understanding," children should be permitted to proceed with mourning at a level and pace appropriate to their development. Children should not be forced to participate in activities when they decline to do so but should be included when they request to do so.

Cohen and Mannarino (2011) indicate that treatment models should include five tasks that incorporate *gradual* exposure to the loss and the traumatic grief:

1. Resilience-building stress management skills help children re-regulate feelings, behaviors, and thoughts related to the traumatic death. Techniques include the use of positive reinforcement, encouragement, and selective attention for positive behaviors by both parents and teachers and teaching relaxation skills such as focused breathing and muscle relaxation to stop and reverse physical manifestations of stress.

2. Affective expression skills development helps children and parents accurately label and express different feelings without passing judgment on negative feeling states. Children should be encouraged to share feelings rather than deny them. At times, both parents and children may be terrified at the variety and intensity of their feelings, so it is important to teach both parents and children affective modulation skills, so they feel confident of not only speaking to their feelings but also controlling them.

3. Cognitive coping skills aid both children and parents in hooking up connections among thoughts, feelings, and behaviors. Children and parents learn how to assess how their thinking is adaptive or maladaptive and to change maladaptive thinking through thought stopping, reframing, and cognitive restructuring techniques.

4. Trauma-specific interventions focus on building a trauma narrative, which is usually started after resiliency skills have been developed in children and parents. This narrative may take several forms, including stories, poems, artwork, and play. The purpose of the narrative is to decrease avoidance behavior, directly confront the feared trauma, make sense of it, and put it in the past. Concomitant with exposure to the feared trauma, safety issues may be dealt with if the traumatic event involved violence in which the child was involved or an observer.

5. Grief-focused interviews help children and parents develop more adaptive grieving processes and include many of the conflicting and ambivalent emotions they may have about the deceased. For children dealing with these issues, play therapy is an ideal, non-threatening vehicle to reconcile loss.

Play therapy can have positive outcomes for grieving children (Salinas, 2021) and has universal cultural adaptability (Gonzalez & Bell, 2016; Hudspeth, 2016).

Webb (2007) recommends directed play therapy as a vital adjunct to cognitive restructuring (Cohen et al., 2006) of the traumatic event in tackling the issue of avoidance. Webb lists the following reasons for doing so:

1. Play therapy provides cathartic relief from tensions and anxiety.

2. It provides ways for the child to symbolically review in play what happened and build an armor plate against the feared feelings of the traumatic event in concrete form through manipulating the play media. Through manipulation of the play material, the child and therapist can safely rehearse plans, problem solve, and gain resolution.

3. It permits role rehearsal to strengthen the child's feelings of competence in handling the future.

4. It can provide a restorative function and transformative experience that moves the child from despair, hopelessness, and lack of self-confidence to reconciliation, hope, and self-confidence (p. 48).

It is also critically important to carry out intervention in a team approach that integrates home and school (Cohen & Marinnarino, 2011). Teachers, school counselors, psychologists, and social workers can all serve as supportive personnel that aid and abet therapeutic endeavors by knowing what is occurring at home and in therapy and by providing backup or, indeed, serving as the primary therapeutic agent.

Bereavement in Adolescence

According to the Childhood Bereavement Estimation Model, by the end of high school, nearly 7 percent of today's students will have lost a parent or sibling (Burns et al., 2020), although the U.S. Census Bureau's (2023) estimation of parental loss by age 17, taking into account the COVID-19 pandemic, was at 4.7 percent. Twenty percent had lost a close friend, and 90 percent said they had lost a significant loved one (Vitas Healthcare, 2023). Besides short-term effects from the loss of a parent, there are long-term effects from childhood bereavement that range from employment issues, lower educational attainment, and more depression (Parsons, 2011).

Adolescents today are encountering death and loss more frequently than ever before, and this presents a challenge to both adolescents and their caregivers. The challenge is to prevent maladaptive grief processes that lead to substance abuse, school problems, aggressive behaviors, and other behavioral disturbances (Hill et al., 2019; Oosterhoff et al., 2018).

Other crises, such as destabilized families and parents' job loss, create in adolescents the feelings of pessimism, futurelessness, confusion, depression, and isolation (Schliebner & Peregoy, 1994). A peer death can be a particularly traumatic experience for an adolescent because it is a nonnormative experience that shouldn't happen, often is violent, and may be seen as preventable. Peer deaths can foster school problems, depression, substance abuse, suicidal ideation, and delayed developmental processes (Balk & Corr, 2001; Balk et al., 2011; Malone, 2011).

Value of Connectedness. Hansen and Frantz (1984, pp. 36–47, 62–72) describe adolescents who are in bereavement as needing to be included (involved) in the family's grief, while at the same time needing periods of privacy. Often, the adolescent may feel excluded, for example, at the sudden death of a grandparent. Bereaved adult family members may erroneously assume that the adolescent's perceptions of events are the same as theirs. At such times, adolescents may not know how to behave because they do not have a sufficient understanding of death, the circumstances surrounding it, the appropriate mourning role, or life experience in general (Brown, 1988, pp. 77–79).

Adolescents may feel a deep sense of pain, fear, anger, guilt, helplessness, confusion, loneliness, and grief (Balk, 2009), yet they may not know how to express or feel comfortable in expressing these emotions. They need opportunities to be included in discussions, planning, mourning, and funeral and commemorative activities (Hansen & Frantz, 1984, pp. 62–67). Guerriero-Austrom and Fleming (1990), researching the effects of sibling bereavement on adolescents, found that physical and emotional symptoms fluctuate over time, showing the most severity at 6 to 12 months following the sibling death and emerging again at 18 to 24 months. Women exhibited more death anxiety and health-related problems than did men. Adolescent grief reactions were documented as long as 3 years following the death of the sibling (p. 11). The problem with these reactions is that death brings a stark reality to already cynical teenagers who may act out their anger and depression in dangerous, life-threatening ways (Brown, 1988, pp. 79–81).

Intervention and Treatment. One of the key components in promoting resiliency to a parent's death has been positive parenting (Sandler et al., 2003; Worden, 1996). While adolescents reported themselves as fearful and anxious over a parent's death (Worden, 1996), they also reported themselves as more mature when assuming parental responsibilities and as growing up faster. Effective parenting cannot be done in hindsight, but interventions that include parents individually or in treatment groups can be effective in supporting both adolescents and surviving parents in moving forward.

While less is known about the effect of good parenting practices on adolescents when a peer dies, parents need to understand and acknowledge the importance of that loss and avoid discounting the loss and turning it into disenfranchised grief. Oftentimes the traumatic death of peers comes from making typically silly teenage decisions: the daredevil stunt that goes horribly awry and results in a broken neck and quadriplegia; alcohol, fast driving, and a victory celebration over an archrival that ends in vehicular homicide and injury to friends; any of a variety of videotaped we'll-put-it-on-YouTube stunts that go wrong, causing injury, death, and lawsuits; or the aftermath of the accident leading to the instigator's depression and suicide. These classic examples of immature adolescent behavior resulting in accidental deaths are vilified by parents, and anger is projected out onto their "stupid" friends and to their children's " senseless" behaviors and "bad" relationships.

When parents dismiss or criticize adolescent peer friendships, first loves, and high school bonds as transitory and insubstantial, they are essentially telling adolescents their friendships don't mean much and their feelings don't count for much either (Balk et al., 2011). Nothing could be further from the truth, and wise parents will react sensitively to their adolescents' grieving over lost friends and relationships.

Finally, school is a major source of support for adolescents (Balk et al., 2011). Chapter 13, "Crises in Schools," provides a good deal of information on the part that schools play in helping adolescents move through the loss of a peer.

Bereavement in Older People

The fact is that older adults may experience considerable difficulties with bereavement (Hansson & Stroebe, 2007; Hinrichsen & Clougherty, 2006). O'Connor and associates (2015) found that when bereavement complications turn into prolonged grief, it may develop into potentiated posttraumatic stress. As medical advances extend life and retirement becomes prolonged, commensurate issues arise involving finances, health, cognitive difficulties, and social support systems that often include the loss of independence. Independence is a precious commodity, and older adults do not lose their desire for it (Langer, 2011), as most children become aware when they deal with aging parents who become obstinate and rebellious over suggestions about quitting driving or going to a retirement center. For older adults, losses of friends are a continual degradation of their support system, and, as these losses pile up, when ultimate loss—the death of a spouse—arrives, the potential for loss to cascade into prolonged grief and bereavement increases exponentially. Indeed, the most profound and devastating loss older people may encounter is the loss of a spouse (Schoenberg, 1980, pp. 211–214). Demographic data indicate that older people, ages 65 and older, are growing at an increasing rate. It is predicted that by 2030 there will be about 70 million older adults, more than double the number now, and that number will represent 20 percent of the U.S. population (Schwiebert et al., 2000, p. 123), so it is clear that this potential problem is going to grow . . . a lot!

From a developmental standpoint, bereavement among older people is compounded by decreases in sensory acuity, a general decline in health, and reduced mobility. Having a lower income and fewer support people available to them than in their younger years also represent changes that are detrimental to their psychological well-being. Older people generally experience more losses than do their younger counterparts: lost independence, social connectedness, financial security, and access to basic necessities and supports (Ishikawa, 2020). Older people might also be experiencing fears about mortality, loneliness, and untreated chronic pain, adding to their grief (Ishikawa, 2020). It appears that advancing age tends to correlate with a decrease in coping strategies, but the relationships of this decrease to greater awareness of impending death, a decrease in physical stamina and function, or other factors is not known (Schoenberg, 1980, pp. 221–223).

Schoenberg (1980, p. 230) summarizes four conclusions that may be drawn from the literature on bereavement and age:

1. Older people present more somatic problems than psychological problems.
2. There is no indication that the intensity of grief varies significantly with the age of the older person.

3. Evidence suggests that grief among older people may be more prolonged than among younger people.
4. Older people tend to be lonelier and have far longer periods of loneliness than their younger counterparts.

Crase (1994) found that the ways the older generation generally deals with loss fall into the following three broad categories:

1. One group totally ignores the inevitability of death and makes no preparation for it. People—especially men—in this category engage in little or no open discussion of death. By ignoring death issues, these elderly individuals attempt to avoid negative feelings, using denial as a defense mechanism. They are vulnerable to being unprepared when struck by disabling disease, crisis, disaster, or the death of their spouse.
2. A second group thinks about death and dying excessively and makes unusual preparations for death's inevitability. These individuals go overboard in making meticulous plans for every detail of their decline, death, and funeral.
3. A third group demonstrates a healthier balance. They are attuned to the developmental implications of total loss, make appropriate plans and decisions, and go on with their normal lives.

The realization of disease, suffering, and eventual loss of life should foster the motivation to look ahead to our death with intelligent preparation, just as we would prepare for any of life's major stages or events (Kaplan & Gallagher-Thompson, 1995). When we don't do this, it is an open invitation for the crisis worker to enter the picture.

COVID Isolation

The COVID-19 pandemic resulted in millions of deaths. The total loss of life caused by this virus will probably never be known. However, another type of loss also took place for many people during the pandemic. This loss involved the experience of isolation and the lack of contact with other people (Khoury, 2022). The realities of isolation many people experienced resulted in loneliness, anxiety, depression, relationship conflict, abuse, increased reliance on alcohol or other substances, sleep disorders, job loss, and myriad other challenges that are taking their toll (Pfefferbaum & North, 2020). These outcomes echo the experience of individuals who grieve and are in the midst of bereavement. The loss of contact for individuals with a chronic illness or other debilitating physical condition was a major loss (Koon, 2022; Robinson-Whelen et al., 2023; Sorscher, 2022). Outside a very few trusted individuals, or even not so trusted, people in this population were particularly affected, feeling a great loss of contact with the outside world.

Job Loss

While it may vary in different cultures, many people are pretty much defined by their jobs. If you don't believe that, consider the first question you might ask a stranger at a party after you find out the person's name. We would wager many times that it's something on the order of "What do you do for a living?" Jobs and one's identity with a job have far more than work and wage ramifications. Besides the fact that jobs determine how much money we will make and what our earning potential may be, jobs structure our day and delineate a regular and required set of activities as we prepare for, go to, and finish our day's work. Our jobs account for our status and identity, our sense of participation and purpose, and the social interaction and network that work brings (Jahoda et al., 1933/1971). While losing one's job under any circumstances can certainly be a crisis, losing one's job for no reason, or one that has nothing to do with job performance, is particularly devastating and a crisis. For those it happens to, what they experience looks and feels very much like grief (Vickers, 2009).

Technological progress and a free-market economy have changed the American workplace dramatically. A major ramification of that change has been the loss of millions of well-paying white- and blue-collar jobs that provided a wage earner with income, job security, and the hallowed, and much aspired to, middle-class existence (Lerner, 2000). In the new economic millennium, the possibility of economic restructuring and job loss is ever present, no matter how diligent and faithful employees are (Newman, 1993).

The ripple effects stretch out to the families of those employees and result in a variety of pathological reactions as the primary breadwinners come to realize that they are now downwardly mobile, with little chance of regaining their former job status. Alcoholism, drug use, battering, child abuse, divorce, suicide, and murder are but a few of the family handmaidens of job loss. On a personal basis, depression, anger, blame, projection, loss of self-esteem, loss of personal identity, lower self-concept, loss of social support systems, stigmatization, loss of control, disintegration of ego integrity, and overall negative mental health are emotional outcomes for someone who may now also suffer secondary victimization not unlike rape or other assault victims (Price et al., 1998).

Secondary victimization may occur at the hands of others who rationalize that people are somehow incompetent, lazy, or otherwise unequal to the job. To acknowledge otherwise would put themselves in peril and say very clearly that they had no control over their own destinies any more than the coworker who was let go (Reichle et al., 1998). Further compounding the problem, the victims often reacts in the same way as the victimizers, casting about in a futile attempt to make sense out of what has happened (Lerner, 2000). When whole industries shut down, outsource, or downsize, entire towns are put at risk, and we now have a systemic crisis.

The negative effects of unemployment on both physiological and psychological well-being are well documented, while job loss as it pertains to grief is relatively new and unknown. Much like those bereaved who suffer traumatic loss due to death, the assumptive world of the newly unemployed is shattered, their view of a just world is challenged, and views of themselves as valuable and worthy are invalidated (Harris & Isenor, 2011). Brewington and associates (2004) studied factors hypothesized to relate to job loss grief. Grief scores correlated positively with time since the job loss and number of dependents. A negative correlation was reported with length of notice of termination. Income loss and lack of perceived reemployment prospects related positively to grief subscales. Donahue (2010) compared a job loss group to a bereaved group. The job loss group demonstrated similar levels of hopelessness, tension, stress, confusion, and physical symptoms and had higher degrees of irritation, guilt, withdrawal from social responsibility, oversensitivity, and brooding than the bereaved group.

Therefore, to say that career counseling is a dull and humdrum job when dealing with job loss is to have one's head stuck in the sand. Vocational outplacement counselors often have to dance between helping individuals look for work and engaging in crisis support therapy for grief, anxiety, depression, and stress (Harris & Isenor, 2011). The ramifications of job loss can be far-reaching and devastating. As we saw in Chapter 8, "Crisis of Lethality," in the example of the outplacement job counseling that turns into a suicide intervention, the potential for crisis when job loss occurs is ever present and often blindsides the unwary human services worker.

Another issue that is often overlooked is how grief is handled in the workplace. Sooner or later, people who lose significant others need to go back to work. Generally, it is sooner; there is nothing comparable to a pregnancy leave of absence for grief-stricken workers. Grieving workers can make poor business decisions, miss business opportunities, have accidents, and cause financial losses (Hazen, 2009). For all these reasons, it is in the best interests of management to pay attention to the human reality of death and bereavement in the workplace (Charles-Edwards, 2009). With increased knowledge about the negative effects of prolonged grief, it should be apparent that businesses need to consider additional support beyond the obligatory floral arrangement for the deceased in making provisions for valued employees who have suffered the loss of a loved one.

Separation and Divorce

In the past few years, the number of people getting married has decreased, and the divorce rate has stayed at a relatively stable rate of around 50 percent (National Center for Health Statistics, 2023). It is devastating to adults and children alike when the relationship dies, but the person is still living (Harris, 2011). It doesn't take an expert in marriage and family counseling or a grief specialist to understand the heartache, sense of loss, and all of the accompanying bad emotions that go with a divorce. The crisis of separation and divorce followed by acrimonious custody fights often places children in untenable positions, causing them to feel confused, insecure, fearful, trapped, angry, unloved, and guilty (Karkazis & Lazaneo, 2000). Bruce and Kim (1992) found that major depression is prevalent among all individuals experiencing marital disruption. According to Johnson (1977), the most common experience that marriage partners have regarding separation is intense and disturbing fear and emotional turmoil.

Almost all separations produce negative feelings and outcomes that were not anticipated by either party. Even when the separation is desired and sought, it precipitates a sense of frustration, failure, loss, and mourning. Schneider (1984) states that people suffering from loss due to divorce or widowhood "show significant and consistently higher vulnerability to almost every major physical and mental disorder, particularly to heart disease" (p. 19). Colgrove and associates (1991) advise that surviving and healing following such loss begin by recognizing and facing the loss immediately and doing the mourning now (pp. 1–2).

Death of a Pet

It is estimated that in the United States, there are 57 million dogs and 62 million cats kept as pets (to say nothing of other pets such as horses, snakes, gerbils, and so on). As many as 63 percent of American households have pets. There are good reasons for pet cemeteries and the expense to which pet owners will go to keep a dying pet alive. The human–animal bond is now recognized as an integral part of pet owners' lives, and it is important for us to recognize and validate the grief that pet owners experience when their beloved companion animals die (Lagoni et al., 1994; Nieburg & Fischer, 1982; Planchon et al., 2002). Weisman (1990–1991) and Reitmeyer (2000) compared bereavement following the death of a companion animal to the experience of the loss of another human. Indeed, the dynamics of the loss of a pet are strikingly similar to the loss of a human (Humane Society, 2023).

Smith (2009) speaks of individuals who have suffered the loss of a pet as manifesting profound grief and depression. Smith notes, somewhat tongue-in-cheek, that there is good reason for such severe reactions. Unlike humans, dogs are absolutely loyal; they keep our secrets, they don't complain, they clearly communicate their needs, and they are pretty patient unless they have to relieve themselves and need to go out or haven't been fed all day.

When pets die or suffer terminal illnesses and have to be "put to sleep," the owners may suffer grief, guilt, and other emotional reactions similar to those experienced at the death of human family members. Hsu (2010) found that the pet owners she examined could be partitioned into high- and low-grief groups. High-grief groups were distressed by dreams of their pets, were distressed by fond memories, kept their pets' belongings, erected shrines and memorials, and felt more social constraints, feelings of alienation, and lack of support for their grief. Low-grief participants, on the other hand, were comforted by dreams of their pets, gave their pets' belongings away, and were comforted by fond memories of their pets. These feelings and responses may be especially acute in the elderly, whose main object of affection is a pet (Brooks & Martinez, 1999), or those who live alone (McCutcheon & Fleming, 2001–2002).

The death of a pet may provide a naturally occurring opportunity for adults in the family to introduce children to the concept and experience of death and dying (Koocher, 1975; Nieburg & Fischer, 1982; Schoenberg, 1980, pp. 203–204). Recently, pet loss counseling has become widespread in the United

States. The Delta Society (2023) publishes a national directory of pet loss counselors at integvrativevetina-raryhealthcenter.com. These counselors are a legitimate and growing occupation and are now affiliated with schools of veterinary medicine, local humane societies, and private practitioners (Reitmeyer, 2000).

Prolonged Grief Disorder, Bereavement, and Mourning Reaction

LO9 When a person is unable to mourn a loss and move on in a context of renewal and growth, the possibility of delayed or chronic grief arises (Middleton et al., 1998; Raphael & Minkov, 1999). Although the purpose of crisis intervention is not necessarily to diagnose, having information on diagnostic criteria is important. As we stated at the beginning of the chapter, many times, unresolved grief lurks around and is the catalyst for other crises. It is a serious mental diagnosis and not something people "just need to get over." It appears to occur in about 10 percent of bereaved persons. It is not only psychologically debilitating but can cause serious medical problems, substance misuse, suicidality, and diminished quality of life as well (Khosravi & Kasaelyan, 2023).

The DSM 5-TR (2022) added Prolonged Grief Response as an official diagnosis in the Trauma and Stress Related Disorder section. The first criterion for a diagnosis of Prolonged Grief Disorder is that the loss must have occurred at least 12 months ago and for children, at least 6 months ago. A second criterion involves the development of a persistent grief response that is shown by an intense yearning for the person who died, a preoccupation with memories and thoughts of the person, or both. The third criterion includes at least three of the following symptoms: (1) feeling that part of the self has died since the death of the loved one, (2) disbelief about the death, (3) avoidance of reminders about the person who died, (4) intense emotional pain related to the death, (5) difficulty resuming typical day-to-day functioning, (6) emotional numbness stemming from the death, (7) loss of meaning for life, and (8) intense loneliness resulting from the death. In addition, to be diagnosed with Prolonged Grief Disorder, individuals must experience a significant reduction in day-to-day functioning in social and occupational life. These are the precursors to prolonged grief and subsequent bereavement and mourning.

The incidence of Prolonged Grief Disorder is difficult to determine since the diagnosis only became official in 2022. However, Kersting and colleagues (2011) found that the incidence of prolonged grief in a representative sample (N = 2,520) was about 3.7 percent in the general population, and the potential for developing it after major bereavement was 6.7 percent. High-risk predictors for developing it were being a woman, low income, older age, having lost a child or spouse, or cancer as the cause of death, although there appear to be limitations to these particular subsets due to small sample sizes.

Some people don't begin to have prolonged grief symptoms until 6 months after the loss. Others experience acute symptoms immediately that continue for a year or more. They also tend to experience co-occurring disorders such as major depression, posttraumatic stress disorder, and generalized anxiety, although researchers contend that prolonged grief is distinguishable from those disorders (Boelen et al., 2010; Neiburg et al., 1997; Prigerson & Jacobs, 2001). People in both time frames do have a higher risk for a major depressive disorder, PTSD, or generalized anxiety disorder than those whose grief runs a more conventional course or who are treated (Kersting & Kroker, 2010; Prigerson et al., 2008; Shear & Mulhare, 2008). More ominously, they have a higher incidence of suicidal ideation and risk of suicide (Shear & Mulhare, 2008). Indeed, people with complicated/prolonged grief appear to have an incidence rate of these disorders and behaviors that is equal to or higher than psychiatric outpatients with other known disorders, those bereaved by suicide, survivors of disaster events, caregivers of people with dementia, and older adults (Piper et al., 2011).

Traumatic Death/Traumatic Grief. When death occurs by traumatic means, such as a vehicle accident, murder, or natural or human-made disaster, the potential for complicated mourning increases exponentially (Figley, 1996; Lord, 1996; Rando, 1996; Redmon, 1996). The degree of trauma is increased by (1) the suddenness and lack of anticipation, (2) violence, mutilation, and destruction, (3) preventability and/or randomness, (4) multiple deaths, and (5) the mourner's own confrontation with death or witnessing of violence or mutilation (Rando, 1996, p. 143). Besides the type and degree of violence in the death, the relationship, both in regard to kinship and emotional connection, and the social support systems that are available are external variables that play a large role in how and whether traumatic grief will turn into complicated/prolonged grief (Hibberd et al., 2010).

Survivors who have not initiated or finished grieving for their lost ones are vulnerable to suffering from residual trauma, transcrisis, impaired functioning, or worse. It is not uncommon in traumatic deaths for the griever to be reexposed over and over to the traumatic death if the legal system becomes involved through either civil or criminal actions (Rynearson, 2010). The differentiating factor between traumatic grief and complicated/prolonged grief appears to be that complicated/prolonged grief is a function of one's degree of emotional relationship with the loss object, while in traumatic grief, the degree of distress has more to do with situational factors such as degree of violence, the extent of maiming of the body, and physical proximity to and witnessing of the death (Holland & Neimeyer, 2011). If the foregoing is now starting to remind you of PTSD stimuli, you are right! In fact, when a complicated/prolonged grief reaction occurs, they may be considered co-occurring disorders, and treatment for PTSD is generally recommended concurrent with bereavement counseling (Figley, 1996; Rando, 1996).

Clues for Identifying Complicated Grief Reaction. Rando (1996) and Worden (1991) have constructed clues for identifying complicated/prolonged grief reactions that may prove useful to crisis workers in cases in which survivors of loss are in serious denial. Examples might be a parent who has experienced the loss of a child and refuses to face the fact that the child is gone, keeping the child's room just as it was years after the death; a spouse or partner whose mate has either died or left for good, and the survivor carries on as if the partner has simply stepped out to the corner convenience store and will return shortly; or adult children angry over the death of a parent with whom they had unfinished business that cannot now be resolved and who project their rage onto everyone else. Rando's (1996, pp. 145–146) and Worden's (1991, pp. 75–77) list of clues may help crisis workers identify and offer help to people who manifest such severe denial or other debilitating reactions.

Crisis workers and other caregivers should take note of and attend to a client when:

1. The person cannot speak of the deceased without experiencing intense and fresh grief.
2. Some relatively minor event triggers an intense grief reaction.
3. The survivor cannot remove material possessions or belongings of the deceased.
4. Loss themes continually come up during interviews.

5. The griever manifests the same physical symptoms that the deceased had.
6. The individual exhibits radical changes in lifestyle following the death or excludes family, friends, activities, or visitation of places associated with the deceased.
7. The person experiences a long history of depression following loss, often marked by persistent guilt and lowered self-esteem.
8. There is a compulsion to imitate the dead person.
9. The person exhibits self-destructive impulses or suicidal ideation.
10. There is unaccountable sadness at certain times of the year.
11. The person has phobias about illness or death.
12. There is definite avoidance of death-related rituals or activities.
13. There is obsessive reconstruction of events surrounding the death.
14. The person focuses on what was happening in the relationship at the time of death (usually negative) to the exclusion of the complete span of the relationship (more positive).
15. Secondary losses, such as the loss of a house or savings due to a lack of planning, impetuous spending, or vulnerability to scams, occur and cause financial problems.
16. There are compulsive and obsessive attempts to fix blame and assign responsibility if the death was caused by humans.

Workers are reminded that relatively few grievers display all of the clues on the list. The value of this list lies in the fact that such grievers are encountered more often than one might think, and workers need to be prepared and not show surprise when faced with such behavior in grievers whom they counsel (Worden, 1991, pp. 65–78). Indeed, many times, clients who have complicated grief reactions have submerged the loss experience from conscious awareness or summarily dismissed it as "part of life." When you are faced with a client who is in crisis for no apparent legitimate reason, you should always assess for unresolved grief and loss issues. These issues may not necessarily have to do with unreconciled loss and sadness over a loved one; they may involve anger over unfinished business with the deceased, the departed lover, or the lost job. Under circumstances in which parting was anything but sweet sorrow, the aggrieved individual must be able to forgive and let go, which is not an easy task (De Moss, 2003).

Intervention Strategies

LO9 If we believe the current research that tells us the stage theories that have held sway for so long in the field of loss and grieving are not very workable, then we are faced with the business of tailor-making and custom fitting an intervention for every person who has a grieving problem. Further, when we dichotomize normal against complicated/prolonged grief, we are faced with another dilemma because they are essentially two different constructs. So how in the world do we go forward? Even though a huge volume of research has been done on the concepts underlying this chapter and on demographics such as age, race, and sex in describing grieving characteristics, the actual testing of interventions as to how effective they are is pretty sparse.

To complicate matters even further, it appears that what is presently being done in the field of grieving and bereavement isn't working very well. Meta-analyses of outcome studies have consistently shown that, in general, grief intervention outcomes don't measure up to outcomes for most other psychotherapy issues, although Neimeyer and Currier's last meta-analysis in 2009 held out some hope for better treatment outcomes, particularly with a constructivist model (Neimeyer et al., 2010). Essentially, most people with grieving problems don't get better as a result of intervention and, in fact, may get worse (Allumbaugh & Hoyt, 1999; Currier et al., 2007; Currier et al., 2008; Kato & Mann, 1999; Neimeyer, 2000; Rosner et al, 2010).

There is a caveat to these findings. While intervention with normal grief reactions is generally unproductive, individuals with complicated/prolonged grief may indeed derive some benefits equivalent to other areas of psychotherapeutic intervention. It also appears that when individuals self-select for intervention, they do much better than do those selected by the researchers (Currier et al., 2008; Rosner et al., 2010). That finding seems to resonate clearly with the entire area of loss; that is, you can't push grieving people into action until they are ready to do something about it.

What we do know about the business of counseling, though, is that more than anything else, the quality of the relationship between a client and a counselor is probably the best basis for determining how effective the counseling is going to be. From that standpoint, we believe that Altmaier's (2011) view of best practices in grief work that focuses on the relationship has a great deal to say about how effective workers can be in dealing with normal grief.

Being There for Grievers: A Worker Imperative

Particularly as the news of a death is received, "being there" is as important as anything the crisis worker does. Being there manifests the qualities of *empathic presence, gentle conversation, providing available space,* and *eliciting trust* (Altmaier, 2011).

Empathic presence involves listening, silence, and support through accepting and encouraging the expression of feelings, allowing pain to be expressed, and responding in a noncritical, nonjudgmental manner in allowing the grief-stricken to tell their story (Altmaier, 2011). Above all else in grief work, empathic listening to the bereaved and their families appears to be the single most useful skill or strategy available to crisis workers (Rando, 1984). Studies by Balk (1990) confirm the value of empathic listening. He found that bereaved college students identify "attentive listening and presence" as being the most helpful to grievers and "avoidance" as being the least helpful.

Avoid cliches, easy answers, and phrases meant to comfort survivors (Altmaier, 2011; Aten et al., 2015). "She's in a better place." "It was God's will." "The good die young." "He's at home now." "You're a strong person." "There's no more pain." "God loves those who suffer most." "Better days are ahead." All these pat phrases are discounting at best and demeaning at worst. They are cliches that people use who are absolutely confounded as to what to say to the griever. What they really mean is: "I haven't a clue as to how to help you assuage this grief and am really embarrassed to try, but I'll mumble this and maybe I'll feel better and can get out of this uncomfortable situation." Trying to smooth things over such as "It could be worse, It'll be OK" are discounts on the depths of feelings. It's up to the survivor to decide when things will be "OK."

Likewise, stay away from "Don't cry! "Don't worry!" Don't be blue!" "Don't feel bad." "Don't swear!" (Aten et al., 2015). Survivors have every reason to "do" all those things. "Don't" generally says more about the anxiety of the speaker than it does about the survivor.

Gentle Conversation. Gentle conversation allows for memory sharing, telling and retelling stories, and owning statements from the worker such as

"I am sorry. I don't have words to begin to touch the feelings you must have, but I am here, and I will stay here and listen if you care to talk." Use active and reflective listening skills (Aten et al., 2015). "I can really sense the caring and feeling you had for your grandfather as you talk about those Sunday afternoon rides down to the lake."

Providing available space has to do with what contemporary research and practice in the field of loss keep harping about—that is, helping the client find support, doing things clients can't do for themselves right now (e.g., pumping gas), but letting them tell us what they can and can't do so they have at least a modicum of control in their lives. Providing available space also has to do with time. Since each client's grieving process marches to its own drummer, patience is a huge virtue for the worker (Altmaier, 2011).

Eliciting trust is a keystone that communicates that clients have the ability to get through tough times, recover, and grow (Altmaier, 2011). It is not cheerleading, but it is gentle encouragement and trust that the client can engage the grief and not avoid it. "I'm in this for the duration as long as it takes. You want to cry, I'm here. You want to swear, I'm here. You want to sleep, I'm here. You want to talk, I'm here. I know you have strength, and I have strength, and we will get through this together." Hughes (1988) believes that grieving clients' expectations of the worker's abilities are crucial in facilitating the healing process. Hughes stated that the worker's expectations are always communicated directly or subtly to the client and that clients heal when they are "informed" by the worker that they are never helpless victims but instead are powerful and capable of healing themselves (p. 77).

We agree that by being there, the crisis worker is an empathic, nonjudgmental pillar of support who provides emotional understanding and allows the client to feel *felt* (Wylie, 2004, p. 33). As odd as that sounds, "feeling felt" ribbon-wraps the total package of "being there." As Schuurman and DeCristofaro (2007) state, "It is that simple, and that complex" (p. 174).

We also believe that a critical component that does much to lend the worker credibility is much like intervention in a disaster area; that is, one builds up sweat equity with clients by doing some very pedestrian and mundane activities. These may include calling relatives, helping make arrangements for organ donation, contacting funeral homes and flower shops, finding legal papers, contacting charitable organizations, and attending to other basic necessities that go with the death of a loved one. If no relatives or friends are present or capable of doing this, it is reasonable and proper for the workers to offer their services in that regard.

Fitting Technique to Style of Grief

The Dual Process Model. When workers operate with contemporary grief models, they are going to have to be nimble, fluid, and adaptable as clients oscillate back and forth between a loss orientation and a restoration orientation. In Stroebe and associates' (2005) dual process model, the griever sometimes confronts and sometimes avoids the stressors of both orientations (Humphrey, 2009, p. 49). In fact, one of the primary jobs of the worker is not only to tolerate but also to encourage such oscillation (Stroebe & Schut, 1999). Humphrey (2009, p. 51) lists the following recommendations for using the dual process model:

1. Identify and explore both loss and restoration stressors and the specific avoidance and confrontation responses the client uses.
2. Keep in mind that an initial period when the client is fixed in a loss orientation is normal. Identify evidence (or lack thereof) of oscillation as time moves forward.
3. Normalize and validate the dual process model by explaining how it works and why it applies to the client's particular situation.
4. Address problematic avoidance such as excessive alcohol/drug use, extreme denial, suppression of emotion, or acting out.
5. Do not push clients toward restoration. Let the oscillation work.

To Humphrey's recommendations we would add another, which we feel is critical to effective resolution of any situation where families or significant others are interwoven in the fabric of the grief. That recommendation is psychoeducation with family and other support systems as to how this model works. Otherwise, there may be some very frustrated and unhappy significant others who, on the surface, see little progress and indeed regression. In that regard, we feel it is highly important to include significant others in progress assessments and support meetings that reinforce them for "sticking in there."

The Adaptive Grieving Model. The same flexibility and ability to operate in a fluid manner is called for from the worker in Martin and Doka's (2000) adaptive model. In our experience, clients seldom remain fixed at one point on the model's intuitive–instrumental continuum. In our opinion, this model calls for a fairly high degree of ability and skill to operate in an eclectic manner across a wide array of therapeutic modalities to fit with the affective, behavioral, cognitive, and spiritual reactions of clients. Note the addition of *spiritual* to the usual triad of intervention strategies. While we don't necessarily believe you have to be able to quote directly from the Bible, Talmud, Koran, or any other spiritual source, we do believe you had better know something about this area and be able to work in it. To not know about spirituality and faith when working with loss, grief, and bereavement or, worse yet, discounting them, is akin to not knowing or discounting any of the affective–behavioral–cognitive triad modalities when involved in other therapeutic endeavors. Given the foregoing admonition, the following strategies from Martin and Doka (2000) can serve as starting points.

Affective Strategies. Affective strategies should initially allow for emotional catharsis through a range of what may be construed as negative emotions from crying to angry swearing. Because emotional dysregulation is seen as a major problem in problematic grieving, setting the stage for emotional exposure is important in regaining regulating abilities. Successive approximation to full emotional regulation through carefully graded, stepwise exposure to experiencing painful feelings is important. Likewise, carefully planning and choosing times, places, and people with whom to field-test affective interaction with others moves the grief from the counseling session into the real world. Assessment and revision of these field experiments is important in determining abilities, skills, and limits and also reinforces the idea that plans fail but people don't.

Behavioral Strategies. Behavior strategies involve a variety of actions that may include substituting a range of positive addicting behaviors, such as running, quilting, fishing, gardening, singing, biking, or building something, for static behaviors, such as sitting trancelike, watching television for hours on end, and ruminating about the loss. Making plans that deal with current problems and tasks, such as disposing of the deceased's belongings, locating a retirement center, starting a job search, and reviewing financial plans, are all examples of concrete, forward-looking behavioral strategies. Confronting and motivating new adaptive behaviors that deal with negative addictions such as alcohol and drug abuse, overeating, anorexic tendencies, or gambling are also part of the behavioral game plan for the crisis worker.

Cognitive Strategies. Cognitive strategies deal with changing maladaptive thinking. Workers help clients create positive counter-injunctions and positive mental billboards in place of negative, self-defeating thoughts. Workers aid clients in reframing and restructuring hot, all-or-none, intolerable, catastrophic thinking into cooler, less absolutistic, more preferable, and tolerable thoughts. They also caringly confront clients on cognitive avoidance, denial, and minimizing or discounting the impact of the loss.

Spiritual Strategies. Spiritual strategies are about transcending the loss through faith-based activities. This is a sensitive and tricky area to operate in because of each person's idiosyncratic interpretation of the part that spirituality and faith play in both the loss and its resolution. This is so because a secondary loss may indeed be a loss of faith over the perceived injustice or the uncaring of God in the primary loss. The worker needs to be extremely sensitive in regard to what will help the client deepen, renew, or discover new or old spiritual wellsprings. So whether through prayer, meditation, reading scripture with a group or on one's own, burning incense at an altar, hugging a large Douglas fir tree, or spending time stargazing, the idea is to activate spiritual resources. The worker does not have to be an ordained minister to do this.

One of the better models for this area is the work of the Christian Stephen ministry, which trains laypeople to administer spiritual psychological first aid to persons who are experiencing all kinds of trouble. Named after Saint Stephen, the first Christian martyr who cared for the poor, they provide a complete system of training and equipping laypeople to provide quality Christian care to hurting people (Stephen Ministries, 2023). We think the analogy of them being the spiritual equivalent of community emergency response workers (CERTs; go to Chapter 16, "Disaster Response") is an apt one, and crisis workers who do not have in-depth spiritual training might do well to go through the Stephen Ministry's workshop or its equivalent with other religions. Barring that, we heavily endorse forming a relationship with a trusted cleric with whom the worker can coordinate this facet of grief recovery.

Cognitive–Behavioral Approaches

Cognitive-behavioral therapies, which focus on changing maladaptive thinking, are the most commonly used therapies for those who suffer from complicated/prolonged grief (Cohen et al., 2006; Humphrey, 2009; Shear & Frank, 2006). Cognitive-behavioral strategies are used in dealing with both loss and restoration orientations (Shear & Frank, 2006). A variety of cognitive-behavioral techniques, including relaxation training, desensitization, thought stopping, cognitive restructuring, depropagandizing and disputing irrational beliefs, guided imagery, and in vivo imagery, are used to deal with the emotional dysregulation, behavioral dysfunction, maladaptive cognitions, and avoidance issues that are characteristic of complicated/prolonged grief.

Constructivist Approaches

Added to basic cognitive-behavioral therapy are the postmodernist constructivist therapies (Neimeyer, 2001, 2010b; Neimeyer et al., 2007) that focus on one of the major tasks of complicated/prolonged grief counseling—meaning making (Slattery & Park, 2015). Meaning making has to do with one's interpretation of reality and truth as the central process of one's life (Humphrey, 2009, p. 62). Certainly, one of the core issues of loss is making sense of it in such a way as to reformulate one's life, develop a new sense of purpose, and move from the past to the future.

Narrative therapy is a social constructivist approach that emphasizes the stories or narratives of people's lives (Humphrey, 2009; Monk et al., 1997; White, 1989). Narrative therapy is particularly important in grief work because it involves the telling and retelling of stories that thematically represent the meaning of the loss in the person's life. It brings to light and helps clients challenge the underlying beliefs and assumptions of dominant, maladaptive narratives that they have created in an attempt to make sense and meaning of the loss and challenges negative descriptions of themselves as guilty, weak, ruined, wasted, broken, guilty, shamed, cowardly and so on, that are often a complicating factor in loss adaption (Humphrey, 2009, p. 175). Narrative therapy also helps reconstruct, rather than relinquish, the relationship of the deceased and gives voice to the unspeakable thoughts and feelings of grievers who perseverate and attempt to reclaim their lives and make meaning of them (Neimeyer, 2010a).

Attachment Theory and Therapy

Attachment theory is one of the oldest theories to deal with grief. While it has origins as a phase theory, it still has a great deal of utility and is a basic premise of grief and loss. Attachment creates bonds that are rooted in the core of our existence, and when those attachments are broken, severe fractures and breaks can occur in the personality. Attachment theory emphasizes separation anxiety arising from the griever's attachment to the deceased, the breaking of bonds of affection, and the need to emotionally detach from the lost object. Attachment theory proposes that human beings form close affiliation bonds (emotional attachments) from birth because close attachment between parent and child is an evolutionary adaption that keeps infants secure and safe, and the resulting close physical contact with the parent enhances physical, emotional, and cognitive development (Bowlby, 1969, 1980, 1988).

The key component in understanding attachment theory comes from Main's (1996, 2000) research on "coherent narrative," which is the way parents told the stories of their lives. It was the most potent predictor of whether their own children would be securely attached to them. In other words, it wasn't what actually happened to them as children but how they made sense of what happened to them. Thus, making meaning of one's childhood, regardless of the actual event, corresponded positively with emotional integration and better parenting (Schuurman & De Cristofaro, 2007). When Bowlby's and Main's research is translated to loss and grief, it is thus not how one actually lived with the deceased, but how one *thought* about how one had lived with the deceased that really matters. As such, how the narrative of that thought process unfolds has a great deal to do with whether one moves through the loss and grief well or not.

If the narrative is maladaptive, then it follows that the griever will be maladaptive as well. At that point, narrative therapy's ability to change the story comes into the therapeutic picture. Thus, attachment theory can blend well with narrative therapy (Dallos & Vetere, 2009).

Dealing With Loss
Sudden Death of a Spouse

LO10 Stuart Wynn, a 44-year-old machinist, his wife Kate, a 42-year-old bookkeeper, and daughter, Anne, an 18-year-old high school senior, were a stable, middle-class family living in a quiet neighborhood in a large city. On her way to work one morning aboard a commuter train, Kate Wynn suffered a severe stroke and was taken by ambulance to a hospital emergency room, where she died. As far as Stuart knew, Kate had been in good health and had had no medical history to indicate that she might have had a health problem.

Sudden deaths have their own constellation of problems, and survivors' ability to use adaptive coping mechanisms is often overwhelmed (Captari et al., 2021). The sudden death is often violent, which means that authorities, autopsies, inquests, identification and return of remains, and a variety of other state and legal activities will often be involved. The news media and the criminal justice system can be intrusive and dramatic in clients' lives. Survivor reactions may be equally dramatic (Cummock, 1996). Because sudden death often occurs when significant others aren't present, questions arise as to how much the deceased suffered. There may be a desire for retaliation and revenge if the death was violent and human caused. The unpredictability of sudden death challenges assumptions about what the world is and how it operates. All of these disruptive negative cognitions can complicate the grieving of sudden losses and leave survivors with unfinished business (Humphrey, 2009, p. 23). Cognitive dissonance in sudden—and, in particular, violent—death is almost always high. The death makes no sense, and the mind cannot comprehend the reality of it. Emotions, and many times behaviors, are completely out of control because of the blame, accusation, and fault finding that the aggrieved erroneously believes will somehow make sense out of this impossible event (Redmon, 1996).

On the Triage Assessment Form, the worker mentally rated Stuart's profile: affective, 5 (emotionally shocked but substantially under control); behavioral, 8 (minimally able to perform tasks relevant to his wife's death); cognitive, 3 (thought processes affected by the crisis but under volitional control and congruent with reality); total, 16 (moderate impairment). Stuart's actions are not atypical in a situation involving sudden death by heart attack or stroke (Hersh, 1996). Despite the immediate disequilibrium following the sudden death of his wife, at that moment, Stuart was maintaining psychological equilibrium; only later would the impact of the loss catch up with him and would he experience severe affective, behavioral, and cognitive impairment. But for the moment, he could cope, even though the help of a crisis interventionist was needed and welcomed.

His daughter Anne was triaged as being much more substantially out of control. Her affect was rated as 10. She was decompensating and highly agitated and could not keep her emotions under volitional control. Behaviorally, she was erratic and unpredictable. She had accused the ER staff of not keeping her mother alive and had to be contained by security. Her behavioral rating was also 10. Her problem-solving skills were barely adequate for the situation. Barely able to contain herself after the intervention of security, Anne was rated 8 on the cognitive scale for a full-scale score of 28. The attending physician suggested that Stuart might wish to have his daughter kept in the hospital overnight and that she be given medication to de-escalate her extreme agitation. It was also recommended that a staff psychiatrist evaluate her due to her extreme agitation and the fact that her triage assessment put her in the potentially lethal range. While Anne is certainly a critical part of the case, here, the focus will be specifically on Stuart as the surviving spouse. The case of surviving children and the problems they may encounter will be dealt with later in the chapter.

The first intervention session was a very brief meeting that included only the crisis worker and Stuart. The second meeting, approximately 20 minutes later, was also a short-term intervention session that featured a meeting between Stuart and his daughter and a multidisciplinary care team consisting of the crisis worker, the attending physician, a psychiatric nurse, and the hospital chaplain. Intervention strategies that were used included Providing Support to help Stuart and Anne as they adjust to Kate's untimely death. Allowing Catharsis was also helpful, but with Anne, the crisis worker was careful not to let Anne's emotions spiral out of control. Other strategies were also used during the session, but these two were relied on as Stuart and Anne attempted to come to some understanding of their loss.

Care teams are important because they are a response to complex biological, psychological, and social problems in sudden death situations that call for experts from more than one profession (Larson, 1993, p. 199). These initial short-term sessions were aimed at providing the following:

1. Empathic understanding and acknowledgment of the special problems related to Kate's sudden death.
2. Assurance to Stuart and Anne that all appropriate emergency medical measures had been attempted in efforts to save Kate.

3. Emotional support for both Stuart and Anne by the worker and by the other members of the multidisciplinary team.

4. Assurance that Stuart and Anne would have time alone with Kate's body prior to it being picked up for autopsy.

5. Referral resources that Stuart needed immediately to make arrangements for the funeral, notification of kin, and other matters.

6. Information about autopsy rights and procedures, in case Stuart requested it (which he did).

7. Contact with the family minister, at Stuart's request.

8. Immediate medical and psychological assistance for Anne.

The care team laid out a long-term treatment plan that included the following intervention strategies to be provided during the initial hours and days immediately following Kate's death. Under no circumstances should you suggest that people immediately seek out a survivors' group or grapple their way through stage models of loss and bereavement. These activities will occur on the person's own mourning timeline and not some "hypothetical" or "scientific" timeline (Humphrey, 2009, p. 6; Shallcross, 2009).

1. **Immediate crisis intervention.** Dealing with the immediate practical necessities of Kate's death, such as autopsies, organ donation, funeral arrangements, contacting her employer, contacting family members. Continued assessment of Stuart's coping ability. Provision of support persons from the hospital, church, family, and friends. Discussion and recommendation to Stuart of immediate temporary hospitalization for Anne due to assessed potential to do injury to herself or others.

2. **Transcrisis individual counseling and intervention.** Identification of Stuart's grieving style on the adaptive model intuitive–instrumental continuum and tailoring the intervention to that style (Martin & Doka, 2000) because research indicates that close emotionally tied marriages like Stuart's tend to result in greater yearning six-months after the loss when they may think they are moving on and then be blindsided as the full impact of their soul mate's loss washes over them (Piper et al., 2011, pp. 97–98). Issues of loneliness and bereavement related to Kate's absence (Giunta & Giunta, 2002, pp. 125–146). Implications for regaining equilibrium and going on with his life.

Identification of functions and roles in the family that were previously carried out by Kate and that must be reevaluated or reassigned. Dependence on the deceased spouse for instrumental tasks increased postloss yearning and anxiety (Piper et al., 2011, p. 97). Grief work regarding Stuart's new identity without Kate: "I, Stuart," instead of "We, Stuart and Kate" (Van Praagh, 2000, pp. 95–153). Identifying and dealing with Stuart's areas of vulnerability created by Kate's death. Assessment of ways to remember and use the positive strengths of Kate's life in a healthy and growth-promoting way for both himself and Anne through the use of attachment theory and constructivist meaning-making strategies.

3. **Spouse-survivor support group work.** Assessment of overall implications of Stuart's widowhood, such as the loss of social connections. Suggested referral to a support group when Stuart and Anne are ready. Group-generated alternatives available to Stuart and others who had recently experienced the death of a spouse. Suggestions from the support group on Stuart's responses to his new single-parent role with his daughter. Groups focus on ways to cope with the loneliness and other emotions brought on by the absence of one's spouse. Most group therapy for loss addresses immediate losses and those who are devoid of clinically significant symptoms (Currier et al., 2008).

4. **Conjoint child–parent sessions.** Given Anne's extremely agitated reaction, she is most likely going to have some severe problems working through from a loss to a restoration orientation. Different family members grieve differently, and they are going to need to negotiate and understand that each person's grieving style needs to be recognized and honored. Differential family member grief, if not dealt with after a traumatic death, can cause severe family problems as the family attempts to reorganize and redefine itself (Humphrey, 2009, pp. 52–53). Both the parent's and child's reorientation may prove to be difficult as they come to grips with a new family system that does not include a wife and mother. To that end, each is going to need to develop loss narratives that move the deceased mother and wife from active presence to bonded memory. While father and daughter may develop their loss narratives individually, at some point, they need to come together in conjoint therapy

and compare those narratives (Cohen et al., 2006, pp. 153–156).

On the afternoon of Kate's sudden death, the crisis worker met individually with Stuart. The following segment illustrates a part of that first intervention session.

CW: (holding Stuart's hand) Stuart, I realize your wife's death has been sudden and overwhelming to you. I want you to know that I am here to help you with whatever you need done. (**Silence. Still holding Stuart's hand.**) I'll be with you as long as needed and assist you in whatever way I can. (**Silence. Still holding Stuart's hand.**)

The crisis worker's assessment is that Stuart's emotional reaction is primarily fear. Behaviorally, he is in shock and immobile, while his cognitive reaction is both loss and threat.

Stuart: (After a long pause, during which the worker waits patiently, Stuart gathers himself and responds.) This is so unreal! I just can't believe she's gone. It's such a sudden blow to me. Right now, all I can think about is Anne, my daughter, and how she is. My God! What will I tell her? My sister-in-law just brought her here.

CW: I will be there with you for as long as you need me. Certainly, we both can talk to Anne and your sister-in-law. We have a whole team that will help you now.

Stuart: I want to be with Kate—to be alone with her some before they take her away. Anne, too, if she wants. Can you arrange for us to do that?

CW: Yes, we'll arrange for that right now.

Stuart: I'm afraid I'm going to be in pretty bad shape after I've seen her. Her sister will be too. I just don't know about Anne. Could you arrange for us to sit in the chapel a while after we get back? And is there a chaplain around who could be with us for a few moments? I left a message with our minister at the church, but I don't know when he can get here.

CW: I'll call Chaplain Gentry again. He's aware of Kate's death, and he said he'd be available anytime, if you want him. I'll go with you and leave you alone with Kate's body and then, when you're ready, I'll go with you to the chapel.

The work with Stuart was immediate and intense. Such a cascade of events, problems, and emotions is typical in a sudden death. Particularly, seeing and/

or touching the body is important to verify that the loved one is actually dead (Hersh, 1996). Stuart manifests very well the initial impact of Stroebe and Schut's (2001) dual process model of an initial loss orientation. Thus, the worker's primary goal was to help Stuart deal with rapidly emerging needs an hour at a time or a day at a time.

The worker kept in mind that as time evolved, Stuart and his daughter would need to start moving toward restoration. But for the moment, the short-term intervention focused on Stuart's need to deal with his initial shock. The worker was also sensitive to allowing Stuart to become aware of his own loss. The worker never tried to or considered trying to manage, defer, speed up, or otherwise intrude on Stuart's grief process. Note the patience and use of respectful silence as a primary intervention tactic and the worker's ability to model strength and acceptance of the client's emotionally distraught state. From that standpoint, while the worker assumed a **facilitator (or a partner... this goes with the chart for high moderate reaction) role** in helping make immediate post-death arrangements, the worker provided only the degree of structure necessary and appropriate to client needs, goals, and preferences. The worker's main function at this time was to serve in a **witness role** to observe, listen, and not do anything other than "be with" the client and allow the client to feel "felt" (Humphrey, 2009, pp. 213–214; Wylie, 2004, p. 33).

About 2 weeks later, after initially taking the death in stride, Stuart was hit with the full impact of Kate's loss. Stuart's grief and his feeling of helplessness regarding emotional support for his daughter were reflected in a rapid escalation of his observed triage assessment scores: affective, 8; behavioral, 7; cognitive, 8; total, 23. This later assessment prompted an immediate referral of Stuart to a long-term therapist for grief work. Such a rapid escalation is a frequent occurrence among clients who have experienced the sudden loss of a loved one.

Stuart's condition concerned the crisis worker. The concern was Stuart developing prolonged grief disorder. The crisis worker was also worried that Stuart showing signs of prolonged grief would affect his daughter. The crisis worker suggested that both needed more than a support group. As a result, both entered a grief group that focused on meaning making. One component of this group was to use narrative therapy to help tell their stories and make sense of Kate's death (Monk et al., 2005) as they struggled to reconcile discrepancies between pretrauma beliefs (this cannot happen) and posttrauma beliefs (This is a bad dream. I can't handle this. I need to move on but can't or won't). This group has two purposes, to help members oscillate between restoration and loss and to start revising pretrauma global meanings (generally very good) and reconciling them with their post-appraisal of the trauma (generally very bad). Such meaning making helps people restore their sense of the world as a meaningful place and their lives as worthwhile and having renewed purpose (Slattery & Park, 2015).

Traumatic Death of a Child

Brad Drake, age 34, a farmer, and his wife Helen, age 30, had twin sons, Gene and Jerome, age 6. Late one afternoon, while Brad was doing the chores at the barn behind their house and Helen was preparing supper, Gene tried to cross the highway in front of their house to catch a runaway goat and was struck by a grain truck. Gene was airlifted to a regional trauma unit hospital 52 miles away but was pronounced dead on arrival. The death of Gene left his parents feeling a soul-deep sense of shock, grief, hurt, bewilderment, guilt, powerlessness, psychological immobility, and vulnerability, and searching for answers and meaning.

The death was ruled accidental; the driver of the grain truck that struck Gene was a local farmer, a friend who was as grief-stricken as the Drakes. Approximately 2 weeks after Gene's burial, Brad and Helen together sought counseling. The crisis worker saw them immediately following the intake interview. During the intake, the crisis worker rated Brad as a 20 overall with an affective rating of 8 because of his limited control of his emotions. The behavioral scale was rated as a 6 due to his behavior being maladaptive but not dangerous, while the cognitive scale was also a 6 because of his overwhelming occupation with thoughts of the death of his son. Helen's overall rating was a little higher and closer to 24 during the intake, with all scales rated at 8. The worker decided that crisis intervention could do four interrelated but equally important things: (1) facilitate the release of their grief energy, (2) reassure them that their feelings were typical, (3) put them into communication with other grieving parents, and (4) assess for post-traumatic stress disorder and complicated grieving and mourning reactions. These goals of intervention, described by Hansen and Frantz (1984, pp. 21–22), Cable (1996), Redmon (1996), and Rando (1996),

formed the basis for starting grief work with Brad and Helen Drake.

This case is an example of long-term intervention. The following strategies were provided and issues explored with Brad and Helen during the days and weeks following Gene's burial.

1. **Assessment for posttraumatic stress disorder (PTSD) and suicide.** Gene's death fit several of Rando's (1996) criteria for traumatic death. It was sudden, it involved a child, there was traumatic and disfiguring physical injury, and it was preventable. These are excellent growing conditions for Horowitz's (1986) stress response syndrome. A very grave mistake in loss counseling is to not deal with the potential for PTSD that arises out of stress response syndrome and overlays mourning. When this occurs, full-scale intervention for PTSD must be instituted before mourning can even begin (Rando, 1996). Thus, assessment for PTSD, as described in Chapter 7, "Posttraumatic Stress Disorder," should be considered. Perhaps more ominous is the research of Zetumer and associates (2015) who found that the death of young children caused more intense increased complicated grief with self-blame and suicidal ideation in their surviving parents.

2. **Couple counseling and intervention.** The situation surrounding Gene's death made it a good bet that one or both parents would blame themselves (Redmon, 1996). Also, the impact of the death on the twin brother, Jerome, would require appropriate parental handling so Jerome would not be neglected as they grieved or overprotected because they feared he would also die (Brown, 1988, pp. 66–68; Silverman, 2000, p. 159). Brad and Helen were reassured that they were not going crazy because for many couples, suffering the traumatic loss of a child, the recrimination, guilt, questioning, vulnerability, and incomprehensibility will make them think they are (Redmon, 1996). They received affirmation that they were the best parents they could be and that their parenting should not be blamed for the accident.

3. **Assessment of family problems and potentials.** This included an assessment of marital and family systems relationships following Gene's death and an exploration of ways to cope with the effects of the bereavement on the marriage and family. When a child dies, there is a high probability there will be serious marital problems within months

following the death (Brown, 1988, pp. 57–65). Parents may attempt to support each other by telling the other person that they were not at fault, only to have the other parent even *more* sure that the spouse is merely attempting to assuage their own feelings and placate them. Or, if blame is assigned, the whole system will deteriorate (Redmon, 1996). A good deal of psychoeducation was conducted with both parents and Jerome. Brad and Helen were reassured that the grief and pain would continue for a long time and that this is normal; that they'll always have memories of the loss; that they will, in time, let go of the pattern of holding onto their grief and move on; and that there is no set timetable for them to finish their grieving.

4. **Parent survivor and support group work.** Brad and Helen became involved in a group whose common focus is the loss of a child. Social support is critical in traumatic loss and needs to remain in place long after the funeral (Henning et al., 2021). Putting the parents in touch with intervention supports such as parental self-help bereavement groups (Snaman et al., 2017) is an important social support. Group-supported talk, reminiscence, sharing, grief, and tears will help the Drakes bond with members who have had similar experiences. It will also give them a point of reference as they see older group members making progress and newer members struggling with issues they have already overcome (Cable, 1996).

5. **Reading and media material.** The Drakes were provided with books, other reading materials, and CDs.

First Crisis Session 3 Months After Gene's Death

The first crisis intervention session with Brad and Helen took place when both were still in a stage of denial, isolation, and depression. They were clearly stuck in a loss orientation and were regressing even further into it. They were given the Texas Revised Grief Inventory, which showed that neither had moved past their initial response to the loss.

Helen: But my words are nothing compared to my thinking since this happened. I'm thinking I may be going crazy or something. I keep going to Gene's side of the bedroom and cleaning it up. I got on Jerome for going over there and messing with Gene's stuff the other day.

CW: Helen, you're not crazy. You're responding in a way that makes perfect sense to me. You have both lost the most important and precious gift a mother and father can lose. It is natural and typical for you to experience unusual feelings and grief. You're doing a very good thing by talking openly about your thoughts and feelings. That's why I'm glad you came and reached out to me today. Nobody can erase your hurt or bring your son back, but I will help as best I can.

Brad: I don't know anything anymore. Everything I knew about dealing with problems doesn't even begin to deal with this.

CW: First of all, there is nothing to compare with the tragedy of Gene's death that you have encountered. As bad and terrible as your feelings are, they are absolutely typical for parents I have dealt with, people who are going through what you are. You are not going insane, and there are things we can do that can help you get unstuck because the inventory you took tells me that you are, in fact, stuck. I want to take some time and let you both tell me the events that got you from Gene's death 3 months ago to my office today. I may ask some questions from time to time, but mainly I am going to listen and understand the emotions, thoughts, and behaviors you are dealing with right now. I want to take time to understand this, so start where you would like.

The crisis worker reaffirms that the abnormality they are experiencing is to be expected. The death of a child has been likened to an amputation. A part of the parent has been cut off much like an amputated limb, and the missing part will always be missed and mourned (Clark et al., 2021). The worker acknowledges this terrible and everlasting hurt and, in the same breath, issues the parents an offer of her help. Later in the same session, the crisis worker facilitated their release of grief energy and suggested that they contact an ongoing support group, the local chapter of Compassionate Friends (2023a), an international organization for parents who have lost a child.

The worker uses basic client-centered therapy. By demonstrating empathy, acceptance, unconditional positive regard, congruence, and concreteness, the worker provides a nurturing, trusting, and safe environment. That environment is particularly important when the griever's reactions are still very strong and they feel anything but safe and in control (Snaman et al., 2017).

The crisis worker noted that they exhibited signs of being physically and emotionally drained; they vacillated between moping and benign circumspection but showed no indication of movement from a loss orientation to a restoration orientation. The crisis worker's goal was not to push them; rather, the aim was to understand their current inner concerns and to provide them with opportunities to identify and express their immediate and deep feelings openly. Narrative therapy calls this listening to the *problem-saturated* story (Humphrey, 2009, p. 180).

CW: (after listening for half an hour to the Drake's story) I get the sense that you are both feeling drained of your emotional energy—like you're stuck there and cannot seem to move on after Gene's death.

Brad: Yes, *stuck* is the word. I don't want to talk about this, just get on with it. Helen talks all the time about it, and I can't stand that. But just sucking it up isn't doing me any good either. (awkward silence) It's like a fog that won't let up that chills you to the bone. It physically hurts and hurts terribly.

CW: So you are hamstrung, Brad. You don't want to hear about Gene's death, but trying to shut it out isn't working either. Where are you with the problem?

Helen: We've just about stopped talking about it. We've become two lonely recluses in the same house. That scares me and hurts almost as much as the accident. I never, ever thought about us ever getting a divorce, but we can't go on like this. This is almost as bad as Gene's death. At least we could put him to rest. We can't seem to do that with this. It just grows and grows.

CW: Helen, what would you like to be doing right now, instead of being stuck and isolated?

Helen: I'd like to be more open. I'd like to know what's going on with Brad, and I'd like to be able to share feelings—even though they may be sad. I have this need to talk about it, but Brad doesn't seem to want to.

CW: If we were to give the problem both of you are having a name, almost as if it were an invasive weed that had come onto your farm, what would it be?

Helen: Paralyzed.

Brad: Stalled.

CW: OK, stalled and paralyzed. How has that kept you from doing something?

Brad: Every time I go out, I seem to just go through the motions. Not getting anywhere or anything much done.

Helen: I get up and do pretty much the same thing every day. Go through the motions. Go to bed. Can't think of anything in between. Neither one of us sleeps much. I know it's bad for Jerome. He has his own problems, he feels guilty over letting the goat get out, but I can't seem to talk to him about it. Whenever I do, he just takes off. (starts to sob)

CW: (hands Helen a tissue) So what do stalled and paralyzed do for you?

Brad: Nothing. We have never been like that. Always faced hard times, drought, floods, hail, wind, insect invasions, you name it. Put your shoulder to the wheel and git 'r done.

Helen: Yes. Nose to the grindstone. Even though it hurts, you move through it, knowing there will be better times. That has always seen us through until now.

CW: I wonder if that's the problem, that you are putting your shoulder to the wheel and nose to the grindstone but it's a pretty immovable object and something you can't sharpen and get an edge on. So how are stalled and paralyzed causing you to be motionless? I want you to picture stalled and paralyzed. What would they look like?

Brad: Just gumbo earth like I can't get through in the south 40 acres. I track the stuff around, can't get it off my boots.

Helen: It's like I have a 100-pound backpack on.

CW: Those are really good examples. Could you see those boots and backpack sitting in the foyer? I'd like you to imagine taking both things off for a minute and just sitting there. How would that feel?

Brad: Different. I dunno. You mean just setting it aside.

CW: Gene will never be out of your life, and I feel like you are trying to slug your way through this and keep him in it in a way that can't be anymore, when it might be OK to just set the stall and the paralysis in the foyer. I wonder if you both could go home and just literally say to one another, boots off here, backpack off here. You might even want to get a backpack and muddy boots to really make those feelings concrete. If you need to pick them up and wear them tomorrow, OK, but right now they are off. What do you think?

Brad and Helen: (in unison) Like it was a dead weight off of us.

The worker's opening statement uses the most profane of contemporary words—"death." Using this word, as opposed to "passed," "went to his reward," or other analogies that deny and soft-pedal the death, acknowledges exactly what has happened (Cable, 1996). The grievers must learn to deal with the painful aspects of the loss, and supposedly kinder, gentler words are a trap the worker must not fall into.

Over the sessions, the TAF for individuals decreased. The crisis worker assessed both Brad and Helen in the mid-teens. This assessment means the worker shifted from partnering with the couple to being more of a guide helping them to move forward. As a result, initially, the worker uses Promoting Mobilization in an attempt to respond in a way that would give both parents the autonomy to experience their current state of bereavement and, at the same time, encourage them to open up and provide mutual support for one another. The worker is also using a series of narrative therapy strategies to help this couple start to oscillate from loss to restoration. After the worker listens to the problem-saturated story, they **externalize** the problem and give it substance by having the couple give names to it (Winslade & Monk, 1999). In most counseling, the last thing we want is to externalize the problem, like the person who misuses drugs who complains that "The crack does this to me" and takes no responsibility for their use of crack cocaine. With the Drakes' grief, however, they are so enmeshed in the problem they need to separate from it. By naming the problem and giving it substance, such as muddy boots or a rock-filled backpack, it is something that can be set down. The crisis worker does not get rid of it because grief is not abnormal nor something to be eliminated (Humphrey, 2009, p. 181). By attaching a name to it, it can be put in its proper perspective as a problem but one that can be set down as well. Notice that the worker says they may choose to put those emotions back on, but they can indeed take them off too.

The worker Provides Support using a constructivist narrative technique by using client-generated metaphors. Metaphors are helpful because they reduce resistance and provide a safe way of talking about

threatening material (Romig & Gruenke, 1991). The worker uses the client metaphors of how they have lived their lives and hooks it to how they continue to strive mightily against the stall and paralysis of their grief but sink deeper in it. The worker explores the metaphors with the clients and attempts to extend them (Humphrey, 2009, pp. 132–133) by changing the metaphors to their antonyms.

CW: Have you ever seen the movie *Always* (Spielberg, 1989)? The characters in the movie are about grieving and processing of bonds when one of the characters dies. Maybe you can stream it. It may be difficult to watch, but I think it is worth seeing and talking about to get this process started. I also think it is critical you get in a support group. There is not one here in Brighton, but there is one in Memphis called Compassionate Friends. There are chapters all over the country and you can google it up to see what they are about, but above all else, the research shows that a support system is critical to your getting through Gene's death, and as tough as it may be, you need to talk about this with other people who have gone through trauma.

Brad: I'm glad we came today. We would like to come in again. The group of parents you spoke about is a good idea. I think we need that now, and we are going to need it more.

Helen: We didn't know about Compassionate Friends. I'll call them this afternoon. It's good to know that such a group exists. It sounds like a wonderful thing.

CW: I think you will both be glad you discovered Compassionate Friends. I'm truly glad you came, and I look forward to seeing you again.

Compassionate Friends is a worldwide organization with over 650 chapters in the United States and Puerto Rico. Other chapters are in Australia, Canada, South Africa, Germany, France, Switzerland, the United Kingdom, and Belgium. The organization exists to support bereaved parents, siblings, and family members in the positive resolution of their grief and to foster physical and emotional health. The Compassionate Friends' credo suggests the unifying sense that bereaved parents can gain from joining a support group: "We reach out to each other with love, with understanding and with hope. Our children have died at all ages and from many different causes, but our love of our children unites us. Whatever pain we bring to this gathering of the Compassionate Friends, it is pain we will share just as we share with each other our love for our children. We need not walk alone" (Compassionate Friends, 2023a).

The worker also gave Brad and Helen *After the Death of a Child: Living With Loss Through the Years* by Ann K. Finkbeiner (1998), one of the best books your authors know in regard to loss of a child, and Harold Kushner's (1983) paperback *When Bad Things Happen to Good People*, which is a classic in the field and a best seller. The two books together represent comprehensive guidelines for surviving the death of a loved one. The crisis worker was employing a strategy of grief bibliotherapy (Becvar, 2001, pp. 237–239), which is an effective way of providing information, reinforcement, and support through reading and other media that can be used to help clients on the path to restoration.

Second Crisis Session 1 Week Later

CW: How are things going?

Brad: It's strange. I did get an old pair of boots and we got one of Gene's old backpacks and set it on the back porch. With mud on the boots and rocks in the backpack. Jerome thinks we have really gone nuts. We finally told him what we were doing. Lo and behold, the goat collar and rope appeared out there yesterday. We didn't ask him why and he didn't tell us, but clearly he is trying to set something down too.

CW: So how does it feel to merely set that stall and paralysis down and watch the world go by and just let things happen?

Helen: You know we went back home and did that after dinner. We went back into the living room and sat down, looked at each other, and sorta goofily smiled at one another.

Brad: Yeah, then we laughed cause we both thought Gene and Jerome would be shocked that we just set the stuff down and didn't work our tails off. We both talked some, did a little reminiscing, and then started to talk a little bit about establishing a scholarship with the Future Farmers of America in Gene's name. Helen knows I want to do that and listened to me. That instrumental thing you talked about, I guess.

Helen: I cried some at the thought, but it is something Gene wanted to be in when he got to high school. I suppose we are getting to understand each other's style of grieving a bit more after what you told us. I do feel like maybe we have started into the restoration part of this wretched business. I slept pretty good that night, and I know Brad did from his snoring. (**smiles at Brad**)

It is not uncommon for two parents to have entirely different views and coping mechanisms (Dias et al., 2021). Helen's need to continuously talk about the accident and weeping at a moment's notice is a common example of catharsis (Lord, 1996). She personifies a largely intuitive grieving style, while Brad's "git 'r done" attitude operates more from an instrumental style. Getting Brad and Helen to understand that they use these different styles is an important issue, so the worker spends time giving them information about adaptive and dual model processes. The change in this session may be considered in terms of the narrative therapy steps of mapping. Mapping the influence of the problem on the person lets clients understand how the problem has been affecting them. The turning point from a complete loss orientation to one that oscillates between loss and restoration is reversing the mapping to focus on the influence of the person on the problem (Humphrey, 2009, pp. 182–184).

CW: So how did all that happen? I mean, I am good, but not *that* good. (**A little self-deprecation and humor when clients are able to handle it is never a bad thing, in our opinion.**)

Helen: Well, I was filling the backpack with rocks and it really felt like I was taking the damn thing off my back, and I dunno... Then Brad said he didn't feel so mired down, and so we decided to go for a walk back to the river, which we used to do a lot, but it kinda reminded us of taking the boys back fishing and we stopped doing that, and we just sorta decided to get out, and I dunno...It just sorta happened.

CW: So taking some time to be with one another, and that hasn't happened for a long time. How did that feel? What was different?

Brad: It felt pretty good, and we talked some going down to the river. Like old times, talking about crops, neighbors, and stuff. Once we got to the river, maybe we put the backpack on and boots on for a while remembering, but we did make the walk, which was impossible before that, and (**smiles sheepishly**) we did hold hands on the way back.

CW: I would really like to have you take those instances apart so you know really clearly what the alternative story line you are now writing is and can continue to build on it. It's called **deconstructing.** Deconstructing means taking apart those disrupted meanings you have created since Gene's death that get in the way of some of the core values you have had up to that time. For instance, when you started to put the boots and backpack on down at the river, you took them off on the way home. I am interested in your holding hands. Could that be a cue that might allow you to refocus when the problem arises and you want to put the boots and backpack on again? Maybe you could think of a new name for yourselves, too, as you work through stalled and paralyzed.

Here, the worker uses constructivist strategies by taking apart (deconstructing) the disruptive meanings (Malkinson, 2007). In crisis intervention terms, the worker is Emphasizing Expansion to help Brad and Helen move from the symbols of the disrupted meanings (boots and backpack). The attempt is to go beyond older core meanings (holding hands)—starting to realize that when they put the disrupted meanings back on, they can use that as a cue to stop the disruption and substitute an old positive behavior. The worker also attempts to install a positive external name for their efforts to readapt.

Third Crisis Session a Week Later

Helen: We have a new name for us. Peace and harmony.

CW: Wow, that is different! So peace and harmony are now in charge. What will that look like in a month? Six months? What would people at your church say about peace and harmony as opposed to what they are saying now about stalled and paralyzed?

Working out the alternative story is not easy. One way of reinforcing the new storyline is to create a support system of significant others to bear witness to the change or to create an imaginary audience to give voice to their efforts at restoration. Indeed, at some point in the future, Brad and Helen may invite witnesses to bear testimony to their change (Humphrey, 2009, pp. 188–189).

Testing One's Faith. Brown (2008) has written at length about the complexity of the relationship between faith, spirituality, and trauma. Faith, or the absence of it, is of critical concern in most traumatic deaths (Aten et al., 2019). Trauma survivors who run into trouble with their faith generally fall into Fowler's (1991) faith

development model stages of **mythical literal**, which is a one-dimensional view of God as an entity that doles out rewards and punishment based on how rigorously one practices one's faith and follows its commandments (typical of children 8–12), and **synthetic-conventional**, which conforms to the community's basic cultural standard of moral behavior, normative beliefs, values, and religious practices (typical of 12 years of age to early adulthood). When losses occur, people in these stages may do three things. (1) They may adhere to these stages and do nothing but pray harder and accept God's will that they are sinners and must atone by hard sacrifices, as their recent loss illustrates. (2) Alternately, they may reject any and all faith, feel that their religion and their God have abandoned them, and become embittered at their faith and the community that supports it. However, through a spiritually focused trauma approach (VanDusen & Courtois, 2015), individuals may move beyond these regressive spiritual states toward Fowler's (1991) stages of **individuative/reflective faith**, where one is able to reflect critically on one's story and values and disregard personal myths about self, God, and one's relationship with the world, and **conjunctive faith** in which an individual can hold two differing beliefs and can deal with the paradoxes and polarities of those beliefs. (3) Finally, they may conduct a critical examination of their religious faith, move into progressively higher stages of introspection, and become even more grounded in their faith.

Brad: We just don't know where to turn. We take our religion seriously, and we've talked to our minister. That doesn't seem to help us. I keep on asking, "Why, why, why?"

Helen: We know the story of Job and such as that. We know tragedy strikes anywhere and anybody. Still, we don't know—we can't see—that a God of love or a God of justice can condone or permit the life of a good and innocent child like that to be snuffed out. I'm amazed at myself for talking like that. There is no justice, no fairness in this. No just God allows a sweet child like Gene to die so horribly.

Attempting to find meaning in the tragic accidental death or murder of a child tests the most dedicated believer. The notion that a life lived according to one's religious precepts, particularly that of a child, is seemingly for naught causes a tremendous amount of anger at God and can cause a severe secondary loss in regard to the person's religious beliefs (Becvar, 2001, p. 235). Religion is not an insurance policy against the outrageous slings and arrows of death, nor does it preclude suffering. Doubting is part of the cycle of faith (Grollman, 1996).

It is not the worker's job to move people from one developmental stage to the next (Humphrey, 2009, p. 30). What discussion of their faith does is allow the worker to assess another significant component of the clients' story and determine whether faith is part of the problem saturation.

CW: I don't begin to have answers, and I would submit that no one but you does have the answers to what part God and your faith play in this tragedy and if you can find solace in your faith. What I might ask you to do as part of the narrative you are creating is to write down your thoughts on these questions that Chaplain Ray Giunta, who is well known for his work in a variety of traumatic events, has posed. You can discuss them with me or your minister or just consider them and talk with one another. At the least, writing this out will allow you to get your thoughts out in the open. These are the questions (Giunta & Giunta, 2002, pp. 13–14):

Think about the loss you have experienced. If you listen to your heart, why did it happen and who is to blame?

What do you think your head might be telling you about your perspective that your grieving heart might not be able to hear?

How do you think God is seeing you in your loss?

How do you see God right now? Do you see him as raising his hand against you or as a loving Father with arms wide open wanting to help your hurt?

Pastoral counselors, in particular, must be very careful how they use their religion and spiritual beliefs to deal with grieving. "It's God's will" or "She is in a better place now" may be very little consolation to a mother whose heart is breaking because she so badly wants to hold her dead 7-year-old daughter again and sit down to tea with her after school. It follows, then, that rather than attempting to provide spiritual answers (which the authors of this book most certainly do not have), our goal must be to find ways of providing encouragement and support in searching for meaning (Wheeler, 2001). Given the foregoing qualifiers, it still appears that there is a tremendous amount of power and healing in prayer, religious ritual, religious ideation, and spiritual faith (Walsh et al., 2002). Your authors firmly believe

bereaved individuals should be encouraged to explore this as one of their options.

Bereavement in Childhood

Thadeus and Latoya Kirk, ages 36 and 38 respectively, were spending all the time, energy, and money they could in their attempts to cope with the terminal illness of their son, Charles, 5 years old. They spent 2 years in and out of the children's research hospital, and the family was exhausted physically and emotionally by the time Charles died. Their only other child, Makeena, age 7, felt sad, bewildered, lonely, and neglected. The whole family was consumed with grief the day Charles died. In addition to grief, Makeena suffered from guilt. She felt guilty because for several months, she had dared to wish that Charles's illness would just end and get it over.

Somehow, Makeena believed that her wish had contributed to the death of her brother (Howard Sharp et al., 2018). She also felt guilty because she was alive and didn't deserve to live as much as Charles. She was also afraid because she was sure she would "catch" the cancer her brother had. Overridden by guilt and fear that she was now an "endangered species" (Becvar, 2001, p. 129), Makeena became isolated both at home and at school, and her grades plummeted. She also started to have physical symptoms similar to those of her dead brother, which is not an uncommon occurrence (Bernstein, 1997). The school counselor, who had a good deal of experience in workshops for trauma and grieving children, was asked to intervene with Makeena. In the initial contact, the school counselor rated Makeena's affective reaction at 5 because of the duration of her emotions and the focus on the death of her brother. Behaviorally, Makeena was also rated at 5 due to her lowered performance at school and the potential of a threat to her health because of neglecting eating and not sleeping. Cognitively, Makeena's rating was higher, rated as a 7. The rating of a 7 was given because her thoughts about the death of her brother are pervasive, and she lacked any problem solving skills. The overall rating is 17, meaning the school counselor should use the "we" approach initially to support and help her begin the process of understanding the death of her brother.

Little attention has been given to siblings, who often get lost in the shuffle—both during the illness and afterward in the parents' grief—to the point that the siblings may feel abandoned (Howard Sharp et al., 2018). Family characteristics discussed in the previous chapter are all affected. Parents may also establish rules that prohibit talking about the deceased sibling because it is too painful. The roles and values of the family are also likely to be changed. Communication and boundaries with relatives or people outside the family may ask siblings how well their parents are holding up and completely neglect how the sibling is feeling. Family discipline may disintegrate, leaving the surviving children with the sense that they really don't count for anything because nobody cares what they do.

Further, if they are afraid they will suffer the same fate as the deceased sibling, they may become paranoid or obsessive in their behavior to "not step on a crack and break my back." Finally, siblings may fear that their parents are too vulnerable and are not able to bear the burden of the surviving child. As a result, they may act out or attempt to become perfect (Becvar, 2001, pp. 129–135). These feelings will almost always be present in such instances. Siblings may have big problems if those feelings are not dealt with in a timely manner, and those feelings may follow them throughout their lives.

Key to addressing the loss is to help the surviving child or children to utilize support systems (Howard Sharp et al., 2018). According to Howard Sharp et al. (2018) the support systems go well beyond the immediate and extended family. These systems include teachers, friends, and peers. These researchers state that guidance may be needed by teachers and peers to provide this support. These nonparental sources serve a buffering role and appear to accentuate the positive effect of parent support in reducing grief.

The following intervention strategies are provided and issues explored with the Kirk family during the days and weeks immediately prior to and following Charles's death.

1. **Individual counseling and intervention.** Assessment of Makeena's concept of death. Ensuring that Makeena has opportunities to participate actively and learn the medical facts relating to Charles's terminal illness in a truthful and realistic manner (Griffith, 2003). Use of child-centered play therapy counseling approaches in helping Makeena deal with and refute her guilt feelings related to her brother's death. Assessment of the impact of Charles's death on both parents and Makeena. Including Makeena in the funeral plans and commemorative activities. Providing opportunities for each family member to release grief energy. Assessment of the impact of Charles's

illness and death on the marriage and provision of individual therapy for Thadeus and Latoya as needed.

2. **Family systems therapy.** Assessment of the family's stress level and coping resources. A variety of toxic responses can come as a result of a prolonged illness of a family member—particularly when it is a child. Scapegoating, stonewalling, detachment, guilt, and masochism are a few of the defensive responses that can occur (Johnson, 1987). Provision of opportunities for the family together to explore the important issues related to Charles's death: the meaning, the good times and memories, guilt, blame, anger, rejection, unfinished business, and new family alignments (Brown, 1988, pp. 74–77; Silverman, 2000, p. 161). Focus on Makeena: ensuring that she knows that she is loved and that the time and energy that Thadeus and Latoya have devoted to Charles in no way diminished their love and devotion to Makeena. Discussion of feelings openly and honestly, keeping in mind the developmental capacity of Makeena (Brown, 1988, pp. 74–77). Ensuring that all family members have permission to mourn openly. Assuming that Charles's death will have a lasting impact on Makeena and will be manifested through her play, her fantasy life, and her relationship to both Thadeus and Latoya.

Play therapy is a way of entering the child's world, and puppets are a primary vehicle into that world. Play therapy can provide the following benefits for a grieving child (Authoracare, 2019; James & Myer, 1987).

1. **It allows for the symbolic expression of feelings.** When vocabulary is limited and mere words can't describe feelings, a child can use a puppet to voice feelings or demonstrate an emotion through the actions of the puppet.

2. **Provides a way to self-regulate strong emotions.** Children may often lack the emotional maturity or the affective regulation to control emotions. Play therapy allows the child to project those emotions through puppets and engage in activities that naturally provide affective regulation common to their everyday play activities.

3. **A way to be in control of a scary situation.** Death or physical or mental incapacitation of a parent is one of the scariest events that can come into a child's life. Using puppets, children can create imaginary scenarios that can put them into

control and allow them to process anxious and scary feelings when in the safe confines of therapy and, with gentle guidance from the therapist, remain in control and safely play out the imaginary scenario.

4. **Experiencing resilience and mastery.** Play therapy provides a vehicle for a child to explore new, unfamiliar, and threatening territory. Manipulating puppets with guided help from the therapist can model and inculcate resiliency and adaptation to new, changing, and unpredictable events that result from the loss.

5. **A safe bonding agent with the therapist.** Puppets on the arm of both therapist and child allow for safe, equitable interchanges between puppets rather than an authoritarian adult–child relationship that can create immediate trust and bonding. It can further allow for direct interchanges between the child's puppet and therapist, the therapist's puppet with the child, and, ultimately, child to therapist direct communication.

Using puppets in crisis counseling with Makeena, the worker was able to help her dispute her irrational and magical belief that her covert wish had caused her brother's death. During two previous sessions with the crisis worker, Makeena had developed a great deal of trust in the worker and considerable facility and ease in using the raggedy puppets. At the third session, there were five puppets: Raggedy Ann, Raggedy Billy (Raggedy Ann's dying brother), Raggedy Mom, Raggedy Dad, and Raggedy Doctor. During the sessions, Makeena's triage rating shrunk to around 10 as she progressed through the grieving process. The overall rating may fluctuate over time, but at this moment, she was able to address the loss in a more productive manner.

CW: (holding Raggedy Billy and Raggedy Mom—Raggedy Billy speaking) Mommy, Mommy, Ann said I'm dying because she had bad thoughts—she wished I would die so you and Daddy could leave the hospital and come back home.

CW: (holding Raggedy Billy and Raggedy Mom—Raggedy Mom speaking) Oh, Billy! Wishing someone is dead can *never, never* make it happen! Your sister, Ann, has a perfect right to wish for this hurting and sickness to end. She is so lonesome for Mommy and Daddy and for you, too. It's normal for her to wish this sickness were ending. But Ann should never feel bad or guilty just because she wished something. Remember, *wishing* doesn't make it happen!

CW: (holding Raggedy Billy and Raggedy Mom—Raggedy Billy speaking) Mommy, I wish I could see my sister, Ann. I'd like to tell her it's OK.

CW: (holding Raggedy Billy and Raggedy Mom—Raggedy Mom speaking) Oh, Billy, my dear son! (Raggedy Mom kisses Raggedy Billy.) I love you, and I love Ann. Here comes your sister now. Why don't you talk to her? She's in the hospital to visit you.

CW: (holding Raggedy Billy and Raggedy Mom—turning toward Makeena, Raggedy Billy speaking) Hi, sister Ann. I'm glad you came to the hospital to see me. I wanted to tell you how much I love you and how much I will miss you when I die. I want you to know that you should not worry about the wishes and thoughts you had. My disease is making me die. Your thoughts cannot make me or anyone else die. I want you to know it's all right. I love you, Mom loves you, and Daddy loves you. We will always love you.

Makeena: (holding Raggedy Ann and Raggedy Dad—Raggedy Ann speaking) I'm sorry. I wish you wouldn't die. I'm very, very sorry. I hope you don't die.

CW: (holding Raggedy Billy and Raggedy Mom—Raggedy Mom speaking) Oh, Ann, we all hope he doesn't die. But I'm afraid he will. Then we will all be sad together. We will miss him. But we will have to learn to live without Billy when he's gone. We will still love him. But we will have each other and love each other. We will never blame you or ourselves for his death. His death will be caused by his sickness, not by your thoughts or wishes, nor by my thoughts or wishes.

Makeena: But then Raggedy Ann could catch what Raggedy Billy caught, and she could die. (lays Raggedy Ann out as if in a casket)

CW: (takes Raggedy Doctor out, who picks up Raggedy Ann and gives her back to Makeena) No, she can't, and I know because I'm Doctor Feelgood. Raggedy Ann could catch some different kinds of bugs and get sick all right, but Raggedy Billy didn't have a bug. He had cancer. You can't catch cancer, so Raggedy Ann shouldn't worry about that. Raggedy Ann could never catch what Raggedy Billy had.

Makeena: (looking wistfully at Raggedy Ann) Well, maybe.

CW: (looking at the doctor puppet) Dr. Feelgood, do you suppose we could talk to that other doctor, who is a real cancer expert? He is a friend of yours,

Dr. Degrott. He takes care of lots of kids who have cancer at St. Jude's.

Makeena: (smiles and hops up) Yes! Let's do that. He took care of my brother. I know him.

CW: OK! I'll go make a phone call and see if we can do that.

Although the segment cannot reveal all the preparatory work and dialogue that preceded and followed this brief encounter, it provides some idea of how versatile and effective puppetry can be. The crisis worker uses directive play therapy, as opposed to the nondirective approach used with most child therapy. The reason is that with the kind of traumatic material being dealt with here, the child may be very reticent to venture into this forbidding territory, and, once there, have no idea what to do. Directive, crisis/trauma-focused therapy can help a child process anxious feelings and learn methods to cope with these terrifying "bad" thoughts (Webb, 2007, pp. 50–51). The crisis worker is focusing here on only two dimensions of bereavement during childhood: Makeena's guilt feelings and her fear of dying from what her brother had.

Once the worker has moved though "forbidden" territory, the child can move forward and grieve the loss. Makeena's grief work could have been processed with equal effectiveness by a crisis worker skilled in using artwork, dolls, storytelling, modeling clay, sand play, or psychodrama (Brown, 1999; Corr & Corr, 1996, pp. 258–261; Johnson, 1987).

CW: (Two pieces of poster board have large word balloons already colored in. A ground line is drawn, with some balloons anchored to the ground and others floating away.) Makeena, I would like you to draw a picture of you and Charles doing something together that was fun for both of you. We can talk about that and other fun things you two did together. When you get done, we are going to put some words in the balloons. The balloons up in the air represent things you have lost with your brother. The balloons anchored to the ground represent all the things you still have of Charles, including your memories.

Makeena: (draws herself and Charles fishing) I like fishing, and Charles would always put the worm on and take the fish off.

CW: So that is something you remember that's really positive. Can you put that in one of the balloons floating away? I wonder, do you remember how Charles did that?

Makeena: Yes. He threaded the worm just on its head and let the rest of the worm dangle. He also pushed down and back on the hook while holding the fish's top fin down so it wouldn't stick him.

CW: So that is something you have learned. You can keep that right here in this balloon that is anchored right by the pier.

The whole purpose of the balloon activity is to contrast what has been and what is: while memories of the positive relationship remain, the real-life experiences of the past are now gone (Stubenbort et al., 2001). From a cognitive-behavioral standpoint, this work is necessary in mentally reworking or cognitively restructuring the loss (Cohen et al., 2006). From a narrative therapy standpoint, it is part of the *restorying* (Zimmerman & Dickerson, 1996) process of creating a new storyline that she feels best about instead of the problem-saturated story she carried into therapy.

We are very big on "anchoring" those positive thoughts in the person's brain with an associated stimulus that is readily available to retrieve memories.

CW: Makeena, you can take this really nice drawing home and hang it up in your bedroom. Now I want you to put these balloons in an imaginary file drawer in your brain that you can pull out whenever you need to remember the good things and times you and Charles had before he died. So, picture a file drawer right up here in your head. Show me where it is. (**Makeena points to a spot behind her right ear.**) OK, that's where it is from the side. Where is it from the top? (**Mekeena points to the left side of the center of her head.**) Excellent, so I am going to take both your fingers from the top and the side and point directly where it is. (**Makeena points so there is an imaginary bisected line in her brain.**) Excellent! You have it right there, and every time you need it, you can pull it out. OK, now just shut your eyes and try it. (**Mekeena smiles and nods her head.**) Good! I believe Charles would be very proud of you the next time you go fishing with your family because you can go right there and get those instructions and tell them Charles showed you how to do it.

Separation and Divorce

When Eric Ishitani, age 32, an automobile salesman, came home and announced to Nancy, age 30, a very successful lumber wholesale manager, that he was in love with another woman and wanted a divorce, it shattered Nancy's world. The marriage had been going downhill for a long time, and during the preceding months, Eric had been staying out nights. Nevertheless, Nancy wanted to patch things up and have a child. But Eric was adamant and left. Nancy was extremely distraught, with feelings of grief, guilt, worthlessness, and failure. She felt her life was meaningless. She didn't want to face life alone; she was stuck in grief and felt that she was doomed to live the remainder of her life unfulfilled, without a husband or a child. She felt like a complete failure and blamed herself for not succeeding in the marriage. Nancy found herself frozen in a state of grief, remorse, guilt, depression, and self-pity.

The following intervention strategies were provided and issues explored with Nancy during the days and weeks immediately following Eric's announcement that he wanted a divorce.

1. **Individual counseling and intervention.** Assessment of Nancy's lethality level. Assessment of her coping skills and resources. Provision of a safe atmosphere for her to talk her grief out and ventilate her emotions. Assessment of available support people. Consideration of her feelings of worthlessness, fear, failure, guilt, anger, depression, self-pity, and lack of self-efficacy and self-confidence. Use of rational-emotive behavior therapy (Ellis & Abrahms, 1978) and behavioral modalities (Williams & Long, 1983) to help Nancy identify and successfully refute her negative and self-defeating beliefs and self-statements and start modifying her maladaptive behavior. Reprogramming her internal sentences and developing positive action steps that she can own, practice, and carry out independently of a helping person. Develop a new restoration narrative that no longer includes her ex-husband.

2. **Support group work.** Identification of divorce self-help groups for Nancy to use as supports. Assessment of her social needs on a time continuum from the present forward for several years. Use of the self-help group to assist her in making realistic plans for her personal and social adjustment to her new situation.

3. **Referral resources.** Assessment of Nancy's need for legal, vocational, and financial assistance. If necessary, identification of specific referral people for her to contact immediately. While interviewing her, careful assessment of statements reflecting her present autonomy and ability to attain her

goals. For example, depending on her husband's attorney, banker, or accountant may not serve her best interests. Many newly estranged wives find that they need a different attorney, banker, and accountant from the ones used by their spouses. They also may need to find employment or training to enable them to become economically self-sufficient. Often, this is a sudden and difficult switch. The worker must be sensitive, supportive, realistic, and assertive because Nancy is so vulnerable during this phase of her separation.

The abrupt termination of a relationship by separation is frequently accompanied by emotional responses that are as traumatic as after the death of a loved one. People who experience the loss of separation may exhibit shock, disbelief, denial, anger, withdrawal, guilt, and depression. Attachment theory indicates that separation and the subsequent feelings of loss can occur in many ways (Bowlby, 1969, 1973, 1980; Shaver & Fraley, 2008), and emotional reactions to a divorce may be very similar to those for the death of a partner. Each person responds in unique ways. Some will cry for several days. Some will verbally ventilate for days on end—to anyone who will listen. Some will go into a state of withdrawal, described by one person like this: "When he came in and told me he was leaving, packed his clothes, and left, I got in the bed and didn't move. I intended to stay there until I died." The loss by separation may be the result of severance of a marriage, a romantic relationship, a long-term friendship, a business partnership, or any other close personal attachment.

Helping people overcome the emotional and behavioral results of losing a relationship requires crisis intervention skills similar to those needed in other types of grief and bereavement. In Nancy's case, the client presented herself for crisis intervention several days after she had stayed in bed with the intention of crying and grieving herself to death. Nancy truly wanted to die after Eric told her he was leaving permanently. At first, her denial was so profound that she thought to herself, "This can never be. I will never be a divorcee. My parents must never know. My friends must never find out." Nancy did not talk to anyone about Eric leaving for several days. There was denial: "He really isn't leaving for good. He will be back. We will work things out." There was guilt: "What did I do to cause this? I must have been a terrible wife. I shouldn't have been so blind to his needs. If I just died in an accident, he could go on and marry the other woman and no one would ever have to know." There was anger: "I've got a good mind to find her and pay her back for all the misery she's caused me." Nancy experienced a flood of negative emotions before she brought herself to the point of presenting her problem to the crisis worker, who was a marriage and family therapist. As she presents herself, her thinking is full of all-or-none, catastrophic thinking. Her sentences start and end with words like "should," "ought," and "must." She believes that the activating event, Eric's request for a divorce, is causing the consequences of her depressed, angry, abandoned behavior, when, in fact, it is her irrational beliefs and automatic thoughts about the event that are causing her distress (Dryden & Neenan, 2004; Ellis, 1973; Ellis & Dryden, 1977; Liese, 1994; Malkinson, 2007).

CW: Well, Nancy, what brings you to see me today?

Nancy: My whole life is a wreck. It's really a mess. The main thing is that my marriage is breaking up. Well, I guess it has broken up. My husband's gone. Been gone for over 3 weeks. I have just got to get him back. That's all there is to it. I am nothing without him. We were high school sweethearts, and this is supposed to be forever.

CW: You're feeling pretty hopeless about the marriage, but you don't want to give up on it. What has happened today, in relation to your marriage breakup, to impel you to come in right now?

Nancy: Well, I was tired of lying around feeling sorry for myself—thinking about killing myself or harming my husband's girlfriend. My intuition told me that neither one of those acts would solve anything, so I've come in here looking for better answers. There should be an answer to this, and I have absolutely got to have some answers to this, or I'll go nuts or wind up alone in some old folks home with no one.

CW: Nancy, I'm really glad you decided to come today. What I want to find out first is whether you are in danger of suicide or homicide now. Is your intuition still keeping you safe? Do you have a means at hand to do it? And how close are you to suicide or homicide now?

The crisis worker's first concern was Nancy's immediate safety. It appeared from her verbal and nonverbal cues that she was hopeful and stable enough to have some mobility. The fact that she came to present her problem was another positive factor. However, the crisis worker still checked out her

lethality level. Then, when Nancy told the worker that she didn't have a definite plan or a definite means to kill herself, the worker proceeded with other steps in the crisis interview. At one point, Nancy appeared to be in a stage of "holding on," which Schneider (1984) describes as having elements of anger, bargaining, and denial, some of the primary stages of Kübler-Ross's stage theory (1969) of loss. The crisis worker rated Nancy between 7 and 8 on each scale, affective, behavioral, and cognitive. Her responses to questions were extremely emotional with almost no ability to control that. The statements she made about her future behavior, while not lethal, were still a concern, and the cognitive reaction also was like her mind was on a merry go round with almost no ability to stop it.

Nancy: I just can't believe this is happening to me. My whole world has caved in on me. This is simply horrible. I just can't stand it. I just don't know what I'm going to do without him. I must be a total loser. I haven't told anybody, but I think everybody in the sales department knows because my sales are way down. Christ! I probably have LOSER tattooed on my forehead. And I am so ashamed to tell my mother, although I think she knows something's amiss. My God! I am so pitiful; I just want to crawl in a hole and never come out.

CW: I want to do a couple things that I think will help you get a handle on the situation. I want to tape-record our session, and I am going to give you a homework assignment that involves some more taping. I think this is a good assignment because I want you to hear what I call *automatic thoughts*. In just the few minutes you have been here, I have heard a dumpster load of them, and those can get you in the kind of hot water you seem to be in now. Automatic thoughts result from people's underlying assumptions and beliefs. The most common type of automatic thoughts involve all-or-none statements like you're making. *Telling yourself* that you can't stand it and *believing* that it's horrible and that you're terrible seem to be exaggerations that are getting in the way. If you listen to all those "musts" and "shoulds," those are also indicators that your belief system is out of sync with what you need to do and is contributing to what I am going to call a problem-saturated narrative you have been building that won't allow you any leniency from all those self-condemning statements your belief system is making. That is different from telling yourself that it is bad, you don't like it, you wish it weren't happening, but that you didn't cause it and that it isn't the end of the world—even though it may make your life very difficult for a while. I want you to see how your catastrophizing, exaggerating, and awfulizing color your thinking and get in the way of you clearly and objectively assessing not only what has happened but also what your real options are. Don't you?

Nancy: Well, I don't know if that's right. I mean, I am pretty logical and linear and rational. I didn't get to be sales manager of one of the biggest wholesale hardwood lumber companies in the world by being a witless twit.

CW: I understand that, but would it be fair to say this is a little different than a sales campaign and the outcomes are a bit different? I have a little exercise I'd like you to do. I'd like you to make a loss and grief map.

Nancy: Well, yes, but . . . OK, I guess that'll be interesting.

CW: Draw a circle in the middle of the page and put your primary loss in it. Think of all your thoughts and feelings associated with it and write them down around the circle. [See Figure 12.1.] Focus on the thoughts, the billboards that pop up when you think about the word D-I-V-O-R-C-E. Once you have the thoughts down, put the feelings down that go with them. Go back and look at feelings. As you think about them, see if others don't bubble up. Lots of times we have a feeling about a feeling. For example, "stupid" might lead to "regret."

Nancy: Yes. I see it. That's pretty bad. I guess I have come down harder on myself and on the problem than is necessary. I know it isn't the end of the world, but I feel, at the time, that it's horrible and awful.

CW: Then you *believing* it's horrible and awful is the real culprit, isn't it? There is a difference between your beliefs and how things really are.

Nancy: You're right! It helps just to look at it differently, even though it doesn't solve my big mess.

CW: You're right. It doesn't solve it. But we can objectively examine it and together begin to figure out options you can choose if we know on the front end, even though you're grieving over your hurt, that we are not dealing with a world-shattering catastrophe.

The crisis worker was intervening by using elements of rational-emotive behavior therapy (REBT) (Ellis, 1973)

and cognitive-behavioral therapy (Meichenbaum, 1977). The worker was attempting to dispute the client's irrational beliefs about the separation and help her begin to direct her emotional energy toward the real issues. Nancy was an intelligent person who quickly responded to the rational ideas presented. But, as is typical in such cases dealing with the emotional state during loss, the worker knew that repetition, practice, support, and encouragement would be needed. A person in Nancy's state must have far more than just a one-shot session using REBT to get her beyond crisis and back to a state of equilibrium.

In addition to using REBT as a crisis intervention strategy, the crisis worker also used a self-managed behavioral technique (Williams & Long, 1983) to help Nancy expend her grief energy over a period of several weeks. What Nancy did was to make a series of audiotapes—alone, at home—in a sequential and systematic manner. The purposes for making the tapes were: (1) to serve as a mechanism for self-catharsis; (2) to present to both her and the crisis worker her full story and form the basis for changing it from a problem-saturated story line to a restoration narrative; (3) to clarify, in her own mind, the loss and movement toward restoration she was going through; and (4) to document her progress in controlling her automatic thoughts and catching her "shoulds," "oughts," and other mustrabatory statements about love, marriage, and her self-concept.

The loss and grief map (Greenspan, 2003) is a concrete representation of all the absolutist, negative, irrational beliefs she has about herself and the divorce. Once she has those in conscious awareness, she and the worker will start working on positive counterinjunctions that cool these hot cognitions off. The worker will also set up a self-managed behavior model with her that will allow frequency counts of the number of times she makes those statement to herself in a day. He will use a thought-stopping procedure and cueing (Dr. James's magical rubber band-on-the-wrist-thought-stopper) to cue her to shift from those all-or-none irrational thoughts to cooler, more positive, self-enhancing counterinjunctions that are designed to start changing her narrative to one of restoration.

The audio recordings were quite useful to the crisis worker in verbally journaling her changing narrative as she worked on her cognitive-behavioral plan. But the main value of the behavioral plan was providing Nancy the purpose and the experience of doing it. She described in detail her thoughts, feelings, and actions throughout several stages: shock and

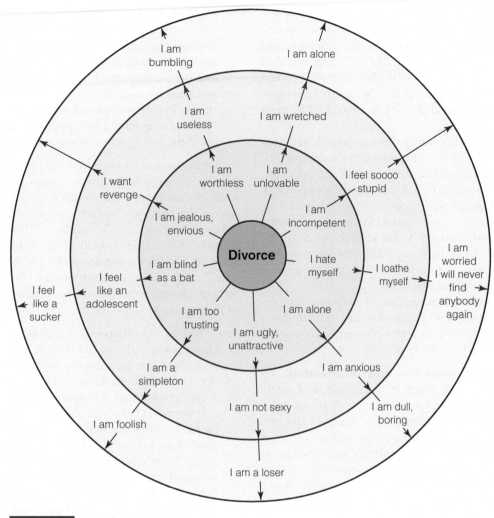

Figure 12.1 Nancy's Divorce Map

disbelief, denial, anger, withdrawal, guilt, depression, searching, and resolution. Nancy made eight recordings. She reported that the most valuable and helpful aspect of the activity was listening to her own recordings, which she found herself doing over and over. Nancy kept the recordings with the stated intention of continuing to listen to them. But she later reported that after her crisis subsided, she didn't need to listen to them anymore.

Nancy also contracted with the worker to go to a divorce support group at a local church. Such groups provide crisis support, role models for survival, adaptation pathways, and new social networks (Raphael & Dobson, 2000). You will note that over and over we advocate the use of these groups as part of a comprehensive crisis and transcrisis intervention treatment model. They are an important part of the response to bereavement, and there is evidence that they are effective as a social and healing process (Kitzman & Gaylord, 2001; Raphael & Dobson, 2000).

Death of a Pet

The Thompsons—Hollis, age 36, Faye, age 33, and their adopted daughter, Dawn, age 5—were grieving over the death of Tincup, their aged terrier. Tincup had been like a member of the family. He had been a faithful companion to the Thompsons since they were newlyweds; he had been the affectionate and protective playmate of Dawn from the day the Thompsons got her through the adoption agency. Lately, he had developed severe health problems, and the veterinarian had finally told the Thompsons that Tincup's medical condition made it necessary to terminate his life. After making the painful decision, the Thompsons decided that they would all be present at his euthanasia.

While on a first reading this may seem horrific for a small child, Butler and Lagoni (1996) make an excellent case that an honest discussion of the pet's condition and the need to put it to death is important. Children respond well to straightforward and concrete explanations. Note that we do not use the more palliative "put to sleep." As Butler and Lagoni (1996) suggest, small children may think that because they go to sleep every night, they may be "put to sleep" if they are bad and never wake up.

The following intervention strategies were provided and issues were explored with the Thompson family during the days and weeks immediately following the death of their pet.

1. **Individual counseling and intervention.** Assessment of the levels of grief, guilt, and stress in each—Hollis, Faye, and Dawn. Assessment of Dawn's understanding of the death of the pet. Provision of a period to grieve and release grief energy. Follow-up play therapy and ceremonial events as outlets for Dawn (Schoenberg, 1980, pp. 203–204) and display of meaningful objects that link Dawn to her deceased pet (Lagoni et al., 1994, p. 265).

2. **Group work.** Providing an opportunity for the family to talk about Tincup's death in a realistic, factual, and honest manner. Using the pet's death to help Dawn begin to develop her concept of death, free of misinformation. Providing opportunities and activities for the family to commemorate the pet's life and to reformulate the death within a context of growth.

3. **Bibliotherapy.** Reading about bonding with pets and coping with crisis and loss.

The pet counselor from the veterinary clinic met with the family 3 days after Tincup's death.

Dawn: I was a little scared, but Dr. Hobbs told me what they were going to do. (whispers) He said it wouldn't hurt but I really wanted Tincup to stay alive. But...but he would yelp every time I tried to pick him up, and I didn't want him to hurt anymore. Dr. Hobbs let me watch and he got Tincup ready, and my parents watched too. He... he just sorta relaxed. I petted him while they put the medicine in him. It was all done in a minute or so, and my parents and I petted Tincup for a while and then we took him home. We buried him in the backyard. (whispers) I go visit him every day. I think I may want a new puppy for my birthday, but right now I just want to go visit Tincup.

As Butler and Lagoni (1996) suggest, getting new pets immediately is not always a good idea. Children, and for that matter adults, need time to grieve the loss of their pets just as they need time to grieve any other important loss. Schoenberg (1980) suggested that families use ceremonial events to help deal with their grief following the death of a pet (pp. 203–204). The Thompsons used a ceremonial event of pet burial to help open up opportunities for discussion, sharing of feelings, and explaining death to their daughter.

Faye: We had a small funeral in the backyard. I helped Dawn invite a few of her close friends to the funeral, and our next-door neighbors mailed us a sympathy card. Hollis and Dawn dug Tincup's grave, and we had a simple but beautiful graveside service. There were flowers and friends, and we paid tribute and said good-bye to him. It was a good thing for our family and for the friends who came. We even had another small ceremony when we put Tincup's collar on the bulletin board in Dawn's room. We're still grieving somewhat over his death, but it has been a learning experience for all of us, and I think Dawn will have a more realistic and healthy view of death, loss, and grief as a result of these activities.

We also got *Zach and His Dog* (Meagher, 2009), which is a story about pet loss and bonding with children. We read that together and had some tears, but it helped put things in perspective too. So Dawn still touches Tincup's collar before she goes to bed, but I think probably by Christmas there may be a new puppy under the tree Christmas morning.

The strategies used in dealing with the loss of pets are aimed at the same goals as those used in any human loss: helping the grievers work through their various stages of grief in healthy and growth-promoting ways. Rituals for pets may seem a bit over the top, but their purpose for children as well as adults is to keep them from getting stuck (Reeves, 2011). It is recommended that people who work with clients who have lost pets read from sources such as *The Human–Animal Bond and Grief* (Lagoni et al., 1994). The Humane Society (2023) has an excellent web page on how to cope with the death of your pet that has a number of activities and support sites, including:

1. The Pet Compassion Careline, which provides 24/7 grief support with trained pet grief counselors.
2. Laps of Love, which provides grief courses and 50-minute one-on-one support sessions with a grief counselor.
3. Everlife Support Groups by state.
4. Association for Pet Loss and Bereavement support groups, available at specific times throughout the week.

Bereavement in Older People

Lenore and Robert Kizer, ages 82 and 85, respectively, had been living in a nursing home for 4 years. Robert had been there more than a year when Lenore had to join him. Their three living children resided in other states and were busy with their own families, so Lenore placed Robert in the nursing home when he was 80 and she was no longer able to care for him because he required 24-hour nursing care. Lenore was in the dining room eating breakfast when one of the medical staff members came and requested that she come to Robert's room because they couldn't rouse him. When Lenore arrived at the room, a staff physician met her and informed her that Robert had apparently died in his sleep. The following intervention strategies were provided and issues explored with Lenore during the days and weeks immediately following Robert's death.

1. **Individual counseling and intervention.** Assessing Lenore's level of grief and coping ability. Providing opportunities for Lenore to release her grief energy. Assessing Lenore's physical and mental capacities to cope. Assessing her children's ability to help. Examining her economic, medical, and legal needs. Using therapeutic strategies such as cognitive/spiritual, reminiscence, and constructive/narrative therapy to help Lenore revalidate herself as a worthwhile person separate from Robert.
2. **Group work.** Groups within the nursing home. Social groups outside the nursing home.
3. **Referrals.** Medical, religious organizations, legal assistance, Lenore's church, her children, and senior citizens' agencies.

Lenore Kizer continued to live in the nursing home following Robert's death. Lenore had several assets, which the crisis worker, a pastoral counselor, used to validate her life as it had been lived and revalidate what her new life would be without Robert. She was physically mobile, she had lots of friends in the nursing home and in the community, she was an outgoing person with an optimistic outlook on life, and her children were supportive. Even with the positive factors she had going for her, Lenore experienced periods of denial, isolation, loneliness, fear, anger, bargaining, and depression that were profound. The crisis worker's goal was to help Lenore achieve a satisfactory degree of reconciliation with and acceptance of Robert's death and to begin to reorient her postcrisis life as a worthwhile person who was not identified as Robert's wife or Robert's widow. The crisis worker did this by first tapping into her strong faith. Cognitive restructuring (Meichenbaum, 1985) and existential therapy (Frankl, 1969) were used to reinvest her socially and inject new meaning into her life. Finally, the worker attempted to change her negative interpretations of the event by using a narrative/constructionist approach (Neimeyer & Levitt, 2000; Neimeyer & Vaughns, 2022; Wass & Neimeyer, 2018).

Lenore: Sometimes I feel it is terrible that I am so alone.

CW: On a scale of 1 to 10, one being absolutely awful and 10 being absolutely wonderful, where would you rate yourself?

Lenore: Probably a 2. Life isn't worth much anymore.

CW: I wonder if you might look back on your strong faith and see and say that a little differently, Lenore. Something like, "Robert is indeed gone, but God is still with me and so are my friends and my children."

Lenore: I know, and sometimes I forget that. God is always here. If I stop and pray a minute, God generally gives me a way to go. I get so moping around I forget that.

Lenore's overall rating on the TAF was 17, with a rating of 6 on the affective scale, a 5 on the behavioral scale, and a 6 on the cognitive scale. Her emotions were mostly under control and focused on the death of her husband, and she appeared very sad. Lenore's behaviors were somewhat unstable, and her daily function was affected, causing her to be immobile. Cognitively, her problem solving was blocked, resulting in her being unable to think about much of anything except the loss of her husband. By reframing and proposing follow-through actions, the crisis worker attempts to cut through the ever-deepening vortex of isolation and despair that assails the grief-stricken when a longtime partner has died. Using the strategies of Providing Support, Allowing Catharsis, and Increasing Expansion, the crisis worker helps Lenore begin the process of moving through her grief. These strategies help her by creating a new resiliency and finding new meaning in life, which is critical for any older person. Many therapists are skittish about bringing spirituality into therapy. However, combining cognitive therapy with spiritual therapy can be extremely powerful (Ramsey & Blieszner, 2000). The worker is also setting Lenore up to engage in solution-focused brief therapy (SFBT) (De Shazer, 1985) for loss adaption (Humphrey, 2009) by using an SFBT scaling technique to lay the groundwork to allow her to reframe her current despondent state and focus on finding positive solutions (de Shazer, 1985).

Lenore: A lot of times I just mope around. Some of the time, I get to feeling sorry for myself. Then sometimes I forget and find myself walking down to Robert's room before I remember that he isn't there anymore. My life seems so meaningless without him.

CW: You're really missing him, and you're having trouble remembering. What would you like to recall most, and when your life is better, how will it be like that? It's certainly fine to do that reminiscing, but also thinking about how you two worked through things together. I wonder how you can use his memories to do that.

While the worker uses reminiscing (described in detail in Chapter 14, "Violent Behavior in Institutions"), the focus is on marshaling positive assets Lenore has used in the past to cope with the present and the future. Together, the crisis worker and the client rewrite the client's story line by deconstructing reality (Humphrey, 2009, pp. 184–185) into more positive self-descriptions that are much closer to her life as opposed to the terrible exception she now faces (Ramsey & Blieszner, 2000).

Lenore: We were very active politically and socially conscious. We were also very active in our church.

CW: So if you were to write those down as the major narratives of your life and have a conversation with the Lord about it, what do you suppose might come of that?

Lenore: Well, it isn't actually in the Bible, but it is a good saying. "The Lord helps those who help themselves." Robert used to say that, and I think it is true. I need to get off my rear end and help myself.

CW: So while this is a terrible exception to how you have generally lived your life, it is indeed an exception and not very representative of the strong and resilient Lenore who forged not only a great married life but also an exceptional independent life of her own.

Lenore: When you put it that way, there is more truth than fiction to it.

CW: So, suppose a miracle happened, and indeed the Lord came down and, in a vision, tonight said, "Lenore, I am about to make a miracle happen with you. Tomorrow you will be as you were before. Robert will not be there, but you will be. What will I see happening, Lenore?"

Lenore: Well, you would see an old woman, but still full of a zest for living, taking the retirement van down to the church and going in the church van out to visit the shut-ins. I suppose you would see me also down at the local Republican Party headquarters doing some things there. I also haven't gone to my quilting group in a while, and I want to make every one of the grandchildren a quilt to remember me by. I have been putting that off, but time is flying by. I guess that is kinda egotistical, huh, Lord? (**A wry smile crosses her face.**)

CW: So, could you do that? And I wonder if you might relate what you have said with the women's group next week.

Lenore: Well, I expect I could do that.

The crisis worker uses the SFBT techniques of the miracle question, exception to the rule, and cheerleading (de Shazer, 1985) in a spiritual format to help Lenore recognize and reinforce the many positive attributes she has had and still has. By having Lenore look at this period in her life as the exception rather than the rule, the crisis worker reframes the loss narrative and seeks to reconstruct her view of life and its meaning. When life stories are rendered chaotic by narrative disruption due to the loss of a lifelong mate, reframing that narrative in more positive terms can foster healing (Neimeyer & Levitt, 2000, Neimeyer & Vaughans, 2021). That healing may be made much more powerful by helping the client form or reform a spiritual foundation.

This narrative therapy technique is called re-membering, which is a way of reintegrating loved ones who have died in a more productive way as opposed to ruminating on the loss alone (Voight, 2017). Retelling her story to her quilting group is another powerful affirming and validating technique that brings a profound sense of meaning not only to the client's story but also serves to strengthen the bond Lenore has with her peer group (Waters, 2022). It may be argued that the foregoing is a "goody-two-shoes" approach to pacify and mollify the aggrieved and that no real change will occur. Further, it may be patently ridiculous to assume that disheartened old people who are only waiting for the grim reaper to appear could be uplifted by reviewing and hearing encouraging and joyous stories. We propose that this view is as negatively stereotypical of the elderly as one can be. Reconstruction of one's self-concept as a primary task of adaptation to spousal loss is a primary task no matter how old or young one is (Lopata, 1996). Research reports that allowing older persons to discuss their thoughts and feelings (Segal et al., 2001) helps reduce a variety of negative thoughts about the loss. Further, older people are not helpless; they have the capacity to adapt and learn new coping responses even after suffering the loss of a mate (Hanson & Hayslip, 2000).

Complicated Grief: Death of a Mother

These case examples end with the most difficult type of grief and loss issue—a complicated grief reaction (Rando, 1993). Ann Marie is a 38-year-old legal secretary who slammed into a bridge abutment but did not die immediately. Her car was totaled. She was unconscious and taken to the hospital for an examination. Luckily, her only injury was a concussion. However, her blood alcohol content was found to be 0.17—twice the legal limit. She was charged with a DUI and was ordered by the court to see a counselor with expertise in addictions.

However, Ann Marie's case is not about addiction to alcohol but about a complicated and chronic grief reaction to the sudden death of her mother after a long bout with lupus. Neither she nor the crisis worker is aware of that at the moment. The crisis worker is a licensed addiction counselor who has also worked in bereavement.

CW: So what was going on before you had the wreck?

Ann Marie: I was angry at my father, and I finally decided to get out of the house and go out to a club with my girlfriend.

CW: Angry! How?

Ann Marie: (**starts weeping**) Look at me. I am 38 and taking care of my father. I never go out. I haven't had a date in forever. I don't know what got into me. I generally don't drink very much at all.

CW: What do you suppose *did* get into you to make you decide to go drinking and driving? As I look at your record, this is your first offense. You don't have so much as a speeding ticket.

Ann Marie: I work all day. I come home at night and cook, wash, clean, and sew for my dad and my brother Ralphie, who is 36 and living at home. I do everything for them. Ever since Mom died, they've expected me to take her place. I even moved back home from Phoenix, and now here I am. It is useless. I am useless.

CW: When you say "useless," I don't like the sound of that. You sound so down and out that I am wondering if getting into that car and slamming into that bridge abutment was not a way of attempting to kill yourself without the stigma of suicide attached to it.

While it may appear that your authors continuously harp on this issue and you are tired of being nagged about assessing for suicide with every client, many suicides are accomplished by automobile. Mustering enough courage to do it by getting intoxicated is another common feature of suicide by automobile. Further, suicidal ideation is one of the markers for a complicated grief reaction. The addiction counselor immediately picks up on Ann Marie's hopelessness and helplessness and pursues it. The addiction counselor has now shifted to crisis mode. Suicidal behavior is one of Worden's (1991, p. 76) complicated grief clues.

Ann Marie: (**cynical laugh**) If I was really serious about that, I'd have knocked Ralphie in the head and stuck him on the front of the hood. Kill myself? Not yet. Drink too much and do something stupid cause I feel sorry for myself? Yes!

CW: OK. I needed to check that out. You mentioned Phoenix. What was that like, and how is this different in Pittsburgh?

Ann Marie: I had a great job with a great law firm in Phoenix 4 years ago. I had a great boyfriend there.

I had a great life. I was going to get married. I just got a promotion to executive secretary. Then Mom got sick. She had always waited on Dad hand and foot. He was useless without her (laughs cynically), about like me now. I started flying home to help out, but the lupus got worse, and Mom went to a wheelchair and then to a nursing home. I got a job out here. The boyfriend said I had to choose. I did. A helluva choice. A dependent father and shiftless brother and a third-rate job. Maybe I did try to drive myself into that abutment. I don't think so, but I don't know anymore. I don't see much of a life for me anymore.

The client's losses are large and many. We know of no rule that says grieving and bereavement must be over a death. The sacrifices the client has made career-wise and in her relationships are profound. The isolation, loneliness, depression, anger, and sadness encapsulate all of the first five of McKenna's (1999) components of survivor grief. While working with Ann Marie, the crisis worker assessed her affective reaction as primarily anger, with a rating of 8. The rating of 8 was given because of her very limited control every time she thought of or talked about her lack of support from her family. The behavioral reaction was also high, rated at a 7 and maybe an 8. Her focus on the lack of her support limited her ability to function on a day-to-day basis. The rating for the cognitive scale was also a 7 and maybe an 8 since her ability to address the situation in a healthy manner was severely compromised. The overall score was somewhere between 21 to 23, meaning the crisis worker will, at a minimum, partner with Ann Marie to help her process the crisis. Crisis intervention strategies would include Allowing Catharsis, Providing Support, Increasing Expansions, and Providing Protection. Other strategies will also likely be used, but these seem critical as Ann Marie works through her loss.

CW: So you have sacrificed your life for your parents. What you have gotten from that is a smorgasbord of bad feelings and bad outcomes.

Ann Marie: (continues weeping softly) My mother died last year. Worked herself to death for them. (clinches her fist and pounds it into her hand) Christ! I wish she were back here. I miss her, but I would give her a piece of my mind for not standing up to those two jerks I am taking care of and making them grow up.

CW: How do you feel about your mother's death?

Ann Marie: Why . . . why . . . what do you mean? Terrible, of course. I loved her. We used to talk at least twice a week when I was in Phoenix.

CW: I am just wondering. You indicated your dad and brother were pretty dependent on her, and now they seem to be that way on you.

Ann Marie: Oh, Dad says he'll get a housekeeper. He's been saying that since Mom got sick, but he won't when he's got his daughter for an indentured servant. And that failure-to-launch brother of mine. "Yeah, I'll pitch in, Sis, right after I get back from the game. Say, mind washing my work clothes? I forgot and don't have any clean for Monday."

The crisis worker's content query moves immediately to the deceased mother. The worker is well aware that what clients say about their dead loved ones may be very different from how they feel. Unfinished business (Attig, 2000, pp. 112–117) can be a major problem in grief counseling. This is particularly true when the death is sudden (Cummock, 1996). Whether that unfinished business is guilt over having or not having done or said something, unfinished business is a common issue that is particularly problematic because of prohibitions against "speaking ill of the dead" or, indeed, the inability to speak to them at all.

In a very odd way, but anything but uncommon, what the client is manifesting is disenfranchised grief. It also has characteristics of rational-emotive behavior therapy's musturbatory behavior (Ellis & Dryden, 1977) in that the client is duty-bound and "must" absolutely take over for her mother no matter the cost to her because that is what "good daughters" do. This **musturbatory behavior** segues into and goes a good deal beyond the client's primary loss of her mother to secondary losses of a love life, career, and independence. When these are piled one on top of the other, they are an excellent recipe for complicated/prolonged grief. Ann Marie meets the proposed criteria (Prigerson et al., 2008; Zhang et al., 2006) for prolonged grief in the following ways:

Criterion A: Yearning, pining, and longing for the deceased to a distressing degree (although she hasn't verbally acknowledged it yet because of her anger).

Criterion B: Experiencing four of the following in the last month as marked, overwhelming, and extreme: (1) trouble accepting the death; (2) inability to trust others since the death; (3) excessive bitterness or anger over the death; (4) feeling uneasy about moving on with one's life; (5) feeling emotionally numb or detached from others since the death; (6) feeling life is empty or meaningless without the deceased; (7) feeling the future holds no meaning or prospect of fulfillment without the deceased; and (8) feeling agitated, jumpy, or on edge since the death. Ann Marie clearly meets Criterion B.

Criterion C: The above symptoms and disturbances cause marked dysfunction in social, occupational, or other important domains. Ann Marie's social and work life have been seriously impaired by the death.

Criterion D: The above symptoms and disturbances must last at least 6 months. A period of 4 years definitely meets this criterion.

Ann Marie: (pounding her fist into her hand) I told Mom again and again to make them be independent. She'd just say, "Oh, you know your dad; he likes to be taken care of, and your brother's had tough luck."

CW: But now it is you who is taking care of them. If you could speak to your mother about what you are now feeling, what would you say to her?

Ann Marie: That's crazy. She's dead. I can't speak to her.

CW: Do you visit her gravesite or memorial?

Ann Marie: I go there every morning and pray in the mausoleum. I am a good Catholic. I also light a candle at Mass. My old girlfriend from high school says I am going too much and can't get over it. It has been almost a year now. She was the one I went drinking with the other night. The only friend I've got . . . from high school! My God, but I am pitiful!

CW: I understand you care very deeply for your mother, but sometimes there are things that are left unsaid or undone. If your mother were sitting right here right now, what might you say to her?

The crisis worker uses a tried-and-true Gestalt therapy technique of the "empty chair" to attempt to allow some of the client's powerful and buried affect about the predicament her mother has left her in to come out (Cable, 1996; Humphrey, 2009, pp. 154–166). While it may seem this technique is used in a lot of situations in this book, it is one of the best for objectifying emotions—and many, many seemingly intractable crises call for just that.

Ann Marie: (tentatively) I guess . . . like always, that I loved her.

CW: Speak to her as if she were here right now in that chair over there!

Ann Marie: I love you, Mom. I wish you were still here. I miss you so much sometimes.

CW: What would you tell her about the situation with your dad?

Ann Marie: Not much, I guess, just I am bearing up.

The crisis worker guesses about her feeling anger that is buried by gently reflecting this and confronting her on her behavior.

CW: I sense some anger about that, not just your dad's demands and needs and your own lack of a life. Bearing up under her load. A load she left you with. Did she ask you to do that?

Ann Marie: Well, sorta. She never asked me to come back home, but she asked me to look after Dad.

The crisis worker now makes an owning statement targeted directly at the anger in an attempt to get the client to speak to the affect. This is not a one-step process; it calls for repeated attempts to uncover the pent-up emotion. This process may take considerable time—or perhaps never happen with some clients who are so deeply mired in it.

CW: If it were me, I might feel a great deal of resentment. I wouldn't quite know how to deal with it, but I would surely feel it. I might even be afraid of some of those feelings that would not seem right, forbidden even. It wouldn't be right to be angry with my mother who died heroically trying to take care of my father, yet I would be angry about the predicament I was in and the loss of my own life—love life, career goals, a chance for a family. I would be very angry about that. If you were that angry, what might you tell her? I have an assignment, if you are up to it. I want you to go back to the mausoleum, and I want you to tell her how you feel. I will go with you if you want, but you need to do this.

Many times, people will go out of their way to avoid returning to the gravesite or memorial site because of the fear of their inability to control their feelings. Or, alternatively, their feelings will be so out of control that they practically deify the gravesite, they are there so often. The client should be willing to make the visit and should never be forced. Having an agenda such as Ann Marie's is important. When the grief is complicated, it is important that the crisis worker be willing to go with the client. While there, the client may write a letter and burn it, or put a message in a helium balloon and let it fly away. After the gravesite visit, it is helpful if the client does something positive, rests, and is reinforced for the accomplishment of the visit. The summation of this visit is to literally put the body to rest and bring closure (Johnson, 1987, p. 181).

Ann Marie: (7 a.m. at the mausoleum by her mother's crypt) I feel so stupid. I . . . I can't . . . I don't know what to say.

CW: Just say what is in your heart.

Ann Marie: (struggles with long pauses) I miss you. I . . . love you. I wish . . . you wouldn't have let Daddy and Ralphie be so dependent on you because they are on me, and I don't know how . . . what to do. I am kinda angry with you about that. . . . In fact, I am VERY ANGRY WITH YOU! How could you have done this? You always encouraged me to go out and be independent. To seek my own life, and I did . . . but then you hooked me and reeled me back in. Damn it! How could you! How could you do that! (leans against the crypt and wails while the crisis worker holds her)

CW: (very gently while holding his arm around Ann Marie's shoulders) Is it possible that underneath that anger is a lot of loneliness for your mom? That the real anger is that she left you without your main support, her wisdom, and the talks you had about your hopes and dreams? I wonder if you can forgive her for that.

Ann Marie: (sobbing) Oh, Momma, I do miss you, and not just for having to take care of Daddy and Ralphie. For always encouraging me and supporting me. I feel so selfish. I do forgive you and hope you can forgive me.

Forgiveness is a difficult thing to do. The anger that overlays her frustration also overlays her fears of now being on her own, of her deep personal insecurity now that her main support system is no longer there. Forgiveness is critical to letting go. By understanding and getting past the subtle fears that prevent forgiveness of real or imagined past indiscretions, injustices, hurts, failures, and insults, clients are finally able to move forward (De Moss, 2003).

CW: (waits for her emotions to pour out) Your mother wanted you to be independent. What do you

suppose she might say to you about exerting some of that independence with your dad and Ralphie?

Ann Marie: (regaining some composure) I guess . . . I . . . guess . . . maybe . . . she would . . . say, "Ann Marie, you know good and well that is not what I meant. You must lead your own life. Now you sit down with them and tell them there are going to be some new rules. I took care of your dad and Ralphie, but I wasn't a babysitter for them. You know I didn't mean for you to do that either." (continues dialogue with her mother)

CW: I would like you to write up a list of "new rules" for your dad and Ralphie and describe how you are going to behave toward them. I would like you to come and visit your mom tomorrow and discuss those rules with her.

While it may seem strange to have a conversation with a dead person who most assuredly will not answer, the fact is that clients may well have a fruitful dialogue and begin to concretize diffuse and abstract feelings that were heretofore unreachable.

We can objectify unfinished business in many ways, such as writing letters, having dialogues, playing music, drawing and painting pictures, creating scrapbooks, sculpting, or creating other symbolic ways to relieve our hurt and anger with the unfinished business (Attig, 2000, p. 116, Neimeyer & Vaughns, 2022). By doing so, Ann Marie was able to start letting go of the complicated grief reaction she had developed and forgive her mother for dying on her so suddenly and leaving her with two dependent men.

While prayer can be positive and helpful in many circumstances, prayer in this case served only to punch back the real feelings Ann Marie was holding toward her mother for having the audacity to leave her with a very dependent father. Until she was able to express her feelings and vent her anger, Ann Marie would continue to have transcrises in her own life, which could indeed become lethal for her. Ann Marie is representative of many people we encounter in crisis who appear to have one kind of crisis yet have a different one underlying it. This underlying crisis is often complicated grief and unreconciled bereavement.

Indeed, while Ann Marie's DUI is most assuredly a problem, and her drinking may be a problem as well, the undergirding crisis is her sense of loss—loss of a job, loss of a romantic relationship, loss of her independence, and finally loss of a parent—none of which she had adequately grieved but over which she had instead built up a tremendous amount of unconscious resentment. Complicated grief is a delicate, sensitive, and troublesome issue that is surrounded by emotional minefields and taboo cultural totems (Rando, 1993). Yet, if a crisis worker suspects an unresolved grief problem, much as our addiction counselor did, then this is the very place that intervention must go. If you do not feel comfortable in doing this, and even we "experts" sometimes don't, then refer the client.

Ann Marie was able to move forward and confront her father and brother. She was also able to engage some effective support systems to help her father and brother become more independent. None of these steps was fast or easy. She no longer visited her mother every day, but still remembered her by lighting a candle for her at Mass once a week. She completed her DUI course and got her driver's license reinstated. At last report, she was actively engaged in a number of community activities and hobbies, and had moved to another, larger law firm with more responsibility. Although she has yet to find true romance, she has accomplished a great deal. She has mourned the loss of her mother, removed the unresolved grief that was an emotional anchor around her neck, regained some of her independence, and started to reinvent and reinvigorate her life.

The Crisis Worker's Own Grief

Before workers engage in grief work with others, they must first take care of themselves. This means becoming proactive in maintaining their own vitality. Failure to do so can result in the phenomenon known as *vicarious traumatization* or *compassion fatigue* (see Chapter 16, "Human Services Workers in Crisis"). Indeed, working with loss and bereavement has a high potential for burnout. The 9/11 World Trade Center (WTC) disaster resulting in a large population of disaster workers needing psychological assessment and treatment is standing testimony to this fact. The traumatic wake of that disaster resulted in the first large-scale screening and use of evidenced trauma practices on disaster relief workers (Olden et al., 2015). The lessons learned from that disaster, the Oklahoma City bombing, and Katrina have led to large-scale development of debriefing, screening, and treatment protocols for disaster workers (found in Chapter 16, "Disaster Response").

Schneider (1984) reminds us that "it is not possible to be a facilitator of the growth aspects of bereavement if the helper is not also experiencing growth

in relation to personal losses" (p. 270). The knowledge and perspective gained from one's own growth following grief should serve as a quiet reservoir of strength for workers. But the worker's own grief experience should not be projected or imposed on clients. Both Rando (1984) and Schoenberg (1980) challenge caregivers to come to grips with their own personal and professional attitudes toward death, grief, and bereavement before venturing into helping relationships with clients who are in grief. According to Rando (1984), there are several reasons why caregivers should ensure that their own grief and attitudes about grief are not allowed to intrude on their strength and vitality for helping others (pp. 430–435).

1. **Emotional investment in the client.** A certain degree of emotional investment in clients is normal and needed. Overinvestment in those whom they help may require crisis workers to expend an inordinate amount of energy on their own grief responses in cases of dying and bereaved clients.

2. **Bereavement overload.** If the worker forms close bonds with several clients, the emotional load may involve too many risks and grief responses on the part of the worker. Workers can deal with their own bereavement overload provided that they are aware of it while it is happening to them and that they act on their internal signals to get help and/or take steps to effect their own renewal before several client losses get them down.

3. **Countertransference.** Sometimes, crisis workers engaged in grief work with others find that such work awakens their own feelings, thoughts, memories, and fantasies about losses in their own lives. Solomon et al. (1998) report on the tremendous countertransference issues that Israeli mental health workers had in dealing with Holocaust survivors and the equally tremendous problems that caused for them and their clients. Workers who experience such countertransference will be severely impaired in helping others. To deal with countertransference, caregivers who regularly work with loss-related clients should be involved in peer supervision, case staffing, psychological autopsies, and debriefing groups for reducing the emotional overload caused by constant involvement with client grief.

4. **Emotional replenishment.** Caregivers in the area of grief and bereavement work must take special care to minister to their own emotional needs. Caregivers need support systems to provide for

their physical, emotional, and psychological well-ness. Emotional replenishment involves both taking care of oneself internally and having environmental supports from significant others—a supervisor, friends, family, colleagues—and meaningful physical and emotional activities that take the person completely away from loss and back into a positive emotional and physical state.

5. **Facing one's own mortality.** One of the important aspects of loss work is that it may arouse existential anxiety over one's own death. Support groups, supervision, inservice training, and reading are suggested coping mechanisms. Spiritual growth activities are worthwhile alternatives for many caregivers.

6. **Sense of power.** Caregivers, like all other people, need a sense of power or control. Working with clients in dying, grief, and bereavement may cause workers to identify vicariously with the losses of their clients. Such identification may result in a sense of loss of power or control on the part of workers. Strategies for preventing feelings of loss of power are essentially the same as those recommended for dealing with countertransference.

7. **Tendency to rescue.** It is essential that workers relinquish the rescue fantasy, especially when dealing with grief and bereavement, because rescuing someone who has experienced or is about to suffer loss is to deny the inevitability of the loss.

The seven proactive points just noted are good starting points for worker vigilance in preventing vicarious trauma, compassion fatigue, and burnout in themselves. It is highly recommended that you thoroughly read Chapter 15, "Human Services Workers in Crisis," for further coping strategies if you are going to do this work.

Humphrey (2009, pp. 218–219) has posed some hard questions for professionals in human services interested in doing this work. They are abridged, encapsulated, and stated here with our own additions. Think carefully about them and reflect on what your answers are!

1. Can I see the differences between my own grief experiences and those of my clients?
2. Am I aware of my own unresolved issues of loss, do I have unfinished business with them, and do they spill over into my work?
3. Do I rescue clients from their grief because it is too terrifying for me or I can't handle their pain?
4. Do I have to expend so much of my energy controlling my own emotions that I am ineffective with my clients?
5. Do I avoid, deny, or otherwise sidestep certain grief-related issues because of my own issues with them?
6. Am I unwilling to let my clients experience the pain of grief because I don't believe they can handle such emotion-laden topics, or is it maybe me that can't?
7. Does the mere mention of the topic of death or dying make me apprehensive or anxious and start dreading the counseling session?
8. Are my own losses so new and raw as to not allow me to work effectively with someone else's loss?

Is There Any Lemonade in All These Sour Lemons?

Of all the chapters in this book, Personal Loss: Bereavement and Grief is one of the most difficult and depressing, at times, to write. The question becomes: Given the overwhelming nature of most losses, can we hope for anything better than just getting back to some level of homeostasis and equilibrium? And if so, then what? Richard Tedeschi and Lawrence Calhoun are two researchers in particular who have been working on this problem for many years (Calhoun & Tedeschi, 2001; Tedeschi & Calhoun, 1995, 2003, 2004, 2006, 2009; Tedeschi et al., 1998). They have been very interested in personal transformation (Tedeschi & Calhoun, 2012) and the potential for **positive traumatic growth** that comes out of any personal transformation that occurs as a result of trauma (Tedeschi & Calhoun, 2010) or the ability to not just survive a traumatic incident, but grow from it (Taku et al., 2008, 2015). One of the keys to understanding how that happens is the ability for individuals to change **intrusive rumination**, unbidden terrifying thoughts entering the person's mind about the trauma, to **deliberate rumination,** wherein the person deliberately thinks about the trauma and attempts to make meaning of it and reconcile it into passive memory (Triplett et al., 2012). Here's the good news: It doesn't happen to everybody, but overall, there is a fair amount of research to indicate that people can grow out of trauma and bereavement and do so for the better (Armstrong & Shakespeare-Finch, 2011; Caserta et al., 2009; Cryder et al., 2006). Zhou et al. (2015) found that intrusive rumination indeed challenged the core beliefs of Chinese middle school students who had experienced a devastating earthquake. On the other hand, deliberate rumination tended to mediate core beliefs toward posttraumatic growth.

Thus, when people are able to start to control their thinking and make meaning of the event, they do better than just adapt, but indeed experience positive growth beyond what and where they were before their losses and the ensuing crises. What is probably most interesting is that the more severe the loss reported, the higher the levels of growth (Armstrong & Shakespeare-Finch, 2011). So take heart! There is lemonade!

It also appears that crisis workers can experience positive growth out of dealing with trauma and loss (Arnold et al., 2005), so we end this chapter by finishing the horrific story of the Wisconsin dairyman you met at the beginning of the chapter. The whole community pitched in to take care of the farm so our dairyman could take his family and get away for a vacation (very hard to do when one milks twice a day and shovels a lot of fertilizer in between). That, in and of itself, was extremely moving and growth promoting for the whole community. One farmer told your author while the two were shoveling fertilizer at the dairyman's farm, "We used to do this a lot. It's the right thing to do, and by God, we did it for Lutherans, Catholics, and even that Methodist family! It didn't make any difference. We helped people when they were down and hurting, no matter who. I personally feel damn good about this, and my guess is everybody else does too."

The dairyman took his family to Disney World, where his deceased son had wanted to go. A week after they returned, your author pulled his truck into the farm lot on his regular Friday route. The dairyman came out of the milking parlor and said, "Ah, come on inside, I got something for you. It isn't much, but it just, umh, ah, my way of, I guess, well, umh, sorta saying thanks for listening to me. It helped a lot." With that, he gave your author a cigarette lighter from Disney World. Your author doesn't smoke anymore, but he still has that lighter, and that was in 1976.

But he got more than that from going into the jaws of this terrible death. He made a decision to get back into the business of counseling, which ultimately led to the University of Memphis, helping give birth to the CIT program that has become international in scope and the gold standard for police training for crisis intervention with the mentally ill, training more than 2,000 police officers from all over the world, 3,500 counselors, and now co-authoring a ninth edition of this crisis book that we humbly believe has affected thousands and thousands of students and, in turn, hopefully has helped them deal effectively with thousands more clients. So, from the dread of walking into that milk house 47 years ago, it is safe to say one of your authors grew more than he could have possibly imagined.

Summary

The stage models of death, dying, grief, and bereavement have become outdated due to a lack of research to prove their viability. Newer models of loss depict grief as highly idiosyncratic, not progressing neatly through linear stages. The adaptive model proposes that grieving over loss occurs along a continuum of styles and that no particular style is the one, right, true path to resolution. The dual process model promotes grieving as oscillating back and forth between a loss orientation and a restoration orientation over an extended period of time. The constructivist model is about making meaning from and building new healthy narratives out of loss.

Several different types of loss typify the kinds of human events or tragedies that might bring crisis workers into contact with persons experiencing grief. All of these losses are the same in that they may strike individuals with grief and all that grief entails. Examples of such losses are (1) the death of a spouse, (2) the death of a child, (3) bereavement in childhood, (4) job loss, (5) separation and divorce, (6) the death of a pet, (7) bereavement in elderly people, and (8) the trauma associated with HIV and AIDS. However, loss is also different in that persons may suffer from a primary loss, secondary loss, multiple loss, ambiguous loss, and stigmatized loss.

Every human being will, at one time or another, suffer personal loss. During our lives, most of us will encounter numerous people who are experiencing bereavement or grief as a result of some personal loss. What may be clearly perceived as a personal loss ranges from a devastating occurrence, such as the death of a spouse or a child, to what many people might view as a minor loss, such as that of a pet or a family heirloom. In any event, it is an important loss if the individual perceives it as such, and workers must treat each client's loss with empathy, caring, and sensitivity. Although the bereaved can never forget the loss and return to a state of complete precrisis equilibrium, they can be helped to reformulate the loss within a context of growth and hope.

Most loss is resolved by grieving and mourning that help the person place the loss in memory and move forward with living. Complicated/prolonged grief is a manifestation of loss that has not been resolved, grief that has gone unreconciled, mourning that hadn't been completed, and as a result is now pathologic.

Complicated/prolonged grief may occur after an extended period of time in regard to a nontraumatic loss and have coexisting disorders such as depression and anxiety. It may also result from a traumatic loss and be classified as traumatic grief with the possible coexistence of PTSD. Complicated/prolonged grief is transcrisis in nature and, if not dealt with, can cause serious to lethal physical and psychological problems for the individual suffering from it.

Intervention strategies, techniques, and skills that crisis workers need for helping people in these categories of grief are focused on cognitive-behavioral and constructivist approaches but may be highly eclectic when interventions are tailor-made to fit the idiosyncratic needs of the individual's grief process.

Crisis workers who work with grieving clients, and particularly clients with complicated/prolonged grief, who do not take care of themselves emotionally, physically, and spiritually become vulnerable to vicarious traumatization and compassion fatigue, particularly if they have not resolved their own losses.

Crises in Schools

13

Learning Objectives

After studying this chapter, you should be able to:

1. Explain the need for and type of security for twenty-first century schools.
2. Explain the purpose of the Clery Act and the lack of its equivalent in K–12 schools.
3. Explain the theories on why youth violence has risen.
4. Identify the types of youth gangs that exist in the United States and programs designed to control them.
5. Explain the role of the school resource officer in dealing with crisis.
6. Identify the dynamics of bullying and bully prevention programs.
7. Identify the three generic types of violence-prone youth.
8. Explain screening techniques to uncover violence-prone youth.
9. Explain the incidence, screening, and use of suicide intervention techniques with children.
10. Explain what Tier instruction is and how crisis intervention is integrated into it.
11. Explain the role of school crisis response teams (SCRTs) and what they do.
12. Explain the role of the school in dealing with grief and memorializing students who have died.
13. Explain how a school crisis plan is conducted and the personnel responsible for it.
14. Explain how a school crisis plan is put into operation and the personnel responsible for it.
15. Explain how a school transcrisis is handled.

The New-Millennium, Violence-Proof School Building

LO1 This chapter might well be called *Preventive Crisis Strategies in Schools*. If you are a school counselor, social worker, behavior analyst, school psychologist, teacher, administrator, secretary, custodian, or a parent, not only are you concerned with progress in school achievement and how to deal with getting schools back in operation after the COVID-19 pandemic, but you are also very concerned with school safety, given the number of school violent acts characterized by mass shootings that make national news and the gang shootings that often don't. Attempts to strengthen your school safety measures while reducing some violent acts by their very presence have paradoxically increased student fears for their safety (Fisher et al., 2020; Laughout & Linear, 2011; Mower & Freng, 2019; Osher et al., 2014; Reingle-Gonzalez et al., 2016). Public opinion about school safety grows dimmer with every school violence newscast. Yet, according to the United States *Report on Indicators of School Crime and Safety: 2021*, criminal victimization of students ages 12–18—including theft, rape, sexual assault, robbery, aggravated assault, and simple assault—has declined since 2009. (Victimization rates dropped from 51 per 1,000 students in 2009 to 30 per 1,000 students in 2019.) Changes to school procedures related to the pandemic coincided with a further 60 percent decrease from 2019 to 2020 in the student victimization rate, down to 11 per 1,000 students in 2020 (Irwin et al., 2021). Further, with the advent of school threat assessment teams, a United States national report on their operation during the 2017–2018 school year indicated that out of 14,869 reported threats, only about 10 percent (1,472) reached a high priority level requiring action, and only 42 resulted in harm occurring (Michaelis, 2019). Still "Too much!" you say. Indeed the "Too much!" is what this chapter is about, and while there are both intervention and postvention procedures in it, prevention is a major component.

The New Millenium School. Welcome to the (pretty much) violence-proof school building of the new millennium. We are not spending any money on landscaping because people can hide behind shrubbery, and we want every square inch of the exterior in plain view of security vehicles that will patrol the perimeter on a 24-hour basis, 7 days a week. We really don't want taggers making their artistic statements on the school or any vandalization, so we have flood-lit the whole facade and built a 10-foot chain-link security fence around the grounds. We maintain a vehicle path around the perimeter so security vehicles or police cars can easily keep surveillance on the building.

We prefer that all students come to school in buses equipped with video monitors and two-way radios. For those few who drive, the student parking lot is enclosed by a 10-foot chain-link fence with razor wire on top. The lot is gated, so all student drivers need passes and hanger tags to get in with video surveillance. A security guard will check all students and parents who come into the parking lot. We also have concrete median dividers angled so there can be no straight-on assault by individuals intent on drive-by shootings or school bombings.

We have only one student entrance into the school, where all students must go through a metal detector. Only see-through backpacks are allowed and will be run through an x-ray machine. School uniforms are mandatory. Once students are in the building, all entry and hall doors will be electronically locked down. Teachers have swipe cards so they can move through the building. Closed-circuit TV

and a call box at the front entrance enable parents to gain access.

Although uniforms are mandatory, you can have your choice of school colors—as long as those colors are not used by any known gangs operating in or around the school. All students must have holographic ID cards attached to their uniforms, as must the faculty. Students also must have global positioning system (GPS) locaters, either carried or skin-implanted. Optical and fingerprint scanners are optional. All faculty are equipped with panic alarms and carry cell phones with speed-dial numbers preset to call security. Armed intruder drills of various sorts are detailed with faculty and simulation drills with role players are conducted and critiques are made on a regular basis. Threat assessment teams meet on an as-needed basis to consider lethality level of threats received and action to be taken.

Kevlar bulletproof vests in the school colors will be issued to all staff. The building itself has almost no windows; the few, very small windows are made of bulletproof glass. Walls are double-brick thick (newer munitions can fairly easily penetrate a single-brick thickness). A central monitoring station is capable of visual, auditory, and motion surveillance of the entire school building—both inside and out. All classroom doors are equipped with timed electronic locks that can be operated only through a computer program or be overridden from the central monitoring station and teacher entry cards. Hallways also have locked electronic doors at strategic locations for crowd control and isolation of intruders.

The real savings is in building architecture. First, we have downsized the gymnasium. We don't need bleachers because crowds are hazardous. Any pep assemblies, sporting events, plays, or pageants will be piped back into classrooms via TV monitors. Athletic events will be played on isolated fields, and spectators can watch via community cable television. As a result, we do not need showers or locker areas. In addition, we have also cut the width of hallways because there are no lockers in this school—lockers are conducive to hiding contraband. There is no need for a cafeteria. Lunches can be either microwaved in classrooms or hot-packed from a central food preparation facility. Cafeterias are places where students congregate, and a congregation of students provides a setting for dangerous behavior. Thus, cafeterias are becoming as extinct as the little red schoolhouse.

There are no faculty bathrooms. Student bathrooms are dangerous settings and must be policed.

So, while faculty are relieving themselves, they can also watch students. Finally, the administrative area is now a command-and-control center that is target hardened with maximum security measures for its protection as the school's nerve center. Because most interaction between administrators and students and teachers is by video, there is little if any need for students or teachers to access this area. Therefore, only staff who require access to the administrative area have electronic key cards. The central staff are a little different from the staff of schools in the last century. Besides the administrative staff, secretaries, and support personnel such as crisis workers, school resource police officers specially trained in dealing with school violence operate from a police-ready room. A central communications staff is in charge of all electronic surveillance and media from the central monitoring station.

The principal in this new-millennium school plays a somewhat secondary role. The co-administrator is the chief of security. That person does not have an education degree or teaching certificate but does have a criminal justice degree and experience in law enforcement as well as a thorough understanding of computer and security systems. In any emergency, the security chief is the primary decision-making authority. This will happen because principals do not have the necessary expertise to coordinate security any more than they would have the ability to operate a nuclear power plant! If you are having trouble picturing exactly what this new-millennium school looks like, a reasonable facsimile would be any correctional facility built in the past 10 years and a number of schools.

Universities will change also in the twenty-first century for those students who actually prefer to come on campus as opposed to taking courses online in their pajamas. Because campuses are spread out over many buildings, the preferred method of security will be a large compound with carefully guarded entrances and high, blast-proof walls topped with razor wire running along the entire perimeter. Access will be carefully controlled; students not only will have to show IDs, but they will also be subjected to iris, handprint, or voice recognition checks. No part of the university campus will be without surveillance cameras, which will be linked to a central command post. If any suspicious activity is spotted, a blue light will start flashing in that area and heavily armed police will be dispatched. Students will also have GPS transmitters that will immediately give their location anywhere on campus to central security (optional at the university level but definitely required in K–12). Students will be required to carry cell phones, and those cell phones must be turned on and keyed to a university threat and warning system that will automatically page the entire student body if a threat is imminent, followed by text message information telling students what to do.

Faculty will not like this safety feature because students' cell phones will often ring in class when students forget to put them in vibrate mode. Loudspeakers and intercoms all over campus will ensure that every person will be warned and receive evacuation instructions. All buildings will have electronic locking systems, which can be centrally activated immediately upon a threat announcement. All faculty and residence hall staff will be trained to recognize any early danger signs and threats of violence and make immediate referrals to the university threat assessment team. There will be few commuter students because of the hassle of getting through the checkpoints at the school compound entrances. Most students who do not live on campus will take courses by distance learning or online. Indeed, cars will be parked at least a quarter mile away from university buildings to reduce the threat from car bombs. The campus police chief will be much higher up in the chain of command and will operate out of a hardened command center with a number of technologists to keep all the security apparatus running.

Are you appalled at the idea of a school that is, in effect, a penitentiary? Although we have not seen a school with every one of the attributes just described, we *have* seen or heard of almost all of the components just mentioned in at least one school building in the United States. In fact, many experts in school safety have recommended the foregoing features (Astor, 1999; Blauvelt, 1998; Brock et al., 2009; Cowan & Paine, 2015; Dorn & Dorn, 2005; Giduck, 2005; Haynes & Henderson, 2001; Jimerson & Furlong, 2006; Nadel, 2004; National Association of School Psychologists, 2015; National Center for Educational Statistics, 2022; Poland, 1999; Schaffer, 2022; Steiner et al., 2021). Suffice it to say that there are numerous companies advertising online that can make the foregoing school building safety improvements happen.

Since the advent of the new millennium, school violence has been a hot topic among the media, politicians, parents, academics, and the general population. During that time, voluminous amounts of research, theory, and debate on both prevention and intervention have emerged on major topics of school violence such as shootings, suicide, and bullying and how to handle them (U.S. Department of Justice, 2022). This chapter is indeed concerned about those "hot" topics, but it is also concerned about the everyday crises that afflict students, teachers, administrators, and parents and how to plan for them.

Our somewhat tongue-in-cheek new-millennium school building or college campus may seem patently ludicrous in Carmi, Illinois; Red Lake, Ontario; Truth or Consequences, New Mexico; or your own hometown or your college alma mater. But to say that such a school building or college campus will never be built is to be so unaware of school violence in the United States and other countries that one would believe you have been living on another planet for the past 30 years. The violence that has arisen in schools is the reason many of these building modifications and security measures are being deemed necessary by more and more school districts and universities. In part, that is what this chapter is about.

Situational crises. School systems are generally able to deal with developmental crises because they are squarely in the middle of one of the greatest developmental crises of all, growing up! But they have not been prepared to deal with situational crises that arise unexpectedly and violently. Why is this so? First, it has simply not been deemed cost expedient to provide all the material and human support needed. These are not just brick and mortar issues either, and they have been going on for quite a while. Updating technology, the use of data analysis, better management and delivery systems for training, communication, and support are all human factors that require time, effort, and expense (Martinez-Prather, 2020; Pitcher & Poland, 1992; Steiner et al., 2021). So, our new-millennium, violence-proof school building is not cheap, and the support personnel to staff it will not be cheap either!

Conflicting Statistics

LO2 The Jeanne Clery Disclosure of Campus Security Policy and Campus Crime Statistics Act (20 U.S.C. 1092(f)), signed in 1990, was named in memory of Jeanne Clery, a freshman attending Lehigh University. On April 5, 1986, Jeanne was raped and murdered by Josoph Henry, a fellow student she did not know. The attack on Clery was one of 38 violent crimes recorded at the university in three years. Her parents argued that, had the university's crime record been known, Clery would not have attended. They sued, were awarded $2 million, and founded Security on Campus, a non-profit group. Her murder triggered a backlash against unreported crimes on campuses across the country.

The goal of the Clery Act is to ensure students, prospective students, parents, and employees have access to accurate information about crimes committed on campus and campus security procedures. The Clery Act requires colleges and universities to annually report all the crime that happens on their campus and distribute the report to current and prospective students and employees or risk getting fined for each undisclosed infraction, losing federal funding, and getting some bad publicity. The report is required to provide crime statistics for the prior three years, how safety and security measures are implemented, crime prevention program descriptions, and what actions are to be taken when alleged sex offenses occur.

The K–12 Equivalent of the Clery Act. So, you might suppose that K–12 schools would have pretty good statistical data on crime as well and provide that to their public like universities do. Not quite! What you are going to read is a best estimate from the annual *National Center of Educational Statistics Crime Report*, but it's probably conservative because K–12 school administrations fearful of bad publicity do not necessarily report all the crimes that occur in their buildings, nor do students who are fearful of their own safety.

Perhaps more problematic is that the high profile crimes, such as those at Columbine, Sandy Hook, Stoneman, Uvalde, and Virginia Tech, get far more attention than the tens of thousands of micro aggressions that occur every day and create a climate of fear and hostility in schools (Irwin et al., 2022). So, a great deal of debate goes on as to whether the 90,000 schools in the United States and the 50 million students who are in them are safe or not. Here are the current statistics. What do you think?

National Center of Educational Statistics Crime Report. The *Indicators of School Crime and Safety* reports on 23 indicators dealing with crime and safety in schools. It includes coverage of violent deaths, nonfatal criminal victimization, and bullying. It further analyzes school conditions, discipline problems, gangs, hate speech, and use and availability of drugs. It finally considers student perceptions of personal safety and the percentage of teachers who reported being threatened or attacked at school.

Incidents of Crime. As previously reported, crime in schools has gone down overall. The rate of nonfatal criminal victimization over the last decade has fallen from an average of 51/1000 to 11/1000 students. This decrease accelerated because of COVID-19 procedures, resulting in a 60 percent decline in the victimization rate in 2019–2021. However, if you put those small percentages into real numbers of victimizations, students ages 12–18 experienced 285,400 victimizations at school and 380,900 victimizations away from school. So put in real numbers, that is a whole lot of being a victim. Perhaps more ominously though, in 2020–2021 there were 93 school shootings with injuries and fatalities, the most since 2001 (Irwin et al., 2022).

Threats to Teachers. Verbal threats to teachers doubled from 2009–2010 at 5 to 10 percent in 2020–2021. Student acts of disrespect for teachers other than verbal abuse rose from 9 percent in 2009-2010 to 15 percent in 2019–2020, and widespread disorder in the classroom went up from 3 percent in 2009-2010 to 4 percent in 2019-2020. In the latest report of confirmed assaults, acts of violence against teachers rose from 4 percent in 2007-2008 to 6 percent in 2015-216 (Irwin et al., 2022). Again, those numbers are probably conservative. A survey done by *Education Week* (Langero, 2022) found that 4 of every 10 educators queried said at least one teacher in their district has been physically assaulted or attacked by a student in the past year. In addition, 10 percent of educators said they personally have been physically assaulted or attacked by a student, according to a survey of 1,042 district leaders, principals, and teachers conducted in 2022. Principals were the most likely to say they have been attacked, with 20 percent reporting such incidents. Eight percent of teachers reported being assaulted, and 5 percent of district leaders said they had similar experiences.

Disciplinary Action. Compared to the previous decade, discipline for student bullying dropped from 23 to 15 percent. There was a small decline in sexual harassment of other students from 3 to 2 percent. However, one wonders if the figures on cyberbullying are a factor in the overall disciplinary action decrease. Cyberbullying increased from 8 percent in 2009-2010 to 16 percent in 2019–2020 (Irwin et al., 2022).

While those are still big numbers, when percentages are changed into numbers for the 90 million children going to school, it really isn't a lot—unless, of course, you or your child was one of those statistics or was subject to a microaggression that was never reported. Schools have a long history of preparing for disasters such as tornadoes and fires that includes standard safety procedures. The situational crisis that involves violence perpetrated by others on students or teachers is not. Homicide is the second leading cause of death of children ages 5-18 in the United States Yet, schools are relatively safe places as far as lethality is concerned. School-associated violent deaths represent less than 1 percent to less than 2 percent of all homicides that occur among school-age children over the past 20 years (Anderson et al., 2001; Centers for Disease Control and Prevention (CDC), 2021).

It is not enough that schools must be prepared to deal with the direct effects of a crisis such as a suicide or homicide. School staff must also be prepared for a variety of metastasizing effects as news of a crisis event ripples out over cell phones and social media. How to deal with huge numbers of other students affected by the crisis? How to deal with critical and concerned parents? How to keep the school safe without trampling on the rights of individuals who may be under suspicion or alleged to have committed violent acts? How to deal with the media that may descend, vulture-like, on the school in the event of a crisis? In short, few if any institutions have as many issues to deal with when subjected to such a crisis as a school district does.

This chapter will not deal with the potential for terrorist attacks on a school or the effects of a terrorist attack on a community, but you should certainly not disabuse yourself of that notion. The parents, teachers, and students of School Number One in Beslan, Russia, know all too well what the ramifications are, and crisis interveners in the United States have certainly been thinking and planning for just such an occurrence (Dorn & Dorn, 2005; Forster, 2006; Giduck, 2005; Jimerson & Furlong, 2006; National School Safety and Security Services, 2013; National Terrorism Advisory System, 2023; Thompson, 2004; Webber et al., 2005) especially since 9/11. So far, the opening of this chapter sounds more like an introductory course in criminology than in crisis intervention. However, you are going to meet some principal players in school crisis intervention who don't look anything like your U.S. history teacher or school counselor or at least have very different roles than teaching you about government branches or filling out course schedules.

Violence and Youth

LO3   Why have today's youth become more violent? Poor parenting practices, an ineffective welfare system, marginalization of underserved populations and other disenfranchised students, availability of high-powered automatic weapons, racism, the growth of gangs, violence in homes, parental neglect and abuse, low academic achievement, bullying, social rejection, neurobiological factors, lack of male role models, hate crimes, physical and sexual abuse, drug and alcohol involvement, and early criminal activity are but a few of the ills that spill over into schools (American Academy of Child and Adolescent Psychiatry, 2017; Blauvelt, 1998; Bushman et al., 2016: Goldstein, 1991; Goldstein & Kodluboy, 1998; Grossman, 1995; Hazler, 1996; Miller, et al., 2003; Office of the Surgeon General, 2001; Pledge, 2003; Poland, 1994; World Health Organization (WHO), 2020).

Media Violence. Dr. James has a birthday t-shirt from his entomologist daughter, Shannon, of two stag beetles locked in deadly combat. Underneath the mortal combat insect scene is the inscription "Peer Review," which aptly characterizes the vociferous debate between academicians on the role of video games in fomenting violent behavior. This is a debate that has gone on acrimoniously in academic circles since the Columbine school shooting in 1999 of "Yes it does!" "No, it doesn't!" That debate has been played out in school PTA meetings, state legislatures, the president's office, and the Supreme Court (Brown, 2010). The United States does not have the corner on this controversy. It also gets played out in Brazil (Beckwith, 2023), Australia (Markey &Markey, 2010), Japan (Shibuya et al., 2009), and Germany (Möller, & Krahé, 2009) as international examples of the furor these games create as a possible causal agent of violent behavior and school shootings.

None other than the American Psychological Association (APA) has gotten involved in the debate, and though vacillating over time, took the position in a policy statement in 2005 (APA Task Force Technical Report, 2015) that "Scant evidence has emerged that makes any causal or correlational connection between playing violent video games and actually committing violent activities." Backtracking somewhat from that statement, the APA 2015 Task Force acknowledged rather equivocally "that violent video games strongly correlate with aggressive behavior, as well as anti-social behavior, but distinguishes between aggression and violence. Their review of current studies in this area described the link between violent video games and aggressive behavior as "both as an increase in negative outcomes such as aggressive behavior, cognition, and affect and as a decrease in positive outcomes such as prosocial behavior, empathy, and sensitivity to aggression."

In another somewhat turnabout, the APA's (2020) resolution on violent video games cited continued equivocal research and then went on to create a laundry list of further research topics to be examined in ferreting out valid outcomes. Indeed, Ferguson and associates (2020) re-reviewed the 2015 APA task force analysis and proposed that even aggression as an outcome should be taken cautiously. So, consider the following theories and decide for yourself. Are violent video games good or bad?

Perhaps the most chilling reasons, though, are proposed by David Grossman in his book *On Killing* (1995, pp. 302–305). He proposes that there are three learning theories at work: Classical conditioning is at work when one sits comfortably in front of a movie or television screen watching mayhem and carnage while eating popcorn and drinking a soda. Operant conditioning thrives at video arcades, which provide immediate feedback and rewards for killing and maiming. Social learning enters the scene when a whole new series of role models, such as Freddy Krueger, do not end up saving the girl and kissing the horse but slash the girl's throat and the horse's, too. Glorification of a thug culture interlaced with weapons, women as sexual objects, and drug use are cornerstones of contemporary music and media that cater to youth. Even the movie and television heroes are antiheroes and operate outside the law because the justice system is portrayed as weak and powerless.

It doesn't take a great deal of imagination after reading Grossman's book to understand why Westside Middle School in Jonesboro, Arkansas, and Columbine High School in Littleton, Colorado, became killing fields and why drive-by shootings occur at any number of other schools across the United States. There is a continuing debate on how much influence experiencing vicarious violence via television and video games has on the manifesting of that violence in children (APA, 2020a, b). That even covers brain imaging studies, some of which show a clear relationship between brain areas that regulate and govern emotion and images of violence (Bailey et al., 2011; Brummert-Lennings & Warburton, 2011; Englehardt et al., 2011; Hummer et al., 2010; Krahe & Moller, 2011; Krahe et al., 2011; Sestir & Bartholow, 2010), although others do not (Szycik et al., 2017). A large meta-analysis of violent media and aggression research by Anderson and his associates (2010) strongly suggests that exposure to violent video games is a causal risk factor for increased aggressive behavior. However, there are enough detractors (Ferguson, 2011; Ferguson et al., 2011; Ferguson & Kilburn, 2009, 2010) that the APA reversed its 2005 (Price, 2007) stand that the research strongly suggested a link between violent media and aggressive behavior (Azar, 2010). It may be that there are mediating factors such as family domestic violence, competition, and different degrees of exposure (Zhao & Jiang, 2010), and older adolescents may not have as much reaction as younger ones (Bucolo, 2011), but the preponderance of research shows that the two correlate, and almost any elementary school teacher can tell when students have been watching *South Park* the night before. In summary, while it cannot be said that media violence causes school shootings, Langman's (2009) in-depth examination of school shooters found that they often have a fascination with violent media and become obsessed with it (p. 8).

Modeling. Modeling is an extremely effective way to reinforce behavior. The field of counseling is a great example. Dr. Whisenhunt wants her students to understand empathic understanding. She first lectures her students on various techniques, such as open-ended questions and reflection of feelings. The students ask questions, and a classroom discussion ensues. However, empathic understanding and the techniques that facilitate it have only been talked about, not demonstrated. So, Dr. Whisenhunt models these techniques in real time in front of the students. The students watch her, ask questions, and then are allowed to try out the techniques for themselves under her watchful eyes and tuned-in ears in the classroom. Modeling also facilitates violence. Peggy Noonan, columnist for the *Wall Street Journal*, put it well when she wrote, after watching the video of Seung-hui Cho, the Virginia Tech murderer, "We'll be seeing more of that from thousands of disaffected teenagers who watched and thought, 'Wow! I could do that! Boy, would that teach them a lesson. Everybody would know me then!'" (Noonan, 2007).

Cho's role models were Dylan Klebold and Eric Harris of Columbine High School infamy. Who will see Cho as a role model to emulate? The showing of Cho's tape by television networks potentially over and over in the view of millions of children set him up as a role model for disaffected, bullied, and socially isolated children. Playing a violent video game such as *Grand Theft Auto*, putting "gangsta" pictures on TikTok, or watching videos of school shooters or slasher movies does not automatically make a child a schoolyard shooter. If that were true, every kid who played *Grand Theft Auto* would go on a murder spree. However, along with other contributing variables discussed later in this chapter, the potential for violence can grow until those biological, sociological, and psychological factors coalesce into a homicidal gestalt, and a meek little second grader turns into Freddy Krueger.

The lethality issues to be dealt with in this chapter include potential physical assault by gang members, bullies, the estranged violent student, and children with suicidal ideations. However, targeted violence against specific students is not the only crisis that schools face. In addition, natural disasters, terrorist assaults, drug misuse, physical and sexual abuse, medical emergencies, and classmate, parent, and teacher deaths are all seen as crises. Crisis in the context of a school, although similar to the definition in Chapter 1, "Approaching Crisis Intervention," has unique features because of the social structure of the school and the sense of community within the school (Allen et al., 2002). As such, a crisis affects more than one student. It has metastatic spreading effects that can tear at the very fabric of the school to the point of destabilizing it (Johnson, 2000, p. 18). Therefore, this chapter will also provide the basic elements of what a school crisis plan should entail as a best bet for prevention, intervention, and postvention, who the players are in that plan, and what their roles are when a crisis of any type strikes a school. To start, let's talk about gangs. Think there are no gangs in your area? Maybe you need to think again.

Gangs

Types of Gangs

LO4 Of all the other contributors to violent behavior, none appears to have the predictive validity and potential for violent behavior in high school as do gangs (Rainone et al., 2006). One piece of good news is that gang activity appears to be down, with only 9 percent of students reporting gang activity in their school compared to 20 percent in 2009 (Irwin et al., 2022). There are basically six types of gangs that human services workers in school districts are likely to encounter.

Homegrown Copycats/Wannabes. There is more than enough media representation of gang members to let every student in the United States who has access to cable TV, movies, magazines, music, or the internet set up a stereotypical Vicelords, Gangster Disciples, Crips, or Latin Kings–type gang (Goldstein & Kodluboy, 1998, p. 5; U.S. Office of Juvenile Justice and Delinquency Prevention, 1995). "Wannabe" status may make them more dangerous in their attempts to prove how tough and cool they are. Generally, they are short-lived. Makeup is composed of any ethnic group resident in the population.

Homegrown Survivalist, Aryan Nation, Neo–Nazi, Extreme Right–Wingers. These gangs are based on political/religious philosophies inculcated by adults and in response to the perceived "browning" of America and the supposed threat that entails. They are often supported both financially and/or morally as "youth corps" by both local and national organizations. Members are typically related to or are friends of adults who espouse such views. They may be transitory or stable in terms of membership, depending on adult support available. They specifically target ethnic/racial minority groups for violence. They are almost always White and "Christian" (Goldstein, 1991, p. 24; Goldstein & Kodluboy, 1998, p. 7; U.S. Office of Juvenile Justice and Delinquency Prevention, 1995).

Transients from Megagangs. Offshoots of megagangs are started by gang members moved to supposedly "safe" rural havens by parents seeking to escape the problems of big-city crime or feeling extreme pressure from law enforcement agencies in their city of origin (Goldstein & Kodluboy, 1998, p. 7; U.S. Office of Juvenile Justice and Delinquency Prevention, 1995). Their children are already members of the gangs they try to escape. These transported gang members start their own gangs in their new location. Racial/ethnic makeup may be mixed, but these gangs are typically ethnic group or race based.

Megagangs Opening New Territory. Increased competition in large metropolitan areas forces gangs to seek new territory to sell their wares (mainly drugs). Interstate arteries and towns adjacent to them are primary targets because of the ease of access (Goldstein & Kodluboy, 1998, p. 7). This is the most formidable type of gang organization. It has older adults who may derive their livelihood from its criminal enterprise. It has a clear hierarchy of members, a sophisticated organizational plan and operating rules, large numbers, recruitment programs, financial backing, and the will to be very violent in the pursuit of its interests. Racial/ethnic makeup of these gangs is predominately African American or Hispanic in the Midwest but may be a variety of nationalities on the east or west coasts. This is the stereotypical street gang of the media (U.S. Office of Juvenile Justice and Delinquency Prevention, 1995).

Smorgasbord Home Boys. Some small gangs are started for a variety of reasons, ranging from instrumental criminal behavior such as theft to expressive behavior such as hate crimes or responses to being perceived as social outcasts. The organizing themes of these gangs range from skinhead neo-Nazism to demonology and devil worship to auto theft to retaliation for perceived social injustices perpetrated on them. This gang type generally is transitory and short-lived, with small numbers of members. Depending on the type, it may avoid violence if theft is its major activity or may be extremely violent and sadistic if it is into racism, Satanism, or a response to social ostracism. It is mostly White in makeup (Goldstein & Kodluboy, 1998, p. 7; U.S. Office of Juvenile Justice and Delinquency Prevention, 1995).

Transnational gangs. With the influx of migrants from central America, the Mara Savatrucha (MS-13) and 18th St. gangs continue to expand their influence in the United States and recruit younger members and are now present in almost every state (FBI, n.d.; ICE, 2022).

Emergence of Suburban and Rural Gangs

Why be too concerned about gangs unless you work in a big, inner-city high school, right? That would be a mistake. Why have gangs or the threat of gang formation become problematic for suburban and rural areas? A variety of trends have emerged that make gang formation a probability for Opie in Mayberry, rural America (Howell, 2015; Watkins & Taylor, 2016). The development of diverse, multicultural communities in the United States will proceed at an accelerated rate in the 21st century, particularly in historically White farming communities of the Midwest (Goldstein & Kodluboy, 1998, pp. 63–91). Like many countries, the United States has generally not had a stellar history of welcoming and integrating newcomers who don't look, talk, act, and think like Americans. The contemporary debate over illegal immigrants coming into the United States from the Mexican border is a prime example. Cable television, the internet, and other electronic information systems make the most pristine and rustic rural areas a part of the global community. The glorification of violence and gangs through electronic media sends children who feel powerless against the world messages about how they can be powerful (Goldstein & Kodluboy, 1998, p. 7).

Chat rooms, websites, and e-mail provide gangs plenty of opportunity to talk to Opie. If Opie is feeling alone and powerless out on 1300 Country Road East, he is likely to talk back. All of the ills that assail dysfunctional families are as characteristic of suburban and rural families as they are of urban ones (DeWitte, 2019; Fernández-Planells et al., 2021) Gang leaders are highly sensitive to these parentless, neglected kids and, like Fagan in *Oliver Twist,* recruit them. The gang becomes a surrogate family (Grossman, 1995, pp. 303–305; Melton, 2001).

Gang Intervention/Prevention Programs

Although this book is about crisis intervention, the fact is that when dealing with gangs, prevention is far more likely to be effective than intervention. After a gang has taken root and grown, fear and intimidation become huge obstacles to constructive change. Changing gang members' attitudes about gang membership is anything but easy. Gang members typically fall into what are called "at-risk" student categories. By definition, "at risk" means that a young person is liable to have underdeveloped academic and socialization skills. when the potential for becoming a responsible and productive adult is limited by barriers at home, at school, or in the community (Fusick & Bordeau, 2004). At-risk students are truant; have trouble with the legal system; are characterized by impulsive behavior, self-doubts, anxiety, depression, drug use, and suicidal ideation; are poor learners; and have few bonds with the culture of the school (National Gang Center, 2021). They are what Melton (2001) calls "phantom students" because, much like the Phantom of the Opera, they wear tough masks to

hide their emotional scars and largely remain in the shadows of the school culture.

Because of the publicized school shootings in recent years, a great deal of interest has been generated in what are believed to be two of its root causes—at-risk students and bullying or being bullied. While not all at-risk students are gang members, many gang members are at-risk students, lost between the cracks and dropping out of school. Not all bullies are gang members, but the reverse is generally true because bullies and gangs both gain power and control over others by fear, threat, and intimidation. Therefore, in discussing intervention methods with "gang" members, the same characteristics and procedures also apply to at-risk students and bullies. Violence prevention approaches are legion; they range from teaching students warning signs of impending student violence (Alvarez, 1999), implementing anonymous warning systems (Hsing-Fang et al., 2022), universal school-based social-emotional development programs, after school, stay-off-the-streets programs, and mentor programs (Ferndon et al., 2016) to teaching body movement exercises for self-control (Kornblum, 2002). The following approaches have all been tried, with varying degrees of success, with children who make up the bulk of gang membership.

Counseling. Counseling, in the sense of having a continuing, person-centered, nonevaluative, nonjudgmental dialogue with a gang member, is one of the least effective intervention strategies (Lipsey, 1992). Given their past experiences with uncaring and punitive adults, alienated and disenfranchised gang members are suspicious and do not establish relationships easily. They are ultrasensitive to perceived threats and insults, and they are manipulative and reluctant to share information (Melton, 2001). Taylor-Austin (2023) makes a strong argument for using reality therapy's (Glasser, 1965) WDEP System. This approach explores the client's wants and needs, direction and doing, evaluation, planning, and commitment. Taylor-Austin maintains that Reality Theory has demonstrated itself to be a concrete approach and one that youth can understand and relate to easily. John and Rita Sommers-Flanagan (1997) propose that challenging such kids in regard to the consequences of their actions is an excellent way to start establishing rapport and trust.

CW: So you don't want to be in here getting this counseling "crap." Is that about right?

Gang Member: Yeah, that's right. I'm outta here.

CW: OK. I'll just call your probation officer, and he can make the arrangements for you to go to the Wilder Youth Facility if you don't want to do this. Now, you are adjudicated here for 12 sessions, but since you don't want to be here, I can see us doing this in, say, 6 sessions, if you are smart enough to catch onto this stuff and not give me a bunch of "crap," as you say, and work hard to get through this stuff. What's your choice?

Counseling that uses reality therapy (Glasser, 1965, 2000) and targets behavior and consequences of actions is more likely to be successful when gang members are constantly confronted with their actions and given choices as to what they want to do (Loeber et al., 1998; Sandhu, 2000; Taylor-Austin, 2023). The same is true of victims.

Lucinda: (Lucinda has been absent from school the last 3 days and is talking to the school counselor about her absences. Finally, she breaks down sobbing and tells the counselor why.) This is the fifth time the Rosebuds have taken my lunch money in the past 2 weeks, but they threatened to break my legs, and they can do that. I've seen Tina do that with a ball bat. She's crazy and scares me to death. They also told me not to snitch or they would hurt my little sister.

School Counselor: Lucinda, I'd really like to get Officer Bates, she's the SRO if you haven't met her, in on this and have you tell her. It is not your fault that you are being mugged. You didn't ask for it, and you don't deserve it. It isn't normal, and it isn't OK. You don't have to face this on your own. I and other people will help you.

Lucinda: No way! No cops! I could get killed.

School Counselor: I understand that it's scary, and there are some real risks. We will keep this confidential, and no one will know but the three of us. But you are not the only one who is getting mugged. You can make a choice about helping to stop this. I have an idea you are pretty tired of getting assaulted. School should be a place to come and have fun with your friends and learn. It is not a place you should be afraid to come to. Officer Bates and I are working with a lot of teachers and other kids. If enough kids like you say, "That's enough!" We can stop this. I won't force you to see the school police officer or even tell her about the mugging. I think your parents need to

know about this though. If you want to have your parents come in and talk, we can do that too. The choice is yours.

The counselor acknowledges the danger to Lucinda as real. Attempts to coerce a student into informing are fraught with ethical peril and quite literally can be dangerous to the student if a great deal of care is not taken to keep the information confidential until the school and law enforcement are ready to act. However, if the counselor feels that the threat to Lucinda is high (see the definitions of low, medium, and high threats later in the chapter), her parents should be informed, and so should the police.

So, what does a comprehensive, school-wide gang abatement program encompass that can alleviate the kinds of problems students like Lucinda encounter?

Guidance Programs. Passive, lecture-based guidance programs that target fear arousal, moral appeal, and self-esteem building have not proven to be highly effective (Gottfredson, 1998) in dealing with gangs or bullying. Active guidance programs that provide direct student involvement through modeling, role play, and behavioral rehearsal in areas such as anger management, bullying, conflict resolution, and peer mediation are more helpful in tackling gang and bullying issues (American School Counselor Association, 2021; Beane, 1999; Coloroso, 2003; Curran & Wexler, 2017; Davis & Davis, 2003; Feindler & Scalley, 1998; Gottfredson et al., 1998; Henebery, 2021; Hazler, 1996; Horne et al., 2003; Larson, 1994; Lupton-Smith et al., 1996; Sexton-Radek, 2004; Walker, 2019). To be effective, these programs must not be a one-shot session but should have continuous behavioral rehearsal and feedback sessions built into them. They must also have clear, easily implemented practices, be intense, and continue long enough with follow-up sessions to reinforce and change some very resistant behaviors in both victims and victimizers (Gottfredson et al., 1998; Sullivan, 2011; Willard, 2007; Zins et al., 1994).

Peer Counseling/Peer Mediation. One of the very *worst* approaches is to use peer crisis workers who are gang members or bullies or for the crisis worker to attempt to run homogeneous counseling groups composed entirely of gang members or bullies (Goldstein & Kodluboy, 1998, pp. 107–110). The gang members or bullies will take over the group. However, there is some evidence that heterogeneous counseling groups, those in which students are chosen from a representative cross-section of the ethnic, social, and economic strata of the school, are useful in helping gang members look at alternative solutions and develop new behaviors. There is also some evidence that a peer counseling/leader program that provides mentoring, tutoring, and support functions keeps at-risk and marginalized students out of trouble and in school (Allen, 1996; Cohen et al., 1982; Fatum & Hoyle, 1996; Scruggs et al., 1985).

Peer mediation (Cassinerio & Lane-Garon, 2006; Day-Vines et al., 1996; Schrumpf et al., 1997; Walker, 2019) is another approach that uses students to deal with other students who have anger problems. While it may seem that the last thing a gang member or bully would be willing to submit to is peer mediation, it should be remembered that peer pressure and the need to conform exert a tremendous amount of pressure on all students.

Further, if students are unwilling to submit to peer mediation, they are ratcheting up the consequences by essentially saying, "I am not willing to try to work this out." Institutional use of these programs should start in elementary schools and be continuously carried through middle and high schools so there is a clear, consistent, and longitudinal approach to providing support to alienated, angry, and disenfranchised students. In fact, elementary schools are the best place to stop bullying, harassment, prejudice, and other forms of problem behavior.

Anger Management. A variety of anger management techniques have been developed to work with adolescents and children (Davis, 2004; Efrid, 2013; Feindler & Weisner, 2006; Nelson et al., 2006; Smith et al., 2006). Most of these approaches involve skill training and behavior rehearsal in prosocial behaviors, the social (reputation) and financial costs (jail and fines), and teaching students cognitive techniques that cool off their hot cognitions about stressful situations. While anger management approaches are effective in reducing abusive verbal and physical responses (Humphrey & Brooks, 2006; Rosenberg, 2004; Sharp & McCallum, 2005; Smith et al., 2006), the problem is their pervasiveness and the environmental variables from both the home and the street that oftentimes see control of anger as weakness instead of strength.

After-School and Community Outreach Programs. As Goldstein and Kodluboy (1998, p. 126) state, "Playing on a basketball team means you are not stealing a car while you're at the game, but it does not prevent you from stealing a car before or after the game." Research indicates that although such after-school programs may have recreational value, they are not highly effective in delinquency reduction. However, programs such as the Boys and Girls Clubs of America that have a comprehensive curriculum integrating recreation with academic and social skill building and career and personal counseling do have high potential for stopping delinquency and reducing gang activity (Sherman et al., 1997).

National Violence Prevention Programs. When violence reduction in gangs has been tried, a major problem has been that gang membership is a proximity and affiliation motivator where the culture and the expectancies of the gang promote and encourage violent behavior (Van Brunt, 2015, p. 126). There are many national and commercially available anger management and violence reduction programs available that specifically target elementary, middle, and secondary school levels (Farrell & Camou, 2006). These programs have ranged from violence prevention curriculums (Prothrow-Stith, 1987) to computer-based conflict resolution (Bosworth et al., 1996) to making physical changes such as brightly lit hallways, limiting access to lockers and keeping graffiti off walls (California Department of Education, 2002), and enlisting coaches in violence prevention programs (Jamie et al., 2015). The U.S. Department of Health and Human Services (HHS) published a highly negative review of school violence programs that a lot of money had been spent on and pessimistically noted that nothing much in the way of manualized programs worked in reducing youth violence (USDHHS, 2001). One of the major problems that Farrell and Camou (2006) report is that little rigorous, evidence-based research has been done that could provide valid information on antiviolence programs in schools that actually work. While this research was reported 10 years ago, as of yet, little in the way of change has been reported. Pretty clearly, programs that appear to work need to have all the trapping of rigorous research such as control groups, reliable and valid assessment devices, and the ability to be replicated. Even then, a one-size-fits-all approach is probably not attainable. It is more likely that successful programs will deal with specific populations and specific conditions and environments within which that population operates (Farrell & Camou, 2006).

Schools. Schools and school districts are not without culpability in the growth and development of gangs, bullying, and violence. Megaschools and megadistricts limit many students' participation in the academic and extracurricular activities of the school; because of the large numbers of students and the criteria that restrict who can participate, relatively few students in very large schools take part in such activities as band or sports or even the chess team (Goldstein & Kodluboy, 1998, pp. 21–22). Schools can play an active role in the prevention and intervention of gang activity. Schools need to set a number one priority of inclusiveness, nurturance, school as community, and the philosophy that no student is left behind either academically or socially (Cypress & Green, 2002). This concept is particularly important in schools where heterogeneity (diversity) of race and culture is the norm. Fairness and consistency for everybody, with open communication among stakeholders, are essential.

Communication flows not only outward from the administration but also inward to them. There must be fair rules and clear sanctions that are enforced evenly in school (Goldstein & Kodluboy, 1998, p. 22). There should be an expectation of success. The total philosophy of the system, starting in kindergarten and working its way up through high school, should not be "If you graduate," but "When you graduate" (Allen, 1996).

Gangs grow in a vacuum. A school is asking for trouble if it has unmonitored areas, such as parking lots and bathrooms; dismisses rumors about planned violence or weapons, drugs, or other contraband brought onto school grounds; excuses the violent behavior of "good kids"; or sees intervention in any of the foregoing areas as "not my job" (Dykeman, 1999; Remboldt, 1994). A school reduces violence when its staff and teachers have high expectations, care about and are involved with their students in inclusive ways, enforce rules and procedures, maintain buildings and keep classrooms neat and clean, and believe it's everyone's job to do so (Stephens, 1997).

School safety goes beyond high-tech security systems. School safety is a sense of not only physical well-being but also psychological well-being. Schools can maintain or take back their turf when they cooperatively develop mission statements; share decisions about school policies; maintain buildings and remove graffiti; organize gang awareness and prevention programs; promote parental and student involvement; allow zero tolerance of bullying, harassment, or gang recruitment; and have school authorities that declare, "This is our turf, not yours" (Blauvelt, 1998; Brock et al., 1996). Instead of asking, "How do I know which students will shoot next?" the question might be, "What is the faculty doing to build quality relationships with students and open lines of communication and to develop the type of climate that will foster a wholesome sense of self in each individual as well as respect for others?" (Cypress & Green, 2002). But preventing gang growth and violence is a task that is much too great for a single school counselor, social worker, psychologist, teacher, or principal—or even a school system.

The Community. It takes everybody in the community working as a team to combat gangs. Cooperation with other agencies such as the courts, corrections, probation, parole, mental health, public assistance, and housing is crucial. Civic and religious organizations must provide personnel and financial support. City and county governments must be willing to put in place ordinances that say there is zero tolerance for this kind of behavior and back it up with law and code enforcement (Bemak & Keys, 2000; Miller et al., 2003; Schaefer-Schiumo & Ginsberg, 2003).

Louvre (2008) makes a compelling argument for integrating community action in school crises. She is puzzled why there is so little outrage over the 97 percent of child murders that occur outside of school walls every year. Louvre argues persuasively that rebuilding trust and a sense of community in a school after a crisis requires the total participation of the community. That is what SARA (scanning, analysis, response, and assessment; Eck & Spelman, 1987), the Justice Department's model for combating gangs, is about. SARA is not about getting rid of gangs in one day. This model is based on the idea that visible signs of crime such as "broken window" or neglected property is tolerated more serious crimes will occur (Ruhi, 2023). The model focuses on little victories, such as getting loiterers off school property and cleaning up graffiti. It gets all of the stakeholders in having a safe community involved in continuous and ongoing linkages that set goals and generate plans to achieve the continuous little victories that make SARA so effective. Turf guarding and political boundaries have no place in a fight to eradicate gangs (Roth, 2000). This approach benefits communities by not letting gangs gain a further foothold in the community, resulting in improved performance by students who went to school in fear each day; decreased teacher stress and burnout; decreased need for security staff/equipment; fewer injuries and lives lost; and most important, renewed freedom in the school and the community.

School Resource Officer

LO5 Along with public outcries against the punitive behavior of general law enforcement, school resource officers (SROs) have come in for their share of criticism in the twenty-first century. Chief among them has been the concept of a school-to-prison pipeline, particularly for students who have been historically systematically excluded, that has been exacerbated by arrest procedures by SROs under zero tolerance programs. Indeed, large cities such as Portland, Minneapolis, and Denver have gotten rid of police in schools. Some research shows that their presence results in increased rates of exclusionary discipline, which disproportionately impacts Black students, especially those in schools with zero-tolerance discipline policies. Exclusionary discipline not only negatively impacts student academic outcomes, but it also increases the likelihood of interaction with the justice system (Perez, 2020). The Brookings research group on criminal justice reform made this statement: "While typically referred to as School Resource Officers, School Police Officers is a more accurate way to describe law enforcement officers detailed to schools based on historical practices. These individuals are trained police officers that function like an arm of local law enforcement rather than counselors or other support services that provide essential resources to staff and students. The "Resource" in School Resource Officers is often a misnomer (King & Schindler, 2021). Thus, we are devoting time and space to this debate because the role of law enforcement is a critical one in forming the cooperative teams and interdisciplinary approach we believe are critical in the promotion of safe schools in the twenty-first century.

Two studies characterize the debate. Theriot's (2009) research findings show that school resource officers (SROs) were not associated with an increase in total arrests when controlling for school poverty, and schools with an SRO had fewer arrests for weapons and assault charges. The results were contrary to the criminalization hypothesis of SRO presence and may even signify that SROs have a positive impact at schools.

Counter pointing Theriot, Na and Gottfredson (2013) found that schools with SROs had more minor crimes, more serious crimes, and higher rates of expulsions than schools without SROs and inferred that SROs were the causative factor in the increased arrest rates at those schools compared to those without SROs. The question raised in this study though is that SROs tended to be assigned to schools that already had significant crime problems as opposed to those who did not, and with higher crime rates, higher arrests would be expected.

Johnson's (2016) review of SRO research found the following outcomes: SROs were no more likely to arrest students than police officers operating on regular patrol, even though they were exposed to more misconduct situations. Further, they tended to downgrade charges from felony assault down to disorderly conduct and were more lenient when misdemeanor and status offenses occurred. Finally, Johnson found that in self-reports by SROs they considered themselves more than just law enforcement but acting at times as social workers, educators, and surrogate parents. The Education Research Center (2018) survey of 400 SROs found similar results in their perceived job roles. While a majority of officers said enforcing the law and safety and security were their primary roles, they also had a role in mentoring and teaching, and over a third interviewed indicated that they fulfilled a variety of other roles participating with students and school activities. The vast majority had received training in active shooters, but fewer than half had received training in child trauma or developmental issues of teenagers, although SROs were more likely to receive across the board training in crisis intervention issues than their peers from school police departments.

The National Institute of Justice review of school policing found the following in their review of school policing (McKenna & Petrosino, 2022). There is consensus that standard police training is inadequate, and specialized training in dealing with students in school settings is highly variable across the country. Little attention is paid to apprenticeship and mentoring from competent veteran SROs when placing new SROs in schools. Overall, research found that school policing was not an effective strategy and is correlated with some harmful effects. The problem is that how school policing is implemented varies dramatically from jurisdiction to jurisdiction and even within schools in the same district.

So why, then, would we be promoting an SRO presence in schools? This issue severely muddles any previous outcomes and results in three of the five major recommendations for school policing programs the reviewers (MeKenna & Petrosino, 2022) made that call for more controlled and rigorous research studies with good control comparisons. That included a recommendation on both practice and research on the selection for school positions. Their fourth recommendation dealt with training specific to working in schools, and their fifth recommendation was implementing and testing a consistent set of implementation measures for setting up and operating school policing programs. They concluded with offering no opinion on whether to limit, expand, or remove police officers from schools.

Yet, the fact is that there are outside lethality threats to schools and indeed problems within schools that go far beyond misconduct and disciplinary referrals. A vivid example is the public outcry for the reinstitution of SROs in the Denver schools after a school shooting that left two deans dead at East High School in Denver and the school board's hasty reinstitution of the SRO program.

We have seen excellent SRO officers in operation, and you will soon meet one. We believe, as with CIT officers, if proper training and support is given to SRO officers, they can have a significant impact on school safety, and training modeled after the National Association of School Resource Officers (NASRO, n.d.) triad model is one way that can happen. NASRO is a not-for-profit organization for school-based law enforcement officers, school administrators, and school security/safety professionals working as partners to protect students, faculty, staff, and their school community. NASRO was founded on the "triad" concept of school-based policing. The triad concept divides the SRO's responsibilities into three areas: Educator, Informal Counselor/Mentor, and Law Enforcement Officer. NASRO (2022) offers basic and advanced courses in implementing the model. Training includes learning how to establish collaborative working relationships with school staff and establish interagency cooperation. There is instruction on school law and ethics to guide legal and ethical decision making while working with children in school buildings. Instructional blocks cover adolescent brain development, establishing and maintaining successful relationships with diverse students, supporting students with disabilities, adolescent mental health issues, substance misuse, suicide, digital culture, and human trafficking. Additional modules cover safety concerns, including de-escalation skills, threat assessment, armed assailant responses, and strategies for planning, preventing and responding to life threatening emergencies in coordination with school staff. While the course is right on target,

cost-conscious departments may not be willing to pay the $500 tuition.

Indeed, we have seen cost-conscious police departments shuffle off patrol officers who are ineffective into supposedly "easy" school officer roles directing traffic and monitoring athletic events. Nothing could be further from the truth. Hiring high-quality personnel for SRO positions is critical, and beyond training, they should have demonstrated the ability to teach and engage youth such as past coaching, mentorship experiences, and excellence in communication skills and interpersonal skills coupled with how students communicate in person and through social media (Hoppe, 2019). Officer Scott Davis, who you are about to meet, has been an effective patrol officer, an effective crisis intervention team officer, and is an effective, trained SRO who brings critical training and those communication tools to crisis intervention in school buildings. But why bring Scott in? Why not just hire additional human service personnel?

The "why" is this. The crisis worker attempts to bring the school resource police officer (SRO) into the crisis because multidisciplinary school pupil personnel service teams that involve the SRO are critically important to stopping threatening and intimidating behavior (COPS, n.d.; James et al., 2011; O'Toole, 2003; Welsh & Domitrovich, 2006). Police in the schools can do much more than direct after-school traffic and monitor ball games. Coordinating intelligence between the police department and the school, working conjointly with school human services workers in gang prevention programs, helping students problem-solve, finding resources and making referrals, deterring violence, obtaining information about illegal activities, role modeling, and mentoring are proactive measures that integrate police officers into the fabric of the school (Dogutas, 2008; Finn, 2006; Finn et al., 2005; Italiano, 2001; James et al., 2011; NASSP, 2023; Petersen, 2008; Vancleave, 2008).

If you read any of the statistics at the beginning of this chapter, it should be apparent why SROs are in school buildings. They are there not only to preserve the peace but also to provide support to troubled students by building rapport with them, serving as empathic listeners, and eliciting information. As such, they are excellent conduits to provide information to school officials that might not otherwise be forthcoming (James et al., 2011). Because many SROs, such as Officer Davis, have training to intervene with individuals with mental illness and/or emotionally disturbances, they make excellent first-line interventionists—particularly when the presence of an authority figure is needed with students in crisis who are emotionally and behaviorally out of control (James et al., 2011). We strongly urge that human services workers and school administrators incorporate these police officers as part of a comprehensive pupil personnel services team that deals with students at high risk for violence because what they do works (Johnson, 1999).

Meet school resource and crisis intervention team (CIT) officer Scott Davis of the Montgomery County, Maryland, Police Department (Personal communication, October 2016). Officer Davis is responsible for policing a high school, a middle school, and three elementary schools. Officer Davis's day starts with roll call at 6 a.m. He patrols the neighborhood and keeps an eye out for people or activities that don't belong and other potential problems. This past month, one of those problems included a very large gang fight that brought a number of police officers to the scene to break up the melee. Because those involved are "his kids," he takes a personal interest in the incident. He follows up with those who were arrested and looks for any others who might have been involved. Occasionally during the day, he will hop in his cruiser and look for students who are truants. He spends about 75 percent of his time at the high school and 20 percent at the middle school, with drop-in visits to his three elementary schools. His first task of the day is to meet with the high school principal in the morning, go over any potential problems that might be occurring before school, and greet the students as they come in the front door. Parents come to his office to talk about problems their kids are having. During the day, he checks out a number of students who have been having problems and promotes his Boy Scout Police Explorer program.

At first glance, his job appears pretty humdrum, but what isn't apparent is that Officer Davis is putting his considerable CIT skills to use every day with "humdrum" stuff and using the same skills when things are boiling over. Laura is 17 years old and has run away. A social worker has been called to the school and is attempting to take her back to a bad home situation. Officer Davis has personal knowledge of the home because he has responded to a disturbance call there. Laura's mother has a drug dependency and is long gone from the home. Laura tried to hit her father with a brick in one argument, so it is clear that home is not very workable. As Officer Davis makes the scene, tensions are rising between Laura and the social worker, who is threatening to have Laura arrested.

Officer Davis: (in a calm but authoritative voice) All right, let's just everybody cool off! First off, you can't have her arrested for a status offense. It's clear home isn't working real well, so Laura, let's you and me go to my office and talk about what's going on and what you think needs to happen.

As Laura explains her situation, Officer Davis asks numerous open-ended questions to allow her to ventilate. He finds out she has a drinking problem but only occasionally uses other drugs. Home is intolerable, but she does come to school. He also finds out she has been diagnosed with Bipolar I but is not taking her medication because of the side effects.

Officer Davis: OK, let's try this. How about going to the crisis center with me. I've got some friends there who might be able to help both in regard to the medication and a place to stay. It may not be exactly what you want, but it beats going home and running away again, 'cause that doesn't seem to be working real well for you. I'll stay there with you and see what they can do. How about it?

Laura: Hey! You're kinda different. Most cops push people around. OK. I'll give it a try.

Officer Davis takes her to the crisis center, where she is evaluated and indeed prescribed different medication. She is also placed in a short-term foster home until her medication can be regulated.

Laura: (a month later, in school, waves to Officer Davis) Hey! Remember me?

Officer Davis: Sure, Laura. How are things going?

Laura: Not real great, but I'm getting by. I went back home. The old man and I are sorta getting along.

Officer Davis: Hey! You're here, aren't you! Best place you can be! Here, you've got options. The more you're here, the less you're at home. Thought about any after-school activities or sports? Get your grades up, and pretty soon the only time you are at home is to eat and sleep.

Officer Davis enthusiastically reinforces Laura for making it to school. Laura's future will be filled with challenges, but at least she is in school, has made contact with somebody, and feels like somebody is really interested in her. These are little victories in the everyday grind of working in a school, but added up, they can win wars for hearts and minds when working with kids who are troubled. But Officer Davis's life is about to take an exciting turn, and we will return to him later in the chapter.

Bullying

LO6 Probably no other topic has received as much attention in the school counseling literature and at conferences in the past 20 years as face-to-face bullying and, more recently, cyberbullying (Chamberlin, 2006; Holladay, 2010; Hornor, 2018; Howe et al., 2013; Munsey, 2012; Paterson, 2010; Sabella, 2010; Suniti Bhat et al., 2010; Swearer & Hymel, 2015)—its causes (Crothers & Levinson, 2004; Espelage et al., 2000), effects (Carney, 2008; Sullivan, 2011; Willard, 2007), and intervention strategies (Bauman, 2011; Burnham, 2011; Burrow-Sanchez et al., 2011; Hicks, 2015; Leo, 2010; Newman et al., 2000; Paterson, 2011; Ratts et al., 2009; Saufler, 2010; Shallcross, 2013; Sullivan, 2011; Willard, 2007). That is particularly true with regard to gay, lesbian, bisexual, and transgender (LGBTQIA+) students (Callahan, 2001; Jackson & Harding, 2010; Jones Farrelly & Robles-Fernandez, 2011; McCollum, 2010; Windmeyer, 2009), who have little power or support systems in most K–12 buildings. Because of bullying, LGBTQIA+ youths' risk of depression and suicide may be greatly increased (Russell et al., 2011), and that becomes even more profound when cyberbullying occurs (Wiederhold, 2014). According to data from the School Crime Supplement (National Crime Victim Survey, 2022), about 22 percent of students ages 12–18 reported being bullied in 2019-2020, which is significantly lower than the 28 percent reported in 2009. Girls got bullied more than boys, at 25 percent versus 19 percent. Middle schoolers versus high schoolers were bullied 27 to 28 percent to 16 to 19 percent. Students of mixed race experienced higher percentages than any other single race children with reports of mixed race, 37 percent; White, 24.6 percent; Black, 22.2 percent; Hispanic, 18 percent; Asian, 13.5 percent. Even more regrettably, students with disabilities are two to three times more likely to be bullied than are their peers without disabilities. Further, bullying is not just a problem in the United States. Every continent in the world reports high incidences of school bullying behavior either in face-to-face confrontations or by cyberbullying, such as in Thailand (Noipom et al., 2023), Brazil (Azeredo et al., 2023), Norway (Fossum et al., 2023), Canada (Vaillancourt et al., 2023), and China (Chan et al., 2023). These studies are capped off by Smith et al. (2023) who surveyed 29 countries from Africa, Asia, and the Americas and found the mean prevalence of bullying to be close to 40 percent on average and

Ioverrno's (2023) survey of LGBTQIA+ youth in 30 European countries that found consistent negative reactions to their sexual and gender identity including sadness/depression, fears for safety, continuing harassment, and physical violence.

The crisis dimensions this problem has taken on culminated in a White House Conference on Bullying in March 2011. That conference sought to establish replicable training and intervention programs that were cost effective and time manageable for teachers already stretched thin (Munsey, 2011). The fact that a number of elementary, middle, and high school students who have died by suicide because of bullying and cyberbullying in the past few years has gotten the attention of the federal government and caused the Department of Education to assist in bullying prevention. In 2010, a technical assistance best practice memo highlighting comprehensive state antibullying laws was sent to state school officers and governors. The Office for Civil Rights at the Department of Education and the Department of Justice are working together and will vigorously pursue complaints of bullying and harassment. This information and much more is available at https://www.stopbullying .gov/ (U.S. Department of Health and Human Services, 2015). This online document is reader-friendly and details cyberbullying, federal laws concerning stopping it, school involvement in stopping it, and what kids can do to prevent it. Besides the veritable tsunami of commercial and professional information online on bullying prevention, the U.S. Department of Health and Human Services (2021) has a community action tool kit available to anybody who wants to start an antibullying program training toolkit at https://www.stopbullying.gov/prevention /in-the-community.

Bullying and intimidation affect large numbers of students. In 2007, 32 percent of U.S. students ages 12–18 reported having been bullied at school that year. In this survey, 21 percent of students said they had been made fun of; 18 percent reported being the subject of rumors; 11 percent said they were pushed, shoved, tripped, or spit on; 6 percent said they were threatened with harm; 5 percent said they were excluded from activities on purpose; and 4 percent said that someone had tried to make them do things they did not want to do or that their property had been destroyed on purpose (National Center for Education Statistics, 2010). That percentage has gone down for face-to-face bullying to about 15 percent (Irwin et al., 2022) although perhaps this is a false negative since a Pew (2022) research study found that 46 percent of teens surveyed had been cyberbullied.

Bullying can take a number of forms (Shallcross, 2013). It can be direct, such as hitting, kicking, or pushing a person. It can be verbal, such as malicious teasing, threatening, or taunting. It can be social aggression, where the leader of a clique influences the group to target a specific individual. It can be overt or covert and involve physical or verbal aggression or more subtle approaches such as rumors, gossip, and social exclusion (Bauman, 2011, p. 18; Shallcross, 2013). It can be relational, in which individuals who have been friends cease to be, and in their acrimony, maliciously attempt to exclude that person from social activities and spread disparaging rumors about the other person (Shallcross, 2013).

Langman (2009) defines bullying as having three components: First, the bully has more power than the victim, because of larger size, greater strength, or greater numbers (clique or gang). Second, bullying involves intimidation through threats to the point that victims are made to fear for their safety. Third, bullying involves a pattern of behavior, not a onetime push (p. 12).

Bullies are proactive aggressors who use aggression methodically, subtly, and with increasing intensity until they achieve their desired goal of personal gain of some kind. Bullying is preplanned and calculated to instill fear and gain control over others with little remorse for its effects on them (Hubbard et al., 2001; McAdams & Schmidt, 2007; Vitaro & Brendgen, 2005; Vitaro et al., 2002). An entire school can be affected by systematic bullying behaviors. If left unchecked, an atmosphere of fear, mistrust, and low morale, along with the academic and behavioral problems that go with a hostile work environment, can create a negative atmosphere for all students (Hoover & Hazler, 1991). Finally, if left unchecked, bullying as a form of aggression can lead to lethal behavior from either the bully or the bullied.

Cyberbullying

Cyberbullying, simply defined, means using technology to harass, humiliate, or threaten someone (Holladay, 2010). Cyberbullying is different from face-to-face bullying. In face-to-face bullying, the effects are immediately known, and the victims know who the bullies are and who their supporters are. Cyberbullying can be far more insidious because the bully can remain unknown (Fortinet, 2023; Shallcross, 2013). Effects can also be more disastrous because the messages can go to an audience literally in the

millions (Bauman, 2011, p. 19). Ominously, research by Nagata et al. (2022) found strong associations between adverse childhood events and cyberbullying, with children who had been physically and sexually abused and suffering from household neglect being high targets for cyberbullying. Research along the lines of cyberbullying as a traumatic causative agent led Vismara et al. (2022) to propose it as a possible mental condition itself.

There are nine types of cyberbullying (Bauman, 2011, p. 57; Fortinet, 2023; Willard, 2007, p. 2):

Flaming refers to angry offensive language. "You are a shit-brained slut."

Harassment is the technology version of discriminatory or hostile behavior toward someone based on gender, race, religion, disability, or sexual orientation. "Jay is a wimpy, gimpy, greasy foreigner."

Denigration is sending or posting defaming information about someone. "Jennifer is screwing every boy on the hockey team . . . and the coach too!"

Masquerading is using someone else's identity to send messages that are rude and inappropriate. "Leslie, you stink! Literally! Get some feminine hygiene products. Signed Phewwwie! Joey" (a guy Leslie is interested in, but so is Devonne, who actually sent the e-mail).

Catfishing is when a person takes information and images, typically from other people, and uses them to create a new identity for themselves. In some cases, a catfisher steals another individual's complete identity—including their image, date of birth, and geographical location—and pretends that it is their own. "Hey Laronda, this is Pierre, we met last summer at the Anglo-French student conference in Montreal. I really missed our conversations en Francais et Anglais. How about we hook up online?" "Pierre" is really George, a 32-year-old cybercriminal who will try and get personal information from the recipient for his personal gain.

Outing or trickery is a way of getting people to reveal personal information that might then be used against them. "Leslie, I really have been thinking you're the fox of the history class. I wonder if you'd like to go out for a pizza and movie Saturday night. INTERESTED A LOT, JOEY." When Leslie replies, Devonne then puts it out on the internet: "Leslie thinks Joey is going out with HER on Saturday night. How delirious and out of touch with reality is she?"

Social exclusion is a means of deliberately excluding someone from a buddy list, chat room, discussion board, or game. "How many of you want Leslie off the discussion board and out of the game? Everybody who does, vote "aye.""

Cyberstalking is the electronic version of pursuing a person who is not interested in the personal attention they are receiving but receiving it anyway. "Don't think I don't know when you come on the discussion board, because I do, and I am going to be here watching and listening."

Cyberthreats are clearly meant to evoke fear and imply that danger is imminent. "It'll be dark by the time you get out of cheerleader practice, and this is the night you always walk home. Have a nice night . . . and . . . oh . . . I'll be watching . . . and waiting."

The crisis worker's intervention with these cyberbullies is difficult and fraught with legal and ethical issues (Stone, 2013, 2015, 2020). Some school counselors and other human services workers in schools have set up websites where students can contact them to deal with bullying and other personal issues in the virtual world that students inhabit (Myer et al., 2022). However, because of the fear of sexual predators, the Missouri legislature attempted to make it illegal for any person employed by a school to have an individual dialogue with a student over the internet. A judge ruled against the law as unconstitutional, but it is a slippery slope and workers can put themselves at risk legally and professionally. The better road to follow, at least at this point, is having clear district policies in place in regard to the use of the internet (Willard, 2007). Those policies should include the following (pp. 195–265):

1. A cyberbullying/cyberthreat and face-to-face bullying review policy for threatening materials sent over the internet or hard copies found at school.
2. School actions and options that are taken in regard to misuse of the internet by students.
3. Incident and report forms that track and record behavior so a chain of continuity can be built.
4. A comprehensive district plan to assess cyber use and misuse.
5. Student needs assessment as to bullying and bullying prevention effectiveness.
6. Teacher needs assessment as to understanding their role in student bullying.
7. District use policy for the internet and agreement signed by students and parents that includes netiquette guidelines, to be given to and discussed with both students and parents.

Systemic Intervention. There have been massive efforts across all school safety issues to strengthen schools, including bullying, yet meta-analyses, though generally favorable, are mixed. The foregoing statistics still indicate it is a rampant problem. Such programs do not succeed because their related cost and requirement of time allocations often get short changed (Midgett, 2016). Further, there is evidence that preservice teachers know little about identifying bullying and how to help stop it (Mahon et al., 2023). To sum this up, just doing the foregoing and calling it "done" won't work. There has to be initiative across the ecological board (Vismara et al., 2022) within the whole community, and that particularly includes parents and is why the *Stop Bullying* (National Institute of Justice, 2015) program has a community planning component. Zero tolerance and one-day "Stop Bullying!" programs don't work (Novotney, 2014). The school's philosophy and policy have to fit with their antibullying efforts, or it is useless. There also has to be a regular evaluation of the program and updating of it, or it will wither and die (Burnham, 2011; Novotney, 2014; Midgett, 2016; Sullivan, 2011). That evaluation should include (Professional School Counseling, 2012):

1. School-wide intervention policies that include peer groups that create a critical mass whereby bullying is absolutely "uncool."
2. Continuous assessment of bullying and dissemination of that data to parents.
3. Gain staff and parent support that ranges from bus drivers to superintendents and community organizations and civic clubs.
4. Form a group to coordinate the antibullying campaign and train them on how to do it, and cycle new members in as older ones leave (both faculty and students).
5. Increase adult supervision in hot spots where it is likely to occur and enforce school rules on bullying and apply them consistently.

Ttofi and Farrington (2011) meta-analysis of school-based programs to reduce bullying found that when the foregoing points are implemented, both bullying and victimization decrease by 20 percent. Note that the best they could do was only 20 percent. Intervention with bullies, first and foremost, should include a strict policy against harassment and intimidation (Kerr, 2009, p. 112), and that policy should be clearly spelled out with no loopholes (McAdams & Schmidt, 2007; Willard, 2007). Sounds pessimistic, doesn't it?

But there are some programs that can be put into operation and be effective.

Remediation. Once a bully has been identified, Sullivan (2011) proposes three approaches to remediation. First is punishment, which can range from dealing with the criminal justice system to expulsion, detention, or other disciplinary procedures. We believe Sullivan's approach should be a last resort because it essentially has no remediation but is used solely to maintain the safety and integrity of the affected students.

Second is a consequences approach. Bullies are generally masters of manipulation and rationalization, so the worker needs to be wary of getting into debates with them or accepting excuses for their aggressive behavior. Bullies don't change overnight, so positive reinforcement needs to be used cautiously and only when prosocial behavior has started to occur consistently (McAdams & Schmidt, 2007). While negative sanctions are involved, they are more educative than punitive in nature. Consequences may be attending an anger management group or working with special education students if that was the target population of the bully; behavioral contracting social skills training can be used (Burnham, 2011).

Third is a feelings approach that focuses on stopping the dehumanization and discounting of target individuals and focuses on building empathy for one's fellow students. Bullies may develop considerable skill in avoiding the consequences of their actions but have much more trouble when the focus is on feelings generated by their hurtful behaviors, so bullies begin to comprehend that there may be consequences when others feel victimized (McAdams & Schmidt, 2007).

Fulton (2015) proposes that separating boys from girls when conducting bully prevention programs is important because males and females experience bullying differently, and a one-size-fits-all approach doesn't work. No provisions were made for students who do not fit these categories. In the first lesson, she uses different film clips for boys and girls to demonstrate the way bullying differs by gender. In the second lesson, she discusses role players such as the bully, sidekick, supporter, disengaged onlooker, possible defender, champion, and target in gender-specific ways. Lesson three focuses on becoming aware of the behavioral impact of bullying and also focuses on gossip and rumors for females. Males learn that teasing can be turned quickly into bullying, and "just joking" is a rationalization of bad behavior that gets reframed by asking them if "just joking" is going to make the target's hurt go away. Lesson four focuses on the actions of the supporters, disengaged onlookers, possible defenders, and champions. For both boys and girls, these roles are examined and specific strategies are discussed that could help target and combat the bullying behavior. An addition for young women is a card game that ends up in the exclusion of one member, and then the effects of the exclusion are processed with the whole group.

Bauman (2011) believes that with minor bullying cases, brief solution-focused counseling can help both victims and bullies. This approach looks at bullying events as exceptions rather than the norm. It builds on both the victim's and the bully's self-identified strengths and develops strategies for similar situations in the future. For more severe cases, she believes support groups can be effective. Supporters of the victim, other individuals involved in the incident, and the main perpetrator can come together to agree on a support plan for the victim. Bauman proposes for the most serious cases that a restorative justice program be undertaken. First, victims are allowed to express how they can be helped. Then, the bully has the option of coming up with a plan to meet the victim's needs in trying to make amends. There is a prescribed procedure and a very formalized structure as to what and when things are done, which most likely takes some additional training. There is a fourth option, and we believe with proper implementation, it can be extremely effective because it applies pressure at its most sensitive point—peer pressure.

Bystander Training

The major problem with bullying is that bystanders do not speak up and, at times, instigate or promote bullying (Feather & Bordonana, 2019). Mobilizing the masses stops bullying and intimidation in their tracks (Charach et al., 1995). Biernesser and associates (2023) conducted focus groups with middle school students. They found that parents and teachers were not confided in or thought to be much help when it came to dealing with bullies, but students felt peers could if they could learn positive bystander intervention strategies. Following is a short synopsis of Midgett's (2016) and Feather and Bordonada's (2019) programs and how we believe they can be incorporated in classroom guidance sessions to become a common cultural standard in the school.

Midgett's (2016) approach involves training students to become "defenders" when witnessing a bullying event and not passive bystanders by using strategies from *Bully Proofing Your School* (National Institute of Justice, 2015). The first step is recruiting students from different peer groups. We cannot over emphasize this point. Our own peer mediator groups came from a cross section of the school population, so it was seen by students as pretty representative of who they were and considered to be fair and trust-worthy. Midgett's training is about 90 minutes long and is composed of three parts. The didactic com-ponent consists of an audio-visual presentation on the definition of bullying, different types of bullying behavior, the roles associated with it (bully, target, and bystander), and the negative consequences asso-ciated with it. The experiential component includes role plays of acting out a bullying situation and using STAC (stealing the show, turning it over, accompany-ing others, and coaching compassion) strategies to stop it. The first strategy, "stealing the show," involves using humor to redirect the focus off the bully, by telling a joke and deflecting attention from the bully-ing comments. The second strategy, "turning it over," involves informing an adult about the situation and asking for help. Note: It is important to clue faculty in so they don't brush off requests for assistance. The third strategy, "accompanying others," means reach-ing out to the targeted student and communicating that what was happening was unacceptable, that the student is not alone, and that others care for and sup-port the bullied student. The last strategy, "coach-ing compassion," means gently confronting the bully that the behavior is inappropriate and asking them to consider what it would feel like if that was happening to the bully. We would segway this last strategy into any action with the offending student in a meeting with the counselor because often, the bully has been bullied and knows exactly what it feels like and needs a chance to talk about it. We would incorporate Midg-ett's plan into classroom meetings throughout all the classrooms in the building.

Feather and Bordonada's (2019) program first apprises students of various types of bullying (i.e., physical, verbal, relational, and damage to one's prop-erty). Discussion then focuses on power differentials and what to do about them (i.e., telling an adult, walk-ing away and ignoring the bully, or avoiding the bully both in regard to the victim and bystanders). Warn-ing signs of bullying are detailed and include physical signs such as scratches or bruising; emotional signs such as social withdrawal, depression and suicidal ideation; behavior signs such as nightmares, eating habits, and dropping school and fun activities where

bullies may be present; and academic changes such as lower grades, not riding the school bus, and isolation at lunch. After discussion of these topics, role plays of the different types of bullying are acted out and discussed. Role plays provide the group with a greater sense of self awareness, self-efficacy, increased social assertion skills, and increased empathy for victims (Feather & Bordonada, 2019).

Glasser (1969) believes that classroom meetings that target real-time school and peer problems are an excellent vehicle for bringing a great deal of peer con-sensus and pressure into play on problems such as the Rosebuds' strong-arm tactics. By combining Glasser with Midgett and Feather and Bordonada's group approaches, a powerful peer antibullying program can be created. Once the majority of students in a school or a classroom decide that a particular behav-ior is "uncool," it tends to diminish very quickly. Fur-ther, by using the democratic, participatory process of Glasser's classroom meetings to problem solve, stu-dents come to feel empowered and are able to stand up to bullying and intimidating behaviors (Glasser, 1969).

Our own experience with a nasty bout of name calling in a middle school class was to have a class-room meeting where everyone wrote a negative nick-name of themselves on a name tag, moved around the circle, and asked the students to say their bad nick-name, why they chose it, and how it made them feel when the counselor called them by it instead of their real name. Teachers reported that the name calling was almost immediately extinguished. Having stu-dents write out experiences with bullying and talk-ing about them in the meetings makes everyone more aware of their own brushes with bullying and how that made them feel and can help make it safe for them to start talking about it.

School Counselor: (Starting a classroom meeting with a sixth-grade class. The objective is to start shining a very bright light on the strong-arm tactics of the Rosebuds, but the counselor does not specifically mention them by name. Indeed, there are two prob-able gang members in the room.) I want you all to write down four stories about bullying, using the following instructions.

1. Describe a time when someone's words or behav-ior hurt you.
2. Describe a time when you said or did something to hurt another person.

3. Describe a time when you saw or heard bullying but didn't do anything about it.

4. Describe a time when you saw or heard bullying and either got help or tried to stop it.

After the students finish writing their stories and share them with the group, the school counselor opens up a discussion centered on how students felt as they heard different stories. What did they think about what they heard? What would they do? And what would the consequences be if they did do something or changed what they did (Beane, 1999, p. 22)? Once students have started openly discussing threatening and intimidating behaviors, the counselor can use the hallmark of the classroom meeting and reality therapy, making a commitment (Glasser, 1969), to make their school a safer and friendlier place by pledging to do so and writing down specifically how that is going to happen (Newman et al., 2000, p. 123). There are a number of effective antibullying programs, and if handled correctly, they can cut bullying and the potential violence that goes with it, but we firmly believe it's a ground up approach, starting with the students and involving the whole educational community of parents, teachers, support staff and administrators.

Finally, Paterson (2011) summarizes a number of researchers and practitioners in advocating for bullies to get counseling. Using peer mediation and self-esteem building will not work because many bullies are very satisfied with their power and control over others. They need to understand that there are consequences for their actions that are bad for them when they make choices to bully and a "No Excuses" Glasser (1975) approach does not allow them to rationalize their behavior away as "just kidding." Other bullies may be motivated by poor social skills and impulse control. For both of these bullying types, empathy is important, but it is also tempered by sticking to a consequences of actions approach that employs reality and cognitive-behavior therapies. It may also be that while bullies see their approach as making them powerful, their thinking is distorted and will invariably get them in deeper trouble. As such, cognitive interventions that reframe their distorted notions of how they obtain and hold power over others may be effective (Health Resources and Services Administration, n.d.). The problem is that for both offender and victim, if things don't straighten out and get better, they run the risk of falling into the next section—and those are the lethal students who make headlines.

Safe haven.   As previously indicated, LGBTQIA+ youth experience bullying at far greater rates than their heterosexual, cisgender peers, and many of those students identify the school counselor as the most likely person they would disclose to and seek support from (Abreu et al., 2018). Our own experience supports Feather & Bordonada (2019) finding's that students with physical and mental disabilities also experience increased bullying. It is easy to speak in terms of social justice for these populations, but it is quite another thing, sometimes in the face of political pressure, to put into place comprehensive programs that entail large-scale, small-scale, and individual interventions for these students (Abreu et al., 2018).

We would like to think that the school counselor's office is a safe haven and welcoming for everyone, but given the issues these two groups face, we believe it is important to develop specific strategies along the lines of Abreu et al. (2018), Feather & Bordonada (2019), and Westheimer (2017) in making extra efforts, loudly and clearly, with both these groups of marginalized students and their parents that the counselor's office is a welcoming safe haven for them.

The Estranged Violent Juvenile Offender

LO7   Although gang violence is a major component of violence perpetrated by and among school-age children and is a major contributor to violence perpetrated by what the following authors (Bilchik, 1998; Hoge, 2008; Loeber et al., 1999) call the serious violent juvenile offender (SVJO), recent school shootings and subsequent homicides and injuries have been perpetrated by juveniles who do not typically fall into the "gang" SVJO category. The purpose of this section is to examine these different, potentially violent juveniles in regard to their psychological profile, screening mechanisms to detect them, and counseling methods to uncover their violent thoughts before those thoughts turn into action.

Peter Langman (2009) has written an excellent in-depth book on school shooters. He believes that most school shooters share some psychological symptoms. He further believes they fall within three general trait categories: psychopathic, psychotic, or traumatized. We believe that these three categories encompass what we call the EVJO. The term *estranged* violent juvenile offenders (EVJOs) is chosen because these juveniles typically are separated from their peers in distinctive ways and harbor a great deal of enmity toward their peers or the school system. We believe these individuals are distinct from their equally lethal SVJO counterparts—gang members. In contrast to a gang culture in which violence is generated to bind its members together in perpetuation of the gang's growth and stature, the EVJO is typically isolated and has no allegiances unless to a very few others who are also experiencing the same estrangement. EVJOs can be partitioned into two major categories, those who are mentally ill and those who are not. Langman's (2009) two categories of psychopathic and psychotic shooter would most nearly fall under our mentally ill EVJO category, and his traumatized shooter would fall under our not mentally ill EVJO category. Although it could be argued that anyone who would shoot a number of their fellow students is "crazy," that does not necessarily make them mentally ill under the APA's (2022) Diagnostic and Statistical Manual of Mental Disorders, Fifth Edition, Text Revision (*DSM-5-TR*) classification system. Therefore, it is also important to discriminate between EVJOs who are and are not mentally ill because of differences in profiles, screening, and intervention. Although we do not arbitrarily exclude the potential for young women in this group, the preponderance of offenders will be young men. As a result, we will use the male gender to describe the potential offender.

A Comparison of Traits, Characteristics, and Behaviors of SVJOs and EVJOs

The following traits, characteristics, and behaviors have been compiled from a number of published sources and interviews with human services workers who deal with both the SVJO and EVJO (Alothari et al. 2019; Carney et al., 1999; Corder et al., 1976; Cunningham & Davis, 1999; Duncan & Duncan, 1971; Dwyer et al., 1998; Fein et al., 2002; Galatzen-Levy, 1993; Hardwick & Rowton-Lee, 1996; Hoge, 2008; James & Dorner, 1999; Lempp, 1990; Levis, 1992; Loeber, 1990; Loeber & Ferrington, 1999; Marohn et al., 1982; Myers & Mutch, 1992; National School Safety Center, 1998; O'Toole, 2003; Sage & Dietz, 1994; Sloan, 1988; Vossekuil et al., 2002; Webster & Wilson, 1994; Zagar et al., 1990). These characteristics fall within what the FBI's Critical Incident Response Group and the National Center for the Analysis of Violent Crime call the four-pronged assessment model that evaluates the likelihood of carrying out a threat of violence. The four-pronged assessment model considers the personality of the student, family dynamics, school dynamics, and social dynamics (O'Toole, 2003).

Understand that there are serious moral, ethical, and legal implications of attempting to label potentially violent students (Simmons, 2000). Mustafa et al. (2022) question its use due to vagueness in methodology, potential race biased profiling, and the credibility and validity of the profilers. A heated debate rages on whether an accurate profile of a school shooter exists. The National Association of School Psychologists (2015) and the U.S. Secret Service (Alotari et al., 2019) emphatically state that no profile exists that can positively identify a school shooter. There is a belief that such profiles are over inclusive, biased, stigmatizing, and can potentially violate the student's constitutional rights (Bailey, 2001; Reddy et al., 2001; Vossekuil et al., 2000, 2002). Mulvey and Cauffman (2001) argue that such profiling is not only unproven but also has limited usefulness and often does more harm than good, particularly when a false positive identification is made and the student becomes labeled as a "homicidal maniac." Therefore, it should be clearly understood that there are serious ethical, legal, and moral considerations about basing action on a profile only. Action should be based on hard evidence to substantiate any threat assessment and not just on an accumulated checklist history of violence indicators.

Langman's (2009) profiling of infamous school shooters in the last 15 years is an eye-opener in regard to some of the stereotypical myths that make for good media sound bites. While the characteristics that follow may be present to some degree in all school shooters, it would be a severe mistake to suppose that any one factor, such as bullying, being a loner, or having a fascination with violence and guns, is *the* factor that causes students to become homicidal, nor is it very likely that the student will have all of the characteristics that profile the school shooter. It is much more reasonable to say that each school shooter has a mix of these potentially lethal ingredients that, when combined in the right amounts and cooked for the right amount of time in the right ecosystem, turn into a recipe for lethality.

Thus, there seems to be enough evidence that, when these traits and characteristics are combined with specific behaviors that indicate an increased threat level, they are at least a preliminary screening device that crisis workers can employ if reasonable judgment and care are used. On the other side of the dilemma, to not recognize that there is a potential threat is also professionally unethical and morally indefensible. More ominously, there are growing legal opinions that unanticipated acts of violence in schools can be anticipated, and courts will expect schools to have prevention programs in place (Capuzzi, 2002).

Summarizing these characteristics of the potentially violent juvenile, your authors would emphatically echo the U.S. Department of Education's *Early Warning, Timely Response: A Guide to Safe Schools* (Dwyer et al., 1998, p. 3) and the Federal Bureau of Investigation's *The School Shooter: A Threat Assessment Perspective* (O'Toole, 2003, p. 30) in their warning that it is important to avoid inappropriate labeling, stereotyping, or stigmatizing individuals based on the following categories. None of the categories by themselves or in combination can absolutely predict who will become violent and who will not. However, if the child fits into multiple categories, the crisis worker should be aware that the *potential* for violence increases and that this is an extremely troubled person. What we are more interested in when conducting a threat assessment are the demonstrated behaviors and communications that are likely to indicate intent (Alotari et al., 2019; Fein et al., 2002; Langman, 2009). Therefore, when reading the following categories, focus not so much on the categories themselves but on what behaviors are being manifested by the individual in his actions and communications. As these behaviors and communications stack up, the potential for violence increases and so do the concreteness and types of threats (O' Toole, 2000)

Types of Threats   The following are types of threat and their degree of intervention (O'Toole, 2000).

   Direct threats identify a specific act against a specific target and may include persons named, time of event, and location. "I'm gonna blow up the #4 school bus tomorrow when school lets out and that lousy driver and all the crummy students in it and I've got the stuff to do it."

   Indirect threats tend to be vague, unclear, and ambiguous. "If I wanted to, I could hurt everyone at school." The threat suggests something could occur, not that it will, and no specifics are detailed. It is typically a low-level threat without clear action to be taken. It could be carried out, but it may not appear realistic as "all the students in the school."

   Veiled threats strongly imply but do not explicitly state violence but leave it to the intended victim to interpret the message. "You cheerleaders wouldn't be so high and mighty if you weren't

pretty anymore." It is a medium level since a specific group is identified, but no clear action is given on how they could become less pretty.

   Conditional threats are often part of an extortion plan that a violent act will happen unless certain demands are met. "If final exams aren't called off, you better get a lot of fire trucks and ambulances ready because there are gonna be a lot of casualties to take care of."

When any of these threats move to a high level, the threat will be specific, direct, and plausible. It will suggest concrete steps have been taken to carry it out. "I will come for Mrs. Seward after school and see if she passes her final exam with my 9mm any better than I passed my English exam."

When this threat is coupled with the background behavioral characteristics of the SVJO or EVJO, then that would place the potential shooter at a high threat level. An absentee triage assessment would undoubtedly mark him in the high twenties and would be a basis for immediate action. The FBI's four-pronged assessment model factors the personality of the student, his family dynamics, the school dynamics and the student's role in them, and the social dynamics and considers each of these domains in assessing the potential for violence (O'Toole, 2000). It should be clear that the more negative assessment of each of these areas, the higher the likelihood of violence. The following characteristics of SVJOS and EVJOS are compiled in a condensed fashion from the references that started this section.

Family pathology. Sexual, psychological, and physical abuses in childhood are fertile fields in which the SVJO and EVJO take root and grow. Exposure to violent role models at home, parental deprivation, frequent moves, loss of a parent, inconsistent and punitive discipline, and rejection are characteristics of both. Home life is turbulent. There are guns or explosive materials in the home available to children and little parental security of them. There is little parental control or supervision of curfews, internet access, or television. Both SVJO and EVJO may rule the roost at home, and parents may be intimidated and afraid of the child. Parent do not react to behavior most parents would find disturbing or rationalize it as just "growing up." For the EVJO who does have a positive and supportive family, his sense of integration into the family likely will be weak and alienated. He will express contempt for his parents and dismiss their role in his life. He will insist on an inordinate degree of privacy, and his parents will have little information about his activities, friends, or school life. Such alienation may be particularly true for the EVJO with mental illness, even though he has an extremely supportive family situation and has received a great deal of nurturing and care. Parents may be in a great deal of denial about the potential for violence in either type.

Academic Problems. The SVJO will probably have a history of school problems that includes truancy, poor grades, discipline problems, and trouble with teachers. There is little bonding to school or school activities, and the student is detached from school, including associating with other students with the possible exception of a small, socially isolated outlier group. He is a bully and gets away with it due to a school culture of silence. In contrast, the EVJO will likely be passively compliant in school and may even do well academically. Unless some traumatic incident causes him to act out, he may well go unnoticed or even be respected by his teachers. Both may have mild to severe language disorders that, when they are placed under stress, will cause them to be more likely to act than talk. The EVJO with mental illness will be likely to experience many academic problems because of his difficulty in maintaining contact with the reality and demands of the classroom.

Altered States of Consciousness. If psychoactive substances are not ingested, their cognitive processes lead both the SVJO and the EVJO to limited reality testing. Typical reports after a violent incident include derealization, decompensation, and depersonalization. Statements such as "I was just seeing red and sort of blanking out," or "It's like I wasn't there, sorta watching a video so it was like me but really not me," are characteristic of both the SVJO and the EVJO. The EVJO with mental illness may operate in a continued state of altered consciousness and have minimum contact with the reality of the situation if not controlled by medication. Misuse of street or prescription psychotropic drugs increases the potential for violent behavior.

Anger/Low Frustration Tolerance. Both types react to stress in self-defeating ways. The SVJO is likely to have a "short fuse" and immediately aggresses in a stressful situation, while the EVJO typically will flee the situation or act in a more passive way. The low frustration tolerance of the SVJO is much more immediate and seen in highly observable ways. In contrast, the EVJO may have less observable behavioral manifestations because his anger is turned inward and sublimated. He may be erroneously seen to have a high frustration tolerance. In contrast, the EVJO with mental illness may have a very low frustration tolerance because of his tenuous grip on reality.

Bully/Bullied. The SVJO is the stereotypical bully. A bully at school, he is most probably a victim at home. The EVJO is the stereotypical bullied child. He may fall into one of two categories, the passive victim or the aggressive victim. The aggressive victim may be hot tempered and attempt to retaliate when attacked. Paradoxically, the aggressive victim may also be seen as a bully. While the passive bullied child is depicted as lonely and socially isolated at school, the aggressive victim is one of the most disliked and notorious members of his peer group. Although the passive bullied child may be much slower to act than his aggressive counterpart, both may bring weapons to school to counterbalance their perceived inferiority to their tormentors.

Chemical and Substance Abuse. Both types may alter consciousness by using psychoactive substances and freeing themselves of psychological restraints to commit violent acts. With the mentally ill EVJO discontinued use of prescribed psychotropic medication combined with illicit drug use has a high likelihood of precipitating a violent episode. Substance abuse markedly increases the potential for violence.

Criminal Behavior. In contrast to the gang member, who probably has a long history of contacts with the police and juvenile authorities, the EVJO most likely does not. The EVJO is as likely as not to be seen as a good and compliant student by his teachers. Comments from his neighbors are typically, "He's a real quiet, polite boy." He may have excellent church attendance and belong to the Boy Scouts or other socially appropriate organizations. If the EVJO has any contacts with the police, it will most likely be of a petty misdemeanor nature and involve passive acts against objects rather than aggressive acts against people. If the EVJO is mentally ill, he may have had contacts with the authorities through domestic disturbance or "mentally ill" calls. He will be on some type of antipsychotic medication and will likely have quit taking it because he doesn't like the side effects.

Delayed Cognitive and Affective Development. Both types may not have reached Piaget's formal operational or even concrete stage of development. Linear and logical thinking is stunted, and short-term emotional gratification overrules long-term behavioral consequences. Their notion of the finality of death or the realness and pain of bodily injury may be very much like a game of cops and robbers in which they are shot and killed over and over in the course of an afternoon. They may not relate their violent actions to any negative emotional outcomes for either their victims or themselves.

Emotional Lability/Depression. While the SVJO demonstrates a quick temper, "short fuse," and rapid mood swings, the EVJO may show depressive characteristics in which anger is turned inward. The EVJO may be serious to the point of sullenness and see little humor in his world, particularly if he has been the object of derisive humor by his peers or significant others in his life. The severely depressed EVJO may see the end point of retaliation against his tormentors as also the end point for himself and may see suicide as a viable option after he has exacted revenge. The mentally ill EVJO may have bizarre thoughts and emotions with correlative mood swings that range from rage to fear. He also may have suicidal ideation, depending on his emotional state and particular mental illness.

External Locus of Control. Fate, a higher power, "The Man," and other external entities play a large part in the behavior of the SVJO and the EVJO. The SVJO may view himself as both the victimizer as a way of gaining power and the victim because of his circumstances. The EVJO clearly assumes a victim status. Both blame others for their outcast state. The EVJO's external locus is tied to a low self-concept that is constantly reaffirmed as being inadequate by the world around him. The mentally ill EVJO may receive "messages" from "voices" that tell him to act against others.

History and Threats of Violence. One of the best predictors of violence is past violence. Particularly when threats of violence are coupled with a past history of violence, the probability of violence increases. While the SVJO will more likely be clear, immediate, and direct with his threats, the EVJO's threats are likely to be more implied, conditional, and veiled for a longer period of time. The mentally ill EVJO may make threats that commingle reality with fantasy such that specific individuals may be symbolized as "monsters" or other objects that are threatening to him.

Hypersensitivity. Both the SVJO and EVJO are hypersensitive to criticism and real or perceived slights and threats. They will both be suspicious, fearful, distrustful, and paranoid in their worldview. While the SVJO will be more overt in his manifestation of these characteristics through name-calling, swearing, and angry outbursts, the EVJO will be more passive. Both are overly sensitive to what they believe others think, feel, and act toward them. They are "injustice collectors"; they harbor resentment over past wrongs and will not forget them or the people believed to be responsible. The mentally ill EVJO will be exponentially more hypersensitive to imagined threats to his well-being and will react angrily to them. Paradoxically, both may have little sensitivity or empathy for others.

Impulsivity. The SVJO is quick to act and wants immediate gratification. He has little consideration for the consequences of his actions, lacks insight, has poor judgment, and has little understanding of how his belief system filters actions and resulting consequences. He habitually makes violent threats when angry. In contrast, the EVJO may be slow to act. He may be hypersensitive as a result of past negative experiences that have been socially and emotionally punitive. His belief system will turn to a "them against me" view that continues to build until his frustration spills out and he aggresses against his real or imagined tormentors. The mentally ill EVJO may fall along a continuum of high to low impulsivity depending on the disorder from which he suffers.

Mental Illness. Hospitalization for mental illness alone is not an indicator of potential violence. However, when hospitalization of the SVJO or EVJO for mental illness is preceded by a history of violent offenses, it is an indicator for more intense and accelerated violent behavior. Violence potential is further exacerbated when psychotropic medication is stopped because of its side effects, the inability to obtain it, or inadequate supervision in administering it.

Negative Role Models. For the SVJO, local and nationally known gang members and movie and music "gangstas" may be role models. The EVJO may be drawn to malevolent historical figures such as Hitler, religious figures such as Satan, and antiheroes in books, videos, and game simulations. The EVJO who is mentally ill may create his own alter ego who tells him to do violent things.

Odd/Bizarre Beliefs. Odd or bizarre beliefs fall into two categories. Schizophrenic-type mental illnesses and personality disorders are defined by odd and bizarre beliefs and behaviors, which would characterize the EVJO with mental illness. The second category more closely typifies the EVJO without mental illness. His thoughts and behaviors may range from an interest in demonology, magical thinking, and satanic cults to extremely rigid political and religious views that promote violent solutions to society's problems, which he knows little about. He disregards facts, logic, and reasoning that might challenge these opinions. Joining splinter groups that advocate such views is a way of achieving the affiliation, status, and power that the EVJO craves.

Pathology and Deviance. A psychological smorgasbord of problems may be exhibited by both types of juvenile offenders. Fire setting, cruelty to animals, defacing and destroying property, temper tantrums, running away from home, and oppositional defiance to authority are some examples. When these behaviors have a long history, they are probably more characteristic of the SVJO. When they seem to occur spontaneously with no prior history or are kept under wraps by parents who are in denial and concerned about the social stigma attached to these behaviors, they more aptly characterize the EVJO. Parents of both groups may be passive in regard to what most parents would find very disturbing and abnormal behavior. If contacted by school officials or law enforcement, parents may respond defensively and minimize or reject reports of obvious misconduct.

Physical Problems. Particularly for the EVJO, physical problems that range from stuttering to severe acne to delayed physical development may contribute to a poor body image and feelings of inferiority. Internal head injuries, congenital brain damage, and a variety of neurological problems may contribute to the potential for violence in the mentally ill EVJO.

Preoccupation with Violent Themes. Both the SVJO and the EVJO may become fixated on movies, books, television shows, videos, and music that glamorize violence. Interest in violent pornography, weapons collections, sadomasochistic paraphernalia, and instruments of torture allow the powerless EVJO, and particularly the mentally ill EVJO who is paranoid, to fantasize about dominance over his persecutors and plot very meticulously how to get rid of them (O'Toole, 1999).

Social Status. The SVJO may be ostentatious and gregarious in his social relations as a means of gaining status. He sees women of all ages as providers of "goods and services" and tends to use them for his own self-gratification. He may display a pathological need for attention and have an overall attitude of superiority and an exaggerated sense of entitlement. A social assessment of the EVJO would generally depict him as a social isolate from the majority of his peers with affiliations that place him in outlier groups. However, there are EVJOs who are popular, participate in extracurricular activities, and would generally be seen as involved in the school community. If asked, his classmates might characterize the EVJO in terms such as "geek," "Goth," "nerd," "freak," "weird," and other terms that clearly set him apart from the social mainstream. His attempts to form relationships with the opposite gender will generally be clumsy and fraught with failure. Women who try to be kind to him may well have their kindness misinterpreted. When the EVJO makes attempts to move beyond "kindness" in the relationship and his romantic overtures are rejected, the isolation he feels is further compounded. Because of his bizarre behavior, the mentally ill EVJO will be extremely socially isolated from his peers and labeled as "nuts," "mental," or "crazy."

Suicidal Ideation. Both the SVJO and EVJO may have severe depressive episodes with significant mood swings. The result may be angry outbursts against others or self, with concomitant threats or attempts of suicide. Such threats or attempts may occur particularly after a real or perceived personal loss. The mentally ill EVJO may consider suicide a very viable option to get the demons out of his head or as a way to keep "them" from getting him and further persecuting him after he does away with his enemies.

Weapons. Both the SVJO and the EVJO may have an undue fascination with and knowledge of weapons. The family may keep guns or other weapons accessible in the home, or the SVJO or EVJO may have easy means of obtaining them on the street. Significant role models may have a casual attitude toward weapons and see them as a useful or normal means of settling disputes. The SVJO may commonly carry or have access to a weapon for both "protection" and "revenge" against other gang members. When the EVJO carries a weapon to school, he is most likely getting ready to act out against his tormentors. The mentally ill EVJO may be much like the SVJO in carrying weapons for both protection and revenge against his imagined enemies (O'Toole, 1999).

Case Study: Seung-hui Cho

Now consider Seung-hui Cho at Virginia Tech in April 2007. How well do you think he fits the foregoing behaviors and characteristics?

Seung-hui Cho, the Virginia Tech mass murderer who committed suicide, is the personification of the mentally ill EVJO. The following behaviors, characteristics, and traits are gleaned from the video he sent to NBC and from a report by Michael Ruane (2007), who interviewed Cho's former suite mate, Andy Koch.

Cho clearly had altered states of consciousness as exemplified by his imaginary supermodel girlfriend "Jelly," whom he claimed he was making out with in his locked room. He had severe ego identity problems, as indicated by his alter ego, Ismail Ax, a name written in red ink on his arm, and by his signature "?" on a class role, which earned him the nickname of the "Question Mark Kid." Claiming to vacation with Russia's president, Vladimir Putin, and to live in the ominous room "666" when his hall only had five floors, boosted his weak self-concept and gave him power. Like most EVJOs, he had no apparent history of direct threats to anyone, but his behavior was most certainly threatening to all around him. His plays were so dark, twisted, and threatening that they caught the attention of his English professors. They are characteristic of the commingling of reality and fantasy for a person with paranoid schizophrenia ideation and behavior and cannot be passed off as the works of "another Stephen King in the making." Cho's stalking behavior, scrawling of scary lines from Shakespeare on a girl's residence hall door, and other antisocial and bizarre behaviors over an extended period of time were precursors of his ultimate acts of violence; those oblique threats would slowly grow and finally take form in the direct and methodical act of mass murder. His hypersensitivities to external threats were legion and ranged from girls to the "rich snobs." He had been involuntarily hospitalized, was found to be depressed but not a threat to anyone else, and was released. Numerous complaints brought

the police to his door. His antiheroes Eric Harris and Dylan Klebold, the mass murderers at Columbine High School, were ideal role models for the rampage he was contemplating. Most likely another role model, Ismail Ax, his imaginary alter ego, urged him along.

Cho's physical problems included not being able to speak well, being small of stature, and being different, although at this writing it is unclear whether "being different" related to being Korean in a school with predominantly White students, bullied, a loner, or some other factor or constellation of factors that set him apart. His writings and Facebook illustration of himself as a Zorro-like figure with only a large question mark in an otherwise blank face portray the graphic images of the violence he was contemplating. Finally and tragically, these characteristics were known to numerous people, from his roommate to professors to the police. The psychological leakage that characterizes a potentially violent student was a veritable flood for Seung-hui Cho.

In summary, if you now refer back through the traits, behaviors, characteristics, and screening factors for the mentally ill EVJO and compare them to Cho's, they should scream at you, "Do something!" However, "doing something" in the case of a college student, even one whose behavior is as blatant as Cho's, is not so easily accomplished, as we shall see in this chapter's section on the legal and ethical issues of potentially violent behavior.

Screening the EVJO

LO8   Langman (2009) emphasizes that the key is early detection and prevention because once an armed suicidal/homicidal student sets foot on the school ground with a plan of action, all the metal detectors in the world are not going to stop him from carrying out his intended plan. The problem with profiling the estranged violent juvenile offender who is not mentally ill is that any staff member in a school could probably identify at least 20 percent of the male population who might fit the foregoing profile and have many of the characteristics described in the foregoing section. How, then, can this population be screened for those students who might have such characteristics and, more important, the intent to carry out a violent act?

Leakage. Leakage occurs when a student communicates to a third party the intent to do harm (Meloy & O'Toole, 2011; O'Toole, 2000). In school, these leakages intentionally or unintentionally reveal feelings, thoughts, fantasies, attitudes, or intentions that signal a violent act. A note given to classmates then dropped and found by teachers, texts and post-its, and social media sites all are possible leakage points. They can be delivered through stories, diaries, essays, poems, drawings, doodles, songs, tattoos, videos, and other media that make boasts, threats, predictions, or ultimatums. Another form of leakage occurs when unwitting friends and classmates are coerced or deceived into helping in preparations for violent acts. Leakage can be cries for help, signs of inner conflict, or boasts that may presage a serious threat. Leakage is considered one of the most important clues that precede a violent act (O'Toole, 2003).

Writings, Drawings, Pictures, Videos, Texts, Social Media, and E-Mails.

The writings, drawings, homemade pictures, and videos of EVJOs are often an open pathway into their troubled minds. In cases of potentially violent behavior, artwork may make the point more vividly than a verbal description. Graphic themes of violence that pervade the writings, drawings, photographs, videos, and e-mails of EVJOs are a tip-off that the student may be contemplating violent action against school staff or fellow students. These hard-copy emotional messages should be taken very seriously when previous incidents of violent behavior have occurred and when such graphic displays of violent ideation are issuing from the "quiet kid" who has no history of disruption in the school. School crisis workers need to apprise teachers of these indicators of predisposition to violence, and such student-generated work should be passed on to the crisis worker (Duncan & Duncan, 1971; Hammond & Gantt, 1998; James & Dorner, 1999).

Being aware of and acting on threats are critical in the prevention of a violent act (Wattendorf, 2002), and leaks are one way of doing so. Training teachers to be aware of and report these types of leakage and not dismiss them as idle, out-of-hand comments is important (Van Brunt, 2015, p. 9). Bondu and Scheithauer (2015) found that when German teachers were trained to detect leaking, they reported improved knowledge about leaking and understanding more courses of action that could be taken once leaks were discovered after training. While this may sound excessive in regard to the cascade of notes teachers find (kids being notoriously sloppy and negligent in the art of getting rid of the evidence), the idea is to turn the leaked material into somebody with threat expertise to determine how valid the threat is.

Peer Referral. There are very, very few instances in which the EVJO does not give some warning of his intentions to harm himself or others. Invariably, in psychological postmortems of situations that resulted in injury or death due to violence by an EVJO, students had heard statements or seen notes from the student indicating his intent to do harm but had generally dismissed them as just "talk" (Hardwick & Rowton-Lee, 1996; James & Dorner, 1999).

However, the problem with peer referral is twofold. First, other students are afraid of and repelled by the notion of "narking" or "snitching" on another student. This reticence to inform on another is particularly true when the student in question may be so threatening that other students fear for their own safety or dismiss the threat of a student they have known for years and, in their opinion, is absolutely harmless. Students need to feel safe in providing information about a potentially dangerous situation (Dwyer et al., 1998, p. 4; Stewart & MacNeil, 2005).

One of the best ways to screen for potentially violent students is through a peer referral and notification system run by peers and coordinated by school crisis workers (Allen, 1996). Conflict resolution, peer mediation, peer leadership, and peer counseling are all programs that allow students to legitimately notify faculty of potentially violent students without becoming informers. Whatever type of peer program is offered should not be operated from the standpoint that its only purpose is to "catch bad kids." The primary purpose of peer programs should be to help other students resolve conflicts, mediate disputes, and provide support, help, and referral for common maturational problems associated with adolescence and acclimation to school. However, when in the course of providing such peer helping services, peer helpers gain information about fellow students in crisis who may be planning to commit violent acts, it is clearly appropriate for them to apprise the crisis worker of the information they have received (James & Dorner, 1999).

Peer helpers need to be carefully trained, monitored, and supervised by crisis workers lest they exceed their limits (Allen, 1996). Peer helpers should be selected from a broad cross-section of the school population (Day-Vines et al., 1996). It has been your authors' experience that students who represent the full spectrum of the student population are much more effective in reaching their peers and being accepted by them. That does not mean that there are lowered expectations of peer helpers either academically or morally. The best peer helpers have been able to demonstrate a willingness to work with and help all of their fellow students. Their very diversity allows the program to reach a broader constellation of students than it otherwise might (Allen, 1996).

Team. The other major step is establishing a threat assessment team much like those that now exist on many college campuses (Lovre, 2013; Myer et al., 2011; Van Brunt, 2015) and now increasingly in K–12 school systems. The team should be composed of at least an administrator, a counselor, an SRO, and enough teachers spread across all grades and all sections of the school to ensure that at least one team member has direct contact with each student. This in-house team would be considered a threat level I team. It meets on a regular basis to filter all potential threats and rate them as to the seriousness of intent. If a potential threat is discovered by the team, then a threat level II multiagency team composed of mental health and law enforcement individuals who are specialists in threat assessment should be brought into the picture. However, assessment is only the beginning of the threat team's job. The real job comes in designing (Lovre, 2013) a plan to not only find potential threats but also to make plans to stabilize and move them away from a lethal thinking and operating mode. As we have discussed in Chapter 8, "Crisis of Lethality," the threshold that an angry person crosses from suicide to homicide can be very easy; thus, the school system should have a comprehensive suicide prevention plan in place. The most effective threat assessment plan does not put that on the shoulders of the school system but sees it as a community problem and brings community resources to bear on it (Lovre, 2013).

Interviewing the Potential EVJO

When interviewing the potential EVJO, the first two tasks of the crisis intervention/prevention model, Predispositioning and Problem Exploration, along with the default task of Safety, are particularly critical in getting the EVJO to start talking about a violent act. The third task, Providing Support, and the default task of Safety are critical in assuring the student that the overriding concern is the student's own safety and well-being and that the

issues that brought him to this point are not going to be shoved in a file drawer and never see the light of day. Coordinated with these preliminary tasks is the three-level threat assessment model provided in *The School Shooter: A Threat Assessment Perspective* (O'Toole, 2003, pp. 8–9).

A low threat is one that poses a minimal risk to the proposed victim. The threat is vague and indirect. The information is inconsistent and implausible, lacks detail, or is unrealistic. The content suggests it is unlikely to be carried out. A *medium threat* is one that could be carried out, although it may appear to be unrealistic. It is more direct than a low-level threat. Wording indicates that some thought has been given to how it will be carried out. There is a general indication of a possible place and time. There is little indication the threatener has taken preparatory steps or made solid plans. There may be a specific statement seeking to convey that the threat is real, as in "I'm serious, and I mean it!" A *high threat* poses an imminent and serious danger to the safety of others. The threat is direct, specific, and plausible. Concrete steps have been taken toward carrying it out, and there is a solid plan with means, opportunity, knowledge, and lethal methodology to carry it out.

Problem Definition. The school crisis worker who interviews a potential EVJO initially needs to proceed with basic listening and responding skills that deeply reflect the student's feelings and allow him to ventilate his angry feelings. It should be understood that other negative emotions are undergirding and supporting the anger the student feels. Suspicion, betrayal, embarrassment, grief, anxiety, inadequacy, threat, insecurity, and particularly, hopelessness and frustration, are but a few of the negative feelings that may be pushing the student toward violence.

Case of John. John is a 14-year-old high school freshman who was referred to the school counselor by a teacher who had screened out John's theme after she had been through a workshop on profiling potentially violent students. The counselor has read John's theme, which is filled with angry and violent threats about a group of girls who have been teasing him.

CW: John, I've read your theme Mrs. Smith sent to me. You seem really angry. Would you like to tell me about what's making you so angry right now?

John: I'm sick of the Tri-Beta Club. Particularly the girls. They ask me to do stuff, and I do it, but then they make fun of me.

CW: Sounds like you're not only angry but hurt too. How do they hurt you?

These feelings and their antecedent causes need to be fully explored by the crisis worker to make a clear determination of what is going on and with whom it is occurring. Exploration is important for two reasons. First, by allowing the student to ventilate, the crisis worker does much toward defusing the potentially violent situation and can start to help the student develop alternative coping and problem-solving strategies. The crisis worker wants to establish an open and trusting relationship with this troubled student. Hearing the student and affirming him, through summary clarification and restatement of the content of his problem and reflection of his feelings, go a long way toward doing that.

John: Yeah. I want to be friends, but I don't think they really want me for a friend. When they need somebody to build a float or put up posters, I'm just fine. But when I asked Sally Johnson if she wanted to go get a soda after the float was done, she laughed at me, said I was a loser, and then told the other girls, and they laughed too. I hate them!

CW: So they really put you down and embarrassed you when you did everything they wanted you to do.

Second, by adequately exploring the affective, behavioral, and cognitive dimensions of the student's problem, the crisis worker may gain valuable information about the *who, what, where, when,* and *how* of the student's proposed course of action. The worker stays away from *why* questions because of their interrogatory nature. John is already defensive, and the crisis worker does not wish to do anything that will further alienate him.

CW: John, it sounds like you'd really like to get back at them for the way they've treated you. How might you do that?

Ensuring Safety. Assessment of lethality is primary in any crisis intervention. Contrary to exploring issues by using open-ended questions, we subsequently assess the potential for suicidal or homicidal behavior by asking specific, closed-ended questions that are designed to get direct answers about the student's threat level. The questions we ask could come straight from a detective's homicide manual and fall within the following areas:

1. Is there a motive?
2. Is there opportunity?
3. What is the method or plan?
4. What are the means?

Most people in psychological crisis who have suicidal or homicidal ideation will talk about what they are going to do, and talking about their plan does not, contrary to popular myth, make them more likely to carry it out. Even though they may believe they have exhausted all other possibilities, their willingness to talk about their thoughts and contemplated actions is a positive sign and an indication that at least some part of them believes there is an alternative. The potential EVJO, in particular, fits this pattern because of his feelings of anger, hopelessness, and frustration and his need to vent those feelings. If questions are asked in an empathic, nonjudgmental way, the individual will be willing to talk about the four points just listed. There is one major exception, and that is the mentally ill EVJO who is paranoid about the behavior of others toward him. He is highly unlikely to voluntarily come to counseling or think that he needs it. After all, he believes it is the others who are all wrong and messed up—not him! Persuading him to talk may best be accomplished by eliciting talk about "them" and displaying a good deal of empathy in regard to injustices perpetrated on him.

As motive, opportunity, method, and means are covered, the threat assessment goes up as each becomes more concrete. The motive of the EVJO is often unclear or muddled, and therefore may be dismissed as inconsequential. It would be a mistake to dismiss such ideation, however, because it is not just the motive itself but the intensity and the lability with which it is discussed that are important. The more emotive the EVJO is about the injustices done him, the more he clarifies and elaborates on his plan and the opportunity to carry it out, and the more lethal his means, the higher the threat assessment (O'Toole, 2003, p. 9).

It should be abundantly clear that if the potential EVJO has access to firearms or other weapons and knows how to use them, the threat becomes critical, and there is increased risk for violence (Dwyer et al., 1998, p. 10; Langman, 2009, p. 182). Thus, the crisis worker should not hesitate to ask the student what he knows about firearms and if he has access to them. If the crisis worker does not know about the types and uses of firearms, the SRO should be consulted.

The following two scenarios, using John as an example, depict low versus high levels of threat.

Scenario 1

John: I wish they were all dead. It'd serve them right!

CW: So if they were dead, it'd pay them back for what they've done to you. How might that happen?

John: Well, I don't know for sure. I'd wish they'd get some incurable disease and really suffer a lot.

CW: So you'd like to see them hurt as much as they've hurt you. How might that happen?

John: Yeah. Well, I dunno for sure. Maybe they'd get that bird flu or food poisoning from the cafeteria.

Here, the student's wish for the death of his tormentors is couched in fantasy with no clear means or method for carrying out his plan. This fantasized revenge would not carry a high lethality level but would certainly indicate that this student is in need of support and continued work with the crisis worker.

Scenario 2

John: I wish they were all dead. It'd serve them right.

CW: So if they were dead, it'd pay them back for what they've done to you. How might that happen?

John: It'd be easy. I'd wait for them after school. When they go out to work on the homecoming float at the bus barn, I'd be behind the incinerator. I could shoot them real easy.

CW: John, do you know how to use a gun?

John: Sure. My dad's got a 9 mm pistol. He showed me how to use it. He says I'm pretty good with it.

CW: Can you get your dad's gun?

John: Well, he's got it locked up in the gun safe, but I know the combination.

CW: John, when are you planning on doing this?

John: I don't know, but if they make fun of me one more time, soon.

In this second scenario, the student's motive, method, opportunity, and access to lethal means are much clearer and better defined. Such a response would indicate a much higher threat level and would call for clear and immediate action on the part of the crisis worker.

Providing Support. In any case in which a student's lethality level is high, we need to provide clear owning statements about what we will need to do to keep the client and others he may intend to harm safe. Parents must be informed, and a clear line of communication needs to be established with the school administration, law enforcement, and other agencies that may become involved (Dwyer et al., 1998, p. 11).

CW: (responding to scenario 2) John, what you have said really concerns me. It sounds like you've really worked out the details, and if you carry this out, I'm afraid for you and the other students. I understand you're really angry and hurt by what they've done to you. I can certainly understand how you could feel that way, but I don't want to see you get hurt any more, either by the other students in what they say and do to you or by the police. I don't want you to shoot anybody, and I don't want the police to shoot you. I need to get some help for you right now, and I need to be sure you're safe. I want you to stay with me until I can make sure you are safe. I need to talk to your parents because I'm sure they would be concerned for you. I also need to talk to the principal to make sure she understands what's going on, so she can make sure that you stay safe. I understand that you might be upset with me for doing this, but I'm really concerned about you right now, John. I understand that right now you think this is the only solution you've got, but I believe there are other ways to handle this, and I want you to understand that I'll help you figure some of those out. I'll stay with you and work with you until we do get things worked out and you are safe.

Many clients will not be happy when they are informed about what is going to happen to them. One of the best responses the crisis worker can make when this happens is to use a combination of what are called "I understand" statements and the "broken record" technique, which continuously and repeatedly acknowledges the client's unhappiness about our decision but also reaffirms our concern and caring for him. If the student becomes angry or enraged over the worker's insistence that help is required and becomes threatening, the worker needs to acknowledge the anger, but also set limits.

John: Hey, everything is supposed to be confidential in here. You tricked me. No way you tell my parents, my old man would beat me to death. Screw this. (**jumps up with fists clenched**)

CW: (immediately rises from her chair as a safety pre-caution) No, I did not trick you, John. You heard what I said about confidentiality when we talked about harming yourself or others. John, I totally get what you say, but don't you want some respect, don't you want to feel better about coming to school? Don't you not want to be tricked and made fun of anymore? These things can happen because you have not acted on that angry notion. So please sit down and let me go to work for you. Nothing has happened so far that says we can't get some more positive results. So please sit down and let me do my job to help you out.

The worker first acknowledges his anger and sense of betrayal. She then uses a series of negative interrogative questions that ask for agreement and attempt to reframe his present cognitive and emotional state to what he desires to have happen. She also uses "these" things to gain psychological closeness as opposed to "that" notion which she wishes to distance psychologically. Finally, she also uses Fauteux's (2010) technique of showing there is still time because nothing has happened yet that would destroy the possibility of John getting what he wants other than revenge.

If these techniques do not get John to calm down, then the worker needs to consider her own safety and follow our recommendations in Chapter 14, "Violent Behavior in Institutions," to get out of the room and/or get help.

At other times, what may at first seem to be a high threat situation may not be and, in fact, may mask other crisis issues. Return now to Officer Davis, whom you met earlier in the chapter and see how his day is going to become very interesting indeed.

Officer Davis receives a call from the school secretary at his home (S. Davis, personal communication, February 17, 2007). She is very distressed. The school has received a phone call from some kind of a psychotherapist in California who has been communicating with and working with a student via the internet, a Goth 16-year-old White male. The therapist is very concerned because the student indicates he is tired of being bullied and is making a bomb to blow up the school. She calls and tells the school secretary this information after the school day is over and the students are gone. The student has put that information on TikTok and indicated he is going to blow up something or somebody. Through some good detective work on the part of the school secretary, she has determined that the boy is Paul Jones. Officer Davis

discretely meets the boy at school the next morning and pulls him into his office.

Officer Davis: Talk to me, Paul. What's going on? You seem kinda depressed.

Paul: Not really. Some kids trash talking me is all, and I'm tired of getting bullied by them.

Officer Davis: Look, you're not in any trouble, OK, but I gotta check this out. It looks like you put some stuff on the net about making a bomb. Want to show me what it was?

Paul: Well yeah! I put some of that stuff on there, but I'm not really making one.

Paul shows him what he put on the net. Officer Davis e-mails this information to the local bomb squad, who are sitting in unmarked cars outside Paul's house. They get very excited over the information and immediately want to search Paul's house for bomb-making material. Officer Davis calls the parents and informs them of what is occurring. A search of the house is quietly conducted, and nothing is found in the way of explosive devices, much to the relief of the parents and everyone else. However, Officer Davis's CIT training kicks in, and he feels something more is going on with this troubled young man. He continues to explore Paul's feelings with him.

Officer Davis: Look, I've done a lot of this stuff, Paul, and I get a good sense when things are really troubling people. You seem really down or maybe something else. I think it's more than getting trash talk for being Goth. You sure you don't want to talk to me about it?

Paul: OK. Look, this is weird. Like I have spiders crawling all over my arms right now. And there is a waterfall right in back of you. Plus, my dad talks to me a lot in class, but like, he's at work and not really there, but nevertheless, he is talking to me, and it really is distracting and scary. See, I scratch my arms, but the spiders still come back.

Officer Davis: (thinking to himself, "Holy mackerel! This kid is having schizophrenic episodes!") Paul, that certainly concerns me. Have you told your parents?

Paul: No, I'm too embarrassed. I don't want them to know. I keep thinking they'll go away. They don't come often, but when they do, it's pretty scary. That waterfall behind you right now is pretty real.

Officer Davis: I don't see or hear it. I know you do, and that needs to get taken care of. I've got a friend at the crisis center who deals with this stuff. I believe after I talk with your parents you need to meet him.

Officer Davis now calls the parents, who are at their home with the bomb disposal unit, and informs them of their son's hallucinating episodes. To say that this is a day they would like to soon forget is putting it mildly. However, Officer Davis calmly talks them though the problem and then drives Paul to the crisis center, where the parents meet him. Whenever Officer Davis has to take someone to the crisis center, he stays to make sure the person is being seen and treated before he leaves. This is particularly true of students, who need a friendly face when they are taken to a mental health facility and are under emotional duress. This tactic allows students to know that he is not abandoning them and pays off down the road when he encounters them again. They know they can trust him and that he really is interested in them as people.

It may be argued that a school counselor, psychologist, or social worker might be the best person to handle this situation. However, when a school resource officer like Scott Davis is also CIT trained, the fact that this is a potentially lethal situation with disastrous ramifications makes him the very best qualified person to deal with Paul. You may wonder whether this is a rose-colored picture of a police officer. With the spread of CIT training across the United States, officers like Scott Davis are becoming more and more common and are, in every sense of the definition, crisis interventionists. Further, they certainly have ample opportunity to ply their trade in 21st-century schools (James et al., 2011).

Acting

How the crisis worker acts depends on a continuous assessment of the student. If the crisis worker determines that the student is indeed a threat, then the worker's response should be to make an immediate referral and notify parents, administrators, and, if necessary, law enforcement personnel. If the crisis worker determines that the student's lethality level is not high, then the worker can move forward in the model to examining alternatives, making plans, and obtaining a commitment to work on positive actions that will help him become less alienated and angry. An investigation might indicate that the behavior was merely a "throwaway" statement that had no meaning other than ordinary misguided playfulness or a

momentary pique of anger. Even then, it would be a proper educative and counseling activity to teach the student not to play this game. However, in today's school environment, threats against others should not automatically be discounted. Thus, the crisis worker needs to keep a record of the encounter and follow up with the student to ensure that those threats do not escalate into action (James & Crawford, 2002).

Punishment by expulsion is not the answer and, in fact, does at least two things we don't want to have happen. First, it likely increases the student's grudge against the school or those in it he feels are responsible for his misery. Second, it is likely to leave the student unsupervised at home and give him free license to plan and assemble the necessary weaponry to pay the school back (Langman, 2009, p. 186). What needs to happen is that the student is evaluated for psychiatric and/or behavioral problems, medicated if necessary, provided counseling, and placed in an alternative school that is well supervised.

A primary consideration is what to do if the student is carrying a weapon. If the crisis worker feels the relationship with the student is positive enough and the student indicates that he has a weapon in his possession, then the crisis worker may ask for it for safekeeping. In taking a weapon, the crisis worker should always be sure it is handed over butt first or, if a knife, haft (handle) first. If the crisis worker is unsure of the student's intent or if the student is resistant, the crisis worker should *immediately seek help and get out of the room*. If the student indicates he has a weapon in his locker or some other hiding place, the crisis worker should have another person go with them to the hiding place. *In no instance should the crisis worker attempt to be a hero and attempt to forcibly take a weapon away from a student* (Crews, 1998). There is no known formula for determining whether to attempt to get the weapon away from the student or leave the premises to get help. Probably the best rule to follow is whatever the crisis worker believes will be the safest course of action for both the crisis worker and the student.

School-Based Suicide Prevention and Intervention

LO9 Because adolescence is the most volatile period of transition in the human cycle of development, factors involving youth who are at risk for suicide are dramatically different from those affecting adults who die by suicide (Berman et al., 2006; Capuzzi, 2009; Maples et al., 2005; Pfeffer, 2006). Suicidal thoughts and behaviors represent the most common mental health emergency among teenagers (King et al., 2013). In the United States, suicide ranks second in 10–14 years old children and third in cause of death for 15–24-year-old adolescents and young adults. Being a young child is no exemption from suicide. It is the eighth-leading cause of death for children ages 2–11 in the United States. For young people between the ages of 10–24, suicide is currently the third leading cause of death. It results in approximately 6,600 lives lost each year (WISQARS, 2021). The United States does not have a corner on child suicide. The WHO (2021) reports that suicide is the fourth leading cause of death in 15–29-year-olds worldwide. Suicide is a global problem, and 77 percent of suicides occurred in low- and middle-income countries in 2019.

But dying by suicide is only part of the problem. More young people survive suicide attempts than actually die. Suicide and self-harm in young people are a major cause of years of adjusting to a disability caused by the unsuccessful attempt (De Silva et al., 2013). During 2019, approximately 1 in 5 (18.8 percent) youths had seriously considered attempting suicide, 1 in 6 (15.7 percent) had made a suicide plan, 1 in 11 (8.9 percent) had made an attempt, and 1 in 40 (2.5 percent) had made a suicide attempt requiring medical treatment. According to data from a nationally representative sample of emergency departments (EDs), in 2019, approximately 95,000 youths ages 14–18 years visited EDs for self-harm injuries (Centers for Disease Control and Prevention, 2020). Breaking down the numbers by gender, in the United States, about one in four women and one in ten men seriously considered killing themselves. By sexual identity, there was a significant difference with heterosexual (14.5 percent), LGBTQIA+ (46.5 percent students), and not sure (30.4 percent). Overall, there was a significant difference in having seriously considered attempting suicide by race/ethnicity (White, 19.1 percent; Black, 16.9 percent; Hispanic, 17.2 percent) (Table 2), with a significant difference by race/ethnicity among male students (White, 13.8 percent; Black, 10.7 percent; Hispanic, 11.4 percent) but not among female students (CDC, 2020).

Given these figures, there is an average likelihood that every year, every teacher in every high school classroom in the United States can expect two girls and one boy to seriously contemplate or attempt suicide (King, 2000), and every principal in the average American high school can expect one death by suicide every 5 years and 170 attempts in any given year, although certainly most of these will never come to the school's attention (Brock et al., 2006). Note that when these articles were published, the suicide rates were lower, at about 4400 deaths a year, so those are conservative estimates (Centers for Disease Control and Prevention, 2002).

Further, unless they are ferreted out, these teenagers are not likely to seek mental health assistance. Husky and her associates (2012) followed up the adolescent supplement national comorbidity study. During the course of 12 months, 3.6 percent of adolescents reported suicidal ideation without a plan or attempt, 0.6 percent reported a suicide plan without an attempt, and 1.9 percent made a suicide attempt. Overall, two-thirds of adolescents with suicidal ideation (67.3 percent) and half of those with a plan (54.4 percent) or attempt (56.9 percent) did not have any contact with a mental health specialist in the past year. Canadian children are resistant as well. Doan et al. (2020) found that high levels of resistance toward help-seeking among youth remained a significant barrier. That resistance was particularly true for those youth who were at highest risk (i.e., with lower support and poorer mental health).

From these figures, it would seem apparent that crisis response programs in schools should incorporate suicide prevention, intervention, and postvention components that are comprehensive and systematic (Austin, 2003; Bray, 2019; Capuzzi, 2002, 2009; Diamond, 2021; Flannery, 2020; Kalafat, 2003; Komar, 1994; Malley et al., 1994; Reis & Cornell, 2008; SAMHSA, 2012; Suicide Prevention Resource Center, 2022; Webb & Griffiths, 1998–1999). To that end, eleven states now require annual training for every teacher on suicide awareness, and twenty other states require it every two to five years (Flannery, 2020). There are any number of excellent state-originated plans on the internet at "school suicide plans." The Suicide Prevention Resource Center (2022) has a shopping list of various school-age target suicide programs at https://sprc.org/populations/adolescents/.

School-based child and adolescent suicide prevention/intervention/postvention should include the following points (Capuzzi, 2002; Kerr, 2009; Malley et al., 1994, p. 131; Maples et al., 2005; SAMSHA, 2012; Suicide Prevention Resource Center, 2022; Thompson, 2004):

1. A written, formal suicide policy statement.
2. Written procedures to address and ensure the safety of at-risk students.

3. Faculty and staff in-service orientation and training in warning signs and referral of at-risk students.
4. Identification and training of mental health professionals on-site or readily available crisis teams.
5. Prevention materials for distribution to students, parents, and the community and for classroom discussion.
6. Procedures for psychological screening, identification, and counseling of at-risk students.
7. Preplanned postvention responses and strategies that occur following any completed suicide.
8. Written criteria for crisis workers to assess the lethality of a potential student suicide.
9. Written policies on how the school-based child and adolescent suicide prevention/intervention/postvention program is evaluated.

Kerr (2009, pp. 24–26) has taken these general procedures a step further and outlined what the response should be to a suicide threat, a suicide attempt on school grounds, a suicide attempt off school grounds or during a school-sponsored activity and reported to an employee, and a fatal suicide attempt.

Risk Factors/Predictors/Cues

How is it that, besides age, young children and teenagers fall into a different risk category than the adults in the Lethality chapter? Almost all adolescent suicide victims have experienced some form of psychiatric illness. Many have suffered adverse childhood experiences including physical and sexual abuse, abandonment, and parental neglect (Kelly et al., 2023; O'Gorman et al., 2023; Wong et al., 2023). These range across affective, conduct, mood, and attention deficit disorders (Baugher et al., 1999; Shaffer, 1988) to antisocial personality, substance abuse, and depressive disorders (Cohen, 2020; Guida, 2001; Hacker et al., 2006; Shaffer, 1988), or the student may have a physical disability (Gryglewicz et al., 2017). Adolescents who have questions about their sexual identity, have recently experienced a loss, suffered humiliation at school or home, been bullied or cyberbullied, had an interpersonal conflict with a romantic partner or a parent, a dramatic change such as the death of a friend or a pregnancy, are heavily into alcohol or drug use, have dermatological problems, have been traumatized by sexual or physical assault, are depressed, have a physical illness, have made a major geographic move to a new school, been placed in foster care,

engage in risky behaviors (parasuicidal), are dealing with hunger, or are petulantly angry and impulsively act out are all candidates for suicidal ideation, threats, and acting (Bartik et al., 2020; Baugher, 1999; Biddle et al., 2018; Capuzzi, 2002; Diamond, 2021; Evans, 2017; Goldbach et al., 2019; Guida, 2001; McIntyre et al., 2013; Mereish et al., 2023; Nelson & Galas, 1994; Ronnstad et al., 2018; Stuart-Maver, 2023). When faced with these conflicts, it appears that a lack of family or peer support is a precipitating factor in generating suicidal ideation (Diamond, 2021; Mazza & Reynolds, 1998). Interestingly, giftedness may also be a contributing factor (Nelson & Galas, 1994). The individual who comes from a home where suicide has been attempted or has had a close friend who has attempted suicide may be at greater risk (Capuzzi, 2002; Diamond, 2021; Nelson & Galas, 1994). To add fuel to a suicidal potential fire, Zuromski and associates (2019) found that children who had dealt with prior interpersonal violence and then went through a disaster had increased suicidal ideation. Once again, as in school shooter profiling, all of these variables have some relationship with suicidal ideation, attempts, and fatal suicide attempts, but they do not predict it will happen. Given all these other variables, probably the best single predictor over time has been a previous suicide attempt (Bostwick et al., 2016; Garcia de la Garza, 2021; Nelson & Galas, 1994; Shaffer et al., 1988).

The clues and behaviors that are commonly found in the suicide indicators in Chapter 8, "Crisis of Lethality," would hold true for most adolescents and children. For children and adolescents, however, warning signs also include a sudden change in friends or dress habits, cutting hair or changing hairstyles, difficulty concentrating, persistent boredom, sudden or increased sexual activity, reversal of valuation of prized objects, use of drugs or alcohol, a loss of interest and decline in school achievement, absenteeism, writings and drawing of death or suicide, dramatic change in eating and or sleeping habits, having a plan to harm oneself, social isolation, dramatic change in dress /physical appearance, and giving things away (Capuzzi, 2002; Diamond, 2021; Greene, 1994; Kaiser Permanente, 2022; Maples et al., 2005; Nelson & Galas, 1994). Copycat suicides are particularly problematic for adolescents, particularly if the adolescents believe there will be notoriety for them. This phenomenon occurs after a suicide when peers, who may have had similar thoughts, also attempt suicide (Austin, 2003). Although most adolescents give cues to their attempts, not all do. Adolescents may verbally indicate their decision to kill themselves in clear terms, or they may be far less direct with such statements as "I wonder what death is like" or "I'm tired of all of this."

Preadolescent Suicide

There is a prevailing notion that young children do not die by suicide. Being a young child is no exemption from suicide. It is the eighth leading cause of death for children ages 2 to 11 in the United States (WISQARS, 2021). Kovess-Masfety and associates' (2017) study of suicidal ideation and death thoughts in young Eastern and Western European children found that suicidal ideation was present in 17 percent of the population, and it ranged from 9.9 percent in Italy to 26.8 percent in Germany, and death thoughts were present in 21 percent of the children with a range from 7.7 percent in Italy to 32.8 percent in Germany. Both kinds of thoughts were found to be more frequent in single parent or large families. So please be disabused of the notion that thinking and attempting suicide in this age group doesn't happen.

Have a conversation with any elementary school counselor, social worker, or school psychologist who has been in the business for any length of time, and you will be quickly disabused of that faulty notion (Diamond, 2021). The problem is that while a ton of work has been done with adolescents, relatively little has been done with young children. Price (2010), in a brief overview, pointed this out. The experts he queried indicated that most young children who die by suicide have some kind of mental disorder and are likely to have been victims of physical or sexual abuse. However, that is certainly not true of every child.

The other major issue is that when children are found to have suicidal thoughts, they tend to be treated as miniature adults rather than in terms of the cognitive and developmental stage they are in. Indeed, because of their level of cognitive development, many young children's thought processes that lead to suicide would not generally be considered reasons to kill themselves if they were adults. But, as with all people who have suicidal thoughts, it makes sense to them. Consider the following reasons: wanting to meet a friend or relative who died; feeling guilty that they are the cause of parents getting a divorce; avoiding punishment or embarrassment they believe is worse than death; wanting to punish someone else (although this can certainly happen with adolescents and adults); believing they will be martyrs for some

cause; and escape from an intolerable situation such as an abusive home or a concentrated cyberbully attack (Diamond, 2021; Muro & Kottman, 1995, pp. 324–325; Padmanathan et al., 2018).

Further, parents and teachers tend to dismiss clues that are common to suicidal ideation. Indeed, it is interesting that most child counseling and therapy books tend to lump a lot of what is known about adolescent suicide into their recommendations and counseling techniques for elementary age children. The bottom line is that young children who emit suicidal clues should be taken seriously, and the child counseling procedures that are depicted in other parts of this chapter and book should be used with them along with the general suicide prevention and intervention techniques that are used with adults. Ominously, van Vuuren and associates (2021) found that suicidal thoughts and behaviors at a young age are not a temporary phenomenon and fade away as children mature but continue on and accelerate in duration and intensity.

Child and Adolescent Cases of Suicidal Ideation

Here are some strategies and suggestions (Capuzzi, 2002; Flemons & Grainik, 2013; Fujimura, 1985; HealthyChild.org, 2022; Nelson & Galas, 1994; Substance Abuse and Mental Health Service Administration, 2020) for anyone (crisis worker, layperson, teacher, school administrator, school custodian, parent) who comes into contact with a child or adolescent suspected of having suicidal thoughts. A worthwhile endeavor is to hold a parent information meeting and provide an army-type wallet-sized smart card with primary suicide indicators on them. Most suicides of children (95.5 percent) occur in the home (National Institute of Mental Health, 2021). Thus, suicidal ideation and attempts do not stop or start at the schoolhouse door, and parents are a critical ingredient in the effort along with school staff to be aware of the following points as to what to do:

1. Trust your suspicions that the young person may be self-destructive.
2. Tell the person you're worried about them; then listen to the person in a nonjudgmental, supportive way.
3. Ask direct questions, including whether the youngsters are thinking about suicide and, if so, whether they have a plan.
4. Don't act shocked at what the youngster tells you. Don't debate whether suicide is right or wrong or

counsel the person yourself if you're not qualified. Don't promise to keep the youngster's intentions a secret. Be calm and supportive and reinforce the person for talking about it.

5. Don't leave the youngster alone if you think the risk of suicide is immediate.

6. Do not be embarrassed or reticent about getting help from a competent counselor, therapist, or other responsible adult.

7. Ensure that the youngster is safe and that the appropriate adults responsible for the youngster are notified and become actively involved with the youngster.

8. Assure the youngster that something is being done, that the youngster's suicidal urges are not being discounted, and that, in time, the emergency will most likely pass. Apprise the youngster that survival is a step-by-step, day-to-day process; that help is at hand; and that calling for help in a direct manner is necessary whenever the suicidal urge gets strong.

9. Assume an active and authoritarian role as needed to protect the child at risk. This is a crisis and calls for applied, directive guidance and management. After the youngster has apparently resolved the high-risk crisis, monitor progress very closely. Many persons have been known to suddenly die by suicide after they seemed to be renewed and strong.

10. Actively acknowledge the reality of suicide as a choice, but do not "normalize" suicide as a good choice.

11. Ask questions about the suicidal ideation, but balance them with interspersed empathic responses.

12. Construct a short-term safety plan. If the youngster is unwilling or unable to comply or there are no parents or guardians available, go to 13.

13. Consider hospitalization if parents are not cooperating, if the youth is highly agitated, or if the student has not been eating, is exhausted or dehydrated, or has some other exacerbating physical condition.

14. Refuse to allow the youth to return to school without an assessment and release by a qualified mental health professional. This assures that the youth will receive the necessary treatment and also protects the school from liability if a suicide attempt or completion takes place.

The following scenarios incorporate many of the suggestions just given.

Billy, Age 11. In a group counseling session, children ages 9 to 12 (including Billy) were engaged in relaxation training, emotive imagery, and self-esteem building. The children were taking turns disclosing a positive image each was experiencing. Billy had been rather quiet and complacent in previous counseling sessions.

Billy: I see myself beside the highway. There's a big 18-wheeler—going fast. I'm feeling like I'm gonna die. I want to die. I see myself jumping in front of it.

CW: Billy, it concerns me to hear you say that! Could you and I talk about that after the others leave? And Billy, I want you to know that I'm glad you didn't keep that image a secret from us.

The crisis worker was shaken and surprised at Billy's sudden description of his images. The worker assessed the suicide risk to be high because of the content and the context of the disclosure (the group activity had been clearly structured to facilitate sharing only positive, growth-promoting images, which other members of the group had done).

Billy's nonverbal body posture and profoundly serious facial expression communicated that he was not fooling. The crisis worker did not deny, refute, or admonish Billy. Recognizing that Billy was taking a great risk by disclosing his thoughts of death, the worker responded by assuring Billy that he had received the message as sent and conveying to members of the group the worker's willingness to attend to and answer Billy's cry for help.

Lester, Age 14. Lester was an intelligent youngster who made good grades in school and had a reputation for being quiet, cooperative, and well behaved. Following his parents' bitter divorce, while living with his mother and a younger sister and brother, Lester began to get into trouble in school because of his overt acting out and belligerent behavior. He lost interest in his studies and school activities, and his grades began to tumble. He became rebellious with his mother, and his appetite decreased to the degree that he just picked at his food. He became very withdrawn, seldom leaving his room, in contrast to his previous behavior of being actively engaged in outside activities whenever possible.

Lester's mother and the school counselor decided to place him in a student support group consisting of middle school students, both boys and girls, all of whom were experiencing severe difficulty following the separation and/or divorce of their parents. At the conclusion of one of the group sessions, Lester asked to speak with the crisis worker.

Co: Lester, sounds like something happened in the group today that got pretty close to you.

Lester: (hesitant, looking down, nervous) I . . . I've been feeling weird lately. Strange. Like I'm somewhere else.

Co: You mean like you're outside your own body observing yourself?

Lester: Yeah. Even at night. I don't understand it. I've even thought I might be going crazy.

Co: (closely observing Lester's body language) Lester, it sounds like this is so serious you may have even been wishing you were dead.

Lester: Yeah. I've been scared. I've just thought about how it would be to just go to sleep and not wake up.

Co: Have you thought about making that happen? Killing yourself, so that you'd never wake up?

Lester: Thought about it, yeah. Thought about it more lately.

The crisis worker had sensed prior to the interview that Lester might be suicidal. At least six indicators on the risk assessment checklist pointed to the conclusion that Lester was at a high risk level: his changing family life, his changing behavior and attitudes, his body language, his eating habits, his social habits, and his grades. Any one of these would have been an important lethality signal (Curran, 1987, pp. 111–118).

Crisis workers and other adults who work with suicidal youngsters must pay careful attention to clues indicating that suicidal ideation is present. Hunt et al. (1991, pp. 20–21) found that classroom teachers who are sensitive to the emotional changes in and have close relationships with their students can be primary identification, support, and referral sources for youth who are suicidal.

Lester's science teacher, Mr. Birch, overheard Lester talking to a classmate about giving him his Bluetooth speaker and the password to his music streaming service. Lester had also taken a pair of scissors and chopped off his long hair. He had gotten into a shouting match with a girl in class and almost come to blows with her before the teacher intervened.

These behaviors were clearly uncharacteristic of Lester. Mr. Birch also knew from a threat assessment meeting with Lester's teachers and the counselor that Lester had thoughts of killing himself. The teacher had a list of warning signs he had received at an in-service training on suicide (Maples et al., 2005). After he became suspicious of Lester's behavior, he looked over the warning signs and made an immediate referral for Lester to the school counselor. The school counselor called Lester's mother, who confirmed Mr. Birch's suspicions. The assistant principal also indicated that Lester had had two disciplinary referrals for fighting after school in the last 2 weeks.

Co: (3 months after the initial intervention) Lester, I asked for this conference because I'm worried about you again. I thought you were doing great! But now, frankly, I'm scared to death for you. Mr. Birch and your mom are worried too and asked me to see you.

Lester: Oh, I'm OK. Things are going great.

Co: (in a calm, soft, caring, empathic voice—not a lecturing or agitated tone) They may seem OK to you, but what concerns me right now is what you've been doing lately. Your mother is very upset and puzzled because you've given your Bluetooth Speaker and music" to a friend, and the principal is livid because you've picked two fights on the way home from school this week. I've noticed that the last 2 days in the hallways and cafeteria you've been like an entirely different person. If these things say what they appear to say, I don't think I can leave here today until I can be sure you're safe. I don't want to wake up in the morning and hear that you're dead!

Lester: It's really not anything you should feel worried about. I'm OK, really I am.

Co: (soft, empathic vocal tone continued) Fine, then you can help me feel OK by discussing with me what's going on. I just want you to know that the clues I'm picking up spell danger and that I'm as concerned for you as I've ever been. And I need to know that you're safe, even though you say you're OK. I really care about you.

The crisis worker was empathic but confrontive and persistent even though it would have been desirable and comforting to believe that Lester was OK. As it turned out, Lester was indeed on the threshold of suicide again. The important thing was that the worker interpreted Lester's unusual actions as clues that called for help—whether Lester overtly called for help or not.

What is particularly helpful for them is decreasing their feelings of isolation and marginalization (Berman et al., 2006). Including suicidal children and adolescents in support groups and other activities that make them feel like valued and contributing members of their school and peer group is an important part of moving them away from suicidal thinking and behaving. Berman and Jobes (1994) found that suicidal adolescents particularly need empathic therapeutic alliances to help them feel affirmed, valued, and understood.

Postvention

Clustering of Suicides. Approximately 1 to 5 percent of teen suicides in the United States occur as part of a cluster (Centers for Disease Control and Prevention, 2022). Cluster or contagion suicides occur when more than one suicide attempt or completion happens within a proximate geographic area, giving the appearance that these events are related. Suicide clusters are defined as a greater-than-expected number of suicides or nonfatal events such as suicide attempts and self-harm occurring close in time or geography. Clusters can also be related to vulnerable individuals from diverse locations who are exposed to a highly publicized suicide and imitate the method of that suicide and are reached by the publicity (Austin, 2003; Gould & Shaffer, 1986; Kalafat, 1990, p. 364); Kirk, 1993, p. 15; Webb & Griffiths, 1998–1999, pp. B43–B48; Niedzwiedz et al., 2014).

Kirk (1993, pp. 15–16) likens such clustering to the infectious disease concept; that is, when a pathogen is introduced into a vulnerable population, the probability of infection is spontaneously increased. Similarly, when an adolescent suicide occurs and is sensationally reported or somehow glorified, other adolescents who may already be in a state of despair, helplessness, or hopelessness may be influenced toward terminating their lives or see it as an excellent way to get a great deal of attention. This can become a metastasizing crisis, a school's worst nightmare.

Contagion. Sandy Austin (2003) reported on a series of four suicides at her school in an 8-month period. The school crisis response team immediately responded to the suicides in the following manner. After each suicide, faculty were called and informed of a meeting the next morning where they were briefed. District mental health personnel were

contacted for support. The principal, counselor, and SRO visited the deceased's family members and asked if a memo could be read that stated the student "took his own life" instead of "committed suicide" to convey the finality of the act and decrease the "glory" of it. Memos were drafted and read in each class. At the end of the day, faculty met for a debriefing to determine how students were doing. Students were invited to come into the counseling office for one-on-one or group counseling or just to come to a "safe room." Parent/community meetings were hosted with an expert to address the suicide issue. The media were asked to construct their stories in a "signs to look for" manner and "how to help someone access resources" to address the contagion effect.

The crisis team was then confronted with another problem. Instead of dealing in typical teenager fashion with the ruts and potholes of adolescence, the students started talking about suicide as a viable option for taking care of problems. The counselor and student representatives visited each English class and asked students to be observant and tell someone if a friend started talking about suicide or showed warning signs. Posters were created on the subject of getting help and watching for clues and placed throughout the community. Crisis line phone numbers were put on cards and passed out. Austin reported that for the rest of the school year, there was at least one tip a day about a potential suicide. The toll went beyond the suicides and the grief felt for their loss. Two peer counselors became suicidal, and one school counselor had to take a month's sick leave due to stress. Thus, you should get a pretty clear notion that vicarious trauma, which you will read about in Chapter 15, "Human Services Workers in Crisis Burnout, Vicarious Traumatization, and Compassion Fatigue," is real.

The school district did everything by the book (SAMSHA, 2012; Suicide Prevention Resource Center, 2022). They did everything they could possibly do and generally did it right, but still, the suicides continued. Shaffer et al. (1990) reported that among adolescent suicide attempters, "talking about suicide in the classroom makes some kids more likely to try to kill themselves" (pp. 3153–3155). Thus, "postvention" classroom programs designed for suicide education and prevention may be appropriate for the majority of adolescents who are not currently at risk but may not be appropriate for the at-risk population. Or at least a massive effort will be needed to get all of the student body involved and willing to tell an adult about a peer's suicidal thoughts or threats without fear of being labeled a snitch.

Publicity and Contagion. Media involvement can help contain or exacerbate suicide contagion. When the media display graphic headlines and images, romanticize the suicide, overstate the problem through emotive words such as "epidemic or "sky-rocketing," repeatedly report on the same suicide or explicitly describe the method or show pictures of the suicide site or grievers, they are aiding and abetting the potential for clustering (Centers for Disease Control and Prevention, 2022; Gould et al., 2003; Niederkrotenhaler et al., 2010; Reporting on Suicide, 2022). Kirk (1993, p. 17), in his investigation about media effects on adolescent suicide, makes three interesting observations: (1) The more sensational the reporting of the suicide, the greater the increase in suicides within the reporting area. (2) There was a significant increase in auto accidents involving teenagers following media reports of youth suicides. (3) There was an increase in adolescent suicides following certain made-for-television motion pictures that focused on episodes showing suicides in the lives of troubled and suicidal adolescents. That's why it is critically important for the media liaison to work closely with the media, as in the case of Sandy Austin's school district. When the media is positively involved, they can provide information on the warning signs of suicide risk, provide sources for help, share messages of hope and resilience, and engage experts to provide facts about suicide and how to prevent it (CDC, 2022; Reporting on Suicide, 2022).

Imperatives for SCRTs in Suicides. School crisis response teams (SCRTs) must be knowledgeable about suicide postvention so clustering does not occur. Crises of suicide are different from other crises because of the self-instigating behavior that goes with them and because so many different emotional evaluations are placed on suicide. If SCRT members do not know about the dynamics of suicidal behavior, they need to get outside consultation that does, and they need to have it available immediately. The worst possible scenario is an insecure SCRT that does not want to "look bad" because it needs outside help to handle the crisis. In our own experience, we have witnessed an SCRT that did not know what it was doing and wound up with three more completed suicides and two attempts on its hands in the space of two months in the same high school! Thus, it is critical that parents, teachers, and students be given notification and information regarding warning signs of suicide—particularly after a completion (Maples et al., 2005).

Jennifer, Age 17. Jennifer was terrified. Although she had suffered from depression, loneliness, and low self-esteem for several years, she had managed to have a satisfactory social life, maintain average grades in school, and regain her equilibrium following each depressive episode. Several stressors during the past year had combined to complicate and disrupt her life. Indeed, one of the major contributors to child and adolescent suicide is the role of the family (Berman et al., 2006; Wagner, 1997). Her parents' separation and divorce were unexpected and bitter. Her maternal grandmother, to whom she had been very close, died from rapidly progressing intestinal cancer. Jennifer was living with her mother and two younger sisters. The mother began dating a single man and permitted him to move in with them. Jennifer changed schools during the middle of the year when her parents' original home was sold. Because of her lack of social adjustment and academic achievement in the new school, Jennifer was placed in a support group at the school and was also seen regularly by an individual counselor.

Following a weekend episode of trauma over the suicide of a friend who attended another school, Jennifer showed signs of being upset, severely depressed, exhausted, and withdrawn. The crisis worker had been notified that Jennifer had missed school on Friday to attend her friend's funeral. Being wary of **contagion suicide** (Centers for Disease Control and Prevention, 2022), sometimes called *copycat suicide* (Gould & Shaffer, 1986), the crisis worker knew that Jennifer's risk level was probably elevated because of her trauma over her friend's suicide in addition to her already stressful family situation.

CW: Jennifer, it frightens me to see you this way. What's happening to cause you so much pain right now?

The crisis worker could see the physical and emotional devastation Jennifer was feeling. It was important to communicate to Jennifer the worker's affective concern and to provide a direct and open opportunity for Jennifer to feel safe and to respond (Patros & Shamoo, 1989, pp. 126–128).

Jennifer: (after a long pause, in a very low, subdued voice) I . . . I've never been this scared before in my life. (pause) All weekend I've been at the end of my rope. I've just thought, there's no use going on anymore. And ever since last Friday at Etta's funeral, I've wondered if it wouldn't be better if I just went like she did. They said such nice things about her. She and I were so close. It was so sad but so comforting to hear all the wonderful things they said about her.

CW: Jennifer, I'm glad you're here now. I can see how the death of Etta and her eulogy really affected you. What frightens me right now is what you just said, that it would be better if you joined her. Does this mean that you're planning to kill yourself over this?

The crisis worker's questioning was aimed at swiftly making a triage assessment of Jennifer's lethality and quickly heading off the idea of contagion suicide. The answer to such a question drastically impacts and changes what the crisis worker does. Even though Jennifer's destabilized family situation would have been signal enough to inquire into any suicidal thoughts and plans she might have, the hint of contagion suicide served as a red flag, alerting the crisis worker to be assertive and direct in asking the suicide question.

The concept of contagion suicide is controversial. Skeptics and critics claim that there is little scientific proof of clustering and copycatting because it is difficult to prove that one suicide attempt or completion directly causes another. There is too much evidence of recent contagion suicides in the United States to ignore or dismiss claims of clustering (Centers for Disease Control and Prevention, 2022; Niederkrotenhaler et al., 2010; Reporting on Suicide, 2022). We agree with these conclusions and believe from our own experience that it is extremely important for school crisis response teams that go into a school after a suicide to know that this phenomenon has a possibility of being activated if postvention is not handled correctly.

There is evidence that providing peer support such as a professionally led peer counseling group can help suicidal teenagers (King et al., 2006). One of the major support systems in schools to prevent initial and contagion suicides is a peer counseling system such as Allen's (1996) peer leader program. Allen's peer counselors meet weekly to talk about issues and problems that are occurring in their high school. They are the eyes and ears of the counselor and are privy to information of a far wider and current scope than school staff will ever be. By relaying information to the school counselor about peers who are severely affected by a school trauma, they enable intervention to happen much more effectively and quickly. As Allen says, "I have no idea what types of drugs or alcohol are currently hot. I don't know who is depressed because he broke up with his girlfriend, but my peer leaders do, and they are not seen as snitches for telling me. It is okay because the rest of the kids see it as the peer leaders' job."

Grief and Mourning After Adolescent Suicide. Kirk (1993, pp. 112–115) found that suicides of adolescents and other youth represent a type of death that severely complicates survivors' mourning and adjustment. He cited the following reasons:

1. The adolescent suicide is generally unexpected.
2. The death of a young person is harder to accept than that of an older person who has lived a full life.
3. To many people, suicide is incomprehensible and perhaps even morally wrong.
4. The suicide completer's family and friends are left with guilt, anger, and a sense of unfinished business with the deceased, which mourners must work through.
5. There is less social support for a suicide completer's family than there may be for other bereaved families because people tend to unjustly ascribe blame to the family.

Kirk also stated that when a suicide occurs in a school setting, grief reaction is often further complicated by the group response of classmates and school personnel. Educators, school crisis response teams, parents, and others involved in designing prevention, intervention, and postvention procedures should be sensitive to the unique grief factors just mentioned. A suicide absolutely must not be glorified or made heroic. That doesn't mean that feelings are ignored or questions concerning the deceased are not answered as truthfully and honestly as possible. Survivors will be seeking answers to why the individual took their life. There will be many questions about who had responsibility or culpability in not preventing it. There will be questioning of oneself as to why it wasn't seen, or if seen, then why it wasn't stopped (Capuzzi, 2009). Empathic understanding of these concerns from students, parents, and faculty is of primary importance, and no questions or comments should be summarily dismissed (Capuzzi, 2002).

As with other traumatic events, a room for counseling students should be set up, factual information should be disseminated, and an SCRT meeting should be held to determine whether other students may be at risk. Maples and her associates (2005) describe an adaption of a four-stage model (Brammer et al., 1993) that can be used to work with teenage survivors of a suicide. In *stage 1,* there will be *shock* and *disorganization.* Typical responses are "It couldn't happen," and "No, not possible!" Initial intervention follows along the lines of the intervention responses described in Chapter 12, "Personal Loss: Bereavement and Grief," and uses basic nonjudgmental listening and responding skills. *Stage 2* is the most potentially volatile stage of this particular grieving process. It involves feelings of *anguish, remorse,* and *guilt* over not having done something to prevent the suicide. "Why didn't I see this coming?" and "I could have stopped it!" are common themes of recrimination. Besides conducting a psychological autopsy on the order of the one in Chapter 8, "Crisis of Lethality," using cognitive-behavioral strategies such as thought stopping and positive mental videotapes may be effective in helping students control their feelings.

Heather: (16-year-old best friend of a suicide starting to shake uncontrollably and with tears streaming down her face) I think I am going crazy. Every time I pass Sally's locker I come apart. We had been best friends since first grade. I could have, should have stopped this, and I didn't even know it. That's some kind of friend.

CW: Remember what we said in the psychological autopsy. It made perfect sense to her. It is a terrible tragedy, but neither you nor I nor anyone else can be, or should be, responsible for her suicide. You have that pink memory band on your arm. Every time you pass where her locker was [note crisis worker's movement to past tense], tap the band and say "STOP!" when those feelings start to flood over you, and remember that one great moment you said when the two of you won the sixth-grade talent show. Smile and remember how deliriously happy and goofy you looked in your Raggedy Ann and Andy costumes. Then move on. You need to do this every time you go by the locker. Don't avoid the locker like you have been, but just make it part of your normal routine. We are going to get that mental image squarely in your mind, so lean back, close your eyes, and let's practice that.

Stage 3 has to do with *reconciliation of the loss.* When faced with traumatic death for the first time, teenagers may struggle with existential questions such as the meaning of life or the futility of everyday living.

"What's it all about?" and "Why bother with school?" are topics for group grief work that helps students reconcile and move on with their lives. Spiritual components of these questions should be considered, and working alliances and referrals to faith-based counseling are good options.

Stage 4 has to do with the *emergence of new goals* for survivors. Recommitment to established friendships or dedication to a worthy cause or a sport season are ways of helping teenagers move past the suicide. Typically, this stage will mark the passing of the friend and recommitment to living by the surviving teenagers.

The suicide of a popular student or teacher is one of the most difficult challenges human services workers in schools face. The potential for interventions to go terribly awry is high, and, thus, interventions must be thought through and carefully applied. One of your authors witnessed one instance in which the faculty of a school assembled after school to engage in a debriefing with the SCRT of the district. The teachers had all sorts of questions and emotions to deal with concerning the suicide of a fellow teacher the previous night. They were told, "If you are having problems with your fellow teacher's death, we suggest you call your behavioral health service provider and talk with them." Then, the SCRT leader dismissed the group, leaving the principal and school counselor to deal with more than 50 enraged and frustrated faculty members.

As in any crisis, being at the school of the completed suicide as soon as possible after notification is critical for planning and for making assessments about the emotional state of faculty and students, quelling rumors, assessing for other possible suicides, and depropagandizing and deglorifying the suicide by debriefing faculty and students. Capuzzi (2009) recommends that a single statement be prepared and read in each class rather than over the public address system so that everyone receives the same message but in the presence of teachers who can be watchful for students who are having a difficult time. It is fruitless and damaging for the SCRT to come straggling in late in the afternoon or the next day. Such dilatory behavior lets rumor and chaos run wild, and makes a statement that there is not a great deal of concern about the health and well-being of the school.

The following points are recommended when the death of a student or teacher is due to suicide (American Association of Suicidology, 1991, 1998; Capuzzi, 2009):

1. Don't dismiss school or encourage funeral attendance during school hours.
2. Don't hold a large-scale memorial to the deceased or dismiss school to do so.
3. Do provide individual and group counseling.
4. Verify the facts, and do treat the death as a suicide.
5. Do emphasize that no one thing or person is to blame for the suicide.
6. Do emphasize that help is available, that suicide is preventable, and that everyone has a role to play in prevention.
7. Don't build a tangible memorial such as a bench or a tree with a marker or dedicate a yearbook to the suicide.
8. Do not release information in large groups such as an assembly. Work by classroom or in small groups.
9. Do be on the lookout for delayed grief reactions.

Do suicide prevention/intervention school-based programs work? Results are variable. Lewitzka and associates (2019) examined national suicide prevention programs in eight different countries over 30 years and found them to be effective but in older age groups. Gijzen and associates' (2022) meta-analysis of school-based suicide prevention programs showed some promise within three months post-test assessments and potentially also have effects that are sustained over time. Katz and associates (2013) found that most suicide prevention programs are designed to improve students' and school staffs' knowledge and attitude toward suicide. Of 16 programs examined, only 2 reduced suicide attempts, although several of the programs did reduce suicidal ideation, improve general life skills, and train gatekeepers to become more vigilant. De Silva and associates (2013) conducted broad-based mapping studies for suicidal and self-harm studies. They found some school-based programs with skills training components to be promising. Zenere and Lazarus (1997) studied a comprehensive suicide prevention and intervention program in a large, urban, culturally diverse school district. Students were tracked over a 5-year period. What they found was that although suicidal ideation remained stable, the rate of attempts and completions was dramatically reduced. Wasserman and associates (2015) conducted a very sophisticated cross-Europe study of 15-year-old students assigned to three treatment conditions. The Youth Aware of Mental Health Programme (YAM) targeted pupils as opposed to screening by professionals and a gatekeeper training program for teachers. YAM was effective in reducing the number of attempts and severe suicidal ideation, although Brent and Brown (2015) noted in a comment that the specific components such as seeking help or using coping were not isolated or discussed. Brent and associates (2013) in their comprehensive review of interventions found that the most effective interventions appeared to have either family interactions or nonfamilial support, so it may be that any school-based program needs to consider the inclusion of support systems outside the school.

Crisis Intervention and the Tier System

LO10 Many of the problems faced in this chapter such as suicide could be ameliorated a great deal if students felt more bonded and affiliated with their school (Erbacher et al., 2015). Alienation from school is a major contributor to school failure and the many negative outcomes that go with it (Morinaj et al., 2017) The innovation of the multi-tiered system of support (MTSS) has been a valiant attempt to overcome such failure by a more targeted, individualized approach to each learner. As the use of the program has become widespread in schools, terms such as tiers, benchmarks, universal instruction, and intensive intervention have become familiar to many teachers. These concepts may also be known by other names. For example, an MTSS might be known by terms such as Response to Intervention (RTI) or Positive Behavior Interventions and Supports (PBIS) in some districts. All of these terms refer to a system of providing all students with the instruction they need at the moment they need it. Most versions of an MTSS include three tiers, or levels, of support whose descriptions follow (Brown, 2016).

Tier 1: Primary—Teaching efforts are applied universally to create optimal learning outcomes in universal or core instruction for all students regardless of learning needs or background. Tiers include not only academic achievement but also social emotional development and classroom behavior management.

Tier 2: Secondary—Teacher efforts are applied for selected students in a targeted manner to reduce or eliminate learning difficulties as soon as they are identified. Secondary prevention typically involves small-group instruction that relies on evidence-based interventions that specify the instructional procedures, Tier 2 is likely to involve small groups of students with similar learning needs who work daily with a teacher using a specific instructional practice or program. Social and emotional development and behavior management needs gain additional focus when warranted in Tier 2. Tier 2 needs to supplement Tier 1 because students who have not yet met learning goals need more time to learn, practice, and review knowledge and skills.

Tier 3: Tertiary—Teaching efforts are applied in response to significant and chronic learning problems to improve student success as much as possible. Tertiary prevention, the third level of the RTI prevention framework, is the most intensive of the three levels and is individualized to target each student's area(s) of need with weekly progress monitoring. These tiers are not just academic but also provide a segway into crisis intervention as preventive procedures at each tier level, with classroom instruction the starting place for Tier 1 classes and Tier 2 small groups (Lerner, 2020).

Lerner (2020) starts each classroom meeting out by reviewing how to submit a request to see the counselor for non-emergencies. Lerner then details her three hurts emergency referral request: physically self-injured or suicidal thoughts; fighting or having homicidal thoughts; or being harmed by someone else, such as bullying or child abuse. Lerner then introduces a variety of crises and techniques for handling them and then role plays putting the techniques in use. Her data count of crisis incidents in her middle school dropped from an average of 200 a year from 2014 through 2018 prior to starting her classroom program to 118 in 2018–2019 and 34 in 2019–2020 after implementation.

Lerner (2021) has also developed a trauma-informed series of classroom meetings. She uses this with Tier 2 students who may need some additional support by using education-based techniques to help group members gain skills and information and develop skills for challenging situations that target goal striving and healthy coping skills. A favorite example is her breathing backward exercise, where students focus on exhaling first and inhaling second, which takes their attention off of negative thoughts while they focus on their breathing.

Tier 3 brings teamwork into play for students who need long term intensive or social and behavioral support (Daigle, 2022). Daigle promotes the school counselor's role as being part of a multidisciplinary team that focuses on strength-based functional behavioral assessment and the instigation of a behavior intervention plan. This approach is a wrap-around service based on home, community services, and the school working together in a culturally competent and strength-based approach.

Jackson incorporates a team approach with Tier 1, 2, and 3 students that systematically delivers a range of interventions based on student needs. Her district teams are made up of school counselors, school psychologists, school social workers, school nurses, drug and alcohol prevention specialists, special education deans, administrators, and school resource officers. These teams meet monthly to review data and discuss programming interventions. The school counselors in each building serve as coordinators of the site-based teams and as a kind of general practitioner, referring students out to Tier 2 supports such as small group counseling and peer metering or Tier 3 supports such as individual counseling, re-entry support, and wrap around services. It should be noted that Jackson's district had both financial and political resources to put this comprehensive effort together. It sounds good, but does it really work? Roesenfeild et al. (2018) conducted an extensive review of research on K–12 school-based problem solving teams and found limited success. Positive outcomes were limited due to gaps in how teams impacted target outcomes and an absence of hard data outcomes to confirm progress. Lack of training in team building and insufficient knowledge of the school culture were also barriers to success.

Planning for a Crisis with the SCRT

LO11 **Federal Emergency Management Agency**. The school crisis events in the 1990s caused a huge change in the way schools viewed security and the need for crisis response. As various state and local education agencies started scrambling to prepare emergency plans that included more than fire drills and tornado warnings, a planning guide for schools was created in 2003 by the U.S. Department of Education. *Practical Information on Crisis Planning: A Guide for Schools and Communities* used the Federal Emergency Management Agency (FEMA) four-stage model for schools—mitigation, preparedness, response, and recovery—as a template for the guide (U.S. Department of Education, 2003).

That guide has been updated by the U.S. Department of Education (2023a) in *Safe and Supportive Schools*, which provides information on grants to support students exposed to violence, school climate, and academic enrichment. It also provides an information hub where stakeholders can access high-quality federally supported information and resources that support student mental and physical health. Of the most importance to school crisis intervention is the **Readiness and Emergency Management for Schools (REMS) Technical Assistance (TA) Center**, (2023). This guide is a comprehensive planning tool for the establishment and implementation of school safety teams in developing comprehensive risk assessment and implementation plans. It also details planning and action steps for active shooter scenarios.

This plan fits with the FEMA national incident emergency model (refer to Chapter 16, "Disaster Response"), which allows for a common language between first responders, school personnel, and the community (U.S. Department of Education, 2020). Having consistency with terms is an important feature because it allows the school districts and the community first responders to speak the same language. Another national school model has been developed by school psychologists.

PREPaRE Model. The PREPaRE (Prevent, Reaffirm, Evaluate, Provide and Respond, Examine) school crisis prevention and intervention model was developed by the National Association of School Psychologists. PREPaRE stands for *prevent* and prepare for psychological trauma; *reaffirm* physical health and perceptions of security and safety; *evaluate* psychological trauma risk; *provide* interventions and *respond* to psychological needs; and *examine* the effectiveness of crisis prevention and intervention. PREPaRE is an evidence-informed school crisis curriculum with a strong mental health component (Brock et al., 2016). While the model is based on the U.S. Department of Education's phases of crisis management and the Incident Command System as proposed by the National Incident Management System, it also incorporates components of Mitchell and Everly's (1995) critical incident stress management (refer to Chapter 16, "Disaster Response"), which introduced "debriefing" and offers both planning for student behaviors in crisis and prevention in school safety (Brock et al., 2011).

PREPaRE follows a planned system to use in a crisis situation, including the assembling of a team, evaluating the potential trauma to students, and

offering crisis services. In addition, the PREPaRE model uses a three-tier approach as all students may receive services following a crisis situation. Tier 1 may be conducted in the form of a classroom meeting, while Tier 2 may advance to a more individual-based crisis intervention. Finally, students who were severely traumatized would receive psychotherapy, which would be categorized under Tier 3 (Brock et al., 2011).

One of the main components in the PREPaRE model is offering training opportunities in order to understand the work of crisis response. Given that the National Association of School Psychologists covers the United States and its members are in practically every school district in the country, it should not be too surprising that many districts use this (Brock et al., 2011). There are, indeed, a number of different models for crisis response in schools, such as the National Organization for Victim Assistance (NOVA) program (2015), the integrated model by Jimerson and associates (2005), and Caplan's (1964) three-tier structure. All these models highlight the importance of tasks that need to be done before a crisis, during a crisis, and after a crisis situation.

Whatever the model, a crisis plan for a school system is not done overnight. It takes a great deal of planning and commitment by the school district and the staff (Brock et al., 1996, 2016; Duncan et al., 2013; Kerr, 2009; Luna & Hoffman, 1999; Maples et al., 2005; Montano & Dowdall-Thomae, 2003; Newgass & Schonfeld, 2005; Petersen, 1999; Petersen & Straub, 1992; Rubin, 1999; Stephens, 1997). Crisis plans are both generic and idiosyncratic. Crisis plans of other schools and consultants can be extremely helpful in making a skeletal outline of what needs to be covered in containing a crisis. No matter whether the crisis occurs in Brooklyn, New York, or Brooklyn, Mississippi, many of the same needs and responses generic to all crises of lethality will be applicable to each. When a disaster hits schools, the federal government encourages schools to follow the National Incident Management System (2023), which standardizes how a crisis response is organized. That's all well and good, but the professional responders will leave after the emergency is over and guess who gets to carry on? Also, they won't be there in the first few minutes or hours of the crisis when the chaos theory you vaguely remember in Chapter 1, "Approaching Crisis Intervention," is running rampant.

Further, each school district and each school building has its own peculiarities in regard to its physical plant, its staffing, its student population, and its community makeup. Each of these variables plays a critical part in how specific planning for a crisis will be conducted. To think that a crisis plan for the Los Angeles school district can be taken wholesale and applied to Waterloo, Iowa, would be misguided, to say the least. A crisis response in a school needs a delivery system. The chief components of any service delivery system are the written policies of what to do when a crisis occurs, the physical resources to carry out the policy, and the trained personnel to implement the service (Nelson & Slaikeu, 1990, p. 339). A crisis plan must cover safety and security; obtaining, verifying, and providing accurate information to the various constituencies of the school; and also dealing with the emotional needs of those constituencies. If these three areas are not addressed concurrently as the crisis unfolds, none will be addressed effectively (Newgass & Schonfeld, 2005). School crisis response teams (SCRTs) have proliferated in the twenty-first century. The *school*-based *crisis response team* provides staff and students with the majority of direct services needed during most *crisis* events such as:

1. Death of a student, a staff member, or a community member whose death affects a significant portion of the school population.
2. Major environmental crises, such as a flood, tornado, earthquake, or fire.
3. A situation that involves a threat to the physical safety of students, such as a school bus accident, even in the absence of injuries.
4. A situation that involves a perceived threat to the emotional well-being of students, such as may be precipitated by hate-crime graffiti or repetitive bomb threats.

One of the primary, initial tasks of the committee is planning for those events (Brock et al, 1996; Duncan et al., 2013; Kerr, 2009; Montano & Dowdall-Thomae, 2003; Newgass & Schonfeld, 2005; Office of Victims of Crime, 2003; Petersen, 1999; Petersen & Straub, 1992; Poland, 1999; Rubin, 1999; Stephens, 1997). A decision needs to be made on the size of the committee. If it's too large, it becomes unwieldy. If it's too small, it's not viable enough to meet a large crisis. The ideal is probably a two-tiered team if the district is large enough to support it and a super-tier regional team outside the district. The first-tier team is a district-wide effort that deals with the big picture of crises. This team should be composed of a wide variety of individuals representing a cross section of social services and government institutions that will have to

respond to the crisis. The second tier is a building response team that is familiar with its physical plant and its constituency. These individuals represent the teaching staff and administration, the parents, and most important, the support staff (failure to include the custodian might mean that nobody knows how to shut off the gas or electricity in the building) (Brock et al., 1996, p. 31; Lovre, 2013; Office of Victims of Crime, 2003). One of the critical ingredients is coordination between these two tiers. If these two levels operate at cross-purposes, not only will they hinder crisis resolution, but they can also make it worse. Coordination should be systemic and integrate partnerships among a variety of stakeholders that work with adolescents (Lubell & Vetter, 2006).

When a crisis is of such magnitude that local staff are overwhelmed or emotionally devastated because of personal involvement, then outside help should be summoned. This calls for a regional team, most typically a state response team. Mobilizing this regional tier should be planned for a long time before the crisis occurs. In small rural school districts where the labor power and expertise for the following positions are beyond the district's capabilities, it is absolutely mandatory that linkages be established between districts and support personnel. It is even more important for these small districts that they have close linkages between county-wide, state, and federal disaster management teams that would compose this super tier.

A needs assessment should be conducted to determine what the school staff needs in the way of training and, even more important, whether the constituency believes in and is willing to support the effort (Davis & Salasin, 1975). One might suppose that few people would be opposed to implementing a full-scale crisis prevention and intervention program in a school given the current publicity about school violence. That supposition may not be true when it comes to the reality of passing a bond issue, providing release time for staff, or disrupting the ease of access to school buildings. Therefore, fully appraising the community and determining their resistance or acceptance are critical to implementing an effective plan (Duncan et al., 2013).

A clear system for dealing with a major school crisis should be established long before the need for intervention. It should ensure that all personnel are clear as to what is going to happen, when it will happen, who will be responsible for each component, how a report is made, who is to make the report, and subsequent follow-up action.

Such planning should include all the school staff and administration. Furthermore, because such interventions will undoubtedly involve law enforcement and perhaps other mental health agencies, they too should be involved in planning for violence intervention and know what part they are to play in it (Blauvelt, 1998; Brock et al., 1996, pp. 33–37; Montano & Dowdall-Thomae, 2003; Newgass & Schonfeld, 2005).

Your authors have seen a number of voluminous crisis plans developed by school systems that are quite impressive. One plan has 29 different leaders, directors, officers, and chiefs, with very detailed roles and functions for each! These plans are gathering dust on the principal's and superintendent's bookshelves. Any crisis plan should be usable, and it should be simple enough that everybody knows their role in implementing it (Blauvelt, 1998; Goldstein & Kodluboy, 1998, pp. 170–171). If staff are not trained to implement the plan, and if a school crisis plan is not practiced, evaluated, critiqued, reviewed, and updated on a regular basis (Brock et al., 1996, pp. 243–248; Duncan et al., 2013; Poland, 1999, p. 4), it is pretty much useless.

The School Crisis Response Team (SCRT)

If the crisis can be handled with help from within the district, the community generally will be better served because these people will be familiar with the setting and their clientele, and the district will know what level of expertise these people have (Brock et al., 1996, p. 61; Rubin, 1999). Not everyone is cut out to do crisis intervention work. Just because a person is a counselor, a social worker, a school psychologist, or a caring teacher or administrator does not automatically make her or him the best person to be involved with the team. Careful consideration should be given to team composition, and people who feel they might not be capable of handling a severe crisis should not be discriminated against because they are truthful about their trepidation (Kerr, 2009, p. 35).

The following roles make up what would be a competent SCRT. There should be redundancy in these roles (Brock et al., 1996, pp. 74–75; Kerr, 2009, pp. 36–45; Poland, 2004). If the crisis response coordinator is a principal who is being held hostage or the intervention coordinator is a school counselor who is injured in an explosion, there needs to be someone else familiar enough with that role to take over.

Poland (1999, p. 4) speaks of three waves in the aftermath of a disaster. The first wave is the medical personnel and police. The second wave is the media. The third wave is the parents. Therefore, it is not just the victims and survivors that a school must be concerned with, but a host of other problems as well. Therefore, an SCRT will need to have a number of other people on it who may not have any expertise at all in crisis intervention but do have the expertise to allow the SCRT to handle the crisis effectively.

Crisis Response Coordinator. This person should be someone with decision-making capability, most likely a school administrator who is knowledgeable about the school district and staff. This person should be highly knowledgeable about the crisis plan and has good communication links within and outside the system. This person is in charge of coordinating, implementing, and evaluating crisis response plans (Brock et al. 1996, pp. 67–68; Rubin, 1999). This role is different from that of the person who would actually coordinate the intervention.

Crisis Intervention Coordinator. This person is responsible for implementing and carrying out the crisis plan. The intervention coordinator should have a thorough understanding of crisis intervention techniques and strategies. This person should have a clear understanding of the objectives and methods of the crisis intervention plan and should be able to deal with a multiplicity of crises that range from individual suicides to natural and human-made disasters. The person also needs to be a good administrator and delegator who can coordinate a number of activities and people under very stressful and chaotic conditions (Brock et al., 2001; Petersen, 1999). It should be readily apparent that time should be allocated for the crisis intervention coordinator to plan and coordinate for crisis events and not just have these "added on" as a supplementary task.

Media Liaison. It is one thing to deal with the local news crew that the SCRT leaders may have developed close personal relationships with over the course of time; it is quite another to deal with national news media. Imagine yourself as a school counselor in Anytown Middle School who has been designated as the SCRT coordinator. An assault at 8:30 a.m. by a person with a personal vendetta after being expelled from the school leaves six children and two teachers dead, the school principal seriously wounded, and nine other children in the hospital with severe gunshot injuries. A panic ensues as frantic parents come to the school to get their children. You are attempting to get information out about who is hurt and dead, trying to coordinate psychological triage of survivors who witnessed the carnage, giving information to law enforcement personnel who are looking for the still-at-large perpetrator, attempting to reunite distraught students with equally distraught parents, plus a myriad of other tasks, when, at 10 a.m., the first national news helicopter lands on the football field and is quickly followed at around noon by a convoy of national news trucks with satellite uplink capability. There is a horde of reporters attempting to interview anybody they can get their hands on. They are particularly interested in getting any school personnel to comment on who is responsible, why it happened, why the school didn't prevent this from happening, what the school is now doing, who the dead and survivors are, and how you personally feel about this, and other intrusive and invasive questions for which they are clamoring for answers.

It should become very clear from the foregoing scenario that dealing with the media is a major responsibility and should be the sole responsibility of one person specially designated and trained for the job. Such a person should be able to keep relationships with the media positive but should also be able to effectively control them by determining how and what information should be shared with them through well-thought-out statements (Brock et al., 2001). One of the worst scenarios in a school crisis is to allow anybody and everybody to talk to the media. The repercussions from the innuendo, rumor, half-truths, and incomplete data can be extremely severe for survivors and further exacerbate the psychological trauma. Media need to be given press releases that indicate how the media can best help and be least disruptive to students. The media liaison provides written notification to parents on what happened as quickly and currently and with as much factual information as possible and also provides helpful literature and directories of support services to deal with the traumatic repercussions of the event (Newgass & Schonfeld, 2005). Kerr (2009, p. 74) has generated a list of media questions that are designed to obtain information that may well be used to cast the district in a negative light. She has also generated a list of dos and don'ts in regard to those questions that any media representative would do well to learn (p. 75).

Security Liaison. The security liaison should have close links with local law enforcement agencies and would coordinate responses to single events such as a bus accident or recurring events such as gang-initiated drive-by shootings. One of the major preventive tasks of the security liaison is training staff in implementing safety procedures across a wide array of potential crisis scenarios (Brock et al., 1996, p. 71).

Medical Liaison. The medical liaison should have established close links between the local emergency, fire, medical, and mental health systems and the school. A critical component of her or his role is planning for the medical triage of victims of a school crisis and communicating to parents and staff the medical condition of those involved in the crisis (Brock et al., 1996, pp. 71–72; Rubin, 1999). If there is a local emergency management agency, the liaison should have a seat on its board so that they know whom to contact and what kinds of resources are available in a disaster.

Parent Liaison. The parent liaison's job is dealing with parents, period! Keeping parents calm, providing them with information, and furnishing them with support are critical in the containment of a crisis. This person works closely with the media liaison in determining what information about the event itself and support services is disseminated to parents and how it gets to them. Where part of the community is not fluent in English, provisions will have to be made for translators, both oral, ASL, and for all written information that goes out to parents. Because parents may need the services of other components of the team, this school official must have a good working knowledge of each member's role (Rubin, 1999).

Community Liaison. This person or persons need to be the direct link to community resources (Kerr, 2009, p. 37). An ideal member may be the local emergency management agency director, the mayor's community action officer, or a high-ranking member of the police or fire department.

Crisis Interveners. While direct service crisis interventionists are most likely to come from the ranks of school counselors, psychologists, social workers, and nurses, it is important to obtain interventionists who are directly linked to children. Thus, it is helpful to include teachers who have direct contact with a broad sample of the students who might be affected.

In an elementary school, at least one primary and one intermediate teacher should be on the team, and in middle and senior high schools, teachers who represent many different subject matter areas or curriculum tracks should be part of the team (Brock et al., 1996, p. 72).

The school and district unit should be capable of handling an isolated, limited crisis such as the suicide of a teacher or a gang shooting. In a more extensive metastasizing crisis such the Sandy Hook Elementary School or Stoneman High School shooting, the crisis interventionists would be an even larger integrated team of school, local, state, and national interventionists. Incorporating students into the team is also a good idea. They can act as messengers, help identify which students are missing, provide information about the status of other students, and function as peer counselors (Rubin, 1999).

Resource/Facilities Person. This member will need to know where a variety of available supplies are and how to get them from point A to point B in a hurry. Depending on the size and type of the crisis, the resource person may need to know how to obtain everything from pencils and paper to a backup diesel generator. This is not a menial job. If the material supplies are not available, including provision of food and drink when a crisis is going full tilt, then everything grinds to a halt (Rubin, 1999). This person also has a working knowledge of building plans and the systems that operate them. Knowing how to shut off gas lines, knowing the location of electrical junction boxes, and being able to show others the opening to steam tunnels can be critical in a crisis where knowledge of building structures is involved (Kerr, 2009, p. 37).

Implementing the Crisis Plan

The following minimum requirements are critical to a school crisis plan (Brock et al., 1996, pp. 75–76; Brock et al., 2016; Brown & Bobrow, 2004; Conoley & Goldstein, 2004; Duncan et al., 2013; Gerler, 2004; Montano & Dowdall-Thomae, 2003; Petersen & Straub, 1992; Rubin, 1999; U. S. Department of Education, 2007; Williams, 2004).

Physical Requirements

Counseling Locations. As many locations as possible need to be identified for crisis counseling offices.

Crisis counseling will involve a wide variety of activities that will require different accommodations. Auditorium-size rooms will be needed to handle large groups of people for briefings of factual information about the crisis as it unfolds and psychoeducational information about what people can expect and need to do in the aftermath of the crisis. Classrooms will need to be designated to administer psychological first aid. Offices will be needed to perform psychological triage and provide individual counseling. If school is in session, a great deal of rescheduling and shuffling of rooms and assignments will be necessary and should be planned for ahead of time, or alternate buildings such as churches will need to be used.

Operations/Communications Center. In a very large crisis, a room that will become the nerve center for a crisis needs to be designated and equipped. All necessary equipment—additional phone lines, supplies, and furniture for additional staff, computers with internet capability, emergency equipment such as portable phones, citizen band and police band radios, and portable generators—should be available here. This nerve center will become the key component of an efficient crisis operation. In it, people will monitor procedures to determine what staff is available, establish procedures for getting written messages to staff, screen outsiders, and disseminate and coordinate media releases and crisis intervention procedures.

Break Room. A place that is private and will allow workers time to relax, eat, and rest; it may also double as a debriefing room for SCRT members and other crisis personnel.

Information Center. A room large enough to handle a number of media personnel, it should be equipped with a sound system and other visual media equipment. It may also double as an information dissemination or briefing room for parents.

First-Aid Room. This room should be stocked with first-aid supplies for minor physical problems.

Logistics

On-Site Communications. Message boards, computers linked to central files, dedicated telephone lines, citizen and police band radios, and walkie-talkies should be accessible. Because telephone lines may be jammed or otherwise inoperable, a central message board should be available for announcements, bulletins, student lists, and other personal information. If possible, dedicated phone lines with the numbers known only to the officials and staff responsible for handling the crisis should be available. Because there may be little or no communication on-site, walkie-talkies are vital. Portable "to-go boxes" provide vital hard-copy data such as updated attendance lists, release cards, emergency numbers, parent/guardian names, and so on and can be moved to an alternate site to check off names of students. All teachers should have a "to-go box" in addition to a master main office "to-go box."

Establishing a Phone Tree Among All Staff. In any size crisis, a redundant phone tree is absolutely imperative. All staff members of a school building need to be informed of a crisis event as soon as there is knowledge of it. The phone tree is critical so all staff members can begin to operate in a crisis mode and assume preplanned positions and duties. Messages about the crisis should be written down by each person on the tree. Relying on memory and verbal transmission will guarantee that facts get commingled with fiction. One of the worst mistakes that can be made is for staff to not be aware of what is happening and go blundering into an ongoing crisis. We have experienced such lack of communication firsthand, and it is, to say the least, a nightmare.

Procedural Checklist. Although it may seem time wasteful to go through a procedural checklist when a crisis is in full swing, not to do so in a chaotic situation is asking for trouble. It is too easy to overlook a critical component of the intervention plan and assume it has been taken care of by somebody else.

Building Plans. Building plans are vital to emergency personnel and police. Blueprints of every building in the district should be quickly available. Someone with knowledge of the building should be available to interpret the plans for emergency personnel.

Provisions. Because crisis personnel may be involved for extended periods of time, food and drink should be provided or be delivered on-site.

Responding to the Crisis

The following points, in linear order, indicate what needs to occur in a crisis response (Brock et al., 1996, pp. 80–104; Gerler, 2004; Kerr, 2009; Petersen, 1999;

Petersen & Straub, 1992; Poland, 2004; Poland & McCormick, 1999; Rubin, 1999). Kerr (2009) has an operational acronym that should be a general overall operating guide to all responders called BE CALM. It stands for:

> **Be**fore you act, be sure you have the facts.
> **C**all for help, communicate instructions, and collaborate with other responders.
> **A**nticipate what could happen next and adjust the plan.
> **L**isten to your audience and learn what they need.
> **M**anage the crisis and maintain the responders with food, rest, water, debriefing, etc., and modify the plan as needed. (p. 9)

Getting the Facts. The ability to quash the rumor mill that invariably starts up in a crisis is critical to calming the fears and anxiety of the public and also to providing valid information to crisis workers on how many and which students were affected, what level of response will be required, what information needs to be disseminated, and to whom it will be given. Facts need to be checked and rechecked. Getting a team member to the scene of a crisis to make a factual report is critical. Distraught parents and children make for extremely unreliable sources of information. Especially in the case of a suicide, getting verification from the medical examiner is a must.

Impact Assessment. As soon as the facts are known, an SCRT meeting should be held and an assessment should be made of the impact the crisis will have on the school. Factors in the considerations to assess the impact are the popularity of the victim, degree of exposure by staff and students, history and recency of similar crises, resources currently available, and timing (a crisis during vacation is likely to be less traumatic than one during school time). At that time, a decision will have to be made as to the degree of mobilization of internal staff and what, if any, outside assistance will be needed.

Triage Assessment. Once the facts are determined and the possible impact of the crisis event is gauged, a triage assessment needs to be conducted to determine those individuals most affected by the crisis. The SCRT needs to compile a list of those who may be directly and indirectly affected and determine who is most in need of acute intervention and who may need less immediate, intensive attention. Once this list is compiled, interviews and paper-and-pencil tests such as those described in Chapter 7, "Posttraumatic Stress Disorder," may be used to further divide individuals into primary- and secondary-care groups.

It should not be assumed that relatives, survivors, witnesses to the event, and close friends within the school are the only people needing immediate and intensive attention. Siblings and close friends in other schools may be just as traumatized, and efforts should be made to assess these individuals as well. Individuals who are known to be at risk due to other factors and students whose reactions are out of proportion to their involvement should also be considered as high risk.

Parents and teachers need to be given checklists and warning signs that will let them know whether their children are starting to develop the symptoms of acute or posttraumatic stress disorder and referral sheets and phone numbers that will enable them to refer those students who may have been missed by the SCRT. Embedded within these referrals should be questions on lethality. Any student who is expressing thoughts about harming themselves or others should immediately be assessed as high risk and in need of immediate crisis intervention.

Psychological First Aid. Psychological first aid (Aguileria, 1997; Slaikeu, 1990, pp. 105–129) is a first-order response that deals with all of the affected individuals no matter what their degree of involvement (refer to Chapter 1, "Approaching Crisis Intervention"). The components of psychological first aid are making psychological contact, exploring dimensions of the problem, examining possible solutions, gaining assistance in taking action, and offering follow-up services. Psychological first aid is intended as a method to provide support, furnish a platform to be heard and valued, dispel rumors, allow catharsis and ventilation of emotions, reactivate problem-solving abilities, reduce potential lethality, and restore general stability to the school. It is probably most easily done in classroom meetings with teachers who are trained and supported by the SCRT. Such classroom meetings are an excellent vehicle for providing factual information about the event, giving students information about the psychological effects they may encounter, and dealing with personal issues and problems students may have as they come to grips with and attempt to resolve the crisis.

The NOVA Model. For older students, the National Organization for Victim Assistance (NOVA, 2016) group crisis intervention model may be used. This model operates along the lines of the critical incidents stress debriefing (CISD) program of Mitchell and Everly (1995). However, it is not as tightly structured as CISD, and the facilitator is a great deal more interactive with participants.

These groups meet for usually no more than 2 hours. The session has a brief introduction detailing safety and security for the participants. Time is then spent on reviewing physical sensory perceptions, going over emotional reactions of shock and disbelief, and giving opportunity for ventilation and validation of these reactions. Typical questions posed are "Where were you when it happened? Who were you with? What did you see, hear, smell, taste, or touch at the time? What did you do? How did you react?" Time is then taken to review the emotional turmoil that has been experienced and to allow ventilation and validation of these feelings.

Questions are asked in regard to the aftermath of the event. "What are some of the memories that stand out in your mind? What has happened in the last 48 hours? What do you remember seeing or hearing during that time? How have you reacted?" The facilitator validates the thoughts and feelings of the group members. No judgments are made as to right or wrong. Where applicable, the facilitator draws comparisons between members to create a common bond and normalize thoughts and feelings that go with the abnormal event (National Organization for Victim Assistance, 1997, pp. 8–10).

Questions are then posed to elicit expectations about the future, what coping strategies can be used, and to help predict and prepare the group for what may happen over the near future. "After all that you've been through, what do you think will happen at school in the next few days and weeks? Do you think your family has been or will be affected? How do you believe you might deal with the problems and issues that have been raised?" As the members identify positive coping strategies, they are reinforced and given alternative strategies if they are generating negative coping methods. Referrals for more in-depth help are suggested. These components are then followed by a summary recapitulation to validate what has been said and reaffirm the validity of the participants' experiences. A postgroup session of about 30 minutes is used to distribute handouts, answer individual questions, and say goodbye (National Organization for Victim Assistance, 1997, pp. 9–10).

Conducting a large assembly of all the school to do this is not recommended. Although a large assembly may be deemed efficient and expedient, it does not begin to address the many personal questions and issues that students may have. Psychological first aid is a two-way street and, to be effective, should allow an interchange of information between staff and students. In and of itself, psychological first aid may be an excellent way of determining who may be in need of more in-depth crisis intervention by observing the reactions of students as they talk about the crisis. This admonition is particularly important in the case of suicide, where other students may have "caught" the contagion and need to be identified.

Crisis Intervention. Any student who is assessed as needing more than psychological first aid should be given a complete screening interview (Aronin & Ransdell, 1994). That interview should consider what the student's exposure and recollection of the events are, whether the event is persistently reexperienced, whether there are attempts to avoid reminders of the event, increased levels of physical and mental arousal, feelings of survivors' guilt, failure of previous coping skills to ameliorate problems, somatic complaints, self-destructive or impulsive behaviors, and pre- and post-event comparisons on the effectiveness of daily functioning. In short, the screening interview should look at the diagnostic criteria set forth by the DSM 5-TR (APA, 2022) for the onset of traumatic stress disorder.

It is important to take the time necessary to completely discuss the crisis, and attempts to immediately reintroduce the academic regimen should be held in abeyance until this task can be completed. Although getting back to the standard humdrum schedule of school is important in normalizing the situation, very few students are going to be academically able to do so if they are struggling with attempts to resolve the crisis.

Classroom meetings can help students move from reaction to pro-action. That is, students can move from talking about the event to planning how they can take action to solve the residual effects of the event. By moving to a proactive stance, students can begin to attain a feeling of empowerment and reinstitute control in their lives. They can also gain closure on the event by cooperatively planning memorials

and memorial services (note the previously mentioned exception of memorializing suicide).

The worker should be especially watchful for client reports that perseverate on special details, worst moments, and violence or physical mutilation. These will be extremely potent points in the crisis and will need to be thoroughly worked through and controlled (Pynoos & Eth, 1986, p. 309). If there are perpetrators involved in the crisis, one of the greatest fears of children is that the perpetrators "will get them." Whether these perpetrators are caught and punished or are still at large makes little difference. The worker needs to take time to clarify what happened to the perpetrators or what is being done to catch them. Feelings of self-blame for not having done enough and an inability to take action, desires to retaliate and punish the perpetrators, and fear that they will be revictimized need to be explored and worked through (Brock et al., 1996, p. 168).

Briefing and Debriefing. Each morning of the aftermath of the crisis, a morning briefing and planning session needs to be held to obtain updated information, review responsibilities, assign tasks, and plan interventions. At the end of each day, actions need to be reviewed, weaknesses and strengths need to be examined, and reviews of referred students, staff, and parents need to be made. Plans are then made for the next day and what staff and resources will be needed to accomplish the goals. Additionally, a nightly debriefing should be held to give the SCRT a chance to exchange information, obtain reassurance, and ventilate feelings (Berman & Jobes, 1991; Rubin, 1999; Williams, 2006). The Missouri School Counselor Association's (2002) *Crisis Manual* makes the following points for SCRT members:

1. Keep your life in balance.
   a. Eat well-balanced meals and get plenty of exercise.
   b. Balance work and rest.
   c. Stick to a schedule as much as you can. It provides stability and the comfort of a normal routine when your feelings are out of control.
   d. Avoid new major projects or decisions.
2. Be realistic about what you can do.
3. Recognize and acknowledge your own feelings of loss and grief. Give yourself permission to mourn. No matter what the nature of your relationship, there is loss. Give yourself the same latitude you give your students. Meet with fellow SCRT

members and be supportive of each other or form a support group.

4. Be kind to yourself. You don't have to get it all together right away. You don't have to do it all, be strong for everyone, or take care of everything. Treat yourself with the same gentleness and understanding you would anybody else.

Demobilizing. Demobilizing occurs when the crisis is finished. It allows the SCRT to integrate the experience into their lives and go back to their regular jobs. An overall evaluation is conducted by the crisis response coordinator with the SCRT. The crisis intervention coordinator writes an after-action report that includes a description of the crisis event and the interventions conducted, an evaluation of the effectiveness of the intervention, and recommendations for future events. As such, it provides the SCRT with a potent learning tool. Furthermore, if questions are raised in the future about what was done or not done, this report documents what happened (Brock et al., 1996, p. 100). You will get an event scenario of an SCRT in action in Chapter 16, "Disaster Response."

Grief and Memorializing Schools

LO12 By age eighteen, one in 13 children will experience the death of a parent or sibling (Nelson, 2022). The COVID-19 pandemic brought the reality of death to every school room in America with the loss of over 200,000 parents and caregivers, which translated into 1 in every 360 children under the age of eighteen in the United States losing a caregiver (DeAngelis, 2022). "While most children adjust and say farewell over time" according to Irwin Sadler, a noted grief expert quoted in DeAngleis (2022), he also maintained "that about 20 percent will experience long-term problems, including long-term development of depression and long-term higher risk of suicide." Such loss can destroy children's sense of safety and upend stability and normalcy in their lives (Nelson, 2022).

While immediate crisis intervention in the aftermath of a school shooting or other traumatic event affecting students is now a standard part of the role and function of school crisis workers and SCRTs, students suffering from individual loss have not been given much attention. While school psychologists, school nurses, school social workers, and school counselors never signed on to be grief and bereavement counselors, the advent of school shootings,

neighborhood drive-by shootings, the COVID-19 outbreak, auto accidents, and other traumatic accidental deaths put those professionals as crisis workers front and center in providing support both individually and in groups for bereaved peers. Nelson (2022) poses an interesting question in that regard. "When we implement programs to identify and support our at-risk students, what are we doing to include the 7.7 percent of our youth who are actively grieving a close family member's death? The chapter on Personal Loss, Chapter 12, "Personal Loss: Bereavement and Grief," deals in general with children and loss, but loss doesn't just stay at home, it comes to school, and this is what this section is about.

Talking about death and survivorship is not easy, and most adults will avoid it when talking with children because they are at a loss as to what to say. That lack of communication can send the following messages to the child: "I don't care, and it isn't important. It's too overwhelming for me to deal with it and I don't think you'd be able to cope even with my help" (Schoenfield & Quackenbush, 2017, p. 22), and that avoidance of the topic can go for school staff as well. However, as indicated from personal anecdotes in the Loss chapter, this is some of the most difficult work a crisis worker can do, but it is also some of the most rewarding.

The sudden death of a student, teacher, or other school personnel may precipitate a bereavement crisis for an entire school or school community, which can lead to posttraumatic stress disorder, high-intensity grief, and complicated mourning. The closer the friendship to the deceased, the more the foregoing is likely to occur. As such, it is important to have a grief resolution program in place (Poijula et al., 2001). Many children will be dealing with the reality of death for the first time. They will also be struggling with the significance of the loss and grappling with the idea that life is no longer predictable or fair. Further, they may have no idea how to grieve and may receive little help if their parents are also grief stricken (Kraft, 2003). Many of the bereavement procedures in Chapter 12, "Personal Loss: Bereavement and Grief," are appropriate for working with children and adolescents. However, because of the social community and culture of schools, there are some specific actions that need to occur when a member of the school community dies.

That being said, you should consider taking on the job as point person coordinating follow-up between home and school (Schoenfield & Quackenbush, 2017), and when you do, it wouldn't be a bad idea to reread Chapter 12, "Personal Loss: Bereavement and Grief," just as a refresher on how you're going to operate. Being point means working with other staff members and apprising them of some of the issues facing the grieving student and coordinating both academic and emotional support when students may experience both academic and behavioral problems.

The SCRT should meet immediately after notification of a death, develop a plan, and assemble all staff and advise them of what is going to occur. One of your jobs as point is in constructing a prepared statement that can be read simultaneously by all teachers along with a letter to parents giving details as to what the school is doing and that crisis teams will be available (National Center for School Crisis and Bereavement, 2020). Template letters are available from the Center at schoolcrisiscenter.org/resources/samples-templates.

One of the major issues in any traumatic event is identifying who is impacted most by it. Teachers should be apprised to watch for nontypical behavior of individuals in response to a tragedy and refer them to the crisis worker. Crisis workers should be available for consultation when teachers have questions about students. Peer group leaders are also an excellent referral sources for classmates who are not handling a peer's death well. Student feelings may range from anger to guilt, and this may especially be true if death is by suicide. Younger student may have more difficulty understanding death and are more likely to have misinterpretations (National Center for School Crisis and Bereavement, 2020).

Individually or in groups, SCRT team members may focus on the grief of a specific grade level, provide group discussion for particular subgroups, temporarily relieve bereaved teachers of classroom responsibilities, staff mini-counseling centers, or work with parents. Two SCRT members may follow a deceased student's schedule. One member will talk with each class, provide factual information, answer questions, clarify misinformation, provide support, provide information on funeral arrangements, explain what funerals and visitations are like and what to expect, suggest what types of things can be said to family members, and encourage students to talk about their memories of the deceased student. While this class discussion is taking place, the other member can assess and identify students who are not coping well and escort them to a support room (Missouri School Counselor Association, 2002).

Assessing students' needs prior to returning to school may help lessen anxiety. A home visit or a phone call that empathically responds to the student's progress can be made. Questions might include "How are you feeling about coming back to school? What is the most difficult thing for you about returning? Is there something you would like me to do to help you? Are you worried about what other students will think?" All these questions are designed to allow students to talk about their fears and trepidation and allow the SCRT member to help them start to feel less anxious. After the student has been back to school a few days, the crisis worker may discuss with the child how she or he is doing with questions such as "Now that you are back at school, what has been the hardest thing for you? What has been on your mind the most? How has the death affected you at school?" These questions allow the worker to determine how well the child is making the transition back into school (Rubin, 1999).

Kandt (1994, p. 207) suggests that school human services personnel working with grieving adolescents should (1) educate themselves about the grief process; (2) give permission to grieve; (3) allow time to grieve; (4) listen, listen, listen; (5) understand that reminiscing is essential; (6) give support for a variety of feelings; (7) know they can't "fix" the pain; (8) draw the adolescents out, keep in touch, and don't abandon them; (9) design a support group; and (10) let them know that they are not alone.

Swihart et al. (1992) surveyed grieving students and listed the following issues that caregivers should be sensitive to:

1. Many students were affected by the loss, even students who were not close to the deceased; therefore, they were reminded of their own mortality.
2. Teachers should not expect peak performance from students who are still too numb the first week following the death.
3. Teachers should be allowed to express their own grief to students who are willing to simply listen.
4. Students should be allowed to grieve in different ways—some in groups, some in their individual ways.
5. After-school activities should be provided for students to work off their grief by expending physical energy.
6. Students should be brought together in commemorative activities so students who were not very close to the deceased one are not excluded.

7. Students should be permitted to discuss grief issues; denial of the opportunity to openly discuss their thoughts and feelings may cut the teenagers off from an open forum of support.
8. School administrators should be cognizant of the deceased student's role in the school; if the deceased was in a leadership role, the school will need to have administrative leadership in filling the role vacated by the deceased.
9. The school should be prepared to respond to the loss for a considerable length of time.

As we have emphasized in the Personal Loss: Bereavement and Grief chapter, one of the best intervention techniques is being there and letting the parents and students know you are there as quickly as they return to school and will be there for as long as they need and will be there for support. There is a fine line between being intrusive and providing support, and it is your judgment call as to where that line is because it will be different for each student. Assure them that there is no right or wrong way to grieve and no timeline set to finish grieving (Nelson, 2022).

Group Work

An accident following the prom in early May resulted in the deaths of four Cedar Grove High School students: Phil, age 16, the driver of the car; Jerry, age 17; LaTara, age 16; and Tracey, age 17. A group of seven classmates at school, representing the four adolescents' closest friends, appeared to be stuck in their grief. Keena, Lee, Samantha, and Rashid, all 17, and Eddie, Amber, and Tarunda, all 16, requested the help of the school counselor in reaching some understanding and resolution of their feelings of anguish and grief.

The following intervention strategies were provided and issues explored with these adolescents by the school counselor during the days and weeks immediately following the burial of the four teenagers who died.

1. **Individual counseling and intervention.** Assessment of individual stress levels. Providing individuals a safe place to release stress energy. Helping adolescents feel comfortable in expressing how they feel. Providing death education for adolescents.
2. **Group grief work.** Providing an atmosphere for the seven adolescents as a group to deal with the deaths of their four classmates in particular and with the area of death and dying in general.

Providing for group sessions and projects that commemorate the deceased classmates. Group exploration of unfinished business through written or role-playing exercises. Provisions for students to deal with the deaths outside the group within the school environment through peer support groups (Samide & Stockton, 2002).

Gray (1988) reported that bereaved teens in support groups found peers to be "most helpful" compared to other school-related workers and that bereaved adolescents did not want to be singled out or treated in special ways (pp. 187–188). In cases of sudden death, grief, and bereavement among adolescents, a great deal of shock, vulnerability, remorse, and other emotions quickly emerge. Because most adolescents lack experience dealing with the deaths of their peers and because social influence is powerful and pervasive in a setting such as a high school, the use of adolescent group grief work is an ideal strategy for controlling distortions and rumors and for helping young people release grief energy and begin to resolve their feelings of loss.

The counselor, meeting with the group in the group counseling room, served as the crisis worker. She met with several grief work groups during the days immediately following the deaths of the four students. The counselor set the tone by introducing the topic and encouraging members to share their emotional responses to the loss. Later, during the session, after the release of students' grief energy, the counselor began to use structured techniques to help them sharpen their memories and focus on reality.

CW: I really appreciate all the expressions of your feelings you've given so freely. Before the session begins today, I asked Samantha to go by the yearbook office and pick up a copy of this year's *Wildcat*. I also asked her to pick up some leftover photographs the yearbook staff did not use. Samantha, would you like to share some of them with the group?

Samantha: I put filing cards in the pages of the annual that I thought we'd like to look at. Oh, and I've got some great shots of LaTara, Jerry, and Tracey. I only found one of Phil, and that was in a group. But Phil's class picture is in there (**pointing toward the yearbook**), and all four of them look so real and alive and so happy in the activities section.

The students in the group showed a great deal of interest and released a great amount of stress energy while examining the photographs of the deceased students. The crisis worker let the students take their own individual time in reminiscing and talking about their grief from 2 minutes to 20 minutes. Because everyone grieves differently, allowing students to take as much time as they need is important in moving beyond the grief (Tillman & Rust, 2011). Later in the session, the group discussed death in general, the impact of death on the living, and their own deaths. The counselor then used a technique called Memory Moments. Students finished off sentences such as "When I heard you died, I . . . ," "Our last conversation was . . . ," "My head feels . . . ," "My heart feels . . . ," "I wish I had said. . . ." All of these sentence stems allow students to openly speak to the wide range of emotions they are carrying (Counce & Sommer, 2003).

The counselor was able to use another technique that is sometimes effective in group grief work—the epitaph exercise. Each group member was given four index cards and was instructed: "If you were given the responsibility for writing the epitaphs for Phil, Jerry, LaTara, and Tracey, write down the exact words on the cards that would appear on their gravestones." The group shared their epitaphs and discussed them. When it is difficult to say or write words about dead classmates, Tillman and Rust (2011) propose making Feeling Hearts by drawing large hearts and having students print their feelings inside it and then pass the hearts around and have the group discuss those feelings.

Eddie: I thought Tarunda's was really good when she wrote—about Jerry—"Here lies the Martin Luther King of Cedar Grove," because he really did like and care for everybody. **(Students nod in agreement.)**

Keena: I *almost* cried when I wrote Tracey's, and then I *did* when Amber read LaTara's. I just felt like I couldn't stand it. It's so true. I'm really going to miss that girl. **(Students nod in agreement. Long period of silence; thoughtful look on all faces.)**

CW: I think what we've done is to write down, in the briefest form, what we want to remember most about each of our beloved classmates.

Before the session ended, the counselor led the group in identifying the positive contributions that each of the deceased students had made and in verbalizing their goodbyes to each of their departed classmates. Grief doesn't always have to be, nor

should it be, only sadness. Having students remember the good times is a powerful way to balance memories of loved ones who have died (Tillman & Rust, 2011). The counselor was attempting to use the power and social influence of the group setting to enhance the emotional impact on each member and to prepare each member to say goodbye, let go of the deceased, and begin to get ready to go on living.

Ending any counseling group after a bond has been formed is difficult. Loss and grief groups are even tougher because they are now truly saying goodbye to the loved one. Saying goodbye should include some simple symbolic ceremony such as releasing balloons, setting small paper boats with candles in them adrift on a river, or writing goodbye letters. Generally, letting the group decide on what simple memorial service to do will work best (Tillman & Rust, 2011). Tillman and Rust propose discussing in age-appropriate terms that endings are a natural part of the life cycle. They further propose that the group summarize and discuss what they have learned from the group. Our own group ending goes something like this: After summaries of the experience have been given, state specifically:

CW: I want all of you to stand up and clasp hands with one another, so we have a circle. This group was about remembering our dead classmates who are gone but not forgotten from our lives. Because we are living, we owe it to them and ourselves to move on with our lives, just as they would if we were gone from theirs. We are going to say one last goodbye in the circle, then we are going to spread the circle until our hands drop, let the spirits of our friends go out of this circle and on their way as we do the same with our own lives.

The counselor's group targeted Worden's (2018) four tasks of mourning.

Task I. Accept the reality of the loss and move past denial. If one can't accept the loss as real, then one can't deal with the affect associated with it and move on to not only intellectual acceptance but emotional acceptance as well.

Task II. To process the pain of the loss. If the pain is suppressed and not adequately processed, it can lead to a delayed grief reaction and somatic manifestations of the grief

Task III. To adjust to an environment where the deceased is missing. There are external adjustments, how has daily living changed, internal adjustments involving the person's self-definition, including one's self-esteem and self-efficacy and spiritual adjustment in regard to one's relationship with their religion, their values, and sense of meaning.

Task IV. To emotionally relocate and memorialize the dead person in a way that one can move on with life.

Defining the Boundaries

Probably one of the toughest jobs of an SCRT and the school administration is to discourage parents, students, or various other interest groups in the community from honoring the death by conducting a commemorative service or other memorial at the school. Unequivocally, suicidal students should not be formally memorialized by the school because of possible copycats (Capuzzi, 2002). It cannot be overemphasized that the school administration and the SCRT should be the ones to make decisions about the response to school tragedies in which deaths occur. *The National Center for School Crisis and Bereavement* (2020) has published an extensive protocol of guidelines for responding to the death of a student or school staff and would do well to follow them. That is easily said but sometimes difficult to follow, given the emotionality and political pressure that can be exerted on a school district to honor a death of a student or staff member. Overall, if possible, it is probably best for the school not to memorialize any kind of deaths in any fashion—assemblies, yearbooks, trees planted, rooms or fields named, and so on—because of the perception of differential treatment (The National Center for School Crisis and Bereavement, 2020).

Bluntly stated, schools are in the education business, not the funeral home or memorial business (Trotter, 2003). The National Center for School Crisis and Bereavement protocol (2020) observes that informal memorials are likely to appear. The SCRT should determine a time period (two weeks) and notify students they will then be removed. Trotter (2003) recommends that after the funeral, all of the drawings and other eulogies and epitaphs be collected and given to the family and not kept on display in the school. She also recommends that the student's chair be left alone until the day after the funeral, but then all chairs in the room need to be rearranged. She proposes that immediately upon notification, a member of the SCRT should go to the student's locker and collect all personal items when students are not present and prevent memorializing the locker. The personal effects of the deceased should be collected and returned to the parent, preferably after school hours and in the school office so they are not faced with the trauma of cleaning the student's desk out (The National Center for School Crisis and Bereavement Protocol, 2020).

The student's locker should be left vacant for the remainder of the year but then be merged into the standard locker assignment for next year's class. Louvre (2002) believes that with younger children, the desk should be left in the room until the other students want it moved out. She further proposes that a suitable memorial be constructed by the children such as positive epitaphs or a signed teddy bear that the class might give to the parents when they come to school to collect the dead child's things.

Finally, in an ever-hungry media world, if a death is dramatic in any way, there is every expectation either professional journalists or social media will intrude (Schoenfeld & Quackenbush, 2017). The focus of all communications, including media coverage, should be on the protection of students and the school environment from unwanted attention. If that happens, it is time to call the SCRT team and have the media liaison field all queries (National Center for School Crisis and Bereavement, 2020).

Transcrisis Intervention with Individuals and the Total School System

LO13 The American School Counselor Association's (2022) position statement on the counselor's role and trauma-informed practice follows: School counselors understand the impact adverse childhood experiences have on students' academic achievement and social/emotional development. Through the implementation of a school counseling program, school counselors strive to identify, support and promote the success of students who have experienced trauma. A trauma-sensitive school is one in which all students feel safe, welcomed and supported (Cole et al., 2013). Establishing a trauma-informed school counseling program paired with a multitiered system of supports (MTSS) and a preventive focus can decrease the effects of trauma exposure (Davis et al., 2022; Martinez et al., 2020; and Rumsey & Milsom, 2019).

For those children who are in need of assistance beyond psychological first aid, traumatic transcrisis intervention uses many of the cognitive behavioral trauma (CBT) approaches (Kataola et al., 2012) detailed in the chapters on posttraumatic stress disorder (PTSD) and sexual assault. The use of drawings, modeling clay, and other manipulative play materials combined with CBT is particularly helpful in empowering young children to take control of a situation that may seem beyond their ability to do. Initially, the child should be allowed to use the materials to construct whatever they desire. The crisis interventionist uses this time to build trust and rapport.

Invariably, the crisis will be manifested in the child's play and will provide clues to the source of the child's anxiety and means of coping (Pynoos & Eth, 1986, p. 307). At some time during the process, a child who has been numbing and repressing the crisis event is going to have an emotional release that may be shocking and unsettling to the crisis worker (Pynoos & Eth, 1986, p. 308). At that point, the worker must be calm, cool, and collected and be able to psychologically comfort the child.

The use of guided imagery and the employment of superheroes as helpers in those images (Lazarus, 1977), conscious dreaming to help stop recurring nightmares (Garfield, 1984), and relaxation and desensitization techniques to teach anxiety control (Thompson & Rudolph, 1992, p. 173) are all potent ways of helping children empower themselves and take back control over their feelings, thoughts, and behaviors.

The Case of Josh

Josh is a 7-year-old second grader who has just recovered from a bite from a brown recluse spider (one of the most poisonous spiders in North America). Josh was bitten in the leg, and the necrosis that developed required reconstructive surgery. He now walks with a cane and a limp. He is afraid of his classmates making fun of him behind his back and feels his classmates are doing so. For a time, it was feared that Josh might lose his leg. What has compounded the problem is that recently, thousands of brown recluses were discovered in the steam tunnels of Josh's school. This discovery set off a panic because the children had seen what happened to Josh and had also viewed news items on television about the brown recluses' movement into their geographic area. Although the school district immediately hired exterminators to rid the school of the spiders, the children's fears were not allayed.

Josh is now hypervigilant in regard to any insects, is afraid to sleep in his own bed, has developed school phobia, and shrieks and screams in terror at going to school. He has recurrent nightmares about hoards of huge, hairy spiders covering his body. He is very sure he is going to die from a spider bite. His academic achievement has fallen, and he is in danger of failing second grade. His parents have talked to him about switching schools, but he is sure that all schools now contain brown recluses. Most of his conversation is centered on insects. He avoids outdoor activities for fear of getting bitten. The duration of his symptoms is now into its sixth week. After an interview with the school psychologist, Josh is given a diagnosis of acute traumatic stress disorder.

Because many other children at the school are manifesting symptoms of traumatic stress due to the brown recluse infestation, the SCRT has a meeting and determines that intervention is necessary with both the student population as a whole and Josh individually. Josh's parents are called, and they agree to individual intervention. The team's media person prepares a number of press releases and goes on radio and television news shows to explain what is being done to control the situation. In coordination with the parent liaison, bulletins are also sent home to all parents.

The medical liaison has classroom meetings with every homeroom in the school. She provides detailed information about what brown recluse bites look like and what medical care is needed and answers the students' questions in a truthful, no-nonsense manner. Another classroom meeting is held with the high school biology teacher, who shows the students what the spider looks like, describes its habits, and also indicates to them that although the brown recluse is poisonous, it is a very shy spider that tries to avoid contact with people. Question-and-answer sessions follow, and students get a good idea of what they need to do at both school and home to avoid being bitten.

Parents are invited to a special parent–teacher meeting where all the SCRT staff are present to provide information about helping children cope with the sudden siege of arachnophobia (fear of spiders and similar creatures). After completing the psychological first aid program, the SCRT staff poll the teachers, who indicate the students seem to have conquered their fears of spiders. But Josh has not!

The crisis worker goes to Josh's home and, after making Josh's acquaintance, sets up the following exercise:

CW: I want you to draw me the feeling of what "scared" looks like, Josh.

Josh: (Takes markers and poster board and draws a picture of a very large tarantula-like spider with huge dripping fangs about to pounce on a small boy cowering in a corner. While drawing, Josh gives the crisis worker a blow-by-blow gruesome description of what the spider is going to do to the little boy.)

CW: Boy! That's scary all right. I wonder what we could do to make that big nasty spider run away and hide?

Josh: I dunno. Nothin', I think.

CW: Well, that is pretty tough with a spider that big, but you know, I've got an idea. It takes a spider to catch a spider. And I've got just the guy to do it. (pulls out a Spider-Man comic book) Have you ever read a Spider-Man comic? He is way cool.

Josh: (eyes light up and takes the comic book and starts looking at it) Yeah, and I've seen him in the movie. He is cool!

CW: So let's get him to help us. Takes a Spider-Man to catch a spider, right?

Josh: Well, I guess that's right.

CW: All right! Let's jump Spider-Man off the comic book and onto your poster board. Can you draw him on there and tell me what's happening?

Josh: Well, OK. (draws Spider-Man casting a big net over the spider) Spider-Man throws this big net over him, see, and the spider doesn't like it. But the more it struggles, the more it gets tangled up. Ha! Ha! Caught in a spider net. That's cool! He can't get out, but he's still there, though. I don't like him right there.

CW: OK! How could we get rid of him?

Josh: Well, we could take him to the bug-man, and let him douse him with bug juice.

CW: Fine. Go ahead and do that. (gives Josh another piece of poster board)

Josh: (continues to draw Spider-Man pulling the spider over to an exterminator who looks very much like Josh)

CW: Now what?

Josh: I'm gonna douse him good.

CW: Good! Do that! What does that spider look like now?

Josh: He's gonna shrivel up and blow away. (Continues to draw the spider all shriveled up; he and Spider-Man triumphantly hold the spider up as a trophy.)

Over the course of the next several sessions, the crisis worker continues to use modeling clay and drawing to give Josh and Spider-Man increasing control over his environment (Webb, 2007). The crisis worker uses the superhero to help empower this frightened and traumatized little boy. The crisis worker now moves further to help Josh regain control over more of his environment by taking him outside to the backyard. Although Josh is somewhat timid about going outside, he goes with the crisis worker, one hand clutching the worker's hand and the other clutching a Spider-Man figurine.

CW: Boy! We're outside here. How do you feel?

Josh: Yeah, I think the backyard is where I got bit.

CW: And you're back out here. That's pretty courageous, almost like Spider-Man.

Josh: Well, it's OK 'cause Spider-Man's here with me. . . and well . . . you too.

CW: Josh, I wonder if Spider-Man could help us with those nightmares too. What I'd like you to do is just sort of have a daydream, you know like let your mind wander like there was sort of nothing to do and you were just kind of relaxing, and just shut your eyes and instead of having a nightmare, just imagine yourself and Spider-Man. Just you and Spider-Man out on patrol, saving the world from those huge spiders. Can you picture yourself and Spider-Man like that? Now just lie back and listen to me and just let yourself relax. (The crisis worker deeply relaxes Josh and then helps him create an image of him and Spider-Man.)

The crisis worker uses a combination of relaxation training and guided imagery to decrease Josh's anxiety and help him build a mental image of himself and his powerful friend taking control of the nighttime environment.

Josh: (with his eyes closed) Yeah, me and Spider-Man are scaling up a tall building, looking for big old hairy spiders. (Josh goes on to explain how they are out on patrol catching all kinds of spiders.)

The crisis worker helps keep Josh on track, and when he gets stuck trying to catch a really huge, fast, fluorescent chartreuse spider, the crisis worker gives him a can of super strong glue, and Josh and Spider-Man spread it out and get the spider stuck in it.

CW: Good. Now what I want you to do is get that image real clear in your mind. You and Spider-Man giving each other high-fives for catching that really monstrous spider. If you start to have that same old nightmare tonight, I want you to change that nightmare, and do just what you and Spider-Man did. That's what I want you to dream. I'll bet you can do that! (gives and returns a high-five from Josh)

The power of suggestion and use of guided imagery to enable a child to change his dreams may seem farfetched, but it must be remembered that children work out their problems through fantasy and play. As the crisis worker continuously reinforces Josh for getting back in control of his environment through the help of the superhero, Josh can start to feel safe not only in his backyard but also in his sleep.

Finally, to expedite Josh's return to school, the crisis worker sets up a classroom meeting with his classmates. Josh tells his classmates about his real spider bite and all the things that happened to him in the hospital. The rest of the children are very curious about all this and ask him many questions. Josh has been embarrassed about his scar and his limp, but now he's in the limelight and eagerly starts to tell them what went on while he was in the hospital and doesn't hesitate to tell them some of the more gruesome details with accompanying "Oohs," "Aahs," and "Ughs" from the class. He also shows them the pictures he drew and tells them, with the help of the crisis worker, how he's "not afraid of any darned old spiders anymore." An examination of Josh's drawings indicates just how potent serial drawing can be (Gumaer, 1984). Over a series of sessions, the spiders get smaller and smaller, and Josh and Spider-Man get bigger and bigger until the spider is in realistic proportion to Josh in the drawings, no more than a spot on the poster board. In the course of 8 weeks, Josh was able to return to school, his nightmares of spiders went away, and he was able to resume the life of a normal 7-year-old boy.

Epilogue

If you are planning on being a school counselor and are reading this book in a formal graduate class, you are probably ahead of most of your peers. That statement probably holds as well for social workers and school psychologists. There is a reason that the Council on Accreditation of Counseling and Educationally Related Programs (CACREP) is mandating crisis intervention in its new standards for school counseling. The American School Counselor Association (2023) has a lengthy resource list of professional development sources, position statements, and articles on crisis and trauma. That has not always been the case, and our own experience in reviewing accreditation for some counseling programs is that they do the bare minimum to meet CACREP standards with no formal course work in crisis intervention. When that happens, Wachter's (2007) comprehensive study on school counselors and their knowledge and ability to practice crisis intervention is sobering. Although school psychologists, school social workers, school nurses, SROs, other in-school staff, and community mental health workers may well be involved in crisis intervention, the typical first responder in a school will be a school counselor. Particularly in a school shooting, school counselors are most likely to become the leaders in their school building. Many are unprepared to take on such a task, but they get it anyway when a building or district has not done the preplanning it needs to do (Fein et al., 2008).

Wachter (2007) found that more than half the school counselors (53.1 percent) reported dealing with all the crises discussed in this chapter plus sexual and physical abuse. About a fifth of the counselors (21.7 percent) reported that they had received no training at all during their master's degree program for any kind of crisis intervention. Forty-four percent reported that after obtaining a master's degree, they had picked up training in areas such as suicide intervention and critical incident stress debriefing on their own. Interestingly, these counselors perceived their on-site staff and resources to be more helpful than external sources of support. The school counselors identified assessment for suicidal and homicidal ideation and the provision of support for students who are at risk for both as critical knowledge components.

To further make the life of a school counselor more exciting, there will not only be the once-in-a-year, or 5 years, or once-in-a-lifetime megacrisis to make one's life more self-actualized. There will also be the daily mini-crisis, the constant transcrisis, and each of these will have the ability to metastasize into really big ones.

To that end, Robertson (2013) provides her counseling interns with a simple SRSR acronym to base their decision making when confronted with a crisis. S is for *safety*. Do I feel safe in this situation? Do I need help maintaining a safe environment? Is this person in danger of hurting themselves or someone else? Do I need to notify anyone else if the answer to the foregoing questions leaves a reasonable doubt in my mind about safety? R is for *role*. Is it within the scope of what I am professionally competent to do? You will be confronted with all kinds of human dilemmas, and many will be beyond your scope of practice. While on the one hand, "It's not my job!" is not acceptable, neither is thinking you are a drug or trauma therapist. Don't be afraid, embarrassed, or too proud to refer.

Interestingly, Robertson (2013) adds *skills,* but emphasizes having faith in and using basic listening and responding skills to defuse and de-escalate most crisis situations. And sometimes, because you do have advanced crisis intervention skills from reading this book and or taking a crisis course, you may even use some of the "stuff" you have learned here. Finally, Robertson speaks to cultivating *resources.* Having a ready list of people and numbers you can call to get specialized help that ranges from getting food and clothing to a burned-out family to finding out someone who knows how to do eye movement desensitization and reprocessing (EMDR) for PTSD should be a first priority when entering new territory.

Crisis and burnout go hand in hand. Fein and his associates (2008) found that, indeed, school counselors suffered from the stress of being leaders in an unknown and chaotic situation where they had to make fast decisions. They learned how to do debriefing on the fly, which would be unthinkable for emergency responders such as police, EMTs, or firefighters. They also engaged in decisions they had never figured they would be involved in doing and suffered traumatic symptoms as a result. While Wachter (2007) found no significant difference in burnout symptoms and individual exposure to crisis, she did find significance in higher burnout rates when physical abuse was the precipitating crisis event. Wachter also determined that master's level training in the kind of course you are now taking with this book is significantly related to *reducing* burnout rates in school

counselors. Finally, Wachter noted that building internal support systems and getting continuing education in crisis intervention is helpful in preventing burnout.

While every school district in the United States most likely has at least some kind of crisis plan that goes beyond fire, tornado, and earthquake drills, and some of those school districts may go to great lengths to detail how crisis teams will operate in large-scale disasters, the simple fact is that school personnel who deal with the day-in and day-out grinding crises that afflict many students don't have a lot of resources to help them (Heath & Sheen, 2005). So, if you are a school counselor or other school professional taking this course, you may find that Heath and Sheen's (2005) book, *School-Based Crisis Intervention: Preparing All Personnel to Assist,* Brock, Sandoval and Lewis's (2001) book, *Preparing for Crisis in the Schools: A Manual for Building crisis Response Teams,* and Kerr's (2009) book, *School Crisis Prevention and Intervention,* would be very helpful in training the people you most likely will have to count on, your fellow professionals. Heath and Sheen's book goes into specific detail about the basic, hands-on crisis intervention skills and activities that teachers, secretaries, custodians, and bus drivers will need to help you out. Brock and associates' book is a step-by-step on how to build and nourish a crisis intervention team. Kerr's book has more to do with laying out the larger operational picture. Along with Scott Poland's (1999) book, *Coping with Crisis: Lessons Learned,* which deals with the logistical, tactical, and strategic problems of a crisis, it is especially appropriate not only for school counselors but school administrators as well. And make no mistake about it, you will need their help. These are all older books, but they have stood the test of time and are still relevant and readable, hands-on tools. Going it alone in a school building when dealing with the kinds of "stuff" this chapter is about will make you an odds-on favorite to be what the burnout chapter in this book is about. So, if you are an aspiring school counselor, be assured that what's in this book is "stuff" you are going to need. The question is absolutely not "if" but "when?"

Summary

The rise of school violence perpetrated by the estranged violent student has caused a great deal of public concern and received widespread media coverage because of its perceived senselessness and its occurrence in communities where residents previously thought they were immune from such horrific events. Although the focus has been on the tragedy of estranged students who act out their frustration and anger in lethal ways, the growth and spread of gang-initiated violence in urban, suburban, and rural communities far exceed the tragedies the estranged juvenile has perpetrated.

Homicides are not the only lethal malady to afflict schools and cause crises. The suicide rate has risen to epidemic proportions among children and adolescents. School personnel face a wide variety of crises that reach far beyond the normal developmental issues and crises of childhood and adolescence. Schools have been called upon to develop wide-ranging prevention strategies for profiling,

screening, and preventing acts of violence both to oneself and to others. Contemporary crisis strategies in schools deal not only with prevention but with intervention and postvention as well. Crisis workers interact with students, faculty, and parents who have been associated with, witnessed, or suffered from traumatic events originating within the school or with students.

Although no known intervention plan will guarantee that tragedies will not take place, there are approaches that hold promise in dealing with a variety of crises that can afflict schools. These approaches call for everyone—community service organizations; child welfare agencies; mental health facilities; local, state, and national governments; the courts; law enforcement agencies; and all of the staff in schools—to work cooperatively in developing and implementing crisis intervention plans. Most importantly, no school should be without a crisis plan and a well-trained crisis response team.

On the Home Front
Crisis in the Human Services Workplace

Part III deals with helping the crisis worker cope with crises that might occur in the human services workplace. The world in which we live and in which crisis workers function is becoming increasingly dangerous and violent for clients as well as for human services professionals. This chapter, on violent behavior in institutions, provides information and techniques to help workers better understand and deal with both the volatile environment and the dilemmas of clients who strive to cope within that environment. prevalent. Chapter 15, "Human Services Workers in Crisis Burnout, Vicarious Traumatization, and Compassion Fatigue," deals with human services worker burnout, vicarious traumatization, and compassion fatigue. These are major crises that directly affect the crisis worker.

Violent Behavior in Institutions

14

Learning Objectives

After studying this chapter, you will be able to:

1. Describe the risks of being employed in the human services workplace and how to take precautions against physical harm.
2. Explain the role the institution plays in violence perpetrated on human service workers and what it can do to mitigate risks to staff.
3. Describe the risk human service workers themselves instigate that cause violence and take precautions to avoid them.
4. Discuss the ethical conflicts and potential legal liability that occurs when violent acts happen against human service workers and precautions to take to avoid legal and ethical dilemmas.
5. Identify methods of assessing for violent behavior and when and on whom to use them.

6. Describe the bases for violent behavior and be able to differentiate types.
7. Explain what intervention procedures are and how they are used with potentially violent clients.
8. Explain what a threat assessment team is and when and how it is used.
9. Describe what kind of training is necessary for violence reduction.
10. Explain the stages of intervention in diffusing an angry client and how they are applied.
11. Discuss issues of violent geriatric clients and specific therapies used with them.

Warning

LO1 Be forewarned! This is not a chapter designed to recruit you into the human services field. Very little class or supervision time in most human service disciplines is given to the topic of dealing with violent behavior in the human services field because of the bad publicity and politics that surround it. We believe, at the very least, that this is morally, ethically, and probably legally wrong. The human service field is one of the most gratifying and rewarding fields a person can be in, but it is also one of the most dangerous. Therefore, training in recognizing and handling violent clients should be one of the highest priorities in this business. Dr. Phillip Kleespies, an imminent researcher, practitioner, and writer on behavioral emergencies, has taken the whole human services field to task in regard to the abysmal teaching and training of health care professionals on how to deal with violence (2014, pp. 47–97). This chapter is an attempt to rectify that a small bit and give you the knowledge to be SAFE! Thus, we believe there is nothing more important you will read in this book that will affect your career in this business.

According to the Bureau of Labor Statistics, 27 out of the 100 fatalities that occurred in health care settings in 2013 were due to assaults and violent acts (Occupational Safety and Health Administration, 2015). That doesn't sound like a whole lot unless, of course, you were one of the 27! Thus, to think that violence against caring and sharing human service workers has never existed or doesn't still exist is to be gravely mistaken (Flannery, 2009; Gabe & Elston, 2009; Slovenko, 2006).

While the following statistics are somewhat dated and merged with health care workers in general, they are a conservative estimate when compared to the advent of the COVID-19 pandemic (McMahon et al., 2022; Rija et al., 2022). From 2016 to 2020, there were 207 deaths due to violence in the workplace in the health care and social assistance industry within the private sector. In 2020, health care and social assistance workers overall had an incidence rate of 10.3 (out of 10,000 full-time workers) for injuries resulting from assaults and violent acts by other persons. The rate for nursing and personal care facility workers was 21.8 (Bureau of Labor Statistics, 2021).

A hospital-specific study generated by the Northwestern University Academy of Quality and Safety Initiatives program surveyed 802 health care workers. The survey inquired about prevalence, location, and type of experience of physical or verbal abuse by patients or families. 34.4 percent of health care workers reported any incident of verbal or physical violence in the preceding 12 months, with 13.5 percent reporting physical assault. Of those with any incident of physical or verbal violence, 60.2 percent endorsed at least one posttraumatic symptom, 9.4 percent missed work, and 30.1 percent had thoughts about leaving their job or career (Rosenthal et al., 2018) Finally, if you graduated with a B.S. in psychology and found work as a psychiatric aide or tech in a mental health facility, good luck with that, and be careful! For psychiatric aides, the occupational injury rate is 69 times higher than the national rate of violence in the workplace and for psychiatric technicians, it is 38 times higher (Bureau of Labor Statistics, 2015).

While the data is more than twenty years old, for mental health workers in particular, the average number of assaults was 68.2 per 1000 (U.S. Department of Justice, Bureau of Justice Statistics, 2001). These results were chilling enough that the Federal Bureau of Investigation sponsored a workplace symposium on violence in 2002. (To put those statistics in terms that tell you how dangerous the mental health services can be, you would be as likely to be assaulted as if you worked in a convenience/liquor store (68.4/1000).

Besides law enforcement and corrections occupations, only bartenders are more likely to be assaulted (91.3/1000) (U.S. Department of Justice, Bureau of Justice Statistics, 1998)! Things haven't changed much since those statistics. The newest reports show that, between 2011–2013, workplace assault averaged about 25,000 annually with 70 to 74 percent occurring in health care settings. Big numbers that don't mean much, perhaps, but note that 10 to 11 percent of health care injuries that required sick leave were assaults, compared to just 3 percent of injuries that occurred in the rest of the private sector (Occupational Safety and Health Administration, 2015).

A best estimate is that the chance of human services workers being assaulted on the job during their lifetime is approximately 50 percent (Turns & Blumenreich, 1993, p. 5). Newhill's (2003, pp. 35–54) comprehensive review of violence studies on social workers in the United States found that between 20 and 50 percent of the professionals studied reported that they had been assaulted. If that isn't enough to make you consider skyscraper window cleaning as an occupation, assaults on human service workers have been found to be a major contributor to burnout (Hensel et al., 2012; Gascon et al., 2013) and added stress, fear, and decreased job satisfaction (Harris & Leather, 2012; Hutchison et al., 2013). Lanctot and her associates (2014) reviewed 68 studies on workplace violence and found that physical, psychological, and emotional wellbeing, effective functioning at work, relationship and quality of care of patients, and general social and financial wellbeing were all affected by violence perpetrated on the workers. The foregoing is, indeed, part of a long list of the reasons human service workers burn out that you will read about in Chapter 15, "Human Services Workers in Crisis Burnout, Vicarious Traumatization, and Compassion Fatigue."

So, being a human service/health care worker anywhere with the possible exception of Antarctica is a perilous occupation. Having a serious mental illness is a major risk factor for both being assaulted and, in a minority of situations, of committing violence across the world (Watt et al., 2018). Countries such as the United Kingdom (Brown et al.,1986; Leadbetter, 1993; Rowett, 1986), Canada (MacDonald & Sirotich, 2001), Israel (Guterman et al., 1996), the Netherlands (Harte et al., 2013; van Leewen & Harte, 2015); Australia (Koritsas et al., 2010), Botswana (Olashore et al., 2018), Nigeria (Ukpong et al., 2018) and the sub-Sahara (El Ghaziri et al., 2014) confirm a high incidence of violence and threatened violence against human service workers. The problem has become so bad in Spain that April 20 is designated a National Day Against Aggression in Health-Care Facilities (Marlasca, 2014)!

Perhaps more ominous is the notion of threat. Newell found in her own study that social workers who do not suffer an assault may experience destruction of property or verbal threats. Those threats are not taken lightly given the violent histories of many of the clients with whom they are dealing (Newhill, 2003, pp. 46–47). Constantly wondering whether an emotionally disturbed or mentally ill client will make good on their threats every time a human service worker walks out of the office is not the way to have a fulfilling and rewarding work experience.

So threat assessment and management is not just the purview of Homeland Security, and to that end, in 2013, the American Psychological Association started the *Journal of Threat Assessment and Management* (Dingfelder, 2013). That journal focuses exclusively on the subject of violence risk. It is applied in nature, dealing with the development, implementation, and evaluation of procedures for assessing and managing violence risk. Finally, it reflects and promotes the values of interdisciplinary cooperation and internationalism, based on the view that preventing violence requires collaborations that cross professional and, in many cases, political boundaries (Journal of Threat Assessment and Management, 2023).

In summary, the foregoing statistics should tell you one thing: Although you may believe that you are some combination of Jane Addams, Carl Rogers, Florence Nightingale and Mother Teresa ministering charitably and caringly to the disenfranchised and outcast, your clients may have a different idea (Newhill, 2003, p. 206)! Why is this so?

Precipitating Factors

A variety of hazards now put human services professionals more at risk of being victims of violent behavior than they have been in the past. This problem has become so pervasive that the American Psychological Association formed a task force to report on education and training in dealing with behavioral emergencies (American Psychological Association, 2000). They found in a survey of the literature that between 35 and 50 percent of psychologists in clinical practice had reported being assaulted. The threat has become so compelling that the American Psychological Association (2002) incorporated in their ethical standards a section to specifically address psychologists' freedom to terminate therapy if they feel threatened or endangered.

The social work profession has become very interested in violence because social workers are invariably in the line of fire as frontline workers attempting to deal with some of the most economically, socially, and emotionally disenfranchised individuals in the human service business (Saturno, 2023). Interestingly, the counseling profession has not seemed as concerned, although high school counselors in particular are in the line of fire with one of the most volatile and violence-prone age groups there is. The amount of violence that now occurs in K–12 schools in the United States is approaching epidemic levels (National Center for Educational Statistics, 2022).

Substance Abuse. Probably the most noteworthy trend in the continuing upsurge of violence has been the increasing numbers of substance abuse clients associated with it (Blumenreich, 1993b, pp. 23–24; Martens, 2023; Occupational Safety and Health Administration, 2003; Monahan et al., 2001; Turns & Blumenreich, 1993, p. 7; Zhong et al., 2020). Intoxication's disinhibiting effect (McNeil, 2009) appears to directly influence violence, particularly in those individuals who are aggressive and impulsive (Chermack et al., 2000) and those with diagnosed major mental disorders (Rach-Beisel et al., 1999).

Deinstitutionalization. Since the "least restrictive environment" movement and subsequent deinstitutionalization of patients in the 1970s, day care centers, halfway houses, and shelters have filled the gap left when the warehousing facilities of state mental institutions were emptied. A lack of facilities for people who are unhoused and/or transients, a shortage of staff, a lack of follow-up care, and an inability to monitor medication closely have created a fertile breeding ground for clients to regress to their previous pathological states (Novella, 2010; Occupational Safety and Health Administration, 2003; Weinger, 2001, p. 4). Any ride-along with a crisis intervention team officer in a major city will tell you all you need to know about deinstitutionalization. Their terminology for the homeless mentally ill whom they encounter again and again is, "Pete and Repeat."

Mental Illness. The role of mental illness in violent behavior has been hotly debated. To say that all mentally ill people will become violent is patently ludicrous. However, there is some clear evidence that a subset of mentally ill people will and do become violent (McNeil, 2009; Newhill, 2003, pp. 96–104;

Treatment Advocacy Center, 2016). Delusions (schizophrenics), hallucinations (multiple disorders), and violent fantasies (sex offenders, multiple murderers) are all cues to possible violence for people diagnosed with a mental health disorder. Organic issues such as internal head injuries, brain diseases, and dementia all have the potential for increased violence (McNeil, 2009; Monahan et al., 2001; Tardiff, 2003). The personality disorders are rife with the kinds of mental disorders that may become violent. Many of the personality disorders are marked by anger control issues, impulsivity, and the inability to regulate or control emotions (Newhill, 2003, pp. 99–104). Most particularly, those persons diagnosed with antisocial personality disorders and those with explosive personality disorders are prime candidates for acute onset of anger and violence (McNeil, 2009). These illnesses manifest in violent behavior not only in mental hospitals but in primary care and community agency settings as well. O'Rourke and associates' (2018) comprehensive review of violence toward metal health workers and mental health settings in England, Ireland, and the United States is pretty sobering.

Furthermore, because society and the judicial system have become increasingly aware of the role that mental illness plays in crime, a number of people who would formerly have been incarcerated are now remanded to mental health facilities (Occupational Safety and Health Administration, 2003). Also, because of prison overcrowding, potentially violent people are released on early parole. Farmed out to halfway houses that are also understaffed and assigned to parole officers who have tremendous caseloads, parolees do not always get the follow-up care and supervision they need. Police now routinely use hospitals for criminal holds on acutely disturbed, violent individuals. Thus, human services workers are now being asked to deal with a wider variety of people convicted of a felony than before (Hartel, 1993; Occupational Safety and Health Administration, 2003; Walker & Seifert, 1994). The Sequential Intercept Model (2022) detailed in Chapter 5 , "Crisis Case Handling," is an integrated effort of law enforcement, criminal justice, and mental health to get this long lasting, catastrophic problem under control.

Gangs. Gang violence can be found in settings ranging from emergency rooms (Wilson, 2017) to juvenile detention facilities (MST Services, 2018). Gang members' extreme violence, either as a rite of passage into the gang or in retaliation for offenses against them, is without fear or remorse regarding any person, time, or place (Kinney, 1995, pp. 168–169; Occupational Safety and Health Administration, 2003). In a process labeled by Albert Bandura as moral disengagement (1999), victims are dehumanized, and inhumane conduct is actively justified as a means to a gang's end in survival and growth. As a result, their violent behavior knows no boundaries. Gang fights that continue into emergency rooms, community mental health centers, churches, and anywhere else where friction against the gang members or purpose occurs are all too common (National Gang Center, 2017). It is further noteworthy that there is a high incidence of mental health problems within individual gang members that make them potential recipients of services in juvenile and adult holding and correctional and mental health facilities (Macfarlane, 2018) and that make mental health workers potential targets.

Required Reporting. The development of child and older adult abuse reporting laws and domestic violence laws throughout the United States have made human service workers into something other than Florence Nightingale in the eyes of those who come into conflict with the social services and legal systems. Most of the time, field staff such as social workers for human service agencies and school counselors and school psychologists become the objects of offenders' ire and retaliation (Guardia & Sippel, 2023; Newell, 2003, p. 81; Weinger, 2001, p. 5).

Older Adults. The increase in the number of older people now institutionalized in nursing homes and hospitals has created a whole new population of potentially violent individuals. Casually dismissed as infirm and incapable of rendering harm to anyone, geriatric patients commit a disproportionate percentage of violent behavior against human services workers. The assumption that older clients are passive recipients of care is misguided. Study after study indicates this clientele to be at risk for behaving violently both in regard to caretakers and other residents (Astroem et al., 2002; Caspi, 2022; Gates et al., 2005; Hillman et al., 2005; Petrie, 1984, p. 107; Puiu, 2022; Snyder et al., 2007; Weinstock et al., 2008). No statistics are readily available on patient-to-patient assaults in nursing homes, but you should be aware that those happen frequently, and if you are considering nursing home care for a loved one, among all the headaches and heartaches that decision means, you should check out their violence prevention protocols and behavior incidents if at all possible.

Institutional Culpability

LO2 By their very nature, most care providers are readily accessible to clientele and have minimal security checks. Often, unrestricted movement throughout a facility may be gained by agitated and distraught family members, gang members, romantic partners, and clients who are frustrated over long waits and a seeming lack of service. Care providers are also at risk to anyone who walks in off the street with intentions other than seeking services and who may believe that drugs or money is readily available (Occupational Safety and Health Administration, 2003; Turner, 1984, pp. v–vi).

Security training and security devices cost time and money. Administrators trained solely in handling the financial, logistical, and personnel functions of institutions with the responsibility of maintaining adequate patient care are unaware of what it takes to provide an adequately secure environment for their staff (Cowman et al., 2017; Dyer et al., 1984; Hallett et al., 2014). Physical features of mental health facilities built to deemphasize security and confinement as a reaction to the "snake pit" mental hospitals of old have paradoxically put the human services workers at greater risk (Turns, 1993). Emotionally "cold and uncaring" settings, unclear staff roles, poorly structured activities, downsizing of staff, and unpredictable schedules are all stress elevators for the potentially violent client (Blumenreich, 1993a, pp. 38–39; Occupational Safety and Health Administration, 2003).

Assessment of the potential for violent behavior should be mandatory in institutions and clinical facilities that deal with the mentally ill and emotionally disturbed (McNeil, 2009). Dismay over increased violence between patients and assaults on staff has caused a shift toward more secure facilities in the twenty-first century (Bayramzedeh, 2016; Bolton, 2016; Bowers et al., 2002; California OSHA, 2018). Instruments are now available that, combined with clinical judgment, do a good job of predicting violent behavior if—and that is a big if—institutions will use them. However, implementation problems are often endemic. Consider O'Rourke and associates' (2018) review of participating risk factors, which detailed the following institutional issues:

1. Poor risk management
2. Communication problems
3. Inadequate care planning
4. Lack of interagency working
5. Procedural failures–both administrative and legal
6. Lack of suitable accommodation
7. Lack of resources
8. Substance misuse
9. Noncompliance with medication
10. Lack of involvement of care providers
11. Minority ethnic issues, e.g., staff being too ready to make incorrect and stereotypical assumptions about minority backgrounds.

Universities and Their Counseling Centers

We have been particularly concerned with safety issues at many university counseling centers we have toured and two we have worked in. In an effort to be open, warm, and accessible, the university counseling center typically has no choke point that controls access to counseling offices. Students are free to roam about the center. Yet, many of the offices are separated from the reception area and are extremely isolated. Even if there are visual, sound, and code alarms, the reaction time for help to arrive will be slow, giving a perpetrator time and ease of egress to escape. Career counseling, academic advising, and personal counseling clients in the university counseling center may all be mixed together in a very egalitarian environment, but it is a situation that has security risks. As evidenced by Seung-hui Cho's rampage at Virginia Tech in April 2007, some of the individuals who frequent the university counseling center may not be there just because they are homesick (Grayson & Meilman, 2006; Myer et al., 2011). They have serious mental health issues and there are a lot of them (Abrams, 2022; Center for Collegiate Mental Health, 2021; Flannery, 2023).

It is a noteworthy anecdote that when the author of this chapter took a faculty development leave and served as a psychology intern in the University of Memphis counseling center, 6 of his first 10 clients in the Personal Counseling Unit were actively suicidal or homicidal.

Numerous studies indicate that university counseling centers are dealing with more acute psychopathology than they have in the past (Benton et al., 2003; Bishop, 2006; Erdur-Baker et al., 2006; Pledge et al., 1998) and that more students are on psychotropic medication (Schwartz, 2006). More than 1 in 10 students sought counseling center services in 2009, which is the highest percentage ever found in the long-running National Survey of Counseling Center Directors. Further, about 48 percent of the students seen in those counseling centers have severe psychological problems (Munsey, 2010). Those shifts appear to be true not only in the United States but in the United Kingdom as well (Waller et al., 2005). Are those changes due to the general population in the United States becoming more pathological or becoming more aware of mental health issues? Or is the on-campus population changing because of the Rehabilitation Act of 1973 and the Americans with Disabilities Act of 1990, which made college campuses more receptive and accommodating to people with existing mental illnesses? This question has become so important that the *Journal of College Counseling* devoted its Fall 2005 issue to the topic of severe and persistent mental illness on college campuses (Beamish, 2005).

The implications for safety issues overall in the university as an institution are sobering. This issue is even more compelling in regard to "chilly" safety considerations in university counseling centers. It is interesting to note that extended searches for any studies analyzing safety issues in university counseling centers turned up no hits.

Rudd's (2004) summary analysis of why college counseling centers are looking more and more like community mental health clinics is sobering. University counseling centers are so overwhelmed they have adopted community health center models of stepped care of treatment (Bailey et al., 2022). Stepped care is a system of delivering and monitoring mental health treatment so the most effective yet least resource-intensive treatment is delivered first. Program intensity can then be either "stepped up" or "stepped down" depending on the level of client need. Why this is so?

1. The majority of college students today meet the criteria for at least one mental health problem.
2. The rates of mental health problems are the same among students of all races, but students of color are less likely to get treatment.
3. Making matters worse, counseling centers are overwhelmed. Waiting lists are long, and many counselors are burned out or contract employees hired part time (Flannery, 2023). Given these issues, overburdened university counseling centers are in crisis (Abrams, 2022; Center for Collegiate Mental Health, 2021; Flannery, 2023)

Counseling centers and universities that do not become proactive in tightening their security, notification, and oversight procedures will put their general populations at risk. Rudd contends that if university administrations have not already identified a risk management officer to place in the counseling center, they will soon have to do so. Comprehensive plans have been generated to violence proof (as much as humanly possible) college campuses (Myer et al., 2011). Chief among these has been the development of multidisciplinary threat assessment teams (Deisinger, & Scalora, 2016; Perione & Pollard, 2016).

In 40 years of counseling in some tough public schools, a state mental hospital, and a federal penitentiary and meeting lots of disgruntled and unhappy consumers with the Memphis Police Department Crisis Intervention Team officers, while the author of this chapter may have a subjective negative bias, he has yet to meet more severely mentally ill and emotionally disturbed individuals who were not incarcerated for their own safety than he has in a university counseling center. Two of the three colleagues he has known who were killed in the line of duty died from assaults inflicted on them by clients at the college counseling centers where they worked. However, I do not think the murderous assault at Virginia Tech in April 2007 was happenstance. Subjective evidence tells us that many of our colleagues in counseling centers around the country still wear rose-colored glasses when it comes to truly appreciating the potentially dangerous people who find their way to a college counseling center and the lack of security that characterizes those centers. Involvement on a threat assessment team can conflict with counseling center staffs' philosophical, moral, and ethical principles. Perione and Pollard (2016) detail the push–pull conflict counseling center staff experience and their reticence to be involved in threat assessment when confidentiality issues come in conflict with safety issues, their competence in making negative judgmental threat assessments, and becoming the point of contact and referral, evaluation, and judgment in regard to a student's continued participation at the school or a mandated requirement to get into counseling.

Denial

Because of the negative publicity that accrues from violent incidents, institutions have been loath to admit that they occur (Lanza, 1985), and it appears that such episodes go largely unreported (California Occupational Safety and Health Administration, 1998, p. 3; Hartel, 1993; Occupational Safety and Health Administration, 2003). Indeed, the reticence of colleges and universities to report campus crime for fear of bad publicity was, in large part, responsible for the Crime Awareness and Campus Security Act of 1990, known as the Clery Act for Jeanne Clery, a 19-year-old Lehigh University freshman who was raped and murdered in her campus residence hall in 1986. A study conducted to determine whether parents were aware of the Clery Act and how to find information on crime statistics found their knowledge of the act to be low (Janosik, 2004). It seems somewhat ironic that the study was carried out at Virginia Tech. One can only wonder if the results of that study would be different today.

Institutional fault lines. For over thirty years, research has continued to target the following problems in health care settings. Understaffing, overwork, poorly maintained physical environments, nonprofessional staff with limited education, high staff turnover, absenteeism, time pressure and deadlines, on-the-job accidents, lack of senior management and staff support; poor or incomplete communication between administration and staff, lack of staff training in recognizing and managing escalating hostile and assaultive behavior, no time for problem solving and debriefing; and the lack of a unifying treatment philosophy allow frustration to build within the staff and disrupt the treatment routine. As the staff transfer their frustration to the clients, the clients, in turn, become more threatened and start testing the limits of what will be tolerated. When staff attempt to impose behavioral limits under these erratic conditions, the outcome is often violent behavior by clients (Blair, 1991; Evens & Petter, 2012; Jensen & Absher, 1994; Lancman et al., 2013; Occupational Safety and Health Administration, 2003, 2015; Piercy, 1984, pp. 141–142). Finally, secondary victimization occurs when, after an injury by an assaultive client, there is the underlying belief that "It wasn't handled right by the worker" (Turns, 1993, p. 131). Thus, not only does the human services worker suffer physical assault and all the psychological ramifications that go with it, but they also become a scapegoat for an administration unable to handle the increased violence (Newhill, 2003, p. 209). From that standpoint, underreporting occurs, and the notion is that the administration discourages it (Anderson, 2011; Spencer & Munch, 2003).

Staff Culpability

LO3 Staff members are also culpable. A prevailing philosophy is that because human services workers are caring, well-intentioned people, recipients of their services will act in reciprocal ways toward them (Newhill, 2003, p. 13; Turner, 1984, p. vii). The ostrich-like assumption that "It can't happen to me, and besides, there are so few violent incidents that I really don't need to be concerned" is fallacious (Dyer et al., 1984, p. 1). Or, if it does, it's just part of doing the job (Anderson & West, 2016). Madden and associates (1976) interviewed psychiatrists who had been assaulted and found that more than half could have predicted the assault based on predictive models but thought themselves immune from the threat.

From the client's viewpoint, becoming violent is invariably seen as a consequence of being provoked by the worker in some way (Rada, 1981; Ryan et al., 2004). Paradoxically, most staff members have little idea what they or the institution do that is provocative (Anderson & West, 2016). For many clients, treatment may be perceived as coercive, threatening, or frightening. When a client feels little control over treatment conducted by an authoritarian staff, the client may feel the only option is to aggressively act out (Blair, 1991). Furthermore, if the staff treatment philosophy includes limit setting such as use of restraints, seclusion, medication, locked units, and assaults as "part of the territory" (Occupational Safety and Health Administration, 2003), then a self-fulfilling prophecy is likely to develop, with violent acting out as the norm and the only way to get attention. Conversely, a staff's failure to set limits in regard to appropriate behavior in a positive, firm, fair, and empathic manner, as opposed to dictatorially taking away privileges without defining how those might be lost or explaining how they can be regained, increases the potential for violence (Blair & New, 1991). The attitude of staff toward clients also plays a part in who gets assaulted. Staff members who are burned out are more likely to be assaulted than those who are not (Isaksson et al., 2008).

Experience also makes a difference. The great majority of assaults occur to people like you who are reading this sentence—that is, rookies in the field who don't know the lay of the land (Flannery et al., 2011). Guy and associates (1990) found, in a national study of psychologists who had been assaulted, that 46 percent of all assaults involved students or trainees and that 33 percent occurred in the first five years of practice. The incidence of assaults decreased the more years of experience workers had. Kleespies and Ponce (2009) report that nearly 80 percent of all assaults on psychologists occur within their first 10 years of practice. So, if you are a student or still pretty new in the business, you might want to personalize the contents of this chapter a little more than usual.

Ethical and Legal Liability

LO4 Although health care providers may be the victims of assaults, they may also become ethically and legally liable for their actions, no matter how well intended those actions may be (Drogin, 2019; Pope & Vasquez, 2016; Remley & Herlihy, 2020). Such liability extends to the institutions and directors of those institutions, who may fall under a heading of "vicarious" civil and criminal liability (Drogin, 2019; Pope & Vasquez, 2016; Remley & Herlihy, 2020). As paradoxical as it may seem, assaultive clients have held institutions and their employees liable for failure of "duty of care owed" to those selfsame clients (Belak & Busse, 1993, pp. 137–143; Packman et al., 2009). Numerous successful lawsuits also have been brought against health care providers for failure to properly diagnose, treat, and control violent clients or protect third parties from assaultive behavior (Felthous, 1987; Packman et al., 2009). The following are some of the knotty issues that are involved in discerning violence according to various (note emphasis on "various" here) state laws.

1. **Requirement of a threat and duty to warn.** Mental health practitioners are not required legally or ethically to take any action until they have reason to know the client is dangerous and, at that time, take any action which is reasonable under the circumstances (Packman et al., 2009). The question becomes what is "reasonable"? Is the statement "I hate him and I'm gonna fix that jerk!" reasonable enough if the therapist knows the client frequents a local gun range?

2. **Requirement of foreseeability.** A therapist's liability is limited to those persons foreseeably endangered by a hospital or an agency's negligent conduct. (Packman et al., 2009). Hey! Your agency was overwhelmed by clients, and you were told to clear 15 percent of your case load. You were very hesitant to do that and quite vocal about it but were called on the carpet for your hesitancy. One case of the 15 percent you cleared from your case load

wound up stabbing his high school math teacher, and siren-chasing personal injury lawyers are now flocking to both your and the agency's door.

3. **Requirement of a reasonable identifiable victim.** So, let's say you were counseling Seung-Hui Cho, and he sorta identified a general population of Virginia Tech students but didn't name anyone in particular, just generally "rich" Caucasian students in general. Is that an identifiable victim? If you were the parent of one of the students killed, you probably thought so. Or how about Stephen Paddock, who killed 58 people in Las Vegas at a country music festival? He told his doctor he was depressed and was offered antidepressants but only took anxiety medication. Even the FBI behavior analysis team couldn't come up with a reason why he became a mass murderer. Could his doctor have foreseen that potential mass murderer and informed authorities?

4. **Breaking confidentiality.** So, you are a school counselor and meet with Jon Q. Junior who is desperately in love with Sally Ann Sophomore who is having none of it but is head over heels in love for Sam Senior. Jon Q states that if he can't have her, nobody will, but when the passing bell rings, he declares he is starving to death, politely thanks you for listening, and leaves for lunch. You jokingly talk about the lovesick younger generations at lunch with other teachers but do not mention names. The principal hears this comment that gets translated as a student who has threatened to kill somebody and calls you into the office and demands to know the student's name with the school police resource officer present to take the individual into protective custody and notify parents of the potential perpetrator and intended victim.

Those issues just begin to scratch the surface of the possible ethical, legal, and professional issues you can be confronted with when the potential for violence surfaces. We will shortly speak about different methods of assessing for violent behavior, but it wouldn't hurt if you'd cruise back to Chapter 3, "The Intervention and Assessment Models," and take another look at the LASER protocol and apply it to those foregoing vignettes as a little wake-up legal and ethical exercise.

Indeed, the field of crisis intervention itself has a major problem with ethical decision making, and it is noteworthy that none of the major mental health and helping professions ethical standards have anything to say about crisis other than reporting abusive and potentially lethal behavior. That is particularly relevant from several standpoints where the major ethical principles of autonomy and maleficence have head on collisions when the potential for violence occurs and create bi-polar dilemmas of being beneficent toward the individual versus looking out for the good of the community (Myer et al., 2022, pp. 85–95)

Thus, what began as a legal duty with the Tarasoff decision and several expansions of it has become an ethical one as well when confidentiality is suspended when there is foreseeable harm (B2.a of the ACA Code of Ethics (2014). But therein lies the conundrum, because it not only breaches confidentiality and the client's autonomy, but it also asks the crisis worker to make a judgment call on level of dangerousness, which is still pretty much a roll of the dice when it gets down to whether a specific individual will be violent or not and when that might happen . . . if ever (Remley & Herlihy, 2020, p.192; Truscott et al., 2019).

Workplace violence has become so serious that the Centers for Disease Control and Prevention (CDC) has declared workplace violence a national health problem (National Institute for Occupational Safety and Health, 1992), and the federal Occupational Safety and Health Administration (OSHA) has come to the conclusion that workplace violence can no longer be tolerated (California Occupational Safety and Health Administration, 1998, p. 5). OSHA has recently started issuing citations to employers who fail to adequately protect their employees from violence in the workplace and have developed a comprehensive violence prevention plan for human service institutions (OSHA, 2015).

Dynamics of Violence in Human Services Settings

There is a long history that proposes actuarial assessments (normed instruments with reliability and validity studies backing them up) are better risk predictors than individual clinical judgment (Meehl, 1954). There are two problems with that conjecture. First, the ability to predict who will be violent, when, and under what conditions has been ongoing and is notoriously unreliable (American Psychiatric Association, 1974; Kirk, 1989; Monahan, 1988; Mulvey & Lidz, 1984; Palmstierna & Wistedt, 1990; Sloore, 1988). Singh and associates (2014) conducted a large

global survey of violence risk assessment. Surveys were completed by 2,135 respondents from 44 countries. Their results seem to support the rather pessimistic meta-analysis of violence prediction by Lam (2010) and Yang et al. (2015) of hit rates in less than 50 percent of respondents. Second, even if the tests were 100 percent accurate, the problem with that piece of information is that many times in crisis, there is no time or inclination on the client's part to sit down and compliantly take a test!

Predictions are especially likely to be wrong when crisis workers have little background information on the clients and may not have time to make more than a rapid assessment of the situation before they have to act. Yet, data do exist to present general profiles of clients who are more likely than others to become violent, given the right constellation of conditions. To that end, accurate behavioral information is the central core in assessment for violent behavior. Cawood and Corcoran (2009, p. 17) propose that the depth and accuracy of behavioral information obtained are directly correlated to the quality and accuracy of assessment of who may become violent, where, and under what conditions. So, with those rather severe reservations, the task of assessment for violence can be placed in five categories: *unstructured clinical judgment, actuarial techniques, structured clinical judgment*, an *interactionist approach* (Jain et al., 2017), and *contextual, real time crisis intervention* (James & Gilliland, 2017).

Violence Potential Assessment Instruments

A great deal of research has been conducted on the prediction of violence and the assessment of it. As a result, Ronan and associates (2014) have compiled a comprehensive book of over 130 scales, questionnaires, and surveys to accurately assess at risk clients. So how to choose what to use? Here are a few representative examples.

The Violence Screening Checklist–Revised (VSC-R) includes checkoff items that review history of physical attacks and fear-inducing/threat behavior during the first 2 weeks of hospital admission, presence or absence of suicidal behavior, schizophrenic or manic diagnosis, and male gender (McNeil & Binder, 1994). This instrument appears to be highly reliable, particularly in regard to the first few days of hospital admission (McNeil et al., 2003).

The Violence Risk Appraisal Guide (VRAG) (Rice & Harris, 1995), combined with the *Hare Psychopathy*

Checklist-Revised (PCL-R; Hare, 1991) is designed to predict whether incarcerated persons who are soon to be released will violently recidivate. It has 12 historical, biographical variables that range across school adjustment to alcohol use and then is combined with measures of psychopathology on the PCL-R.

The Broset Violence Checklist (BVC; Linaker & Busch-Iversen, 1995) checks for the presence or absence of six factors that are frequently seen as a prelude to violent incidents on acute psychiatric wards: confusion, irritability, boisterous acting out, verbal threats, physical threats, and attacks on objects. This device has been shown to have good predictive validity during 24-hour follow-ups if two or more of these items are checked. A large-scale study of older patients who were violent as opposed to those who were not found the BVC to be a good predictor of violent episodes and a good discriminator between those who would and would not become violent (Almvik et al., 2007).

Structured Professional Judgment

While all of these instruments would seem to do a good job of predicting both short- and long-term violence risk in psychiatric populations, the problem is still predicting when it is happening "RIGHT NOW!" and doing something about it. From that standpoint, knowing the verbal and physical cues and using visual and/auditory analysis are still the best bet for staying out of harm's way. Understanding and knowing the observable risk factors for violence you will read in the following section are known as **decision support tools** when combined with actuarial techniques (Kleespies, 2014, p. 109). These are not standardized psychological tests but risk factors that have been assessed to have high reliability and predictive ability in regard to violence risk.

In that regard, Kleespies (2014, pp. 108–109) has critically reviewed an alternative to either instant eyeballing or four hours of sit-down testing which involves what Borum and associates (2010) have termed **Structured Professional Judgment (SPJ)**. SPJ combines the art of clinical judgment with the science of actuarial predictors. Van Brunt (2015, pp. 121–137) details the following steps to arrive at a structured professional judgment decision about an individual's potential for violent behavior:

1. Gather information via clinical assessment and comprehensive background information from family, school, community, law enforcement, and the workplace.
2. Determine the presence of risk factors (as detailed in this chapter) as they apply to the present situation.
3. What are the potential motivators, disinhibitors, and destabilizing elements present in the current environment that could turn potential violence kinetic.
4. Given that the foregoing variables have reached a critical mass, develop potential scenarios as to how the violence might potentiate.
5. Construct case management of the individual based on the foregoing potential violent scenarios.
6. Communicate these findings to all of the parties that will play a part in the case management and have the formal report on file and readily accessible.

SPJ is now a well-established approach to risk assessment for violence and is used in psychiatric hospitals, forensic mental health services, and criminal justice systems (Webster et al., 2014). As an example of how these go together, *The Dynamic Appraisal of Situational Aggression (DYAS)* checks for immediate risk of violence and is also a treatment plan aid that helps in reducing the risk of violence. When combined with professional observation, the DYAS was found to be a better predictor than clinical judgments alone (Ogloff & Daffern, 2006).

In arriving at a decision of potential risk of violence, the clinician uses evidence-based risk factors combined with clinical opinion. These risk factors have been reduced to manual form in such instruments as the *Historical-Clinical–Risk Management 20* (HCR-20; Webster et al., 1997). Singh and associates (2011) did a comprehensive meta-analysis of nine of the most commonly used structured violence assessment instruments. Out of the 68 studies they examined, they found the HCR-20 to be one of the better decision support tools for predicting who will and who won't become violent. The HCR-20 is a violence risk assessment rating device that asks clinicians to rate clients on 20 variables based on a variety of questions concerning clients' history of violence, clinical mental health status, self-management, and degree of risk upon return to society.

The ratings show good reliability in predicting who among forensic psychiatric clients will become violent both in the long term (Douglas et al., 2003) and in the short term (McNeil et al., 2003), although it fared poorly when assessing incarcerated women in regard to who might commit a violent crime and had an inverse ability to predict which women had been convicted for murder (Warren et al., 2005)! So, it is also not a perfect predictor. However, one of the interesting assets of the HCR-20 is that a *Violence Risk Management Companion Guide* has been developed (Douglas et al., 2001) that offers suggestions on treatment approaches based on the constellation of elevated clinical and risk factors presented.

TRAP-18. If you are in homeland security and are searching for terrorists, then the *Terrorist Radicalization Assessment Protocol-18* (TRAP-18) (Meloy, 2017) is your ticket. Or wait a second! You are a psychologist in a college counseling center, and you are talking to a radicalized student who is also quite possibly suffering from paranoid schizophrenia who is ranting and raving about the godless government. The TRAP-18 is designed to work with just such a client as a lone actor terrorist threat (Meloy & Gill, 2016). This is not a "Yes/no, got so many checked off so you're in or out!" assessment device but calls for knowledge and expertise with both law enforcement and forensic experts in making structured clinical judgments. To be most reliable, it needs three sources of data. A direct interview, collateral interviews with acquaintances, and public records including law enforcement. (Meloy, 2017, 2018).

The instrument is composed of 8 proximal and 10 distal signs of potential violence (Meloy, 2017; Meloy & Gill, 2017). Proximal signs (Meloy & Gill, 2016) you should be checking on: Is there a *pathway of planning* to the violence? Is there a *fixation and preoccupation* with a person or cause? Is there *identification* with other supposed "martyrs" or identifying oneself as THE agent to cause change? Is there *novel aggression* in unrelated acts of violence which are a testing ground in preparation for "the real deal." Are there *energy bursts* of behavioral increases in activities toward the target, although such activities may appear to be benign. Is there *leakage* in communication to do harm to a third party via personal communication or more publicly through the internet?

Now combine these with ten distal characteristics. *Iron clad ideology* that supports the belief for violence with the extremist group or rejection of the group by the individual as being too weak and a "I'll show you" attitude takes place. *Dependence on the virtual community* to express radical beliefs, find like-minded groups, or gather information on needed supplies, tactical skills, timelines, geographical layouts

and other target specific needs. *Thwarted academic/careers goals* through major setbacks or failures. *Creativity* in development of the violent act that is "outside the box" in relation to similar acts. A past history of *criminal behavior. Changes in thinking and affect* where thoughts and emotions become more strident and simplistic. There is no room for discussion. It's "my way or the highway" if you don't adhere to my beliefs. *Failure of sexual intimate pair bonding* is replaced by sexualizing of violence thorough guns, fantasizing afterlife sexual gratification, or use of sex workers or pornography in place of a significant other. *Diagnosed with a mental disorder* which may be exacerbated by the distorted ideology.

Do you think the TRAP-18 is way out there and would be of little use to you? Refer back at the Lethality chapter and image you were counseling Seung-Hui Cho and compare the way the TRAP-18 fits him. Collins and Clark (2021) report that one proximal sign warrants active threat management and clusters of distal characteristics merit threat monitoring. Ashley and Wicks (2022) review of 17 empirical and case studies found the TRAP-18 to be a useful tool in forecasting violent behavior in the aggrieved loner. Yet, there's another kind of specific violence potential problem and an assessment device that fits that for the stalker.

CTAP. The *Communications Threat Assessment Protocol* (CTAP) is a structured professional judgment tool for initial threat assessment of scary and threatening personal communications to famous people. They generally deal with unrequited love or boiling anger. The majority of such inappropriate, aggressive, or threatening communications are harmless, but some are not. The problem is how to separate the two (James et al., 2022). Taylor Swift's publicity manager would probably be in need of this assessment device a lot. The device grew out of the Fixated Threat Assessment Center in Great Britain, which was established in 2006 to assess and manage the risk to dignitaries from isolated loaners pursuing them with malevolent or misguided attention (James et al., 2013). The CTAP has two levels of assessment. The first level concerns those who initially open the communication. This first level, called the *Quick Correspondence Screen (QCS)*, is a simple screening process for deciding which cases to refer to risk managers or law enforcement. It contains an 18-item checklist, and if any item is checked, a referral is made. The CTAP contains 25 items, each of which is associated with an increased risk of violent behavior. Five of the factors are "red flag" items, such as a threat to kill, associated with a high risk of violence, and the presence of one item alone is sufficient to trigger a high alert until proven otherwise. Thus, the second level concerns the determination of threat level by the risk managers, security staff, or policing teams to which such cases are referred and who will decide what action needs to be taken (James et al., 2022).

The assessment device has shown good inter-rater reliability, but as of this writing, only one outcome study (James et al., 2023) has been published, although it showed an extremely accurate correct classification of 85.5 percent of cases with a positive predictive rate of 81.8 percent and a negative predictive value of 86.4 percent. So why might such a test be relevant to you?

Let's go back to our harried school counselor who was being pressured by the school principal to give up the name of a "homicidal" student. Suppose that Jon Q. Junior wrote a rather lengthy hard copy e-mail to his buddy that got misplaced and was found by the art teacher, who turned it over to the counselor. In it, Jon Q. said some nasty things about Sally and was plotting some ways to get even. Now how handy do you think the CTAP might be in helping the counselor decide to turn it over to the school threat assessment team and how helpful would that be to them to make a decision on how to manage the threat? But given all of the foregoing devices, critics still see shortcomings in these approaches (Jain et al., 2017).

An Interactionist view. One of the issues with the foregoing methods is that none of these approaches provides much consideration to the cognitive and interpersonal processes that lead to violent incidents (Jain et al., 2017) nor the context in which they are likely to occur (Myer & Moore, 2006). Toch (2017) proposes that individual intrapersonal personality factors such as motivation and inhibition, interpersonal variables such as lack or availability of support systems, and environmental variables such as poverty and drug cultures are all critical parts in predicting violence. To bring out these interactive variables, Jain and associates (2017) propose that knowing the individual's intrapersonal, interpersonal, and environmental factors are critical in making sound judgments as to intent to commit violence. They propose three operating variables that are critical in assessing how individuals operate and react and that can lead to violent behavior.

Construct of intent and cause. We need go no further than gang culture in regard to the potency of this approach. Meaning making of a slight on an inner-city street corner can have a very different outcome than a slight at a bar or a university recreation center. While laughed off at a bar or university recreation center, the street corner slight can easily turn into acute embarrassment or a challenge that ends up in a gun battle. So what happens with a slight remark has a lot to do with what the particular culture views as "normal" behavior.

Normative reference points refer to what the expected and normal reaction to that slight on the corner might be. The reaction is sudden and spontaneous violence. In the gang subculture, this would be highly valued, and anything less would be received with disdain, ridicule, and possible banishment.

Emotional dysregulation is the harbinger of crisis (Ford, 2021, Kleespies, 2014). From an intrapersonal standpoint, it is how individuals regulate the cascade of emotions that occur when placed under threat and normal, stable emotional control goes flying out the window. Domestic violence calls are probably the poster child for emotional dysregulation for police when reasonable people can go berserk and run violently amok. It stands to reason, then, that SPJ analysts would do well to integrate those components into any interview process.

Given all of the foregoing models that work reasonably well when administered in closed, secure environments, we are still left with the prediction problem when individuals are free and at liberty to act in any manner they choose. That's why, along with knowing some of the major variables that can precipitate violent behavior, we built the Triage Assessment Form you were introduced to in Chapter 3, "The Intervention and Assessment Models." We believe it is absolutely critical for you to understand how it works, practice using it, and incorporate it into your crisis skill set.

The following are some of the critical variables that are used as a basis for judgment in predicting risk of violence.

Bases for Violence

LO6 Keeping in mind the terms "general profiles" and "right conditions," the following bases for profiling violence are "best bet" predictors of "RIGHT NOW!"

There are biological, psychological, and social bases for violence. Biologically, low intelligence, hormonal imbalances, organic brain disorders, neurological and systemic changes of a psychiatric nature, disease, chemicals, intense and chronic pain, or traumatic head injury may lead to more violence-prone behavior (Fishbain et al., 2000; Hamstra, 1986; Heilbrun, 1990; Heilbrun & Heilbrun, 1989; McNeil, 2009; Newhill, 2003, pp. 107–108). Psychologically, specific situational problems, certain functional psychoses, and character disorders are predisposing to violence (Greenfield et al., 1989; Heilbrun, 1990; Heilbrun & Heilbrun, 1989; Klassen & O'Connor, 1988; McNeil, 2009; Newhill, 2003, pp. 94–106). Socially, modeling the violent behavioral norms of family and peers, homelessness, lack of social support, relationships with potential victims, and the milieu within which one lives can exacerbate violent tendencies (McNeil, 2009; Nisbett, 1993; Tardiff, 1984a, p. 45; Wood & Khuri, 1984, p. 60).

Finally, specific on-site physical environmental stressors such as heat, bad lighting and decor, crowding, noise, conflict, and poor communication can trigger violence (Anderson, 2001; Jensen & Absher, 1994; Newhill, 2003, p. 190; Valler et al., 2005). The problem is that when all these ingredients are mixed together, the results start to resemble the kinds of people and environments with which the crisis worker is likely to come in contact (Tardiff, 1984a, p. 45)!

Age. Men between the ages of 15 and 30 continue to be the most violent subgroup (Blumenreich, 1993a, p. 36; Fareta, 1981; Shah et al., 1991; World Health Organization, 2023). The American Psychological Association (2020) has developed a long rogue's gallery list of potential contributors to becoming violent in youth. Some signs of potential for violence may be historical or static (unchangeable) factors like:

- A history of violent or aggressive behavior
- Young age at first violent incident
- Having been a victim of bullying
- History of discipline problems or frequent conflicts with authority
- Early childhood abuse or neglect
- Having witnessed violence at home
- Family or parent condones use of violence
- A history of cruelty to animals
- Having a major mental illness
- Being callous or lacking empathy for others
- History of vandalism or property damage

Other signs of potential violence may be present over time and may escalate or contribute to the risk of violence given a certain event or activity. These might include:

- Serious drug or alcohol use
- Gang membership or strong desire to be in a gang
- Access to or fascination with weapons, especially guns
- Trouble controlling feelings like anger
- Withdrawal from friends and usual activities
- Regularly feeling rejected or alone
- Feeling constantly disrespected

Some signs of potential violence may be new or active signs. They might look like:

- Increased loss of temper
- Frequent physical fighting
- Increased use of alcohol or drugs
- Increased risk-taking behavior
- Declining school performance
- Acute episode of major mental illness
- Planning how to commit acts of violence
- Announcing threats or plans for hurting others
- Obtaining or carrying a weapon

This bulletin from the APA cautions that these dynamic points are more predictive of short-term risk for violence than the more static historical factors, which are more indicative of long-term risk (American Psychological Association, 2020). It should not be surprising that the last set of new behaviors should particularly be a cause for concern if you are a school counselor, social worker, or psychologist.

Next come older clients, who are disproportionately represented in the population that may become violent (Astroem et al., 2002; Bourbonais et al., 2019; Caspi, 2022; Hindley & Gordon, 2000; Petrie, 1984, p. 107). Crisis workers tend to dismiss this group as being harmless, but in a study of 200 cases of assault at the Cincinnati Veterans Administration Medical Center, Jones (1985) discovered that 58.5 percent of the assaults took place in the facility for geriatric patients. This statistic is noteworthy because the institution also had a large psychotic and substance misusing population.

Substance Misuse. There is probably no psychotropic drug, either legal or illegal, that does not correlate with violence when it is misused. Whether the drug misuser is going on a meth high, coming off Valium, or experiencing the withdrawal of heroin, violence and drug use have a strong relationship (Blumenreich, 1993b, p. 24; Piercy, 1984, pp. 131–135; Rada, 1981; Simonds & Kashani, 1980). Add young men into the drug/alcohol mix, and they are far greater risk factors for violence than mental illness (Treatment Advocacy Center, 2016). The foregoing statement most certainly includes alcohol. Alcohol has been associated with more than half of reported cases of violence in emergency rooms and one-fourth of reported cases in psychiatric institutions (Bach-y-Rita et al., 1971). The potential for violence is further increased when individuals who have a history of psychosis engage in alcohol or drug use (Klassen & O'Connor, 1988; Yesavage & Zarcone, 1983).

Predisposing History of Violence. A history of serious violence, assault and damage to property prior to admission, attempted homicide, sexual attacks, assault, or threat of assault with a deadly weapon are some of the best predictors of future violence (California Occupational Safety and Health Administration, 1998, p. 3; Campbell & Messing, 2017; Fareta, 1981; Gumber et al., 2020; Meehan et al., 2016; Monahan, 1981; National Collaborating Center for Mental Health, 2015) and is included in every assessment device checkoff list. Any background that includes contact with the criminal justice system for aggravated felonies, weapons possession, threats against prospective victims, or a history of assaultive behavior while hospitalized should automatically put the human services worker on notice to be extremely cautious with the client (Blumenreich, 1993a, p. 37; Klassen & O'Connor, 1988). Of all the predisposing clues for violent behavior, there is probably none better than being brought to a facility for violent behavior as a part of emotional disturbance or mental illness.

Psychological Disturbance. A variety of mental disorders may be predisposing to violence: the person diagnosed with antisocial personality disorder who has a history of violent behavior, emotional callousness, impulsivity, and manipulative behavior; the person diagnosed with borderline personality disorder who lacks adequate ego strength to control intense emotional drives and repeatedly exhibits emotional outbursts; the person experiencing paranoid delusions who is on guard against and constantly anticipating external threat; the person with a manic personality disorder experiencing elevated moods, hyperactivity, and excessive involvement in activities that may have painful consequences; the person diagnosed with intermittent explosive disorder who has sudden escalating periods of anger; the person with schizophrenia who is actively hallucinating and has bizarre or grandiose delusions; the panic attack victim who is

fearful, dissociative, and has extreme fight-or-flight reactions; and the depressed and suicidal person who is hopeless, agitated, and acting out suicidal plans (Blumenreich, 1993b, pp. 21–22; Grassi et al., 2001; Greenfield et al., 1989; Gumber et al., 2020; Heilbrun, 1990; Heilbrun & Heilbrun, 1989; Klassen & O'Connor, 1988; McNeil, 2009; Meehan et al., 2016; Murdach, 1993; Newhill, 2003, pp. 96–104).

Social Stressors. Loss of a job, job stress, breakup of a relationship, a past history of physical or sexual abuse, and financial reversals are a few of the social stressors that cause acute frustration and rage in an out-of-control social environment that leads to violence (Blumenreich, 1993a, p. 370; Campbell & Messing, 2017; Munoz et al., 2000).

Family History. A history of violence within the family is often carried into other environments. An early childhood characterized by an unstable and violent home is an excellent model for future violence (Wood & Khuri, 1984, pp. 65–66). A history of social isolation or lack of family and environmental support also may heighten the potential for violence (Campbell & Messing, 2017; Heilbrun & Heilbrun, 1989; Munoz et al., 2000). A nasty predictor of future criminal and violent behavior is cruelty to animals (Felthous & Kellert, 1986; Hellman & Blackman, 1966). It doesn't take too much imagination to predict that children who set cats on fire or do other cruel things to pets are capable of a lot of violence as they become adults. Predisposing family histories of witnessing family violence, being abused, enduring excessive physical punishment, abandonment, deprivation, and neglect, as described in the chapter on partner abuse, are all predisposing to adult aggression (Eddy, 1998).

Work History. A history of fractiousness and problems at a worksite is another correlate with violence (Newhill, 2003, pp. 110–111). Being fired at the post office is not the only situation in which workers exact revenge. Job loss and economic instability easily translate into paranoid "they did me wrong" thinking, which can then transfer over to social workers in unemployment offices and vocational counselors at employment services.

Time. In relation to a person's admission and tenure in a facility, time is critical. Admission on Friday or Saturday night during "party hours" significantly increases the potential for violence. In geriatric and mental hospitals, the evening hours, with the onset of darkness, change of shift, and decrease in staff, often lead to client disorientation and states of confusion (Occupational Safety and Health Administration, 2003). The effects of this time period have become so notorious that they have been labeled the **sundown syndrome** (Cleveland Clinic, 2023, Piercy, 1984, p. 139). Mealtime, toileting, and bathing are also prime times for violent outbursts (Barrick et al., 2008; Jones, 1985). Patients in both general and forensic psychiatric hospitals are more likely to be violent immediately after admission to the hospital (McNeil et al., 1991), if they have been readmitted, have a longer stay, and were a nonvoluntary admission (Gumber et al., 2020). McNeil et al. (1988) found that recent violent acts in the community are highly associated with violent acts in the first 72 hours of inpatient care. For most patients committed involuntarily, the possibility of assault is significantly increased during the first 10 to 20 days after admission, and for individuals dealing with paranoia, it remains high during their first 45 days (Rofman et al., 1980).

Presence of Interactive Participants. Violent behavior may be contingent on those who bring the person to the institution (Occupational Safety and Health Administration, 2003; The Joint Commission, 2018). Family members or friends who bring patients in for treatment often interact in a volatile manner with admitting staff, particularly if the staff are seen as abrasive and callous (Ruben et al., 1980) and treat either the patient or support persons in a curt or uncaring manner (Wood & Khuri, 1984, p. 58). Arguments that may occur between the client and support persons are easily transferred to staff. Furthermore, when admonitions by distraught or intoxicated supporters to "fix" the client are not given immediate attention, they or the client may express grievances against the institution and staff by acting out. Any client who is accompanied to the institution by a police officer should be viewed as potentially violent (Kurlowicz, 1990; McNeil et al., 1991; Piercy, 1984, pp. 140–141).

Motoric Cues. Close observation by the human services worker of physical cues will often give clues to emergent states predisposing to physical violence (Kurlowicz, 1990; Petrie, 1984, p. 115; Weinger, 2001, p. 24). Early warning signs include tense muscles; bulging, darting eye movements; staring or completely avoiding eye contact; closed, defensive body posture; twitching muscles, fingers, and eyelids; body tremors; and disheveled appearance (National Institute of Occupational Safety and Health, 2020; Tardiff, 1989, p. 98; Wood & Khuri, 1984, p. 77). If the client is pacing back and forth, alternately approaching and then retreating from the worker, this may be a sign that the individual is gathering courage for an assault (Dang, 1990). The agitated client may have an expanded sense of personal space up to 8 feet in radius, instead of 3 to 4 feet, and may be extremely sensitive to any intrusion into that space (Moran, 1984, pp. 244–246; National Institute of Occupational Safety and Health, 2020).

A number of verbal cues are precursors to violent action by the client. Heightened voice pitch, volume, and rapidity of speech may occur, particularly if the client has been using amphetamines or other psychostimulants. Confused speech content can reflect confused thoughts and psychotic breaks. Clients may use profanity or verbally threaten significant others, the worker, or the world in general. Note that there is a high correlation between threats of violence and acting on those threats. The more specific the threat is to the person, method, and time, the more seriously the threat should be taken (Blumenreich, 1993a, p. 37; National Institute of Occupational Health and Safety, 2020; Tardiff, 1989, p. 99).

Multiple Indicators. The more the foregoing indicators are combined, the higher the potential for violence becomes (Klassen & O'Connor, 1988; Campbell & Messing, 2017). Tardiff (1989) indicates that, if possible, the human services worker should attempt to assess all these factors; if they are present, the worker should clearly note the potential for violence on an intake form (p. 97) or on one of the violence prediction instruments previously mentioned. Tardiff further proposes that whether or not this information is available, one of the better verbal assessment techniques is to ask, "Have you ever lost your temper in a violent manner?" If the answer is "Yes!" the worker should proceed to ask how, when, and where this happened and then perform an assessment much like that for suicide (p. 98). If any of the foregoing factors are apparent or are stated by the client, no matter how calm the client may appear to be, then a triage assessment of 10 on the interpersonal behavioral dimension should be made, the client's record should be flagged, and caution should be used in regard to the potential of the client to harm self or others.

Does this mean you should not go into the human services business and go into something less stressful, like hauling explosives? Your authors would propose not, because about 85 to 90 percent of violence is preventable (Mack et al., 1988). The rest of this chapter will attempt to demonstrate how that percentage can be achieved.

Intervention Strategies

LO7 Because the institution itself plays such a large part in the who, what, why, how, and when of treatment, it may be viewed as an equal and contributing partner in resolving problems with clients disposed to becoming physically and verbally assaultive. No two institutions are alike with respect to a number of variables that affect what the institution can do about the problem of violence. Yet, when confronting clients who may be distraught, angry, fearful, and experiencing disequilibrium, all institutions have a common core of problems. Given the financial, legal, treatment, organizational, and philosophical limits idiosyncratic to each setting, the following intervention strategies should be viewed as a best "general" approach.

Security Planning

No antiviolence program can be accomplished without the commitment and involvement of top management, so everybody in the institution or agency or an individual in private practice understands that preventing violence is an absolute top priority (Barret et al., 1997; California Occupational Safety and Health Administration, 1998, p. 6; Emanuel, 2013; Ford, 2021; Kleespies, 2009, 2014; Munsey, 2008; Newhill, 2003; Weinger, 2001). The five main components of any effective safety and health program also apply to the prevention of workplace violence. These components are management commitment and employee involvement, worksite analysis, hazard prevention and control, safety and health training, and record keeping and program evaluation (Myer et al., 2011; Occupational Safety and Health Administration, 2003, 2015). The OSHA *Guidelines for Preventing Workplace Violence* (2015) have very specific criteria and checkoffs for each of these general areas, and if these criteria are followed and implemented, there should be very little opportunity for workplace violence to occur.

Commitment and Involvement. One of the first steps in preventing violence is understanding what precautions the institution has taken to ensure the safety of clients and staff. The Canadian Patient Safety Institute has created a model template for mental patient safety (Emanuel et al., 2013), which any mental health facility could profit from adopting. Management

leadership and commitment and employee involvement in a safe workplace are critical (Hallett et al., 2014; Occupational Safety and Health Administration, 2003, 2015). The institution should have a zero-tolerance policy for violence for both clients and providers (Wilson, 2017). It should assign clear responsibility to all staff members so they know what is expected of them, along with adequate resources to carry out those responsibilities, and make them accountable for doing so (The Joint Commission, 2018).

Certain precautions can be taken to ensure that workers are not put at extreme risk by their clientele. First and foremost, management should conduct a security management analysis with experts in the security field and overall enhancement of access to enhanced security measures in the facility (Ishimoto, 1984, p. 211; Kinney, 1995, pp. 47–50; The Joint Commission, 2018). Kinney (1995) and Wilson (2017) urge that management recognize that the people with the most knowledge are the frontline workers who deal with the institution's clientele on a day-in, day-out basis, even though management may not want to hear from these workers for fear of what they might say. There should be channels for employees to bring their concerns to management and receive feedback without fear of reprisal or censure; this is critical in implementing measures to reduce violence (Occupational Safety and Health Administration, 2003; The Joint Commission, 2018).

Worksite Analysis. A worksite analysis involves taking a step-by-step approach to addressing potential hazards, focusing on areas in which they may develop, and reviewing procedures put in place to curtail violence (Occupational Safety and Health Administration, 2003, 2015; The Joint Commission, 2018). This questionnaire analyzes and tracks records, generates screening surveys, and reviews workplace security (Occupational Safety and Health Administration, 2003, 2015). If such a survey is not taken, not only does the facility risk outbreaks of violence but the staff will also perceive management as not being greatly concerned about what happens to them (Lewellyn, 1985). Once the results of the survey are compiled, the organization should institute planning in hazard prevention and control.

Hazard Prevention and Control. All staff should have input into these questions, and a comprehensive security plan should be worked out and disseminated

(California Occupational Safety and Health Administration, 1998, p. 8; Occupational Safety and Health Administration, 2003, 2015; The Joint Commission, 2018). Such a plan should be comprehensive and simple, detailing who is responsible for what and under which conditions. The plan should cover the entire domain of the institution, starting with the parking lot, moving through the front door to admissions, and proceeding through the building to encompass day treatment facilities, staff offices, food services, pharmaceutical dispensaries, and client rooms (Ishimoto, 1984, pp. 209–223). Although the administration may view the initial costs in time and money for this service as burdensome, net cost will be minimal if this action avoids just one lawsuit by a client or staff member (Moran, 1984, p. 249). It is of more than passing interest to note that Cowman and associates (2017) study of violence problems covered 2,809 participants in 17 European countries. Besides an overwhelming request for training in violence prevention, respondents felt management issues far outweighed clinical issues as the greatest challenge to violence reduction. Staff management and coordinated teamwork with direct providers was identified as the major challenge. So, it shouldn't be too surprising when you read the Human Services Workers in Crisis chapter about institutional problems that contribute to burnout.

Threat Assessment Teams

LO8 Threat assessment has become big business and has now achieved enough critical mass to be formed into an international organization called the Association of Threat Assessment Professionals (2023). You can apply for membership, go through training, take an exam, and become a certified threat professional (Association of Threat Assessment Professionals, 2023).

So, what exactly is a threat assessment and management team (TAMT), and what do they do? TAMT's are multidisciplinary in nature and are made up of a cross section of professions that may include social services, mental health providers, human resources, medical personnel, faith leaders, law enforcement, management staff, and others depending on the situation and the context (Center for Prevention Programs and Partnerships, Homeland Security, n.d.). While consultants with different areas of expertise in violence containment may be helpful, planning should start by forming a threat team composed of a cross section of the staff and by naming a violence prevention coordinator. TAMTs aim to assess dangerousness, not to predict violence. They focus on analyzing the contextual behaviors of possible perpetrators and any potential victims with which they intersect (Albrect, 2010). Tied to TAMTs' concentration on behavior, threat assessment is not static and changes as time and conditions change so that, much like the TAF in use in this book, a TAMT is not static in its analysis but is dynamic. TAMTs serve five functions:

1. Information gathering: What does the team know about the threatener and the targets?
2. Interviewing: What can TAMT personnel learn from anyone personally or professionally connected to the threatener and victims?
3. Evaluation: What does all of this information mean in terms of threats of violence to people and the organization?
4. Decision making: What should the team do now and in the immediate future? Who will take the lead role in managing the subject's behaviors or actions (e.g., human resources, law enforcement, security, campus police, EAP, mental health clinicians)?
5. Follow-up: If the emotional temperature has cooled around this situation, how will the TAMT continue to monitor the people and behaviors involved so it does not reescalate?

Given these five guiding points, the duties of this team and coordinator will be to (1) outline the scope and activities of a threat management policy; (2) issue a clear and publicized statement against violence, even if the statement simply says, "This organization will not tolerate violence and aggression either from within or from outside the organization"; (3) identify a location and person for reporting threats; (4) determine when threats are serious enough to convene the team; (5) set training for all staff; and (6) establish a protocol for violence reduction that addresses unacceptable types of behavior as well as appropriate sanctions for that behavior (Kinney, 1995, pp. 73–80; Myer et al., 2011; Newhill, 2003, pp. 189–199; Nicoletti & Spooner, 1996; Weinger, 2001, p. 53).

Establishment of a threat assessment team is particularly critical on a college campus (Myer et al., 2011, pp. 256–267) and K–12 schools (Michaelis, 2019). Virginia Tech is a classic example where, for various political, logistical, legal, and ethical reasons, a silo mentality occurred, and critical information was kept in separate units and never shared. It should be clearly understood that Virginia Tech was no different from any other institution in regard to the barriers erected and communication channels that were effectively blocked that could perhaps have mitigated the effects of a mass murderer before he got to the tipping point. In fact, thanks to changes in Virginia law, institutions of higher education and mental health facilities in Virginia are now better able to communicate and exert sanctions and exclusions on individuals who fail to cooperate in assessment and treatment programs than in most other states (Mandatory Treatment of Mental Health Patients, 2007; Threat Assessment Team Formation, 2008; Threat of Violence, 2008).

Individuals such as Seung-Hui Cho may come to the attention of a variety of people, entities, and departments but never be so blatant and labile that they come to the attention of anyone who can make a decision to place them in a psychiatric legal hold, and nothing is done to proactively contain them until a tragedy occurs. That's why a cross section of campus representatives from housing, recreation, food services, academic departments, the counseling center, and law enforcement all need to be part of a threat assessment team that meets regularly and sifts through all incident reports that occur on campus. The same holds true in other institutions where a cross section of workers are used. To that end, the administrative assistant, because of their central location, or custodians, because of movement throughout the building, should not be overlooked as possible members of the team. That threat assessment team also needs a common language such as the TAF (Myer et al., 2007), discussed in Chapter 3, "The Intervention and Assessment Models," so they have a common set of terms and behavioral anchors to use in making dispositions of individuals that come to their attention (Myer et al., 2011, pp. 233–270).

Precautions in Dealing with the Physical Setting. Safety precautions should be taken to deal with the physical settings of the institution in which staff members are most likely to become involved in potentially violent situations with clients. Two critical areas important to all crisis workers are the admissions area and the worker's office. Entry should be locked, visible by video, and clients buzzed in (Munsey, 2008). The reception area or waiting room should offer a television set, reading material, and accessibility to snack areas. Availability of entertainment and food and drink gives clients and visitors an opportunity to engage in a pleasurable activity that can offset the hostile feelings that may be engendered by the problems they are facing and can defuse the stressful situation of admission (Somers-Flanagan & Somers-Flanagan, 1997; Wood & Khuri, 1984, pp. 79–80). One admonition is necessary with regard to food and drink: Clients who are extremely rebellious about entering the institution may attempt to choke themselves on food or even swallow pull tabs from metal cans. The admissions staff should carefully monitor clients if they are allowed to eat or drink (McCown, 1986).

The admissions area should be clean and well kept, with furniture, carpet, and wall coverings well maintained. First impressions are lasting. If the client's first impression of a facility is that staff have little regard or respect for the facility, the client will have little reason to respect what goes on there either (Marohn, 1982). Subdued painting and decorating and comfortable, relaxing furniture do a lot to alleviate anger, tension, and pent-up agitated feelings and thoughts. No sharp, movable objects, including furniture, should be available as potential weapons (McCown, 1986). Clients should be given lockers in which to put their belongings (Munsey, 2008).

The area should be set up so that it is a choke point: only one way into the rest of the facility should be available from the admissions area. Video surveillance should be kept on this area to record everybody who comes in and out, along with a sign-in sheet that records everyone coming in and is checked to make sure that everyone has gone out (Annis et al., 1984, p. 30). There should, however, be another way out for workers, and a panic room where workers could secure themselves from intruders is not a bad idea (Munsey, 2008). Depending on how much security is needed, the reception area may also have electronically locked doors that separate it from the rest of the facility, identity check procedures, curved mirrors, and metal detectors (California Occupational Safety and Health Administration, 1998, p. 10; Munsey, 2008; Occupational Health and Safety Administration, 2015). Clients who are waiting for service should be treated in a courteous and friendly manner and updated on interview delays. Waits should be kept to a minimum (Weinger, 2001, p. 53). In that regard, is it any wonder that people become agitated and enraged in most hospital emergency rooms?

The admissions worker will make the first contact with the client and will engage the person during one of the most potentially violent moments the institution is likely to encounter. The admissions worker should be highly skilled in crisis intervention techniques and should have one primary job—*staying with and attending to the client being admitted*! Under no circumstances should a secretary, receptionist, or any other support person who is not professionally well versed in crisis intervention or who has other tasks to perform, such as typing letters or answering the telephone, be delegated to handle this important assignment. The admissions worker should not leave the client until all admitting procedures have been accomplished and the client is safely settled (McCown, 1986).

The admissions worker should also never be left in a position of isolation from the rest of the staff (Turnbull et al., 1990). Security support equipment such as a body alarm (a button-activated device that, when triggered, will automatically send an alarm and position fix to security), an automatic dialer preset to in-house security and 911, convex mirrors to monitor the whole waiting area, panic buttons, closed-circuit television monitoring equipment, button locks on elevators, and a metal detector at the entrance should be available. Initial interviews are critical in setting the tone for what will occur behaviorally. Therefore, the interview area should be open, yet afford privacy. At times, if the client is very agitated, other staff or, indeed, a police officer may need to be present (Doms, 1984, pp. 225–229; Jones, 1984; Munsey, 2008; Weinger, 2001, p. 53; Wood & Khuri, 1984, pp. 79–80).

This is the setting to wear sensible clothing with freedom of movement! Care must be taken when wearing clothing clients can use to harm you in some way, such as neckties, necklaces, some earrings, and so on. The reason is some clients have real boundary problems (Newhill, 2003, p. 191), and here is not the place for their impulsivity to take over and for you to wind up being sexually or physically assaulted because those assaults on staff do happen. Alink and associates (2014) investigated the amount and kind of violent acts perpetrated on 178 workers in youth facilities. Eighty-one percent experience violence. There was no difference in assault rate by gender. Put on professional work clothes that say, "I am here to help you, but I mean business!" Conversely, you don't need to look as though you stepped out of *GQ* or *Vogue* magazine, but not looking like a professional conveys the impression that you aren't. It is called **face validity**. If clients don't believe you look as though you know what you are doing, you will probably not get the chance to demonstrate that you do.

Personal work environments should also be safe. Desks should be set up so they allow for separation of client and worker, even though communicating across a desk is not the most desirable counseling setup. Furniture should be heavy and difficult to move. Space should be arranged to permit both the worker and the client clear access to the door and to allow the worker to leave the room without having to confront the client or cross the client's personal space. No potential weapons such as paperweights, letter openers, and sharpened pencils should be openly displayed or within easy reach of the client. The same personal warning devices and procedures recommended for the reception area should also be in place in workers' offices (Jensen & Absher, 1994, 1998; Munsey, 2008; Occupational Safety and Health Administration, 2015; Tardiff, 1984a, p. 50).

The receptionist or others in the building need to be able to warn the worker if danger is imminent and vice versa. There should be a common code word that is understood to mean a summons for immediate help. A panic button and a telephone that the worker can use to get in touch with the outside world should be available. These last two points are particularly critical because of the typical isolation of the human services worker with a client in a therapeutic setting (Jensen & Absher, 1994, 1998; Munsey, 2008; Occupational Safety and Health Administration, 2015; Tardiff, 1984a, p. 50).

Training

LO9   Planning is of little consequence if no training follows. Staff who have been trained in the appropriate methods, techniques, and procedures have increased confidence in their ability to de-escalate violence and have reduced assaultive behavior (Emanuel, 2013; Thomas et al., 2005; Turnbull et al., 1990). Training should include both knowledge and skill building and should be ongoing, with immediate training for new members of the treatment team and continuing education for veterans (Cowman, 2017; Dyer et al., 1984, pp. 12–15; Newhill, 2003, p. 207; Turnbull et al., 1990; Weinger, 2001, pp. 52–53; Wilson, 2017). Every employee should understand that violence should be expected but can be avoided or reduced through preparation (Newhill, 2003, p. 206; Occupational Safety and Health Administration, 2003, 2015).

Training should begin with the crisis intervention skills listed in Chapters 3, "The Intervention and Assessment Models" and 4, "The Tools of the Trade," and additionally cover legal aspects, theories of aggression, reporting and recording of incidents, assessment of contextual and environmental variables, verbal defusing techniques, triggers of aggression, warning signs, use of safety and alarm devices, self-defense and restraint techniques, behavioral observation, consultation, follow-up staffing procedures, and debriefing (Blair, 1991; Kinney, 1995; Munsey, 2008; Murray & Snyder, 1991; Occupational Safety and Health Administration, 2003, 2015; Turnbull et al., 1990). A critical component of training is not just talking about problems but gaining practice in solving them (Kleepies, 2014). There is no better way of doing this than in role-play and incident simulation situations, which can be videotaped for analysis and feedback by instructors and peers (Forster, 1994; Turnbull et al., 1990).

Anti-Violence Intervention. Most approaches to anti-violence prevention in institutions involve the use of behavioral (token economies, shaping, modeling, contingency contracting) or cognitive-behavioral intervention methods (reframing negative attributions, thought stopping, relaxation training, positive counter injunctions) (Douglas et al., 2009).

The **risk-needs-responsivity (RNR) model** is a procedure that is taken from the corrections field (National Institute of Corrections, n.d.). The risk component proposes that high-risk individuals get more targeted, specific, and tailored therapeutic inputs before they go critical. The needs component focuses on the dynamic risk factors that, when changed, reduce recidivism. This procedure has been applied to anti-violence programs with people diagnosed with severe mental illness who are experiencing acute emotional disturbances. RNR usually incorporates cognitive-behavioral therapy, social skills training, anger management, and behavioral techniques that apply role rehearsal, modeling, and shaping to prosocial behavior (Douglas et al., 2009). While not perfect by any stretch of the imagination, it appears that RNR is at least somewhat effective with people fitting the above description. (Lovell et al., 2001; van den Brink et al., 2010; Wong et al., 2008; Yates et al., 2005) who present with very tough, intractable, and chronic issues that are generally resistant to change.

Assumptions. Adequate training should endow the crisis worker with the ability to make certain assumptions and take certain precautions when dealing with potentially violent clients (Kleepies and Richmond, 2009; Newhill, 2003, pp. 121–165; Turnbull et al., 1990; Weinger, 2001, p. 45; Zold & Schilt, 1984, pp. 98–99).

1. Assume the potential for anger, suspicion, and disorganized thought. Maintain a calm, professional,

this is business attitude. Do not attempt to use logic to counter arguments in response to the disorganized thoughts. Maintain a professional, confident, and calm demeanor with angry responses and set limits and provide clear instructions with options that define what positive and negative consequences will occur if anger escalates.

2. Assume the client feels a number of debilitating emotions such as fear, depression, anxiety, helplessness, anger, rejection, and hopelessness, and demonstrate concern by encouraging verbal ventilation through *how* and *when* questions, showing empathic concern by restatement and reflection of the client's feelings, and reinforcing appropriate behavior and communication of feelings.

3. Assume frustration of normal activity and boredom when the client is in residence and provide activities to keep the client fruitfully busy.

4. Assume a threat to the client's self-esteem, independence, and self-control, and provide choices and opportunities to help in carrying out medical and psychological activities with a "we as team" approach to solving problems.

5. Assume tension and arousal, and provide a calm and relaxing atmosphere, particularly in high-tension periods, by manipulating environmental variables and using a cooperative "we" approach.

6. Assume that there will be confusion and provide a careful explanation of all procedures to be employed, being particularly sure that all staff are operating from the same frame of reference.

7. Assume responsibility and provide for one primary staff member to act as chief caretaker and advocate of each client.

8. Assume disconnectedness and rootlessness if the client is to be institutionalized for any length of time and provide familiarity and psychologically calming anchors associated with pleasant memories.

Precautions. While providing support through the preceding proactive behaviors, the wise human services worker should observe a number of precautionary measures (Blair, 1991; Forster, 1994; Greenstone & Leviton, 1993; Kleespies, 2014, p. 26; Moran, 1984, p. 244; Munsey, 2008; Piercy, 1984, p. 143; Turnbull et al., 1990; Weinger, 2001, pp. 33–48; Wood & Khuri, 1984, p. 69). There are a lot of "Don'ts" to follow, but reviewing them every once in a while may save you a trip to the emergency room!

1. Don't deny the possibility of violence when early signs of agitation are first noticed in the client, such as restless pacing, grinding teeth, clenched fists, swearing, muttering threats, loud agitated responses, etc.

2. Don't dismiss warnings from records, family and peers, authorities, or fellow workers that the client is violent.

3. Don't become isolated with potentially violent clients unless you have made sure that enough security precautions have been taken to prevent or limit a violent outburst.

4. Don't engage in certain behaviors that may be interpreted as aggressive, such as moving too close, staring directly into the client's eyes for extended periods of time, pointing fingers, or displaying facial expressions and body movements that would appear threatening.

5. Don't allow a number of the institution's workers to interact simultaneously with the client in confusing multiple dialogues.

6. Don't make promises that cannot be kept.

7. Don't allow feelings of fear, anger, or hostility to interfere with self-control and professional understanding of the client's circumstances.

8. Don't argue, give orders, or disagree when not absolutely necessary.

9. Don't be placating by giving in and agreeing to all the real and imagined ills the client is suffering at the hands of the institution.

10. Don't become condescending by using childish responses that are cynical, satirical, or otherwise designed to denigrate the client.

11. Don't let self-talk about your own importance be acted out in an officious and "know-it-all" manner.

12. Don't raise your voice, put a sharp edge on responses, or use threats to gain compliance.

13. Conversely, don't mumble, speak hesitantly, or use a tone of voice so low that the client has trouble understanding what you are saying.

14. Don't argue over small points, given strong opposition from the client.

15. Don't attempt to reason with any client who is under the influence of a mind-altering substance.

16. Don't attempt to gain compliance based on the assumption that the client will share your rationale regarding your approach to the problem.

17. Don't keep the client waiting or leave a potentially violent client alone with freedom to move about.

18. Don't allow a crowd to congregate as spectators to an altercation.

19. Don't use *why* and *what* questions that put the client on the defensive.

20. Don't allow the client to get between you and an exit.

21. Don't dismiss increasingly vociferous client demands as merely attention-seeking, petulant, or narcissistic behavior.

22. Don't enter a room ahead of unknown clients. Stay behind and visually scan them as you go into the room.

23. Don't remain after hours with a potentially violent client unless proper security is available.

24. Don't fail to make contingency plans for violent incidents. Take your personal safety seriously by playing "what if this happens" scenarios in your mind and with others.

25. Most importantly, *don't attempt to be a hero.*

Outreach Precautions. In the rapidly changing world of mental health, much crisis intervention now occurs on-site (refer to Chapter 16, "Disaster Response"). With the passage of the *Patient Protection and Affordable Care Act of 2010,* traditional health care delivery is increasingly shifting to private settings, and in those settings, home health care workers experience one of the highest rates of client violence (Campbell et al., 2014). Although outreach and "mobile go-out" teams give the crisis interventionist far more mobility and rapid response capability, on-site intervention also has the potential to put crisis workers in extreme danger as they operate in violent neighborhoods and households (Burry, 2002). Besides the foregoing warnings given for in-house operation, the following injunctions generated by your authors and a variety of others (Cawood & Corcoran, 2009; Greenstone & Leviton, 1993, pp. 31–33; Jensen and Absher, 1998; Kleespies, 2014, pp. 146–148; Newhill, 2003, pp. 199–204; Occupational Safety and Health Administration, 2015; Weinger, 2001, pp. 56–59) should be added to the repertoire of the crisis worker who operates outside the walls of the institution. Again, checking this list every once in a while before you make a home visit may save you a trip to the emergency room.

1. If you are not familiar with clients, check records before ever making a home visit for incidents of violent behavior. If they are present, do not go by yourself.

2. If at all possible, go with a partner, or at least have a cell phone or other means of communication to get help in a hurry with a code word indicating you are under threat and need help.

3. Let someone else in the office know where you are going and when you will be back. Log in and log out with specific name and place of client visited, scheduled time and expected duration of visit, your car description and license on file. Office contact after visit termination and management procedures when no log in occurs.

4. Check out your surroundings. Although time is of the essence in most crisis intervention, move into the situation slowly and carefully, and be fully aware of what is going on in the environment around you.

5. Plan what you are going to do before you go. Take time to gather in-depth and accurate behavioral information on the client and family. Note any incidents of violence, drug misuse, or other potentially threatening behaviors in the client's folder before the visit. Our Crisis Intervention Team officers for the Memphis Police Department rendezvous and plan who is going to do what before they enter a hazardous situation whenever possible. You should do the same.

6. Don't park directly in front of the place where the crisis is occurring. Check out the area as you drive by, and park just beyond it. If you have to leave in a hurry, this position allows you to leave without crossing the line of sight of a person who may be able to harm you.

7. Before knocking on a door or entering a building, listen carefully for a few seconds for clues as to what may be going on inside.

8. Never stand directly in front of a door. Knock and, as the police do, stand aside, so you are not assaulted or shot through the door. If the client hesitates in opening the door, be very wary of going inside. If you think that something is happening that is suspicious or that could be hazardous to your health, politely terminate the appointment and leave.

9. Consider what you are wearing from a safety viewpoint. A tie or a choke chain may make you look more professional, but it can also be used to strangle you. High heels are elegant, but you can't run in them. Loose-fitting, mobile, and nonflashy clothing is the watchword.

10. Once the door is open, immediately scan the room to determine who is in it and where they are. Compare these visual data to information you may have received previously on the situation. Don't take anyone for granted, particularly older people who may look harmless. Ask if there are other people in the house and who and where they are. If they are not supposed to be there, politely postpone the appointment and leave.

11. Monitor the verbal and nonverbal behavior of all the people in the room. What are they doing, and what must you do to stabilize the situation? If there are intoxicated people present, politely postpone the appointment and leave.

12. Enter the room only a short distance so you can first assess what's going on and can get out quickly if you have to.

13. Don't let a crowd of bystanders gather or let neighbors "drop in" to see what's going on. Politely ask them to leave. If they won't leave or refuse to disperse, get out or get the police!

14. Alert the client you are coming to visit, find out who else will be there, or if you are in a housing project, alert the building captain or housing authority police.

15. If a verbal dispute is going on, first and foremost consider your own safety. If necessary, leave and call the police. If you believe you can control the situation or don't seem to have any other choice, attempt to take control as quickly as possible. Separate disputants and have them sit down. Stay calm, and make clear, concise, assertive statements about what you want them to do. If that doesn't work, get their attention by making a tangential request: "Stop that! I need to use the telephone to call in." If all else fails, a police whistle gets everybody's attention.

16. Sit in a chair where you can observe what's going on. Seat yourself so you're leaning forward and can easily get out of the chair quickly! If you sense that the situation is deteriorating, leave. *Don't be a hero!*

17. Leave your credit cards, purse, jewelry (except a wedding band, which can be a deterrent to sexual advances), and most cash at the office. Carry only your identification and driver's license. You don't want to get mugged.

18. Stay out of kitchens. They have knives and other things that can hurt you. Interview in the living room.

19. Check and see if the client has used firearms. If there are firearms present, leave immediately.

20. Remember that you are not on your own turf, and the unexpected can happen at any time. Stay alert from the moment you enter the neighborhood until the moment you leave the neighborhood.

These injunctions are not a recipe for avoiding violent confrontations, but they are general working procedures that will help the human services worker move adroitly with the client through the intervention stages.

Record Keeping and Program Evaluation

You will soon meet Jason as he is adjudicated to an inpatient mental health facility. As per Van Brunt's recommendation (2015, p. 137) a threat analysis and management structured professional judgment report should be on file and available to all the staff that will come in contact with Jason. Incorporated in that should be a lethality assessment and a first order of business in an intake interview if violence toward self or others is indicated (Kleespies & Richmond, 2009). This report should be reviewed as soon after Jason's arrival as possible so a threat management plan is in operation. Thus, employees follow a procedure that provides for reporting *all* incidents, with or without injury. They participate in a safety and health committee that receives information and reports on security problems, makes facility inspections, analyzes reports, and makes recommendations for corrections. Regular case conference meetings are used to identify potentially violent clients and discuss safe ways of handling them (California Occupational Safety and Health Administration, 1998, p. 7; Newhill, 2003, pp. 205–213; Occupational Safety and Health Administration, 2003, 2015; Weinger, 2001, pp. 49–55). Most importantly, good records allow for program evaluation.

Stages of Intervention

LO10 On the Transtheoretical Stages of Change Model (DiClement & Prochaska, 1998), Jason is barely in the *Precontemplation* stage. In this stage, Jason does not intend to take corrective action in the foreseeable future (defined as within the next 6 months). He is in denial and pretty much unaware that his behavior is problematic or produces negative consequences other than getting him caught and remanded for treatment. In this stage, people often underestimate the pros of changing behavior and place too much emphasis on the cons of changing behavior. It would be ideal and hitting the psychological power ball if Carol could move him all the way to the *Action* stage (DiClement & Prochaska, 1998) where he changes his antisocial behavior to pro-social behavior and keeps moving forward while testing these new behaviors out. The reality is if Carol can move him into the *Contemplation* stage (Di Clement & Prochaska, 1998) where he sees the possibility of positive change, she will have done an outstanding job with this resistant and troubled young man. To do that, and depending on Jason's behavior, she will operate on Piercy's nine-stage violence prevention model.

There are three primary levels of intervention (dos Reis et al., 2003) within the model. At level 1, the primary objective is to prevent further escalation. Level 2 intervention aims to reduce the target symptoms. Level 3 intervention maintains the safety of the clients and staff. Within these three broad levels, management of potentially violent situations should proceed in a sequential manner, based on a nine-stage model developed by Piercy (1984, pp. 147–148). The stages are (1) education, (2) avoidance of conflict, (3) appeasement, (4) deflection, (5) time-out, (6) show of force, (7) seclusion, (8) restraints, and (9) sedation. The cardinal rule for all of these stages, as stated by Larry Chavez (1999)—a noted authority on violence prevention in the workplace—is "Never, ever deprive another human being of personal dignity, respect, or hope nor allow anyone else under your control to do so." For each of these stages, personal responsibility is paramount. Furthermore, whether by circumstance or design, the first person who comes in contact with the problem is the one most likely to be the agitated client's focus of attention (Moran, 1984, pp. 233–234).

Stages 1 through 5 all rely heavily on talking instead of acting, in accordance with one of the primary goals of crisis intervention with violence-prone individuals: getting them to talk it out rather than act out. This approach may seem obvious, but it is difficult to achieve. The agitated client clearly has a limited ability to talk and think through problems as opposed to acting on them and giving little thought to the consequences (Tardiff, 1984a, p. 52). While the immediate goal is to defuse and de-escalate clients' rapid movement toward violence, the overall end goals are to alter violent clients' motivation so they can utilize nonviolent ways to reestablish their lost sense of control; monitor them and preempt their reengagement of violence; and model for and assure significant others such as peers, family, fellow patients, and staff that calmness and serenity will prevail and violence will not be tolerated (Cawood & Corcoran, 2009, p. 8).

As we move through the nine stages, we will follow Jason, a 16-year-old White male client, and Carol, a therapist who by most standards is an old pro. She has been at Seashore Village, a comprehensive mental health inpatient treatment facility, for 4 years. Jason is new to the business of institutions. However, he is not new to being angry, which he is right now as he sits with a deputy sheriff in the reception area waiting for Carol to come through the door.

Jason's teen years have been filled with petty larceny, truancy, conduct problems at school, alcohol and drug use, and parents who have gotten him out of one scrape after another. He is impulsive, has anger management problems, and has difficulty controlling his emotions. His latest escapade of stealing a car landed him in front of a juvenile court, and he was sent to Seashore as an alternative to the state juvenile correction system. His father, fed up with Jason's behavior and over the objections of Jason's mother, has pushed for this placement. Jason feels betrayed and is extremely angry at his father for doing so.

Seashore itself is representative of a broad sample of institutions. It is neither the best nor the worst in terms of clients, staff, resources, and security measures. The endeavor here is to paint as representative a picture as possible, so please withhold judgments about the efficacy and appropriateness of these strategies in every institution. Our hope is that the procedures used in the case of Jason will make you think carefully about your own present or future role in an institution, compare the ideas proposed here with the requirements imposed on you, analyze the procedures used, and thoughtfully compare these techniques and the real world within which you operate.

Jason: (thinking to himself, hands sweating, slight tremors racing through his body) Man, this place is scaring the hell out of me. How'd I ever get in this fix? What are they gonna do to me? I'll be at the mercy of the rest of the crazies in here. I'll really go nuts if I stay here. I gotta get out of this place if it's the last thing I ever do.

Jason is extremely angry and anxious about what will happen to him, frustrated that he has lost control of his life and that what he has considered to be normal activity is going to be severely curtailed. He also feels extremely vulnerable, confused, bewildered, and alone. Jason's feelings are typical of those of a client who is being introduced to a long-term treatment facility for the first time (Blair, 1991; Zold & Schilt, 1984, p. 96). Anger generally comes out of frustration or hurt and is one way of creating an emotional wall that protects us from being vulnerable

(Fauteux, 2010). To say that Jason is feeling very vulnerable right now is a big understatement.

As soon as Jason enters Seashore, someone from admissions immediately calls the adolescent unit. Carol comes quickly to the reception area and meets Jason. As she enters the room, she makes a fast visual assessment of Jason's verbal and nonverbal behavior and monitors Jason closely to see what his reaction to her initial query will be.

Carol: (thinking to herself) What's going on with this kid? Any signs he is agitated? Yes! He's pacing around, eyes darting to and fro, keeps cracking his knuckles, looking at the door and the cop. He'll run if he gets the chance! Muttering to himself. Who brought him in? Nobody else here but that cop over there. He keeps watching him. Must be an adjudication. If a cop brought him here, be careful.

Carol picks up the file the deputy has brought, quickly looks it over, and finds the boy's name and rap sheet. A fast review tells her that Jason has been in a series of escalating scrapes with the law, that his parents are fed up with his behavior and feel he's out of control, and that he has been involved in fights when his explosive personality got out of control. Carol then talks briefly with the deputy and finds out what kind of a trip Jason had from the juvenile detention center.

Carol: (thinking to herself) OK! Check him out and see how stabilized he is, and let him find out what's going to happen to him.

Stage 1: Education.   Clients need to be educated about what is happening to them, and why and how it is happening, through reasoning and reassurance. One way of doing this is to assume the role of the client's advocate (Pisarick, 1981). As in most all crisis interventions, first contact is important (Kleespie & Richmond, 2009; Somers-Flanigan & Somers-Flanigan, 1997, p. 35).

Owning statements that indicate concern over the client's welfare are a good opening gambit. It must be assumed that in this new, strange, and alien environment, the primary feeling of the client will be fear and anger (Rada, 1981). Open-ended questions and reflection of the client's feelings are crucial to conveying that the client's feelings count for something and are being taken into consideration (Turnbull et al., 1990). Carol sees how unenthused Jason is about being at the facility and uses sarcastic empathy (Newman, 1994) to try and ease a hostile situation.

Carol: Hi! My name's Carol, and you must be Jason. I'm the person who'll be working with you. I'll bet you've been really looking forward to that!

Jason: **(Gives a menacing look.)** OH Yeah! So what? **(Points to officer.)** The cop got me in here, but I ain't gonna go any farther.

Carol: I understand how you feel. Most people who come here feel about the same way. Seems like everybody's against you, telling you what to do. I'd be angry too! I want you to know, though, that here at Seashore, you're going to have some options about what happens.

Jason: Screw your options. I ain't stayin' here. **(Makes a menacing move toward Carol.)**

Carol: **(Senses move and moves back and a little to Jason's left, giving him some increased space.)** One of your immediate options is that I'd like you to come with me and meet some of the other kids here and have them tell you what's going on and see if what they have to say fits with what you're about. On the other hand, the court sent you here, and if you don't like the first option and want to fight it out, you could be carried back to the unit, and we can wait until you've got yourself together. I understand you're angry, and I'd be angry too, but I'd like to know if you feel that fighting or running is gonna make it better for you and improve your situation rather than checking things out. So you've got a choice. I think you might be interested in meeting some of the other kids, but you'll have to show me you can handle that, starting right now.

In this initial meeting, the worker uses the technique of providing options (Newhill, 2003, p. 158; Turnbull et al., 1990). This opening statement includes acknowledging the client's feelings but also conveys expectations that the client can control himself. By doing so, Carol sets the tone for what the behavioral expectations are in a clear and caring, yet firm, way (Steveson, 1991). She is letting the client have some semblance of control of the situation but is also clearly outlining what the consequences of his choices are. As soon as possible, she is going to model option therapy (McCown, 1986). Option therapy, in simple terms, says, "You always have a choice. You need to start deciding as soon as possible who's going to have control over those choices, you or us."

The staff has reviewed Jason's records and their Threat Assessment and Management Report (Van Brunt, 2015, pp. 124–130) and determined the motivators (arousal and adrenaline rush via bullying), disinhibitors (negative attitude that sees the world as a hostile place and lack of integration socially with peers) and destabilizers (disturbed attention span, difficulty staying on task, obsessive thinking that misattributes blame with a tunnel vision view of the world and racing thinking where thoughts can't be controlled and jump to incorrect and paranoid conclusions) that are likely to instigate violence. Therefore, scenarios of his initial interactions with his peers would predict watchfulness and early intervention at the first sign of trouble.

Jason: Well . . . all right . . . lady, I'll give it a look-see, but I ain't promisin' nothin' after that.

Carol: I don't expect any more than that at the moment. What I want most for you is to see what's going on here and what some of the other kids think about what we do before you make any kind of promises. We don't lie, and we don't make promises we can't keep.

The worker has to make a quick judgment about how directive or nondirective to be. Telling Jason he needs to calm down is not an option. How do you react when you are upset, and somebody tells you "Just calm down"? Doesn't work very well, does it? And it probably upsets you even more, and goodness knows you handle your emotions pretty well. That statement would be telling the client he is not in control but someone else is, which affirms for him that he isn't in control, so the behavior escalates even more (Fauteux, 2010).

Carol is directive only to the extent of setting boundaries equivalent to how out of control the client is. Her other mission is to establish rapport and credibility with the client. She does this by accepting and acknowledging the client where he is and in turn stating the same from the institution's perspective. She offers no platitudes or false promises (Turnbull et al., 1990). Jason has a chip the size of Mt. Rushmore on his shoulder, so he is always looking for an excuse to argue and bully his way through life. Carol will assiduously avoid arguing with him so as not to reinforce his behavior (Van Brunt, 2015, p. 178) Her technique of letting the client talk to other people on the unit is designed to let the client hear and see with his own ears and eyes what is going on without feeling he is getting a lot of propaganda. However, she will not provide a forum for him to act out, and, if in her judgment Jason is not controlled enough to make a tour with her, she will summon assistance, and Jason will be escorted to an observation room (McCown, 1986).

Carol: We have a lot of activities, so if you don't clearly understand what's happening or you want to know some more about it, just ask. **(Carol outlines Jason's schedule.)**

Very little free time is available. For most people who enter a facility such as Seashore, a major problem has been too much free time and the inability to handle it well. Structuring the environment brings some badly needed discipline back into their lives. Particularly for adolescents, burning up energy in constructive ways is of paramount importance. Furthermore, too much free time is a fertile breeding ground for acting out behavior (Jensen & Absher, 1994).

Seashore is also on a behavior management program that makes use of levels. Part of that behavior management program is a risk-need-responsibility component (National Institute of Corrections, n.d.) that will be used to help Jason to learn how to control his emotions. Jason will start at entry level. Depending on how Jason operates in his environment, he will go up or down on the level system and will concomitantly receive more or fewer privileges. At an entry level, he will have few privileges—early bedtime, no passes—and will be under fairly close supervision. By conducting himself in a responsible manner, he may increase his level designation and gain access to a broader array of recreational activities, later bedtime, ground privileges, and weekend passes. The system is explained to Jason in a careful and clear manner, with emphasis on the fact that whether or not he moves to higher levels is his responsibility.

Educating a client about what is to happen medically and psychologically needs to be done slowly, methodically, and in nontechnical terms with numerous perceptual checks. Keeping explanations simple and helping the client gain understanding ameliorates the situation, whereas complexity only increases the chance for violent behavior to occur (Jensen & Absher, 1994; Moran, 1984, p. 234).

Jason: **(somewhat belligerently)** Like, what's this group meeting?

Carol: The group meets every day. The group decides how to tackle a community problem and then collectively makes a commitment to do something about it. Second, when problems between people

arise, we all put our heads together and see how those problems can be solved. You don't necessarily have to accept an idea, but you must listen to what's being said.

Jason: I don't think I got anything to say to these nerds.

Carol: Maybe you don't. However, a lot of kids here do. Your behavior and your willingness to work say how long you're going to be here or be in a juvenile detention facility if you don't work. My guess is you want to get out of here as quickly as you possibly can. Right?

Jason: You got that right lady.

Carol: So are you willing to cut a deal with me? We look pretty hard at what's going on with you right now as you deal with other people here, how that behavior may or may not cause you problems, and what's down the road for you if you do decide to change some things in your life and what's likely if you don't. We don't ask you to love everybody here, but we do ask you to respect what they're trying to do, just as we ask them to respect you. You do that and I move you through levels faster than that Joey Logano #22 NASCAR T-shirt you have on.

The human services worker's responses are from Glasser's reality therapy (1965, 1969) and focus on the issues of becoming involved, looking at alternatives, making value judgments, accepting no excuses, and assuming responsibility and consequences for one's actions. They also use Somers-Flanigans' (1997) motivational technique of "cutting a deal." You do what I want, "Work hard!" and you get what you want "Outta here faster!" In this manner, Carol goes over the entire schedule with Jason. While she explains the content of the program, she also makes sure to assess and reflect the emotional content of Jason's responses, again and again reinforcing the idea of options, responsibilities, and commitments.

Stage 2: Avoidance of Conflict. Conflict and confrontation are avoided whenever possible. Matching threat for threat is likely to obtain for the human services worker exactly the opposite of control and containment of the situation (Dubin, 1981; Fauteux, 2010). Workers who delight in continuously pushing and escalating issues are not practicing good therapeutic intervention techniques and are clearly asking for trouble (Blair, 1991). One week has elapsed since Jason's admission.

Jason: (standing in the hallway, shouting, shaking, and trembling, face flushed) If you think you or anybody else can make me stay in my room or in this place, you're crazier than I am. I just wanted a drink of water, and Mr. Richardson started yelling at me that it was past quiet time. Just try stopping me and see what happens.

Carol: (quietly and calmly) Jason, OK, sounds like you feel he put you down, but if it's a drink you want, then return to your room, I'll bring you a cup of water. Please go into your room. You can have your drink, and we can talk about it. While I do that, I'd like you to be doing a little thinking about what you really want and how to go about getting it.

The worker reflects his feelings, which have now probably become more important than the drink he was going to get. However, by offering to get him a drink if he complies, the worker is giving him an honorable way out, reinforcing prosocial behavior, and also offering to listen to his concerns (Fauteux, 2010). If the client is fast approaching a point of no return, let them ventilate feelings. Although shouting, cursing, and yelling are not pleasant, they are better than hand-to-hand combat (McCown, 1986; Vinick, 1986). The worker rolls with the resistance (van Brunt, 2015, p. 179) and does not meet it head on but instead encourages the individual to start thinking in new ways about the situation.

The worker should attempt to remove the agitated client from the vicinity of other residents, who may aggravate the situation (Chavez, 1999; Turnbull et al., 1990). This is best done by immediately asking the client to go to an area that is away from the other residents (McCown, 1986). If the client retains some semblance of control, the client's own room may be an appropriate place. If the client is fast losing control and cannot calm down, a better choice is a room devoid of stimuli. Such a place should be specifically prepared and reserved for this sort of occurrence.

Carol: What are you angry about?

Jason: (still standing in the hallway, quite agitated) He was treating me just like my old man, just making me feel like a baby.

Carol: And what were you doing?

Jason: Hey, I was just going to get a drink of water. I still had 2 minutes until quiet time. He made me so mad I wanted to pick up a chair and bust him. I still feel like going after that jerk.

Carol: What will that accomplish?

Jason: It'll show him he can't push me around like my old man does.

Carol: If you do that, it'll just confirm that you need to be here, that you can't control yourself. Is that what you want?

Jason: Maybe I just don't care.

Carol does not display anger or fear, even though the situation is potentially volatile. She speaks in a calm, controlled voice, lower and slower than Jason. She is setting the example and controlling the dialogue (Chavez, 1999). For those clients who do not respond to verbal attempts to defuse the situation, the next step for the human services worker is to give assurance that violent behavior by anybody, including both staff and clients, is unacceptable and then to indicate what the person's choices and consequences will be if the behavior persists (Kinney, 1995, p. 49; Wood & Khuri, 1984, pp. 67–68).

Carol: You can choose to pick up a chair, Jason, but that'll mean a number of things will happen. First, nobody is allowed to hit anybody else here, and that goes for both staff and kids. If it comes to that, we will restrain you, something I'd not like to see happen. Second, if you choose to do that, no one else will get to hear your side of it, and we won't have a chance to work your problem out with Mr. Richardson. Another choice would be to go back to your room and then ask for a drink. If you do that, I will get Mr. Richardson and we'll all sit down and work this through. Would you be willing to do that?

Carol is absolutely truthful about what will happen to the client. At this stage, loss of credibility would be catastrophic (Chavez, 1999). Clients should be confronted with their inappropriate behavior but in a caring, supportive, and problem-solving way that is not tinged with sarcasm or challenge. If the situation is deteriorating so rapidly that the worker no longer feels that communication can be maintained, it may be fruitful to have someone else enter the scene whom the client will perceive as a neutral party (Lakeside Hospital, 1988). This tactic is risky and involves a judgment call on the worker's part. Allowing clients to be rewarded for acting out by getting other people to come to the scene may reinforce inappropriate behavior and lead clients to believe that they and not the institution control the situation. Carol uses a combination of confrontation and empathy. She also provides options for Jason and sets limits as to what will be tolerated (Newhill, 2003, p. 158).

Jason: It ain't just Richardson. This whole place sucks. They won't let me do nothin'. And you don't understand either. Chaplain Gentry's the only guy who I can really talk to.

Carol: I understand that you're really disappointed and mad that you couldn't get a drink. I also know you're pretty angry at me and everybody else right now, and about the last thing you want to do is go peacefully back to your room. I know that you and Chaplain Gentry are pretty close. Would you be willing to go to your room and wait quietly while I get him?

If the client does not choose this option, then the worker will have to move the client to a safe place, which will be a time-out room. A show of force may be necessary to send a clear message: "If you can't handle yourself, we will."

Carol: Jason, I want you to go down to observation for 15 minutes and think this out. (**speaking to technicians**) Bob and Jerry, will you see that Jason gets to observation? In 15 minutes, I'll be down to see if you're ready to talk this through.

Stage 3: Appeasement. Stages 3 and 4 are probably most appropriate in emergency situations in which the worker has little basis to judge the client's aggressiveness and violence and is unable to obtain immediate assistance. Appeasement is not applicable in a number of settings under ordinary circumstances, and if Jason had reached the point of being removed to involuntary time-out, appeasement or deflection of feelings (Stage 4) would be highly inappropriate and run counter to good therapeutic practice.

However, generally it is better in all situations to err on the side of humility than to project a "tough guy" image, regardless of the client's verbal barbs, threats, and exhortations. This recommendation does not mean that the human services worker should become a doormat to be walked all over by the client. It does mean that by operating in an empathic mode, we can recognize just how frightening and alarming the situation is to the client. The reason threats are made is mostly because clients are scared, frustrated, and at a loss as to what to do over situations they can't control (Newhill, 2003, p. 175). Any attempts by the workers to counter threat with threat in an emergency

situation are likely to confirm the client's suspicions that bad things are going to happen.

Appeasement can be attempted if the client's demands are simple and reasonable, even if those demands are made in a bellicose manner. Early on, it is better to grant demands and to defer until later worry about what "lessons" need to be taught (Piercy, 1984, p. 148). This approach may be difficult for some human services workers to accept because it is based on the idea that there is no winner or loser in a potentially violent confrontation between an agitated client and the institution (Moran, 1984, p. 234). In Jason's case, when he feels that his use of anger to make his point is ignored, that makes him more aggressive, and his anger moves up to hostility and threat.

Jason: (**Barges into the human services worker's office, fists clenched, and starts shouting in an agitated, high-pitched voice.**) Listen, big shot! I wanted to mail this letter to my girl. She doesn't know what's happened to me, and that jerk Richardson won't give me a stamp. I could bust all yer heads!

Carol: (**in a calm, collected voice**) He's going by the rules, but I understand you're being hot under the collar. Please sit down at the table here, and I'll see what can be done about getting a stamp.

The human services worker meets this demand because it is easily done and does not seriously conflict with institutional rules. She is also alone with an extremely agitated client who may or may not act out. There may be a discussion afterward with the other worker who gave the original order, but there needs to be a clear understanding among all workers that in emergencies, judgment calls may bend the rules a bit or countermand orders of others.

Stage 4: Deflection. Deflection of angry feelings is attempted by shifting to other, less threatening topics. Deflection acts as an emotional buffer. We do not have to deal with feelings directly when we focus away from the thing making us feel uncomfortable. While it is usually seen as a defense mechanism, it can also serve as a counseling technique when emotions are heating up to move away from the hot topic to cooler ones. This may be done in a variety of ways. Asking the client to take a physically less threatening position shifts the focus away from agitated motor activity to problem solving (Wood & Khuri, 1984, p. 68).

Carol: (repeating her statement patiently, firmly, and respectfully) Jason, I understand how important it is for you to be able to write to your girlfriend and how it frustrates you when things don't seem to go your way, but getting in my face won't get you what you want. Please sit down. I'm going for my mid-morning snack. Since you're in a writing mood, if you can write out how to replay this meeting with Mr. Richardson and handle your feelings when you feel like the rules are unfair, then maybe a snack shows up for you too while we talk about and see if we can iron out this problem, and if that happens, then maybe a stamp shows up too.

The human services worker literally and figuratively gets the client off his feet and in a less threatening operating mode (Epstein & Carter, 1988). The worker is also quietly but firmly setting limits by asking the client to sit and write. When clients engage in bullying behavior, it is important for the worker not to threaten the person's critical need to get control, but it is equally important to let the client know you will not be intimidated by it (Fauteux, 2010). Because agitated people seldom listen closely to requests for compliance, Carol acknowledges Jason's feeling state and then uses the broken record routine (Canter & Canter, 1982) of repeating her request. The Somers-Flanigans (1997, pp. 69–74) make an eloquent case for using food as a mood-altering device. It's a lot more difficult to be angry when you're eating an ice cream bar. She is also employing another behavior management technique: By making a reward contingent on a compliant behavior, Carol is using "Grandma's law" (Becker, 1971), which basically states, "First you eat your spinach, and then you get your ice cream." By using problem-solving techniques, no matter how small the real or imagined injustice is, the human services worker conveys to the client an interest in the client as an individual and not just another name in the institutional computer (Wood & Khuri, 1984, p. 71). Parceling out the problems into workable pieces, the worker removes them from the realm of the enormous and makes them solvable (Weinger, 2001, p. 45).

Having the client write down problems also defuses angry feelings and acting out. In many instances, the client may just be testing limits. Testing limits is a given with a client such as Jason, and the human services worker can be expected to be tested over and over again (Poliks, 1999). To write down clearly and logically what the problem is calls for time and effort, which very few clients will invest if the problem is not important (Epstein & Carter, 1988). Writing down the particulars of the problem is also cathartic for clients, allowing them to gain some emotional distance from it and view the situation in a more objective light (McCown, 1986).

Jason: I can't get nothin' done here. Everything's screwed up. School, home, people, the food, my freedom. It's a prison.

Carol: OK. There seem to be at least three things that are really bugging you right now. Not being able to get a pass yet, the way your dad got angry in family therapy, and your problem with the math assignment yesterday. Together, I can see how it'd become overwhelming. Let's take them one at a time and see what can be done about each. Let me take some notes so I can keep all this straight. (Jason goes into a long-winded explanation while Carol listens and takes notes.)

Until absolutely sure what the problem is, the human services worker should never make promises about what can or cannot be done when attempting to calm an agitated client (Newhill, 2003, p. 210; Wood & Khuri, 1984, p. 71). By allowing Jason to ventilate and by taking notes, Carol affirms that what he has to say is important and plays up rather than down the client's concerns (Chavez, 1999).

Carol: I know that weekend pass is really important. A pass is based on good behavior and your level status. If you feel like you've gotten jerked around, griping about it won't help much. Very specifically, write down why you think you deserve the pass. I'll take it to the staffing this afternoon.

When other, more overt ploys are ineffective, the client may use manipulation and threat to obtain demands.

Jason: If you don't get that pass for me, you ain't much of a counselor, and they'll be real sorry they didn't give it to me.

Carol: When you try and lay that guilt trip on me and make threats about what you'll do if you don't get your way, that's a pretty good indication that the staff's judgment was right and makes it even more difficult to act as your advocate. It's not so much any of the demands that you want, but more like pushing the limits to see how far you can get by manipulating and threatening me.

The response the human services worker makes is one from Adlerian psychotherapy called "avoiding the tar baby" (Dinkmeyer et al., 1979, p. 118). By responding directly to the client, the human services worker does not allow herself to be caught up in the manipulative trap the client lays for her. Although the response is confrontive, it is exceedingly effective with manipulative individuals because it deflects them from their game plan and causes them to consider the consequences of their actions (Wood & Khuri, 1984, p. 71).

When clients become agitated, deflecting anger through physical activity can be helpful (Frey, 2021). Clients can take out their frustrations through activities that range from pounding on a heavy bag (Vinick, 1986) to tearing up telephone directories (McCown, 1986). At the same time, the human services worker can reinforce the client for acting in more appropriate ways (Jensen & Absher, 1994). Although teaching anger management skills may be more effective in the long run (LeCroy, 1988), appropriate and safe physical exertion to burn up angry feelings is an effective short-term solution (Frey, 2021).

Jason: (tearing up the Yellow Pages) Umphf! I . . . get so mad . . . I . . . Arggh! I . . . wish this phone book was that no-good SOB's face.

Carol: But in fact, you haven't torn anybody's face off. You've made a good choice. Much better than when you were going around clobbering people. You don't have to pay any consequences at all for tearing up the phone book. You get it out of your system and get back in control.

Jason: (Continues ventilating, until finally he runs out of energy and lets his arms hang limply at his side.)

Carol: (Continues to reinforce Jason for acting appropriately and within limits.) Look at what you could have done. You could have swung a chair at Richardson, which would have gotten you into hot water. The very kind of thing that got you here in the first place. But you didn't do that. What you did was perfectly acceptable and within the limits here.

Stage 5: Time-Out. When clients cannot contend with the emotion of the moment, they are asked to go to a reduced-stimulus environment to be alone and think things out. A clear assessment of how agitated the client is needs to be made at this point. Is the client able and willing to leave a high-stimulus situation for a few minutes to rest and think things over? If the client is not overly reactive, then the worker may ask the client to take a minimal time-out in living quarters.

Jason: I don't want to sit, talk, or be reasonable. I want this scumbag place to do something!

Carol: Right now, I can see there's no way this is going to get solved. You can go to your room and think things over. Go for 15 minutes. If you can come back and show me you're in control, that's it, no reduction in level, no write-ups, and it's forgotten.

When a clear threat is made, there is still a possibility of reducing the tension by telling the client that threats will not work, but the client has still not done anything wrong, so there is still time to work things out (Fauteux, 2010). However, if the client can't calm down and start to work on the problem constructively, then time-out is the next option (Vinick, 1986).

Carol: I've tried to work this through with you, and you clearly don't want to hear it. When you continue to make threats, you're saying to me you're not willing to abide by the rules and are choosing to have rules enforced. I want you to go to the observation room for 30 minutes right now. At the end of that time, I'll be around to see you. If you don't feel like talking, you don't have to, but you can go back in the room for another 30 minutes. You can continue to do that until you're willing to talk to me about how you think you've been treated unfairly.

The human services worker states these conditions in a matter-of-fact manner and does not press the issue (Vinick, 1986). If the client is so agitated as to be beyond the grasp of reality and is unwilling to be compliant with the human services worker's request, then the worker needs help to contain the situation.

Stage 6: Show of Force. If the client is unable to proceed to time-out or is otherwise noncompliant or acting out, then a show of force is needed (Piercy, 1984, p. 148). If the client is already agitated enough to warn the human services workers that help may be warranted, the interview should be carried out in an open hallway or large meeting room where the participants are in plain view of other staff members and the client can be restrained easily (Viner, 1982). The show of force indicates that any display of violence or threat of violence will not be tolerated and often helps disorganized clients regain control of themselves (Wood & Khuri, 1984, p. 68). If this stage is reached, the potential for violence is high, and the worker should not attempt to deal with the client alone (Munsey, 2008). Either by paging help through an emergency code or by having assistance readily available, the worker needs to be able to summon enough help to demonstrate that compliance is now required (Lakeside Hospital, 1988).

However, there are times when, through no fault of the worker, potentially violent situations occur when the worker is alone and not immediately able to call for assistance. The following procedures may keep the worker out of harm's way (Chavez, 1999; Epstein & Carter, 1988; Lakeside Hospital, 1988; Moran, 1984, pp. 238–248; Morrison, 1993, pp. 79–100; Thackrey, 1987; Turnbull et al., 1990).

1. **Stay calm and relaxed.** Tensing of muscles and agitated movement only fuel the situation and cause the client to expect that something bad (for the client) is about to happen. Relaxation techniques such as simple deep breathing are extremely helpful, allowing one to stay loose, anticipate client responses, and move quickly.

2. **Practice positive self-talk.** Even in the worst situations, running positive "billboards" through the mind's eye will help keep control of the situation.

3. **Do not stare at the client.** Keep casual eye contact because the eyes of the individual will typically move to where a blow might be struck. Focus on an imaginary spot on the client's upper chest, about where the first button on a shirt would be, occasionally glancing at the eyes and other parts of the individual's body. Keeping focus on the centerline of the client's body will also let the human services worker avoid being faked out by extremity movements.

4. **Stay an arm's length away or more.** Make a judgment about how long the client's arms are, and stay an arm's length and a bit more away. Remember that agitated clients generally have an expanded sense of personal space and feel threatened when that space is entered.

5. **Stay on the client's dominant side.** Know which of the client's hands is dominant and stay close to the client's dominant side. Especially on men, the watch hand typically indicates the client's weak side. If you cannot determine this for sure, stay on the client's right side since most people are right-handed. In an aggressive stance, a person invariably places the foot of the weak side forward. If the worker keeps to the dominant, or right, side of an assailant, any blow aimed by the assailant is likely to have less power and be a glancing one because the assailant will have to pivot to get workers back on their left to hit workers more easily. Staying on the right, or dominant, side means the assailant will have to take time to move into a more favorable position and will not be able to use their strength as effectively.

6. **Keep arms at sides and hands open.** Folded arms or hands on hips are bad for two reasons. They imply hostility or authority, and they put the worker at a distinct disadvantage because of the time it takes to unfold them and defend oneself.

7. **Assume a defensive posture.** Stand with feet slightly spread, face to face with the client but tending a bit to the client's weak side. Move the dominant leg slightly to the rear with the knee locked ready to pivot and run. Move the other leg slightly forward of the body and bent slightly at the knee. This position will allow the worker the best chance to stay upright, and staying upright is the best safeguard against being hurt.

8. **Avoid cornering.** When the client is placed in an angle formed by two walls or other objects, with the human services worker directly in front of the client, the only way out is through the worker.

9. **Avoid ordering.** When a client is threatening violence, attempting to order or command a client to do something is likely to aggravate the situation further. Staying with the basic empathic listening and responding skills used throughout this book is far more likely to lead to satisfactory results.

10. **Do perceptual checks.** Ask for the client's help. If current verbal responses are merely agitating the situation, ask the client what solutions or techniques might calm things down.

11. **Admit mistakes.** If you've made an error in judgment, admit it and make an apology. If things have gone this far, do not be afraid to lose face.

12. **Do nothing.** If doing something will make matters worse, do nothing. If the client is determined to leave and help is not immediately available, let the client go. *Never* attempt to touch a client under these circumstances without first indicating what you are about to do and getting the client's agreement to do so.

13. **Give validation.** In a sincere and empathic manner, acknowledge that the person has a good reason for feeling that way and let them leave.

All human services providers and especially crisis workers should undergo training in simple self-defense and takedown procedures (Blair, 1991; Morrison, 1993, pp. 79–100; Thackrey, 1987; Turnbull et al., 1990; Wilson, 2017). Gately and Stabb (2005) found restraint and defensive training topics least attended to by training programs. Numerous facilities provide such training for little or no charge. Local community centers and college continuing education courses may offer such instruction, or the local high school wrestling coach may even be prevailed on. Instruction should be a priority of the institution, and *all* personnel should receive training. The organization should certainly provide self-defense training. If it doesn't, and you have decided to work there, you absolutely need to get training yourself.

Stage 7: Seclusion. Seclusion may be generally differentiated from time-out by its length, its setting, and its involuntary nature. Seclusion is a severe type of limit setting for the client in a safe and secure environment where the client can reorganize thinking, feeling, and behavior (Mattson & Sacks, 1978). Cowman et al. (2017) found in their survey of European practices of reducing violence that seclusion, along with medication and restraints, was a default solution to violent patients. Hallett's (2014) literature review of U.K. practices echoed the same finding that seclusion and restraint were the primary means of handling violent clients. Seclusion along with restraints and medication at times is the least harmful option. Yet, such action clearly runs roughshod over patient autonomy, and to that end, careful use of it is warranted. When seclusion or physical or chemical restraints are used, federal and state guidelines must be followed. They should be used only when there is imminent danger to the client or others and no safer or more effective alternatives are available (dos Reis et al., 2003). There is a great deal of controversy as to whether seclusion or restraints should be used, given the potential for physical and psychological harm (Glezer & Weintrab, 2010; Kumble & McSherry, 2010; Mohr, 2010). However, in some cases, there is no other option if self-harm or harm to others is imminent.

There are a number of reasons for seclusion: (1) the client is agitated, hyperactive, verbally threatening, or damaging property; (2) the client is impulsive or intrusive and does not respond to limit setting; (3) the client is making suicidal gestures and is unable or unwilling to make a verbal contract about controlling behavior; or (4) the client must be protected from possible harm by others (Baradell, 1985; Lewis, 1993, p. 105). This intervention still allows the client some control over mobility, thinking, and autonomy. Seclusion may be of greater benefit to clients who are overstimulated by social contact (dos Reis et al., 2003).

Negative emotions such as anger, guilt, confusion, helplessness, and loss of control are typical client responses to seclusion (Outlaw & Lowery, 1992). Given these negative feelings, it is more than likely that the client may not willingly go to seclusion. In the confrontation with Jason, a response team has been called and is ready to take Jason to seclusion.

Carol: I'd really like you to go on your own down to time-out. It's up to you. You can go on your own right now, or the technicians will take you to seclusion.

Even at this late hour, the worker is still attempting to allow Jason to exercise options and make choices (Baradell, 1985).

Jason: I ain't gonna go nowhere 'ceptin' outta here.

Carol backs away, and the response team moves in. On a predetermined signal by the leader, they quickly take Jason down. One member holds his head, and the other four carry him to seclusion. Once placed in seclusion, the client is oriented to what is going to occur, and a staff member is assigned to monitor the client. Checks are made at 15-, 30-, or 60-minute intervals, depending on the client's mental status. Copies of nursing and general care orders are given to both staff and the client. Seclusion has a low level of sensory input—no radio or television, no visitors—and the emphasis is on biological needs. "Low level" does not mean that the client is sensorially deprived; it is important to prevent feelings of abandonment. The client is shown acceptance by the human services worker and reassured that seclusion is necessary and temporary and that the client can return to normal routines when the behavior calms down (Baradell, 1985).

Carol: I'm sorry you chose to go to seclusion, Jason. You decided to exercise that option, but when you can agree to not make threats, control your behavior to the point you can talk this through, and make a written contract as to what you will do, you can come back out.

In an acute stage of agitation such as Jason has just experienced, it is no longer appropriate to explore conflicts or feelings (Ruesch, 1973). Carol's communication with the client is brief, direct, and concrete but kind. Given the client's sensory overload, sleep is an excellent therapeutic modality, and the client should be allowed to use it (Baradell, 1985).

One negative footnote is appropriate here: A few clients may use seclusion as a way of achieving notoriety and a macho image (Gutheil, 1978). If such a hidden agenda is suspected, the human services worker should thoroughly discuss this problem with the other residents and obtain their help in being nonresponsive to the client's "tough guy" behavior.

Stage 8: Restraints. Restraints are most often employed in psychiatric facilities and are used in conjunction with a request from the nursing staff and backed by a doctor's order. When a client is placed in restraints, close observation is absolutely necessary. Under no circumstances should clients be restrained without such guidelines and available professional medical staff. If the client is acting out and will not go to seclusion, restraints will have to be used. Restraints might be either physical or chemical. Restraints are controversial, and their use is closely regulated in both a legal and an ethical sense (dos Reis et al., 2003). The Canadian Patient Safety Institute position on use of seclusion and restraints is blunt. Restraint and seclusion are behavioural management interventions that should be used as a last resort to control a behavioural emergency. Behavioural emergencies are often the result of unmet health, functional, or psychosocial needs, and you can often reduce, eliminate, or manage such emergencies by addressing the conditions that produced them.

Restraints are employed when it is evident that the client may be harmful to self or others (Stilling, 1992; Tardiff, 1984a, p. 48). If the client is to be restrained, then adequate staff should be available, consisting of at least one person for each limb and another person who serves as leader, for a total of five members. Written guidelines and constant rehearsal of procedures with observation and critique should be used to keep the team's skills well honed (Tardiff, 1984b).

Seclusion and restraints should *never* be used as a way of controlling clients, making life "easier" for the custodians, or as punishment. These are truly last-resort measures because their use can cause a host of other problems for the client (Morrison, 1993, p. 105). If at all possible, the crisis worker should not be involved in the episode because involvement may erect barriers to future therapeutic endeavors.

Stage 9: Sedation. If all else fails, the client needs to be chemically restrained by a doctor's order (dos Reis et al., 2003). The problem now becomes clearly medical, and until the medical staff believes that medication is no longer necessary, there is little the human services worker can do. If sedation is needed with Jason, it does not mean the end of Jason's story. Stage 9 is essentially a complete time-out for both Jason and the staff. For Jason, it will allow the sensory overload he is experiencing to diminish and return to normal limits. It will give the staff members time to reorganize their thoughts on how best to deal with this highly agitated adolescent. When Jason comes out of sedation, the staff will start down the treatment road with him again and will have developed a new plan to deal with this angry young man.

The Violent Older Client

LO11 Although medical science has been able to prolong the lives of Americans, treatment for neuropsychiatric disorders concomitant with increased longevity remains beyond the reach of medical science at present. Accompanying the neuropsychiatric problems of the older client are reduced judgment and increased impulsivity, limited mobility, drug dependency, multiple personal loss, financial problems, and limited social supports, which all potentially contribute to violent behavior (Caspi, 2021; Mentes & Ferrario, 1989; Petrie, 1984, p. 107). Nursing home staff are at high risk for assault by patients, and they need to be trained to be aware of and respond to potential threats of physical assault (Gates et al., 2005; Hillman et al., 2005; Newhill, 2003, pp. 91–92; Tak et al., 2010; Tardiff, 1989).

The case of Cliff demonstrates how the agitated and mildly disoriented older client can be stabilized without medication. Reality orientation (Osborn, 1991; Heerema, 2022; Taulbee & Folsom, 2006), reminiscence (Butler, 1963; Klever 2013; Liu et al., 2021), and remotivation (Garber, 1965; Janssen & Giberson, 2013) techniques are workable options for the mildly disoriented older client. The case of Grace shows how validation therapy (Feil, 1982; Neil & Wright, 2003) may be used with the severely disoriented older adult. These cases illustrate that psychologically infirm elderly clients need not always spend this final stage of their lives in chemically induced compliance.

Mild Disorientation: The Case of Cliff

Cliff Hastings has lived a full and eventful life, but now, at the age of 74, he is a resident of a skilled nursing care facility. He was a strapping man who had worked all over the world on big construction projects until he was 72. He invented many engineering techniques in steam fitting and chilled water-cooling systems. He lost his wife to cancer 10 years ago but submerged himself in his work and lived a highly productive life as a widower. He has had excellent relationships with his two children, Jan and Robert. Although they and their families live geographically distant from Cliff, they love their father very much and are very concerned about him.

At age 73, Cliff got up one morning, prepared to go to work, and fell flat on his face with a stroke. Although he recovered to the extent that he was able to shuffle around the house, lung complications set in. He was diagnosed as having emphysema and went on oxygen. Six months later, he was no longer able to take care of himself physically, was starting to have memory lapses, and was moved to Hursthaven Nursing Home by his children. At Hursthaven, he has become progressively more confused about people, places, and times and, when asked to do something, has been either rebellious or passively resistant.

A crisis was precipitated when he knocked over an oxygen tank in the middle of the night because the "Arabs were after him" and broke the nose of a male attendant who tried to calm him down as he attempted to struggle out of his bed. Cliff is about to meet Marilyn, a gerontological counselor. She has just been retained by Hursthaven to deal with crisis situations such as Cliff's.

Assessment. Marilyn has thoroughly reviewed Cliff's chart and has discussed his case with the medical and primary care staff. Many of the primary care staff members maintain that Cliff is noncompliant, badly disoriented, and dangerous, and they would like to keep him heavily sedated. Cliff's stroke, his unplanned aggressive outburst, his hostile and uncooperative behavior, his fear of the medical equipment, and his depression, plus the fact that his outburst occurred at night, all support the staff's contention that little but chemical restraint is left for Cliff.

Marilyn decides to conduct her own assessment by interviewing Cliff. She has three purposes in mind: (1) to determine Cliff's degree of disorientation and agitation, (2) to use her therapeutic skills to reduce his disruptive behavior and help him return to a state of equilibrium with as little reliance on medication as possible, and (3) to help Cliff use whatever resources he has to live this final stage of his life as fully as he is able.

Marilyn: Hello, I'm Marilyn. I don't believe I've met you. You seem pretty angry about something.

Cliff: (suspiciously) Who the hell are you?

Marilyn: I'm new here, part of the staff, and I'm getting around meeting all the residents. Sorry you're so angry. What can I do to help?

Cliff: I'm Cliff Hastings, and I'm mad as hell. Look at what those SOBs have done to me. I pay $12,000 a month for this place to strap me down. I'll kill the bastards if I get a chance. Can you get me out of here?

Marilyn: (speaking in a strong but soft and empathic voice, while pulling up a chair and sitting down directly in his line of sight) No! I can't right now. I guess I'd be mad too if I were strapped in like that. Do you know where you are?

Cliff: I'm in Hell, and these people are all devils.

Marilyn: It may feel like that right now, but this is Hursthaven Nursing Home. Do you know that?

Cliff: Too damn well.

Marilyn: Do you know what day it is?

Cliff: Who cares? They're all the same in here.

Marilyn assesses Cliff's degree of contact with reality by determining how well oriented he is to person, place, and time. Although he does not give specific, concrete responses, his retorts indicate that he is fairly well in touch with reality, given his present agitated state.

Marilyn: I'm sorry you're feeling so angry. Can I get you a drink of water?

Eliciting Trust. Offering clients food or drink tends to defuse the situation and make them more accepting of initiating overtures the worker may tender (Wood & Khuri, 1984, p. 67). Marilyn also sits down by Cliff and meets him at eye level. She places herself on his physical level and in his direct line of sight. Standing over a client who is confused tends to distort the caregiver's image in grotesque ways and may be very threatening (Wolanin & Phillips, 1981, p. 106).

Cliff: (Takes a sip of water from cup Marilyn offers.) Yeah, that's the least somebody around this place could do for the money I pay to be doped up and trussed up like a pig.

Marilyn: How do you feel?

Cliff: How the hell do you think I feel, young lady?

Marilyn: I guess I'd not only feel like a pig all trussed up, but mad as a wildcat in a gunnysack as well. How did this happen?

Marilyn matches the vernacular of the client and interjects a bit of humor (Tomine, 1986). She is interested in knowing what happened, but her major concern is to continue posing open-ended questions to assess how much in touch with reality Cliff is and to let him know she is interested in and concerned about him. Marilyn manages to gain a working rapport with Cliff and explores last night's incident.

Marilyn: So what happened last night that got you in that fix?

Cliff: The Arab, he was after me. He was gonna strangle me, but nobody believes me. (Points to attendant.) That guy said it was one of the guys that work here at night. Said I busted his nose. Well, it was the Arabs.

Marilyn: Why do you think it was the Arabs?

Reality Orientation. Marilyn is taking a first step in attempting to relieve Cliff's confusion by using reality orientation (Taulbee & Folsom, 1966), which has been shown to have some success with people experiencing dementia (Spector et al., 2003; Onder et al., 2018). Reality orientation focuses on anchoring clients to who they are, where they are, and why they are there. When a client's response or behavior is out of touch with reality, the worker asks the client a why question, in an approach contrary to that of most therapeutic interventions (Taulbee, 1978, p. 207). Marilyn does this because she is trying to find out the reason for the behavior. Once she knows that, she can start to reorient Cliff.

Cliff: I spent a lot of time in the Arabian Pennisula, you know. Worked in construction. Put up a lot of refrigeration plants and steam systems. Hard to believe you'd need steam in that hothouse. Sometimes I wish I was back in Arabia. I loved that wild country and made some good friends there. By and large great people. But then there were the radical Jihadists we had to watch out for

that hated Americans. So that doesn't mean any damn terrorist can come in here in the middle of the night and kill me and steal my stuff for their crazy causes.

Marilyn: (genuinely interested) Hey! That sounds pretty exciting. I've hardly been out of the Midwest. I'll bet you've seen some pretty hair-raising things, and I can guess how you might think somebody was an Arab, being in a strange place like this.

Cliff rambles on for quite a while about his experiences there, with Marilyn listening and responding using person-centered techniques of attending, affirming, restating for clarification, reflecting feelings, and asking open-ended questions.

Pacing. Cliff's response about working in Arabia gives Marilyn a clue about the image Cliff saw attacking him in the night. However, she does not try to change his mind about what happened. She keeps pace with Cliff. She lets him tell his story without hurrying or trying to persuade him that he was mistaken last night. Patience is of maximum benefit in gaining the trust she will need if she is to accomplish anything with him (Taulbee, 1978, p. 210).

Reminiscence Therapy. Marilyn's approach in urging Cliff to talk about his past is contradictory to most standard operating procedures and generally accepted counseling techniques. Most therapeutic systems try very hard to keep clients in the present time and view trips to the past as counterproductive to changing real-time problems. However, allowing older clients to ruminate about past experiences can be therapeutically effective and, although inconsistent in outcome studies, have some lasting effects on quality of life, cognition, communication and mood (Brooker & Duce, 2000; Buchanan et al., 2002; Cully et al., 2001; Ebersole, 1978a, p. 145; Hsieh & Wang, 2003; Hyer et al., 2002; Woods et al., 2018).

Reminiscence therapy (Butler, 1963; Osborn, 1991; Society of Clinical Psychology, 2012) is a nonthreatening experience designed for older adults with mild to moderate depression. The therapy aims to reduce depression, improve self-worth, increase life satisfaction, reduces unwanted behaviors such as stress, anxiety, and agitation, improve self-esteem, encourage participation, and provide opportunities to connect with others (Bridges, 2023). It further helps older adults cope with crises, losses, and life transitions by allowing older clients to reflect on their lives and restore credibility to them (Miller, 1986). Webster's (1993) Reminiscence Functions Scale (RFS) includes eight reasons why people reminisce: boredom reduction, bitterness revival, prepare for death, conversation, identity, intimacy maintenance, problem solving, and teach/inform. Reminiscence therapy has become one of the standard treatments for the depressed older adult and has been successfully used worldwide in both individual and group formats (Ando, 2005; Cappeliez & Watt, 2005; Haber, 2006; Jo & Song, 2015; McKee et al., 2005; Melendez et al., 2013; Spar & La Rue, 2006; Van Puyenbroeck & Maes, 2006; Wang, 2005) and has been adapted to the computer with touch screen technology with the Computer CIRCA-BC Interactive Reminiscence Conversation Aid (CIRCA) program (Purves et al., 2015).

Memory dysfunction and personality disorganization are central to Cliff's current crisis and confusion. Reminiscence helps in personality reorganization and increases self-confidence because it draws on aspects of long-term memory that have been imprinted and can be recalled easily (Singer et al., 1991). Reminiscence can be therapeutic and healing for the client; it is a simple, enjoyable sharing of anecdotes that allows the worker to form a close affiliation with the client (Ebersole, 1978a, p. 145).

Individuals may use reminiscing to reconcile and put to rest bitter memories, reconstruct and enjoy pleasant memories, reduce boredom, and prepare for death (Cully et al., 2001). Further, if reminiscence is used in groups, interpersonal bonds can be increased as clients relate to historical benchmarks, personal achievements, objects, locations, and people. Older clients regain a sense of empowerment as the "experts" on the times they have lived in. Self-esteem is enhanced through recall of past achievements in the face of declining physical capacities (McMahon & Rhudick, 1964, pp. 292–298). "Unfinished business" from the past may be identified and handled (O'Leary & Nieuwstraten, 2001). It also offers the opportunity for physical contact and validation for what older adults have done with their lives (Baker, 1985) and helps them cope with grief and depression through social interaction and renewed social skills (Hsieh & Wang, 2003; Singer et al, 1991).

Cliff: Yeah . . . (**Voice trails off.**) . . . I used to be hot stuff . . . but I'm not so hot now. Hell, half the time I don't even know who, what, or where I am.

Marilyn: (**Touches client's arm lightly with her hand.**) It sounds like that's pretty scary, having run things most of your life, and now things are out of control.

Cliff: I hate to admit it, but that's right. Now I got to have help getting to the john! How'd you like that? It embarrasses the hell out of me. They treat me like a 2-year-old.

Marilyn: So being embarrassed and not being treated like a man are the worst parts of being here. I wonder what we might do to change that?

Anchoring. Marilyn uses a reflective statement of feeling to integrate Cliff's past with his present. By bringing up past incidents and hooking them to the present, she attempts to reinforce and help Cliff reassert his competence. Marilyn also uses touch to anchor him psychologically to someone in the institution (Wolanin & Phillips, 1981, pp. 105–106). Prior to the assault, a kind but sterile atmosphere had existed for Cliff at Hursthaven.

Like most human beings, Cliff has not responded well to living in an emotional vacuum. Since the attack, the atmosphere between Cliff and the staff has become adversarial in nature. Marilyn needs to change Cliff's view of the staff as being against him and the staff's view that Cliff is to be avoided. Staff members who have hands-on contact with Cliff on a regular basis need to be given training in the approaches Marilyn is using. Staffing and case review are particularly important for coordinating the different staff members who will deal with Cliff in a 24-hour period. All staff members who come in contact with him during the course of the day will introduce themselves, call Cliff by name, state the date, give a short preview of the next few hours' activities, and also explain any procedures, medical or otherwise, that they are carrying out. By consistently orienting the client, the staff takes a first step in treating confusion (Taulbee, 1978, p. 209).

Marilyn also picks up on Cliff's fear of losing control. Being wildly out of control is completely out of character for clients like Cliff, who are frightened at the prospect of losing their minds. Even more fears are generated when older clients sense someone is afraid of them or avoiding them because of fear of violence (Lion & Pasternak, 1973). Marilyn engages in a number of activities in this dialogue. The most important is that she has made a small but significant change in the interactional system that currently exists between Cliff and the staff by representing herself as an empathic, caring spokesperson for the institution and as an advocate for him (Fisch et al., 1983). Second, she reflects Cliff's anger, fear, and loss of control. She acknowledges and validates his experiences, but she is not just mouthing platitudes. She knows that the more he lacks current orientation, the more the staff will tend to avoid him. The more he is avoided, the less contact he has with people, and the more out of touch and disoriented he is likely to become (Petrie, 1984, pp. 114–115). The cycle can become deeper and deeper if uninterrupted and may cause even more disorientation and aggressive acts in the future (Miller, 1986).

Distinguishing Between Illusions and Hallucinations

Marilyn understands that what agitated Cliff was probably not a hallucination, as the staff thinks, but more than likely an illusion. While piecing together the tale of the night before, she determines that one of the nurses who works at the nursing home and made rounds about the time Cliff became agitated is an Indonesian Muslim who wears a hijab. That may have made Cliff perceive her as an Arab person in the dim light. Thus, what Cliff saw was probably an illusion based in fact, not fiction.

By proposing an explanation of the event, Marilyn allows Cliff to understand that he was not delusional but was misperceiving reality. The two problems are very different, and the difference is of great significance in calming Cliff. Although this conclusion may sound very pat, such happenings are all too common among mildly confused and disoriented clients. Very definite, concrete stimuli often create illusions that disrupt peace of mind for older clients, leaving them to doubt their own perceptions. It is extremely important for the worker to relate such a hypothesis to mildly confused clients such as Cliff who are very much concerned about keeping in touch with reality (Wolanin & Phillips, 1981, p. 107).

Marilyn: (Relates her hypothesis to Cliff.) So I believe that you weren't really crazy last night, but actually saw Naomi making rounds. If you think about it, it makes sense. If you'd like, I'll bring her around to meet you. She usually works in the other wing but sometimes subs down here in the east wing.

Cliff: I don't know. I guess so. I still really believe there was an Arab bandit with a big knife in here trying to get my stuff.

Marilyn: From all you've told me about your experiences there, I can understand that. But I also know that when you're zonked out in a strange place with the medical equipment around and strangers passing to and fro, suddenly waking up and seeing things differently is not uncommon and doesn't mean you're nuts. I'll bet if you think about it, it has happened before. I know it has happened to me. There's a big difference between misunderstanding what you see and seeing something that isn't there.

Sundown Syndrome. Because the event happened in the early evening, the sundown syndrome must be considered. Events that accompany the end of the day in an institution are strange and unsettling to residents who have been used to a regimen of activities based on their own time and the security of their own home. Unmet toilet needs, absence of a snack, staff members' attitudes, different noises, decreased light, effects of sedatives, and the presence of fewer personnel all add up to fear and strangeness without the support of another human being. These conditions can lead the client to act out (Blair & New, 1991; Stilling, 1992; Wolanin & Phillips, 1981, p. 107). Given the need to further assure Cliff about the reality of the situation, Marilyn relates the problems that occur with the approach of evening in the institution and makes some suggestions about how things might be changed to make this time less threatening.

Marilyn: If you could make things here a bit more like home, what would they be?

Cliff: Well, I used to put my earphones on and listen to some country music and have a beer before I hit the hay. I don't know much else, just watch TV and stuff. No special furniture or anything. I lived in apartments and hotels most of my life.

Marilyn: I notice that there's not much of you in this room. It looks like a hospital room instead of Cliff's room. You mentioned a lot of items you collected over the years and picture albums of all your travels. Where are they?

Cliff: Oh, my kids just stored them away.

Marilyn: I'd like to see if we couldn't get some of those in here, dress the place up a bit, so when people come by they'd know it was Cliff Hastings, world-class engineer, who lives here.

Security Blankets. Marilyn proposes that articles familiar to Cliff be brought into the room for two reasons. First, creating a familiar environment may go a long way toward creating a basis in reality for the fact that this is now Cliff's home and reconciling him to this stage in his life (Petrie, 1984, p. 116). Second, suddenly awakening in a medical environment with a variety of strange machines and tubes running in and out of one's body is extremely threatening because such foreign objects alter a person's body images and surroundings in a very negative way (Wolanin & Phillips, 1981, p. 106). Having familiar objects immediately visible can help Cliff reorient without becoming agitated in the process. Marilyn will check with administrative staff to see whether Cliff's sound equipment can be brought into his room. She will also check with medical staff to see whether a bottle of beer in the evening will confound his medication. If possible, providing these amenities will further approximate Cliff's routine at home and provide orientation and security (Miller, 1986).

Remotivation. Remotivation therapy is designed to stimulate and reinvigorate individuals who have lost interest in their environment, past interests and activities, other people, and the future. Individuals are remotivated by encouraging them to describe themselves as concretely as possible (Dennis, 2013). Remotivation attempts to persuade clients that they are accepted by others as individuals who have unique and important traits that make them distinguishable from everyone else (Garber, 1965). The idea is shift from a "sick" identity to a "healthy" one by tapping into skills and abilities that have become latent though disuse. The therapist's attempt to reawaken those functions in life that have been substantiating by detailing past experiences doing those activities and realizing that only part of them is "sick" and those latent skills, abilities, and creative components of their personalities are still alive and healthy (Dennis, 2013; Dyer &Stotts, 2005). Finally, Marilyn will use remotivation therapy in an attempt to involve Cliff in the activities of the institution by actualizing some of his latent abilities, albeit in very different ways. It is important to involve clients interpersonally and have them become physically and psychologically active in their environment. For people like Cliff who have been highly active throughout their lives, it is critical to fill idle time in meaningful ways to keep such clients from drifting into depression (Donahue, 1965). This does not mean forcing and cajoling clients into doing something contrary to what interests them. Playing bingo might be fun for many people, but forcing a person to engage in such an activity is inappropriate (Miller, 1986). After listening to Cliff, Marilyn makes a proposal designed to reinvolve him with other humans.

Marilyn: I'd like you to consider a proposition I have to make. Hursthaven has an alliance with St. Peter's Orphanage. None of those kids have anybody to care about them. I have a couple of boys in mind that I think you could do some good with. You've got some great stories that they'd love and probably some wisdom that could be helpful to those guys. They just mainly need a man to talk to, and I wonder if you'd be willing to help out. They also love baseball and I know you mentioned you were a Cardinal fan—followed them all over the world. I know you'd like to go see the Triple A Redbirds down at Autozone park but can't physically. Those boys would love to go to a game, and they could help you get into the park and sit in the accessible section. Our limo service would take you down there and you've been complaining about being cooped up in solitary here. So, I wonder if maybe a deal can't be worked out.

Cliff: (Hrrrummpf). I dunno. They're probably Cubs or worse yet Braves fans.

Marilyn: Well then you'd have some ground to convince them otherwise. Maybe I was wrong and you're not up to the challenge of mentoring two boys like the Cliff Hastings I've been talking to (**Big sigh**).

Cliff: (Hrrrrmpf) Don't try that reverse psychology stuff on me. I'm not promising anything, but have the juvenile delinquents come over after lunch and we'll see.

Marilyn's agenda is twofold. She is truthful in what she tells Cliff. She also knows that the two boys will have a positive effect on Cliff in turn. Older people seem particularly interested in sharing their experiences with the young (Ebersole, 1978b, p. 241). Cliff's candidness, wisdom, and trove of stories are likely to have a positive effect on two boys who are as anchorless as Cliff. She focuses on Cliff from a strength perspective (Newhill, 2003, pp. 160–161) and uses baseball as a common ground they can start to relate to one another. Rather than focusing on what is wrong with the client, she capitalizes on the client's strong points, positive qualities, and overall potential for controlling his behavior.

Outcome research on remotivation is slim. Dennis (2013) reports a number of older studies that have positive outcomes such as more daily participation, increased friendships, renewed interest in activities, and more social awareness. Calhoun's (1975) small study supports those types of positive outcomes. However, numerous other studies found no differences over a number of different treatment comparisons.

Disorientation with Dementia: The Case of Grace

The standard regimen for working with older clients has been to attempt to "reality orient" them to the present. Such an approach becomes problematic for moderately confused clients and profoundly so for those who have almost entirely retreated from the reality of the present. Attempts to orient moderately to severely confused very old clients to person, place, and time are generally futile. For many of these clients, nothing could be less worthwhile, for there is clearly not much in the present worth remembering (Miller, 1986). Seizing on this notion, Naomi Feil developed validation therapy (Feil, 1982; Feil & deKlek, 2012). Validation therapy is a successful way of communicating with older adults with dementia. Because validation therapy provides techniques for approaching and communicating with a person with dementia, it is particularly helpful in preventing a reaction in the person with dementia that might escalate into an unwanted behavior. It is also useful for calming and diffusing challenging behaviors. Her thesis is to acknowledge the feelings of the person, no matter how irrational they may seem to be. By dignifying feelings, the worker validates the person. To deny the client's feelings is to deny past existence and thus deny the personhood of the individual.

Feil also believes that validating early memories enables clients to resolve the past and justify their role in old age. Positive outcomes from using the approach are restoring self-worth, reducing stress, justifying life, resolving unfinished conflicts, restoring dignity, and establishing a better and more secure feeling for the client (Feil, 1982, p. 1). The worker continuously validates the client as a first step in restoring self-worth and affirming that at least one person is interested and concerned enough to listen to what the client's life has been. Anyone overhearing a dialogue between a worker and a client who has severely regressed into an irrational past would probably wonder at first whether the worker had also become senile. For validation therapy to be effective, the worker must have some creative insight into the verbal meanderings and repetitive behaviors of the client (Miller, 1986).

Listen to Marilyn as she attempts to convince an 83-year-old woman to go to dinner. Grace is standing in the hallway refusing to be moved. She is engaging in a rocking motion with her arms and softly humming to herself. The staff's efforts to get her to go to dinner have been fruitless, and she is becoming increasingly agitated and threatening as a number of staff members are attempting to orient her and get her to comply with their requests. Marilyn enters this scene and asks the rest of the staff to leave them.

Grace: There, there! Don't you cry.

Marilyn: I see you're really concerned about your baby.

Grace: Yes, I've been up all night with Ellen. She must have colic, but I can't seem to get her to settle down. I need to get Dr. Heinz, he's our family doctor, but I don't have anyone to drive me to town.

Marilyn: It really worries you that Ellen doesn't seem to be getting any better. You must be awfully tired and hungry!

Grace: Even though Ellen's cranky, she's no bother. She's really a beautiful baby. It's just that her father isn't around much. He works on the railroad, and I could use some help sometimes.

Marilyn: You must love her very much. Maybe we could go down to dinner together, and you could tell me some more about her.

Grace: She's got to have quiet to get to sleep. It's too noisy there.

Marilyn: It's important to you that she gets to sleep. Perhaps we could have dinner served in your room. It'd be quiet there.

Grace: Well, I suppose, if you'd really like to.

In this short exchange, the worker demonstrates two critical components of validation therapy. The client may well have lost the ability to comprehend and reason with any degree of complexity. By keeping communication short and simple, the worker avoids losing the client in a variety of ideas that may rapidly become overwhelming. The worker also responds directly and continuously to Grace's feelings, validating to her that the symbolic act she is engaging in is highly important (Miller, 1986). Genuine, deep, empathic responding is critical to doing validation (Feil, 1999). Although the purpose of validation therapy is not to manipulate or lie to the client (Feil, 2004), the worker's approach is far better than forcibly taking the client to the dining room, where she will probably be so distraught over having to neglect her baby that she will not eat anyway.

Whether Grace has ever had a baby named Ellen or whether she is trying to resolve some shortcoming she has long felt in regard to mothering is of little concern in the present moment. What is of concern is that the worker treats the situation as if it were real and of importance to the client and acknowledges the client's scattered thoughts and feelings in a congruent, empathic manner. Feil and Altman (2004) are adamant that validation therapy is not a "therapeutic lie," as some propose that is meant only to humor those with dementia. Feil proposes that all people with dementia deserve to be treated with dignity and respect, and to listen to them is an excellent way of doing so. She believes it is absolutely normal for older adults to return to the past to attempt to resolve unfinished business before they die. When these emotions are expressed and someone listens with empathy and unconditional positive regard, frustrations are eased.

Validation therapy is not intended to return the client to reality. However, for the human services worker who has to intervene in a crisis situation with the severely disoriented older adult, it does have the potential to calm them down, avoid situations conducive to acting out, and provide an effective therapeutic technique in an area where few have been found (Miller, 1986). Jankowski and Frey (2012) have pointed out that with the "silver tsunami" of older adults coming and the dementia that comes along with them, this neglected therapy needs to be taught to the students who'll be needed to work with this population. Even though Grace appears to be a senile, frail, and confused woman who is easily handled by the crisis worker, don't be misled. The very person Grace represents, if thwarted and frustrated, is the reason that assaults against geriatric workers who discount the "old, senile, fragile fool" Graces are so high.

Hard evidence of the effectiveness of validation therapy is slim. Neal and Wright in 2003 reviewed outcomes studies for validation therapy and found only three randomized control studies which had varying results. Their conclusion back then was that there was insufficient hard evidence to tell if it worked. A later study by Erdmann and Schnepp (2016) of a somewhat hybrid German form did have positive outcomes. It is regrettable that any of the foregoing "best" practices of working with older clients are not strongly evidence based and have lasting effects over time. Yet, for temporary relief and diffusing oppositional behavior, they do seem to have utility, and that may be sufficient for crisis intervention.

Follow-up With Staff Victims

LO12 Follow-up after an assault is critical to both the person assaulted and the rest of the staff (Kleespies & Ponce, 2009; Kleespies, 2014; Wilson 2017). Workers may brush off assaults as just part of the business and then find out that the psychological ramifications are far greater than they imagined (Fauteux, 2010; Wilson, 2017). Workers who are victims of violent attacks by clients may have emotional responses that include hypervigilance, startle responses, intrusive thoughts, unresolved anger, and poorer overall mental health and anger control (Lenehan & Turner, 1984, p. 256; Wilson, 2017; Wykes & Whittington, 1998). They may look much like the victims of posttraumatic stress disorder (PTSD) (California Occupational Safety and Health Administration, 1998, p. 17; Murray & Snyder, 1991; Wilson 2017).

Practitioners who experience assault feel disempowered, anxious, depressed, and fearful (Littlechild, 2002). Their job performance suffers as they lose confidence to carry out their work roles, question their competence, feel less caring and attachment to clients, and experience self-blame, guilt, and anger about the incident. Further, they fear for their future safety, fear reporting future episodes that would label them as incompetent, and fear that their fellow employees and managers will not see them as dependable (Flannery et al., 2001; Littlechild, 1995; Wilson, 2017).

Bard and Sangrey (1986) found that workers go through three stages of trauma resolution after a physical assault. First, they experience a **disorganization of self** that includes feelings of shock. They may dissociate from the experience as unreal, as if it didn't happen or they viewed it as a video of themselves. They may blame themselves and start having peritraumatic stress disorder symptoms involving sleep disturbances and emotional outbursts. The second stage, **period of struggle**, is characterized by anxiety attacks, intrusive thoughts, hypervigilance, and psychosomatic symptoms, which are characteristic of acute stress disorder. The third stage is **readjustment of self**. If the worker is able to move forward, then the incident is integrated into the self and the worker becomes the wiser for it, comes to see that clients can be dangerous, and takes more precautions. However, if the worker does not integrate the incident, then the possibility of PTSD looms large.

Lanza (1984) and Wilson (2017) both found that nurses who had experienced such attacks had negative emotional, cognitive, and behavioral reactions up to a year afterward. It is extremely important to work through the aftermath of violent behavior suffered by staff for two reasons: first, so the victim does not become debilitated personally and professionally by the incident, and second, so other members of the staff will perceive that the institution takes such events very seriously and is concerned for their safety as well.

After an attack, staff members initially may ascribe blame to the victim to ease their own fear and trepidation about the possibility that it could happen to them (Wilson, 2017). Under no circumstances should this be allowed to happen. Sympathy and support for the victim are vital. Pity, condescension, or subtle implications about provoking the assault should be avoided. There should be acknowledgment that the attack occurred, and crisis intervention should be started immediately. Normalizing the situation is imperative and lets the worker know that others would feel the same way that they are feeling (Wilson, 2017).

Psychoeducation should be conducted with workers to familiarize them with some of the psychological reactions they may have and what strategies they may use to alleviate them (Weinger, 2001, pp. 66–67). Institutional support groups for victims of violence should be available (Busch et al., 2021; Hallett, 2014; Stortch, 1991), and staff should be prepared to give immediate help with problem solving and decision making, such as determining injuries, providing medical transportation, staying with the victim, providing moral support, and helping with medical, legal, and police reports (Lenehan & Turner, 1984, pp. 255–256). Unit staff should also receive counseling to prevent "a blame the victim attitude" from developing (California Occupational Safety and Health Administration, 1998, p. 17; Occupational Safety and Health Administration, 2015; Wilson, 2017) We enthusiastically agree with the foregoing. As soon as the victim is able, a psychological autopsy should be performed on the incident. A **psychological autopsy** (Schneidman, 1987) examines in detail the situation that led to the violent episode. (Refer to Chapter 8, "Crisis of Lethality,"

for a complete description of this procedure.) Having the worker and others write a report as soon as they are able may be helpful in allowing workers an emotional outlet and to further understand and conceptualize the incident. *This report should not be seen as a scapegoating or blame-fixing exercise and should be clearly stated as such by the administrative head.*

All staff members who are involved with the client should attend the autopsy. It dissects what the staff and the client did behaviorally before, during, and after the incident. *It is also not about fixing blame but finding out what caused the incident to happen so it won't happen again.* Further attention should be given to the environmental setting to determine whether it played a role in instigating the aggressive behavior. Hopefully, the autopsy will provide clues as to the *whys, hows*, and *whats* of the incident so it does not recur. The victim's opinions should be solicited and should be used as expert testimony. Staff should gather to discuss what happened, work through feelings about the event, and generate options for preventing a recurrence. Reviewing the traumatic experience also enables the victim to deal with feelings of loss of security and control (Lenehan & Turner, 1984, pp. 254–259).

In the past, mental health institutions have left worker recovery from a client assault pretty much to chance, with a "Suck it up, it's part of the job!" approach (Wilson, 2017). That is now patently unacceptable. Some form of debriefing should be conducted simultaneously with the psychological autopsy in helping the assaulted human services worker attain precrisis equilibrium and homeostasis (California Occupational Safety and Health Administration, 1998, p. 17; Fauteux, 2010; Kinney, 1995; Mitchell & Everly, 1995; Spitzer & Burke, 1993; Spitzer & Neely, 1992; Vandenberg, 1992). Debriefing seeks to alleviate the acute stress crisis that workers experience when they are traumatized by an event such as a physical assault on them. Generally, debriefing should occur as soon after the event as is reasonably possible, but it should also take into consideration the worker's ability to go through it. Dr. James Cavanaugh of the Isaac Ray Center for Rush–Presbyterian–St. Luke's, a pioneer in development of debriefing critical incidents such as assaults on staff, cites compelling evidence that immediate posttrauma care can be very effective in helping both individuals and organizations become stabilized after a crisis (Kinney, 1995, p. 188). Kleespies (2014, pp. 163–170) advocates using the Assaulted Staff Action Program (Flannery et al., 1991), which is a system wide, peer-help program to assist staff in coping with the traumatic wake of an assault.

The Assaulted Staff Action Program (ASAP, Flannery et al., 1991) is a combination of the foregoing. When an assault occurs, a staff member responds to offer support, is available to deliver basic psychological first aid, and determines whether additional medical or psychological care is necessary. The responding ASAP member queries the victim as to whether they feel able to manage their feelings and whether they are able to return to work. The ASAP member keeps up with how the member is doing for up to 2 weeks post-incident. ASAP also offers support groups for assaulted staff members.

The question is, "do these follow-ups work?" Busch et al. (2021) conducted an extensive review of two peer support program at the University Missouri's Health Care Center for YOU team and Johns Hopkins Hospital's RISE (Resistance in Stressful Events) team. Their 10-year study found both teams to be very busy with YOU having 834 peer interventions and RISE having 367 peer interventions, but no follow-up appears to have occurred in regard to alleviating or reduction of any type of emotional dysregulation. The professionals in the field believe that some kind of peer after-action support is critical to not catching PTSD or burning out. The problem is that, much like the Busch and associates' study, we don't know if there is hard evidence measuring outcomes, and therein lies the conundrum for most crisis intervention work since it's a little difficult to get control groups and also do follow-ups.

Finally, Gately and Stabb's (2005) survey of doctoral-level counseling and clinical psychology students should serve as a bellwether. Students overwhelmingly reported that their training to deal with violent clients was inadequate and their confidence in working with these clients was low. Weisman (2011) reports that while mental health staff generally get minimal training in violence prevention, mainly in restraint and seclusion protocols, they don't get training where it matters, and that is protecting themselves in offices, home visits, and street encounters. Since it is beginning practitioners who are most likely to be assaulted, it is your authors' considered opinion that to not train human services students to understand and deal with violent clients in the contextual situations within which they operate, given the degree and knowledge we have today of violence in the human service workplace and techniques to handle it, is unethical and immoral.

To learn more about what an overview of assessing for violent behavior looks like, the Association of Threat Assessment Professionals (ATAP) has published *Risk Assessment Guideline Elements for Violence: Considerations for Assessing the Risk of Future Violent Behavior* (2006) available at www.atapworldwide.org, although you'll have to join to get to know all about the business.

Summary

Violence in the human services setting has increased exponentially in the past three decades. Increased abuse of drugs, the closing down of large state mental hospitals, child and adult abuse reporting laws, gang violence, increased adjudication of felons to mental health facilities, and increases in the older adult population have been major contributors to this phenomenon. The problem pervades all parts of human services, and institutions as well as workers may be culpable in allowing violence against staff to proliferate. Both service providers and their staff have largely looked the other way, and when violence against staff has occurred, either it has been seen as going with the territory or the victim has been blamed for being incompetent, stupid, and careless.

Human services statistics indicate a strong likelihood that sometime during workers' careers, they will become a victim of violence. Given that high probability, it would seem mandatory that both workers in the field and students in human services be educated about the potential for violence and taught defusing and de-escalating skills to be used with potentially violent clients. Techniques ranging from option therapy to validation therapy are intended not only to help the client stabilize but also to prevent the human services worker from being the object of an assault.

Finally, the worker who has been assaulted should be given immediate support from the administration and fellow workers. Incident debriefing and psychological autopsies should be mandatory after every assault on staff.

Human Services Workers in Crisis Burnout, Vicarious Traumatization, and Compassion Fatigue

15

Learning Objectives

After studying this chapter, you should be able to:

1. Explain the dynamics of burnout.
2. Describe the myths surrounding burnout.
3. Explain the host of behavioral, physical, attitudinal, and interpersonal symptoms that indicate burnout.
4. Identify the levels of burnout when encountered.
5. Explain the stages of burnout and be able to ascertain them when present.
6. Explain the interrelationships and differences among burnout, compassion fatigue, secondary traumatic stress, and vicarious traumatization and be able to ascertain them when present.
7. Explain that compassion satisfaction is a buffer against compassion fatigue and burnout.
8. Identify the role of organizations in perpetuating and preventing burnout.
9. Identify individual intervention strategies for burnout and how to use them.
10. Explain both individual and organizational assessment devices for uncovering burnout.
11. Explain culture's influence on burnout.
12. Describe impairment as an ethical issue.

Burnout

Respond to the following questions with a yes or no.

1. Have you left parties early because the occasions offered you no opportunity to counsel?
2. Do you continue to counsel even though it interferes with your earning a living?
3. Do you sometimes have the "shakes" in the morning and find that this unpleasantness is relieved by counseling a little?
4. Do you repeat everything you hear? I mean, do you repeat or paraphrase everything you hear?

These questions are part of Adam's (1989) humorous, satirical test of counseling addiction. Yet the questions may not be too far off target when viewed in terms of another severe problem that strikes many professionals in the human services business—burnout—and its handmaidens, compassion fatigue and vicarious traumatization. Burnout has become part of lay nomenclature, but what exactly is burnout? Maslach and Leiter (2016) define burnout as "a psychological syndrome emerging as a prolonged response to chronic interpersonal stressors on the job," which is characterized by three dimensions: "overwhelming exhaustion, feelings of cynicism and detachment from the job, and a sense of ineffectiveness and lack of accomplishment" (p. 103).

So, you are a brand-new human services worker with a diploma fresh off the presses and ready to go out and cure the world. You are full of vim and vigor and one salty dog! What's with burnout? That's just old dudes that are washed up! Apparently, since the last edition of this book went to press in 2015, the 6,518 peer-reviewed articles and 1,769 dissertations or theses on burnout retrieved from the American Psychological Association (2023) search engine, *PsychInfo*, suggest otherwise. They also seem to be talking about you, young grasshopper! Research indicates that if you are a younger woman, you are more likely to wind up in the burned out category of human services workers (Baum et al., 2014; de Figueiredo et al., 2014; Star, 2015; Volpe et al., 2014). There are likely multiple explanations for this gender difference.

In their analysis of burnout in female physicians, Templeton et al. (2019) discuss a number of factors that may contribute to the disproportionate burnout experienced by women. These may include difficulty managing the competing demands of work and family life, being on the receiving end of gender-based bias and discrimination, experiencing sexual harassment, and having limited control over their schedule and workload (Templeton et al., 2019). It is also interesting to note that researchers have found female medical providers experience greater expectations regarding their willingness or ability to address psychosocial matters with their patients (Linzer & Harwood, 2018; Templeton et al., 2019), which may contribute to higher levels of emotional burnout. It would be reasonable to assume that similar expectations may hold for female human service workers outside of the medical profession. To be sure, there are varied reasons, including socioculturally nuanced reasons, for the patterns in burnout. However, burnout affects people worldwide and from all walks of life.

If you were a teacher from Ireland (Foley & Murphy, 2015), a Chinese civil servant (Hao et al., 2015), or a Peruvian correctional officer (Clemente et al., 2015), there was some concern you might be burning out. Indeed, it appears that about every country and occupation in the world is concerned about burnout, and it is far from humorous. Burnout is not just some pop psychology term designed to elicit sympathetic responses from one's coworkers or spouse. It is a complex individual-societal phenomenon that not only affects human service workers but also their clients (Bottini et al., 2020; Kitchingman et al., 2018; Montgomery et al., 2022; Salyers et al., 2015; Salyers, Fukui et al., 2015; White et al., 2015).

Put in economic terms, billions of dollars are lost each year because of workers in all fields who can no longer function adequately in their jobs. Signs and symptoms of burnout include turnover, absenteeism, lowered productivity, and psychological problems (Golembiewski et al., 1986; Leiter & Maslach, 2005, pp. 3–9). Yet, if burnout has been discussed in all occupations, why should it be endemic to the helping professions?

Helping Professionals: Prime Candidates

The bulk of writing and research that has been done on burnout has come from the helping professions because of its poorer job satisfaction and higher turnover and burnout compared to other occupations (Coates & Howe, 2014). The very nature of the job is to be intensely involved with people, and generally, these are people who are, by the nature of the crisis event, not presently at the highest levels of self-actualized behavior (Maslach, 1982b, pp. 32–33). Burnout tends to afflict people who enter their professions highly motivated and idealistic and who expect their work to give their lives a sense of meaning (Pines & Aronson, 1988, p. 11). When many of the clients do not make progress or their symptoms worsen instead of improve despite all of the workers' skill and effort, burnout becomes a high probability for these idealistic people.

Compounding the harsh realities of historically low success rates, the human services business is becoming more difficult. Human services workers are likely to intervene with people with severe psychological and physical traumatic problems connected with trauma, addiction, and persistent and chronic mental illness. Because of managed care and restricted budgets, human services workers are expected to handle larger caseloads in shorter time periods. Particularly when dealing with high caseloads and challenging work relationships, mental health providers tend to have a high risk of burnout (O'Connor et al., 2018). These traumatic problems call for tremendous amounts of the worker's energy, resilience, and hardiness. Day in and day out, the severity of these problems and their duration can wear down any worker's optimism and motivation (Luther et al., 2017; O'Connor et al., 2018; Yang & Hayes, 2020).

The foregoing problems are at the core of the helping professions, making them not just some of the most challenging but also some of the most stress-prone occupations. Thus, human services professionals must be able to tolerate a variety of complex problems that are generally couched in ambiguity, deal with conflict from both clients and institutions, and somehow meet a myriad of demands from the ecological framework in which they operate (Paine, 1982, p. 21).

For the crisis worker, this is true many times over. Crisis center work settings are notorious for long and erratic hours, low pay, poorly functioning clients, immediate deadlines, a lack of control over when clients will arrive or phone, few second chances, repeat callers with chronic problems, hostile and emotionally "raw" clients, and interagency red tape. These are only a few of the stressors that assault crisis workers, making them prime candidates for burnout (Distler, 1990). Because the crisis worker is exposed to a high incidence of trauma for extended periods of time, phrases such as "compassion fatigue" (Figley, 1995, 2002), "traumatic" or "event" countertransference (Dahlenberg, 2000, pp. 12–13), "vicarious traumatization" (McCann & Pearlman, 1990; Pearlman & Mac Ian, 1995; Pearlman & Saakvitne, 1995a, 1995b; Saakvitne, 2002), and "traumatoid states" (Thomas & Wilson, 2004) have found their way into the literature to describe what happens when workers are faced over and over with unspeakable trauma. Through their professional exposure to high levels of client distress, crisis workers are prone to develop vicarious traumatization, stress, burnout, and other psychological disorders that not only cause them personal distress but may also limit their professional efficacy (Kitchingman et al., 2018).

However, a question arises about whether burnout and its derivatives are really dynamically identifiable. There is a lively ongoing discussion in the professional literature at this writing as to whether burnout is an identifiable, stand-alone malady or is really just clinical depression dressed up in work clothes and struggling through a workday (Bianchi & Laurent, 2015; Bianchi et al., 2015; Chiu et al., 2015). Indeed, Hafkenscheid (2005) proposes that the term *vicarious traumatization* is no more than a fancy term made up to excuse therapeutic failure. Paine (1982, p. 11) and Maslach (1982b, p. 29) report that critics propose that burnout is "part of the job," so if a human services professional "can't stand the heat, then they ought to get out of the kitchen" because there "always has been stress on this job and always will be." Such cursory dismissal of burnout does not consider the major personal, social, and organizational costs that accrue when job stress turns into crisis (Paine, 1982, p. 11). Indeed, job stress is connected to absenteeism and turnover (Daniel, 2019); loss of job productivity (Daniel, 2019; Iskamto, 2021); medical issues (Daniel, 2019); mental health concerns, such as depression and anxiety (Harvey et al., 2017; Poursadeghiyan et al., 2016); and interpersonal issues (Ayadi et al., 2016; Repetti & Wang, 2017). Moreover, there is ominous research that indicates people who experience high levels of job stress may be more prone to cardiovascular disease and type 2 diabetes (Kivimäki & Kawachi, 2015). Burnout is not just part of the territory; it has major ramifications for both individuals and institutions (Maslach, 1982b, p. 39).

Dynamics of Burnout

LO1 A historical definition of burnout places it as a child of the 1970s. The term comes from the psychiatric concept of patients who were "burned out" physically, emotionally, spiritually, interpersonally, and behaviorally to the point of exhaustion (Paine, 1982, p. 16). It was first coined as a workplace term by Herbert Freudenberger to describe young, idealistic volunteers who were working with him in alternative health care settings and who started to look and act worse than many of their clients (Freudenberger, 1974, 1975). Yet, defining burnout adequately is not simple.

A very broad definition depicts **burnout** as an internal psychological experience involving feelings, attitudes, motives, and expectations (Maslach, 1982b, p. 29). Being burned out means that the person's total psychic energy has been consumed in trying to fuel the fires of existence. This energy crisis occurs because the psychic demand exceeds the supply (Tubesing & Tubesing, 1982, p. 156). It is experienced as a state of physical, mental, and emotional exhaustion caused by long-term involvement in emotionally demanding situations. It is accompanied by an array of symptoms including physical depletion, feelings of helplessness and hopelessness, disillusionment, negative self-concept, and negative attitudes toward work, people, and life itself. It represents a breaking point beyond which the ability to cope with the environment is severely hampered (Pines & Aronson, 1988, pp. 9–10) and the inability to work effectively (Stamm, 2010).

Put in plain language, burnout is lost energy. You are exhausted. A good night's sleep is out of the question, and sleep aids (including alcohol) don't help much. Brief getaways don't help, and you come back feeling worse than ever. Work is demanding beyond reason and exceeds the best of your available resources. Burnout is also lost enthusiasm. You despise your bosses and the clients, and you aren't overly thrilled with your coworkers either. All the zeal, energy, creativity, expertise, and enthusiasm you brought to the job are long gone. Going the extra mile has turned into wondering whether you can go the few yards to the break room. Finally, your confidence has gone out the window. The less effective you become, the more your self-worth shrinks. Why keep going (Leiter & Maslach, 2005, p. 2)? Indeed, you are now a candidate for the long shopping list of maladies you'll soon learn that come out of this thing called *burnout!*

Burnout is not generally perceived as a crisis event because its onset is slow and insidious. There is no one point or incident that is readily identifiable as the instigating trauma. Rather, it is a slow and steady erosion of the spirit and energy as a result of the daily struggles and chronic stress typical of everyday life and work (Pines & Aronson, 1988, p. 11). Because of the difficulty in identifying burnout, it becomes much easier to chalk it up as a character deficit. A crisis appears only when people are so defeated and exhausted by the environment that they take extraordinary means to find relief, such as quitting a job or occupational field, developing a serious psychosomatic disease, using substances to problematic degrees, or attempting suicide. What is even more problematic is that recovery from burnout is not always linear and tends toward chaos and crisis as the individual tries to come to grips with core issues of vocation, personality, and relationships (Kesler, 1990). As a result, the precipitating crisis of job burnout may move toward a more global, existential crisis wherein the person is in a state of crisis over living or finding purpose in life.

Occupationally, burnout occurs when past and present problems from the job continuously pile up. Leiter and Maslach (2005, pp. 14–19) propose that there are six major sources of burnout: **workload**, when the work is too complex, too much, too urgent, or just too awful; **control** issues from being micromanaged or having ineffective leaders or teams; lack of **reward** in the form of compensation, recognition, or pleasure; an **absence of community** that provides social support; lack of **fairness**, with little justice and lots of arbitrary and secretive decision making and favoritism; and **discordant values** that indicate you and the organization are severely at odds regarding your belief in the validity and worth of the organization and the organization's belief about your validity and worth. The foregoing problems may vary in degree and kind, but the result is a continuous and

grinding interface between the person and the work environment (Pines & Aronson, 1988, pp. 43–44; Riggar, 1985, p. xvi). From the worker's standpoint, no short- or long-term relief is forthcoming.

The body's nonspecific response to any demand is stress. Humans need some stress for optimal performance. However, there comes a point of maximal return for each person. That point is a function of genetic, biological, behavioral, and acquired physiological factors. Beyond that point, stress is harmful (Selye, 1974). Environmental events may either "cause" the activation of the stress response or, more often, set the stage for it through cognitive-affective processing (Everly, 1989, p. 45). The stress response itself involves enervation of neurological, neuroendocrine, and endocrine systems either singularly or in tandem with one another, which, in turn, activates various physiological mechanisms directed toward numerous target organs (p. 47). In Selye's (1956) **general adaptation syndrome (GAS)**, overstimulation and excessive wear of target organs lead to stress-related dysfunction and disease. If the stressor is persistent and there is a chronic drain on adaptive energy, eventual exhaustion of the target organ will occur. The end result physiologically may be as dramatic as a heart attack or as common as a headache. Indeed, where GAS is found, burnout may not be far behind, and it has been linked to a wide range of both physical and mental illnesses (Maslach et al., 2001).

Stress occurs when there is a substantial imbalance (perceived or real) between environmental demands and the individual's response capability. Burnout occurs when the stress becomes unmediated and the person has no support systems or other buffers to ease the unrelenting pressure (Farber, 1983, p. 14). The outcome is a person affected in every dimension of life by unlimited combinations of symptoms. Such a description very adequately meets the crisis conditions of being in a state of disequilibrium and paralysis.

Cornerstones of Burnout

Let us now examine two human services professionals who are experientially and professionally different but by almost any definition are in the process of burning out.

Mr. Templeton. Mr. Templeton has worked as a school counselor at Central Middle School for 2 years. In that time, he has instituted some sweeping changes in a counseling program that was, before he came, notorious for running attendance checks and not much more. Mr. Templeton's counseling approach changed all that. Formerly, the last place that students would have gone for help with personal problems would have been the counseling office. By getting out and explaining what his job was all about to students, faculty, parent groups, civic organizations, and anybody else who would listen, and indeed making good on his promises, Mr. Templeton has turned the counseling office into a hub of mental health that sparks envy among other school counselors in the district. His principal would now fight a circular saw to keep Mr. Templeton around.

What the principal does not know is that Mr. Templeton has fantasies about sending the entire eighth grade to an Outward Bound camp in the Sahara Desert. He has not had a new idea about how to improve the counseling program in six months and is wondering if maybe that stockbroker's job that he so capriciously turned down last year was not such a bad idea after all. As he considers all this, he wistfully looks at his wristwatch, then at the eighth grader sitting across from him, and wonders whether she is in his office because of grade problems or a problem at home. She has been talking for 30 minutes, and he cannot remember two sentences she has said.

Josaline Josaline is a social worker at an outpatient clinic for a community mental health center. She has worked there for five years. Her patient load resembles something on the order of bus traffic to Mecca. She has just received a memorandum from the director further increasing her caseload by 20 percent, along with a rather curt directive to move on some of those old cases and get them off the clinic rolls. Josaline is sitting in her friendly local tavern quietly getting drunk and wondering how she is going to put 20 people out on the street with no support. She is also mulling over what response she will make to her spouse, who just this morning asked for a separation. Among the complaints her spouse voiced, Josaline's job was prominent: the lousy pay for somebody with a master's degree, the long hours with no compensatory time, the emergencies in the middle of the night, and particularly forgetting she is the mother of their two children and a marital partner. Josaline stares across the bar and orders another drink. While waiting for her order, she swallows an antacid tablet for the dull, burning pain slowly working its way outward from the pit of her stomach.

What do these two human services professionals have in common? They are alike in that they are empathic, sensitive, humane, idealistic, and people-oriented and have been highly committed and dedicated to their profession. However, like others prone to burnout, they also tend to display higher levels of neuroticism and lower levels of agreeableness, conscientiousness, extraversion, and openness (Angelini, 2023). Moreover, they tend to experience countertransference with their clients, which, when combined with other job stress factors, can lead to burnout in mental health professionals (Yang & Hayes, 2020). For both of them, one or more of the following foundation blocks of burnout have been laid (Borritz et al., 2005; Farber, 1983, p. 6; Hamois, 2015; Lee & Ashforth, 1993; Olivares-Faundez et al., 2014; Powell, 1994; Rupert, 2015).

1. **Role ambiguity.** They lack clarity concerning rights, responsibilities, methods, goals, status, and accountability to themselves or their institutions.
2. **Role conflict.** Demands placed on them are incompatible, inappropriate, and inconsistent with their values and ethics.
3. **Role overload.** The quantity and quality of demands placed on them have become too great.
4. **Inconsequentiality.** They have a feeling that no matter how hard they work, the outcome means little in terms of recognition, accomplishment, appreciation, or success.
5. **Isolation.** They have little social support either in the institution or outside of it.
6. **Autonomy.** Their ability to make decisions as to what they will do and how they will deal with their clients is co-opted by the bureaucracy of their place of employment.

These foundation stones are not thrown down haphazardly. They are built up slowly but surely over time through a variety of dynamics.

Research on Burnout Dynamics

The following points have been supported to varying degrees by research on burnout (Angelini, 2023; Ayadi et al., 2016; Baird & Jenkins, 2003; Bianchi et al., 2014; Borritz et al., 2005; Carroll & White, 1982; Cook et al., 2021; Daniel, 2019; Decker et al., 2002; Golembiewski & Munzenrider, 1993; Golembiewski et al., 1986; Golembiewski et al., 1992; Grossi et al., 2005; Grouse, 1984; Hasan Bozgeyikli, 2012; Hoeksma et al., 1993; Koeske et al., 1993; Lee & Ashforth, 1993; Lee et al., 2010; Linley et al., 2005;

Lizano, 2015; Lyndall & Bicknell, 2001; Oerlamans & Bakker, 2014; Maslach, 1982a; Maslach & Leiter, 2016; Mather et al., 2014; Melamed et al., 2006; O'Connor et al., 2018; Piedmont, 1993; Pines & Aronson, 1988; Powell, 1994; Rupert et al., 2015; Salston & Figley, 2003; Talavera-Velasco et al., 2018; Toker et al., 2005).

1. All stressors are cumulative and can help lead to burnout.
2. Burnout is psychobiological.
3. Environmental factors other than work can be contributors.
4. A lack of effective interpersonal relationships contributes to burnout.
5. Signs of burnout will occur, but recognition of them depends on the observer's astuteness.
6. Symptoms sometimes appear quickly, but most usually occur over time.
7. Burnout is process oriented rather than event oriented.
8. Burnout varies in severity from mild energy loss to death.
9. Burnout also varies in duration.
10. Burnout and resulting crisis can occur more than once.
11. Awareness varies from complete denial to full consciousness of the problem.
12. Burnout is infectious in that it puts additional stress on other workers.
13. Burnout is greatest for beginning and long-term workers and least for mid-duration workers.
14. Those who are single experience the most burnout, while those with families experience the least. However, stressors that enter family life can exacerbate burnout.
15. Restorative and preventive measures have to be individually tailored because of the idiosyncratic nature of burnout.
16. Burnout has progressive phases that can be identified by the varying degrees of depersonalization, personal accomplishment (or lack thereof), and emotional exhaustion the individual exhibits.
17. Burnout is not a disease, and the medical model is not an appropriate analytical model.
18. Burnout should not be confused with malingering.
19. Progressive deterioration in physical and mental health occurs as burnout increases.
20. Job autonomy, sense of coherence, and social support buffers are critical to preventing, containing, and reducing burnout.

21. Making time for leisure and using it wisely are as important as any job variable.
22. Burnout can lead to personal and professional growth as well as to despair and trauma.
23. More education, training specific to trauma work, supervision, and institutional support are all related to lower burnout rates.
24. A personal history of trauma is a contributing factor.

This long, exhaustive list of causes for and buffers against burnout should give you a pretty good idea that burnout is the real deal. When we talk about safety, it isn't just physical safety; we're talking about your psychological safety as well. That's the reason this chapter is in this book.

Myths That Engender Burnout

LO2   Candidates for burnout believe a number of myths about themselves and how they must operate in their environment (Everly, 1989; Friedman & Rosenman, 1974; Kesler, 1990; Maslach, 1982a; Pines & Aronson, 1988; Rodesch, 1994). They tend to distort the reality of the situation in typical type A personality patterns (Friedman & Rosenman, 1974), generating a variety of irrational statements about themselves and their work. These statements are modeled after Albert Ellis's (James & Gilliland, 2003, pp. 232–265; Patterson, 1980, pp. 68–70) unhealthy *musturbation* (Ellis's term for continually harping and brooding on what MUST be done) thoughts people say to themselves about their predicaments.

1. "My job is my life." This means long hours, no leisure time, and difficulty delegating authority. Anxiety, defensiveness, anger, and frustration are the result when things do not go perfectly.
2. "I must be totally competent, knowledgeable, and able to help everyone." Unrealistic expectations of performance, a need to prove oneself, a lack of confidence, and overriding guilt occur when one is not perfect.
3. "To accomplish my job and maintain my own sense of self-worth, I must be liked and approved of by everyone with whom I work." Such workers cannot assert themselves, set limits, say no, disagree with others, or give negative feedback. Therefore, they get manipulated by others in the work setting—including by clients. Self-doubt, passive hostility, insecurity, and subsequent depression are the reward.

4. "Other people are hardheaded and difficult to deal with, do not understand the real value of my work, and should be more supportive." Stereotyping and generalizing about specific problems and people occur, and lack of creativity, wasted energy, and decreased motivation result. The person has a defeatist attitude and a passive acceptance of the status quo.

5. "Any negative feedback indicates there is something wrong with what I do." The person cannot evaluate their work realistically and make constructive changes. There is a great deal of anger with critics, which may manifest itself in either passive or aggressive hostility, depending on the person toward whom the anger is directed. Frustration and immobilization are the outcomes.

6. "Because of past blunders and failures by others, things will not work the way they must." Old programs are not carried to fruition, nor are new ones created. Stagnation and decay in the work setting are the result.

7. "Things have to work out the way I want." The person's behavior is, thus, characterized by working extra hours and checking up on staff members' work, an inability to compromise or delegate, over-attention to detail, repetition of tasks, impatience with others, and an authoritarian style.

8. "I must be omniscient and infallible." The person can never be wrong. The very act of doing therapy with humans in all their infinite ways of behaving means fallibility for the worker, particularly when the client is in crisis.

These dynamics lead to a wide array of symptoms.

Symptoms of Burnout

LO3 Burnout is a multidimensional phenomenon consisting of behavioral, physical, interpersonal, and attitudinal components. Table 16.1 is a ready reference. While the list is lengthy, it is undoubtedly not all-encompassing. Certainly, not all human services workers in crisis manifest all the symptoms listed. Yet for the watchful observer, many will become noticeable, particularly if one looks back in time and notes any pronounced changes in the worker.

Levels of Burnout

LO4 Burnout can be categorized as occurring at one of three levels: *trait*, *state*, and *activity* (Forney et al., 1982). At a trait level, it is all-pervasive,

encompassing every facet of the worker's life. The worker is completely nonfunctional in regard to person, place, and time. The trait level of burnout is extremely serious and calls for immediate intervention in the worker's life. At a state level, burnout may be periodic or situational. An example is what occurs after media coverage of the suicide death of a prominent celebrity, such as Robin Williams. Following Williams' death in 2014, calls to suicide hotlines (Pirkis et al., 2020) and suicide rates in the United States increased significantly (Fink et al., 2018). After a period of a few weeks, the increase in calls wanes (Pirkis et al., 2020), and the crisis line worker returns to some semblance of normalcy. However, over the long term, such state events contribute mightily to anticipatory anxiety, which, if not managed, can precipitate total burnout.

Finally, burnout may be activity-based. Any activity that is performed over and over at an intense level, as in encounter group counseling with individuals who have substance misuse disorders or serving as a chaplain to the grief-stricken in a trauma center, will invariably wear the armor off the most emotionally bulletproof crisis worker. A simple way of decreasing the chances of burnout when the stressor is activity-based is to change the routine. However, such change is not always easily accomplished or even recognized as needed.

Stages of Burnout

LO5 Another way of characterizing the road to burnout is by stages. Edelwich and Brodsky (1982, pp. 135–136) delineated four stages through which the typical candidate for burnout goes.

Stage 1: Enthusiasm. The worker enters the job with high hopes and unrealistic expectations. If such idealism is not tempered by orientation and training programs that define what the worker can reasonably expect to accomplish, such a rose-colored view of human services work will inevitably lead to the stage of stagnation.

Stage 2: Stagnation. Stagnation occurs when the worker starts to feel that personal, financial, and career needs are not being met. Awareness may come from seeing people perceived as less able moving up the career ladder faster, pressures from home to meet increased financial obligations, and lack of personal intrinsic reinforcement for doing the job well. Astute

Table 16.1   Symptoms of Burnout

Behavioral	Physical	Interpersonal	Attitudinal
Reduced quantity or efficiency of work	Chronic fatigue and exhaustion	Withdrawal from family	Depression
Use and misuse of alcohol and illicit drugs	Lower resistance	Compulsion to do all and be all at home	Feeling of emptiness, meaninglessness
Increase in absenteeism	Maladies occurring at organ weak points: ulcers, migraines, gastrointestinal upset, facial tics, etc.	No mature interactions—keeping hidden agendas	Ranging from omnipotence to incompetence
Increase in risk taking	Colds and viral infections	Keeping others subservient	Cynicism
Increase in medication	Poor coordination	Feeling drawn to people who are less secure	Paranoia
Clock watching	Insomnia, nightmares, and excessive sleeping	Reduction of significant others to status of clients	Compulsiveness and obsessiveness
Complaining	Muscular tension	Breaking up of long-lasting relationships	Callousness
Changing or quitting the job	Addiction to alcohol and/or drugs	Becoming therapeutically minded and overreacting to comments of friends	Guilt
Inability to cope with minor problems	Increased use of tobacco and caffeine	No separation of professional and social life	Boredom
Lack of creativity	Over-or undereating	Allowing clients to abuse the privacy of home by calls or visits at any time	Helplessness and/or hopelessness. Suicidal/homicidal ideation
Loss of enjoyment	Hyperactivity	No opportunity for or enjoyment in just being oneself	Terrifying and paralyzing feelings and thoughts
Loss of control	Sudden weight gain or loss	Loneliness, trust issues	Stereotyping
Tardiness	Flare-ups in preexisting medical conditions: high blood pressure, ulcers, asthma, diabetes, etc.	Loss of authenticity	Depersonalizing
Dread of work	Injury from high-risk behavior	Loss of ability to relate to friends, family, or clients	Pessimism
Vacillation between extremes of overinvolvement and detachment	Missed menstrual cycles	Avoidance of close interpersonal contact	Air of righteousness
Mechanistic responding	Increased premenstrual tension	Switch from open and accepting to closed and denying	Grandiosity
Accident proneness	Injury from accident	Inability to cope with minor interpersonal problems	Sick humor, particularly aimed at clients
Change in or cessation of religious affiliation	Rapid heartbeat	Isolation from or overbonding with staff	Distrust of management, supervisors, and peers
Errors in setting therapeutic boundaries	Breathing difficulties	Increased expression of anger and mistrust	Hypercritical attitude toward institution and coworkers
Errors in judgment and strategy in and outside therapy	Anxiety and panic attacks	Increased vigilance and safety issues for self and loved ones	

(continued)

Table 16.1 (continued)

Behavioral	Physical	Interpersonal	Attitudinal
posttraumatic stress disorder (PTSD)-like symptoms of intrusive thoughts, numbing of affect, sleep disturbance, nightmares, and hypervigilance	Dizziness	Overprotection as a parent	Entrapment in job and relations
Regression	Impaired immune system	Decreased interest in intimacy or sex	Free-floating feelings of inadequacy, inferiority, incompetence, and survivor guilt
Impatient and irritable			Self-criticism and perfectionism
Withdrawn			Rapid mood swings
Losing things			Loss of faith, meaning, purpose
Suicide attempts			Change in religious beliefs
Homicide attempts			Sense of grounding, inner balance lost. Increased sense of vulnerability to the world at large

management policy will head off stagnation by providing a variety of incentives that clearly say to the worker, "You're doing a good job here, and we appreciate it." If intrinsic and extrinsic reinforcement does not occur, the worker will move into the next stage, frustration.

Stage 3: Frustration. Frustration clearly indicates that the worker is in trouble. The worker starts questioning the effectiveness, value, and impact of their efforts in the face of ever-mounting obstacles. Because the effects of burnout are highly contagious in the organizational setting, one person's frustration is likely to have a domino effect on others. One appropriate way of meeting frustration is to confront the problem head-on by arranging workshops or support groups to increase awareness of the burnout syndrome and generate problem-solving as a group to bring about changes within both the institution and the individual. Catching the problem at this stage may well lead back to a more tempered stage of enthusiasm. If the problem is not resolved, then the final stage, apathy, is reached.

Stage 4: Apathy. Apathy is burnout. It is a chronic indifference to the situation and defies most efforts at intervention. Apathy is truly a crisis stage: The person is in a state of disequilibrium and immobility. Further compounding this stage are denial and little objective understanding of what is occurring. At this point, psychotherapy is almost mandatory for reversal to take place.

Worker–Client Relationships

LO6 **Compassion Fatigue, Secondary Traumatic Stress, and Vicarious Traumatization.** As crisis intervention has spread to more and more areas of psychological trauma, interest in what happens to the workers who deal with these clients has led to the development of concepts that describe "empathy-based stress" reactions, such as **compassion fatigue (CF)**, **secondary traumatic stress (STS)**, and **vicarious traumatization (VT)** (Rauvola et al., 2019, p. 297). These concepts and their distinctions (or lack thereof) have been the subject of debate for decades. As such, we introduce each of these terms, but readers should know that expanding research in this area may change the way these concepts are defined and measured.

CF is defined as "disengagement of caregivers from their patients, which culminates in a reduction or inability to feel empathy and compassion toward patients and an inability to provide the patient care that is deemed appropriate," which results in diminished "meaningful and purposeful" interactions between clients and their providers (Coetzee & Laschinger, 2018, p. 4). The exact relationship of

CF to burnout is unknown, but there appears to be some inherent interaction between CF and burnout (Henson, 2020). CF is generally thought to emerge from providers demonstrating high levels of empathy. However, Coetzee and Laschinger (2018) posit that a combination of "lack of resources, an absence of positive feedback, and the response of personal distress" collide to form the basis of CF (p. 14).

STS is described as "natural and consequential behaviors and emotions resulting from knowing about a traumatizing event experienced by a significant other (or client) and the stress resulting from helping or wanting to help a traumatized or suffering person" (Figley, 1995, p. 7). STS is a consequence for health care professionals who are frequently exposed to the stress and trauma of others in the course of treating them (Hensel et al., 2015), and individuals who develop STS may begin to display some symptoms of post-traumatic stress.

STS is akin to what McCann and Pearlman (1990) call vicarious traumatization (VT), or the "transformation in the inner experience of the therapist that comes about as a result of empathic engagement with client's trauma material" (Pearlman & Saakvitne, 1995, p. 31). VT is based on a constructivist model in which the individual's experience and worldview are changed as a direct result of secondary exposure to trauma through crisis work (Pearlman & Mac Ian, 1995). For this reason, STS may be conceptualized differently from VT, wherein VT may be a more severe type of stress reaction. However, both STS and VT involve the transformation that occurs when an individual begins to change in a manner that mimics a client's trauma-related symptoms. CF, STS, and VT are the very real, concrete negative effects that occur when human services workers have prolonged exposure to traumatized clients who are in crisis.

Research indicates that mental health services workers experience more negative effects from crisis work than other types of health services workers (Arvay & Uhlemann, 1996; Blanchard & Jones, 1997; Charney & Pearlman, 1998; Johnson & Hunter, 1997; Smart et al., 2014). The potential for STS is even more pronounced in crisis workers who work with long-term disasters. Wee and Myers (2002) conducted a study of mental health workers who did long-term follow-up in the Murrah Federal Building bombing in Oklahoma City, and they found that about half of the respondents reported being more stressed than doing normal mental health work and being at high risk for both compassion fatigue and burnout. Why is this so?

It is so because trauma work and crisis intervention are so potentially addictive and, at the same time, so potentially destructive! Much like the "rush" that law enforcement officers, paramedics, and other emergency workers experience from being in the middle of traumatic events, crisis workers feel the "adrenaline high" of successful crisis intervention, and this can become highly addictive. As an example, psychologists who worked the aftermath of 9/11 in New York City reported more positive than negative feelings regarding their work (Eidelson et al., 2003). Yet the constant exposure to the "highs" that come with dealing with traumatic events also means that the crisis worker is exposed to a constant barrage of some of the most graphic and horrible physical and psychological ramifications that nature or humankind can visit on people. Along with CF, STS, and VT, while doing crisis work, the potential for countertransference is constantly present and high.

Countertransference. Whenever therapy becomes intense, as in crisis work, the potential for countertransference rises dramatically. Countertransference is the attributing to the client, by the crisis worker, of traits and behaviors of past and present significant others or events in the crisis worker's own life. Countertransference responses may be positive or negative, spoken or unspoken, conscious or unconscious. They may include physical, psychological, social, gender, racial, moral, spiritual, cultural, or ecological factors that have impacted the worker through past experiences and are manifested in the "here and now" of therapy by the client. At times, the client's emotional aspects may agitate feelings, thoughts, and behaviors that are deeply buried within the worker's own personality.

When confronted with their own shortcomings, fears, faults, prejudices, and stereotypes as mirrored by the client, human services workers may begin behaving in inappropriate ways. Workers may act in ways designed to meet their own needs and not the client's. The result is that clients are made to fit neatly into the workers' preconceived patterns for the way things "ought to be," and not necessarily in reference to the client but how they "ought to be" for the crisis worker (Freudenberger, 1977).

The general axiom of psychoanalytic therapy is that countertransference needs to be guarded against. The therapist's refusal to recognize countertransference and deal with it can, at the least, inhibit the therapist's effectiveness and, at the most, be destructive to the relationship (Dahlenberg, 2000, pp. 1–6). If the phenomenon of countertransference is not recognized and dealt with in positive ways, the human services worker ends up feeling guilty about having negative feelings toward the client and is not even sure why those feelings are occurring. Such feelings are antithetical to what the worker has been taught and believes, and those feelings can significantly compound the occupational stresses that lead to burnout.

However, Pearlman and Saakvitne (1995a, pp. 22–24) propose that if crisis workers are to deal successfully with and understand the pain of their clients in deeply empathic ways, then countertransference is inevitable and necessary. Particularly emotion-laden issues such as physical and sexual abuse of children, terminal illnesses, and chronic suicidal ideation are prime examples of content that may be exceedingly stressful to the worker because of strong feelings and experiences the worker may have about the problem (Dahlenberg, 2000; Fox & Cooper, 1998; Pearlman & Saakvitne, 1995a). The pluses and minuses of countertransference as it applies to trauma appear to balance precariously on a very thin psychological high wire. Main's (2008) study of sexual offender treatment providers found that, although the providers manifested disruptions in cognitions, emotions, and behaviors consistent with those that characterize compassion fatigue and vicarious traumatization, they also possessed many of the components for **compassion satisfaction** (the positive feelings and intrinsic rewards one feels from helping others who have experienced a traumatic event) (Stamm, 2010) and reported that their child sexual abuse histories were an advantage in the treatment of sex offenders. As such, one of the critical components to handling countertransference effectively would appear to be close and competent supervision.

Worker Vulnerability. Maslach (1982b, pp. 36–37) states that the only human services workers who burn out are the ones who are on fire. For such workers, Saakvitne and Pearlman (1996, pp. 26, 49) and Figley (1995) believe that the deep empathy needed to deal with the heart-wrenching situations that often accompany crises makes workers vulnerable to intense and overwhelming feelings and profound disruptions in their beliefs, which assaults the very core of their hope and idealism. Over time, such assaults lead to compassion fatigue (Figley, 1995),

wherein the crisis workers' energy is literally wrung out by the incidence and amplitude of dealing with the horrific problems that trauma clients face.

Between a very real dedicatory ethic and at times an insatiable need to assist everyone with any type of problem, idealistic human service workers see their job as a calling. In an imperfect world, such an idealistic outlook can lead to over involvement and identification with the client—often to the worker's detriment (Koeske & Kelly, 1995). As the human services worker becomes more deeply enmeshed in the helping relationship, the worker's strong need to be accepted and liked makes it harder and harder to say no to the client's demands. At this point, the worker has started to take on responsibility for the client.

The worker's over involvement with the client may be manifested in a variety of ways. Some of the many indicators that the worker is not paying attention to their own needs, or frankly to the client's, include extending the session beyond its usual time limit; taking and responding to phone calls at home at all hours of the night; experiencing hurt feelings over client failures; attempting dramatic cures on impossible cases; becoming panic stricken when well-laid plans go awry; refusing to withdraw from the case when it is clearly beyond the worker's purview; becoming angry, sarcastic, or bored with clients; changing the subject and avoiding the topic, providing pat answers; discounting the client's problems and minimizing distress; not believing clients; fearing what the client will say; silencing client trauma talk; wishing or suggesting the client would "just get over it"; feeling numb or avoidant; not being able to pay attention; being constantly reminded of one's own personal trauma events; hoping the client won't show up; becoming frustrated over lack of progress; and losing one's sense of humor over the human dilemma (Baranowsky, 2002; Dahlenberg, 2000; Van Auken, 1979). The foregoing are all indicators that unresolved countertransference and vicarious trauma/compassion fatigue issues are flourishing.

Under these circumstances, the worker comes to see the helping relationship as a chore, and the client may regress and act out as a way of announcing the client's awareness of the worker's apathetic attitude. As this psychological vortex continues to swirl and the worker becomes even more overwrought and discouraged, the client is likely to terminate the therapeutic relationship (Dahlenberg, 2000; Watkins, 1983). Such negative reinforcement does little to mollify the worker's already bruised ego and may lead to a further downward spiral into burnout. Whether exposure to these occupational hazards has negative or positive outcomes depends a great deal on how both the individual worker and the human services institution deal with them in proactive ways (Dahlenberg, 2000; Deiter & Pearlman, 1998; Figley, 1995; Pearlman & Saakvitne, 1995a; Saakvitne & Pearlman, 1996).

LO7 **Positive Responses to Counseling Practice.** There are three commonly recognized potential positive responses to counseling practice, particularly trauma and crisis work. These include compassion satisfaction, vicarious resilience, and posttraumatic growth. This is not to say that counselors do not grow in other ways through their work. But, in looking at the particularly demanding subfields of crisis intervention and trauma therapy, these three concepts seem most applicable to describe the positive effects on mental health professionals.

Stamm (2005) describes compassion satisfaction (CS) as simply the pleasure you derive from being able to do your work well. The reason CS as a construct has gained notoriety is that it appears to be an extremely effective buffer against burnout. Factors that tend to increase CS may include having specialized training in trauma therapy (Sprang et al., 2007), cultivating high levels of professional self-efficacy (Hasan Bozgeyikli, 2012), engaging in mindfulness practices (Martin-Cuellar et al., 2018), and strengths-based supervision (Treworgy, 2010). Moreover, human services workers who are satisfied with the effect they have on clients consistently show low levels of vicarious traumatization and burnout (Conrad & Keller-Guenther, 2006; Eastwood, 2007; Killian, 2008; LaFauci Schutt, 2009; Lawson & Myers, 2011; Ling et al., 2014; Ringenbach, 2009; Sullivan, 2004).

Vicarious resilience (VR) is defined as the "transformations in the therapists' inner experience resulting from empathetic engagement with the client's trauma material" (Hernández et al., 2007, p. 237). Hernández et al. (2007) posit that various elements are necessary for the development of vicarious resilience:

> witnessing and reflecting on human beings' immense capacity to heal; reassessing the significance of the therapists' own problems; incorporating spirituality as a valuable dimension in treatment; developing hope and commitment; articulating personal and professional positions regarding political violence; articulating frameworks for healing; developing

tolerance to frustration; developing time, setting, and intervention boundaries that fit therapeutic interventions in context; using community interventions; and developing the use of self in therapy (p. 238).

According to Hernández et al. (2007), therapists who experience VR tend to demonstrate an "increased understanding of the therapeutic process, increased understanding of the resiliency process, and an increased sense of efficacy in their work" (p. 238). These changes manifest within the context of observing clients' growth and therapists recognizing their own contributions to the clients' growth (Hernández et al., 2007). Further, it is likely that VR and VT may occr as mechanisms of the same processes (Hernández et al., 2007). In short, VR seems to reflect ways in which trauma professionals grow through their work with trauma survivors, drawing upon the resilience they observe and help foster in others. Killian et al. (2017) have developed the *Vicarious Resiliency Scale*. It has seven factors: "changes in life goals and perspective, client-inspired hope, increased recognition of clients' spirituality as a therapeutic resource, increased capacity for resourcefulness, increased self-awareness and self-care practices, increased consciousness about power and privilege relative to clients' social location, and increased capacity for remaining present while listening to trauma narratives" (p. 23). If you are curious about your resilience, consider taking the *Vicarious Resilience Scale* (Killian et al., 2017) to discover if and how your work with trauma survivors has had a positive effect.

Posttraumatic growth (PTG) is defined as the "experience of positive change that occurs as a result of the struggle with highly challenging life crises" (Tedeschi & Calhoun, 2004, p. 1). Individuals who experience PTG tend to manifest changes in multiple dimensions of functioning, which Tedeschi and Calhoun (2004) describe as an "increased appreciation for life in general, more meaningful interpersonal relationships, an increased sense of personal strength, changed priorities, and a richer existential and spiritual life" (p. 1). Individuals who experience PTG grow through the trauma and experience pronounced positive changes as a product of their recovery from the trauma. This is not intended to diminish the negative impact of the trauma or to invalidate the survivor's struggle (Tedeschi & Calhoun, 2004). Indeed, individuals who experience PTG endure immense pain en route to their healing. However, PTG represents the potential for growth that some individuals experience following the experience of trauma.

Although the traditional concept of PTG applies exclusively to clients and survivors of intense trauma, vicarious PTG has garnered attention as a transformational growth experienced by some trauma professionals. Vicarious PTG can be conceptualized as the growth in mental health professionals who work with trauma clients and, as a product of their work, experience pronounced positive effects, such as "living life more fully, treating others differently, or becoming more emotionally expressive in their relationships due to indirect trauma exposure" (Deaton et al., 2021, p. 26). Tsirimokou et al. (2022) further describe the growth experienced by mental health professionals who experience vicarious PTG. They discuss positive changes mental health professionals experience across various domains, such as self-perception (e.g., confidence, pride in their work, resilience, empowerment), worldview (e.g., appreciation, adaptability, perspective), and relationships (e.g., intimacy, respect, assertiveness, anger management) (Tsirimokou et al., 2022). Vicarious PTG is not just a manifestation of quality therapeutic work therapeutic work. Tsirimokou et al. (2022) discuss the importance of other factors to support the development of vicarious PTG, such as having and using a solid support system, engaging in quality trauma-informed supervision, utilizing effective self-care strategies, developing empathetic rapport with clients, engaging in meaning-making processes, and finding opportunities to express humor. Indeed, it is evident that mental health professionals can experience tremendous growth through their trauma work with clients as they concurrently support growth in their clients. The dynamic exchange certainly has risks, such as empathy-based stress reactions, but the therapeutic process can also yield significant benefits for both providers and clients. With these things in mind, it seems reasonable to assume that organizations would make intentional efforts to provide trauma training, require ongoing clinical supervision, support wellness and mindfulness practices, and provide feedback to affirm the important work mental health providers are doing to support clients. Regrettably, that is often not the case and, as we will discuss next, organizational issues can account for a large portion of job stress and empathy-based stress reactions.

The Culpability of Organizations

LO8 Much of the responsibility for burnout and empathy-based stress reactions rests with the employing agency and its inability to either recognize or do anything about organizational problems that lead to burnout (de Figueiredo et al., 2014; Everly, 1989, pp. 295–297; Kulkami et al., 2013; Pines & Aronson, 1988, pp. 97–111; Shinn & Mørch, 1983, p. 238). Savicki and Cooley (1987) compared degree of burnout with work environment and found that the workers who scored highest on burnout indexes felt they had little impact on procedural and policy issues, lacked autonomy within the guidelines of the job structure, were unclear about agency objectives, had a high intensity of work assignments over extended periods of time, were highly restricted in how they could deal with clients, and felt generally unappreciated by their coworkers or supervisors. Leiter and Maslach (1999) identified six core organizational contributors to burnout. They agreed that a heavy workload, lack of control, and minimal reward or appreciation are characteristic of organizations that tend to produce burnout in their employees (Leiter & Maslach, 1999). However, to that list, they added a lack of social and communal support, a perceived lack of fairness in how employees are treated, and a mismatch between the organization's values and its employees' values (Leiter & Maslach, 1999). Over the years, some combination of these factors has been demonstrated time and again to lead to burnout in employees.

Additionally, and of major relevance to mental health professionals and crisis workers, handling client verbal and physical aggression is a major mediating factor in burnout (Gascon et al., 2013; Hensel et al., 2012; Ho et al., 2013; Yung, 2013). And, when workers feel management is not responding to their safety concerns, the threat level increases (Evans & Petter, 2012), along with the potential for burnout. Naturally, there are also factors related to the employees, such as their personality (Angelini, 2023), ability to handle stress (Mullen et al., 2017), and history of mental health issues (Yang & Hayes, 2020) that affect the development of burnout.

In contrast, those agencies that allow input into the mission of the organization, are flexible in providing instrumental and emotional support to workers, generate support groups, provide consultation, have job clarity, promote managers with social leadership styles, retain realistic expectations for the progress of their clients, and furnish supervision to help workers solve problems associated with the high stress of their jobs report workers with lower indexes of burnout (Everly, 1989, pp. 299–309; Kahn, 2005; Melchior et al., 1997; Pines & Aronson, 1988, pp. 107–111; Savicki & Cooley, 1987). One of the critical support mechanisms for crisis workers is easy access to consultation, support, and supervision (de Figueiredo et al., 2014; Handran, 2014; Ling et al., 2014; Salloum et al., 2015). Crisis intervention should never be done in isolation, and the case example presented in this chapter is an excellent example of why that is so.

Self-Recognition of Burnout

Whatever the degree of burnout, human services workers and their organizations have a notorious blind spot. What they can detect in others and change by therapeutic intervention, they are generally unaware of in themselves. Skewed by perceptual bias and "stress-induced cognitive deficits," mental health professionals may have difficulty recognizing the signs of burnout in themselves (Ledingham et al., 2019, p. 125). Further, in the absence of recognizing the signs of burnout in themselves, mental health professionals may not implement the needed measures to address the burnout, thereby perpetuating the cycle and potentially leading to progressive impairment. When they are finally confronted with the fact that something is terribly wrong in their professional lives, their initial maladaptive response is likely to be "What's wrong with me?" rather than "What can I do to change the situation?" Their typical operating mode is not to change the situation but rather to see themselves as professionally inadequate; they may question their professional competency and career choice (Cook et al., 2021).

Before delving into assessments and intervention, your authors want to be very clear that they agree with Watkins (1983) that no one—and we would go a step further and state that *absolutely* no one—who practices in the human services professions is immune to burnout. Furthermore, it has been our experience that human services workers who, like some of you who are reading this passage, think "It'll never happen to me" are invariably the kinds of fellow professionals we end up treating; or, in the absence of treatment, become those who can no longer stand to ply the trade and quit; or, at the extreme, become reliant on substances or suicidal or homicidal. In these circumstances, the outcomes range from bad to worse: bad for the profession and worse for you, the professional.

Assessment

LO9   Three types of instruments are important in determining burnout and compassion fatigue.

Burnout. The first type has to do with determining the degree of burnout in the individual. The most widely used instrument is the Maslach Burnout Inventory–Human Services Survey (MBI-HSS; Maslach & Jackson, 1981a), which is a valid cross-occupational and cross-cultural (Bakker et al., 2002; Gorter et al., 1999) instrument that measures three symptom patterns associated with burnout. The Emotional Exhaustion scale assesses feelings of being emotionally worn out by work. The Personal Accomplishment scale measures feelings of competence and achievement with work. The Depersonalization scale measures unfeeling and impersonal responses toward clients. The scales can also be combined to produce a total frequency and intensity score for burnout. A variation of the scale for professional burnout in general (MBI-GS; Maslach et al., 1996) measures exhaustion, cynicism, and reduced personal efficacy, three components that parallel the original MBI-HSS. There is also a Maslach Burnout Inventory for educators (MBI-ES; Maslach et al., 1996), which uses the foregoing components to measure degree of burnout in educators.

Golembiewski et al. (1986) used the Maslach Burnout Inventory's three domains to develop a progressive phase model of burnout. In their model, depersonalization is seen as the least potent and initial burnout phase. It must occur prior to any substantial reduction in feelings of personal accomplishment, which they see as a secondary response and more potent level of burnout. Emotional exhaustion, the third and most potent indicator of burnout (Lee & Ashforth, 1996; Wright & Bonett, 1997), would follow heightening of the prior two stages.

Lee and associates (2007) have developed the Counselor Burnout Inventory. This instrument measures five burnout dimensions: exhaustion, incompetence, negative work environment, devaluing client, and deterioration of personal life. This instrument attempts to integrate both personal and organizational components of potential burnout factors and determine how much workplace factors contribute to overall burnout. They have attempted to determine what particular patterns of these scales best classify levels of burnout and pattern clusters (Lee et al., 2010). Their research, which sampled counselors who worked in a variety of settings, identified three sets of counselor profiles. A cluster they called "Well-Adjusted Counselors" (WACs) had low scores and flat profiles across all the scales. WACs also reported high job satisfaction, good self-esteem, and decent pay. Their MBI scores correlated with their CBI profiles, with low scores on Emotional Exhaustion and Depersonalization and high scores on Personal Accomplishment.

Lee and his associates (2010) found a second cluster they called "Disconnected Counselors" (DCs), who had medium-level scores on Exhaustion, Negative Work Environment, and Deterioration in Personal Life with high Incompetence and Devaluing Client scores. DCs' scores on the MBI paralleled their CBI scores, with a very high Depersonalization score, low Personal Accomplishment, and midrange Emotional Exhaustion scores. They reported low job satisfaction, poor self-esteem, and low pay.

A third cluster, which the researcher named "Persevering Counselors" (PCs), was characterized by high Exhaustion, Negative Work Environment, and Deterioration in Personal Life, but low scores on the Incompetence and Devaluing Client scales. Of the three groups, the PCs scored far higher on the MBI Emotional Exhaustion scale, in the midrange on Depersonalization, and high on sense of Personal Accomplishment. They reported the most counseling experience, highest positive self-esteem, and highest pay of the three groups, even though they reported the most dissatisfaction with their jobs. The PC cluster is interesting in that they are still performing well, but all the indicators are there for burnout. As such, it would appear that this instrument could identify not only workers who were functioning well as opposed to those who were burning or burned out but also those who were moving in that direction. Further research has substantiated good reliability and validity of the CBI among both professional counselors and school counselors (Bardhoshi et al., 2019).

Compassion Fatigue and Compassion Satisfaction. The Compassion Fatigue Self-Test (Figley, 1995) specifically targets different facets of secondary stress. From Wee and Myers's (2003) preliminary work with this test, it appears that satisfaction with doing crisis intervention work is indeed a counterbalance to compassion fatigue. What they found was that although approximately half the workers sampled had high compassion fatigue scores, almost 90 percent had high satisfaction scores and low burnout scores. The belief is that compassion satisfaction can act as a protective buffer against compassion fatigue and burnout (Collins & Long, 2003; Ray et al., 2013).

The Professional Quality of Life Scale (ProQOL; Stamm, 2002, 2005, 2010) measures compassion satisfaction, compassion fatigue, and burnout. It is a test for workers in the human services field but is particularly designed for first responders such as police, EMTs, firefighters, and ER personnel. The Compassion Satisfaction and Fatigue Test is of particular interest because it factors in the worker's satisfaction and therapeutic fatigue with clients. Certainly not all crisis workers manifest STS many workers are resilient, hardy, and continuously involved in crisis work over long terms with no ill effects. Stamm (2002) hypothesizes that it is because their satisfaction with doing the job counterweights and compensates for the heavy fatigue factors they experience. Therefore, this test gives scores for compassion satisfaction (CS), compassion fatigue (CF), and burnout (BO). Research indicates that, indeed, compassion satisfaction is an ameliorating factor in both compassion fatigue and burnout (Ray et al., 2013).

Work Environment. The third type of instrument measures the work setting. Typical of this type of assessment device is the Work Environment Scale (Moos, 1981), which measures 10 different dimensions of an organizational component named "social climate." These dimensions are job commitment, support from coworkers, management support, independence in decision making, efficient and planful approaches to tasks, performance pressure, role clarity, degree of control by management, variety and change in job, and physical comfort. Taken together, these various instruments provide a way of examining the degree of burnout in relation to environmental factors within the organization, yield a fairly comprehensive picture of how burned out the worker is, and indicate the degree of intervention necessary (Savicki & Cooley, 1987).

Intervention Strategies

LO10 Because burnout is related to and may be a first step in the development of empathy-based stress reactions, we focus on burnout intervention and prevention in this section. Intervention with CF, STS, and VT may have similarities, although traumatic responses, like those seen in STS and VT, may require the use of specific skills such as those addressed in Chapter 7, "Posttraumatic Stress Disorder." We believe the foregoing information is a good starting place to prevent and intervene with burnout, which might help to reduce the likelihood of developing more severe and longer-lasting empathy-based stress reactions.

While there is a great deal of literature on self-care and balancing other life experiences against work as a buffer against burnout (Ling et al., 2014; Oerlemans & Bakker, 2014), there have been few protocol and hard data studies to identify specific treatments that work with those who are experiencing empathy-based stress reactions and are burned out (Bercier & Maynard, 2015).

Practitioners on the road to burnout typically are perfectionistic workaholics (Falco et al., 2014) who push relentlessly toward emotional exhaustion, becoming more inefficient and unhappy as they do so. Note the "aholic" component because our experience is that burning up professionals are much the same as persons who experience substance misuse disorders in their vehement denial that things are going badly awry until a severe crisis of their own is created that it finally gets their attention. Thus, when we consider individual crisis intervention with an impaired fellow professional, emphasis in applying the crisis task model in this book will usually focus on the directive end of the continuum because of the depth of the crisis and an "I know more than you do, and I'm not nuts" fellow worker. The crisis interventionist who helps a burned-out human services worker typically must proceed in a very directive manner while confronting the client's irrational beliefs, proposing definite alternatives, and getting the client to commit to specific action steps that will get the person out of the state of immobility. Put in simple terms, fellow human services workers are some of the most stubborn and denial-prone clients there are when they have reached the later stages of burnout.

Intervention for the human services worker suffering from burnout may best be considered in three distinct dimensions: intervention through training and/or supervision, intervention with the organization, and intervention with the individual. Triage assessment of the level of burnout is important in determining the type of intervention to be used. At a trait level, individual therapeutic intervention will clearly be warranted. At a state or activity level, training or organizational intervention may be sufficient. When the organization itself becomes a client, triage assessment would clearly include the administering of both burnout and work-setting instruments to all members of the organization and following up that administration with individual interviews.

Intervention Through Training and/or Supervision. Although burnout and empathy-based stress reactions affect workers across all fields of practice, human service work is replete with factors that may increase the risk of burnout, CF, STS, and/or VT. This may be particularly true for trauma professionals (Maslach & Leiter, 2016; Ray et al., 2013) and new professionals (Craig & Sprang, 2010). Although Saakvitne and Pearlman (1996, pp. 25–26) argue that the deep empathy needed for trauma work inevitably begets countertransference and the possibility of vicarious traumatization, at least a part of training should focus on increasing therapeutic detachment and moderating idealism (Warnath & Shelton, 1976) and learning to practice emotional and physical separation/compartmentalization from work (Figley, 2002). A delicate balance exists between providing empathy and manifesting sympathy for a client. To that end, trauma-informed worker development training has been found to be a strong predictor against burnout (Handran, 2014; Salloum et al., 2015).

In an effort to both prevent and ameliorate the symptoms of burnout, human service workers can make efforts to practice holistic wellness (Coaston, 2017), including mindfulness (Martin-Cuellar et al., 2018) and self-care, bolster the development of self-compassion (Coaston, 2017), pursue continuing education and supervision to promote self-efficacy (Bozgeyikli, 2012), utilize socially-based art therapy or other creative strategies to address compassion fatigue (Reim Ifrach & Miller, 2016), and participate in individual counseling to address unresolved issues and obtain support for navigating stressful work conditions (Govindu, 2023). There is also some evidence to suggest that using evidence-based practices may reduce the likelihood of developing burnout and/or empathy-based stress reactions in trauma professionals (Craig & Sprang, 2010). Naturally, each person's self-care plan will differ, but the point is to not forsake one's own self-care in response to work demands. Lax self-care is often a formula for burnout and empathy-based stress reactions and, as a result, may actually lead to diminished performance. Supervisors play an important role in supporting and monitoring supervisees.

Supervisors can help support wellness in their supervisees through modeling wellness practices and intentionally discussing wellness within the supervisory context (Coaston, 2017). And, due to the increased risk of developing emotional exhaustion and CF in mental health professionals who have a trauma history (Ray et al., 2013), supervisors may take special precautions to provide trauma-informed supervision and monitor supervisees for countertransference (Pearlman & Saakvitne, 1995) and other potential indicators of diminished functioning. Further, considering that CF and burnout tend to be positively correlated with imposter syndrome (Clark et al., 2022), supervisors can work with supervisees to foster CS, recognize therapeutic successes, normalize feelings of inadequacy, and generally support appropriate therapeutic confidence.

Although all mental health work includes some measure of trauma therapy and crisis intervention, specialization in these fields is not for the faint of heart. Not all students in the human services field are psychologically equipped to go into trauma therapy or crisis work. Although this work is absolutely some of the most gratifying and reinforcing there is in the human services field, it is also some of the most gut-wrenching and heartbreaking. Students who are not exposed to realistic field experiences and good supervision may go blindly into one of the most stressful occupational fields known.

Intervention with the Organization. Organizations play a central role in preventing burnout (Moss, 2019). According to Moss (2019), burnout is a costly problem that can be averted "if only leadership started their prevention strategies much further upstream" (p. 4). Human services organizations are notorious for being "high in demands and low in resources" (Maslach & Leiter, 2016, p.103). Lack of physical, human, and financial resources militates against comprehensive service provision and long-term planning. Organizations that face crises such as funding and human resource cutbacks often cope with problems by unwittingly adopting crisis characteristics and operating in a state of disequilibrium and immobility. Just letting the crisis "run its course" is no more appropriate for organizations than for individuals in crisis (Devine, 1984). Therefore, from an ecological standpoint, the organization needs to move away from piecemeal interventions and apply techniques that have general inputs to the total organization rather

than just inputs focused on individuals (Paine, 1982, p. 25). Ideally, interventions should be multifaceted and take into consideration both individual and environmental issues in a balanced and sensitive fashion (Carroll & White, 1982, p. 53).

We spoke earlier about Leiter and Maslach's (1999) six areas of work life that contribute to burnout: workload, control, reward, community, fairness, and values (p. 472). Using this model, an important first task is for organizations to work toward setting realistic expectations regarding employee *workload* (Leiter & Maslach, 1999). However, following recent economic declines, workforce shortages, and diminished financial resources, organizations face challenges in finding a balance between sustaining suitable operations and supporting employees. Failing to effectively balance employee workload, though, ultimately results in lower productivity, diminished effectiveness, and increased turnover (Maslach & Leiter, 2016). Moreover, individuals who experience burnout and remain in the organization may have a contagious effect on others, promoting burnout in colleagues (Maslach & Leiter, 2016). Secondly, in the area of *control*, organizations should work to empower employees and minimize role conflict (Leiter & Maslach, 1999). When employees perceive conflicting or ambiguous demands from various authority figures, they cannot effectively prioritize their tasks or adequately practice autonomy in their role (Leiter & Maslach, 1999). Working in an organization characterized by this type of dysfunction can feel a bit like living in a game of whack-a-mole; the targets keep moving, and it's impossible to get ahead. The third area of work life is *reward* (Leiter & Maslach, 1999). When employees feel inadequately compensated, insufficiently supported, or socially isolated, they may be more prone to burnout (Leiter & Maslach, 1999). It should be emphasized that reward is not just about financial compensation; recognition from supervisors and peers goes a long way to helping employees feel valued. Moreover, having supportive relationships with both supervisors and peers can help employees feel a sense of belonging that may insulate them against burnout. The social dimension characterizes the fourth area of work life, which is *community* (Leiter & Maslach, 1999). Indeed, social support from colleagues and loved ones can create a "buffer" against feeling the strain of work demands (Leiter & Maslach, 1999). The fifth area of work life is *fairness* (Leiter & Maslach, 1999). Leiter and Maslach (1999) describe fairness as "the spirit of mutual trust among people in an organization" (p. 481). Fairness is associated with equitable, transparent, and respectful decisions and allocation of resources (Leiter & Maslach, 1999). The sixth and final area of work life is *values*, and is characterized by congruence between the individual's and the organization's values and mission (Leiter & Maslach, 1999). When employees' values match the organization's values, employees tend to be productive and fulfilled in their work. When organizational values and/or mission change due to shifts in leadership, previously engaged and committed employees may find themselves questioning their commitment to an organization that does not embody their personal and/or professional values. Transparent conversations about values can go a long way in building trust and commitment among employees. Attention to these six areas of work life can go a long way in structuring organizations that are characterized by high employee productivity, engagement, and efficacy and low in turnover.

It is well known that systems resist change, though. So, when trying to intervene in an organization that is characterized by poor employee management and high levels of burnout, leaders may face numerous setbacks. Most attempts to deal with the organization by people who are burned out are typified by passively hostile actions that include physical, emotional, and mental withdrawal from problems the organization faces (Pines & Aronson, 1988, pp. 91–93). However, effective organizational change rarely is generated solely by the administration or by the individual. Both parties must decide that stopping burnout in its tracks is a good thing to do. To effect change in the organization, each individual must recognize that there is an institutional problem and be responsible for doing something about it. Likewise, administrators and boards of directors must be constantly vigilant and not deny these kinds of problems exist in the organization. Beginning to take responsibility for effecting change in a difficult situation is therapeutic in and of itself simply because it reduces the debilitating effects of the feeling of helplessness.

Yet, workers who believe that everything about an organization is wrong and should be changed are the most likely to be burnouts, and administrators and boards of directors who believe the same about their workers are likely to go out of business. Some aspects of the bureaucracy cannot be changed short of destroying it. Thus, workers need to develop the ability to distinguish between those aspects of the organization that can be changed and those that cannot (Pines & Aronson, 1988, p. 29).

Burnout-Proofing an Agency. Probably one of the very best organizations at preventing burnout your authors are aware of is the Exchange Club–Carl Perkins Center for the Prevention of Child Abuse in Jackson, Tennessee, which is used as an example of an exemplary child abuse treatment program in Chapter 9, "Sexual Assault." We first encountered Carl Perkins over twenty years ago when we were doing research on burnout (East et al., 2001). We were struck then by what in Chapter 1, "Approaching Crisis Intervention," we characterize as a small agency start-up to meet a local need that grew and evolved from its base in Jackson, Tennessee, to presently covering all the counties except Shelby (metropolitan Memphis) in the Third Grand Division of West Tennessee. In essence, they are the golden rule of how an agency thrives, evolves, grows, and prospers.

One of the reasons for the Carl Perkins Center's excellence is that its directors attempt, to the best of their ability, to burnout-proof the agency and the people in it. Consistency and longevity in excellent leadership are the primary reasons any organization grows and prospers. Pam Nash, the CEO, and Delaine Bottoms, the Vice President for Operations, have been with the program from the start. As described by East et al. (2001), they use several strategies to prevent burnout, STS/VT, and CF that are recommended by many of the researchers in this chapter. In June 2023, Dr. James met with the Carl Perkins case manager, Chase Sanders, in a follow-up interview (Sanders, 2023) to validate how well the Carl Perkins Center continues to implement the following points. The result of that interview follows.

1. Nobody works more than a 40-hour week. Although emergencies may arise, workers will immediately take comp time off after the emergency has passed. Nobody works through lunch; lunch is downtime and is expected to be taken.

Chase Sanders: Forty hours is it! I've worked in places where 55 hours and up is common. It doesn't happen here. Sometimes an emergency arises, and we have to put extra time in, but it gets compensated. And you and I are going to lunch. Thanks for the invite.

2. The center takes quality time to promote in-service education as a way of continuously updating staff on the most effective and innovative practices available in the field. Quarterly in-services combine staff development, organizational issues, and fun events on skill building.

Chase Sanders: We constantly train. We don't stand still. An example is that we are experiencing a big uptick in child-on-child sexual assault (e.g., 9-year-old on a 6- year-old). Probably due to access to porn on the internet. This is not your normal kid's curiosity about sex. Our therapy protocols are built around teen-age to child, adult-to-child aggression, and it's not working well with kid-to-kid. We've got a new program coming that we're going to implement in the Fall. The world changes, and we've got to change with it.

Dr James' note: The supervisory and executive staff constantly trains as well and gets new training themselves. Vice President Bottoms was in Kentucky when this interview took place.

3. Supervision is continuous and supportive. Each worker has a weekly session with a supervisor. The role of the supervisor is to listen, provide empathic support, consult, and plan cases.

Chase Sanders: We've gotten a lot bigger, so we meet about every two weeks. My job is to provide psychological support, case planning, and follow through.

4. The center expedites logistical problems. Work areas are clean, well lit, with cheerfully decorated offices and meeting rooms. Therapy rooms have brightly colored carpets and colorful children's murals on the walls. There is a well-stocked resource center with videos, instructional programs, and reference books. There is adequate office and clerical help for all workers, so they do not drown in paperwork. Supplies are adequate and readily available.

Chase Sanders: We moved into the old Union University campus, so we have a lot more space for the main office. There is some variance in capabilities and ambience in our satellites, but they are pretty decently housed.

Dr. James' note: The main office is a cheerful building with clean, bright, positive décor and well-equipped therapy meeting and office areas. Clerical and reception staff were friendly and available for help. The one satellite office he visited was smaller but definitely was in excellent building condition and had the necessary rooms and equipment to do the work.

5. Case staffings are carefully constructed in a comprehensive manner with team inputs. A clear treatment plan is laid out. There is little confusion about mission goals. There is a definite feeling of "we" between the administration and the staff. All supervisors have worked their way up through the organization, so they are acutely aware of the problems and issues staff face.

Chase Sanders: The state Department of Human Services will pay for a maximum of 12 therapy sessions. If needed, we will exceed that, although this isn't "therapy forever." We operate from an evidenced-based trauma cognitive therapy protocol but will bring play therapy techniques in to help bond and gain trust with kids. We also work with parents, but how that happens is on a case-by-case basis. So, while we operate from a standard therapeutic protocol, we still vary that on a case-by-case basis.

6. There is a clear delineation between work and home. Home and family are an overriding priority, and the directors of the center are adamant that families come first, and work comes second.

Dr. James' note: Chase was asked specifically what he does to keep Carl Perkins and home separate.

Chase Sanders: First of all, I live in Huntingdon, so I'm not stuck in an office day-in-day out. I travel all over the Third Grand Division from the Mississippi river to the Tennessee river and from the Kentucky line to the Mississippi state line. I enjoy that. I like to stay busy and see things accomplished. In this business, you never finish things off. Believe it or not, I like to mow the lawn and do yard work. I can see when it's finished, and that's satisfying. I also have an antique military firearm collection I can go get lost in when I need to put work aside. When at home, my family is most important and comes first, my wife and I talk a lot about "stuff" and so that's a way of getting it out of your system.

7. Faith-based renewal and spiritual growth are encouraged. As one worker stated, "I can't do this alone. I have to give it over to God." This approach is encouraged without regard to denomination. Prayer is a powerful tool for these people, and they use it. There is a saying in war that there are few atheists in foxholes. A parallel can be made to the trauma and crisis business. Finding a sacrosanct spiritual center that one can believe in and retreat to is paramount, given the often-heinous nature of crisis work (Collins, 2005; Kennedy, 2006; SAMHSA, 2023). Because Jackson, Tennessee, is in

the "Bible Belt," you may suppose that the staff's deep reliance on faith is a Southern cultural artifact. You would be wrong. A good deal of research (Harrison & Westwood, 2009; Lawson & Myers, 2011; Reese, 2009; Simpson, 2006) demonstrates that spirituality is a key component in keeping the nastiness in this chapter out of your life. Short of proselytizing, your authors believe that anybody in this business needs to find some spiritual rock or belief in something greater than themselves to anchor them.

Chase Sanders: I'm not so sure we're in the Bible Belt anymore. The COVID-19 pandemic changed that. Also, I may not be a good common example since I am also a Church of Christ minister to a small congregation near my home, but I do think most of the staff here have some religious connection that they lean on.

Dr James note: I know from over my years of working with Carl Perkins staff members that a spiritual taproot runs deep for many of them, and it nourishes them in a business that can be pretty poisonous to the human spirit.

8. Debriefing is used continuously. Whenever a tragedy occurs, such as a child's death or other traumatic event, workers are debriefed, and it is done as expeditiously as possible.

Chase Sanders: Thankfully, child deaths are rare for us to directly encounter. Our workers do receive vicarious trauma intervention regularly. We also have a few local therapists who will work with our workers on an individual basis if there is an especially traumatic event.

9. The center does not work on an assembly-line basis with repetitive, day-in-day-out work assignments that grind staff down. Workers are expected to schedule variety into their days.

Chase Sanders: Our workers largely make their own schedules. We encourage them to break up tasks such as sessions, documentation, training, supervision, etc. throughout the day so that they do have variety. Session schedules are largely dictated by the needs of clients.

10. The center provides technical support. All of the staff have offices, computers, cell phones, video recorders, and other equipment necessary for optimal performance.

Chase Sanders: We try to update particularly technologically. For example, you wrote previously about our one-way mirror viewing rooms when we do forensic interviews. Everything now is video recorded and goes to a central viewing room where law enforcement and social service staff can watch.

11. Workers use a team approach. No one is above getting their hands "dirty," and everyone pitches in when something needs to be done. It is not frowned upon to ask for assistance. The center does not deify go-it-alone, heroic martyrs.

Chase Sanders: While everyone has a specific role within the agency, we do approach everything as a team. We rely on each other to do our specified tasks, but we help each other as well. A therapist will often need an advocate's help to transport a family to and from their therapy appointments due to lack of reliable transportation. A therapist may assist a family in court accompaniment if an advocate has multiple victims with appearances on the same day.

12. Safety is the most important product of the center, for both its clients and staff. Clear-cut safety procedures are constantly taught and reinforced to ensure the workers' well-being both at the center and during home visits.

Dr. James' note: I was met at the front door of the center by Chase. Keypad entry access to the building. The waiting area is open and observable by reception staff with all offices and therapy areas accessible but secure. A sort of security blanket is that the center is directly across and 100 yards away from Juvenile Court, which has a quick response capability nearby.

Chase Sanders: Most of our buildings are controlled access or will have a worker stationed near the front door. Children are never left alone in buildings, and they are never alone with only one worker in the building. Alleged perpetrators of sexual abuse are never allowed on the premises. Interaction between families is limited when possible. All clients complete a safety plan at the beginning of treatment to assess for any specific safety issues. In the rare event of a significant safety issue at the Center, our relationship with law enforcement means that we usually get an extremely rapid response.

13. The workload is "doable." Over the years, the center has lightened workers' caseloads. As the

total number of cases rises, more workers are hired. The center has been able to increase staff because its administration is very adept at convincing its constituency that it is doing a great job and should be given the financial support to continue to do so. The administration works very closely with its board and continuously educates it regarding the financial and staffing needs of the center.

Chase Sanders: Our therapists are in a rather unique position since their entire caseload consists of intense trauma cases. These cases also may require some degree of case management, travel to provide therapy, and other tasks that are not accomplished in the clinical session. We have found that most therapists begin to feel stretched thin around 20 cases. Unfortunately, there are always more victims needing therapy. There is an acute lack of mental health services in many communities within our service area. It is not easy to refer victims to another provider. Over the years, we have added additional therapy positions to accommodate the needs of clients in our community. This has also allowed us to increase the quality of our work experience by limiting travel between locations. The center has been able to increase staff because its administration is very adept at convincing its constituency that it is doing a great job and should be given the financial support to continue to do so. The administration works very closely with its board and continuously educates it regarding the financial and staffing needs of the center. The executives and the board spend a great deal of time on fund raising through charitable giving, charity events, writing grants, and state contracts.

Dr. James note: To be able to do what they have done, it still boils down to, "Where's the money coming from?" Pam Nash and Delaine Bottoms, the two long-term founders and executives have had years of practice in raising money and they are extremely good at showing how that money is spent and the results it gets.

14. The center does an excellent job of networking. It serves a large geographic area and, therefore, has established relationships with other social services agencies (such as schools, law enforcement, and state welfare agencies) in outlying counties. The center also goes out of its way to provide support for other agencies within its service area. This not only increases the center's credibility with the agencies and institutions, but it also allows for reciprocal perquisites: center employees can utilize office space and the support of staff in other agencies when the employees are far away from their home office. There are 21 counties in the Third Grand Division of West Tennessee, and some of those counties define "RURAL" in capital letters in regard to geographic isolation, small population centers, and lack of social and mental health services.

Chase Sanders: We continuously work closely with police departments, schools, and county social service and mental health agencies throughout the Third Grand Division by providing them updated abuse information, service, and training. It is noteworthy that in some of our more rural and isolated counties, we are pretty much it for mental health services. The Center serves 20 counties in West Tennessee. We have physical locations in 17 of those counties. We currently have 19 full-time therapists, 11 victim advocates, and four forensic interviewers. Additionally, each county is served by an executive director, office manager, and other support staff.

15. The administration is very thorough in its hiring selection. Candidates are carefully screened to determine how well they will fit into the overall scheme of things.

Chase Sanders: I can tell you pretty quickly whether someone's gonna hack it here. We are pretty good at selection. Particularly, some of the candidates who have been completely educated online don't measure up. I can generally tell within a month whether a person is cut out to do this work.

16. Staff are positively reinforced both intrinsically and extrinsically on a consistent basis. Workers are told they are doing a good job in specific behavioral terms, and they are told often. After a particularly horrific incident in which three sexually abused children all died in a house fire at a foster home, the associate director went to the field office and picked up the workers who had been engaged nonstop in dealing with this tragedy. She piled them into her van and, without a word, took them to a local spa, where they spent the day getting makeovers, massages, aromatherapy, yoga lessons, and a nice lunch. While a day trip to a spa can in no way assuage the grief and stress these workers felt, it does say very clearly,

"We care about you!" and that message comes across loud and clear to all of the staff.

Chase Sanders: While the spa treatment is not a typical response, we do try to provide our workers with downtime and fun activities. The Carl Perkins Center sees its workers as its most important asset and understands the perils of the kind of work it does.

17. Does all this work?

Chase Sanders: In fiscal year 2022, we reviewed 2,334 individual cases of abuse. Of those cases, we provided 924 forensic interviews, 144 forensic medical exams, 1,093 were assisted with victim advocacy, and we provided 8,051 mental health sessions. Here are the results from our outcome survey questions (Carl Perkins, 2023), which says we're doing something right, I think.

1. My immediate sense of safety and security has increased as a result of the services I received from this agency. Ninety-two percent Agree
2. I am more knowledgeable of the services and community resources available to victims. Ninety-seven percent Agree
3. I am more knowledgeable about the criminal justice system. Eighty-seven percent Agree
4. I am satisfied with the services I have received at this agency. Ninety-seven percent Agree
5. I know more ways to plan for my safety. Ninety-three percent Agree
6. My crime-related symptoms are less frequent or less severe since I became involved with this agency. Ninety-six percent Agree

The Carl Perkins Center sees its workers as its most important asset and understands the perils of the kind of work it does. The outcomes are proof positive that a proactive program to prevent burnout works. The attrition rate is extremely low. Because this is a fairly young and rapidly expanding agency, many of the workers are young. Research indicates (Meyers & Cornille, 2002) that the demographics and job role of this group would cause them to be at high risk for burnout. They were and are not!

Chase Sanders: Our case workers tend to stick around; I think the average "life" expectancy in the child abuse business is about 16 months. Most of our caseworkers have been here five or six years or more.

Although the Carl Perkins Center previously administered a variety of assessments to measure employee burnout and related constructs, the Center does not currently engage in assessment of their employees. However, the stability and thoughtful practice of burnout proofing the agency has clearly continued with powerful effects. Employees are encouraged to focus on their emotional health, and it is not frowned upon for employees to acknowledge when they experience burnout. The climate is accepting rather than shaming.

In conclusion, the administrative staff at Carl Perkins understand the effects that vicarious traumatization, compassion fatigue, and burnout can have on their organization and set aside time and resources to deal with it. In providing support to staff, the Carl Perkins Center follows very closely the six points proposed by Pines (1983), listed and described in the next section. It would thus appear that even in one of the most stressful of all types of crisis agencies—one that works with traumatized children (Meyers & Cornille, 2002)—the institution can stop burnout dead in its tracks if it has the will to do so.

Intervention with the Individual. Mental health providers are notoriously guilty of selfless giving until all of their resources are depleted. Coupled with the erroneous notion that we should be able to help ourselves rather than allowing others to help us, mental health workers are prime candidates for burnout. When burnout reaches a critical level in which the mental health worker's quality of life and/or therapeutic efficacy are diminished, outside support and changes to the workplace and/or workload may well be needed. Maslach and Goldberg (1998) talk about changing work patterns that can be implemented to address burnout, such as taking breaks or vacations, not working long hours, reducing caseloads, and generally trying to achieve work-life balance. However, many recommendations for intervention at the individual level focus on prevention in the form of wellness practices and social support. Maslach and Goldberg (1998) also talk about the utility of developing coping skills, including cognitive-based skills; employing social support; using relaxation strategies; practicing good physical health and exercising; and increasing self-awareness, including personal counseling. To that end, let's delve deeper into wellness and social support.

Wellness Practice. Burnout is an ethical matter for mental health workers (Simionato et al., 2019), and the utilization of self-care and wellness practices is an ethical obligation. These points are affirmed by the inclusion of self-care and monitoring for impairment in Section C of the American Counseling Association Code of Ethics (2014) and SAMHSA's (2019, 2023) self-care for disaster workers, which certainly fits here as well.

There are various established methods for fostering wellness: practicing mindfulness (Harker et al., 2016; Thompson et al., 2014), mindful self-compassion (Coaston, 2017), and spirituality (Lizano et al., 2019); exercising (Chirico et al., 2021; Govindu, 2023) and interacting with nature (Govindu, 2023); and using cathartic techniques, such as journaling (Roux & Benita, 2020) and art (Reim Ifrach & Miller, 2016; Roux & Benita, 2020), to name a few. The aforementioned are effective strategies to prevent burnout and address burnout at low or moderate levels. However, we would be remiss if we did not mention the critical role of play in achieving overall wellness.

In William Glasser's reality therapy/control theory (1985), one of the central axes on which his theory revolves is engaging in positive addicting behaviors, and central to those positive addicting behaviors is having fun. The whole notion of Glasser's theory is that when you engage in these positive addicting behaviors, your personal world grows much larger, and so does your social world as you interact with it.

Nobody can make you get out of your rut, and it is extremely easy to stay in it. The word *recreate* makes a lot more sense when you break it down into *re-create*. So meditate, play rugby, work up your fantasy football team, make a quilt, run a marathon, shoot some pool, play bridge or poker, master your skills in an MMORPG, go fishing, see a ballgame, weed your flower garden, go snorkeling or SCUBA diving—any of those will do as long as you are having fun, enjoying it, and it has absolutely nothing to do with anything in this book. Just remember, you cannot use this directive to recreate as an excuse for failing to finish this chapter and flunking your Crisis Intervention course.

Social Support Systems. Social support systems act as buffers for the individual and help maintain psychological and physical well-being over time (Ling et al., 2014; Oerlemans & Bakker, 2014; Pines, 1983, p. 157; SAMHSA 2019, 2023). Social supports, whether personal or professional, are critical to avoiding burnout (Bray, 2018; Chirico et al., 2021; Govindu, 2023; Maslach & Leiter, 2016; Reim Ifrach & Miller, 2016; Rupert et al., 2015; Thomas et al., 2014); Reim Ifrach & Miller, 2016; Rupert et al., 2015; Thomas et al., 2014. Family systems are major sources of support (Killian, 2008; Lawson & Myers, 2011; Sullivan, 2004) and can

help insulate workers against burnout (Bakker et al., 2005; Halbesleben, 2006; Maslach & Jackson, 1981b). However, it is impossible for one's spouse, partner, family, or friends to fulfill all the support tasks a crisis worker who engages specifically in trauma work will need (Pines, 1983, p. 172). Clearly, the worker needs to have functioning support systems at the job site (Handran, 2014; Li et al., 2014; Maslach & Leiter, 2016), and it would behoove organizations to focus on socialization strategies in the workplace (Avanzi et al., 2018; Thomas et al., 2014).

Social support systems have six basic functions: listening, technical support, technical challenge, emotional support, emotional challenge, and sharing social reality (Pines, 1983).

1. **Listening.** Periodically, all workers need someone to listen actively to them in an empathic manner without giving advice or making judgments (p. 158).
2. **Technical support.** When confronted with complex client problems, all workers need someone who can affirm confidence in their endeavors. Such a person must have the expertise to understand the complexities of the job and be able to give the worker honest feedback (p. 158).
3. **Technical challenge.** If workers are not intellectually challenged, they will stagnate. Intellectual contact with significant others stretches the worker in a positive way. Such challenges can come only from people who do not intend to humiliate or gain an advantage and who have professional expertise equivalent to that of the worker (p. 158).
4. **Emotional support.** Workers need someone to be on their side in difficult situations, even if the significant others do not necessarily agree totally with the workers. Professional expertise is not necessary for this function (pp. 158–159).
5. **Emotional challenge.** It is comforting for workers to believe that they have explored all avenues in attempting to resolve their problems. Support persons serve a valuable function when they question such assumptions and confront the worker's excuses. This function should be used sparingly; otherwise, it may be construed as nagging (p. 159).
6. **Sharing social reality.** When workers become unsure of the reliability of their own perceptions about the reality of the situation, they need external validation. This function is especially important when workers feel that they are losing

the ability to evaluate what is happening with their clients and with the organization (p. 159).

Support groups. Within the organizational structure, time should be set aside for formal, structured support groups. Structurally, a support group resembles a problem-solving discussion group. The goal of such a group is to build a sense of competence and help workers feel they can deal with the stresses they encounter in their work situation. A support group is a safe place for workers to disagree and challenge feelings of helplessness.

The group serves as a cathartic agent for releasing pent-up emotions related to the job. Once catharsis occurs, members can realistically examine feelings associated with job stressors. By providing feedback, the support group validates for members that they are not alone in their feelings and reassures them that they are not abnormal in their response to the situation (Sculley, 1983, pp. 188–191).

To do this effectively, a support group not only needs the support of the administration but also must have a consultant/facilitator who is sensitive to the issues involved and can walk a tightwire between allowing the group to vent feelings and keeping the group in a problem-solving model. The buffering effect of a third-party consultant/facilitator can help reduce conflict stressors (Giebels & Janssen, 2005). The consultant/facilitator also needs to be in a position to provide the administration with information from the group that will allow for effective organizational change without becoming a "snitch" in the process (Sculley, 1983, pp. 193–194).

Finally, for those members suffering from vicarious traumatization, compassion fatigue, and the later stages of burnout, referring them for personal counseling should be done with the understanding that these outcomes are indeed occupational hazards no different from carpal tunnel syndrome for keyboard operators or arthritis for concrete finishers. In that regard, organizations must be careful not to secondarily victimize such people as being of weak character or lacking in the "right stuff."

The Individual and the Organization. Vocationally, there are four major maladaptive responses to the onset of burnout. As the level of burnout increases, so does escape avoidance behavior (Thornton, 1992) and employee turnover (Gharakhani et al., 2019; Perrone et al., 2019). Workers may attempt horizontal job

mobility. They continuously look for the "right" boss or organization when it is the job they are in that is causing their unhappiness.

Others tire of the constant interaction with clients and decide to move vertically up the job ladder into administrative positions. What they fail to realize is that their cynical and jaundiced view of the system will not be left behind but will be carried with them into a whole new set of stresses. It is an understatement to say that these people do not make very good bosses.

There are also people who become what Pines and Aronson (1988, p. 18) call "deadwood." These people have long ago decided that their best bet is to not "rock the boat" so they can make it to retirement. If you have ever read the comic strip *Dilbert*, Wally best represents these individuals. When asked to do something, they politely indicate they are too busy, or agree with every idea put forth but venture none of their own, or contribute only what is minimally necessary to escape notice or censure, or turn the tables and cast incompetence on others to cover up their own failings. Finally, some people quit their job and the vocation, and in some instances, this may be the wisest choice of all.

At this stage of frustration, choices may seem to be limited to job change or job stagnation, but the individual does have other options. First, clearly defining one's role within the organization is a high priority (Kesler, 1990). The worker should conduct a job analysis and determine which tasks are necessary, which are self-imposed, and which contribute to role overload (Pines & Aronson, 1988, p. 109). Through assertive negotiation with the administration, the worker needs to define a reasonable work level and commensurate financial or other rewards for the work performed. Clients should be clearly apprised of the limits of service regarding time as well as the amount and kind of service to be provided. Although service to clients needs to be a high priority, other tasks should be clearly prioritized. If chores that do not have a high priority cannot be delegated, then serious consideration should be given to dropping them (Leiter & Maslach, 2005).

Finally, if it is apparent that the organization is so entrenched and regressive that little change in policies and programs can be affected, it is probably time to look for greener occupational pastures. It would behoove a worker who is in the frustration stage to consider what a near-future job change entails and start planning for it before reaching the apathy stage.

Knowing company severance policies and state unemployment benefits, updating a resume, saving money, and commencing a job search are examples of prudent measures workers may take before they are so mentally, physically, and emotionally exhausted that there is little energy left for a major shift in one's life.

LO11 **Cross-Cultural Comparisons.** This chapter is not just for human services workers in the United States. If you are reading this book in Germany, Scotland, Brazil, Australia, Poland, India, Canada, Denmark, China, Korea, Egypt, Israel, Japan, or some other country, this chapter is also for you. Victor Savicki (2002) conducted a landmark study of child care workers, culture, work environment, and burnout across the United States, Australia, a number of European countries, and Israel and compared them on Maslach Burnout Inventory subscales (Maslach & Jackson, 1981a). What Savicki found when he compared 13 different cultures was that all of you out there don't do well and tend to burn out when there are heavy workloads, unsupportive middle-level managers, an atmosphere in which new ideas and practices are restricted, and inefficiently organized work. Conversely, when the work environment offers encouragement for new ideas, a team of coworkers lends support, and managers set the stage for positive feelings of goal attainment, low burnout scores are the result (Savicki, 2002, pp. 80–87).

However, when culture is factored in, Maslach's three components of burnout change dramatically. For example, Danish and both French Canadian and English Canadian workers have low emotional exhaustion, low depersonalization, and high sense of personal accomplishment scores. Child care workers in what was formerly West Germany have high burnout profiles with a low sense of personal accomplishment and high emotional exhaustion and depersonalization scores. Interestingly, in what was formerly East Germany, respondents had very little sense of personal accomplishment, yet they were not emotionally exhausted, nor did they feel much depersonalization. Clearly, even though those are both German populations, the political cultural artifacts left over from what was formerly a communist country seem to play a role in how child care workers operate and what their culture expects from them, in contrast to the democracy of the former West Germany. Now, compare the German scores to those of the Israelis, who had very low depersonalization and a very high sense of personal accomplishment but were at the median on emotional exhaustion. Then, refer to the United States, whose workers scored extremely high in sense of personal accomplishment but unhappily also had high emotional exhaustion and high depersonalization scores (Savicki, 2002, pp. 78–79).

Both general environmental work measures and individual cultural conformity measures showed significant relationships to the burnout subscales (Savicki, 2002, pp. 88–89). For example, the concept of **power distance** means the amount of control that bosses feel they have over workers and vice versa. High power distances mean that bosses believe they can dictate the behavior of their subordinates. It should come as no surprise that high power distances lead to burn out. Likewise, the **uncertainty avoidance principle** is the degree to which cultures establish rules, procedures, and rituals to compensate for uncertainty and chaos (Savicki, 2002, pp. 38–41). Again, it should be no surprise that those cultures with high uncertainty avoidance and many rules to guide the bureaucracy tend to have high burnout scores.

The implications of Savicki's (2002) work would seem to be that not only are the individual worker and the work setting complicit in whether burnout potential is high or low but also that the overall culture may be a factor as well. If that is true, changing the cultural factor is a tall order indeed! Savicki's (2002) study examines countries whose cultures are generally seen to be more individualist as opposed to collectivist, although arguments could certainly be made for a more collectivist Gestalt in what used to be East Germany and other former Soviet bloc countries of Eastern Europe. It would be interesting to see how child care workers from Middle Eastern, African, and Asian cultures that tend to operate more on the collectivist end of the cultural continuum would fare on the Burnout Inventory. Much like avian flu, burnout circles the globe, and you can catch it pretty much anywhere.

Private Practitioners and Burnout

The occupational dream of many of our students is to start their own private practice. They fantasize that they could do the kind of therapy they wanted with the clients they selected, be rid of overbearing supervisors and be their own boss, not be bothered with bureaucratic hassles and avalanches of paperwork, set their own hours, and make lots of money! Indeed, some research suggests that those in private practice may have lower incidence of burnout (Lent, 2010). Although, to some degree, private practice practitioners have more control over their work life, working in isolation and with the looming stress of making a living can carry its own burdens.

Although the aloneness that pervades a private practice is not the same as the isolation that agency workers sometimes impose on themselves when placed in high-stress situations, it can be more complete. Fenced off from other professionals by ethical and ecological boundaries, the private practitioner has few others with whom to discuss client problems. More important, there are few other individuals with whom they can discuss their own personal problems, and colleagues are not readily available to bring attention to the private practitioner's behavior when signs of burnout or other empathy-based stress reactions emerge.

Private practice is clearly a business. As such, working in private practice can be challenging due to various demands associated with billing, working with insurance companies, and maintaining a caseload (Bray, 2021; Mishna et al., 2015). Determining one's fees, number of sliding scale or pro bono clients, and overall caseload can be a complex endeavor—one that requires the practitioner to examine their financial needs and expenses (Bray, 2021). Further, handling client non-payment presents additional concerns, such as imposing cancellation fees (Bray, 2021) and dealing with collections agencies. Every client termination raises questions: "Will there be someone to take her place?" "Will he pass the word along that I did him some good?" When one's way of life depends on their own work, and there is no steady paycheck coming from an employment agency, concerns about performance can easily become more pronounced than concerns about therapeutic efficacy.

Starting and maintaining a private practice also calls for maintaining a public presence. Whether such a presence involves making speeches to the Rotary Club on stress and the businessperson, consulting with the oncology staff on death and dying at the local hospital, or giving a workshop on discipline for Parents Without Partners, the continuous pressure of needing to be seen as active, abreast of current developments, and visible is part of a sales program that must constantly be maintained and upgraded. In the age of telebehavioral health, the importance of a positive online presence cannot be overstated. Clients can easily search for their counselors online and access reviews from angry clients and the counselor's social media profiles. To be sure, as we discussed in Chapter 6, "Telephone and Online: Crisis

Counseling," "Telephone and Online: Crisis Counseling," navigating online presence is a unique challenge and a requisite skill for modern practitioners.

Although the private practitioner is their own boss, being an independent businessperson also means being completely responsible for maintaining the practice. Long hours and difficult work periods are the rule rather than the exception. Because most clients work regular hours, private practitioners devote many evenings and weekends to their work. Usually, there is no one to pick up caseloads, so vacations or even short respites are few and far between. Private practitioners can easily get caught in a way of thinking in which they calculate the financial cost of vacation days, making it harder for them to justify taking time away from their work due to financial incentives. Certainly not all private practitioners suffer from burnout; many are enriched and energized by their work and their occupational independence. However, when burnout does occur with human services workers who are in private practice, it is accelerated by the foregoing problems and issues.

Intervention with the Individual: A Case Study

Direct action, in which the worker tries to master the environmental stressors, and palliative action, in which the worker tries to reduce disturbances when unable to manage the environment, are the two positive ways to cope with stress (Pines & Aronson, 1988, p. 144). Direct action is applied externally to the situational stressor in the environment, whereas palliative action is applied internally to one's cognitions and emotions about the stressor. Social support groups, workshops, assertiveness training, flextime, taking time off, salary increase, and role shifts are all examples of direct action. Mindfulness, meditation, relaxation techniques, biofeedback, physical exercise with no ego involvement, adopting positive cognitions, engaging in leisure-time pursuits, utilizing expressive and/or art techniques, and adding more humor and joy to one's life are all palliative "decompensation activities" that allow the worker to put stressors aside (Chirico et al., 2021; Govindu, 2023; Harker et al., 2016; Maslach & Goldberg, 1998; Reim Ifrach & Miller, 2016; Roux & Benita, 2020; Thompson et al., 2014)1998; Reim Ifrach & Miller, 2016; Roux & Benita, 2020; Thompson et al., 2014.

While workers who are at the frustration stage may well be helped by being involved in self-initiated directive and palliative actions, those at the more serious stage of apathy will not be (Edelwich & Brodsky, 1982, p. 137). In such cases, individual counseling is more appropriate (Baron & Cohen, 1982). Kesler (1990) proposed using Arnold Lazarus's (1976) BASIC ID (behavior, affect, sensation, imagery, cognition, interpersonal relationships, and drugs/biology) paradigm as a treatment approach to burnout. To this formulation, Kesler adds an *S* for setting. Given the interactive effects of burnout across multiple facets of the individual, the BASIC IDS approach seems valid for attacking burnout in a comprehensive way.

The following case illustrates the crisis worker using combinations of direct and palliative actions in an abbreviated BASIC IDS approach. It should be clearly understood that neither symptoms nor intervention procedures are all-inclusive. For example, Tubesing and Tubesing (1982, p. 161) listed 36 possible intervention strategies that cover physical, intellectual, social, emotional, spiritual, and environmental components of burnout, and those are not comprehensive by any means. If the client is identified as having more compassion fatigue or vicarious traumatization, a more specific program that focuses on STS symptoms may be used, such as the Accelerated Recovery Program (ARP; Gentry et al., 2002). The case presented is that of a professional with a doctorate and many years of experience, but neophytes should understand that Dr. Jane Lee is genotypical of any human services worker. Her case clearly points out that no worker is immune to burnout, no matter how much experience or expertise that worker may have.

The Client

Dr. Jane Lee is a striking, raven-haired, 43-year-old woman with aquiline features, a low, melodious voice, aquamarine eyes that twinkle, and a smile that could serve as a toothpaste commercial. She is extremely witty and incisive of intellect, is widely read, and can talk as easily with truck drivers as she can with lawyers. At any social function, people gravitate toward her. She seems to have been born with the natural empathy and easy familiarity that many people consciously work their whole lives for yet never quite attain. Divorced for 10 years, Jane has raised her only son while carrying on an exceedingly successful professional life.

Jane has a thriving practice in marriage and family therapy. She has a heavy client load and is clearing approximately $150,000 a year. She is seen by her peers as extremely capable, and her clients speak highly of her. Jane has been in private practice for eight years. Prior to entering private practice, she worked in a community mental health facility. She was so skillful at therapy there that she rose to the directorship of the clinical program.

Jane graduated from a major university with a doctorate in counseling psychology and completed her internship in a VA hospital. She then successfully completed an American Association of Marriage and Family Therapists internship at a private clinic. She has written and published many articles on therapy for individuals living with anorexia and the families of individuals suffering from catastrophic illnesses. She has also given many in-service programs and presentations at national human services conferences.

By any criteria imaginable, Jane appears to be a highly competent, successful therapist and an exceptionally endowed woman overall. Her ability and demeanor have made her a role model that many in her community aspire to emulate. As Jane sits down with the crisis worker, she is seriously considering drinking a good deal of wine, closing her garage door, climbing into her new Lexus, turning on the ignition, and killing herself.

Jane: I came here today because of what you said to me the other night when we were having a drink. You pretty much have me pegged. I'm burned out even more than what you think, more than what I like to admit. Today I had a decision to make, whether to kill myself or come here. I came here, but I'm not sure it's the right decision. If I killed myself, it seems like it would just be over and done with. I've taken care of everything concerning Bobby, my son. He's practically through with college, and even though we're very close, I really think it'd be better for him if I were gone.

He wouldn't have to put up with my lousy behavior, and believe me, it's lousy right now. There's enough in the bank account to get him finished up in school, and he could sell the house. He's the only one that really matters besides my clients, and right now I'm not doing worth a damn with them. I'm probably hurting more than I help, and I'm just not up to it anymore. So much pain and so damn little I can do about it. The only thing I can think about now when I go into a cancer ward is how bad the patients smell. Whoever said "You don't have to smell them. All you gotta do is help them!" sure wasn't in this end of the business. I'm also starting to behave like those screwed-up anorexia clients I work with, too. It's starting to seem pretty reasonable to me that they aren't eating. Why the hell should they? Why the hell should *I*? Just sort of fade away and look thin while you're doing it. At least I'd make a great-looking corpse. Anyway, the main reason I came over today was to see if you'd be willing to take my clients. I've thought this over, and you've got what it takes. I think you could help them, and if you agree, I'll start talking to them about coming over to your practice.

CW: What you just said scares the living hell out of me. There's a part of me that wants to run right out of here, because what you're saying is really hitting home with the way I feel at times. There's another part of me that wants to tie you up in log chains until you come to your senses. Finally, there's another part of me that cares for you so much that I'm angry that you've let yourself get into this predicament. Most of all, though, I'm glad I made that reflection the other night and that it finally sank in. I've seen you going downhill for quite a while now. My guess is that you didn't even know it was happening or just laid another piece of armor plate over yourself and said something like "I've got to gut this through" or some of that other irrational garbage I hear you unload on yourself. First of all, I won't even consider what you said about the clients until we agree on one thing, and that is you don't do any harm to yourself until we talk this through. So, I want an agreement both as your therapist and as your friend that we shake on that before anything else happens. I won't take no for an answer. If that's not acceptable, we'll negotiate it. No matter what, we're now in this together.

Ethical Issues

LO12 The crisis worker is in a difficult position as the client's friend, fellow professional, and now as a therapist dealing with another human being in crisis. When a human services professional who is a colleague becomes impaired, it is the ethical duty of the fellow professional to do something to prevent harm to clients (Harrison & Westwood, 2009; Thomas & Levitt, 2010), and there is research that impaired therapists can hurt clients (Lawson et al., 2007). The overall principle of nonmaleficence (do no harm) comes into play. It is simpler if impairment is due to drugs or alcohol abuse that can be readily observed or if the professional works in a setting where other professionals can observe the behavior, but it becomes much more difficult when the professional is in private practice or the impairment is burnout, which cannot be smelled or seen in slurred speech or unsteady walking.

Oftentimes, close friends and colleagues of burned-out professionals are the first to notice the impairment. Clearly, there are many personal and social dilemmas about "snitching" out one's colleague. The question then becomes: Should colleagues report the impaired professional to the state licensing board, supervisors, or attempt to intervene and help the person by themselves (Myer et al., 2023)? It is a slippery slope, and, as with many ethics questions, there is no clear answer.

Although there are ethical issues in treating a friend and a colleague, when a client is in crisis and lethality is involved, the primary concern is keeping the client safe and returning the individual to a state of equilibrium (Myer et al., 2023). Depending on what comes of this crisis intervention, if Jane can regain her psychological equilibrium and manage her own self-care, the crisis worker may do nothing more. If Jane doesn't, the worker is ethically bound to notify a licensing board or supervisor, although that might well spell the end of the friendship (Myer et al., 2023; Thomas & Levitt, 2010).

The nuances of this ethical dilemma can be argued after the fact, but right now, the crisis worker needs to act. Particularly in small towns where there are essentially no other professionals with the necessary expertise to provide immediate assistance, the appropriate ethical response would be to provide the best level of care as quickly as possible. In that regard, it is most likely that the crisis worker will have some personal or professional relationship with the client.

Because the crisis worker knows the client, she feels free to make some initial owning statements that let the client know exactly how she feels about the situation without becoming sympathetic in the bargain, which she could easily do because she has felt much the same way at prior times in her professional life (countertransference). The crisis worker also makes an initial assessment of the lethality level of the client. Her reflective statement to the client a few evenings earlier was not idle conversation. The crisis worker has seen a slow but steady change coming over Jane in the last three months, and as she thinks about it, she sees that it was coming a good while before that. Jane has been keeping a stiff upper lip, but there have been indicators that all has not been well lately. She has been rather cynical about clients, as evidenced by her comment about how they smell. She has been suffering a variety of physical maladies that have ranged from unending colds to some severe gastrointestinal problems ominous enough to indicate that surgery might be needed in the near future.

As the crisis worker continues to assess the situation, she further realizes that Jane has truncated relationships with most of her acquaintances and has done this lately with the crisis worker on at least two occasions. Their relationship had been characterized by an easy rivalry, good comradeship, and just generally a lot of good times together without ever engaging in one-upmanship. Lately, though, the crisis worker has had the feeling that Jane has treated her more as a client than as a friend and has attributed some deeper psychological meaning to even the most innocent conversation.

Assessment

Behaviorally, Jane is in serious trouble. Her performance of daily tasks has become seriously compromised. Her uncharacteristic behavior coupled with her suicidal thoughts places her at a triage level of 7 to 8 on behavior. The only positive behavior she is currently exhibiting is seeking out her colleague. Even though she says she is doing that only to transfer clients, dynamically, she is making a clear call for help.

The rather detached, mechanistic way that Jane has reported all this and her blank, hollow look are completely at odds with Jane's usual sparkle, which has been absent the past few months. Performing a quick synthesis of all this background knowledge, what Jane is saying, and the depressed way she is looking and behaving, the crisis worker makes the assessment that Jane is not kidding about killing herself and that the threat must be taken seriously. The crisis worker immediately goes into a suicide prevention mode and institutes a verbal contract with Jane not to kill herself. Even though Jane is a practicing therapist, she is no different from any other client in this regard.

Besides the threat of suicide, a triage assessment of Jane by a worker unfamiliar with burnout might cursorily dismiss her problem as typical whining about one's work. However, the difficult clients she deals with, the amount of time that she has done so, the isolation she has imposed on herself, and the absence of social support systems in her work and at home all lead to a hypothesis of vicarious trauma/

compassion fatigue that is rippling out into every component of her life (Figley, 2002, p. 7). Research clearly indicates that the more traumatic clients are and the more often they are seen, the more likely it is that the therapist will experience compassion fatigue, vicarious traumatization, and burnout (Simpson, 2006). In short, Jane is fitting many of the behavioral, attitudinal, emotional, and interpersonal descriptors mentioned earlier in this chapter regarding symptoms of burnout.

Triage assessment for affect is 7 to 8. Although her outward demeanor is calm and collected, her affective responses are uncharacteristically angry and hostile for someone in the helping professions. Jane is using considerable effort to control her feelings. Coupled with the emotional exhaustion that is the most salient factor of burnout, she is close to being acutely depressed. This should come as no surprise, because depression and burnout often go hand in hand (Koutsimani et al., 2019; Richardson et al., 2020).

Cognitively, Jane is operating at a triage level of 6 to 7. Although Jane is thinking in a linear manner, her logic is twisted, and her belief system is severely compromised by obsessional self-doubt. She is manifesting a great deal of Ellis's (1973) "musturbatory" thinking and demonstrating another hallmark of burnout: a severe decline in her belief in her personal competence, along with depersonalization of her clients. Her complaints go beyond her job and indicate problems with social relationships, physical health, personal integrity, professional identity, belief system, and her total environment. Jane's total triage assessment scale score of 20 to 23 places her in the low to moderate marked impairment range. She is currently functioning between the frustration and apathy stage of burnout and is at a trait level where burnout has become pervasive across her environments. Without intervention, she is likely to move quickly into severe and lethal impairment.

Jane has done one thing right. She has gone to a significant other and is using that trusted other to self-disclose in a very intimate way some of her most troubled feelings (Maslach, 1976; Watkins, 1983). Because Jane's problems have spread out across her environment, the crisis worker will do exploratory counseling across BASIC IDS (Lazarus, 1976) components with the idea that no component of Jane's life is immune to the burnout currently assailing her.

Jane: All right, I can agree to a safety plan. I know that's part of the procedure. Hell, I guess I knew you'd do that when I came in here. Maybe I'm only kidding myself about all this anyway, just a bit of the blues, feeling sorry for myself, and all that crap.

CW: I'm glad you came here, for whatever reason, and I'm also glad you agree to our verbal contract even though you know it's part of the program. I also don't believe that about having the blues, either. I think it's much more than that. I believe right now you're hurting quite a bit. But first, I'd like to hear what you think and feel is going on in your life right now.

Intervention

While the crisis worker is acknowledging her regard for Jane, she is also doing quite a bit more. First, she has decided to take a pretty directive stance with Jane for the time being. The worker balances between making emotional challenges to the client and listening closely and accurately to Jane's problems. She also knows Jane is extremely astute at the business they are engaged in, as evidenced by her comment about the safety plan. She is not going to let Jane play the game ahead of her. Her analysis is that Jane is out of control right now. The crisis worker is therefore going to take control of the situation and will not sit back in a passive mode.

Jane: I don't know. I've dealt with all kinds of problems in my life, and right now there's nothing I can really put my finger on. In comparison to what is going on now, I can tell you that going through the divorce with Jeff, taking off on my own to finish up the doctorate, fighting my way up the ladder in the agency, and then finally making a decision to go out on my own while raising Bobby make what's happening to me now seem like peanuts.

CW: Right! Those were really tough times, and you went through those like Superwoman. But that was then, and we're right here, right now, and from the looks of it, you don't much feel like you're Superwoman, and what's happening in your life surely isn't peanuts, or we wouldn't be having this talk right now. So what do you feel like right now?

The crisis worker acknowledges how tough the client has been but will not let her get stuck in the past. The crisis worker wants to find out what is happening right now. What is more important about this now than it was a year ago? Furthermore, the crisis worker will not let the client discount the problem. It is interesting that if Jane were the counselor here, she would probably ferret out what she has just done—retreating into the past—in a second. The difference is that Jane has really become a client, and she is as unaware of the way she talks, thinks, and behaves as any other client. Jane being a therapist gives her no edge in dealing with her own problems. In fact, her own expertise may militate heavily against her (Kesler, 1990).

Jane: All I can tell you is I'm washed out. Like I get dates and appointments all mixed up. Last week topped that all off. I saw 44 clients last week. I think I got about a dozen appointments mixed up. My appointment book was really screwed up. It was a madhouse, and some of the people got agitated. Nothing like that ever happened before.

CW: Never?

Jane: Well, to a far lesser extent. I've been strung out before, but I could always get it straightened out.

CW: How?

Jane: About every 3 months things would start to get out of hand. I'd just sit back and say, "Janie, old girl, you've got to get out of here for a while." I'd just hop in the car and take off for a weekend in Chicago. Check into a hotel, take in a show, eat some really special meals, and use about half the hotel's hot water washing the clients off of me. Seems like that would clear the cobwebs out of my head.

CW: When was the last time you did that?

Jane: (wistfully) About 9 months ago.

CW: Why so long?

Jane: Well, I bought that new office and went in and remodeled the whole thing. I cut the contractor a deal. If I could work on it too, he'd reduce the price.

CW: So being the omnipotent individual you are, you threw out at least one thing that keeps you on an even keel. In fact, rather than getting away from the office, you've been spending almost all your time there. Let's see, we've got a couple of characters running around inside of Jane—Dr. Jane, healer to the world, and Jane the carpenter. Wonder who else is inside there?

The crisis worker is looking for a link between the past and the present. If Jane had some coping mechanisms in the past, what were they? She is specifically looking for coping mechanisms in the past that can be linked to the present and what is happening in the present to keep those coping mechanisms from being put into place. She is also beginning to build a character repertoire with Jane in the hope that Jane can start to see all the various aspects of herself that are now motivating her to do some of the things she does (Butts, 1996). To set the stage for the client regaining control of her life, the crisis worker proposes a positive character in Jane.

CW: I also heard a character that I'd call Janice, a person who knows when her stress bucket is full and is practical and smart enough to get away from the crap that goes on at that office. Where have you stuck her?

Jane: Back up on the shelf with Janie?

CW: Who's Janie?

Jane: She's the gal who is a little crazy, who can joke with her clients and get up in the middle of the night and go out and start seeding her lawn and sing Chuck Berry songs while she's doing it. (**embarrassed**) There's just no time for them right now. It's not just the new office, but I also needed another car, and since Bobby has changed schools there were a lot of added expenses in that. So, I really needed to devote my time to building my caseload up. If I can get through the next two years, I can breathe easier.

CW: Well, I'm sure glad to hear you're planning on being around for the next two years, anyway. But that's not the question now, is it, because right now it sounds to me as if you're wrung out. You don't have any more energy to give, and you've set up on the wall a couple of people who are pretty important in recharging your batteries. Do you see how important they are and what it has cost you to do that?

The crisis worker is not yet making direct suggestions as to what Jane needs to do; however, she is hoping to raise Jane's consciousness to the fact that she has unconsciously changed her operating method. The crisis worker attempts to get her to recognize this by describing what these very positive characters have

done for her. By doing so, the crisis worker is attempting to reintroduce some very healthy defense mechanisms that have previously helped Jane cope well with the stressful life she leads. Three major pathways that keep Jane in equilibrium are currently missing from her life: resiliency, self-management and self-care, and connection with others (Gentry et al., 2002). The crisis worker will attempt to reintegrate those into Jane's life.

Jane: I guess so, but I don't know how to get out of it.

CW: What will happen if you don't work on the office this next weekend?

Jane: The new plumbing isn't in. Clients wouldn't be able to use the bathroom. I'd also feel guilty for not working on it.

CW: (**laughing**) Well, the first part of that problem is pretty easily handled. Call the Porta-Potty people. I can imagine a sign that says, "The crap stops here," hanging from the door as clients walk in. (**Jane starts to smile and giggle for the first time since walking in the door.**) The other part of that is, who's the character laying a guilt trip on you? Tell me some more about her.

The crisis worker takes a little bit of a well-gauged risk here by injecting some humor into the situation (Moran, 2002). She does this because humor has been important in Jane's life, is helpful to her in coping, and turns her away from some of the cynicism she feels toward her clients and starts to allow her to laugh at herself a little. The ability to laugh at one's own foibles and some of the bizarre and ridiculously funny things that happen in our clients' lives cannot be overemphasized (Pines & Aronson, 1988, p. 154). Van Auken (1979) extols the judicious use of humor even in the most pathetic of situations. Getting a smile or a laugh from clients is a direct intrusion into the depressive thought processes and behaviors in which they are mired.

The crisis worker also starts to hammer a bit on Jane's guilt. Generally, the crisis worker sees guilt as a pretty useless emotion, consumptive of energy that could be used in other, more positive ways. Guilt is invariably an emotion of the past, and whatever was done can never again be retrieved. It is one thing to learn from one's past mistakes and quite another to carry past, unfinished business into the present, particularly when one is feeling guilty about not measuring up.

Jane: That's Mother Superior. I get all kinds of lectures from her. (**bitterly**) She's just like Sister Angeline at St. Mary's, where I went to school. "Say your Hail Marys and Our Fathers. Get your homework done. God doesn't like a shirker. Watch how you dress." Jesus, I hated that!

CW: You hate it, but it sure sounds like you're living it. Small wonder you're feeling so lousy.

The crisis worker starts hooking up feelings with thoughts and actions. The response the crisis worker gets indicates that the burnout has spread out into the client's family life.

Jane: You know, I think that's maybe why Bobby and I are having problems right now. I really sound and act like a Mother Superior to him. My Lord! He's 21 years old, and I've started treating him like he was a 6-year-old. He's about like some of those clients I have to lead around by the nose.

CW: Did you hear what you just said? "He's about like some of those clients I lead around." First of all, I didn't know that was the business you were in. Sounds like Jane the handywoman. Fix 'em up the way you do your office. Second, I wonder how many people outside the office you've decided to fix up and look out for. I have to tell you that's one of the kinds of feelings I've had around you lately.

With this information, the client gives the crisis worker a chance to plunge into some core issues that have definable behavioral outcomes. By stating how she deals with Bobby, Jane is manifesting another of the typical signs of burnout: trying to treat significant others in her life as if they were in a therapeutic situation (Van Auken, 1979). Her relationship with Bobby is extremely important because one way of decreasing burnout is to have a satisfying family life (Bakker et al., 2005; Halbesleben, 2006), especially with one's children (Forney et al., 1982). Worse yet is that she has become autocratic in the therapeutic situation, so it is not surprising that a major component of her life that has been highly reinforcing to her is no longer so and, in fact, has taken on some very negative connotations.

The crisis worker lays that squarely on her. She is mixing up her characters and has replaced Dr. Jane with Jane the handywoman. This state of events is not so surprising since both characters are working in the same office. Jane needs a break in her day-to-day activities and needs to get away from the office to do it (Forney et al., 1982).

Finally, the crisis worker relates and owns her own experience of having been treated the same way by Jane. She tries to make Jane aware that, like rings on a pond, the ripple effect from her burnout goes far beyond her immediate line of sight (Kesler, 1990).

CW: Indeed, I wonder about your relationships other than those with Bobby, myself, and your clients. Anyone else you're trying to control right now?

Jane: (**frostily**) If you mean men, absolutely no. When I get home at night, I'm so bushed all I want to do is fall asleep, but then all those clients go tumbling around in my head, and I start thinking about car payments, mortgage payments, how to straighten things out with Bobby, and I wind up getting about 2 or 3 hours of sleep a night.

CW: So right now you're so exhausted that you'd just rather be alone.

Jane: That's right, but I feel like I ought to be out mingling with people. I'm so damned isolated anyway.

CW: OK! I can understand that, and I'd agree with you, but let's look at right now. Seems as if you really need some time to just curl up in the fetal position, turn the electric blanket up to nine, and get your batteries recharged. Could you just go home and go to bed, put the answering service on until Monday, and not get up for the whole weekend?

Jane: I suppose.

CW: No supposes. If you don't want to do that, we'll look at something else. But right now, you look like *The Grapes of Wrath* and just seem to really need to rest before you think about doing anything else. Are you willing to call the contractor up and tell him you won't be there Saturday and Sunday without feeling guilty about it?

Jane: I could use the rest. All right! I'll give it this weekend.

CW: Fine. But there's one more thing. If you really get to feeling blue, plug the phone in and call me at home. I also want a report next week, so what time do you want to come in?

Jane: Sounds like I'm a client.

CW: Sounds like you're right. (**laughs**)

The crisis worker is basically assisting Jane to make a simple commitment to do one thing—get some rest. A critical component in treating burnout is revitalization (Tubesing & Tubesing, 1982, p. 160). Jane is physically fatigued, and the first order of business is to get her physical batteries recharged. A number of other options are available at this juncture, but the crisis worker follows Tubesing and Strosahl's (1976) advice to let the client make the choice of what treatment is appropriate. Keying on the client's own words about needing sleep, the crisis worker follows up and gains commitment to a specific behavior that the client will engage in over the short term. This is not a dramatic first step, but considering the least dramatic steps first is probably the way to go (Van Auken, 1979). The most important objective of this initial encounter is finding some short-term intervention techniques the client is able and willing to use (Freudenberger & Robbins, 1979).

A particular behavior the crisis worker touches on is the use of the telephone. Private practitioners are notorious for taking phone calls from clients at all hours of the night and on weekends. Van Auken (1979) urges human services workers not to let clients run—or, for that matter, ruin—their personal lives. The crisis worker makes sure that Jane follows this dictum, even though the crisis worker herself doesn't practice what she preaches, which leads one to wonder whom the crisis worker may soon need to be talking to about burnout. Finally, the worker provides emotional support, but once Jane is able to ventilate her feelings, the worker moves into a problem-solving mode.

The Next Week

Jane: I'll have to admit I do feel better. Couldn't sleep at all Friday night, but I got 10 hours in Saturday. I can't believe it! I woke up, and I was all curled up in the fetal position. The clients looked somewhat better this week. I can't say it was wonderful, but at least I wasn't an ogre to them. I guess what bothers me most about that is that I've lost all my creativity.

CW: OK! Let's talk about that a bit. You haven't been paying very much attention to the right side of your brain, so what do you expect? What could you do creatively that isn't client involved that'd get the right side of your head going again?

Jane: I've got a couple of articles I've been putting off—how about that?

CW: Got anything to do with clients?

Jane: Yes.

CW: Is that going to help you out?

Jane: I don't guess so, the same old stuff, only I'm writing about it.

CW: What else, then?

Forney et al. (1982) propose that a variety of professional activities may be an excellent coping mechanism; nevertheless, the crisis worker confronts Jane about this suggested alternative. The crisis worker is fairly sure that the client's stress bucket is full to the brim professionally. Jane needs to become less, not more, involved in her professional life.

Jane: Well, there is something else. I bought this sailboat for Bobby and me. The Coast Guard Auxiliary is putting on a sailing class. It would sure surprise Bobby if the next time he came home I could handle that Y-Flyer.

CW: Is that something you want to do? Would like to do it, not need to do it?

Jane: Yes!

CW: And not pile it on top of everything else. Really reserve some time for yourself to enjoy it.

Jane: You sure drive a hard bargain, but I can do it.

This is a wedge in the behavioral repertoire of the client that the crisis worker has been looking to find. Writer after writer in the burnout literature has promoted the use of leisure, particularly physical exercise, as a way of breaking up the dogmatic, work-brittle behavior of just going through the motions that often characterize the burned-out human services worker (Hoeksma et al., 1993; Melamed et al., 1995; Oerlemans & Bakker, 2014; Savicki & Cooley, 1982).

By proposing for the client a combination of leisure, physical exercise, and quality time with her son, the crisis worker has neatly integrated a number of positive interventions. The crisis worker is moving methodically around Myers and associates' Wellness Wheel (Myers et al., 2000; Myers & Sweeney, 2005), which has at its center spiritual self-direction, and which Dr. Jane is now mostly without. Specific spokes that radiate out from that wheel that the worker is attempting to put back in place in the client's life are nutrition, exercise, self-care, stress management, a sense of control, realistic beliefs, a sense of humor, renewed creativity, and awareness and coping across her entire ecosystem. With that many spokes missing, it is no surprise that Dr. Jane's psychological vehicle has about lost its spiritual axle as it careens down a crisis cliff that has become a burnout landslide of behavioral, physical, interpersonal, and attitudinal problems.

The crisis worker now takes on the main issue of the client's private practice.

CW: Fine. Let's talk about your practice for a while.

Jane: You know as well as I do about that. Sure, I've got a great caseload now. But who knows, it might dry up next week, and then where would I be?

CW: Has it ever dried up? Even in the last recession?

Jane: No, it hasn't, but I keep expecting the worst.

CW: You've been in private practice 8 years now, right? Has it ever been such that you didn't have enough clients to keep the wolves away from your door?

Jane: No. I guess there's something else. I feel a little foolish saying this, but it's almost like if I don't live up to my reputation and take on those really tough cases, I start feeling like I'm not the queen of the mountain. I mean, in the past I've been real proud of that, but now I don't seem to feel anything but that there's an albatross around my neck.

CW: Sounds like Superwoman again. I frankly admire you for dealing with those terminals' families, and you're right! Not many could do that. But if there's no intrinsic payoff, why are you fooling yourself into thinking you can heal the whole world? See the trap you've put yourself into?

Jane: Well, no! I guess I don't.

CW: OK! I want to try something. Maybe you've used it on some of your clients before. It's a game of "Who Told You?" I want you to move over to my chair and ask that empty chair, which will represent Jane, some questions. I'm going to stand aside and process as we go along, but it'll mostly be up to you. I want you to use all your insight as a therapist and really bore in and go to work on Jane's fictional goals, those crazy things she tells herself that have no counterpart in reality.

Jane as CW: (shifts chairs and gets a glitter in her eyes) OK, toots! Who told you you had to be Superwoman?

CW: Now shift back.

Jane: Nobody, really, I've just got a lot of responsibilities.

Jane as CW: Responsibilities, my foot! You've been going up that success ladder so fast you've scorched the rungs. Always got to show them. Be number one. My God! You little twerp. You're 43 years old, and you still think you're back on the VA ward.

Got to show them you're better than any man. Volunteer for the worst cases. Scared to death you won't succeed. And when you did, you were scared you wouldn't succeed the second time. Who told you that?

Jane: Nobody! It was reality. I had to be better than the men there.

Jane as CW: That was 20 years ago, nerd! The only men you deal with now are your clients. And that's another thing. Is that why you're so afraid of going out with any other man? And don't give me that stuff about getting burned again. You know why that divorce happened, and it sure doesn't have anything to do with having good social relationships now.

Jane: It's just that with the financial obligations for Bobby, I really don't have the time.

Jane as CW: (really angry and shouting) I won't have that! How long will you be responsible for him? He's 21 years old. Who supported you when you were 21? I'll tell you who. You did! You just use that as an excuse. Just like you use all those clients as an excuse. You don't fool me, you little martyr. Oh, sure! You get those strokes. (*dripping sarcasm*) Just like Annette here said, "I really admire you, Jane." You go around fooling everybody, but worst of all you fool yourself. Look at you. Sitting here the pathetic little wretch. You don't fool me. You're not little Miss Goody Two-Shoes. Behind all that depression is a really angry, bitter bitch who's always going around being everybody's servant. So just who told you you had to be that?

Jane: (Breaks and sobs. The CW goes to Jane, gathers her into her arms, and hugs her for dear life. Five minutes elapse.) Good Lord! I didn't realize that was all in there. I really got on a roll.

CW: Neither did I, but I figured if anybody could get it out, you could. What have you got out of that?

Jane: Besides spilling my guts, which I haven't done in 25 years, I see now how I got into this. I really set myself up.

CW: What do you want to do?

Jane: Well, I'm not going to kill myself, literally or figuratively. I've got some living to do, and although I'm not going to quit the practice, there sure are going to be some limits put on it.

The "Who Told You?" technique is a combination of Adlerian, rational-emotive behavior, and Gestalt therapy that is extremely powerful. Given a person with the kind of insight Jane has, it often has dramatic results in pointing out the way clients delude themselves. By using Jane as her own therapist, the crisis worker provides no one for the client to rationalize to, attack, manipulate, or otherwise attempt to fool but herself. For a person with Jane's abilities and insight, that seldom happens for very long. Underneath most depression lies anger. If that anger can be mobilized, then the client has taken a major step toward getting back into control of the situation. By putting Jane in a position to view her behavior from outside herself and also giving her a stimulus to attack her irrational ideas by the "Who Told You?" technique, the crisis worker provides an arena in which Jane can combat the apathy she is experiencing.

Such a dramatic shift to being mobile is uncommon among the general populace, and Jane's case is a condensed version of what may generally happen. The crisis worker often must provide the stimulus statements that are the core of clients' irrational ideas because of clients' poor cognition of their own negative self-talk. However, in dealing with highly trained professionals, it is not uncommon for such rapid shifts to occur.

Given the initial stimulus, they may pick up on the technique and provide their own dialogue with little or no help from the crisis worker. When emotional catharsis occurs, the crisis worker then takes a nondirective stance and serves as little more than a sounding board as their fellow professionals put reasonable parameters back into their lives. At that point, human services workers as clients tend to be able to make good decisions quickly about the behavioral, emotional, and cognitive aspects of their lives.

Indeed, if burnout syndrome is successfully overcome, it is not unreasonable to expect that human services workers will come back to their profession with hardier personalities, stronger commitments to self and profession, better self-temperance, a greater sense of meaningfulness, and increased vigor toward their environment (Kobasa, 1979). Furthermore, new coping styles that include greater self-awareness, increased self-insight, and a more direct approach to problem solving are likely to result for those who successfully navigate these treacherous waters (Cooley & Keesey, 1981). Finally, it is our own observation that human services professionals who have successfully conquered burnout respond not only to their work but also to their daily living with calmer and wiser choices, behaviors, and work style.

Vignette Summary

In this vignette the crisis worker uses the BASIC IDS model to deal with multiple, overlapping issues in the client's life (Kesler, 1990). Jane's workload affects her relationship with her family and friends. Her role as a mother affects her image of herself. Her image of herself affects her beliefs about her abilities as therapist and mother and, finally, affects her coping behaviors across the board. The crisis worker links all of these dimensions into a unified whole because each modality interacts with other modalities and should not be treated in isolation (Cormier & Cormier, 1985, p. 153). Jane's sailing expeditions not only will provide her with fun, relaxation, and togetherness with her son but also are as necessary to her therapeutic functioning as her doctoral training. Achieving balance among the various parts of her life and compartmentalizing them to the extent that they do not start to run into or over one another allow Dr. Jane Lee to be fully functioning in all of them and, at the same time, limit the stresses inherent in each (Pines & Aronson, 1988, p. 152). Oerlemans and Bakker (2014) have conducted a one-day-at-a-time plan that focused on physical vigor and cognitive liveliness through low-effort social and physical activities and got positive results on burnout reduction indicators. In other words, don't take your work home with you, and follow Glasser's theory (1985) and have some fun!

Webb (2007) has listed the following points that can help crisis workers who deal with traumatized children stave off vicarious traumatization, compassion fatigue, and ultimately burnout.

1. Pursue training and professional activities that promote learning. Keeping up in this business is important not only for the knowledge gained and skills learned but also for meeting other professionals and continuing to build a professional support system.

2. Work with a variety of clients and limit exposure to trauma in general. It is tempting to specialize in trauma work. Many crisis workers take pride in doing work not everyone can do. It is also an adrenaline rush and addictive. However, the old saying "Pride goeth before a fall" is true here. Varied client issues are not only a good way to keep the worker on their game but also provide relief from the constant grit and grind of trauma work.

3. Create boundaries between work and home, and maintain a personal identity. One of your authors is married to a middle school counselor. Do we

talk about our work? Yes! Do we talk about it all the time? Absolutely not! We leave most of it at the door. "It'll be there tomorrow" are words to live by.

4. Find professional friends who understand the stress of this business. You can't have too many professional friends and colleagues. One of your authors makes regular dates to watch baseball games with a psychologist who works at a VA hospital. We talk not only about psychology, but we also discuss theology and politics, watch baseball, eat peanuts, drink adult beverages, and sing "Take Me Out to the Ballgame" during the seventh inning stretch.

5. Spend time with people who are not in the throes of trauma recovery to maintain a balanced perspective of humanity. That's why it is important to get into a church, civic organization, fitness center, bridge club, model train club, or benevolent organization where there are just "regular" folks engaged in just "regular" activities.

6. Confront intrusive images and work through them. After reading this chapter, you should understand full well that if you start having pop-ups in your mind of the bad stuff you deal with or have nightmares about the stuff, don't punch it back as part of the job. Go get help.

7. Engage in activities that promote a sense of efficacy and empowerment. You may not decide to run for office as a U.S. senator, but getting involved in a community action program or government committee is an excellent way of feeling empowered and helping promote causes that give you a sense of self-esteem.

8. Engage in your own psychotherapy. While we do not advocate becoming your own "shrink," what is meant by this point is knowing yourself. Knowing your psychological strengths and weak points

is critical in this work. Practicing **mindfulness** techniques by increasing awareness and acceptance of feelings and body states and gently letting go allows one to preempt stress as it starts to arise and ameliorate it when it's present. Research (Decker et al., 2015; Felton et al., 2015; Thieleman & Cacciatore, 2014; Thompson et al., 2014) has shown that practicing mindfulness has positive effects on decreasing CF and increasing CS.

9. Get supervision from somebody who knows their business about crisis and trauma work. Your bartender, hairdresser, minister, golfing buddies, or book club members are fine to talk with, but they are the "regular" folks up in point 5. You do need somebody who knows this business and how to effectively supervise you as you do it.

The foregoing is all well and good at prevention, but what if you wind up with a good dose of burnout? In the case of Dr. Jane, you can see the interventionist using an integrative approach with a variety of therapeutic techniques tailored to major maladaptive behaviors that drive the burnout. The question becomes then, do you have to be a master of all these different therapeutic approaches, or is there a magic bullet therapeutic approach that will get the job done? The majority of current research studies on treatment of burnout have been on the use of Acceptance and Commitment Therapy and Mindfulness techniques to reduce burnout symptoms. Studies employing mindfulness (Kinnunen et al., 2020; Sopezski et al., 2020) and Acceptance and Commitment therapy (Ahola et al., 2017; Oro, 2021; Perski et al., 2017; Prudenzi et al., 2021; Towey et al., 2022) seem to support a reduction in stress symptoms, but the overall ability to reduce burnout symptoms is less clear. So, we can finish this chapter by saying the old proverb that an ounce of prevention is probably worth a pound of cure.

Summary

Burnout is not simply a sympathy-eliciting term to use when one has had a hard day at the office. It is a very real malady that strikes people and can have extremely severe consequences. It is prevalent in the human services professions because of the kinds of clients, environments, working conditions, and resultant stresses that are operational there. Because of the intense and stressful nature of crisis intervention, a major contributor to burnout is constant exposure to clients who have had horrific experiences.

Prolonged exposure can induce what is variously called *vicarious traumatization, compassion fatigue, or secondary traumatization* in the crisis worker. No one particular individual is more prone to experience burnout than another. However, by their very nature, most human services workers tend to be highly committed to their profession, and such commitment is a necessary precursor to burnout. Private practitioners may experience burnout even more severely than their counterparts in organizations because of their professional isolation. All human services workers, public or private, tend to be unable to identify the problem when it is their own. No one is immune to its effects.

Burnout moves through stages of enthusiasm, stagnation, frustration, and apathy. In its end stage, burnout is a crisis situation. The crisis takes many forms. It can be manifested behaviorally, physically, interpersonally, and attitudinally. It pervades the professional's life and can have effects on clients, coworkers, family, friends, and the organization itself.

Recognition of the beginning symptoms of burnout can alleviate its personal and organizational ramifications. Raising consciousness levels in regard to the dynamics of burnout in training programs and conducting on-the-job workshops are important ways of halting and ameliorating its effects. Support groups within the organization that provide instrumental and emotional resources to victims are important. In the past, burnout has been regarded as a malady that resides only within the individual. That view is archaic. Burnout should also be viewed in a systems perspective and as an organizational and cultural problem. At its end stage, burnout is a crisis situation that calls for immediate, direct, and reality-oriented therapeutic intervention. Given corrective remediation, victims of burnout can return to the job and again become productive.

No Man's Land
Facing Disaster

The last part of this book refers back to the World War I term used to describe the desolate land between the two opposing armies. In a similar way, the chaos that greets survivors and first responders of disasters is very much like the desolate, wrecked landscape that lies between two battle lines in trench warfare. Pictures of the wildfire that swept over Maui in August 2023 and obliterated the historic town of Lahaina show the destruction that results from disasters. Well more than 100 people died; burnt out cars on the streets and buildings with nothing left except a few cinder blocks stacked together show an almost total devastation. Undoudtably by the time you read the following chapter other disaster such as earthquakes, tornadoes, and mass-shooting will have occurred. Some will involve destruction of property and others loss of life. Another disaster always seems to be just around the corner in a manner of speaking.

The final chapter of this book is divided into two parts. The first part deals with how the system operates in response to a disaster. Large-scale crises can never be taken out of the context of their systemic impact. The second part deals with the people who go into that no man's land and the survivors who are there to greet them. It is our belief that a lot of you who aspire to a career in this field will be going into wrecked landscapes like this. The experiences of several professional counselors are used while responding to several disasters for which they provided services. Although other disasters have occurred since then, their feelings, behavior, and thinking are still relevant.

When a disaster occurs, many of you using this book will want to respond. You got into this business because you are caring and want to share that with those in need. Before jumping on the band wagon and traveling across the country to assist survivors, we encourage you to reflect on yourself. Not everyone is cut out to provide services in the aftermath of disasters. Likely, you will encounter many problems you had no idea even existed. Some may be mental health in nature while others logistical. Logistical issues generally involve day-to-day functioning. You might be sleeping in a gymnasium on a cot with a 100 other people in the room. Shower facilities may not be all that private. What about meals? Well let's say you will not be eating at five, four-, three-, two-, or one-star restaurants. Maybe not much better than what you get at a local fast-food restaurant drive through. When talking with survivors, you probably will not be in a room with four walls and comfortable chairs. In fact, at times, you may find yourself at a picnic table listening to survivors. And there probably will not be any tree shading it. We say this not to scare you off but to help you be prepared for this type of crisis intervention. Key to doing this work is being prepared and taking care of yourself. The common-sense advice of eating properly, getting enough sleep, and finding time to relax is critical. Make sure you do this.

Disaster Response 16

Learning Objectives

After studying this chapter, you will be able to:

1. Identify the types of disaster and general crisis response to them.
2. Describe the history and development of disaster mental health relief in the United States.
3. Discuss the status of disaster mental health in the world.
4. Identify the part ecosystems play in crisis intervention.
5. Explain what National Crisis Response Teams are and do.
6. Explain what a disaster mental health plan entails.
7. List what crisis workers do in a disaster.
8. Explain how multiculturally competent crisis workers operate in a disaster.
9. Describe how the crisis worker handles spiritualism and religion in disasters.
10. Discuss the principles and techniques of debriefing.

Types of Disasters

LO1 Throughout this chapter, we will be referring to many different disasters. Some disasters have occurred in the past few years, while others occurred over a decade ago. Although somewhat dated, a good portion of the chapter focuses on the terrorist attacks on 9/11 and Hurricane Katrina. The two disasters, each in their own way, brought out the best of people wanting to help survivors but also some of the failures and cracks in the way systems respond. The systemic breakdowns were a catalyst to learn and do better the next time a disaster occurs.

The human impact of every disaster is unique, and the destruction distinct. Some disasters are natural, resulting from hurricanes, earthquakes, floods, tornados, and so on. Other disasters are caused by humans and are commonly referred to as manmade disasters. Examples of these include mass shootings (which seem to occur almost daily in the United States), building collapses, bombings of buildings, and accidents involving trains or airlines. Finally, in this section, we discuss what is considered a megacrisis. This type of disaster is so devastating it changes the way the world, and we mean everyone in the world, functions on a day-to-day basis. Understanding the types and general reactions helps in providing services in the wake of disasters.

Natural Disasters. Natural disasters are many times unpredictable and come with fierce quickness with little to no warning. The series of catastrophic tornadoes that hit the Southeast United States on April 27, 2011, is an example. These tornadoes caused 316 deaths, 2,400 injuries, and over $4.2 billion in damages (Hayes, 2011). Earthquakes also happen suddenly and without forewarning but are over quickly, many times resulting in injury, property damage, and, unfortunately, sometimes death (Mirhashemi et al., 2007). The Napa Valley earthquake of August 24, 2014, is a perfect example, causing an estimated $352 million in damage. Survivors of this disaster had to navigate streets worried about trees falling, power lines snapping, lack of water and sewage facilities, and continued anxiety and stress about earthquake aftershocks. A more recent example is the September 2023 earthquake in Morocco resulting in over 2,000 people dying and another 2,000 injured. The recovery from this disaster will take years as the people adjust and adapt to their new reality.

Other natural disasters like floods seem to creep up slowly, resulting in billions of dollars of damage each year. Survivors of this type of flood have commonly said that initially, they were not worried. However, as the water continued to inch higher and higher, they became increasingly scared and even panicked, worried that their home would eventually be swamped, and rescue would be impossible. Adding to their fear was a sense of helplessness to do anything. To the contrary, flash floods range from Southern New England into Tennessee, as far north as Minnesota, and all the way to Arizona. Other floods come suddenly, like the Buffalo Creek Flood of 1972 in West Virginia (Rosenfield et al., 2010) and the Johnstown Flood of 1977, which was caused by over 11 inches of rain falling in 10 hours, resulting in six dams collapsing (Spencer & Myer, 2007a). Each flood took its human and physical toll, causing many people to lose their homes, numerous businesses to cease to exist, and mass financial strain to be put on families (Spencer & Myer, 2007b). Li et al. (2022) predict that the number of flash floods will increase in the foreseeable future, meaning you may be asked to provide services helping survivors of those floods, such as the current inundation of Vermont as of this writing.

Hurricanes are another disaster that, because of advances in radar, can be predicted (La Greca & Prinstein, 2002). Hurricanes start slowly with wind and rain then build in strength, seeming to arrive abruptly with a furious brutality unmatched by other disasters. Hurricane Maria pummeled Puerto Rico in September 2017. Numerous federal agencies and nongovernmental organizations were called on to help in the recovery process (McLeod, 2022). Hurricane Fiona hit the island in 2022 and staggered the recovery process both in terms of physical and emotional recovery. Hurricanes disrupt families' lives, and the property damage from these storms is almost unimaginable (Rosenfeld et al., 2010).

The perception is that natural disasters are "Acts of God" for which only the minimum can be done in the way of prevention (Myers & Wee, 2005), leaving people with a sense of helplessness (Halpern & Tramontin, 2007). Granted, earthquake proof buildings can be constructed, homes erected outside of flood plains, and infrastructure created that mitigates the effects (Dass-Brailsford, 2010). Yet, these efforts only lessen the effect; they do not prevent the disaster. Being aware of this reaction is key to providing services (Myer, 2015). Survivors' experience also has a direct influence on reactions to disasters. For example, even though Hurricane Ian was predicted to be a Category 5, "Crisis Case Handling," in 2022, many people who had been through storms previously refused to leave their homes, instead deciding to ride out Ian. Typical comments discounted the potential danger, saying, "I've been through this before," "It will not be that bad," or similar comments. Ian did monstrous property damage, and 27 people lost their lives. Age also influences survivors' reactions (Myers & Wee, 2005). Children might become preoccupied with details, while teens can be overlooked because they react with a sense of invulnerability (Rosenfeld et al., 2010). Adults might feel more of a sense of responsibility resulting from natural disasters. For disaster counselors, these issues should be addressed as part of the process for helping survivors.

Humanmade Disasters. Disasters resulting from some type of human error, action, or inaction have historically been referred to as "Manmade Disasters." These disasters result from human decisions or negligence (Myers & Wee, 2005) and come as a surprise with little to no warning. Individuals failing to turn on or off a gas line or coolant system might cause pressure to build, resulting in an explosion. Other decisions made months and even years before may result in a disaster (Shaluf, 2007). An example might be cutting corners on materials, making a building unsafe after being used for a period of time. Experts state the Champlain Tower South building collapse in Surfside, Florida, was a "progressive collapse," occurring because of numerous factors, including design flaws and less robust construction codes in effect at the time the building was built (Glanz et al., 2021).

Negligence also carries with it the potential for disasters. Two examples are maintenance schedules being ignored or production procedures not being followed. Carelessness of this nature hypothetically can be the root of some humanmade or technological disasters. Although the investigation is not complete, preliminary evidence for the May 28, 2023, collapse of the building in Davenport, Iowa, in which at least three people died, suggests negligence in maintenance was a factor.

A distinctive attribute of manmade disasters is their unpredictability. Transportation accidents or toxic spills, airline accidents, nuclear catastrophes, dam breaks, and other similar events do not occur on a set schedule. Humanmade disasters have a strong possibility of leading to linked disasters that may be years in the making. The Chernobyl and Fukushima nuclear accidents in 1986 and 2011, respectively, have affected and will continue to affect the regions in which they occurred for years. Nuclear accidents and other toxic spills might cause cancer years after the disaster (Halpern & Tramontin, 2007).

Drawing conclusions about the psychological effects of manmade disasters is difficult because each is so different (Myers & Wee, 2005). While debated, many people believe that manmade disasters have the potential to cause more distress than natural disasters (Halpern & Tramontin, 2007). The speculation is that the reason for the increased distress is that the disaster could have been prevented (Myers & Wee, 2005). For crisis intervention, helping survivors search for explanations while finding meaning in what happened prior to, during, and after the disaster is paramount (Webb, 2004). For many survivors, finding meaning will be like trying to fit a square peg into a round hole or the other way around. No matter what explanations are used, a perfect fit will never be found. A critical factor for survivors making meaning of the disaster is time (Myer & Moore, 2006). Making meaning does not happen overnight, rather, this process evolves over time. As a crisis interventionist, you may be involved at the start but not the end of the process.

Megacrisis. Megacrisis is like a disaster on steroids, blanketing the world with changes in the way everything is done. Boin et al. (2021) write that the way people work, play, interact with others, shop, travel, and just about anything else you can imagine, change as the result of a megacrisis. Although not the first megacrisis, in 2020, the unthinkable disaster of the COVID-19 virus changed the world (Helsloot, 2021). Other megacrises of this magnitude are the Black Plague in 1347, the flu epidemic from 1918 to 1920, and the 1952 polio epidemic. Each of these changed the way people lived on a day-to-day basis. Some megacrises are not health-related but still change the way the world

functions. The much-debated climate crisis is an example. Weather patterns are changing. Tornadoes now regularly strike in places that, 50 years ago, never or rarely experienced them. Droughts, excessive rain, and hurricanes are intensifying. Earlier, we reported about the increase in flash floods in the United States, causing devastation. Wildfires are at an all-time high. The smoke from Canadian wildfires in May and June 2023 blanketed the Eastern coast of the United States, resulting in sporting events being canceled, schools going back to remote learning, and people being cautioned to stay inside because breathing the smoke for a day was comparable to smoking from a half to a full pack of cigarettes per day. Whether or not climate change is permanent or will fade is not the issue. The drastic changes in weather patterns are changing people's lives.

The field of mental health drastically changed as a result of the COVID-19 megacrisis (Costa et al., 2021). Providing services transitioned from mostly in-person to mostly using technology, including phones, video conferencing, texting, and other communication platforms. This shift meant developing protocols ensuring client confidentiality and changing assessment techniques and intervention strategies (Emergence Health Network interview, November 2022). The effect on crisis intervention mirrored the changes in providing everyday mental health services. During this time, personally distancing was observed whenever possible, and face masks used. It is unlikely you will be called and asked to volunteer by the Red Cross or other organizations that respond to a megacrisis. But you will encounter clients in crisis that are linked to the megacrisis.

A Brief History of Disaster Mental Health Provision

LO2 When the first edition of this book was published in 1988, it didn't have a chapter on disaster response. The simple reason was that we would have been hard pressed to fill up three pages of print on theory, research, or practice with regard to the provision of mental health services after a large-scale disaster. Although the federal government has been involved in disaster relief since the nineteenth century, until recently, it has paid very little attention to the psychological aftershocks of a disaster. It wasn't until 1974, as part of a major overhaul of disaster policy, that the Disaster Relief Act was passed. In that bill was section 413, which authorized the National Institute of Mental Health (NIMH) to supply counseling services to victims of disasters and also provided funds to train professionals in the provision of mental health services to disaster victims. The need for services in the aftermath of disasters has steadily increased over the years. In 2022, the death toll worldwide from natural disasters was 3,100, while in the United States, the toll was 474 (Statista, 2023: USA Facts, 2023). Hundreds of thousands of other people surviving the disasters were affected. These staggering numbers reveal the overwhelming need for support during the recovery period.

We believe the notion that people would need mental health assistance after a disaster has roots similar to those of the crisis movement itself. It appears that at least four distinct variables fell into place prior to 2000 to make this happen. First was the birth of community mental health, authorized by the Community Mental Health Act of 1963, which put mental health workers in underserved areas like Rapid City, South Dakota; Wilkes-Barre, Pennsylvania; and Logan County, West Virginia. These were "hometown" folks, not bureaucrats in some far away capital city, and they would give voice to the misery, both psychological and physical, survivors were suffering after a large-scale natural disaster.

Second was the classification of posttraumatic stress disorder (PTSD) as a personality disorder in the DSM-III in 1980. That medical classification acknowledged and legitimized the concept of people suffering enduring mental problems after direct exposure to a life-threatening event. That diagnosis can admirably fit survivors of disasters.

Third was the American Red Cross's decision in the early 1990s to establish a mental health certification program after Hurricane Hugo and the Loma Prieta earthquake in 1989. Indeed, the American Red Cross separated out disaster mental health from its disaster nursing mainly because of its workers breaking down from prolonged field placements in the back-to-back disasters of Hurricane Hugo and the Loma Prieta earthquake (Morris, 2011).

Fourth was the women's movement during the 1960s and '70s, which brought increased awareness of how often trauma strikes families and what its aftershocks do to a family whose entire belongings have been swept, blown, or burned away. When combined, these variables would play a major role in moving the concept of disaster mental health from an idle backwater into a tsunami of disaster mental health assistance in 2011. Given that movement, you are now going to read a whole lot more in this ninth edition

than the few pages we might have scraped together in the first edition back in 1987.

If you harken back to Chapter 1, "Approaching Crisis Intervention," where we talked about the coalescing of grassroots movements into a large voice that attracts attention from the media and, soon after, legislatures, you will begin to understand why specific places like Rapid City, South Dakota; Wilkes-Barre, Pennsylvania; and Logan County, West Virginia, became important players in the birthing of disaster mental health. All three of these places suffered terrible flooding in 1972, and Logan County became particularly notorious because of a mining company's failure to maintain the Buffalo Creek dam, which ruptured. The resulting flood waters at Buffalo Creek killed 125 people and wrecked or badly damaged 1,500 homes. To make matters worse, God or Mother Nature didn't cause the disaster, but the coal company did, so there was someone to focus attention on that could have prevented the disaster.

Local mental health providers were overwhelmed by survivors needing psychological assistance in all three places, and both state and federal officials were slow to react in providing help. This issue caught the eyes and ears of reporters, and a great deal of publicity was garnered in support of providing mental health assistance to disaster survivors. So, legislators who were already attuned to the notion that survivors would need psychological help thought it made good common sense (and particularly good reelection sense) to include mental health funding in the 1974 bill.

Although now we know that psychological intervention would be helpful, 50 years ago, research on the need for psychotherapy or counseling following disasters was minimal. But that made little difference given the publicity these three floods received. The few mental health workers that were on scene and their cries for help made good subjects for interviews. One of the best examples of how well disaster mental health assistance could be played in the media was the San Fernando Child Guidance clinic that decided to treat trauma after an earthquake struck the San Fernando Valley in California in 1971. The clinic announced that they were offering counseling services for children who had been in the quake area. Over the next few weeks, they counseled more than 500 children in the quake area and got the attention of the national media, which generated headlines like "Quake proofing kids." Dr. Stephen Howard, director of clinical services, got nationwide attention when he declared in an interview with the *New York Times* that the American Red Cross's attitude of "keeping a stiff upper lip" wouldn't work and that survivors needed to "talk about their issues" (Morris, 2011).

Return now to Rapid City, South Dakota. The local government's small number of overwhelmed mental health professionals and the federal government's lack of interest in the survivors' plight prompted a call for help from a steering committee organized by the local mayor that reached all the way to the Denver, Colorado, office of the National Institute of Mental Health (NIMH). The NIMH finally responded by sending psychiatric help to the beleaguered city. The problems of adequate mental health provision that were uncovered at Rapid City motivated U.S. senators from the state to become very active in funding these provisions for the Disaster Recovery Act.

In Wilkes-Barre, a model program developed by local community mental health providers and the NIMH served as a blueprint for the creation of disaster mental health programs. Called Operation Outreach, one component of this program was the training of outreach workers to go out and meet survivors as they tried to reassemble their lives and provide basic mental health services. Their initial attempts to provide those services were not accepted kindly by the survivors until the workers started giving them assistance in getting the basic necessities of living back in their lives. Then, the survivors started to take them into their confidence. Please note that this is a hard lesson to learn for zealous mental health practitioners who volunteer to go to a disaster. Like the workers at Wilkes-Barre and Dr. Holly Branthoover, whom you will get to meet later in the chapter, it is about moving boxes, procuring lice kits, and having your underarm deodorant fail before you ever get to the counseling stage.

Finally, rescue workers in the Buffalo Creek dam failure in Logan County noticed many of the symptoms in survivors that would later be formalized into PTSD criteria. The resulting lawsuit against the mining company whose failed dam had caused the Buffalo Creek disaster brought a number of famous mental health experts into the courtroom. One of them was Robert Lofton, a psychiatrist from Yale, who had done extensive study on Vietnam veterans and would later lay the foundation blocks for what would become PTSD from his work with them. He recognized some of the same pathology in the flood survivors and testified that everybody in Buffalo Creek was affected (Morris, 2011).

A group of people from all three of these disasters were gathered by the medical advisor to the Office of Emergency Preparedness (then the leader in disaster mitigation). There was general agreement that there was not a large outbreak of mental illness, but it was acknowledged that the emotional security of a large number of individuals had been compromised (Morris, 2011). Thus was born the Disaster Relief Act of 1974. This act then evolved into the Stafford Disaster Relief and Emergency Assistance Act of 1986, with section 416 providing for enhanced mental health services to disaster survivors.

To really understand why mental health generally did not get front row status for a long time, you need to understand that the U.S. government's historical approach to disasters was piecemeal and spread over a variety of agencies. It wasn't until 1978 that the Federal Emergency Management Agency (FEMA) was authorized. It absorbed a variety of agencies that ranged from insurance to weather prediction to civil defense to dam and building safety to counterterrorism. It essentially became a catchall for everything that might create some kind of disaster in the United States. After 9/11, FEMA itself was absorbed into the Department of Homeland Security, becoming the Department of Emergency Preparedness and Response Directorate, which pretty much put FEMA in the back seat politically, financially, and prioritywise. After the debacle of Hurricane Katrina, FEMA once again regained stand-alone status as a department. So, it is not just mental health that has been given short shrift, but the overall coordination of natural and human-made disasters in the United States. So, why has all this now changed?

Since 1974, there has been a huge change as the human impact of disaster is better understood (Mageletta et al., 2022). Today, psychological services and the people who provide them are seen as an integral part of disaster intervention by the federal government (Dodgen & Meed, 2010). The trauma business meandered along in the 1990s, but school shootings such as Marjory Stoneman Douglas High School in Parkland, Florida, and Sandy Hook Elementary School in Newtown, Connecticut, along with the Virginia Tech University massacre, highlighted the need for intervention services. The 2012 Colorado movie theater shooting in Aurora focused attention on disaster in suburbia, and the carnage of 9/11 put trauma back in the limelight on the national marquee. The horrific foul-ups by FEMA during Hurricane Katrina sealed the notion that mental health would be an important part of any disaster in the twentieth century in the United States.

In the aftermath of Katrina, the government poured $52 million for mental health support into Project Recovery in Mississippi, Project Rebound in Alabama, and Louisiana Spirit in Louisiana. That sum of money was second only to the $132 million that went in to mental health services after 9/11 (Morris, 2011).

The emerging concern is how very large intervention systems interact with one another to deal with large-scale crises and megacrises that may arise at the national, state, or community level and directly or indirectly affect neighborhoods, families, and, ultimately, the individual. Part of the problem is that crisis response systems have not been upgraded along with the times. Remember from Chapter 1, "Approaching Crisis Intervention," that large disaster relief systems in the United States that are designed to physically aid communities after catastrophes are about 100 years old (Echterling & Wylie, 1999). The field of individual crisis intervention as it is applied in a scientific and systematic manner is about 80 years old (Lindemann, 1944). Systematic and comprehensive intervention by the United States government is about 45 years old (FEMA, n.d.). The addition of psychological crisis intervention systems and their incorporation into those large macrosystems is about 35 years old—if we are very generous in our time estimation.

While there has been a great deal of research since 9/11 on the kinds of mental health interventions and techniques that work on individuals (Watson et al., 2011; White et al., 2022), very little research in large-scale **ergonomics** has been conducted. Cognitive and organizational ergonomics is the rather interesting scientific discipline concerned with understanding the interactions among humans and other elements of a system. It is the profession that applies theory, principles, data, and methods to product design to optimize human well-being and overall system performance—which also applies to coordinating, collaborating, and allocating resources after a disaster.

System interfaces with individuals and ergonomics are pretty cerebral as well as seemingly unusual and not likely to be the topic of discussion over coffee at Starbucks or beer at a sports bar. Therefore, understanding how those systems work, the effects they have in the fight against terrorism, in large-scale natural disasters, and the mental health issues that go with them is critically important (Nickerson, 2011). In a compelling article on this subject, Nickerson (2011) points out that his literature search turned up very little on how ergonomics could help deal with the effects of terrorism when they occur. That research is compelling because, over and over, communication between human beings operating in different systems becomes problematic.

Former members of the 9/11 Commission, meeting on the 10th anniversary of that act of terrorism, stated that there were still problems of communication among first responders (Callahan, 2011). Although much progress has been made since that report, these issues remain a concern. Take, for example, the failure of communication in Uvalde, Texas during the shooting at Ross Elementary School. First responders were notified and responded very quickly, yet communication on the scene broke down and over an hour went by before any action was taken. In most disasters, communication has improved, but there is always more that can be done when going back and analyzing what worked and what could be improved.

Further, research is sparse on the way large systems work—or, in fact, whether they do work—in a palliative psychological manner with various subsystems or individuals (Dziegielewski & Powers, 2005; Litz & Gibson, 2006). Some research is beginning to be conducted on vicarious victimization on the responses by first responders (Gho et al., 2020; Hallinan et al., 2021; Molnar et al., 2017). Other research is examining the need of wireless methods and social media for communication to prepare for and in the aftermath of disaster (Aten et al., 2011). However, the manner in which systems communicate with one another and understanding the effects of rapid changes in technological, geophysical, and societal forces on prevention, intervention, and postvention are key issues in the mitigation of a disaster (Aten et al., 2011; Stokols et al., 2009).

To the contrary, research into evidence-based posttrauma practices for individuals has exploded since 9/11 in the quest to find the best way to help people with mental health issues postdisaster (Watson et al., 2011; White et al., 2022). The acronym PTSD was known to very few people in the first edition of this book in 1988—including our students! PTSD has become a household abbreviation used by traumatized individuals and has become a well-known go-to label by people outside the human service field. PTSD is thought to explain any and all ill effects following a crisis or traumatic experience. This misuse has been a catalyst for professional organizations to ramp up their focus on trauma. Public news media uses the term at the drop of a hat following almost any traumatic experience, such as mass shootings, hurricanes, floods, tornadoes, building collapses, and so on. Division 56, Trauma Psychology, has been formed by the American Psychological Association and is one of its fastest-growing divisions. The Council on Accreditation of Counseling and Related Educational Programs (CACREP), the accrediting body for counselors, has mandated crisis intervention as part of a required curriculum, as has the National Association of School Psychologists. Many professional organizations have published psychoeducational materials that range from mental health reactions after a disaster to providing schools with memorial guides. Substance Abuse Mental Health Services Administration (SAMHSA), has numerous resources available to the public addressing mental health issues related to disasters (SAMHSA, 2023).

Where the World Is

LO3 The United States is not alone in its changed attitudes toward mental health provision after a natural disaster. Australia has been one of the leaders in the area because of the many natural disasters it has faced. Beverly Raphael, a professor of psychiatry in Australia, has been at the forefront of disaster research and practice with her landmark books *The Anatomy of Bereavement (1984), When Disaster Strikes* (1986), and *Disaster Response Handbook* (2000), and dozens of research articles, chapters, and edited books on trauma and disaster.

Europe has established the European Network for Traumatic Stress (TENTS, 2011) in response to a need for consensus on what evidenced-based outcomes work. TENTS has been funded by the European Union (EU) and has built Europewide networks of expertise in the psychosocial management of victims of natural and other disasters. It provides services, expertise, and support to areas of the Union that lack resources and the availability of trained personnel (TENTS, 2011).

Internationally, the United Nations' Inter-Agency Standing Committee (IASC, 2007) has published *IASC Guidelines on Mental Health and Psychosocial Input Support in Emergency Situations*. Those guidelines are being used by countries as small and remote as Nepal to put into operation their disaster responses (Jordans et al., 2010).

International Terrorism and Human-Made Disasters

The ecological, contextual model of crisis intervention, based on the ecosystem theory that has emerged on the international scene, is characterized by continuously accelerating events in dynamically changing cultures and environments (Conyne et al., 2003; James et al., 2003; James & Gilliland, 2003, pp. 341–342; Myer & Moore, 2006; Norris et al., 2006). Foremost among these events in the United States has been the September 11, 2001, hijackings and terrorist attacks, the destruction of the World Trade Center (WTC) towers in New York City, the attack on the Pentagon, and the crashed airliner in Pennsylvania. These tragedies caused untold grief, loss of property, loss of life, economic damage, and a change in the attitudes of most Americans regarding safety and security (Bass & Yep, 2002; Pyszczynski et al., 2002). The actions following 9/11 also set in motion other unprecedented events, such as the passage of the Homeland Security Act by the U.S. Congress and the invasions of Afghanistan and Iraq, and placed security in the United States at wartime levels. Practically every American had the feeling of having been individually attacked (Brainerd, 2002) and that many were, indeed, at war.

Add to 9/11 other terrifying events—the bombing of the Murrah Federal Building in Oklahoma City, the mass shooting in Uvalde, Texas in which 19 children and 2 adults lost their lives, the shooting at the Pulse Nightclub in Orlando with the loss of 49 lives, the shooting in Pittsburgh that killed 11 at the Tree of Life synagogue, the Monterey Park shooting in which 12 people were killed, the Route 91 Harvest music festival in Las Vegas where 60 people were killed and another 400 plus were injured, and the killing of students at too many universities to name. There is good reason for most Americans to think the United States is no longer a sanctuary but a battleground. Across the world, events such as the taking of hostages by Chechens and their resulting deaths in a rescue attempt in a Moscow theater and a southern Russian school, Palestinian suicide bombings in the streets of Israel, Muslim radicals' bombing of a nightclub and hotel in Bali and Jakarta and trains in Madrid, the Charlie Hebdo magazine attack in Paris, the assassination of armed services recruiters in Chattanooga, Tennessee, drug cartel wars in Mexico that approach total war, embassies and nightclubs blown up in Africa and Asia by al Qaida, and the postwar chaos in Iraq and Afghanistan, all send clear messages that the world is a dangerous place where terror may strike unannounced anywhere and at any time. As a result, the hypervigilance of being constantly on guard, the economic loss because of these attacks, and the social and financial expenses of guarding against them cause a variety of previously unknown stressors to appear that impact and crosscut entire nations, cultures, and ecosystems.

Disaster in the form of terrorism has its own special brand of traumatic wake for survivors and has the potential to have metastasizing effects across large systems (Lee et al., 2022). This is true because of the unpredictability of when, where, and to whom it will happen. Further, the seeming randomness creates fear and anxiety because there is no assurance that it will not happen again, and where it could happen is anybody's guess. The use of insidious means such as poison gas, germ warfare, or nuclear arms causes horror and incredulity at their seemingly immoral use in the business of mass murder. Information is often inaccurate or highly controlled by the government, which creates uncertainty and anxiety. Increased, constant hypervigilance creates constant and heightened anxiety, which causes both immediate and long-term physical health problems.

Media coverage enhances the horror of gruesome death, and injuries have increased during the past 20 years (Felix et al., 2020). Constant viewing of scenes of death and destruction increases trauma risk. Further compounding the trauma is the aftermath of the terrorist attack with ruinous financial loss and frustration and anxiety at the government's inability to act or bring the perpetrators to justice—particularly when they are outside the country's borders. Finally, there is the added difficulty of finding victim services and mental health professionals who have the know-how to deal with the unique issues that terrorism victims bring with them (Dziegielewski & Sumner, 2005; Myers & Wee, 2005, pp. 247–248). Pastel and Ritchie (2006) aptly call these weapons of mass *disruption* because of the profound psychological ripple effects they cause.

The Israelis are no strangers to terror. Practically all Israeli children carry cell phones so they can immediately contact their parents and let them know they are safe after bombings or rocket attacks. It is somewhat chilling that one of the favorite children's costumes during the Israeli Purim holiday among ultraorthodox Jews was a replica of the "Zaka" uniform. Zaka is an ultraorthodox volunteer organization dedicated to ensuring proper burial according to Jewish rituals. In the immediate aftermath of a terrorist attack, they search for body parts to bring as much of the body as possible to burial (Galai-Gat, 2004). After Galai-Gat delivered the paper just cited at the Annual Convening of Crisis Intervention Personnel, she related how amazed she was that people could come and go so freely from the downtown Chicago hotel where the convention was being held. Thus, in a changing world, the question arises, "As go the Israelis, shall the rest of the world go also, and does our mental health system go with it?"

Terrorism brings unique challenges to mental health professionals when weapons of mass destruction are used (Lee et al., 2022; White et al., 2022). The ratio of physically dead and wounded to psychologically afflicted is astounding. Obhu and associates (1997) found that in the Tokyo subway gas attack, 11 people died, but up to 9,000 people sought medical care because they *thought* they had been gassed. There is also the potential for organic mental disorders along with standard stress reactions given the type of weapon used. Medical isolation and quarantine can create additional stress in individuals who may not be able to receive support from their social systems and in fact may be seen as "lepers" to be avoided (Flynn, 1998; Minihan et al., 2023).

The worldview of individuals subjected to terrorist-generated disasters may be very different from others' (Lee et al., 2022). There is a good deal of evidence to indicate that these individuals experience PTSD, panic and anxiety disorders, and depression at a far greater and more intense rate than others who are subject to "natural" disasters (U.S. Department of Justice, 2000). While there has been progress, with the counseling field becoming more trauma aware (Mirick et al., 2023) and the Red Cross making concerted efforts to provide crisis intervention training to wider segments of first responders, there is as yet little unified training for the sheer number of mental health providers needed in *any* large-scale disaster or megacrisis. This issue is even more pressing with the lack of expertise to deal specifically with terrorist acts and the hesitancy of and barriers to survivors seeking help (Ghurman et al., 2014; Myers & Wee, 2005, p. 251; Overmeire et al., 2021; Roberts, 2005; Vandentorren et al., 2018).

Lastly, the mental health infrastructure itself may be destroyed or disabled by human-made or natural disasters or simply be overwhelmed by the staggering volume of people it will be expected to service (Myer, 2015). In her pictorial representation of early interventions with survivors of terrorist attacks, Galai-Gat (2004) showed a Gary Larson cartoon of a crisis center going over a waterfall while on fire—a good analogy for the worldwide state of crisis intervention and the kinds of chaos ecosystemic crises can bring to local agencies, as witnessed by New Orleans mental health facilities attempting to get back into operation after being completely shut down by Hurricane Katrina (Shraberg, 2006).

New Directions and New Visions

LO4   Crisis intervention is no longer just a one-on-one proposition. We would like to introduce you to what we and some others (Collins & Collins, 2005; Cook, 2012; Gist & Lubin, 1999; Kilmer et al., 2010; Myer & Moore, 2006; Stokols et al., 2009) believe will characterize more and more of what crisis intervention will become in the twenty-first century—ecosystemic crisis intervention in the wake of a large-scale crisis or megacrisis (Helsloot et al., 2012; James et al., 2003; Lagedec, 2009). An ecosystemic crisis is one that reaches out and pervades, at a minimum, the community and perhaps whole regions or nations. If it turns into a megacrisis, it becomes "The embedded engine of chaotic world that evolves and mutates through global dynamic whose texture is made up of complex, unstable webs of constant, global, major dislocations of resource" (Lagedec, 2009). If that jawbreaking definition sounds a lot like the business of Chaos Theory described in Chapter 1, "Approaching Crisis Intervention," you would be on target. It may be immediate and horrific, like 9/11, with a relatively small loss of life, but have immense ramifications and spread shockwaves around the world. It may slowly and surely spread out across whole continents and have the potential for a tremendous loss of life, such as the COVID-19 pandemic. It may be human-made, occur dramatically, and then have long-lasting environmental effects that span thousands of years and destroy the social and governing infrastructure of an entire region, such as the Chernobyl nuclear power plant explosion and contamination (Bromet, 1995). It may be malevolent terrorism, creating widespread fear and anger, such as 9/11. It may be a smorgasbord of natural disasters, such as the 2019/2020 wildfires in Australia or Hurricane Maria in 2017, that drastically alter the landscape and the lives of those in the surrounding area (Mellish et al., 2022; Montero-Zamora et al., 2023).

The megacrisis created by the COVID-19 pandemic added a distinctive twist to the discussion of crisis intervention. The pandemic seemingly caught the world by surprise, resulting in changes in the way people, governments, and private organizations function (Boin et al., 2021). Think back to the first of January 2020. News outlets began reporting the spread of the virus, but at that time, business was as usual. People were traveling, stores were open, sporting events were taking place. In February, news media started reporting the increasing spread of the virus and possible

lethality if you were infected. Some alarm was given about the need to be careful by washing your hands and possibly considering wearing a mask. However, the warning was mixed, with some people saying not to worry while others sounded the alarm saying the virus had the potential to infect millions and to kill thousands. That message changed only marginally until late March 2020. In the final week of March and the first few weeks in April, everything, and we mean everything, changed. The world pretty much shut down. Only essential services and stores such as grocery stores and hospitals remained open. Of course, first responders (i.e., law enforcement, firefighters, and so on) remained on duty. Granted, some people and regions discounted the recommended safety measures and went about as if nothing had changed. But for most of the world, everyday life had changed. In varying degrees, an ecosystemic crisis does all of the foregoing. An ecosystemic crisis not only creates victims who directly experience the traumatic event in widespread numbers, but it also creates potential victims because of their vicarious experiencing of the event—even though they may be some geographical or psychological distance from the event itself (Chung et al., 2003; North, 2004; Shallcross, 2011).

This is particularly problematic because often, insurance or other mental health care providers do not recognize these groups of survivors as being in need of assistance (Galai-Gat, 2004). Therefore, the definition of an ecosystemic crisis used in this chapter is somewhat different from the definition of crisis as it applies to individuals that is used in the rest of the book. An *ecosystemic crisis* is any disruptive or destructive event that occurs at a rate and magnitude beyond the ability of the normal social process to control it. Unless dedicated resources are brought to ease the crisis, the integrity of the social fabric is generally degraded in the course of the event such that it becomes very difficult, if not impossible, to sustain the way of life as it was before the crisis occurred (Hilsloot et al., 2012; Lagadec, 2009; Ren, 2000).

Although a number of theorists and researchers have examined wide-scale disasters and the collective experiences of the populations who experience them (Freedy & Hobfoll, 1995; Gist & Lubin, 1989; Hobfoll, 1988; Hobfoll & deVries, 1995; Kaplan, 1996), most of the literature focuses on a dissection of the individual's psychological responses (North, 2010). Kaniasty and Norris (1999) propose that the individual's psychological response to disaster cannot be understood without considering the collective response that interacts with the political, cultural, environmental, and social realities of the ecosystem as it operated before and after the disaster.

Alternatively, on a very pragmatic and mundane level, the FEMA and its various departments spend a great deal of time and energy on providing education, information, and direct service in regard to operational responses to disasters of all kinds (FEMA, n.d.). However, what FEMA—or anyone, for that matter—doesn't do is determine how these all go together and, as you will read in a short while, that had ominous implications when Hurricane Katrina came ashore. What one also does not find is a way of making sense out of how crisis intervention strategies interface with the community-wide stressors people experience after a disaster and the various agencies that respond to help them.

Although the impacts of community-wide and national traumatic events date back historically at least as far as Pompeii being buried by a volcanic explosion nearly 2,000 years ago or the Black Plague killing millions of Europeans in the Middle Ages, the knowledge of those catastrophes and their resulting impact was slow to be felt because news of the disaster traveled only by word of mouth. Likewise, help could come only as fast as responders could spread the word and bring together resources that might arrive in horse-drawn carts or be carried on one's back. Often, help was simply unavailable, as there was no known way to mitigate the spread of disease.

Communities were isolated, and when a natural or human-made disaster struck, it was typically felt only at the local level. Further, at the local level, the constituents were essentially of the same race, tribe, clan, or other social identity and commonly held the same cultural, moral, and religious values. In short, until the 20th century, if Haiti suffered an earthquake, it was known and dealt with by the local community and perhaps the regional ruler. The prevailing philosophy was that people took care of themselves because they were the only ones affected by the traumatic event. In fact, if "strangers" had come to offer help, they probably would have been viewed with distrust and suspicion, given the insular cultural values of the time. The best that could be done proactively was to build cities that wouldn't be washed away by flood or blown away by winds, or to quarantine cities infected with disease. Historically, then, most crisis responses were by passive, preventive means that were meant to minimize the damage before it occurred.

Little could be done after the fact to minimize the deaths, economic loss, or societal disintegration.

It should also be understood that there is a rather spirited debate today in world health circles as to whether there is in underdeveloped countries any need for a Western world mental health disaster mitigation plan as opposed to the need to obtain basic necessities for survival. PTSD is seen as a Western cultural artifact contrived to justify and propagate the medical mental health model (Summerfield, 2005). On the contrary, others do not see PTSD as a cultural artifact but as a phenomenon that is cross-cultural in nature and that to deny it would be a terrible professional error and subvert the prevention of suffering (deVries, 1998; Dyregrov et al., 2002).

With the advent of the industrial and information ages, active crisis intervention came to mean that a whole society could be rapidly mobilized and coordinated to reshape the total dynamics of a crisis by using the machines and the command/control/communications/intelligence systems that have evolved in the last two centuries (Ren, 2000). With the condensing of geographic and communication distances, a fundamental but essential trend is that a crisis can no longer be contained within an enclave. The interventionist must necessarily function within and become an integral part of an ecological system that is continually and often richly interwoven with environmental components in the immediate neighborhood, town, district, borough, city, county, parish, canton, state, province, country, continent, hemisphere, and, ultimately, the world.

This fundamental trend is a melding of systemic crisis intervention strategies that interact in the total environmental and multicultural context of a pluralistic and dynamically changing world. Yet, this view is clearly not shared by everyone and may be seen by some as a pretext to impose Western medical practices on the rest of the world. Thus, in the early edition of the Sphere Project world health working paper on disaster response ("Humanitarian Charter," 1998), mental health was not even covered. Indeed the term **psychosocial** (having mental distress as a result of social upheaval) has been coined to take away the stigma that a person is mentally ill (Van Ommeren et al., 2005). Note what the International Interagency Standing Committee on Mental Health and *Psychosocial* Support calls itself to make it more palatable to some parts of the international community (IASC, 2023). Indeed, most survivors of a catastrophe may only need social support, and "psychosocial support" is a lot more psychologically palatable than the designator of being "mentally ill." You should thus understand that what is being proposed in this chapter is not universally loved and admired, or even thought to be necessary or right by a number of people.

To that end, this chapter deals with an emerging **ecosystemic** view of what crisis intervention is becoming as it operates in large systems and deals with metastasizing, large-scale crises and megacrises. **Metastasizing** crises are those that start small but, if not contained both physically and psychologically, can quickly turn into large-scale crises (James, 2006). **Large-scale** crises are those that, at a minimum, affect whole communities or regions either directly or vicariously. **Megacrises or ecosystemic crises** are defined as those that affect entire countries or the world, either directly or vicariously.

System Overview

The ecological, contextual crisis intervention approach that is described in this chapter reaches far beyond the relational interactions between and among the various members of the crisis client's family or individuals in the client's workplace and immediate surroundings. Essentially, it is a dynamic, sociocultural, and multicultural view of all ecological influences that impinge upon the individual. It consists of five environmental systems, ranging from the fine-grained inputs of direct communications with social agents (individuals capable of interacting directly with crisis clients) to the broad-based inputs of local community agencies as well as the widespread influences of national imperatives and the attitudes and ideologies of the cultures within which these systems operate (Santrock, 2021). Cook (2012, p. 5) defines the term **ecosystem** as "The total sum of the interactive influences operating within an individual's life in varying degrees of proximity ranging from their biologically determined characteristics to the broader sociocultural context which structures human interactions." The approach is continually changing, emerging, evolving, and developing to accommodate the ecological and multicultural contexts within which it exists. It represents a paradigmatic shift: a newly emerging ecosystem that encompasses an interdependency among and within people at all different levels of the total environment. This is not some static amorphous entity. It is very much alive, and as one part is impacted, other parts react.

This ecosystemic view of crisis intervention is adapted from Uri Bronfenbrenner's (1986, 1995; Bronfenbrenner & Morris, 1998; Santrock, 2021) ecosystemic theory of human development, and our own (James et al., 2003; James & Gilliland, 2003, pp. 336–337, 341–342) and other psychotheorists' (Cook, 2012; Conyne & Cook, 2003; Conyne et al., 2003; Klotz, 2003) views of ecosystems as they apply to psychotherapy in general and crisis in particular (Collins & Collins, 2005; Norris et al., 2006; Vernberg, 1999). In crisis intervention terms, not only is the individual in crisis affected, but the client's total environment also becomes the context that must be considered by crisis workers (Myer & Moore, 2006). Bronfenbrenner (1986, 1995) identified the five environmental components as the microsystem, mesosystem, exosystem, macrosystem, and chronosystem (see Figure 16.1).

Microsystem

The microsystem is the setting in which the person in crisis lives. The microsystem setting's contexts may include the individual's family, friends, coworkers, peers, school, neighborhood, and usual haunts. It is within the microsystem that the individual in crisis experiences the most direct social interactions and communications with others. In the microsystem setting, whatever difficulties individuals experience tend to spill over into the family constellation and compound the difficulties caused by the disaster (Green & Solomon, 1995). In the traumatic wake of a disaster, many previous relationships, alliances, partnerships, bonds, and agreements in the microsystem, which were held together in the immediate aftermath as a means of mutual survival, crumble under the weight of compound stresses (Smith & Belgrave, 1995).

The crisis worker adhering to the ecological, contextual, and multicultural approach views the person in crisis not as a passive recipient of experiences in those microsystemic settings but as an individual who actively participates in the construction of the settings (Santrock, 2021). Reciprocally, the settings have a positive or negative effect on the individual and family and may ameliorate or exacerbate the crisis depending on the person's proximity, relationship to, and perception and meaning of the event (Myer & Moore, 2006).

Mesosystem

In Bronfenbrenner's (1995) developmental system, the mesosystem serves as the communications channel, pathway, or interactive mechanism between components in the microsystem and the exosystem. The mesosystem is essentially the total communications

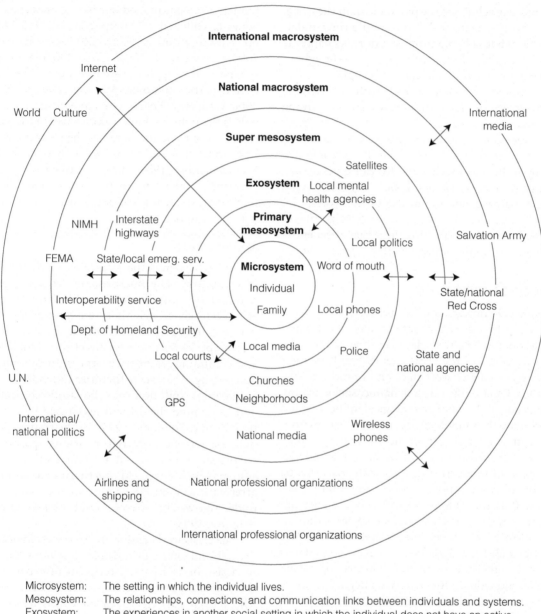

Microsystem: The setting in which the individual lives.
Mesosystem: The relationships, connections, and communication links between individuals and systems.
Exosystem: The experiences in another social setting in which the individual does not have an active role; the exosystem does influence the individual's experiences in the immediate context.
Macrosystem: The national and regional systems, attitudes, and ideologies, behavior patterns, beliefs, and other products that are passed on from generation to generation and make up the fabric of the larger culture.

Figure 16.1 Adaptation of Bronfenbrenner's Ecosystemic Model for Crisis.

network that allows all individuals and groups within each ecological system to exchange information. It includes every form of communication—from word of mouth to the most sophisticated electronic technology— and is far more than cell phones and television news announcements. In terms of crisis and crisis intervention, the mesosystem and its function as the command-and-control structure of the total system are critical. The COVID-19 megacrisis proved multiple forms of communication are invaluable to alert the public to the threats posed by the virus. (Shao et al., 2021; Wittenberg et al., 2021)

The crisis mesosystem is interspersed not only between the microsystem and exosystem (primary mesosystem) but between the exosystem and the macrosystem as well (super mesosystem). Both the primary and super mesosystems play critical roles in resolving ecosystemic crises. These two systems are extremely fluid and may expand very rapidly during a crisis. Think of a lava lamp where, as the oil heats up, there are rapid and nonsymmetrical movements of the colored oil. This analogy carries over to a rapidly heating and expanding crisis. (Whether this expansion alleviates or exacerbates the crisis depends a great deal on how and what is communicated by whom and under what circumstances.) One of the major failures in the aftermath of Hurricane Katrina was the breakdown of this system at both the primary and super levels. It should be understood that disaster mental health systems are complex mesosystems (networks of other systems) in and of themselves, and what makes them even more complex is that they will be imposed on to host micro- and exo-mental health systems that have their own agendas, vary in preparedness for a disaster, and may well suffer severe disruption themselves due to the disaster (Norris et al., 2006).

Local emergency management agencies (LEMAs) expend a great deal of time and effort conducting tabletop and on-scene exercises to determine the most effective way of handling a crisis, dealing with logistics, and field-testing communication links (Freeman, 2003; Lane, 2003). These systems directly link crisis interventionists with emergency management agencies. Human service workers trained by NOVA, FEMA, the American Red Cross, and state and local mental health agencies are on call for emergencies, and when a disaster of a magnitude greater than what the local authorities can handle is encountered, these crisis teams are called up and go into action. In the United States, calling up the National Guard is a fair analogy to what happens when a call goes out for crisis workers. Hurricane Katrina is an excellent example of the need for both.

Primary Mesosystem. Communication in the primary crisis mesosystem means having translators to speak to victims whose native tongue is not the national language. It means having ham radio operators and trained weather spotters with two-way radios and crisis response teams and search-and-rescue teams with walkie-talkies to communicate with one another in wrecked buildings or in a blown-down forest. It means establishing clear links from emergency management agencies to media outlets. It means creating integrated communication networks between emergency management agencies and a wide variety of supportive agencies that range from law enforcement and fire departments to heavy equipment operators and mental health professionals.

A primary **mesosystem** is everything from sign language for a person who is deaf or hard of hearing to the most high-tech wireless computer satellite uplinks to state and FEMAs (Freeman, 2003; Lane, 2003). It maintains connections and communications within and among workplaces, schools, religious institutions/organizations, families, peer groups, and local social, medical, and governmental services (Bronfenbrenner, 1995; Freeman, 2003; James & Gilliland, 2003, pp. 341–342; Lane, 2003; Santrock, 2021).

For crisis intervention agencies, fast, effective, clear communication is at the center of everything they do. Communication redundancy is critical because if one system fails, another can be substituted. For example, during an electrical storm, the emergency management director of Nassau County, Florida (Jacksonville area), was in her car and attempting to communicate with a member of her staff about storm damage. But she quickly found that communication was impossible because of electrical interference. Despite all of the sophisticated equipment the county EMA had, the only thing that worked was leaving messages on each other's voice mail (Freeman, 2003). It is not accidental that Jerry Lane, the former emergency manager of the city of Sycamore, Illinois, is a licensed advanced-class amateur radio operator (Lane, 2003). One of the more aggravating problems of Hurricane Katrina was that various local agencies used different radio frequencies and could not communicate with one another, nor could they communicate with the super mesosystem. Thus, a recurring theme throughout disaster intervention is that communication is vital to the ability to respond in a disaster (Rebman et al., 2008).

Super Mesosystem. Interlinking the macrosystem with all interior systems is the super mesosystem. The super mesosystem that connects the exosystem and the macrosystem serves many of the same coordinating functions but on a national level. The super mesosystem is composed of information systems that range from the postal service to national commercial radio and television corporations and from the internet and its websites, e-mail, instant messaging, and chat rooms to satellite communication and global positioning systems. Federal agencies such as FEMA and its parent, the Bureau of Homeland Security, are linked with other governmental agencies such as the Bureau of Justice and private agencies such as the Red Cross and National Organization of Victims Assistance, National Oceanic and Atmospheric Administration weather satellites, the U.S. Weather Service storm prediction centers, supercomputers at national agencies that model and predict disaster scenarios and relief efforts, and the National Emergency Broadcast systems for the public.

National agency and federal department interlinks and downlinks to state EMAs and agencies are all part of the super mesosystem for crisis intervention that operates in the United States. It has major command-and-control centers that can be linked to state communication and control centers, which, in turn, are linked to local emergency operations centers. These national organizations and agencies have complete mobile command, control, and communications centers that can be rapidly moved on tractor trailers by highway, rail, or ship or flown into any disaster site. This system was so devastated during Hurricane Katrina that the base of operations for repairing the levees and pumping systems in New Orleans was situated in the U.S. Army Corps of Engineers' office in Memphis, Tennessee, more than 400 miles up the Mississippi River!

Therefore, the **mesosystem** is of primary concern to crisis interventionists and the crisis intervention process because it coordinates and drives dynamic linkages among all components (people, groups, contextual connections, ecological resources). The crisis interventionist—in the role of consultant, collaborator, coordinator, and communicator—is a key resource person operating within the mesosystem.

The advent of smartphones with multiple applications has enhanced the potential of both the primary and super mesosystems' ability to communicate in a variety of ways (Wang et al., 2020). Aten and associates (2011) and Wang et al. (2020) detailed a number of applications made possible by this new technology:

1. Texting takes far less bandwidth than talking. When other phone systems are plugged up, text messages are likely to get through. Many universities now have text warning systems that can get to any student who has a cell phone on.

2. Smartphone users with weather and news apps can access outside information when they might not otherwise have access to current conditions that affect the crisis.

3. Social networking sites such as WhatsApp, Facebook, Threads, X (formerly known as Twitter), Flickr, and LinkedIn allow people to stay in synchronous contact with other internet users. Clearly, these sites can be used for organizing activities of large groups of people, as witnessed by the recent revolutions in Egypt and Libya which used these devices to organize large demonstrations and avoid police dragnets. These sites would seem to have the same applicability in organizing people during disasters.

4. Global positioning systems (GPS) have proliferated both as hardwired applications in automobiles and trucks and in portable systems such as smartphones. These have tremendous applicability in a disaster for directing traffic, giving directions, providing alternate routes, and locating people who don't know where they are. OnStar is a satellite communication, GPS, and emergency notification communications system hardwired into new General Motors (GM) vehicles. GM has teamed with the American Red Cross to provide information on shelters, medical services, safe routes, food sources, and other services. Aten and associates (2011) reported that OnStar's usage rate went up 30 percent during Hurricane Gustave, which is a pretty good indication of how much its subscribers relied on it during what they considered to be an emergency.

5. When super mesosystems use systems like OnStar, a great many people can access these systems in a hurry, and they don't need an electrical transmission line to do it. The Centers for Disease Control and Prevention (CDC) have picked up on this technology and made podcasts that provide "what to do and what to know" information about disease epidemics, safety tips, and other health-related information that can be used by people in disaster areas with no electricity who might otherwise be cut off from critical health information (CDC, n.d.).

6. Many smartphones now have emergency calling capabilities. For example, newer iPhones and Apple watches also have SOS and fall detection capacity. These can be used in health emergencies, automobile accidents, and other emergency

crisis-like situations. Other smartphones have similar capabilities or apps designed for emergency notifications that can be added.

The point of all this new technology is that for many people in the primary mesosystem, using it daily is standard practice. Thus, super mesosystems like those operated by the federal government or international charitable organizations can use them not only with their own workers when standard communication links are down, but also with a large number of primary system users who are not mystified by the technology and can then spread the information by word of mouth. If these new devices and systems are put to use wisely, they may do much to push the communication problems that have plagued relief efforts into the dustbin of history.

Exosystem

The **exosystem** exposes the crisis client or clients to experiences in a wider social setting than those encountered in the microsystem context (Bronfenbrenner, 1986, 1995). The exosystem reaches much farther out into the community and may even include state or regional entities. Legal and social welfare services, local mass media, and all governmental agencies and programs that are in a position to impact the individual and to assist persons, families, or groups who are in crisis are part of the exosystem. Crisis workers who live in other parts of the state or province may be called in to help. Typically, in the United States, each local EMA has backup personnel who are in place or on standby support if a crisis arises that temporarily exceeds local capacity to handle the situation.

How effective the exosystem and macrosystem are in providing services depends in large part on how well information passes back and forth through the primary and super mesosystems and how well resources are allocated, delivered, and used based on that information. The FEMA on-site, one-stop-shop for all related disaster assistance to individuals is an excellent super mesosystem example of direct communication between victims in the microsystem and national providers in the macrosystem.

Macrosystem

The **macrosystem** includes the national government and all its agencies and national charitable, religious, service, professional, and benevolent organizations. It encompasses the national rail, air, marine, and highway transportation modalities and food, fuel, and energy transmission systems. The macrosystem encompasses the total culture in which people live (Bronfenbrenner, 1995). Total culture refers to the behavior patterns, traditions, beliefs, mores, historical artifacts, legal constructs, and all other traits and pursuits that are endemic to a group of people and that are passed on from generation to generation (Santrock, 2021). The macrosystem has importance in crisis intervention for two reasons. First and foremost, when a disaster exceeds the normal coping capacity of the disaster impact area, the macrosystem is most likely the place from which help and resources will flow. Second, if the crisis is of a national magnitude, such as 9/11, it will be important to do a triage assessment of the national psyche to determine what, if any, intervention needs to occur with the entire ecosystem.

Disasters do not have to be large in geographic scope or have large numbers of fatalities to be considered macrosystemic. The killing rampage in Uvalde, Texas at Robb Elementary School reverberated through the entire United States. Although 19 children and 2 adults tragically died, that number pales in comparison to the number of dead on 9/11 in 2001. By all objective measures, the Uvalde deaths did not compare to 9/11's loss of life. Yet, the fact that the tragedy occurred in this quiet Texas town, in a place where one's children are supposed to be safe, upset the nation's sense of control. The heartbreak in Uvalde was as great if, not more so, as what was experienced from the shooting at the high school in Parkland, Florida, and the elementary school in Sandy Hook, Connecticut. The shooting at Robb Elementary School quickly turned into a metastasizing crisis that carried far beyond Uvalde, Texas. These types of disasters result in telephone connections being overwhelmed and text messaging skyrocketing. Facebook and other social networks are also used to relay the news of the tragedy as these incidents occur and caution people to get out of and avoid danger zones (Aten et al., 2011).

Most particularly, parents who had sent their children off to school became very concerned about their children's health and well-being, no matter what K-12 school, university, or college they attended and no matter what part of the country it was in. Those parents immediately began sending a deluge of phone calls, letters, and e-mails across the country (a national macrosystem), demanding to know what safety measures were in place to protect their children from distressed politically motivated gunmen and other potential predators.

Perhaps even more importantly, the constituency in the education system, students, staff, teachers, administrators, and professors, were highly capable of communicating across the super mesosystem via e-mail, blogs, cell phones, and text messages. That rapidly expanding super mesosystem put the information, conjecture, hypotheses, and rumors about the massacre at Robb Elementary School out into the international macrosystem within hours of the shootings. The manifestos often left behind by the perpetrators of shootings of this type are chilling and filled with hate messages that raise concern in the mesosystem.

While your cell phones are almost an Aladdin's magic lamp that will tell all and do all with the right apps, they have a ways to go in emergency management. The major problems that afflict the use of this modern technology are threefold. Information can't be collaborated (Valecha, 2020), so its validity is open to question. Second, information gaps and gathering significant data shackles the practical use of emergency management information systems (Ghosh et al., 2018). Third, data reflecting human behaviors on a large scale needs to be prompt and timely to support the variety of emergency management systems in making corresponding correct and accurate responses (Wang et al., 2020).

Chronosystem

The Individual. The chronosystem is identified by Bronfenbrenner (1995) as the patterning of environmental events and transactions over the life span as well as the social and historical circumstances that influence the individual, family, peers, coworkers, and others. The essence of the chronosystem is the dynamic influence that time has on events, and time, with its movement, is an absolutely critical variable in regard to disasters. The crisis chronosystem starts with the birth of the traumatic event and not the birth of the person. Although the crisis chronosystem starts with the event, if possible, the crisis interventionist needs to backtrack over the personal developmental chronosystem of the individual to determine what, if any, precursors may have contributed to the incident's impact and what antecedent events may cause it to be exacerbated.

In crisis intervention, understanding the part the chronosystem plays in exacerbating or ameliorating the crisis is particularly important. There are two types of disaster trauma—individual and collective (Erikson, 1976). **Individual trauma** hammers the individual psyche and breaks through the person's defenses so forcefully and suddenly that reaction is impossible. **Collective trauma** does the same thing, only it does it across the microsystem (the community) to the extent that the social bonds that connect people are torn apart, and the community is rent asunder. The chronosystem is important for both individual and collective traumatic responses and can be marked in phases that are generally linear and progressive in nature (see Figure 16.2). The following are brief descriptions of those phases.

Impact phase. The first few minutes and hours during and immediately after the crisis are critically important. While fear and shock are common, most people behave adaptively and take action to protect themselves and their loved ones. Time may become disoriented and slowed down, with disbelief and denial at what has happened. However, while a good deal of collective chaos may ensue, people react mainly in proactive ways (Myers & Wee, 2005, p. 20). Maslow's hierarchy of needs comes into operation, particularly when the crisis is a disaster that leaves people without food, shelter, or clothing. As the crisis plays out in the traumatic wake of the next few days, the resolution of problems ranging from having a roof over one's head to communicating or being physically reunited with one's family becomes critical.

Emergency/acute Heroic/rescue Phase. Immediately after impact, people spring into action to save others and to save property and regain control of the situation and environment. During this heroic or rescue stage (Myers & Wee, 2005, pp. 20–21; NIMH, 2002; Pennebaker & Harber, 1993), individuals are generally highly energized physically and emotionally, have great morale, cognitively perseverate on the event, and gain relief by talking about their anxieties surrounding the crisis and their responses to it. While individuals are highly energized, problem solving and priority setting are often compromised by the sheer magnitude of the disaster, which many times translates into lots of activity and low efficiency. Seeking or finding out that family members are safe and can be reunited is critical.

Inventory/recovery Phase. At some point between the impact and the heroic stage, an inventory and initial attempts at the recovery phase occur. People conduct an appraisal of the situation and start to plan what they are going to do (NIMH, 2002). They engage in information seeking in regard to finding loved ones, determining whether they are safe or injured,

Time

	Event occurrence	**Impact**
Individual/systemic traumatic onset of a crisis event		
	First hours	Emergency/acute heroic phase
	First days	Inventory phase
Shock, denial, hysteria, anger, grief (peritraumatic symptoms)		
		Honeymoon phase
	First month	Avoidance phase
Acute stress disorder		
		Adaptation phase
Chronic posttraumatic stress disorder	3 months	Disillusionment phase
Delayed onset posttraumatic stress disorder	6 months	
Anniversary of crisis; regression to event	1 year	Pathogenic to salutogenic shift
Transcrisis-complicated grief, delayed PTSD, chronic drug use, anniversaries, etc.	More than a year	Restabilization/reconstruction

Figure 16.2   Pathological Chronosystem of a Crisis Event.

and finding out how well their homes and places of employment have fared (Myers & Wee, 2005, p. 21). Typically, there is frustration with the inability to find loved ones or anger at authorities for not letting the survivors back into their neighborhoods to find out about their homes.

Honeymoon phase. There is a collective "we are in this together" attitude. The phrase that seems to have become the mantra during this phase is "City name"

Strong. Examples are El Paso Strong following the Walmart shooting or Fort Myers Strong in the aftermath of Hurricane Ian. This may last anywhere from 1 week to 3 months post-impact. The community pulls together. There is optimism about recovery, and the belief that there will be full restitution of financial loss is high. There is a great deal of media coverage and high-level political attention. Public outpouring in the form of physical and financial donations gives the community a sense of hope for rebuilding, and there is a strong sense of having shared a horrific experience but having prevailed over the worst of it (Farberow & Frederick, 1978).

At any time from 2 weeks to 2 years, depending on the severity and scope of the event, individuals will experience reintegration and return to a pre-event level of functioning or better, or they may not.

Avoidance Phase. As individuals work their way through the next few weeks, the kinds of physical and psychological support systems that are provided affect whether acute stress disorder will arise and whether it will eventually turn into PTSD. As time passes, an avoidance phase generally emerges (Pennebaker & Harber, 1993). People stop talking about the event, but the images and thoughts about it continue to dominate cognitive functioning.

Adaptation Phase. Whether the pathology of the event continues and the individual enters the adaptation phase (Pennebaker & Harber, 1993) depends a great deal on the resiliency of the individual and the crisis worker's ability to institute a salutogenic model (Antonovsky, 1980, 1991) that emphasizes health and wellness over sickness and pathology. The salutogenic concept affirms what we historically know about people and crises. Stress is ever present, and severe stress is going to occur, but people are resilient, recover, and can thrive and grow from it. If people can come to grips with the financial, emotional, and environmental problems they will invariably face and come to see that, no matter what they do, things will never quite be the same as they were before, but they can move forward, they will have adapted and move on. However, for many, adaptation will be difficult because of the disillusionment that sets in.

Disillusionment Phase. Disillusionment may begin several days or weeks after impact and may last for years, depending on how individuals adjust to their new environment. Disillusionment occurs because the media and politicians go home, bureaucratic red tape slows recovery, insurance money doesn't pay out as much as thought, and multiple other problems arise that suggest that recovery will be slow, if at all. Fatigue finally sets in, and the individual is emotionally and physically exhausted from extended psychological and physical stress (Rosenfeld et al., 2010). Survivors begin to wonder why someone is getting assistance and they do not. Survivors are often frustrated during this phase because each time they

contact the insurance agency or government relief organization, they talk to another person and must tell their story again or worse, get different answers to their questions. A variety of public health problems may arise from poor living and sanitary conditions, environmental pathogens, and communicable diseases. Stress-related health symptoms, ranging from high blood pressure to exacerbation of preexisting health problems, may occur. Disaster relief workers ironically refer to this period as the second disaster. Psychological problems may range from PTSD to panic and anxiety disorders to depression and suicidal ideation (Myers & Wee, 2005, p. 23).

Anniversary Phase. As time moves forward into the next year, the anniversary of the occurrence may become significant (Cohen et al., 2006). After a year or more has passed since the incident, a transcrisis state may be reached, depending on whether the individual has resolved the trauma or not. For some victims, the need to talk about and seek help validating their experience will go on and on, much to the dismay of others. This continuing need for catharsis and rumination about the crisis may be met with disapproval and outright anger by others in the victim's support system who seek to distance themselves from it (Smith & Belgrave, 1995). The result is often a perception by the victim of secondary victimization.

Pathogenic to Salutogenic Shift. Around the time of the first anniversary of the traumatic event, a benchmark is usually reached. If individuals have put the traumatic event into past context, mourned their losses, and started to rebuild their lives, then they have made a salutogenic shift in their lives (a shift that is healthful, wholesome, and promotes psychological growth) (Antonovsky, 1980; Mittelmark et al., 2017). They have met the challenge the traumatic event posed for them and are able to move on with their lives. In contrast, if individuals have remained mired in the traumatic event long past the acute stage, then they may be said to have made a pathogenic shift (diseased, unwholesome, and psychologically debilitating) that may become residual and chronic, bringing on a host of physical and psychological maladies. A continuing and contentious issue in the field of trauma therapy is how individuals attain and retain a salutogenic state and if they do or do not need assistance in doing so (Mittelmark et al., 2017; Stuhmiller & Dunning, 2000). Antonovsky (1991) has demonstrated that the stronger people's sense of coherence (the extent to which the stress is deemed manageable, coherent, and meaningful), the more likely they are able to cope with life's stressors. If that model is adopted, then much of the role and function of the crisis worker ceases to exist because in a salutogenic model, stress is universal, humans have adapted to it, and they do not necessarily crumble under traumatic stress (Mittlemark et al., 2017; Stuhmiller & Dunning, 2000).

Restabilization/Reconstruction Phase. As time passes, decisions have to be made as to whether to rebuild one's life in the same environment or move on to a different place. Rebuilding is not just putting a new house up after an earthquake. It is also about rebuilding and restabilizing one's emotional and social self. Even though there are setbacks, with denied loans, divorce papers, homes that are a total loss, friendships that have been lost, or friends who have died in the disaster, somehow, over the months and perhaps years, stabilization and new constructs replace the old.

Therefore, as time moves forward, the survivor needs to engage in a process that is much like Schneider's (1984) transformational model of grief. Monitoring and following up on this transformational process to the client's final acceptance and putting the disaster in perspective may require tracking the client for a year or more. Richard Tedeschi and Lawrence Calhoun have been hard at work on the concept of posttraumatic growth (Taku et al., 2015; Tedeschi & Calhoun, 2009, 2010, 2012; Triplett et al., 2012). These two researchers have developed different inventories: Post Traumatic Growth Inventory (Taku et al., 2008); Post Traumatic Growth Inventory for Children (Kilmer et al., 2009); Short Form of the Traumatic Growth Inventory (Cann et al., 2010); and The Event Related Rumination Inventory (Cann et al., 2011) to assess people's ability to discover new possibilities such as better ways of relating to others, new personal strengths, positive spiritual changes, and stronger appreciation of life in the wake of a crisis (DeAngelis, 2011). One might say they are putting the empirical test to the Chinese Kanji characters indicating both crisis and opportunity.

The Society

When we move from the individual to the society at large (the micro-, exo-, or macrosystem), the chrono-system also plays an important part in what is going to happen systemically. In the immediate hours and days in the aftermath of the crisis, all of the resources, agencies, and personnel needed to bring control and equilibrium back to the community are brought to bear, and time becomes acutely important. During this heroic stage (Raphael, 2000), the system responds with unselfishness, self-sacrifice, and heroism in its attempts to rescue people and provide shelter and emergency assistance. Indeed, if there is forewarning, such as the landfall of a hurricane, timelines will extend backward to precede the occurrence.

As an example, the Nassau County Florida Emergency Management Department has an activation emergency model. County officials use a three-level activation model to assess situations and take appropriate action. Level 3 involves County Watch Officers monitoring local, regional, and world events while Emergency Management and Planning Professionals collaborate with partners and stakeholders to develop plans, conduct training, and drill/exercise plans to improve disaster preparedness throughout the county. Level 2 indicates a threat is looming that could adversely impact the county. Officials work to identify trigger points and consult with subject matter experts to respond to questions from the public. Level 1 is a full activation and is declared when the disaster is imminent. Representatives from each emergency response and support specialty (e.g., law enforcement, fire rescue, transportation, utilities, health, animal care, business, and industry, etc.) report for duty (Nassau County Florida Emergency Management Department, 2023). These individuals are expected to be available 24/7 to respond to any situation needing their expertise.

During the immediate aftermath, a psychological honeymoon stage (Raphael, 2000) occurs in which there is a great deal of attention by the media, massive intervention by disaster relief agencies, and the notion that things will be set right and services quickly restored. There is an overall "We're all in the same boat, and everybody is equal" attitude.

After all of the emergency crews have finished getting power and phone lines back on, the wonderful outside assistance and resource support have gone home, and the media have moved on to the next disaster, the long-term degrading effects of the disaster are still there and consuming additional resources. When physical facilities—such as churches, schools, parks, and community centers—are gone, activities and interpersonal contacts that were taken for granted may be lost. State and federal bureaucracies and insurance companies seem to have miles and miles of red tape and may deny requests for compensation and support for the reconstruction of basic infrastructure. Both for individuals and communities, this phase has often been called the "second disaster" (Myers & Wee, 2005, p. 29).

Losing access to community gathering places has symbolic, social, spiritual, and psychological meaning and may have long-term toxic effects on the community. Rebuilding these structures and reestablishing social links that were severely fractured take a great deal of time and effort (Kaniasty & Norris, 1999). At this point, a disillusionment stage may emerge (Raphael, 2000). There is a sense of frustration, hopelessness, and abandonment that things will never be the same. Widespread posttraumatic stress and depressive symptoms are likely to appear if continuous and long-term mental health assistance is not available. Thus, a very real question arises as to the "when" of the provision of services. It is not nearly as glamorous 6 months after a disaster strikes to appear on the scene "ready to help," but it may be as critically important to provide mental health services in the long term as it is in the short term.

The megacrisis of COVID-19 meant most people's connection with their community changed (Boin et al., 2021). Video conferencing became the go-to method for work, pleasure, education, and many health appointments (Elbaz et al., 2022; McCabe et al., 2023; Shao et al., 2021). Even if individuals ventured out, they were encouraged to stand at least six feet apart, wear masks, and interact as little as possible. Many restaurants, if they had not already, started delivering meals with no-contact deliveries, and grocery stores and other retail outlets did the same.

Community resilience has become a key component in federal emergency plans. Whether a community rebirths or dies after a disaster has a lot to do with how well it plans for disaster by building community resilience through both individual preparedness and establishing a supportive context within that community (Plough et al., 2013). That supportive context particularly speaks to providing social justice for vulnerable populations that typically experience short shrift in the provision of goods and services in the aftermath of a disaster (Baker & Cormier, 2015; DeAngelis, 2014; Royiscar, 2013; Roysicar et al., 2013).

The chronosystem, then, represents the development of events in individuals' lives and larger social systems over time, and crisis interventionists need to be aware of how important time and timing are in responding to crises. The phrases "Time changes everything" and "Time is of the essence" appear to capture the flavor of the chronosystem (James & Gilliland, 2003, p. 342).

Defining Principles of a Crisis Intervention Ecosystem

Coming to grips with complex ecosystem service delivery issues is daunting, to say the least. The key ingredient here goes far beyond just social services or first responders to a crisis but is interdisciplinary, with a wide variety of professions involved (Iikevich & Shiapak, 2014). However, Coyne and Cook (2003) and Norris and her associates (2006) have generated the following principles for bridging disaster response gaps.

1. **Systems must be interdisciplinary.** No single discipline or "ology" has a corner on this market. No one can be the solitary hero when offering services after a disaster. Emergency management agencies and crisis intervention systems must rely on a broad spectrum of people, ranging from sanitation workers and electrical linemen to civil and logistical engineers to medical emergency staff and communication workers to law enforcement and fire and rescue personnel to sociologists and psychologists to bankers and economists to religious leaders and social workers. And most often, a pecking order and rules exist when working with emergency management systems.

   The Red Cross is an example of an organization with an organizational system that volunteers are asked to follow. We say this not as a criticism, because order is needed in the midst of chaos, but rather as information to be aware of when volunteering. Further, all of the people in these skills, crafts, trades, and professions must work in an integrated manner. The competent crisis worker integrates seamlessly into this smorgasbord of "ologies"; the pretentiousness sometimes associated with a college degree and the egotism of a particular profession have no place in an ecosystemic crisis. Ecosystemic crisis intervention is the most egalitarian of all mental health endeavors, and layperson volunteers may be just as effective as psychiatrists. Anyone with an inflated ego will soon be humbled in a large crisis.

2. **The system must be multitheoretical.** If we examine only the psychological component of

wide-scale crises, no single psychological theory is presently adequate to deal with the complex swirl of human dynamics that comes out of a crisis. It should be stated absolutely and unequivocally that nobody has a theoretical corner on this market. That includes proselytizers for any of the "alphabet" techniques such as CISD, EMDR, TF-CBT, or, alternatively, those who would rail against them. It especially includes the authors of this book! When dealing with large-scale crises or megacrises, psychological theory must, at the very least, harmonize with logistical, medical, communications, economic, and political theory. To further complicate matters, it is not just which psychological theories and techniques are used but also when and how those services are delivered.

3. **Individuals are part of the ecosystem.** Like it or not, unless we can somehow find a place in the desert or mountains to become hermits, we are part of the total ecosystem of the world. Our biological makeup, interpersonal relationships, physical environment, and sociological context are all becoming more tightly interwoven into the total ecosystem of the world. An appreciation of your context and the context in which you are providing services is a must.

4. **Multiple contexts must be considered.** Micro-, meso-, exo-, and macrosystems are all components of the total ecological system that impact the individual when a megacrisis occurs. To deny that these systems are vectors and forces that impinge on the individual is to have a very parochial view of what this business is about and be doomed to fail.

5. **Time is of the essence.** If we believe any of the PTSD research about the deleterious effects the passage of time has on the individual if nothing is done to alleviate the possible effects of the trauma, we need to understand that what occurs in the chronosystem is critical. The availability of adequate physical and psychological resources to deal with a crisis in a timely manner is paramount.

6. **Meaning is important.** What sense we make of the crisis from a broad systemic view is as important as what sense we make of it individually and has much to do with how quickly and effectively it is resolved for both individuals and society.

7. **Parsimonious interventions are needed.** Concordance and coordination within various systems are needed if large amounts of precious time and energy are not to be wasted. At the federal level, sufficient funding and information resources must be generated and disseminated. At the state level, preparedness plans should address multiple levels of the response across relevant jurisdictions, which includes clear plans on how the state agencies will communicate with the public and providers. Optimal utilization of resources is critical, and collaborative relationships and understanding between agencies need to be formed in advance. Intervention in large-scale crises is extremely expensive in terms of person power and material resources. One of the major balancing acts of local EMAs is to have just enough resources available to bring maximum effort to bear at just the right time to experience maximum effect.

8. **The process is cooperative, collaborative, and consultative.** Just as no single discipline holds sway in a large-scale or megacrisis, cooperation, collaboration, and consultation within, among, and between systems and individuals are paramount. The provision of mental health services is important, but so are getting communication and power systems back on and determining where there is available shelter and whether buildings are safe. The ethics of the manner in which these resources are distributed comes into play (Myer, 2015). The timing and amount of the allotment of these resources can be a problem. No matter the decision, someone will be left out. Although this decision is above your pay grade, you will feel the fallout from the decision. Using a "utilitarian" approach means resources are sent where they do the greatest good for the greatest number of people.

9. **There is a full range of targeted interventions aimed at individuals, institutions, and communities on up to the national level, depending on how widespread the crisis is, and they are ongoing in response to longer-term needs.** Each involved system component, from the individual to the nation, needs to be triaged. Based on that assessment, target-specific interventions need to be made. How things will wind up after a disaster is not just determined in the days after it but in the months after it. The infrastructure and community as a client are as important long range as are individuals.

10. **The service characteristics of credibility, acceptability, accessibility, proactivity, continuance, and confidentiality should be adopted**

as "cast-in-stone" goals for service delivery in disaster-stricken areas. Norris and her associates (2006) found adherence to these characteristics to be one of the most impressive of her findings of the 9/11 response in New York City. Meeting this gold standard of service delivery most likely means that the whole disaster mesosystem is integrated with host systems and running well. To do that effectively requires a variety of organizations and individuals who operate with a high level of cooperation to make that system work.

Overarching all of the foregoing points are planning, more planning, practicing, critiquing, evaluating, and yet more planning. The necessity for vertical and horizontal links in the ecosystem of disaster planning cannot be overemphasized. The result of not having such links became clearly evident after Hurricane Katrina. One of the critical components of planning is making sure that disaster mental health planning and activities do not take a backseat to security and safety concerns; people who can make clear decisions must be in place and have the authority to make those decisions (Flynn, 2003). That issue became abundantly clear in the aftermath of Katrina, with local and state leaders bickering about plans that should have been carved in stone long before the hurricane made landfall (Flynn, 2003; Gheytanchi et al., 2007).

National Crisis Response Teams

LO5 Perhaps the most important outreach approach has been taken by a group of national agencies for training in on-site delivery of mental health services at major disasters and the coordination of these services with other relief efforts (Pfefferbaum et al., 2010). Because of past criticism of how both charitable and federal agencies have handled major disasters, those agencies have done a great deal of work to better coordinate their efforts in providing comprehensive disaster relief that cuts across the survivors' total environment (Bass & Yep, 2002; Pyszczynskl et al., 2002; Smith, 2002). Mental health support does little good when people don't have a roof over their heads because it has been blown away in a hurricane. However, it also does little good for survivors to obtain housing but be so traumatized and depressed from the disaster that they cannot begin to regain control over their lives. From plane crashes to university campus shootings, to floods, to post office shootings, to forest fires, to train wrecks,

to building bombings, to earthquakes, to school shootings, and to 9/11, some of the most potent and appropriate examples of the ecological nature of crisis interventions have occurred in the United States in the last 10 years, as has a large mobilization, training, and response effort to provide emergency mental health services to victims and survivors of any type of imaginable disaster.

An enormous number of mental health workers from throughout the country, working under the auspices of the American Red Cross, NOVA, FEMA, and state and local EMAs and supported by the major professional mental health organizations in the United States, have contributed monumental services to the thousands of clients affected by those disasters (Bass & Yep, 2002; Gladding, 2002; Hayes, 2002; Juhnke, 2002; McCarthy, 2002; Pyszczynski et al., 2002; Riethmayer, 2002a, 2002b; Smith, 2002; Sullivan, 2002; Underwood & Clark, 2002). Among the comments of hundreds, perhaps thousands, of mental health workers over dozens of major crises, the following from Samuel Gladding is perhaps both descriptive and representative:

> In that capacity, I was an escort who walked with families from the front of the building to the back and talked with them about what they were feeling, what they had felt, or what they anticipated doing in regard to the emotions that would be coming. I also accompanied families to Ground Zero so they could see for themselves the horror and finality of the event. The view from the site helped many individuals begin the process of grieving in-depth, as they realized in a stark and striking way that those they had loved and cherished in so many ways were indeed dead and would not be coming back to be with them. (Gladding, 2002, p. 7)

Development of Crisis Response Teams (CRTs). The Oklahoma City federal building bombing, the shootings at Columbine High School and Sandy Hook Elementary School, and the 9/11 attacks felt like a punch in the stomach for many, if not most, people in the United States. The massive amounts of media coverage of those traumatic experiences and the disaster relief that followed in their wake brought graphic attention to how disasters are handled, including the work of immediate follow-up rapid response teams. These teams did not just spring up full-grown at the time of those disasters. Rather, throughout the late

1980s and 1990s, rapid response teams were developed to handle numerous tragedies and disasters, including hurricanes (Shelby & Tredinnick, 1995), serial murders (Wakelee-Lynch, 1990), plane crashes (Modrak, 1992; Shafer, 1989a), bank robberies and hijackings (Brom & Kleber, 1989), campus shootings (Guerra, 1999; Guerra & Schmitt, 1999; Sleek, 1998), and train explosions and post office shootings (National Organization for Victim Assistance, n.d.).

National Organization for Victim Assistance (NOVA) CRTs. The rapid crisis response team movement received impetus and support on a national level with the establishment of the National Crisis Response Project by the National Organization for Victim Assistance (NOVA) in the late 1980s (Young, 1991). Originally established to help victims of crime, NOVA, a private, not-for-profit organization, has branched out to offer help to victims of all kinds of disasters through the National Crisis Response Project. It has state and local affiliates throughout the United States. The project set up national crisis response teams (NCRTs) to assist communities following community-wide crises or disasters. One of the first major organized national responses of an NCRT for the specific purpose of providing mental health assistance was on August 20, 1986, when an Edmond, Oklahoma, postal worker shot and killed 14 coworkers and himself.

The main objective of an NCRT in dealing with a local community disaster is to form local crisis response teams that are in a position to deal with the community's grief reactions, stress effects, and PTSD resulting from the disaster. According to Young (1991), the "project is based on the premise that disasters can cause individual and community-wide crisis reactions and that immediate intervention can provide communities with tools that are useful in mitigating long-term distress" (pp. 83–84).

NCRTs are dispatched at the request of leaders in the affected community. "When a disaster occurs, NOVA is placed in contact with the community in one of two ways: either the community calls NOVA, or NOVA, on hearing of the tragedy, calls the community and offers assistance" (Young, 1991, p. 95). Three types of disaster service are available: (1) providing written material giving details on how to deal with the aftermath of a disaster; (2) providing telephone consultation to leading caregivers in the area affected; and (3) sending in a trained team of volunteer crisis workers to assist the community.

The Red Cross. The American Red Cross, like its Red Cross and Red Crescent counterparts around the world, is tasked with dealing with all kinds of disasters. Founded by Clara Barton, the American Red Cross has been in business for about 120 years. It is a private organization that has close ties with local, state, and federal governments. It helped the federal government start the FEMA. It is a major contributor to crisis intervention in the wake of large-scale disasters and megadisasters through its training of mental health professionals as members of rapid response teams (Red Cross, 2023). Professional organizations in counseling, psychology, and social work are closely linked with and provide candidates for its mental health training program.

Federal Emergency Management Agency (FEMA) and the National Institute of Mental Health (NIMH). FEMA was born in 1979 as the result of complaints about federal agencies' slowness, bureaucratic red tape, inefficiency, ineptitude, and duplication of effort in responding to a disaster. Several different agencies were merged into FEMA, and it is now housed in the Department of Homeland Security. FEMA has numerous responsibilities. Among them are education about all kinds of disaster preparedness and coordination between federal, state, and local emergency management agencies in regard to preparedness, training, and disaster mitigation. It provides disaster assistance that ranges from debris removal and rescue efforts to disaster loans for rebuilding and on-site mental health crisis response teams. Its Emergency Management Institute at Emmitsburg, Maryland, is a virtual university of emergency preparedness courses. Courses range from training community emergency response teams (CERTS), made up of ordinary local citizen volunteers who provide support to first responders to aid in rescue efforts, to colloquia with state mental health service providers on the latest techniques for providing mental health services after a large-scale disaster (FEMA, 2023).

Sometimes, more than one agency of the federal government coordinates the work of crisis response teams. Several instances of events during modern times that triggered such a coordinated effort were the earthquakes in both the Los Angeles and San Francisco areas; Hurricanes Hugo, Andrew, Floyd, Katrina, Rita, and Ian that brought devastation and flooding to large parts of the southeastern United

States; the nuclear accident at Three Mile Island; and the Love Canal contamination. The response teams were sent in by the NIMH and sponsored and funded by FEMA. In all such national disasters, FEMA and NIMH provide the widely affected areas with instruction, consultation, and expertise in developing local and regional support systems to cope with the enormous aftermath of these disasters (Shafer, 1989b).

Professional Organizations. Professional organizations, such as the American Psychiatric Association, the American Psychological Association, the American Counseling Association, and the National Association of Social Workers, provide volunteers for the Red Cross and NOVA CRTs. These organizations also provide a variety of publications for both professionals and laypersons that can be obtained on their websites or ordered from them. Their conferences and conventions provide formats for discussion and dissemination of the theory and practice of crisis intervention.

The American School Counseling Association and the National Association of School Psychologists are involved in providing crisis intervention services to school children and adolescents in the face of a large-scale disaster. The American School Counselor Association lists numerous resources for children and adolescents to deal with disasters (American School Counselor Association, 2023). The National Association of School Psychologists also lists many resources for helping children and adolescents cope in the aftermath of disasters (National Association of School Psychologists, 2023).

The National Association of School Psychologists has national emergency assistance teams (NEATs), which are tied in with NOVA. The mission of NEAT is to develop policies and procedures, disseminate information, provide consultation, and facilitate the training of school-based crisis teams in response to significant emergencies affecting children and adolescents (National Association of School Psychologists, 2023). These NEAT teams go to the scene of school disasters and provide support for local agencies. They are composed of nationally certified school psychologists who have expertise in crisis prevention, intervention, and postvention. The intention of the NEAT team is to help save lives, reduce trauma and injury, facilitate the psychological well-being of students and staff, and allow schools to return to regular activities as soon as possible (Zenere, 1998).

Faith-Based Organizations. Many faith-based organizations also respond during and after a disaster. The Salvation Army has been providing support since 1917 for disaster recovery (Dass-Brialsford, 2010). The Brethren Disaster Ministries helps survivors of disasters rebuild storm-damaged homes (Brethren Disaster Ministries, 2023). The Salvation Army provides food services, spiritual care, communication assistance, and social services (Salvation Army, 2023). The Southern Baptist Disaster Relief also offers disaster relief providing food, water, supplies, and comfort to people in need (Southern Baptist Denomination, 2023). The Samaritan's Purse provides international disaster relief in the form of food, water, medicine, shelter, and other supplies as needed (Samaritan's Purse, 2023). Many other faith-based organizations provide a wide range of services to assist and support survivors of disasters.

Constructing an Outreach Team. Depending on the nature of the crisis and the ecological setting, outreach teams generally have a diverse occupational range: from psychiatric nurses, paramedics, emergency workers, and psychiatrists to social workers, volunteers, rehabilitation counselors, police officers, and psychologists. These outreach teams are characterized by their multidisciplinary team approach, strong social and community networks, user participation in policy and service delivery, and egalitarianism in the workplace (Gulati & Guest, 1990). Alise Bartley, a private practice licensed professional counselor, describes her experience as a volunteer worker following Hurricane Katrina. Based in Gulfport, Mississippi, she slept in a large Navy Seabee storage facility with 600 other volunteers. She slept two feet from a retired nurse on one side and a Vietnam veteran on the other, both of whom she had just met for the first time in her life (Kennedy, 2007).

Integrative-collaborative teams have a distinctive operational setup and are characteristic of many geographical areas where financial and human resources are not sufficient to form freestanding, specialized crisis units. They are not an ad hoc group collected after a crisis but rather are trained prior to the crisis. Each member has different skills that, combined, allow the team to respond to a variety of crisis situations. They operate much as a volunteer fire department does. Members typically have primary jobs in other settings, but when a crisis call comes in on a hotline, they immediately leave their regular job, form a crisis team, and go to the crisis site. They are identifiable within the community as the crisis response team and are a cost-efficient and effective way to provide generic crisis intervention (Silver & Goldstein, 1992).

Vertically and Horizontally Integrated Local Emergency Management Systems.

Overarching all local agencies involved in a crisis after a disaster are the local emergency management agencies. They are the offspring of the old Civil Defense system of the Cold War. The examples that follow refer to Florida and Illinois, where local agencies are linked to the state emergency management agency. In turn, the state agency is linked to FEMA (Freeman, 2003; Lane, 2003).

Role of Local EMA Directors.

Local Emergency Management Agencies are the frontline of assistance following a disaster. Staff in these agencies are responsible for planning and coordinating to prepare, respond, and recover from natural and man-made disasters. Directors of these agencies work in consultation with state and federal emergency agencies to coordinate efforts. To say the least, the task is complicated but also different from city to city and region to region. Plans must take into account the possible disasters, both natural and man-made, that might occur in their location. For example, in Florida, plans must include maps for evacuation routes in case of hurricanes. In the farmlands of Illinois, directors must be concerned about chemical spills of agricultural products, intentionally or accidentally. In 2023, local emergency management agencies are working with state and federal agencies as they face water shortages due to a drought. Each city and region must tailor responses based on the likely disasters that might occur.

Local emergency managers are a breed of technocrat that are being placed in charge of coordinating a welter of activities, agencies, and logistical problems in regard to managing every conceivable emergency you might imagine and then some. If you'd like a job like this, a major aspect of this job is the use of acronyms, so be prepared. Want to be able to do an HHVA (hospital hazard vulnerability analysis) or get a RACES (radio amateur civil emergency system) up and running? Are you curious to know what the differences among cold, warm, and hot zones are, or whether you need a Level A protection suit when you venture into one of them? Does that sound like an interesting job? Think you'd like to do that?

Background and Training.

What are the qualifications? You may ask. What university do I need to attend to major in that "stuff"? The answer to that question now is, "About any place in the world." Several universities have stepped up to the challenge to train students specifically in disaster mental health. Other universities may offer an emphasis in a program, such as certificates or individual courses on the topic. You should understand that the content of these programs varies quite a bit because, as of yet, there is no clear consensus on what all that "stuff" should be. If you sought to earn a bachelor's degree with a major in Emergency and Disaster Management from Western Carolina University, for example, your courses could range from Social Dimension of a Disaster to Principles of Hazard Mitigation to Crisis Communications (Western Carolina University, 2023). If you already have a bachelor's degree, the University of Denver offers a master's degree in Security Management with a concentration in Emergency Planning and Response (University of Denver, 2023). Not interested in all that other "stuff," just want to stick to mental health? The University of South Dakota offers a 12-semester hour graduate certificate in Disaster Mental Health (University of South Dakota, 2023). So there's something for everyone who wants to get into this field.

There is a national certification process and an International Association of Emergency Managers. In Florida, emergency managers must be certified through a combination of coursework, training, and work experience. They must also take continuing education courses every four years to retain their certification. There is continuous ongoing training in management tools, resources, new technology, and communications.

If you want a professional emergency manager's job and certification in Florida, here are the requirements as of 2024: (1) Prescribed training and educational criteria plus 4 years of work experience in comprehensive emergency management, 2 years of which must be in Florida. (2) Working knowledge of basic tenets of emergency management, including mitigation, prevention, protection, response, and recovery. (3) Experience and knowledge of interagency and community-wide participation in planning, coordinating, and management functions designed to improve emergency management capabilities. (4) Ability to effectively accomplish the goals and objectives of emergency management in all environments (Florida Emergency Preparedness Association, 2023). Qualifications a little daunting? Maybe you want to start out as an assistant manager, which cuts your experience time in half. The point here is that while not every state, county, or municipality has such stringent requirements, the times of obtaining a job like this due to one's political patronage are pretty much gone.

What Do Emergency Managers Do? Certainly, disasters don't happen every day. Does that mean that emergency managers sit around playing video games, drinking coffee, eating doughnuts, testing their skill at Wordle, and polishing the fire engine, waiting for something to happen? Local EMAs are in the business of preparing for, preventing, intervening in, and mitigating the effects of any and all kinds of disasters. To do that takes a great deal of planning and coordinating. Direct your attention to the matrix of city and county agencies and the support functions they engage in as primary or secondary supports in a disaster (see Figure 16.3). While you might think of roads, bridges, potable water, and sewage disposal as being critical, the last thing you might think of would be animal issues. But if you had severe flooding after a hurricane, animals—both alive and dead—would be a very real problem.

Planning for Disasters. There are two types of disasters, those that have prior warning time and those that do not. As a result, local EMAs have various disaster plans that are implemented in stages. Although there might be very little warning in the case of a tornado or a chemical spill from a derailed train, hurricanes and forest fires generally do have a lead time for preparation. Generally speaking, plans are laid out in identifiable stages. A sample plan for hurricanes described below provides the blueprint and can be adapted for other disasters. This plan was originally developed by Nassau County in Florida (Nassau County Emergency Management Department, 2003). A brief description of those stages follows to give you an idea of the complexity of any plan. For each stage, a particular action is noted, and the responsible section is designated to implement it. Those sections are emergency operation center (EOC) command, planning, logistics, operations, administration, recovery task force, and elected policy makers.

   Awareness stage. 72–60 hours Estimated Land Fall (ELF) of a hurricane. In this stage, the Emergency Command Center is activated, and communication is established with the National Weather Service, the state department of emergency man-

agement, surrounding counties, media, utility services, law enforcement, and fire agencies. While that sounds straightforward, plans must be made for maintaining that communication during the duration of the hurricane. This is the time to also test EOC communications equipment. An initial vulnerability analysis is conducted, including monitoring primary evacuation routes. Notification is made to all gas and diesel wholesalers to restock retail outlets within 12–24 hours.

   Standby stage. 60–48 hours ELF. The emergency broadcast system is activated, and amateur radio groups are notified to go on standby. Local media and National Weather Service bulletins are used to advise boat owners, homeowners, drawbridge operators, and motel and hotel managers and detail causeway and bridge closings and evacuation routes. Emergency worker shelters are created, along with stocking supplies and other resources. EMS ambulances, transport vehicles, oil spill trailers, and heavy equipment are advised to be ready to respond when the need arises.

   Decision stage. 48–45 hours ELF. Emergency transport is secured, and a traffic control plan is started. A state of emergency is declared, and the emergency plan triggered. Advisories are broadcast for non-essential businesses to close. Decision-making shifts to an emergency model that bypasses typical bureaucratic roadblocks. All municipalities, law enforcement agencies, fire districts, utility companies, hospitals, and medical care facilities with the State Division of Emergency Management and the National Hurricane Center are informed to be on standby and ready to respond in appropriate and safe ways.

   Preparation stage. 45–36 hours ELF. Plans for "at risk" populations such as those living in mobile homes, people with physical or developmental disabilities, tourists, campers, people without transportation, and low-lying areas are activated. Activation of all EOC communication systems is started. Announcements of public closings are made. 24-hour operation of fleet management garage and fueling resources is implemented. Emergency transportation plans and shelters are activated.

   Evacuation stage. 36–4 hours ELF. Identification of and areas at risk evacuation orders issued. Public announcement of shelter open-

Agencies (P = Primary, S = Support)	ESF 1 Transportation	ESF 2 Communication	ESF 3 Public Works	ESF 4 Fire Fighting/Emerg. Medic	ESF 5 Information & Planning	ESF 6 Mass Care	ESF 7 Resource Support	ESF 8 Health and Medical	ESF 9 Search & Rescue	ESF 10 Hazardous Materials	ESF 11 Food & Water	ESF 12 Energy	ESF 13 Military Support	ESF 14 Public Information	ESF 15 Volunteers & Donations	ESF 16 Law Enforcement	ESF 17 Animal Issues
All local media														S			
Amateur Radio Emerg. Serv.		S			S									S			
Acme County Medical Center				S	S			S						S			
Goodwill Industries Center														S	S		
Midville City Public Works Dept.	S		S		S		S						S	S			
Midville City Fire Department		S		S	S				S	S				S			
Midville City Police Department		S			S									S		S	
Midville City Planning Department					S									S			
Civil Air Patrol		S			S									S			
Contracted Medical Examiner								S						S			
State Dept. of Law Enforcement													P	S			
State Highway Patrol													S			P	
State National Guard Forces													S	S			
State Power and Light Dept.												S		S			
State Public Utilities Dept.												P		S			
Animal emergency care centers														S			S
Home Health Care Agencies								P						S			
Regional Electrical Authority		S					S					S		S			
Medical Supply Companies								S						S			
Acme County Building Dept.		S			S		S							S			
Acme County Cattleman's Assoc.														S			S
Acme County Clerk of Court							S							S			
Acme County Coordinator														S			
Acme County Council on Aging	S				S		S	S						S			
Acme County Emergency Mgmt.				S	P	S	S	S		S	S		S	P	S		S
Acme County Engineering Services				S	S		S							S			
Acme County Extension Agency						S	S				S			S	P		S
Acme County Facilities Maintenance		S			S		S							S			
Acme County Fire/Rescue		S		P	S		S		P	P				S			
Acme County Geog. Info. Systems					S		S							S			
Acme County Health Dept.						S	S	P						S			
Acme County Humane Society														S			P
Acme County Jail							S							S			
Acme County Library System														S			
Acme County Planning Dept.					S		S							S			
Acme County Risk Management								P			P			S			
Acme County Road & Bridge Dept.	S		P		S		S						S	S			
Acme County School Board	P				S	P	S	S						S			
Acme County Sheriff's Office	S	P		S	S		S	S	S	S	S			S		P	S
Acme County Solid Waste Dept.			S		S		S							S			
Acme County Veterinary Society														S			S
Acme County Volunteer Center							S							S	S		
Regional American Red Cross						P		S			S			S	S		
State Parks & Recreational Services													S	S			
Private businesses												S		S			
Salvation Army						S						S		S	S		
Mental health centers								S						S			
Volunteer organizations												S		S			

Figure 16.3   Midville City/Acme County Emergency Support Function Matrix

Source: Adapted from Nassau County, Florida, Emergency Management Department (Freeman, 2003).

ings and transportation pickup points are made. Requests are made to the National Weather Service to broadcast information on road closures. The shutdown of electric power services is activated/coordinated. Communication with public shelters, emergency worker family shelters, special care centers, emergency transportation, area hospitals, animal emergency care facilities, power, water, sewage, utilities, fire districts, law enforcement, and public works is continuous.

Storm/emergency stage. There is constant monitoring of storm/emergency characteristics. Pre-planning post-storm activities and communications with other agencies is nonstop.

Immediate emergency stage. Local emergency response activities are ongoing as permitted, ensuring the safety of responders. Assessment begins for long-term human service needs, including mental health care counseling. Information and referral services are determined. Temporary housing needs are assessed. Resources such as food, water, clothing, and cleanup kits are distributed. The recovery task force is activated, and a review begins for reporting damage. The implementation of appropriate moratoriums and the adoption of emergency resolutions and ordinances are recommended. Public health conditions are monitored, and a curfew is implemented on an as-needed basis.

Evaluation stage. Establish if the primary threat still exists, and conduct/coordinate initial impact assessment efforts. Reaffirm and/or reestablish communications with all shelters, hospitals, towns, state emergency operations, law enforcement, public works, fire districts, and surrounding counties. Enact emergency resolutions. Determine initial mutual aid requirements and request assistance from state EOC. Discuss emergency ordinances to be enacted. Issue news media releases. Establish times for briefings/planning meetings. Report accidents to date, update statuses. Assess damage to areas with existing or potential hazardous materials. Summarize the current operational activities underway. Begin a review process of the plan and its effectiveness. Determine if additional resources are needed. Implement rest and rotation policies for emergency workers. Assess the logistics of the transportation routes opened, distribution sites,

feeding procedures, and available sleeping facilities.

Reconstruction stage. Perform long-term activities or projects focused on improving or strengthening the community's economy. Complete the restoration of services. Dispose of debris and allocate resources to cleanup chores. Focus on community recovery planning, building and construction issues, and environmental/ecological issues. Continue/complete human service delivery assistance of information and referral, resource distribution, health care delivery, mental health care counseling, and transportation assistance. Complete activities for a presidential disaster declaration. Perform hazard mitigation projects to reduce the community's susceptibility and vulnerability to hurricanes. Repair, replace, modify, or relocate public facilities in hazard-prone areas.

Restoration stage. Perform an assessment of community needs and economic damage. Address the following restoration issues: economic and job base assessment, community recovery planning, building and construction issues, public information and citizen outreach, environmental issues, and ecological concerns. Provide health care delivery for both pre- and postdisaster needs, including home health care management and case referral. Put mental health care counseling into operation. Determine victims' counseling needs by triage assessment. Determine training needs for mental health professions on disaster-related issues. Place mental health professions/CISD team members on community assessment teams. Determine where counseling services will operate. Determine the transportation needs to public feeding sites, shelters, and disaster service sites. Reestablish and implement public transportation service. Complete chore service needs assessment for cleanup. Determine needs and coordinate with volunteer groups for debris cleanup, interior home cleanup, window repair, etc. Coordinate with FEMA to set up a Disaster Field Office and Disaster Application Centers. Assist in establishing temporary housing sites. Establish a federal public assistance office to coordinate all disaster relief efforts to clients. Participate in interagency hazard mitigation team and hazard mitigation survey activities. Complete after-evacuation report and county incident report. Critique the management of the storm emergency.

Throughout the unfolding stages of the disaster, constant needs assessment should occur. A community mental health needs assessment formula (Flynn, 2003, p. 23) that constantly updates the dead, hospitalized, non-hospitalized injured, homes destroyed, homes with major and minor damage, unemployed due to job loss, and other losses will give a good indication of the potential numbers of people in need of crisis counseling services. The same community-wide assessment should continuously occur in regard to mental health (Katz, 2011).

As we stated, the foregoing plan for hurricanes can be tailored to any kind of disaster, whether natural or human-made. While timelines may be very compressed or, in some instances, operations may start at the emergency stage, the format is replicable with just about any kind of community-wide crisis. Although local EMAs have very little preparation time for other types of disasters, they do not stand idly by waiting for something to happen. Continuous interagency tabletop exercises give them practice in responding to a variety of potential disasters. Assessment of particularly vital and vulnerable public sites, ranging from water treatment plants to nursing homes, is made to determine what needs and weak points there may be. Emergency managers generally spend a fair amount of time working with individual agencies to develop their own internal disaster plans to fit with the overall one the local EMA has.

Mental Health Components of Local EMAs

LO6   Any local mental health clinic should have a prototype disaster response plan (Lane, 2003). While each community will have variations due to its own particular regional and state systems of mental health delivery, geographic locale, and population differences, they should generally follow along with what Hartsough (1982), and SAMHSA's (2021) *TAP 34: Disaster Planning Handbook for Behavioral Health Systems* has outlined for mental health agencies' typical response to a disaster.

The following points are abstracted from Hartsough (1982), Lane (2003), and SAMHSA (2021). First of all, the centers must have a plan that assumes they may be victims themselves and have breakdowns in communications; loss of or inability to find staff; loss of equipment, supplies, and records; inability of staff to cope with loss; and problems recognizing their functional limits. The mental health center must be prepared to provide services in two situations—a localized but traumatic event and a large-scale disaster. A

localized event can be responded to without affecting operations to any great degree. A disaster will most likely disrupt operations to some degree, while drastically increasing the demand for services. This may happen in two distinct ways. If the disaster is local, dealing with their own residential population is the primary focus. If in an evacuee center, dealing with guest evacuees plus handling their own client population, becomes the dual focus.

A clear chain of command with redundancy features is mandatory. There should be an assessment of population groups in the area with regard to high-risk groups such as children, English language learners, older adults, people with physical or developmental disabilities, and low socioeconomic groups. Interagency cooperative agreements should be made in regard to backup resources in regard to treatment, habitation, medical supplies, and personnel. A specific mental health liaison person should be named to the local Emergency Management Agency.

Predisaster training encompasses the development of outreach programs that target "average everyday people acting normally in an abnormal situation." Risk and threat assessment teams should be formed if they are not already in place. Training specifically targets practitioners who have not had formal training in outreach or who historically perform poorly when they have to rely on their formal training in individual counseling and not on-the-spot creative thinking and decision making. Consideration should be given to sending local clinicians to Red Cross training. Drills and tabletop exercises should be developed and conducted in coordination with the local Emergency Management Agency.

Personnel. Volunteers who would function as reserve crisis counselors should be recruited and trained in crisis intervention skills. Specified workers should be selected for multidisciplinary crisis response teams. A chief of operations should be nominated and will be the individual actually running the disaster response. There should also be an emergency preparedness coordinator who will be responsible for planning and preparation prior to a disaster and will function as a consultant to the chief of operations during an actual emergency. This person will be the liaison to the local emergency management agency. There should be back up available to these critical positions. The SAMHSA disaster mobile app (SAMHSA, 2021) should be in the hands of these critical staff. This tool offers first responders immediate access to SAMHSA operational procedures for any type of traumatic event at every phase of response, including pre-deployment preparation, on-the-ground assistance, and post-deployment resources.

An outside clinical consultant should be retained to assess the physical and mental condition of the staff. A command-and-control and communications center should be established and staffed by a team leader and other staff necessary for it to function effectively. A historian should keep an ongoing journal of activities that occur as a result of the disaster. The decisions, events, problems, and information should include details, names and addresses, times, and issues that can later be used for debriefings, psychological autopsies, system improvements, grant requests, or reimbursement.

A personnel liaison will assist the chief of operations in assessing, making, and tracking staff and volunteer assignments. A media/information liaison will provide information to the media and local government, develop press releases, and distribute general information regarding service delivery. Staff may be made available to the local EOC to provide psychological support.

Transdisaster (0–14 Days). The mental health unit needs to initiate immediate mental health services when the disaster occurs; restore services to clients served during normal times; provide service to any evacuees with a particular emphasis on methadone and buprenorphine treatment provision; act as the disaster mental health advisor to the local government; provide outreach programs and coordinate resources for the delivery of disaster mental health services from the Red Cross, NOVA, FEMA, and other religious and philanthropic organizations; coordinate the responses of any contractors for services with a particular emphasis on the evacuation of residential facilities; target specific areas, such as evacuation centers, emergency relief centers, and FEMA "one-stop" service centers; provide support services for disaster workers; and assist with mental health emergencies in hospitals with victims requiring medical or psychiatric care. Contingency plans should be made for resupplying medication, security, and dispensing of medication in sometimes chaotic conditions. Client records should have safe storage and retrievable sites. Confidentiality is at risk of being compromised, so efforts to keep records secure should be considered in where and how they are stored

Postdisaster (15–365 Days). Evaluate and assess the need for postdisaster services; implement prepared

immediate services grant and prepare regular services grant if a presidential disaster is declared; establish linkages with American Red Cross mental health workers to hand off clients requiring longer-term care; monitor for long-term psychological effects; educate the public regarding disaster-related psychological phenomena; evaluate the program response, both short and long term; perform a psychological autopsy on the total crisis response; and debrief workers.

In the foregoing sections of this chapter, you have read about the overall composition of disaster planning and infrastructure. In an ideal world, even in a world of disasters, all of this runs smoothly. While 9/11 certainly had its share of chaos and confusion (Halpern & Tramontin, 2007, pp. 171–197; Kaul & Welzant, 2005; Norris et al., 2006), order came out of that maelstrom fairly quickly, and everybody thought they had learned a lot of lessons. Then along came Hurricane Katrina, and everything got turned upside down.

What Happened With Katrina?

In any disaster, there is invariably an attempt to fix blame. If blame can be fixed, then people may start to believe that the impossible, out-of-control, unbelievable, chaotic, and unfathomable event can be contained, made sense of as to the reasons it occurred, and a sense of control regained as to what went wrong and how it can be made right the next time. In that sense, Hurricane Katrina is no different from the multitudes of other natural disasters that have hit other countries. Indeed, in comparison to typhoons and earthquakes that have plagued Asia and the Middle East, it is a relatively small event, and certainly so in regard to loss of life. Yet, the recriminations from Hurricane Katrina are unending and rub raw nerves from the standpoints of socioeconomic, racial, political, and even interstate rivalries. It is expected, rightly or wrongly, that disasters will occur in other countries that are not likely to happen in the United States. Most people in the United States pride themselves on controlling their destiny through science and industry, up to and including controlling nature. After Katrina, apparently not!

This is not an exposition about who's to blame or what's to blame. The emerging facts suggest that there is plenty of blame to pass around and share. However, what Anahita Gheytanchi and her associates (2007) have compiled is worth reporting as a way of looking at how the various systems within a disaster ecosystem operate or, in the case of Hurricane Katrina, . . . don't! Gheytanchi and her associates report 12 key failures of response.

1. **Lack of efficient communication.** The sine qua non of disaster mitigation is communication. Both within and between the primary and super mesosystems, communication failed. At least four separate command structures were operating in Katrina's aftermath: two command structures in FEMA and two military command structures. That's at least two too many and resulted in crossed communications, duplicated or incomplete efforts, and generally clouded decision making.

2. **Poor coordination plans.** Coordination is about moving assets to where they are most needed. The inability to coordinate relief efforts ranged from not utilizing one of the finest hospital ships in the world, the U.S.S. *Bataan,* which sat idly offshore, to the inability of FEMA to find buses and drivers and move people out of the Superdome, to hundreds of trucks filled with ice sitting idly in Memphis freight yards with no place to go, to thousands of house trailers sitting in Arkansas when they were desperately needed in Mississippi and Louisiana.

3. **Ambiguous authority relationships.** The Department of Homeland Security remained on a "pull" basis, which means the state had to request federal assets rather than a "push" basis, which means that assets would be immediately made available to the state. The National Response Plan Catastrophic Incident Annex (NPR-CIA) should have been invoked prior to landfall but, in fact, was never invoked. The prevarication and waffling by Louisiana state and local governments on instituting mandatory evacuation because of the cost, even though they were getting intense pressure from federal authorities to do so, caused severe problems that culminated in the Superdome fiasco.

4. **Who's in charge?** Factious political fights plagued relief efforts. The shifting of blame from the mayor of New Orleans to the governor of Louisiana to the president of the United States settled nothing. Lessons from previous hurricanes about coordination among federal, state, and local governments had not been learned or at least not been put into practice. Laws that govern the use of the armed forces in the continental United States also severely hamstrung efforts to quickly deploy military personnel and needed to be changed.

5. **Counterterrorism versus all-hazards response.** Money, staff, and other assets had been drained out of FEMA and moved to Homeland Security's efforts to combat terrorism. A natural disaster the size of Hurricane Katrina compares to any terrorist attack up to a nuclear detonation or release of the plague. Yet, Homeland Security funded disaster preparedness for terrorism as opposed to natural disaster at a 7-to-1 ratio pre-Katrina.

6. **Ambiguous training standards and lack of preparation.** Across the board, training and experience with disasters were lacking. While the aforementioned FEMA training to become a certified LEMA manager sounds good, the reality is that the training requirements to become an emergency manager and become certified were cumbersome and difficult to complete. Standards for the accreditation of response agencies were also vague and not tied to any performance-based evidence.

7. **Where is the "learning" in lessons learned?** A multiagency hurricane exercise that very closely resembled Katrina was completed prior to the storm. Outcomes closely paralleled what actually happened. Yet, the failure of local and state governments to follow up and take advantage of the exercise doomed it to collect dust on the shelf. This is not the first instance of failure to heed learning from the past. Putting into practice all of the procedures necessary to stave off a disaster like Katrina is difficult, costly, and time consuming; it demands expertise and interagency cooperation at the local level and vertical integration with state and federal agencies. Tackling the logistical and tactical problems involved in implementing those procedures takes a backseat when the danger is not imminent.

8. **Performance assessment was not integrated into the process.** In an evidence-based world, continuous performance assessment should be built into disaster relief efforts, but that is not the case. Performance evaluation is especially lacking in mental health provision. An assessment device that provides benchmarks and rubrics to gauge how relief is proceeding and how well it is going is sorely needed so best practices models may be generated. However, the uniqueness of disasters makes developing performance assessment processes difficult at best and impossible at worst.

Although disasters have common elements, the individuality of each must be accounted for.

9. **The geography of poverty.** Are race and socio-economic status response factors? While race became a factor because the majority of people in the lowest income bracket in New Orleans were African Americans the fact is that disaster plans as they are currently formulated put the poor, older adults, people with disabilities, and other disenfranchised individuals who are not financially or physically able to evacuate, relocate, or rebuild at extreme risk without regard to race, creed, color, national origin, religion, sexual preference, or any other distinctive human quality.

10. **Rumor and chaos.** Urban legend and rumor, the bane of any disaster, ran rampant in New Orleans. No clearly designated official spokesperson appeared, giving clear, unconflicted, factual messages that could be believed. Exaggeration by elected officials of armed violence was given airtime by the media, and these rumors then turned into "facts" and took on a life of their own. At its best, the rumor served to warn people and put them on their guard. At its worst, it turned into a self-fulfilling prophecy that slowed rescue efforts. Concrete, factual, up-to-the-minute information by an official spokesperson with both face and content validity was essentially absent. Above all else, an ironclad rule in any disaster is that one highly valid, knowledgeable spokesperson gives facts out in a timely manner and dispels rumors as they arise.

11. **Personal and community preparedness.** There was clearly a sharp divide between what happened in Louisiana and Mississippi in regard to recovery efforts. Both states suffered an equal amount of catastrophic devastation along their coast. However, for whatever reasons, and there are many variables to be examined, Mississippi was more resilient. Whether the majority of its people had better resources and support systems is a different question from whether they were prepared. However, that question needs to be examined carefully, for both physical and psychological differences. Cultural differences that heavily influenced long-term outcomes in the two states must also be taken into account.

12. **Disaster mental health and the role of mental health professionals.** What actually works for reducing mental health problems in people afflicted with a disaster like Katrina is still not clear, and a great deal of research needs to be done to find out what evidence-based practices do work. Critical incident stress debriefing (CISD), which has been used and most certainly abused as a panacea, appears not to be the ultimate answer. Further, attributions that label survivors as suffering from a mental illness don't work very well either. The preferred operating mode now is the use of psychological first aid and social support (Watson et al., 2011). Self-efficacy models that foster self-reliance, coping, and problem-solving skills, focus on individual needs, seek to extinguish PTSD at early onset, and concentrate on functional recovery rather than looking for pathology seem to hold promise (Ruzek, 2006).

What about COVID-19?

The unthinkable became thinkable when the COVID-19 pandemic spread across the globe (Boin et al., 2021). Emergency management agencies ran as fast as they could in attempts to respond, keep up with, and provide services. The mental health field was no exception. The COVID-19 pandemic caused a drastic shift in the manner services were provided (Emergence Health Network interview, November 2022). Experiencing and struggling to manage fear and anxiety, not to mention the other mental health issues related to the spread of the virus that could lead to a higher risk of suicide was an issue (Shah et al., 2020). The stress produced during the pandemic resulted in shattering social cohesion in terms of trust, threatening its sense of collective efficacy (Tabernero et al., 2020).

Tayyib (2022) suggests five strategies needed to address the mental health effect of the COVID-19 pandemic and possibly new megacrises. Each builds on the others, developing a comprehensive plan to mitigate the mental health issues in the midst of megacrises. The first strategy is to engage and partner with community leaders and community-based organizations. This strategy creates the communication, cooperation, and coordination line needed when a disaster happens. The second strategy involves establishing or re-establishing community support networks, including self-help groups. The third strategy involves conducting community outreach, education, and training on the signs and symptoms of mental health issues. This training involves ways to access mental health resources and effective supportive and coping skills during the disaster. Strategy four is the deployment of community health workers to access, engage, and educate community members. Finally, the fifth strategy uses a community capacity-building and community empowerment-oriented approach. Tayyib (2022) adds that religious/spiritual leaders can be particularly useful to engage and strengthen their communities during an infectious disease outbreak by building a sense of community solidarity and resilience.

Psychological First Aid and Psychosocial Support as Applied to Disaster Survivors

As detailed in Chapter 1, "Approaching Crisis Intervention," the NIMH (2002) defines psychological first aid (PFA) as establishing safety of the client, reducing stress-related symptoms, providing rest and physical recuperation, and linking clients to critical resources and social support systems. Psychological first aid has now been adapted and modified from its initial use by Raphael (1977) into a first-order, evidence-based approach to working with survivors of mass disasters (Brymer et al., 2009; Hobfoll et al., 2007). It may be taught to paraprofessionals and nonprofessionals. For example, it is one of the training modules (CERT, 2011) that volunteer CERT workers get as part of their search and rescue work training.

Psychological first aid as it is applied in a disaster is designed to reduce distress, generate short- and long-term adaptive functioning, and link survivors with additional services (Megaletta et al., 2022). *The Field Operations Guide for Psychological First Aid* developed by the National Child Traumatic Stress Network and the National Center for PTSD (NCTSN/NCPTSD, 2006) is considered state-of-the art in that regard (Webber et al., 2010). Delivery of PFA includes a number of core actions (NCTSN/NCPTSD, 2006): make initial respectful contact by a warm, engaging presence; gather and provide information in regard to supports needed to deal with immediate physical and safety concerns; provide and direct people in regard to practical assistance needed; provide for their safety and comfort both from a physical and psychological standpoint by linking them with social services; teach them basic coping skills if requested; get information and help that will connect them to social supports, such as reuniting them with family and other social groups with which they are involved.

The job of CFA workers is not to attempt to engage in therapy or elicit details of the tragedy; rather, it is to reduce acute psychological distress by their supportive and compassionate presence through basic active listening and responding skills (Everly & Flynn, 2005). Initiating contact involves the notion of "just being there" or "compassionate loitering" (Webber et al., 2010), which emphasizes careful observation, a nonintrusive presence, and caring, respectful contact. One example is the crisis workers who were available in the dining halls of Virginia Tech residence facilities and classrooms immediately after the shootings there. Volunteers had handouts on common reactions to tragedies, self-care tips about trauma, and resource lists. Workers were instructed to engage and support students who seemed to be struggling by a respectful, nonintrusive introduction as a way to offer their support. They wore purple armbands to identify their presence. They reported that students initially would not speak to them, but as time went by and students started coming to terms with their grief, they would stop by and thank them for being there (Lawson et al., 2010).

Even doing the foregoing may not be necessary as most people are pretty resilient after a disaster (Hobfoll et al., 2007). As indicated in Chapter 2, "Culturally Effective Helping in Crisis," insistence on participating in "psychotherapy" may be met with anger and extreme resistance. In support of the concept of voluntary participation, Bonanno et al. (2011) found that a "one size fits all" intervention might hold no advantage over, and could even undermine, the self-efficacy and resiliency of survivors. For many others, PFA may be both necessary and sufficient. Finally, for a few others, PFA may be necessary but not sufficient.

When More Than PFA Is Needed

It was first thought that the severity of exposure to the event and the severity of postevent stress and adversity would be the greatest factors indicating the need for more in-depth intervention for serious and chronic psychological problems (Norris, 2006). However, since 9/11, it is clear that the degree of exposure or proximity to the attacks does not explain all of the persons presenting with severe psychological problems after a disaster. An individual waving an American flag for hours and hours over an interstate highway 1,000 miles from the impact sites and refusing to come down for safety is one example among literally thousands of individuals across the country who were so distressed after 9/11 and needed something more than PFA. In other words, vicarious traumatization through exposure to merely seeing or hearing about disaster events could instigate maladaptive psychological responding. As a consequence, Watson et al. (2011) have compiled a laundry list from their own and a number of other researchers that total 22 risk factors for adults and 13 for children. We believe it doesn't make a lot of sense to try to go through that list and winnow out significant variables. What we do believe in is knowing how to use the Triage Assessment Form (TAF) in this book. People scoring 20 or more are going to need something more than PFA for sure; they are going to need someone to monitor them closely until they regain some precrisis equilibrium and are able to make healthy constructive decisions. People in the high 20s, who are potentially lethal to themselves or others either by intended commission of unsafe acts or unintended omissions of activities needed to keep them safe, should not be turned loose. People in the high teens will most likely profit from PFA *and* a good deal of on-site psychosocial support so they don't escalate into the 20s. People in the low teens are probably ideal candidates for PFA. Anyone in the single digits on the TAF probably needs to counsel us!

The Current State of Affairs

The problem with this latter approach, however, is twofold. First, it assumes that a large enough number of practitioners have the necessary crisis intervention skills to do this. If mental health practitioners are not available, then paraprofessionals or laypersons like those who operate in Community Emergency Response Teams (CERTs) and are taught psychological first aid as part of their training may be initial providers of psychological support. That may be stretching it a bit. With all due respect to CERT volunteers, we spend a lot of time teaching these "first aid" techniques to graduate students. They are not easy to implement, particularly when faced with a person in crisis, and we wonder if the estimated learning time of 1 hour and 15 minutes (including video) will be sufficient (CERT, 2011).

You will soon hear from a licensed professional counselor who was deployed in Louisiana post-Katrina. This counselor has extensive training and practice in crisis intervention. She is still the exception rather than the rule. Given her background and training, she struggled and reevaluated her therapeutic worldview as she went through her tour of duty. Her story is not much different from that of many others who were there with her. While the American Red Cross crisis counseling training program has trained thousands of practitioners, that resource was clearly not enough for Hurricane Katrina. The Red Cross and government agencies were forced to suspend their standards and bring in any licensed counselor, psychologist, social worker, psychiatric nurse, or psychiatrist they could get their hands on.

FEMA's crisis counseling assistance and training program (CCA-TP) is available to state mental health authorities once an area has been declared a disaster area by the president. That is a lot like closing the barn door after the horse has escaped. Way too many things are happening to stop and say, "OK, we now have a large, metastasizing disaster on our hands; let's do some training!" This training occurred in Memphis approximately a month after Katrina when the city was full of evacuees. To say it was mostly useless is being kind. We believe that training should come prior to any catastrophic event and follow-up refresher courses should go with it. After a congressional inquiry into this program's problems in south Florida, a critical review of it was instigated, and a number of worthwhile recommendations were made to tighten it and beef it up—particularly in regard to coordination activities (Department of Homeland Security, 2008). None of those recommendations made it clear whether a municipality can actually get training prior to a disaster, though.

Young and his associates (Young, 2006; Young et al., 2006) have developed a comprehensive predisaster training program that holds much promise. It has a conceptual framework that differentiates natural and human-caused disasters and examines effects on both individuals and communities. It has both practitioner and administrative training components and specific modules on high-risk client populations and interfaces with other organizations. This fine program is time consuming, most likely expensive, and requires trainers who have expertise in both disaster mental health practice and administration. Those are difficult commodities to find. The same criticism can be leveled at employing SAMHSA's (2021) training manual. While the content is fine, it boils down to finding the funding and expense as to who will do it and when the time will be set aside in typically understaffed and overloaded client community mental health facilities for it to happen.

Consistent and comprehensive training for mental health providers in crisis intervention as they matriculate through professional training programs has been piecemeal at best (Coke-Weatherly, 2005) as clearly described by Roberts (2005). That appears to be changing to some extent. The Council for Accreditation of Counseling and Related Educational Programs and the National Association of School Psychologists both require the teaching of crisis intervention in their accrediting criteria. While that may now be seen as necessary, it remains to be seen whether what is taught will be sufficient. Other professional accreditation agencies appear to make the provision of crisis intervention training voluntary.

Most certainly, Katrina was a natural disaster that had metastasizing effects far beyond its geographic landfall and a physical scope that had never before been experienced, with disenfranchised people shipped all over the United States. The terrorist attack on 9/11 probably had the widest range of vicarious psychological effects ever experienced in the United States, with the possible exception of the Japanese attack on Pearl Harbor. A number of national committees issuing from both 9/11 and Katrina have made numerous recommendations in regard to the provision of crisis services to individuals following these human-made and natural disasters. These recommendations have been summarized by Watson et al. (2011) in their article on postdisaster psychological intervention since 9/11, supplemented by our comments.

1. Be proactive ahead of time with pragmatic, flexible plans that match appropriate services to each phase of the recovery period. They don't need to be expensive, but they don't need to be cheap either.

2. Promote a sense of safety, connectedness, calm, hope, and efficacy. We operate with a salutogenic mind set which means a "can do!" attitude.

3. Participate in groups with stakeholders to coordinate and learn from others, minimize duplication, and mend gaps in service and take the time to do it right.

4. Be culturally sensitive and consider human rights. Chapter 2, "Culturally Effective Helping in Crisis," details some pretty hard evidence that disenfranchised people, including those who are older and have a disability, can be given short shrift in disaster relief efforts.

5. Be willing to undergo evaluation and open to scrutiny of practices. Debriefing should not be person but product and service centered.

6. Stay up to date on evidence-based practices. Read journals, go to conferences, have informal focus groups as to what's new and try new procedures out.

7. Maximize participation by local populations and find and use local resources and capabilities. The real estate sales pitch is, "Location! Location! Location!" Yours should be, "Network! Network! Network!"

8. Integrate activities and programs into larger systems to reduce stand-alone services, reach more people, and be more sustainable over time and space. Network means other folks in other professions as well.

9. Use a stepped approach that focuses early efforts on practical help and pragmatic support, with psychological first aid for a generally resilient population. Use the most minimal and efficient approach you can. If it isn't working, step it up ... some!

10. Use triage assessment and focused care for those with specialized needs who require increased levels of intervention. Trust your TAF assessment ability.

11. Provide technological assistance, consultation, and training to local providers and build alliances and network with them while you are at it.

12. Conduct needs assessment of the community with ongoing monitoring of services and program evaluation. Time passes and things change. Keep up with the times.

13. Support community-based cultural rituals, memorial services, and spiritual healing practices. If you are a newcomer to the community, talk to people who are in the memorial, funeral, and spiritual business and find out how the community responds to loss.

Priscilla Dass-Brailsford's book *Crisis and Disaster Counseling: Lessons Learned From Hurricane Katrina and Other Disasters* (2010) examines many of these recommendations, and the lack of their in-depth implementation. The book places particular emphasis on cultural variables (Boyd et al., 2010; Boyd-Franklin, 2010; Dass-Brailsford, 2010) that affected mitigation efforts post-Katrina. How the worker interacts in the first few minutes and hours of contact will most likely determine how effective intervention is and can profoundly affect the recovery course of survivors (Miller, 2010). You should understand that this is why we included a chapter on multiculturalism in this book because this is one of the most important variables in disaster crisis intervention.

You should also understand that, as yet, we believe the foregoing 13 principles are neither well known nor practiced regularly by a sufficient number of folks in this business to handle a disaster. That is particularly true of pandemics, in which the needs will be exponentially greater than in a local disaster like Katrina (Webber & Mascari, 2010).

Crisis intervention is not the major occupational definition of most of the people who are called to a mass disaster, nor are you going to find it named in the Dictionary of Occupational Titles. Until that happens, there are likely to be, both on an individual and systemic basis, problems from people attempting to ply this trade who don't know what they are doing or, worse yet, think they do but don't. Frankly, the mere fact that you are reading this book most likely makes you more knowledgeable about crisis intervention than a lot of other professionals who hold PhDs in the helping services fields. The recent birth of Division 56 (Trauma Psychology) of the American Psychological Association and the requirements of counseling and school psychology accrediting agencies for the provision of crisis intervention are a start, along with the American Red Cross's view to expand its psychological intervention curriculum and conduct outreach to more constituencies. Evidence-based treatment practices are starting to be published, but the real-time chaos of disasters makes it hard to do much other than do ex post facto studies. We agree with Silverman et al. (2010) that with all due respect to PFA, which appears to have replaced CISD as the treatment de jour, we would like to see a whole lot more outcome studies on its effectiveness, particularly in regard to whom it is applied, by what kinds of people, under what kinds of conditions. Please forgive us for being flinty-eyed about panaceas, but 130 collective years in this business have seen a lot of cure-alls come and go.

The People of Disasters: Responders and Survivors

Crisis Workers at the Disaster

LO7 Crisis workers have a wide range of duties after a disaster. Foremost is simply being available for survivors to talk with, listening to their experiences, empathizing, and processing with them as they attempt to make sense of it. These activities fall mostly within the provision of psychosocial support services and psychological first aid. Workers may help survivors locate significant others, help relatives with the identification of victims, or help make arrangements for the deceased. They may provide information on the affective, behavioral, cognitive, interpersonal, and physiological responses to traumatic events (Friedman et al., 2006).

Crisis workers may help relatives through the grieving process, promote social support systems for survivors, and devise a plan of action to mobilize the survivors' resources. They may make appropriate referrals and provide follow-up services. They may also provide debriefing to other emergency service workers (Walker, 1990), prepare food, find clothing, wash dishes, move rubble, help people find lost puppies, talk about how a family who has just lost everything is going to get their 17-year-old into the private college they had planned sending her to but now have no money to do so, administer first aid, help people figure out insurance and FEMA claim procedures, help determine what to do with a grandmother whose nursing home is now full of black mold, conflict-resolve angry feelings between tired, hot, smelly inhabitants of a disaster shelter, and do a thousand other things that lend physical and psychological support—all while dining on military MREs, contracting head lice, going without a bath for a *very* long time, getting bitten by fire ants, and seeing a dermatologist for an unknown skin condition after their tour of duty. The following are some reflections by Dr. Holly Branthoover (personal communication, October 18, 2006) on her experience post-Katrina.

Thoughts of a Mental Health Worker on Katrina One Year Later

Dr. Holly Branthoover, Licensed Professional Counselor and Associate Professor of Counseling, Indiana University of Pennsylvania.

I was recruited by the National Board for Certified Counselors via e-mail on Sunday, September 4, 2005, to respond to hurricane Katrina for the Red Cross. I filled out the application packet immediately, faxed it back, and expected to hear from them in a few weeks. The Red Cross contacted me 2 days later, on Tuesday, September 6, asking, "When can you leave?" I garnered permission from the university, prepared coverage for my classes, and flew out on Saturday, September 10. Preparation for the trip included a Red Cross phone orientation and faxed material providing me instructions.

I flew into Baton Rouge, Louisiana, and completed my "in processing" with the Red Cross. I slept in a staff shelter in Baton Rouge that evening and received my assignment the next morning. I was assigned as a part of a team of three mental health workers—a team leader who was a licensed clinical social worker and another team member who was also a licensed professional counselor. We drove to Covington, Louisiana, to the regional Red Cross headquarters for the eastern region of Louisiana. At Covington, we were given our field assignment—to live and work with evacuees at Pearl River High School in Pearl River, Louisiana (275 residents), and to also service three other shelters: Riverside Elementary (25 residents), 6th Ward Elementary (36 residents), and Abita Springs Middle School (35 residents). We also added 5th Ward Elementary (50 residents) when we got to the field.

I stayed in Louisiana for 2 weeks, leaving on Saturday, September 24. However, my departure was very stressful as Hurricane Rita arrived on Friday, September 23, closing the Baton Rouge airport and necessitating a drive to Jackson, Mississippi, to catch a flight. Here are some of the points I feel are important if you decide to do disaster mental health work:

In addition to my initial mental health team of three, we received another mental health team member and heavily utilized some local mental health people who had volunteered. The local people were very important in that they were a potential constant in people's lives, whereas we could only be available for a short time. So we had them handle people or families that were potentially staying in the area. It worked very well. I believe this use of local resources is paramount to a successful operation on this scale.

Another thing that I feel very strongly about after my experience is that roving teams may work for medical personnel, but they do not work for mental health. You must join the system. My team lived in the shelter. We ate from the ERV (emergency response vehicle). We showered (or didn't, in some cases) in the same showers as the residents. Although we certainly did not share their experience of loss, we did share their experience of the frustration of living in a shelter, and I believe it helped them to develop a rapport with us that facilitated assistance.

When we first got to Pearl River High School, we were assigned a counseling room in which to see people. How many people came to that room? Not one! People in crisis do not present for counseling; they are not looking for self-actualization. We had to be out there, in the shelter, sitting with them, talking to them, listening to their stories. As previously mentioned, our team was covering several other shelters, not just Pearl River High School. Our team leader made a wise decision that we needed to provide a constant presence there, as well, so the same people traveled to the same shelters on a daily basis.

One of the things that crisis textbooks talk about is that crisis responders should have the quality of flexibility—I never realized the importance of this until my experience in Louisiana. I had no idea where I was going when I boarded the plane to Louisiana. I had to call a phone number when I landed to get more information. Talk about an adventure! After I reached my assignment in Pearl River, communication was terrible. Even 2 weeks after the storm, cell phone service, landline phone service, TV, internet, electricity, and so on were all unreliable or nonexistent. Information was carried by courier in some instances, and by the time a directive reached us, it could be wrong or changed.

Misinformation was rampant. We spent some time on rumor control. We actually traveled by car to sites that we "heard" were providing services—like water, cleaning kits, food, blue roofs (tarpaulins to cover damaged roofs), and so on. We tried to confirm what information was factual and pass that to our residents. Who would want to use the last of their gas to drive to a site for assistance and find there is no assistance available? We also acted as a liaison with FEMA representatives in the area, getting accurate information and facilitating services. Much of our time was spent in linking clients to assistance—more social work than counseling.

Medical services are also a part of what the Red Cross provides during a disaster. The mental health staff worked closely to assist the medical staff. Some people were in crisis because of their injuries (e.g., a woman with a severe vaginal infection from being in the floodwater who thought she was dying). Some were in crisis because they could not get their medication (everything from life-sustaining medication to methadone). We detoxed half a dozen people from their methadone in the shelter. Lack of medication was a big issue. Since we, as a team, had a car, we tried to barter and borrow supplies and medication when we came into contact with staff at other locations or on trips to regional headquarters. Things like hand sanitizer and lice kits were quite a commodity.

Working with the children in the shelters was another important activity that we engaged in. One of the members of my team was the head of a day care center in New York, so she was very invested in setting up children's programs. Again, we did very little counseling here. Our team member set up children's activities three times per day at Pearl River. Activities included arts and crafts, games, movies, and the like. This served two positive purposes: providing structure to the children's day (the shelter is a boring place) and giving parents a break. We had to put boundaries on the parent break because some took advantage. For example, we had to make a rule that parents could not leave the shelter while children's activities were going on (so they could be available if there was a problem). Although it varied by developmental level, children began to express their feelings about the hurricane and their current life situation via the artwork and games.

When we first arrived, and periodically throughout, we worked with disaster relief services staff a great deal. Staff were stressed and burned out. At some of the smaller shelters, we were the only professional mental health service providers that the disaster relief staff had seen since the hurricane. At one shelter, several medically needy residents had died, and staff needed to talk about and process this experience. They were angry at the lack of supplies and communication—so much food was available that it was sometimes thrown away, but there was a great lack of medical supplies. At times, staff members got into arguments, and we would mediate. Sometimes, the staff was just stressed and needed to talk. Our team leader consulted often with the shelter manager, assisting in administrative decisions about shelter services. I believe this was a strength of our shelter manager—getting mental health input on shelter operation. In one instance, I was asked to talk with a staff member who had violated Red Cross policy and was going to be relieved of her duties and sent home early.

In the shelter, we had National Guard protection for only the first 2 days. From then on, we had 24-hour protection from local law enforcement—parish sheriffs, with at least two on duty at all times. We worked closely with the sheriffs—assisting with resident arguments, and so on. There were two cocaine arrests at the shelter, with those residents being taken to jail. We had two domestic violence incidents—we worked with security to come up with a safety plan for all residents (this meant moving the two offending husbands to a different shelter). I spoke personally with a least two people at high risk of suicide, and we worked with security to observe them since there were no inpatient mental health facilities available.

Another incident that was particularly scary happened two nights before I left. When hurricane Rita was coming, a mandatory evacuation of New Orleans resulted in our shelter numbers swelling to close to 500 people. Many were Hispanic workers from construction crews who spoke little or no English. A local person and a worker got into a fight in the cafeteria, and a gun was pulled. Although security directly dealt with the gun issue, we assisted with crowd control and calming everyone down afterward—including staff!

Some of my philosophies of crisis intervention were challenged as a result of this experience. The goal of crisis intervention is to return clients to their precrisis state of functioning. In this case, the majority of the clients in the shelter had a precrisis state of functioning that was dysfunctional! By two weeks poststorm, most of the residents left in shelters were people who had little before the storm in the way of resources—both personal and financial. People with family support systems or money were already gone. The majority of our residents had supported themselves via public assistance or SSI disability. Many were involved with community mental health, child protective services, and the legal system. Several were inmates from the county jail who had been released as the storm approached. Drug misuse, child abuse, and domestic violence were prevalent. Given the demographics, it was hard to tell when crisis intervention should end! I also found it important to help people problem-solve within the context of their culture. One man felt trapped about making a decision to go back to work. He did not want to leave his wife alone at the shelter, as he felt it was his duty to protect her. His wife had been called back to work, too. However, he did not want her working while he was not (who would watch their stuff?), and his duty as a man was to provide. I had to work within these values—not my own.

My last two thoughts are related to actually being a part of a team response. Just because you are "mental health" doesn't mean that you are not part of the entire shelter team. Pitch in! I did kitchen work, carried and moved things, and cleaned. Each night, after residents went to bed (curfew at 10 p.m.), the whole shelter was disinfected. I helped with this every night. Working alongside someone can give a great opportunity for them to share their feelings or vent. It also allowed us to be part of the staff—not separate. This said, I do not minimize the benefit of doing mental health things for staff. The second week I was there, a local pizza place opened. The mental health team organized a pizza party for staff after residents went to bed. It turned out to be a great stress reliever.

Last, all of the things I have talked about occur while you are living the experience of a disaster and trying to help people at the same time. I slept on a cot, showered only once the first week, and tried to avoid getting lice (which I did, luckily, because the thought alone freaked me out!). In our travels, we saw the horrific devastation in Slidell, Louisiana, which borders Pearl River and was where the eye of the hurricane passed through. We also traveled, on our day off, into New Orleans, again witnessing the loss and devastation of the storm. During our trip to the city, we got free pizzas from Dominos (they were passing them out) and water. We drove around the city to different National Guard troops, firemen, and EMS companies, passing out pizza and water, and spent time just talking to them—something they were grateful for when they found out we were "mental health." It was scary to be in a city that looked like a ghost town, patrolled by military personnel with M16s. We got to see the Superdome and the Convention Center. I believe it was important to have this R&R even though we were still, in a way, doing our mental health job. There were several times in the two weeks when I got really stressed out (like when I asked for lice kits at headquarters and was told we couldn't have lice at our shelter—because they hadn't gotten a report of it!). So it is important to find a way to take care of yourself—phone calls home, camaraderie with other staff, watching a DVD (after the power is back on!), and so on. You can't help others if you are a stressed-out, burned-out mess!

Now switch to Memphis, Tennessee, 450 miles away.

Lessons I Learned From Katrina

Dr. Richard James, Licensed Professional Counselor, Psychologist, National Board Certified School Counselor, Department of Counseling, Educational Psychology and Research, University of Memphis.

When Katrina hit the Gulf Coast, little did mental health providers in Memphis, Tennessee, realize that they also would be in the eye of the hurricane. As the magnitude of the disaster started to become clearer and the flow of evacuees moved away from the coast, one thing became very clear in a hurry. We were not prepared for the onslaught of people with wide-ranging mental and medical problems that were about to descend on us. Compounding the problems those medically and mentally fragile people brought into our community were 13,000 individuals who were essentially living out of their cars or motels for the first two weeks post-Katrina. As it became clearer that these people were not going back home immediately, a variety of crisis situations arose.

Three anecdotes will give you a pretty good idea of how ill prepared the city of Memphis and Shelby County, Tennessee, were to deal with a major disaster as far as provision of mental health service was concerned. This is probably more ominous when

considering that the scene of the actual disaster was more than 400 miles away from us.

On September 3, 2006, I was helping my daughter and her fiancé load my truck with gasoline, Coleman stove and cooking fuel, lanterns, cooking equipment, firearms, meals ready to eat, sleeping bags, and other supplies as they prepared to go back to see what was left of their home in Long Beach, Mississippi, after Hurricane Katrina sent a 5-foot wall of water through it. At 10:00 a.m., I received a phone call from a harried Shelby County Red Cross director of medical services who had located me by word of mouth and was told I might be able to help since "I knew everything about crisis intervention." He asked if I could provide assistance to the crew of the *American Queen* sternwheeler passenger liner that was docked in Memphis with a crew of 250 very agitated individuals. The boat and crew all shipped out of New Orleans, and they had no word of their families or homes because they had been on the Mississippi River since Katrina hit. The problem was that no one could find this 400-foot-long boat—in Memphis, not even the police. Finally, the riverboat was located at 5 p.m. I got another counselor and headed for the boat. Now the problem was that the boat was set to sail at 6 p.m., passengers were filing on board, and dinner was being served, so no one could come to talk to us. That was the start of what came to be a deluge that we were ill prepared to handle and caused us to reevaluate every facet of our disaster preparedness and mental health provision system in Memphis.

The bishop of the Memphis Catholic diocese had witnessed Katrina firsthand from a hotel room as he saw his car go floating away in Bay St. Louis, Mississippi. He immediately flung open the doors of all the Catholic schools in Memphis and welcomed any and all families from the coast to enroll their children tuition free in the Memphis Catholic school system. Many of these children came from very low-income families with extreme deficits in their educational backgrounds. A lot of these kids were the toughest of the tough to teach and found their way into new Catholic inner-city Jubilee schools, which operate on very tight budgets with little support staff. Since I was "the guy who knew all about crisis" and was also a school counselor educator, I was asked to put a workshop together for the private schools in Memphis on dealing with traumatized children. On September 10, together with Dr. Jo Epstein, a National Certified School Counselor and an elementary school counselor with the city of Memphis, I delivered a workshop at the University of Memphis that was attended by 31 counselors and teachers from 19 private schools. After we finished delivering a 3-hour workshop on trauma and what they might expect to see in their school buildings, I looked out over the room and saw that many of those faces looked like deer caught in the headlights of an oncoming truck! I immediately knew that I would need help in dealing not only with evacuees but also with teachers and counselors, who would be suffering from secondary traumatization from helping those children. For the next 6 months, these teachers and counselors met with me for supervision as they valiantly worked with these children who were traumatized and staved off compassion fatigue and burnout.

It quickly became apparent that we didn't have enough mental health professionals to deal with the people coming into our city with a host of medical and mental issues. We also did not have anyone in charge of handling these people. The coordinator of the local crime victims' assistance center, a licensed clinical social worker, and another LCSW at one of the local mental health clinics stepped into the breach and started to make order out of what was rapidly turning into a classic example of chaos theory at work (go to Chapter 1, "Approaching Crisis Intervention"). Picture your author sitting in a reception center talking with a person on methadone maintenance who had been addicted to heroin from New Orleans.

Client: "Hey, man, they won't give me any methadone, say I got to have a prescription. If I don't get some methadone pretty damn quick, I'll go rob a liquor store and get the real deal!"

By the middle of September, we had approximately 13,000 expatriates from New Orleans and the Gulf Coast in our city. All thoughts about licensing and certifying mental health workers for disaster work went right out the window with Katrina. The faculty at our university mobilized 200 students in the counseling, school psychology, and social work departments, and with faculty supervisors, they started working in the shelters. These students and faculty served up to 2 months in this capacity until some semblance of order could be restored.

The bottom line was that we too were not prepared for this disaster. The outcome of this disaster was the establishment of a planning committee for the Greater Memphis Area Emergency Preparedness for Mental Health. That committee's composition ranges from mental health personnel from hospitals, community agencies, and human service provision organizations to religious leaders, school system personnel, city and county officials, the police, fire, and EMT departments, charitable organizations, homeland security, medical facilities, and universities. This is certainly a work in progress. Will we be better prepared than we were for Katrina? That's a good question! Wherever you are in this country, or any other country for that matter, you might ask yourself the same question.

9/11 What No Class Prepared Me For

Dr. Rick A. Myer, a licensed psychologist and a retired Counselor Educator, University of Texas El Paso. At the time of 9/11, I was an Associate Professor at Duquesne University, Pittsburgh, PA.

I vividly remember the day of 9/11. I was in my office when another faculty member came in and said you need to come now to see what is happening. I watched in horror seeing the live pictures on national news about the terrorist attacks in New York City. I shuddered when the first tower collapsed and wondered just how bad the destruction and loss of life would be. That evening I talked with my family and said I wanted to help. Of course, most people that day wanted to help. The next morning, I contacted the Red Cross and volunteered. I had previously gone through the Red Cross mental health training and thought if I could just get to New York City I might be able to do something, just if only to provide support.

As it turns out about 3 days later, I received a call from an insurance company asking if I would be willing to travel to New York City and do CISD with a large international business located across the street from the WTC. Since I had not heard from the Red Cross I immediately agreed. Seven days after 9/11 I was on a train to New York City choosing not to fly because of concern over safety.

My work began by providing services at a drop-in center for the organization. After a week I was asked to do group work using CISD. To be honest, CISD did not seem to be working after about 10 minutes into the first session. Maybe I was not doing it correctly. I switched to what I knew much better and that was crisis intervention. That worked. As the days, weeks, and months went by I spent a great amount of time in New York City with that organization. Initially, I did group work and then talked with individuals. However, after about two months my role began to transition to providing consultation with management about human impact issues and concerns. They sought my consultation on ways to support the employees. I remember one specific question was literally a $40 million question. I was asked about what would happen if the organization moved to another location or stayed in lower Manhattan. If they moved that meant losing $40 million and if they stayed, employees would have to relive the trauma experienced on that day. I gave by best advice on the way relocating or staying in lower Manhattan would affect employee retention. The decision was to renovate and remain in lower Manhattan.

After about two weeks, another task was to accompany employees returning to the building they abandoned in fear of their lives a few days before. The purpose was to gather personal items and business documents needed to maintain business. Usually about 20 employees would gather at a specified location with myself and the facilities manager. We would form a line and snake our way through three to four check points, each checking IDs with the facilities manager leading the parade and me at the end. When entering the building everyone would immediately go to the west side to look out the window at the rubble. At that time smoke and a few little fires were still visible. After about ten minutes the employees drifted off to collect what they came there for. At that time there was still no cell phone service, so I was given a walkie talkie for communication. In the three to four hours in the building I would be asked to go to a specific floor in the southwest corner, or another place because someone was not doing well. I would arrive and start doing crisis intervention.

I learned a great deal about crisis intervention during the 13 months I worked off and on with that organization. I had done a lot of crisis intervention prior to 9/11 but nothing like that. No class, no training had taught me what to do after a terrorist attack in which over 2,000 people lost their lives. I learned to rely on what I knew using intervention strategies I felt were effective. I learned to be adaptable to the current situation. I learned to be caring and simply be me. These lessons have worked well in the crisis intervention I have done. In addition to my work after 9/11 I have provided services for four, and arguably five mass shootings. The fifth incident involved a murder suicide in which a man murdered his wife and two children before he took his own life. Finally, I was honored and felt privileged to provide services in all these situations.

The ripple effects of disasters this large flow far out from the epicenter. Disasters that affect such a great number of people need all of the professions mentioned above if successful crisis intervention is going to occur, as you will soon see.

Case Study of the Benefield Family

Now meet the Benefield family, who are about to experience the crisis of their lives. The Benefields typify, in an encapsulated way, how the ecosystemic crisis intervention model *should* (note the emphasis on "should") operate when a large-scale disaster afflicts a family.

Tuesday, April 21, 14:00 Hours Military Time (2:00 p.m. CDT)

An F4 tornado has hit Midville, Tennessee, a town with a population of approximately 40,000 in the south-central United States. The storm cut across the town and left a path of destruction about one-quarter to one-half mile wide for a distance of more than five miles. It effectively cut a path through the industrial park, damaging numerous buildings but particularly wreaking havoc on the automotive plant, which employed more than 1,000 people. The plant was close to a total loss. The storm continued through several residential areas and a housing development, hopscotched, and then hit the main elementary school of Midville and reduced it to rubble. All 600 students were inside the building at the time, under cover in the hallways.

The water plant received a direct hit from the storm and can no longer keep water pressure up or produce potable drinking water. The power grid has been disrupted by downed power lines and wrecked substations, and the city is currently without power. Both cellular and landline telephone systems are inoperable because of downed towers and lines. The local hospital has received minor damage but is still in operation. Local fire, police, and emergency services have emerged largely unscathed and are close to fully operational. There has been a significant loss of life in addition to injuries that appear to be in the hundreds.

The Benefield family includes Travis Benefield, age 33, a machinist at the local automobile plant; his wife Sara Lee Benefield, age 32, a dental assistant; their children Jason Benefield, age 13, an eighth-grader at Midville Middle School; Lou Ann Benefield, age 11, a sixth-grader at Midville Middle School; Shawn Benefield, age 6, a first-grader at Midville Elementary School; and Loretta Benefield, age 54, the mother of Travis.

April 21, 14:15 Hours Military Time (2:15 p.m., 15 minutes After the Tornado)

Travis Benefield is emerging from the rubble of the automobile plant. He has no major injuries, just minor cuts and bruises from falling and flying debris. While frantically helping dig others out, he is also attempting to reach his wife on his cell phone, but it is not working. Sara Lee Benefield is currently upside down in her van in a water-filled ditch. She is there because she heard the tornado siren and, instead of taking cover in the dentist's office where she worked, she became emotionally distressed and was on her way to school to pick up her children. She is semiconscious, bleeding, and clearly in need of rescue and medical assistance.

Jason Benefield is currently looking for his sister, Lou Ann, in the melee that is now Midville Middle School. No one was hurt in the middle school or high school, and neither school was significantly damaged. Everyone in both the middle and high schools had been protected in the hallways; however, chaos now reigns as teachers attempt to control panic-stricken students who heard the tornado go over and can now see the destructive path it has made. Lou Ann is likewise attempting to find her brother Jason. She is also hysterical because she has seen that the tornado essentially destroyed the elementary school that her brother Shawn attends. Shawn is currently missing, probably buried somewhere under the rubble of the elementary school. Loretta, the grandmother who resides with the family, is currently lying in a field, dead from a broken neck and back, about one-quarter mile from where the family lived in a manufactured home that has been blown away and no longer exists.

April 21, 14:25 Hours, Emergency Command Center

LEM director, Thaddeus Washington: (on short-wave radio to all ham operators and state police emergency and state emergency broadcast systems) It appears we have had a major tornado disaster here involving most of Midville. We currently have no power or cellular or landline telephone communication. It appears that there is a large path of destruction throughout the city, and there is also a very high casualty rate as we had less than 15 minutes'

warning time. We have ruptured gas lines and water lines and have no ability to pump water. We have at least two fires. We are requesting immediate assistance from the region IV and state emergency management network. We are making a damage assessment now. Instructions will follow in about 30 minutes.

As the reports from police cars and ham radio operators start to come into the center, the director has to make several quick decisions about the magnitude of the disaster. From the initial reports, he decides to alert the regional and state emergency management coordinators. He also needs a better assessment of what is going on in the community. He therefore asks for a state police helicopter and instructs his emergency preparedness manager to get airborne and conduct an assessment.

April 21, 14:35 Hours, Midville Middle School, School Crisis Response Team Meeting in Cafeteria

Linda Gidcome, Assistant Superintendent, Crisis Response Coordinator: It appears that we have a major crisis involving not only the elementary school but the whole town as well. The police are over at the elementary school, but we have many children trapped in there. Undoubtedly, there are casualties in that building. Jackson Little, the elementary school counselor and our crisis intervention coordinator, is not yet accounted for. Until he is found, Jim Constansis, the high school vocational coordinator, is his backup and in charge of intervention. We also have some other missing people, so, Jim, I want you to get backups for them. I am going to turn the meeting over to Jim.

Jim Constansis, Crisis Intervention Coordinator: We also have to deal with our children here and in the high school to be sure they are safe. We need to get everybody back in their rooms and run the roll. Right now, we don't have any good information about where "safe" is. As such, we are going to hold all middle and secondary school students in their respective buildings. It appears that right now there is no way into the school from outside due to debris on the roads. I want to get backups for all the missing members of the team. Our first priority is to run the rolls and see who is missing. So we need to take the TO GO boxes' primary hard copy and send three teams (Red, Blue, Green) over to the elementary school, while the Orange Team stays here, and the Purple Team stays at the high school to start receiving kids. We will bring K through third grades here and fourth and fifth grades to the high school. Red has K and 1, Blue has 2 and 3, and Green has 4 and 5. They are going to need medical assistance over there, so I want the Orange Team to pull all of our available medical supplies out of the sports facility storage and set up a dispensary in the cafeteria.

Luda Sarapokin, our school nurse, will be running that. We're going to get on the radio and let OEC know what our condition is just as soon as the building engineer can get the generator hooked up to it and running. All of you pick up your two-way radios. Things are going to get pretty hectic, so remember your radio manners and protocol. We have done this in an exercise; the only difference was that the middle school was the target. We can do this. Let's go to work!

The Incident Command System has been in place for 2 years in the Midville School District. It has a clear incident command system (Nickerson et al., 2006; Thomae, 2002) that has been activated on the tornado's departure. Its first and primary job is to account for all the children. Any parents who could somehow manage to get to the school would be taken to a waiting area before any children would be released. The parents have been informed of this plan and know what to expect and what to do.

April 21, 15:05 Hours, above Midville in a helicopter

Saria Wickeramasaka, Emergency Preparedness Coordinator: (in a state police helicopter above Midville, on the radio speaking to the LEM director) The Packard engine plant is completely ruined; the total building is involved. I can see human movement, but there are undoubtedly people trapped in the plant. I do not see any evidence of fire. We will need heavy equipment including cranes and hoists. We will need EMTs and rescue equipment and units. The Hi Power petroleum bulk plant got hit and there is leakage from their storage tanks. It appears both gasoline and fuel oil are being discharged, although the berms seem to be containing the fuel at present. We will need a containment and cleanup crew there along with fire equipment and spillage trucks. I see no evidence of fire. The

elementary school has received a direct hit. The middle of the building has sustained a great deal of damage and the east wing has collapsed. I can see movement, and it appears the school CRTs are working at the elementary school. There are undoubtedly many casualties.

The roads to the school are currently impassable. We will need heavy equipment including teams with chain saws to get in there. I would recommend this as our first priority. We do have two house fires, one on Appleton at Branch and one on Sycamore past Hoover. The one on Sycamore is in danger of involving an apartment complex. It should be fought immediately. The street is blocked from the north, but trucks can come in from the east side and through the apartment complex.

The waterworks is a total loss with the pumping station and filter house completely wrecked. You can probably assume that the available water supply is what is currently in the two north and south standpipes, which appear to have sustained no damage. The sanitary works is operational. The path of the tornado is pretty steady from southwest to northeast approximately one-quarter to one-half mile wide running from state highway 37 to just south of I-69 for a stretch of about 5 miles. There are some skips, but it has pretty much gone through Midville from the industrial park on the southwest side of town through the west side of town. Before it went back up in the air, it got the mobile home park on Breezemore Road. There are mobile homes blown apart and on top of one another. I can see human movement here also, but there are going to be lots of casualties here as well.

I estimate about 200 homes destroyed or heavily damaged and 600 more with some damage. We need to notify Midville Central and St. Andrews hospitals that they need to go to Code Red [highest emergency status]. We are going to need Tennessee Valley Power to do the same, as it appears we have a complete power outage across the city. Midville Power and Light will not be able to handle this outage alone.

As this assessment comes into the emergency operations center (EOC), information is relayed through the regional EOC coordinator and transmitted to the state EOC. As the magnitude of the disaster unfolds, the governor is notified and mobilizes National

Guard units. Word goes out to FEMA, the Red Cross, and the Salvation Army, and these groups begin mobilizing human resources to go to Midville. Within 1 hour and 10 minutes, a massive mobilization effort is underway. Food, drinking water, medicine, medical supplies, emergency medical personnel in the form of EMTs and fire departments, rescue teams, and heavy equipment all move toward Midville.

As Lane (2003) indicates, if roads are impassable and it is possible, someone with the Emergency Management Agency needs to get airborne and conduct a visual assessment of the extent of the damage and relay information to the center about what and who are going to be needed where and under how high a priority.

April 21, 15:21 Hours, Command Center

As the LEMA director sends out mobilization orders, a number of workers you will soon meet swing into action. In these first few hours and days, they will be administering what is generally construed to be psychological first aid as they attempt to gain control over the chaotic scenes and traumatized individuals who are survivors of the disaster. As they enter the setting, they will be sensitive to the culture and diversity of the populations they are serving. They will also be aware of and looking for at-risk populations. They are, first and foremost, interested in the immediate physical safety of survivors. To that end, they will attempt to provide a sense of predictability, control, comfort, and safety to survivors by providing straightforward and easily understood information about disaster response activities and services. They will attempt to protect survivors from additional traumatic experiences and trauma reminders while they go about their work. Major tasks will be reuniting children with their caregivers, stabilizing emotionally overwhelmed survivors, and providing support for acutely bereaved persons (National Center for PTSD, n.d.a).

To accomplish the foregoing tasks, the workers will engage in a great deal of information gathering in regard to current needs and concerns about the following:

1. Nature and severity of experiences during the disaster
2. Death of a family member or close friend
3. Concerns about immediate post-disaster circumstances and ongoing threat
4. Separations from or concern about the safety of loved ones

5. Physical illness and need for medications
6. Losses incurred as a result of the disaster (home, school, pets, personal property, etc.)
7. Extreme feelings of guilt or shame
8. Thoughts about causing harm to self or others
9. Lack of adequate supportive social network
10. Prior alcohol or drug use
11. Prior exposure to trauma or loss
12. Prior psychological problems (National Center for PTSD, n.d.a)

When the workers have the foregoing information, they will identify and clarify the most immediate needs of the survivor, discuss an action plan with the person, and then act to address the identified needs. Integral to this process is providing information on traumatic stress and coping mechanisms to help alleviate the stress and linking the individual with the disaster relief services they will need (National Center for PTSD, n.d.c). Follow these crisis workers now as they put the foregoing points into action.

April 21, 15:51 Hours, Midville Elementary School

Jack Tankersly, School CRT Blue Team member at Midville Elementary: (helping a dazed boy with some cuts and blood on him out of the rubble of the east hallway of Midville Elementary School) I'm Mr. Tankersly from the middle school. How are you doing?

Shawn: Iah guess Ah'm okay, Iah dunno. . . . Whaaat happened?

Jack: There was a tornado, but you are going to be all right. If you can walk okay, we are going to take you to the middle school and get you checked out. Can you do that?

Shawn: Yeah, I guess. I just got some little cuts on my arms. There's some other kids hurt bad back in the hallway, though. Jamie's eyes were shut and he wasn't talkin' even when I shook him. He was hurt real bad, maybe even dead or something.

Jack: Yes, I know, and we will get them out. So don't worry about that. Right now let's focus on you. Can you give me your name and tell me who your teacher is?

Shawn: Shawn Benefield. Ah'm in Mrs. Cruz's first-grade class.

Jack: (Checks over the two-way radio with the documentation leader on the student in the central

elementary To Go box.) Good. You have a brother and a sister in the middle school, Jason and Lou Ann, right?

Shawn: Yes.

Jack: I am going to have someone take you up to the middle school and get those cuts cleaned up and check you out. I'll let them know you are coming, so your sister and brother will know you are okay.

One of the critical components in any disaster in a school is keeping track of and accounting for children. Nowhere is the concept of the school as *in loco parentis* (in place of the parent) more important. Portable, centralized, and redundant To Go boxes (Thomae, 2002) are critical to such an endeavor; they hold classroom lists, student names, addresses, telephone numbers, medical issues, release forms, and parent and guardian names. Moving a school full of injured, confused, and terrified students is an undertaking that must be done carefully and precisely so no student is lost or unaccounted for. While there is a school Critical Incident Stress Management Team to deal with students' psychological concerns, it is separate and distinct from the incident command system and will not come into operation until the physical safety of the students is assured. Particularly important staff members on this team are bus drivers, secretaries, and custodians who have knowledge of children and building facilities that educators do not (Allen & Sheen, 2005). Reuniting missing children with parents is a critical component and one of the highest priorities in any disaster (National Center for PTSD, n.d.a). As an example, one of the Herculean efforts accomplished by the National Center for Missing and Exploited Children after Hurricane Katrina was reuniting all 5,192 children reported missing with their families (Missing Children, 2006).

April 21, 15:30 Hours, EOC Command Center

Thaddeus Washington: (addressing command center staff) We have a Class One disaster. We are going to be overwhelmed with dead, wounded, and people needing shelter, food, water, clothing, and mental health assistance. We are setting up a shelter at the National Guard Armory. We are going to set up a morgue at the Seabrook Packing Plant. The high school and the middle school are going to be reception and clearing centers, so we can get people sorted out and families reunited.

We may have to turn them into shelters too. As soon as we get that done, we will probably set up for the Red Cross and FEMA teams here at the Civic Center. Our first priority is to get the kids out of the elementary school. Preliminary reports indicate that there are a number trapped in the building.

We need to get the roads opened so we can get heavy equipment in there. The EMAs from Sawyer, Plainfield, and Cumberland are sending fire and rescue units. The state EOC has been notified and informed the governor, who is going to call for a presidential disaster order. We need to get the road opened, so get all of Howell Paving and Construction and the State Highway department equipment on the road and heading in that direction, and get three of our CERT teams to help them clear trees, so let them know we have to have chainsaws. Saria landed and says we will need at least one and possibly two tracked cranes.

Our second priority will be the Packard plant. I want Cassius Mendoza, the construction superintendent for Norton Metal Frame Buildings, to go out there and tell us what we need. We also need to get people out there to help organize them—although Joel Pickard, the plant superintendent, and I have gone over their emergency plan and they seem to be functioning pretty well given the way the whole thing came down. Get the rest of the CERT teams spread out along the line from state route 37 up to I-69. Be sure we get one team up to the mobile home park on Breezemore. We need to get the water system back on line. It appears most of our staff at the waterworks, including Joe Mulvidge, the chief engineer, and Hack Townsend, the superintendent, have been injured. I have asked staff from the Sawyer water system to come and give us an assessment. Until further notice we will ration water and put a boil order out because we are bound to lose pressure on the system. I have a feeling that this is going to be really bad. I hope our practices have paid off. Dr. Benjamin, we are going to need to get your mental health team assembled. I am afraid there is going to be work for them. OK, everybody, you know your jobs, let's go to work!

April 21, 15:35 Hours

Dr. Yolanda Benjamin, Executive Director of Hatchie County Mental Health Center and mental health liaison to the Midville EOC: (speaking to Esther Carey, her secretary, at the mental health center on an emergency band radio) How many staff have we got that are at the center? OK, good! They know what to do. We are going to need counselors at the National Guard Armory and out at Seabrook Packing. We are also going to need to send counselors out to both hospitals to work with the chaplains out there. As soon as they open the road to the schools, I'll go out there and see what kind of assistance they need there. There are going to be Red Cross counselors coming in, but right now we are it.

Both Washington and Benjamin are going to have to balance between being responders and coordinators. For the present, they are in the responding business, but as more outside assistance arrives, their job will change to consulting and coordination with the external support systems that are going to flood into the area (Lane, 2003). It is critically important that integration of mental health services with other disaster responders occurs and that it is recognized as a critical component to overall relief efforts, as exemplified by Mr. Washington and his immediate referral to Dr. Benjamin and her mental health teams (Ørner et al., 2006).

April 21, 17:12 Hours

Juanita Sanchez, leader of Community Emergency Response Team (CERT) 10: (Looking for survivors, she clambers down a steep ravine into a muddy creek bottom where Sara Lee Benefield's SUV is upside down. Sara is barely conscious and keeps rambling incoherently about needing to get her kids.) (speaking into her two-way radio) Jake, notify the medical and rescue LEMA that CERT 10 has a woman pinned in her car at the bottom of Rutledge Creek at the Brunner Street Bridge. We are going to need medical assistance, a wrecker, and an extraction team. (speaking to Sara Lee) Can you hear me? I want you to talk to me. OK? We are getting help here for you. Can you tell me your name? Mine is Juanita. I am on a CERT team. I found you down here where the tornado blew you and your car. We are going to get you out of here.

Sara Lee: I . . . need mah children . . . Shawn and . . . I cain't remember . . . (Eyes roll back.)

Juanita: OK, I understand that is what you need to do. Now you stay with me. Stay awake! We will help you with that. Do you hurt anywhere?

Sara Lee: (slow, measured, and staggered speech in a low voice) Mah . . . legs . . . are . . . numb and mah

chest hurts. Iah cain't move. Iah need to git mah kids. Where . . . are . . . mah . . . kids? Iah need . . . some . . . hep!

Juanita: There are people at the school right now taking care of all of the kids. Good! Great! You are talking to me! Stay awake! (Radios information back to the team.) I am not going to leave you. My name is Juanita Sanchez. Can you say my name?

Sara Lee: Juanita . . . Juanita Ramras.

Juanita: Close enough! (Starts to conduct a head-to-toe basic medical assessment. Covers Sara and keeps her talking to postpone shock and unconsciousness.)

CERT volunteer teams are common everyday citizens who have undergone FEMA training as a rapid and immediate reaction force to help save lives. The FEMA training teaches volunteers skills needed to assist before, during, and after a disaster, such as fire suppression, diagnosing and dealing with the three major killers of the injured—airway obstruction, bleeding, and shock—first aid, light search-and-rescue operations, disaster psychology and team organization, and disaster simulation exercises (FEMA, 2015). Juanita is a volunteer who has gone through CERT training. Her occupation is a bookkeeper at a local auto dealership.

April 21, 18:23 Hours

Allie Tran Nyguen, CERT Team 4 member: (in a field 300 yards northeast of the Breezemore Mobile Home Park, speaking into his two-way radio) I have a female, approximately age 50, who is unresponsive and who has no pulse, lying about 150 yards north of Breezemore Road. We need to get her IDed. She has no identification on her. Can we get her transported? We will need a four-wheel drive.

Carl Hanratty, Team 4 leader: I'll send Sheila, Jon, and Jerry over there with the 4 × 6 ATV. LEMA is setting up a morgue at the Seabrook Packing Plant. We'll get her out of the field, and then they can pick her up. Write down her description and the details of where she was found, and we'll attach that to her bag.

April 21, 19:02 Hours, Midville Civic Center

Travis Benefield: (at the Civic Center, stunned, irate, and half-hysterical, speaking rapidly and loudly to Kate McClain, mental health counselor) I NEED SUM BY-GOD HEP HERE AND RITE NOW! I cain't git to mah house. Iah heared that everything in the Breezemore Park has done blowed away. Mah momma was at our home there sleepin'. I don't know where mah wife is, there weren't no one at the dentist's office 'cause it was all beat up from the twister. Iah heared that everybody at the elementary school done got kilt, and Iah got kids there, but they won't let me near there neither. Iah walked and hitched a ride into here 'cause Iah ain't got no vehicle 'cause part of the Packard plant's on top of it. And Iah cain't find mah dad-burned tools.

Kate: (deescalating Travis) I see how upset you are. I am Kate McClain. I do not know your name.

Travis: Ah'm Travis Benefield. Iah work out to the Packard plant and mah wife's Sara Lee and she works at Doc Collard's office. She's his dental assistant, and Iah got three kids out to the schools— Shawn, Lee Ann, and Jason, and then there's mah momma, Loretta, and Iah been out at the Packard plant pullin' folks outta there, and there's a lotta people bad hurt, and Iah lost all mah durn tools, and Jim Houston, the other millsetter, is dead under a stamping machine, and . . . I'm ahm ABOUT TO GO NUTS AND AH NEED SOME DAD GUM HEP! (Rapid, panting breathing, eyes rapidly moving back and forth, fists clinched pounding hand in fist, rapid, random pacing verging on hysteria.)

Kate: (Gently interrupting his continuous, escalating, out-of-control verbiage, she starts with enough command in her voice to get Travis's attention, then rapidly diminishes her voice level.) TRAVIS! T-R-A-V-I-S. IF I AM TO HELP YOU, I NEED YOUR FULL ATTENTION. (Travis gives a startled look but slows down and attends to the worker.) Thank you, Travis. I want you to take a deep breath and just listen to me for a moment. Good. Just take a deep breath. Again, I understand all the confusion. It is a mess, but we will get it straightened out. I hear how concerned you are about all your family and how terrifying that is not knowing anything. I need you to get grounded here so I can be of the most help. To do that, I need for you to have your wits about you. OK! So humor me here a moment. Tell me where you are right now, tell me what time it is on that clock behind me, and tell me what they're doing over there in the corner?

Travis: Ah, well, we'uns are here into the com-mun-it-ee center and it's ah well . . . I think that thar clock has done stopped. Them ladies is settin' up what

looks like some sammiches 'n' sodas 'n' water and what-not.

Kate: Excellent. I just wanted to get your feet planted back on the ground here so we can make some headway. OK?

Travis: (rather sheepishly) Yes'um, I do indeed have my wits about me now. I do apologize for my unseemly behavior thar.

Kate: Thank you. You have every right to be upset. That is normal. But we will get this squared away. I am a counselor here, and I am going to help you. Right now I need you to help me, though. How about let's go over here and sit down and let me get Jodell Brown over here. She is one of the coordinators, and we will see what we can start to find out, and get you reunited with your family. I bet you haven't had anything to eat or drink since the tornado hit. I need you to be calm and collected, so we can get the information we need, so do you suppose you could sit here and maybe eat a sandwich and have a soda and tell me and Jodell what we need to know to help you?

Travis: Well, OK. Ah'm jest so scared, though. It were purely awful out there to the plant, and Iah cain't find out nuthin'. Iah done pulled people out of there as much as Iah could until they done got there with the heavy equipment, then Iah didn't want to leave but Iah had to find out about mah family.

Kate: So you did what you could out there. It is certainly understandable that you want to find out about your family and get them together. Not knowing is really the worst part, but here is Jodell, and she is going to get the information she needs from you, and then we will be able to tell you something. And that's really what you want to know, isn't it? Let me go get you a sandwich and a soda and just tell Jodell.

In the preliminary stage of a crisis, mental health counselors need to understand that they can best help by providing very practical support (Myer, 2015; Ørner et al., 2006). A central information area will be a trip into chaos and confusion with people attempting to reunite with families. Getting order and direction is a first priority. This is not a time to attempt to do "counseling." Help is what is needed, and the mental health crisis worker can best do that by calming and defusing people who are very distraught, angry, grief stricken, and in shock.

Kate is helpful in deescalating and defusing a very distraught individual who has been severely traumatized and is now terrified that his family has fared even worse. She uses two standard techniques with excitable and distraught clients. Kate rated Travis overall as 22 on the TAF with an 8 on the affective scale, a 7 on the behavioral scale and his cognitive reaction as 7. The rating meant that Kate would at least partner with Travis and possibly even use a more direct approach to support him as he struggles with his reactions. First is **entrainment** (literally synchronization of the organism [Travis] to an external rhythm [hers] here slowing Travis down by use of verbal calming techniques) and then **grounding** (a reality orientation technique that helps keep someone in the present and helps reorient a person to the here-and-now and in reality) (Webber et al., 2010). She raises her voice in a command level manner, but not quite as loud as the client's; she then tails off her decibel level and speaks more slowly. This tactic catches the client's attention, but then hopefully models for him to tone down and slow down. She uses simple calming techniques of introducing herself and asking for his name. She then asks him to take a deep breath to slow him down. She does a quick reality orientation that refocuses him into his present environment. She then offers him food and drink and a place to sit. All of these are basic calming and grounding techniques that are simple but effective. Her negative interrogative question is generally a very bad counseling technique because it implies agreement, but in this case, Kate specifically uses it to get agreement and further stabilize and get Travis under control.

April 21, 19:22 Hours, Civic Center Reception and Clearing Area

Jodell Brown, clearing coordinator: (Kate McClain, mental health crisis worker, is also present.) Mr. Benefield, here is what I have. All of your children are safe. Shawn had some minor cuts and bruises, but he has received medical attention for those and is fine. They are all at the middle school. They are getting supper served to them. We will relay to them that you are safe also. Your wife is in the hospital. She was pinned in her car, but they got her out. She had to have one leg operated on because it was fractured. She has two fractured ribs, but she is okay and in stable condition. She already knows the children are safe, and we are now relaying to her that you are safe. From what

we now know, I am sorry to tell you that there are no homes left standing in Breezemore Park. There were many people who were killed, and there were many injured out there, and presently it is off-limits as they sort through the debris looking for survivors. We have no one identified as Loretta Benefield at any hospital. As of now, we are listing her as missing. We will have transportation here to take you to the children. If you do not have any friends' or relatives' home you can go to, then we can take you to the National Guard Armory for tonight. There will be a FEMA field office set up tomorrow, and there will be all of the major insurance carriers here in mobile disaster units by tomorrow morning. As soon as we have any word about your mother, we will let you know. Now Kate will go with you and get you out to the children. Do you have any questions for me?

Travis: (Dazed, taking in all of that information, hesitates and thinks. The crisis worker waits patiently.) Well, no, I don't rightly guess. I guess mah sister over to Crowley could take we'uns in, but I don't know how to git word to her. I guess fer tonight we'uns just best go to the Armory. Ah'm sick to death about not knowing about momma. But I do thank you for findin' out all the rest. I 'preciate it most kindly, ma'am.

Jodell: You are welcome, Mr. Benefield. If you will give me her phone number and address, we will try to get in touch with her. Just so I can be sure that you have gotten all that, could you sort of summarize it so I'm sure that I haven't left anything out or have been unclear?

The crisis worker very carefully and specifically goes through the items she needs to cover. She then asks Travis to recapitulate what she has said so they all have a clear understanding of what has been covered and what is going to happen. Kate will see that Travis and his children are reunited and will hand him off to another crisis worker at the shelter. This is basic psychological first aid that is designed to slow things down, get some control back in the situation, provide support and reassurance, and improve short-term functioning (Halpern & Tramontin, 2007, pp. 203–218).

April 22, 08:35 Hours, National Guard Armory Disaster Shelter

Ollie Naifeh, MSW, Red Cross disaster counselor from Memphis: Mr. Benefield, hello, I am Oliver Naifeh, a Red Cross counselor from Memphis. You can call me Ollie. I just got your name as one of my people. How did your night go?

Travis: Well, not real well, sir. Iah didn't sleep much, but the kids did. Iah'd like to git over to see Sara Lee. And Iah'd shore like to find out about momma.

Ollie: We have contacted your sister, and she is on her way over here now. The whole city has been declared a disaster area, so it is going to take her some time to get here. I do not have any good news to tell you about your mother, Travis. She was not among the survivors. I am sorry to tell you that a woman answering the description you gave us was found in a field about 300 yards from your home, and she was deceased when she was found. She is at a temporary morgue. This is a terrible task, but we need you to go down there and see if the person is your mother. There will be another counselor there. His name is Jeffrey Chung. He knows you are coming, and he will be there to help you if indeed it is your mother. I will stay with you until your sister comes, and we will talk about what you will need to do about housing and insurance and any other assistance you may need. There will be counselors at the FEMA One Stop to help you with any questions you may have or assistance you may need.

April 22, 09:42 Hours, Seabrook Packing Plant Temporary Morgue

Travis Benefield and Jeffrey Chung, Licensed Professional Counselor from Hatchie County Community Mental Health Center and grief specialist, look on as a medical assistant gently unzips a body bag.

Travis: (**Recoils in shock, then gently touches his mother's cheek.**) Oh Lordy, momma! You have done gotten yourself kilt dead. I told you and done told you to go to the shelter if'n a twister was comin', but you didn't never pay no mind to me. Oh, dear God! Mah momma is dead! (**Starts sobbing.**)

Jeffrey: (**Nods to the attendant and gently turns Travis away.**) I am terribly sorry for your loss. Come on, let's go outside and sit down and talk.

Travis: (**crying**) Did she . . . do you . . . know . . . ah . . . suffer much?

Jeffrey: The field report said she was dead when they found her, and the autopsy shows she died of a broken neck, so I would say no. (**The counselor waits patiently while Travis weeps.**)

Travis: (**head in his hands**) Iah jest . . . it is jest too much. Iah don't know . . . cain't think. Too much.

Jeffrey: (**Uses STOP technique. Slowly and easily puts his hand on Travis's shoulder and gently guides him out of the morgue and over to a chair, where he sits down with him. After a while of letting Travis sob quietly, he begins speaking very gently and slowly while making eye contact.**) It is overwhelming, and that's why I am here. I would be happy to get the paperwork together and move your mother to a funeral home if you would like. Or we can keep her here for a while and give you some time to decide what kind of arrangements you would like to make. Oliver Naifeh is your counselor, so he will work with me. Given all you have gone through, it is understandable that you feel overwhelmed. Anyone would. It is a common response to an awful, abnormal situation. You may feel guilty about not doing enough to get your mom to go to a shelter, but that was her choice. (**Sits patiently and gently touches Travis's forearm while he silently sobs.**) Do you have a minister or anybody else I could call?

Travis: Oh . . . OK. If'n you could do that. Our family has always done gone to Kittinger's Funeral Home. Iah guess you could call them up. Iah hadn't even thought about church. We'uns go to the First Baptist Church. Pretty near every Sunday. Reverend Dehl is the minister, but I 'spect he is right busy about now. I guess he'd like to know 'bout Loretta 'cause she sang in the choir and was a pretty staunch member. If'n you could take care of it, Ah'd 'preciate it most greatly. Seems like Iah cain't take care of mah family what's alive right now hardly a'tall, let 'lone what's done and gone.

The morgue counselor does three things. First, he implements the STOP technique, which for a morgue counselor is standard operating procedure given the further trauma people will experience when they identify loved ones. **STOP** is an acronym for Sit, Think, Observe, Plan (Webber et al., 2010). The counselor slowly moves the client away from his mother and guides him over to a chair where they sit down. He gauges that it will be okay to put his hand on Travis's shoulder given what he has observed about the cultural norms of the area in times of grief. He observes that indeed Travis will need basic assistance and starts to plan out what he will need to help him with. Being in charge of a morgue at a disaster site takes a great deal of compassion and sensitivity, and the STOP system is a sort of default way of slowing things down and gently moving the bereaved in helping them to get mobilized.

Second, he offers to provide very specific help with details concerning Travis's mother's death. Jeffrey's triage rating of Travis is in the low 20s. He sees a person who is cognitively overwhelmed and behaviorally and emotionally exhausted, has narrowly escaped death, as has the rest of his family, and now has to identify his mother's body. As a result, Jeffrey needs to gently but firmly provide support and direction. How access to the dead is provided to loved ones and the interaction that occurs while this is happening are often critical to the survivors' ability to integrate the traumatic event and avoid further psychological injury (Shalev et al., 1998).

Finally, the worker suggests help from his church. Faith-based organizations play huge roles in disaster relief (David et al., 2019: Park et al., 2019). The worker is fairly sure that, given the culture of the area, Travis's church and minister can and will provide a great deal of support to him. Thus, he asks if he can contact his church.

The morgue counselor is further aware of the stages of survivor grief (go to Chapter 12, "Personal Loss: Bereavement and Grief") and empathically responds to Travis's shock, sadness, anxiety, and guilt without judging Travis's ability to "handle" all of it. Further, Jeffrey does not judge what Travis has or has not done, nor does he offer meaningless platitudes about Travis's losses. The scenario is played out over and over with other families in the immediate aftermath of a disaster. Local crisis workers work closely with Red Cross, NOVA, and FEMA crisis workers to provide an integrated, efficient, and seamless operation. While these crisis workers will provide immediate mental health assistance, it will be most often in terms of support. This support provides for both the family's survival needs and emotional needs.

April 24, 11:00 Hours, Hatchie County Mental Health Center

Sara Lee Benefield: Well, we'uns are in a fine fix right now. We are both out of work and livin' with Travis's sister, and we still have funeral arrangements to make fer Loretta. It's like we don't know where to start. We did have some home insurance, but Iah don't think it will be near enough. There isn't

a thing left of our home, so we'uns have to start all over again. About what we've got is the clothes on our backs and $437.12 in the bank. Travis hasn't even got his tools, which he cain't seem to quit worryin' about all along with the other stuff.

Ollie Naifeh, social worker: OK, I am going to drive you over to the Civic Center, and we will go to the Disaster Recovery Center. I am going to introduce you to some people I know in the Red Cross and the Salvation Army. They can help with immediate assistance for food and shelter and maybe even tools. We can go to the FEMA One Stop and see about getting you a home loan to get you back on your feet and a roof over your heads. They will send an inspector out there really quickly and get the ball rolling, and they will work with your insurance company. They will also work with you on what is called disaster unemployment compensation. It is not quite your paycheck, but it will help out a good bit. Jeffrey has gotten your mother taken care of, and we can talk about funeral arrangements for your mother, Travis. I am guessing that money may be a problem?

Travis: Well no, momma had one of them universal burial policies, although I don't have no idea where it is, and she had about $5,000 put back. Reverend Dehl said he would be proud to preach momma's funeral as soon as we let him know, and there was Wednesday night services, and everybody done gave us their condolences and said what a fine person Loretta was and not to worry over much, that they would hep take care of things.

The crisis counselor does very little mental health counseling at this juncture. He is far more concerned with just getting the basic survival needs of this family met (Ruzek, 2006). There will be time enough for the other later on. As soon as external crisis workers help the community regain control after the immediate aftershock of the crisis, they will leave and turn their clients back over to the local mental health unit.

April 25, 18:00 Hours, High School Gymnasium

Eva Jane Walters, Superintendent, Midville Public School District: (speaking to about 500 parents) Thank you for being here under the tough circumstances you are facing. I know many of you have lost your homes or have your home heavily damaged. I know this because I have been sleeping with many of you at the National Guard Armory as my own home is heavily damaged. We are now four days post-tornado. It is Friday. It is time to get your children back to learning. I also know we are going to have school Monday morning, and that includes all the elementary school students. We have been working this week to make those arrangements happen. At the end of my talk, there will be a number of teachers in the cafeteria with homerooms, children's names, and new attendance centers for them. St. Benedict's Catholic Church and Midville First Baptist have graciously opened their doors to us, and we are going to hold classes there. That will be in walking or carpooling distance, and we will have buses at the shelters for those children still housed there. Some of your children will have different teachers because their teachers are dead or injured. We are going to have school counselors trained in crisis intervention from Saline, Wahatchie, and Forked Deer counties' schools here working with our counselors, school psychologists, and school social workers from the Tennessee River Special Education District will be here as well, and teachers to deal with any emotional issues children have. We are composing a series of classroom guidance meetings, which should go a long way toward helping us identify and work through problems that children are having. We are going to work very closely with you in this regard, and we want you to work very closely with us. We know this community does not lack for courage and mental toughness, and we know you and your children are tough-minded and resilient, but there is toughness, and there is smartness, and we want to be smart about taking care of your children's academic, social, and emotional needs because we know if those other needs are taken care of, we get better academic results, and in the end, that is what we are about, the best academic success we can get. Midville schools have long been outstanding, and part of the glue that holds this city together and gives it pride. We are not stepping back from that one inch, but to do that, we are going to need all of the cooperation this community can bring to bear on getting these schools up and running. If you have any questions, I will be happy to take them now or talk with you individually later on.

I also want to say something about our loss, not only of a building but also of teachers and students who made it into the viable academic community it was and will be again. We are now planning with the PTA a commemorative memorial service in the Civic Center that will take place before school is out at the end of May. We understand that many of you are dealing with your own personal grief and loss right now, and we want to give you time to work through that. We want to be supportive of you in any way we can because we know it is important to you and your children. The Hatchie Mental Health Center and grief counselors will be available if you or your children have need of them. You can call the Hatchie clinic or call us at the high school counselor's number. All the calls will be kept confidential. Thank you for coming. If you have questions now, there are teachers who will bring you a microphone so everybody can hear. I have the rest of the schools' administrative staff here, so if I don't have the answer, one of them probably will. When we are done here, we'll exit toward the cafeteria, where you can pick up your child's school, room, and teacher assignment. We will have e-mail as power becomes available again but are not sure when that will happen. So we've resurrected some old mimeograph machines, and you grandparents will recognize the purple bulletins. Welcome back to the 1950s, but we'll get information to you, rest assured. This is not going to be easy, but with your help, we will get the Golden Eagles back up and running.

The superintendent does five things that are critical when a school suffers a calamitous event. First, the "whole child" is the focus. Academic, social, and emotional components are all targeted. Second, she is intent on moving the school and the community as quickly as possible back to day-to-day living and a sense of "normalcy." Third, she seeks to develop a strong sense of community with the families whose children attend the school. Fourth, she has the school function as a valid and reliable source of information by telling parents specifically what is happening and keeping a communication line open to them so that they know there is a centralized and trusted source of information that they can go to when the rumor mill gets going (Kilmer et al., 2010).

The superintendent also does something else that is critical in the face of a disaster in which children's lives are lost. Students' ability to work through the grieving process is, in part, a social phenomenon that is anchored in their peer group when friends are lost (Worden, 2002). Therefore, school needs to get started again to serve as the place where they come together to grieve friends' loss. Providing not only counselors to deal with adjustment problems but also grief counselors who can work with the whole family to help them come to terms with their loss is not an easy sale at times. However, providing the common ground of the school as a brokerage for such deeply personal issues can go a good way toward easing the stigma of having to seek help with one's loss. Even if parents have not lost a relative, many people will have lost houses, places of employment, or social gathering places such as churches, clubs, and organizations that play integral parts in their lives, fracturing both their microsystem and, to a large extent, their exosystem supports. We are fully aware that a school system should not get into the funeral business (refer back to Chapter 13, "Crises in Schools"). However, when faced with a large magnitude disaster that affects the whole community, the school system certainly needs to provide a process for students to grieve and move on. It also needs to take part in memorial exercises that are inclusive of all students and parents as a way of acknowledging the loss, allowing expression of feelings, and effecting reengagement with school (Kerr, 2009, pp. 130–132). You may wonder why we included this piece about schools here and not in the school chapter. It is important to understand how critical a school is in the fabric of a community and its recovery from disaster (Kilmer et al., 2010). To not have one example of the part the school plays in disaster mitigation is to leave out a critical part indeed of the exosystem of a community.

April 30, 16:00 Hours, Hatchie County Mental Health Center

Kate McClain, licensed professional mental health counselor: How are things going? I spoke with Ollie before he left, and he said things were moving along. How do you feel about that?

Sara Lee: Well, we have done got the loan approved, and the insurance company has been real good about things. We have got us temporary housing assistance and have a place over in Crowley. The kids want to stay here with their friends, so we'uns are gonna bring them over here every day. Mah dentist office is gonna open up next week. But we don't know when or if the Packard plant will reopen, so Travis is gonna be on unemployment.

Travis: Maybe y'all could talk to Shawn some. He is wakin' up at night screamin'. Iah don't think he is near over the school fallin' in and his best friend

gittin' kilt. It was tough buryin' momma, but we got that done, and the church really hept.

Sara Lee: And maybe you could talk to Travis here too about him feelin' so durn guilty about leaving the plant to come look fer us. And Iah don't suppose it would hurt for me to talk some too, seein' as how I feel so stupid about runnin' off like a chicken with mah head cut off and makin' things even worse, durn fool that Iah am.

Kate: OK, I will be glad to do that. I think you are making progress and showing me that you have some strong fiber, that you are moving forward rapidly to getting things back to some kind of normalcy. Maybe your minister has told you, but there is going to be a community-wide meeting put on by NOVA. It's called "Y'all come" for all those who were in the tornado or affected by it, kind of a community memorial, talking, and bonding service. That might be something you would want to go to. That really sort of helps when people come together to talk about their experiences. I would also like our psychologist to give you some tests that will tell us how much this is affecting you. Those will help me better plan what we might want to do. Some of what you are experiencing is quite common. We just don't want it to turn into PTSD. **(Explains the difference between ASD and PTSD and what they are all about. She puts a positive view on the disorders by explaining that while most people start out with these symptoms, they tend to go away, particularly when people are proactive about doing things like what she is proposing to the Benefields.)** We are having some small support groups meet, and you are welcome to join them immediately.

I will also contact Shawn's school counselor, Janet Beverly from the middle school, who is filling in there since Mr. Little is still in the hospital, and see if we can set up something for Shawn. We have worked pretty closely together. We might want to have you all in as a family. I know she is starting some family groups there for people whose kids are having some problems. I also want to tell you that I really respect your observations and request for help about your children. That tells me you are truly caring parents. That is going to be really important in the days and months ahead.

The counselor does some psychoeducation with the Benefields in regard to ASD and PTSD. While there is limited evidence about the benefits of psychoeducation, particularly self-help materials regarding trauma, Wessely and associates (2008) recommend that any psychoeducation should promote resilience and adaptability rather than pathology. Therefore, the counselor de-escalates the situation by assuring the Benefield's their reaction is to be expected and attempts to allay fears that this means they are losing their minds rather than having a naturally occurring response to what they have been through. For many people, the psychological symptoms of hypervigilance, startle responses, nightmares, and the like, are as scary or more so than what they have just been through. While the education does not make the symptoms disappear immediately, it is calming to know they are common occurrences and that these survivors are not losing their minds.

The counselor also seeks to get them involved in a group. It is one of the best ways to share experience, bond with other survivors, and start back on the road to recovery. Finally, the counselor reinforces the mother for thinking about her children and husband. It is extremely important that caregivers provide a supportive, understanding environment in which children may manifest symptoms, can process thoughts and feelings without fear of recrimination, and otherwise attempt to integrate the trauma into their lives and come to terms with it (Gil-Rivas et al., 2010). Many times, caregivers' ability to support their children will be compromised by their own trauma-related issues (Gil-Rivas et al., 2007).

May 8, 09:00 Hours, Midville Baptist Church (Temporary Site for Midville Elementary School)

Janet Beverly, elementary school counselor: Shawn, I wonder how you are getting along?

Shawn: Yes, ma'am. All right, I guess.

Janet: I looked at some of your drawings you made when we had the classroom meeting about the tornado. (**Shows him one of his drawings.**) I wonder if you could tell me about this?

Shawn: Yes, ma'am. That's me and that there's Jamie and that's Leotis. They were mah best friends. Jamie was right next to me in the hall when the tornado hit, but he's dead now. Ah'm red 'cause I thought I was all bloody, but it was really his blood. Leotis was with Mrs. Cruz. He and her both got kilt, and Iah don't know why. Ma says it was God's will, but Iah jest don't rightly know. Iah don't think much of God if he done let this happen, to tell the truth. Ma wouldn't like me sayin' that, but Iah reckon that's how Iah feel. Iah don't sleep too good at night neither, and Iah shore don't like storms. Sometimes Iah think Iah hear Jamie and Leotis. We used to play a lot together, soldiers and stuff down by Brunner's Creek. Iah miss them somethin' terrible.

Janet: I wonder if you might like to come to a group I am starting, Shawn. It is for a bunch of kids who have friends who died or got hurt or lost other things, who just plain feel sad and maybe a little lonely right now.

Shawn: Yes, ma'am. Iah guess that'd be OK. Iah sure wish Jamie and Leotis could come. Iah miss mah grandma too. She used to have cookies made when Iah'd git home.

As indicated throughout this book, when children are involved with traumatic events, as Stacy Overstreet, a Tulane University school psychology student who worked with post-Katrina students in the New Orleans schools, stated, "There are two vital keys to recovery: social support and putting experiences in context" (Dingfelder, 2006). This is exactly what the school counselor is doing with Shawn when she uses expressive arts and group counseling to help him start to come to terms with his traumatic experiences, put them in his past, and grow from them (Malchiodiel et al., 2008, p. 299). Groups are powerful ways to bring children together to share commonality of experience, own feelings that range from scared to angry to guilty, decrease isolation, enhance coping and adaptation, seek commonalities, build cohesion and trust, and help members cope with those negative feelings (Nisivoccia & Lynn, 20007). There is not a lot of outcome evidence on postdisaster groups for children, but at least two studies indicate they do help to reduce posttrauma stress symptoms (Chemtob et al., 2002; Salloum & Overstreet, 2008).

A child with traumatic grief can get "stuck" on the traumatic aspects of the death, which then interferes with the normal grieving process (DeAngelis, 2011). The fact that Shawn was covered with the blood of his close friend and lay there with his friends' bodies admirably fits such criteria. Chapter 7, "Posttraumatic Stress Disorder," describes how, by using trauma-focused cognitive-behavioral therapy in creating a trauma narrative using a combination of stress management, play therapy, and cognitive behavior techniques to monitor and control emotional dysregulation, children can move through both their grief and the post trauma stress symptoms that often accompany it (Cohen et al., 2006). Indeed, if intervention is used as indicated in Chapter 13, "Crises in Schools," the school can become a post disaster anchor for children (Munsey, 2006).

May 15, 16:00 Hours, Hatchie County Mental Health Center

Kate McClain, licensed professional mental health counselor: (meeting with Sara Lee and Travis) I have talked with Janet Beverly, the school counselor. She is recommending that Shawn go into one of her counseling groups. Her report and what the psychologists report is that he has had a pretty rough time and is suffering from what we call acute stress disorder. **(Reiterates what ASD is and why it is important for it to be dealt with before it becomes PTSD.)** I am also going to recommend that you all come to the clinic as a family. I think it will be helpful for all the kids to talk about some of this stuff and see that, even though you have suffered some severe losses, your family is still together.

Sara Lee: I 'spect you're right. I don't suppose Travis will own up to it, but he's not the same, and neither am I. Shawn isn't the only one havin' nightmares. I jump near outta mah skin every time there's a thunderstorm. Travis and I have never had a hard word with one another, but the other night we done had a huge fight over nuthin'. It was jest nuthin'. **(Tears start to well up in her eyes.)** It was awful. It was in front of his sister's family and the kids. **(Starts to cry.)** He went and apologized, and so did I, but that is not like us a t'all. I don't know what we're becomin', and it scares me half to death.

Travis: (Puts his arm comfortingly around his wife.) Iah "spect you're right, honey. Iah still cain't git them durn tools off mah mind, and that is plumb ridiculous. Iah got a whole new set, though. The church has really hept out and all, but it jest seems like things keep tumblin" through mah mind, and Iah cain't git no peace with them. That's why Iah got mad "cause Sara Lee kept tellin" me to git over it, that we had other things to think about. And Iah got mad. Iah don't like it much neither.

Kate: I want to assure you that those are perfectly normal responses to an abnormal situation. But that doesn't make them any easier to bear. I would really like you to go to the NOVA "Y'all come"

meeting. The ministerial association is going to put on some stuff along with it. I think you will find it helpful to hear and share some of the things you have gone through. You are strong folks, but everyone could use a little help and support, and I think this would be good.

The counselor is very interested in how her client family is dealing with the traumatic wake of the disaster. She coordinates her efforts with the school counselor and the clinic psychologist. The NOVA meeting and the church provide community support, but there are specific individual mental health issues that assail this family that need to be worked on so the family does not fracture (Myers & Wee, 2005, p. 33). While most people are resilient in a disaster and will recover (Aldwin, 2007), it is critically important to intervene when there are indicators things are not going well (Ruzek, 2006). This emergency mental health intervention process is set up on a Family Assistance Center model (Halpern & Tramontin, 2007, pp. 190–191; Leskin et al., 2006), in which one person acts as a broker and communicator to deal with the many social, psychological, and financial issues that will assail them. Getting all the family into therapy is a positive move because no one then feels the stigma of being the identified "sick" person when everybody else is doing well.

May 22, 16:00 Hours, Hatchie County Mental Health Center

Travis: Well, we went to that "Y'all come" meeting, and I would say it was helpful. Sort o' gives you a sense of pride 'n' hope, I guess. Kinda like we'uns are all in this together. They had a pretty good community church memorial service and all afterward. Eighty-three dead and over 600 hurt. Lord A'mighty!

Sara Lee: Iah'd agree. But what Iah really liked was our first family meeting. Iah talked to the kids afterward. Lee Ann and Jason both didn't want to come, but they both said afterward they wouldn't mind coming again, which means they really did like it. Iah jest feel a little more peaceful somehow. Like we'uns are on the right track.

Travis: Iah guess it is like gittin' back in control. Ain't felt like that much.

Kate: I am glad to hear that. We will take this slow and easy. We have plenty of time. We will work on this as long as you feel the need to.

Travis' and the other Benefields' TAF ratings have obviously decreased. Now, the overall rating is in the low teens. Kate continues to support the family now in more of a consultant role. Kate, the counselor seeks to reinforce the Benefields for their courage and willingness to commit to some pretty arduous mental health work in addition to all the other challenges they face. She reemphasizes that there is no rush to work through their problems. Kate is now working on what is called *second phase* crisis intervention in the crisis chronosystem. The immediate crisis is over. Basic physiological needs have been met. At this point, the crisis worker is more concerned about possible long-term effects on the whole family; therefore, she is treating the family system as a client. She seeks to coordinate her efforts with other human services workers both from an individual perspective, as in the case of Shawn, and a wider community perspective, such as helping support the NOVA and the community church program. The more social support that can be generated, the more likely the victims are to use it to help with the distress (Yates et al., 1999).

April 25 (1 year and 4 days after the tornado), 16:00 Hours, Hatchie County Mental Health Center

Sara Lee: Iah guess we'uns are ready to say goodbye, Kate. We'uns really 'preciate what you have done fer us. We'uns couldn't have done this a t'all without you. We all went to the big memorial service last week out to the Civic Center. It'll always be part of our lives, but it's behind us now, and we kin go on. Shawn is really doing well. He is off antidepressants and has a couple of new friends. We'uns couldn't go back to Breezemore. Jest too many bad memories, but we done got a lot out south o' town and put our new manufactured home on it, and there are some new kids out there Shawn met at Southside Elementary. None of us are having any nightmares either, although Iah still don't like thunderstorms, and we have a tornado shelter by our home now.

Travis: Iah guess Ah'd agree. Iah shore do appreciate what y'all have done fer us. It was tough, but Iah think we'uns are better fer it as a family. We're a whole lot tighter than before. Iah don't even think about mah tools no more, and even though Iah got mah head shrunk it feels better. (**Laughs.**) Durndest thing about them tools. We got momma buried beside paw out to Big Prairie Cemetery. Got her

a nice stone, too. Pink marble. She always liked pink. She's at peace . . . and I guess fer that matter, so am Iah—as fer as one could be, given the circumstances. We are about ready to reopen the engine works, and Iah been workin' gittin' the machines all set up.

Kate: I am glad to have worked with you. I agree. I think we are ready to get divorced. (**Everybody laughs.**) I expect I will see you around town, so I look forward to seeing you out and about. I also want to tell you I really respect you for what you have done. I have learned from you, probably as much as you have learned from me, and I appreciate you coming into and touching my life. It makes me feel even more sure that this is the business I was meant to do.

Sara Lee: Well Iah think the good Lord put you in the right job. Thanks, and goodbye.

Travis: Amen to that. (**Both hug Kate and go out the door and on with their lives.**)

Over the long haul, most people, even when they suffer comprehensive and horrific loss like the Benefields, are resilient and equal to the task of moving on with their lives (Gist et al., 1999). What the crisis counselor provides is not so much therapy as information and programs that help families like the Benefields normalize an abnormal situation and address their material resource losses (Farberow & Frederick, 1978). The crisis worker also takes precautionary steps to monitor this family very closely for a while. While people sometimes do develop delayed PTSD, the vast majority are amazingly resilient and do not (Drabek, 1986).

The major role that the crisis worker initially plays is one of victim advocate by facilitating the return of basic services to survivors (Salzer & Bickman, 1999). The crisis worker then shifts from problem-focused to more emotion-focused coping (Lazarus & Folkman, 1984) and seeks to help the family move forward and reframe the crisis and distance themselves from it through preventive and supportive therapy (Chemtob, 2000).

Often, the lack of use of mental health services by families like the Benefields is not happenstance (Norris & Alegria, 2006). There are many reasons, some good and some bad, why mental health services are underused after a disaster, and stigma, no matter how great the emotional distress and turmoil, is a leading cause (American Psychiatric Association, n.d; Center for Disease Control, 2023; NAMI, n.d.; Yates et al., 1999). Some individuals see the use of such services and facilities as a sign of mental illness and, therefore, a major character flaw that would label them as "nut" cases. To avoid being perceived as outcasts by their peers, these individuals may be very loath to use mental health services (Bethel & Oates, 2007). If such services are poor, uncoordinated, culturally insensitive, and intrusive, they indeed may do more harm than good. In this instance, good mesosystem coordination and communication among a number of local and national agencies in the micro-, exo-, and macrosystems worked to provide nonintrusive help and support. The sensitivity, caring, support, and unconditional positive regard of a variety of different helping professionals working in close coordination—including social workers, psychologists, licensed professional counselors, school counselors, and "just plain folks"—helped make the Benefields' experience with mental health services a positive one.

The anniversary of the disaster is a benchmark for positive resolution, and like most people, the Benefields are resilient and capable of moving forward with a little help. The tornado has left an indelible imprint on their lives that will never go away, but like the Chinese symbols that start every chapter in this book, they have found opportunity in the crisis and have come out of it stronger than they were before.

Multiculturalism at Work

LO8 While the Benefields represent the stereotype of a White, fundamentalist Christian, blue-collar family in the south-central United States, you might gather from the surnames of some of the people who came to their assistance or who worked on the overall disaster that they represented a rainbow coalition of Americans of all races, ethnicity, and cultural backgrounds. That was not done to be politically correct. The fact of the matter is that even in rural west Tennessee, we are becoming a melting pot of races, ethnicities, and divergent cultural backgrounds. As such, a multicultural perspective is critical to any crisis intervention—and, indeed, people with just such divergent surnames work on crisis teams with which we are involved.

A top down-bottoms up cultural approach. This crisis team operates on Wei Chen Hwang's (2012) Psychotherapy Adaptation and Modification Framework (PAMF) and Formative Method for Adapting Psychotherapy (FMAP). While Hwang generated these approaches with Chinese Americans in mind,

we believe these approaches have universal transferability to any culturally different environment crisis workers enter. The PAMF has a top-down, three-tiered approach of domains, principles, and rationales. Domains are general areas that practitioners should consider when modifying therapeutic approaches to clients. Principles involve more specified recommendations of adapting therapy for specific groups. Rationales are corresponding explanations for why these adaptations may be effective when used with the target population. This paradigm serves two critical purposes when applied to the real world of crisis intervention with people whose culture is very different from our own. PAMF seeks to build evidenced-based therapies (EBTs) and manualized treatments that can be used universally and help practitioners shift from the abstract notion of being "multicultural sensitive" into being concretely multicultural competent in real time under crisis conditions.

The FMAP is a community-based bottom-up approach that consists of five phases: generating knowledge and collaborating with stakeholders, integrating generated information with theory and empirical and clinical knowledge, reviewing the initial culturally adapted clinical intervention with stake holders and revising the culturally adapted intervention, then testing it and finalizing it. The FMAP was developed to generate ideas for culturally adapted EBTs, while the PAMF was designed to improve the cultural competency of clinicians (Hwang, 2012). It appears that Goodman and associates (2014) successfully used an approach that closely resembles Hwang's FAMP model in their work with Haitian communities in Florida after the 2010 Haiti earthquake. During peer supervision sessions, they used content information on the community's culture, strengths, and sociopolitical issues to conceptualize the community's needs and informed their outreach process. Their success appears to be in stark contrast to a number of international programs that offered help after the 2004 Indian Ocean tsunami, which was not well received in the Indian state of Aceh because sensitivity to and building intervention strategies with the local culture didn't happen (Fananay & Fanany, 2013).

As these two concepts are integrated, they can be used to build EBTs that are custom-made to different cultural groups, whether they be Chinese Americans in San Francisco or Southern Whites in Appalachia. We would propose that using this protocol is critical in crisis intervention and should be operationalized in real time in conjoint dialogues between leaders in the local population and crisis team leaders in the daily debriefings that occur in the context of a large-scale disaster. This approach fits admirably into contextual/ecological models of crisis intervention (Cook, 2012; Myer & Moore, 2006).

A final word on multiculturalism. Crisis workers should also understand that their own cultural biases have an even higher potential for surfacing when faced with oppositional defiant clients who may not think, talk, act, look, or even smell like the worker. For example, more than one of the editors of this book has queried the author when reading the dialogues of the Benefield family.

Editors have questioned words such as *we'uns* (which literally means "we ones") and *fer* (meaning "far" or "for") because they were unsure themselves of the meaning and were equally unsure that you, the reader, would understand what was being said. Those words were intentionally used in the dialogues to test readers' responses to the deep southern rural dialect of Travis Benefield and his family. If you were put off by that dialect, found it hard to understand, and knew it was not standardized English, then you might be put off by Travis as an "ignorant redneck" as well. Despite all your good works and good intentions, you might then unintentionally treat him with less respect than you would a person who talked like a 6 o'clock network news broadcaster. As a result, do you suppose Travis's reaction to you would be different than it was to the social workers, licensed professional counselors, and other crisis workers who were culturally sensitive to him and treated him respectfully despite his language? Cultural sensitivity is displayed when the worker translates into primary language that the client can understand (Myers & Wee, 2005, p. 62), whether that be Spanish, Urdu, or English with a deep southern accent.

Although you might think that Travis's obsessive concern about his tools is somewhat bizarre, in fact, it has a deep cultural basis. Bethel and Oates (2007) have found that an Appalachian man like Travis, the patriarchal head of his family, is expected to be a good "hunter" who provides for and takes care of his family by supplying them with food, shelter, and clothing. The loss of his tools strikes at the very heart of who Travis is and how his culture defines him as an independent, hardworking, self-reliant provider for his family. In Travis's world, a blue-collar job in which a man can be skillful with tools may be more valued than a white-collar job. It is no accident that Travis persists in brooding on the loss of his tools, for those tools are, in fact, symbolic of his very identity as a man. The wise and culturally sensitive crisis worker will understand that the loss of his tools is as critical to Travis as the loss of his house, and that worker will be empathic and supportive, placing a high priority on helping Travis get his "durn" tools replaced.

Spiritualism/religion

LO9 Aten and associates (2015) report a great deal of research on the central role of religious institutions and prayer in recovery from a disaster and maintain that one of the most critical components for the recovery of a community is through the religious organizations that support it. Spirituality and faith roles in recovery following disasters have been found to be beneficial in individuals and families recovering and finding meaning following a wide range of disasters, including hurricanes, floods, mass shootings, and the COVID-19 pandemic, to name a few (Davis et al., 2019; Park et al., 2019; San Roman et al., 2019; Zang et al., 2021). The deep roots that the Benefield family has in their religion and spiritual values should also be understood as a significant part of their life and culture. Religion and spirituality help buffer individuals from the negative emotional and physical consequences that happen after a disaster. Ai and associates (2005) found that stronger faith, hope, and spirituality staved off the depression and anxiety that was related to exposure of those who experienced 9/11. Conversely, that lack of religious faith exacerbated poor physical and mental health following a disaster (Zang et al., 2022). Given that support is one of the most critical components to moving through any crisis, to not use and honor their religion and spiritual values to help salve the wounds of their losses would be a grave mistake indeed (Bethel & Oates, 2007; Stambor, 2005). Graham (2014) proposes that the provision of "pastoral" care is a critical part of a community's recovery after a disaster and occurs in three parts: sharing the anguish with God or a higher being, examining the causes from a spiritual perspective, and reinvesting in hope and rebirth. Graham also maintains that organized religion plays a critical part in the political aftermath of a disaster in the process of ensuring solace and safety, along with guidance and influence in helping rebuild the community and its sense of coherence and meaning.

In that regard, any crisis worker who enters a disaster area would be well advised to follow Aten and associates' (2015) general guidelines for how to handle spiritual issues in a crisis aftermath.

1. If you don't feel comfortable discussing religious issues say so and refer the person to another worker.
2. Do not argue with or try to persuade a person that your spiritual beliefs are better.
3. Let people tell you what their beliefs are. Don't assume anything.
4. Help people use their spiritual beliefs to cope.
5. Assure individuals that it is normal to ask questions about God/higher being and/or their beliefs.
6. If they are angry with God/higher being, let them cathart.
7. Do affirm the injustice and wrongness of what has happened.
8. Encourage people to use the spiritual writings in their religion to find answers, solace and peace.

Focus on the Worker

Debriefing Models

LO10 "Debriefing is an intervention designed to assist workers and survivors in dealing with intense thoughts, feelings, and reactions that occur after a traumatic event, and to decrease their impact and facilitate the recovery of normal people having normal reactions to abnormal events" (Myers & Wee, 2005, p. 173). There are three general types of debriefing as described by the National Center for PTSD (U.S. Department of Veterans Affairs, n.d). They are:

1. **Operational debriefing** is a routine and formal part of an organizational response to a disaster. Mental health workers acknowledge it as an appropriate practice that may help survivors acquire an overall sense of meaning and a degree of closure. Currently, many mental health workers consider some form of stress debriefing the standard of care following both natural (earthquakes) and human-caused (workplace shootings, bombings) stressful events.
2. **Psychological or stress debriefing** refers to a variety of practices for which there is little supportive empirical evidence. It is strongly suggested that psychological debriefing is not an appropriate mental health intervention.

3. **Critical Incident Stress Debriefing (CISD)** is a formalized, structured method whereby a group of rescue and response workers reviews the stressful experience of a disaster. CISD was developed to **assist first responders** such as fire and police personnel; it was not meant for the survivors of a disaster or their relatives. CISD was never intended as a substitute for therapy.

Probably no emergent technique in crisis intervention has created more controversy than debriefing procedures. The attacks on debriefing psychotherapy (Gist & Lubin, 1999) have been some of the most vituperative we have seen in 50 years in the field of counseling, and while there are several different models of debriefing (Armstrong et al., 1991; McWhirter & Linzer, 1994; Myers & Zunin, 1994), these attacks have been especially virulent in regard to Mitchell and Everly's (1995a) critical incident stress debriefing (CISD) model and their lack of hard research evidence to demonstrate its effectiveness (Gist, Woodall et al., 1999). Further, like most wishful searches for a panacea in dealing with an intractable problem, debriefing has been hailed as a potent vaccination against PTSD. However, research indicates it is not (Bisson & Deahl, 1994; Bisson et al., 1997; Deahl, 1999; Hobbs et al., 1996; Kenardy et al., 1996; Lee et al., 1996; Raphael et al., 1995). Van Emmerik et al.'s (2002) meta-analysis on its utility in decreasing PTSD symptoms found it to be ineffective. It has come to the point that psychological debriefing cannot be endorsed for use with survivors (Brymer et al., 2009; Gray & Litz, 2005).

In fact, Mitchell and Everly have not been able to provide scientific evidence that CISD does much of anything beneficial for workers or victims (Gist, Woodall et al., 1999), and at least one study found it to be harmful (Avery & Orner, 1998a, 1998b). Further, caustic rebukes have rained down on CISD as a get-rich-quick scheme for "quack" therapists and a "get out of jail free" (or almost free) card for businesses and insurance companies who can claim it is an effective vaccination against PTSD and therefore do not have to pay for much more expensive rehabilitation procedures to employees who come down with PTSD symptoms (Gist, Woodall et al., 1999; Raphael, 1999). CISD has also been roundly criticized for mandating that all workers who were victims of the crisis obtain CISD, even though it may be personally or culturally inappropriate (Silove, 1999; Weisaeth, 1999). Finally, there is a serious ethical question as to the blanket use of CISD for all kinds of populations for all kinds of trauma under all kinds of conditions (Raphael, 1999). At the NIMH consensus conference, the following recommendation was approved:

Early intervention in the form of a single one-on-one recital of events and expression of emotions evoked by a traumatic event (as advocated in some forms of psychological debriefing) does not consistently reduce risks of later developing PTSD or related adjustment difficulties. Some survivors (e.g., those with high arousal) may be put at heightened risk of adverse outcomes as a result of such early interventions (NIMH, 2002, p. 8).

On the other side of the debate, adherents absolutely believe in its effectiveness, and there are studies to support that (Chemtob, 2000; Jacobs et al., 2004; MacDonald, 2003; Pender & Prichard, 2008, 2009; Robinson et al., 1997; Wagner, 2005). Many of its adherents tend to be frontline workers. Their responses to those who would vilify CISD are that it does work—if the procedure is used correctly and if the people who do it are trained to use it the way Mitchell and Everly (1999) propose (Freeman, 2003; Lane, 2003; Montano & Dowdall-Thomae, 2003). One of the major issues has been its profligate use for *anybody for any kind of traumatic event.* Mitchell and Everly (1999) never intended it to be that. It was intended to be applied directly to emergency service workers, firefighters, and police officers to help them quickly integrate feelings and thoughts so the experiences would lose their potential to become disturbing. Part of why it has been so successful (and so abused and misapplied) is that, at face value, it *should* work; survivors appreciate that someone cares enough about them to listen, and talking bad stuff out is a good way to get rid of it (Halpern & Tramontin, 2007, pp. 265–266).

Sharing experiences is one way of bonding through an adverse experience. If you don't believe that, get invited to an American Legion bar and talk to some ex-marines, or spend some time with police officers at "choir practice" after a tough drug bust where shots were fired. Debriefing objectives of ventilation of feelings, reordering and reorganization of cognitions, normalization of experience, increased group support, verbal reconstruction and integration, and screening for traumatic stress referral would seem to be laudable goals for postintervention with any disaster worker (Halpern & Tramontin, 2007, pp. 267–268; Myers & Wee, 2005, pp. 172–174).

Your authors tend to be in guarded agreement with the use of CISD for specific populations of first responders. We have seen this technique work

in powerful ways with some very cynical and tough police field commanders who were very much in need of debriefing a multitude of traumatic events and the stress and pent-up emotions that went with them (Addy & James, 2002). It is also worth noting that when we do role-play CISD shooting scenarios with our students (Dr. James is certified as a CISD-trained debriefer), they almost universally agree that they thought the debriefing was helpful.

The issue remains muddied. Tuckey's (2007) critique of debriefing focused on methodological and conceptual shortcomings that have prevented research in this area from progressing. Tuckey proposed an organizing framework of research within which the key issues would be identified, clarified, and linked to guidelines for future research, which should foster greater understanding about the empirical side of the debriefing debate. Extensive review of the research since Tuckey's article has not found that has happened. It appears that the previous debate has lost traction and is no longer a hot topic. Having presented the foregoing arguments for and against, the fact stands that different types of debriefing strategies still predominate in the field of trauma and disaster work. For that reason alone, the following description of debriefing emergency workers is presented.

Debriefing Emergency Workers

Critical Incident Stress Debriefing (CISD). CISD was developed by Jeffrey Mitchell, a firefighter and paramedic in Baltimore County, Maryland, as a result of his own responses to the traumatic incidents he continuously witnessed. Originally designed to deal only with firefighters and EMTs who were first responders to fires, accidents, and other events where they saw and dealt with horrific sights, sounds, and smells, CISD is now used with a variety of people who have suffered trauma (Morrissey, 1994). CISD teams are typically composed of two members who must hold a minimum of a master's degree in the mental health professions and who have undergone training and received certification in CISD. Debriefing is designed to mitigate the psychological impact of a traumatic event, restore homeostasis and equilibrium, prevent PTSD from developing, and identify people who will need professional mental health follow-up (Mitchell & Everly, 1995a, p. 270).

Informal Defusing. Informal defusing is a first-order intervention following traumatic incidents and is typically performed by CISD-trained on-site personnel. The goal of defusing is to lessen the impact of a traumatic event and accelerate the normal recovery process by providing a brief, time-limited format to air feelings and thoughts of the event (Myers & Wee, 2005, p. 167). This three-stage intervention is a shortened version of a full-scale debriefing and usually takes about one hour. First, team members introduce themselves and then explain the process and delineate expectations. Second, the traumatic experience is explored via participants' disclosure of facts, cognitive and emotional reactions, and finally symptoms of distress related to the traumatic event. Third, participants receive information to normalize the dissonant cognitions of the event and educate them with regard to stress, stress management, and trauma (Mitchell & Everly, 1995a, p. 275).

Formal Debriefing. The formal debriefing process has seven stages and typically takes place within 24 hours to seven days after a traumatic event. It is generally two to three hours long. It is a combination of psychological and educational elements formatted in a structured group setting, and it involves personnel who have been directly affected by a traumatic event such as police officers, firefighters, EMTs, and ER staff. It is not intended for use with the general public (Pender & Prichard, 2008). Debriefing helps make the transition from processing facts about the event to emotional responses to the event and, finally, back to cognitive information about reactions and coping with traumatic experiences. It is not psychotherapy but rather a controlled meeting that allows participants to discuss their emotions and thoughts about the event in a nonthreatening environment (Mitchell & Everly, 1995b).

The seven stages are described as follows:

1. **Introduction.** The introduction is crucial to setting the tone of the debriefing. Besides introducing team members and explaining the process and guidelines for the CISD, the introduction also seeks to lower resistance and motivate the participants by discussing sensitive issues such as confidentiality (Mitchell & Everly, 1995a, p. 271).

2. **Fact finding.** Facts are discussed first because they are easiest to deal with and are typical of what may be discussed with emergency workers after a traumatic event. The leaders typically start by making statements such as "We only have a sketch of what happened. We'd like you to fill us in on what happened. So we can get an overall picture, we'd like everyone—no matter what

part you played—to give us your perspective on it. If you don't feel ready to do that, that's OK too. Just shake your head, and we'll move past you. We need to know who you are, what your involvement was, and what happened from your point of view." Order doesn't matter; the episode will sort itself through the facilitative ability of the CISD leaders (Mitchell & Everly, 1995a, p. 272).

3. **Thoughts.** The CISD leaders ask the participants for their initial or most poignant thoughts about what happened. Moving from facts to thoughts starts to personalize the event and allows emotions to surface. As participants voice their thoughts, the leaders should elicit those emotions that come naturally with their thinking about the situation and that allow for movement into the next phase, reaction (Mitchell & Everly, 1995a, p. 272).

4. **Reaction.** This phase is the most emotionally powerful for participants. Questions that elicit responses are variations on a theme of "What about the situation was most bothersome to you? If you could change one part of it, what would it be?" Leaders will act more as passive facilitators at this point, as participants spontaneously speak to their affective responses to the event (Mitchell & Everly, 1995a, pp. 272–273).

5. **Symptoms.** The symptom phase is used to shift the group back to more cognitive material. The discussion deals with what went on both during and after the event. The leaders ask the group to describe their experience in terms of affective, behavioral, cognitive, or physical experiences they had. To get the group going, the leaders may give examples such as "My whole body was shaking for 5 minutes after the firing quit; I was under control, but I kept thinking I can't stand another minute of this; I wanted to say something, but my tongue was tied; I'm scared to death, but I know I have to go back into that building so my feet move me there somehow" (Mitchell & Everly, 1995a, p. 273).

6. **Teaching.** Leaders may point out that what the participants have talked about fits precisely into the symptoms of acute stress. The leaders let the participants know that these are normal, typical reactions, that they are not losing their minds or otherwise somehow not equal to the task. The participants are instructed in how to recognize and understand symptoms that might not have surfaced yet. Participants are also given information on stress management techniques. This phase moves the participants even farther away from the

emotional content they have worked through in the reaction phase (Mitchell & Everly, 1995a, p. 274).

7. **Reentry.** The reentry phase is a final opportunity to summarize and bring closure to all the issues that have been discussed. The CISD team's job at this time is to answer questions, provide reassurance, reflect on any agendas they believe have not been brought out, dispense handouts, and provide referral sources for extended psychological work (Mitchell & Everly, 1995a, p. 274).

In summary, the CISD derives its effectiveness from early intervention, the opportunity to experience catharsis in safety, the opportunity to verbalize the trauma, a definite behavioral structure, group and peer support, and a provision for follow-up if needed (Mitchell & Everly, 1995b, p. 41).

Debriefing Crisis Workers

Whether one buys the CISD model or not, it seems abundantly clear that *some* kind of debriefing process is indispensable in assisting crisis workers themselves to regain a state of emotional, cognitive, and behavioral equilibrium following their intensive intervention work in the aftermath of a chaotic crisis (Alavi et al., 2022; Hanna & Romana, 2007). The detailed procedures that follow are provided because it is essential for crisis workers to know how to debrief disaster workers as well as to understand the value of being debriefed themselves. The techniques and perspectives offered here may even enable the crisis worker to debrief the debriefers.

The Need for Debriefing. Throughout this book, crisis intervention is often depicted as complex and chaotic. Natural disasters, mechanical or human-caused large-scale accidents, mass murders resulting from terrorism, or death and destruction from floods and tornadoes all create the confused and chaotic disorder that, much like a battle, is so disorienting that for crisis workers, there are no scripts and little time for reflection, planning, or rehearsal. It is not surprising that crisis workers themselves tend to suffer psychological problems from the same trauma they are trying to alleviate in others. What the crisis worker sees, hears, smells, and touches may also rattle long-buried skeletons in the worker's own emotional closet. This phenomenon is known as vicarious traumatization (Saakvitne & Pearlman, 1996) or compassion fatigue (Figley, 2002), wherein the worker unwittingly absorbs and internalizes the very trauma that the client

manifests (see Chapter 15, "Human Services Workers in Crisis Burnout, Vicarious Traumatization, and Compassion Fatigue," for more on this phenomenon).

CERT team members are all citizens with different occupations. They are not therapists, and they do not receive supervision. Corey-Souza (2007) conducted a study of 96 members of the Florida Crisis Responses team on measures of compassion fatigue and compassion satisfaction. She found a strong negative correlation between compassion fatigue and compassion satisfaction and that burnout is one of the strongest predictors of compassion fatigue. So put yourself in the place of Jeffrey Chung, the Midville morgue counselor, or any of the CERT team members who found Loretta Benefield. Do you think you would be up for some kind of psychological debriefing? Finally, compounding it all, mental health crisis workers may be called on to debrief other emergency personnel who have been up to their arms in blood, gore, wreckage, and a panoply of human tragedy. It is important, then, that crisis workers themselves go through debriefing and that certain precautions are taken to arm them against the multiple stressors they will face when doing disaster work (Armstrong et al., 1991). As an example, Leffler and Dembert (1998) conducted a study of U.S. Navy divers involved in the recovery of wreckage and passenger remains from TWA Flight 800, which crashed en route to Paris in 120 feet of water off the coast of Long Island, New York. They reported that divers who were exposed to human remains, especially those of children, found that experience to be far more stressful than the safety hazards they encountered.

First responders to the twin towers of the WTC manifested all of the themes of what Robert Lifton (1983) calls the psychology of survival—psychic numbing, guilt over having not done enough or living when others did not, paranoia over attempts to provide psychological help, vivid death imprints, and futile and abortive attempts to make sense out of what they saw, heard, smelled, and touched (Henry, 2004). If this sounds to you suspiciously like PTSD or the vicarious traumatization you read about in Chapter 15, "Human Services Workers in Crisis Burnout, Vicarious Traumatization, and Compassion Fatigue," on burnout, you are correct. Compound this with Henry's (2004) and Addy and James's (2002) research, which found that responders such as police officers tend to be very wary of "head shrinkers." If you are an EMT, firefighter, or police officer, just to admit you may have some kind of mental problem puts you at risk because your partners may fear that your inability to function under pressure may harm them (Henry, 2005). So what is to be done? Above all else is self-care (Merlino, 2011), which means knowing you are not a super crisis worker, nor is anyone else, and having enough sense to look out for yourself and your team both physically and psychologically.

Precautions. First of all, crisis work of this kind is done in teams. Whether at the actual scene of the crisis with a number of specialists or in an after-action debriefing, workers do not act in isolation. Using the buddy system allows workers to rotate with difficult clients, ventilate to one another, check out perceptions, watch each other for signs of fatigue, and give each other a break (Hayes et al., 1990; Mitchell & Everly, 1995b; SAMHSA, 2003; Talbot et al., 1995, p. 286; Walker, 1990).

Second, crisis workers in a disaster need to take time off to sleep and decompress. An 8-hour shift under disaster conditions is a long time (Hayes et al., 1990). Crisis workers need to be rotated out of high-stress jobs, such as body identification and survivor notification, on a regular basis and be given less stressful duties (Walker, 1990). They also need time off between crises to rest and recuperate physically and psychologically (Talbot et al., 1995, p. 293). The U.S. Department of Mental Health proposes a maximum of 12-hour shifts followed by 12 hours off. They also propose that work rotations should change from high-stress to lower-stress functions (SAMHSA, 2003), 2021).

Third, as trite as it sounds, it is important to have plenty of water and nutritious food at the scene (SAMHSA, 2003, 2021). One of your authors has been in a crisis negotiation situation in which he and two police officers were unable to get food or water. The salvaged contents of the lunchbox of one of the officer's children that had been left in the backseat of her squad car was a lifesaver after we had been there from 5 p.m. until 3 a.m. without food and with very little water!

Fourth, have a clear chain of command with clear role and function statements. Nothing is worse or potentially more lethal than going into a disaster without a clear understanding of what one is going to do and to whom one is going to report. Correlative to the foregoing is having adequate and timely supervision to process what one is doing (SAMHSA, 2003, 2021).

Fifth, on-site crisis workers should not debrief one another (Spitzer & Neely, 1992; Talbot et al., 1995, p. 286). Another team of crisis workers who have not been at the scene should be brought in to lead debriefing. In this manner, the leaders cannot be construed as engaging in recriminations, second-guessing, or accusations about who did or didn't do what.

Sixth, the debriefing should be held away from the crisis scene if possible (Talbot et al., 1995, p. 286). Moving away from the scene physically allows the crisis workers to move away psychologically.

Seventh, the organizational context within which the group operates should be taken into consideration because it too plays a part in how the group is affected (Talbot et al., 1995, p. 286). The way the organization—and this includes even charitable organizations such as the Red Cross—runs its disaster relief program is critically important to how the individual handles stress at the disaster site.

Eighth, the crisis workers need to be in excellent physical and mental health themselves. From both a physical and mental standpoint, they will be stretched to the limit. Diving into the wake of a traumatic event is no place for someone who is out of shape, either physically or mentally (Walker, 1990). But even if a crisis worker is in excellent physical and psychological condition, no one is immune from the cumulative and acute onset of stress (see Chapter 15, "Human Services Workers in Crisis Burnout, Vicarious Traumatization, and Compassion Fatigue").

Although overuse of the procedure and policies requiring mandatory CISD attendance can create passive participation and even negative resentment, it would seem that a standing operational order for all emergency workers and crisis workers should be some kind of regular debriefing (not necessarily the CISD model). There are a variety of models that focus on different aspects of the event, such as positive reframing (Charlton & Thompson, 1996), group processing (Dyregrov, 1997), intensive follow-up after the debriefing (Solomon, 1995), multiple stressor debriefing (Armstrong et al., 1991), dynamic understanding of the event (Talbot et al., 1995), and disaster debriefing (Myers & Zunin, 1994).

While there are concerns that traditional CISD may sabotage personal integrity in favor of victim status by emphasizing pathology over resiliency and trauma over strength, Echterling et al. (2000) believe that linking people in crisis, hearing one another's crisis stories, normalizing reactions, and facilitating the group's coping are positive outcomes that are critical to resolution. Your authors absolutely agree. Debriefing should be the natural and final act of the emergency and crisis workers' job and should be no less expected than that of a first responder returning from a call.

Dynamics of Debriefing. The debriefers of crisis workers are dealing with a matrix of issues: the crisis event and its victims, the response to that event by the crisis workers, the individual crisis worker's personal and professional response to the survivors, the dynamics of the group as it goes through the debriefing process, and developing a collective plan for handling the next crisis (Echterling et al., 2000; Silove, 1999; Talbot et al., 1995, p. 286).

From a professional standpoint, crisis workers need to understand and evaluate the usefulness of their interventions, explore alternatives, and plan future courses of action. Focusing on survivor aspects rather than victimization is important in refocusing the individual on perseverance, creativity, and sensitivity, which often fade into the background in the face of the pain, anguish, and helplessness that the worker feels (Echterling et al., 2000). Individual crisis workers also need to look at how they operate as members of the group. Group dynamics and cohesiveness impart a powerful influence on each worker, so the group as client may need to be examined. Such dynamics may, in fact, parallel the dynamics of the victim group and are referred to as **parallel processing** (Talbot et al., 1995, p. 291).

On a personal basis, the debriefers need to explore with workers their own personal issues that may intrude into their crisis intervention work. Particularly, parallel processing and countertransference issues need to be examined. As opposed to the CISD approach of Mitchell and Everly (1995b), which does not delve into the personal dynamics of emergency workers, Talbot et al. (1995) believe that psychological understanding and integration are exceedingly important to crisis workers because this is the stuff they are made of and how they operate. The personal history of the individuals in the group and of the group itself may also be of importance. Past baggage of the group, or the individual workers' issues with the group, may carry over into the present, and everyone needs to acknowledge that baggage and be helped to set it down and leave it.

Confidentiality. A continuing issue in debriefings centers on ethical concerns about acts of commission or omission, issues of responsibility or integrity, and even larger questions concerning life-and-death decisions (Walker, 1990). In that regard, all debriefings of emergency workers or mental health workers should be absolutely confidential, and that fact should be stated and enforced from the beginning (Mitchell & Everly, 1995a).

Understanding. One of the main tasks of the debriefer is to make psychological sense of what is going on and

help the crisis workers absorb that knowledge. Thus, debriefers should be well grounded in group dynamics, group functioning, and group counseling skills. They need to be able to compliment workers on their respective strengths—accentuating the positive rather than the multitude of negatives that can easily pervade a crisis (Echterling et al., 2000).

The debriefer needs to summarize, and allow people to verbalize, what they have learned from the crisis and the debriefing to minimize workers' vulnerability to the phenomenon of vicarious traumatization (Saakvitne & Pearlman, 1996). Crisis workers need to have a sense of mastery over what they have done as well as to feel positive about themselves as they take leave of the traumatic event and the debriefing (Echterling et al., 2000; Silove, 1999; Talbot et al., 1995, p. 296).

Qualifications to be an excellent debriefer do not come from one weekend workshop such as one of your authors went through. An excellent debriefer, according to Jordan (2002), will have experience not only in crisis intervention but in trauma counseling as well. Jordan proposes that those who do trauma supervision need to have not only an excellent understanding of what trauma is about but also an understanding of themselves as they operate in a traumatic situation both with people who are suffering from trauma and with those who are intervening with the traumatized. Knowing how secondary traumatization affects first responders and mental health workers is critical. Also, knowing what to do about secondary traumatization and how to convince hardheaded veteran first responders and mental health workers is the zenith of this business, and not many achieve those heights.

In summary, the combined processes that Mitchell and Everly (1995a), Echterling et al. (2000), and Talbot et al. (1995) describe derive their effectiveness from:

1. An early intervention before the trauma is concretized and becomes a disease reservoir
2. An opportunity for catharsis by ventilating emotions in safe surroundings with a structured environment and a knowledgeable and trusted facilitator
3. An opportunity to verbalize the traumatic event and the parts played by reconstructing it, making sense of it, and integrating it into awareness
4. The provision of structure through the debriefing procedure of a definite beginning and a definite end that provides a clear, linear sequence of events

that leads to closure as opposed to the chaos so recently encountered

5. The dispelling of myths that one must be able to "handle" all things and that emotions are liabilities

6. Peer support from others who belong to the same "club"

7. Provision of follow-up if the traumatic stress and the symptoms are not decreased

8. Education about the effects of stress and the concept that it is a naturally occurring process and not a "weakness"

9. Dynamic understanding of both past and present motivators and causative factors that actuate specific responses in each individual

10. Reframing and emphasizing the positive outcomes and strengths demonstrated by the worker

11. The knowledge that such debriefings allow individuals not only to survive job stress but also to do their jobs better.

However, when debriefings don't work and crises move beyond acute stress disorder into PTSD territory, then we revert back to the heavy-duty prolonged exposure and cognitive behaviors therapies you met in Chapter 7, "Posttraumatic Stress Disorder" (Olden et al., 2015).

Final Thoughts

It has now been 35 years since we wrote the first edition of this book. Burl Gilliland, an original coauthor of the book, died in 2003, so these final thoughts will be those of the other original coauthor, Richard "Dick" James. Claire Verduin, our editor at Brooks/Cole at the time of the first edition in 1988, remarked with some humor and some cynicism that it would probably be a nice one-time edition that would wind up gathering dust on library bookshelves, and that would be it. At that time, there were three or four books on crisis and very little research or theory that made it into professional journals. Burl Gilliland started a crisis class at the University of Memphis back in 1975 with little more than pamphlets, mimeographed handouts, and guest speakers from various grassroots organizations that were doing crisis work of different kinds. Crisis intervention was a psychological backwater that had few adherents and even fewer practitioners. Almost none of the material that appears in this closing chapter was in existence at that time. In fact, most of the material in the entire book was not! That should give you an idea of how much this field has grown in that short time.

The past 35 years have seen crisis intervention become a specialty field. No longer is crisis intervention viewed as only talking with individuals considering suicide and talking them out of jumping off the bridge in a manner of speaking. Many books, probably hundreds, are now available. We are still learning, revising, and perfecting techniques. Our training and experiences have informed much of the content of this book. Many of those experiences were learned by being dumped into the deep end of the pool and having to sink or swim. Each time you sit or stand across from someone in crisis, you will learn something. We say this because we are still learning.

Summary

This chapter is predicated on emergent trends that encompass the total ecological and cultural environments in which we live and work. It is a multisystemic approach to crisis intervention. The five-dimensional circle and cylinder of systems that impact crisis workers and the individuals and groups who are their clients include the microsystem, mesosystem, exosystem, macrosystem, and chronosystem. These five systems, based on the Bronfenbrenner model, make up the arena in which crisis workers intervene in situations that may include individuals, families, groups, and organizations in a variety of crises at the local level as well as in widely dispersed geographical areas and cultural settings.

The rise of the FEMA and the various state and local emergency management agencies has given a great deal of impetus to the integration of emergency services and the crisis intervention that goes along with them. The case study of the Benefield family as a model of integrated crisis intervention services is the ideal and demonstrates how these various systems interface and act on individuals in the microsystem. Given Hurricane Katrina's traumatic wake, it appears that the ideal state of service has not yet been reached.

Crisis workers and first responders to disasters and other traumatic events themselves need a format to air their thoughts and feelings, to ventilate and decompress from the intense work they engage in. In response to this need, defusing and debriefing strategies have been developed. Chief among them has been critical incident stress debriefing (CISD). CISD, in particular, has come under sharp criticism as being not helpful and, in some cases, harmful to go through. However, adherents just as vehemently state that it is absolutely necessary to keep them sane. From that standpoint, it appears that some model of debriefing for crisis workers is imperative. However, in the twenty-first century, one thing is abundantly clear: Crisis intervention is a growth industry, and it is here to stay.

References

Aakvaag, H. F., Thoresen, S., Wentzel-Larsen, T., & Dyb, G. (2017). Adult victimization in female survivors of childhood violence and abuse: The contribution of multiple types of violence. *Violence Against Women, 23*(13), 1601–1619. https://doi.org/10.1177/1077801216664427

Abbas, M, & Hoyt, W. T. (2014, August). *Virtual reality exposure treatment to PTSD: A meta-analysis.* Paper presented at the 122nd American Psychological Association. Washington, D.C., the United States

Abd El Moez, K., Elsyed, M., Yousef, I., Waheed Eldeen, A., & Ellithy, W. (2014). Psychosocial characteristic of female victims of domestic violence. *Egyptian Journal of Psychiatry, 35*(2), 105–113. https://doi.org/10.4103/1110-1105.134197

Abei, E., & Kruger, M. L. (2009). The widowhood effect: A comparison of Jews and Catholics. *Omega: Journal of Death and Dying, 59*(4), 325–337.

Abel, N. J., & O'Brien, J. M. (2015). *Treating addictions with EMDR therapy and the stages of change.* Springer Publishing.

Abram, S. V., Batki, S. L., & Pennington, D. L. (2021). Working memory and alcohol demand relationships differ according to PTSD symptom severity among veterans with AUD. *Experimental and Clinical Psychopharmacology, 29*(2), 166–177. https://doi.org/10.1037/pha0000463

Abrams, Z. (2022). Student mental health is in crisis: Campuses are rethinking their approach. *Monitor on Psychology, 53*(7), 60–64.

Abramson, A. (2021). Building mental health into emergency responses. *Monitor on Psychology, 52*(5), 30.

Abramson, L. Y., Alloy, L. B., Hogan, M. E., Whitehouse, W. G., Gibb, B. E., Hankin, B. L., & Cornette, M. M. (2000). The hopelessness theory of suicidality. In T. Joiner & M. D. Rudd (Eds.), *Suicide science: Expanding the boundaries* (pp. 18–32). Kluwer Academic.

Abreu, R., Mceachern, A., Geddes Hall, J., & Kenny, M. (2018, October). Promoting LGBTQ students' well-being in schools. *Counseling Today.* 33–37.

Achenbach, T. M. (1991). *Manual for the Child Behavior Checklist/4-18 and 1991 Profile.* University of Vermont, Department of Psychiatry.

Ackerman, P., Newton, J., McPherson, B., Jones, J., & Dykman, R. (1998). Prevalence of posttraumatic stress disorder and other psychiatric diagnoses in three groups of abused children (sexual, physical, and both). *Child Abuse and Neglect, 22*(8), 759–774.

Adams, C. (2013). Millions went to war in Iraq and Afghanistan. https://www.mcclatchydc.com/news/nation-world/national/article24746680.html

Adams, K. B. (2006). The transition to caregiving: The experience of family members embarking on the dementia caregiving career. *Journal of Gerontological Social Work, 47*(3/4), 3–29.

Addy, C., & James, R. K. (2002, April). *Lieutenants in the crosshairs: Alternative approaches in the treatment of crisis and trauma in field command level staff.* Paper presented at the 25th Annual Convening of Crisis Intervention Personnel, Chicago, IL, the United States.

Addy, C., & James, R. K. (2005, May). *Finding the best CIT practices across the country.* Paper presented at the First Annual National Conference on Crisis Intervention Team Convention, Columbus, OH, the United States.

Adler, A. B., Bliese, P. D., & Castro, C. A. (2011). *Deployment psychology: Evidence-based strategies promote mental health in the military.* American Psychological Association.

Adler, N. L. (1997). *International dimensions of organizational behavior.* South-Western.

Adlington, J. (2009). *Online therapy: Reading between the lines.* MX Publishing.

Adúriz, M., Bluthgen, C., & Knopfler, C. (2011). Helping child flood victims using EMDR intervention in Argentina: Treatment outcome and gender differences. *International Perspective in Psychology, Research, Practice, Consultation, 1*(S), 58–67.

Aguilera, D. C. (1998). *Crisis intervention: Theory and methodology* (8th ed.). Mosby.

Aguilera, D. C., & Messick, J. M. (1982). *Crisis intervention: Theory and methodology* (4th ed.). C. V. Mosby.

Aguirre, R. T. P., McCoy, M. K., & Roan, M. (2013). Development guidelines from a study of suicide prevention mobile applications (Apps). *Journal of Technology in Human Services, 31*(3), 269–293. https://doi.org/10.1080/15228835.2013.814750

Ahmad, A., Aziz, M., Anjum, G., & Mir, F. V. (n.d.). *Intimate partner violence and psychological distress: Mediating role of Stockholm syndrome.*

Ahmadabadi, Z., Najman, J. M., Williams, G. M., & Clavarino, A. M. (2020). Income, gender, and forms of intimate partner violence. *Journal of Interpersonal Violence, 35*(23–24), 5500–5525. https://doi.org/10.1177/0886260517719541

Ahola, K., Toppinen-Tanner, S., & Seppänen, J. (2017). Interventions to alleviate burnout symptoms and to support return to work among employees with burnout: Systematic review and meta-analysis. *Burnout Research, 4,* 1–11. https://doi.org/10.1016/j.burn.2017.02.001

Ai, A., Cascio, T., Santangelo, L. K., & Evans-Campbell, T. (2005). Hope, meaning and growth following the September 11, 2001 terrorist attacks. *Journal of Interpersonal Violence, 20,* 523–548.

Akan, M., Ayaz, N., Taşkapan, M. Ç., Bulut, N., & Erbay, L. G. (2021). The relationship between suicide attempt and gonadotropins, gonadal hormones, and cortisol in females. *Alpha Psychiatry, 22*(5), 230–236. https://doi.org/10.5152/alphapsychiatry.2021.21237

Akl, S., Temares, A. E., Diaz, B. N., & Walker, L. E. (2023). Psychological testing in forensic evaluations of battered women who kill. *Journal of Aggression, Maltreatment & Trauma, 32*(1–2), 148–166. https://doi.org/10.1080/10926771.2022.2068391

Al, C. M. W., Stams, G. J. J. M., van der Laan, P. H., & Asscher, J. J. (2011). The role of crisis in family crisis intervention: Do crisis experience and crisis change matter? *Children and Youth Services Review, 33,* 991–998.

Alatheri, L., Drysdale, D., Driscoll, S., Blair, A., Mauldin, D., Vinyard, N., Foley, C., & Bullwinkel, J. (2019). *Protecting America's schools: A U.S. Secret Service analysis of targeted school violence.* U.S.

Secret Service. https://www.secretservice.gov/sites/default/files/2020-04/Protecting_Americas_Schools.pdf

Allen, M., Burt, K., Rashid, E., Carter, D., Orsi, R., & Durkan, L. (2002). School counselors' preparation for and participation in crisis intervention. *Professional School Counseling, 6*(2), 96–103.

Alavi, S. M., Kia-Keating, M., & Nerenberg, C. (2022). Secondary traumatic stress and burnout in health care providers: A post-disaster study. *Traumatology*. Advance online publication. https://doi.org/10.1037/trm0000418

Albrecht, A. (2010). *Threat assessment teams: Workplace and school violence prevention*. Federal Bureau of Investigation. https://leb.fbi.gov/articles/featured-articles/threat-assessment-teams-workplace-and-school-violence-prevention

Aldrich, R. S., & Cerel, J. (2022). Occupational suicide exposure and impact on mental health: Examining differences across helping professions. *Omega: Journal of Death & Dying, 85*(1), 23–37. https://doi.org/10.1177/0030222820933019

Aldwin, C. M. (2007). *Stress, coping, & development*. Guilford.

Alexander, P. C., Teti, L., & Anderson, C. L. (2000). Childhood sexual abuse history and role reversal in parenting. *Child Abuse & Neglect, 24*(6), 829–838. https://doi.org/10.1016/S0145-2134(00)00142-3

Alexy, E. M., Burgess, A. W., Baker, T., & Smoyak, S. A. (2005). Perceptions of cyberstalking among college students. *Brief Treatment and Crisis Intervention, 5*(3), 279. https://doi.org/10.1093/brief-treatment/mhi020

Alfaro-Velcamp, T. H., McLaughlin, R., & Schumacher, U. (2019). Rape without remedy: Congolese refugees in South Africa. *Cogent Medicine, 6*(1), 1–9. https://doi.org/10.1080/2331205X.2019.1697502

Ali, S., Haykal, H. A., & Youssef, E. Y. M. (2023). Child sexual abuse and the Internet—A systematic review. *Human Arenas, 6*(2), 404–421. https://doi.org/10.1007/s42087-021-00228-9

Alink, L., Eusei, S., Bakermans-Kranenburg, M., & van IJendoorn, M. (2014). A challenging job: Physical and sexual violence towards group workers in youth residential care. *Child & Youth Forum, 43*(2), 243–250.

Aliouche, H. (2022). The role of crisis teams in mental health management. *News-Medical*. https://www.news-medical.net/health/The-Role-of-Crisis-Teams-in-Mental-Health-Management.aspx

Allam, A., Kollareth, D., & Russell, J. A. (2022). On judging the morality of suicide. *Journal of Experimental Social Psychology, 103*. https://doi.org/10.1016/j.jesp.2022.104384

Allan, J., & Berry, P. (1987). Sandplay. *Elementary School Guidance & Counseling, 21*, 300–306.

Allen, B. A. (2020). *An exploratory analysis using the MMPI-2 versus the MMPI-2-RF in assessing personality characteristics of alleged intimate partner violence perpetrators—ProQuest* [Alliant International University]. https://www.proquest.com/openview/d7930f0cafacc35ca4236db07d60cc45/1?pq-origsite=gscholar&cbl=18750&diss=y

Allen, B., Wilson, K. L., & Armstrong, N. E. (2014). Changing clinician' beliefs about treatment for children experiencing trauma: The impact of intensive training in an evidence-based, trauma-focused treatment. *Psychological Trauma: Theory, Research, Practice, and Policy, 6*(4), 384–389.

Allen, J. G. (2001). *Interpersonal trauma and serious mental disorder*. Wiley.

Allen, M., & Sheen, D. (2005). *School-based crisis intervention: Preparing all personnel to assist*. Guilford Press.

Allen, R. S., Haley, E., Roff, L. L., Schmid, B., & Bergman, E. J. (2006). Responding to the needs of caregivers near the end of life: Enhancing benefits and minimizing burdens. In J. L. Werth & D. Blevins (Eds.), *Psychosocial issues near the end of life: A resource for professional care providers* (pp. 183–201). American Psychological Association.

Allen, S. (1996, November). *The rural school counselor*. Paper presented at the Tennessee Counseling Association Convention, Memphis, Tennessee.

Allumbaugh, D. L., & Hoyt, W. T. (1999). Effectiveness of grief therapy: A meta-analysis. *Journal of Counseling Psychology, 46*(3), 370–388.

Almvik, R., Woods, P., & Rasmussen, K. (2007). Assessing risk for imminent violence in the elderly: The Brøset Violence Checklist. *International Journal of Geriatric Psychiatry, 22*(9), 862–867.

Alsaleem, S. A., Alsabaani, A., Alamri, R. S., Hadi, R. A., Alkhayri, M. H., Badawi, K. K., Badawi, A. G., Alshehri, A. A., & Al-Bishi, A. M. (2018). Violence towards healthcare workers: A study conducted in Abha City, Saudi Arabia. *Journal of Family & Community Medicine, 25*(3), 188.

Altmaier, E. M. (2011). Best practices in counseling grief and loss: Finding benefit from trauma. *Journal of Mental Health Counseling, 33*(1), 33–42.

Aluko, O. E., Beck, K. H., & Howard, D. E. (2015). Medical students' beliefs about screening for intimate partner violence: A qualitative study. *Health Promotion Practice, 16*(4), 540–549. https://doi.org/10.1177/1524839915571183

Alvarez, T. (1999). APA and MTV launch youth anti-violence initiative. *Practitioner Focus. May–June 1999*. American Psychological Association, Public Relations and Communications Practice Directorate.

Amado, B. G., Arce, R., & Herraiz, A. (2015). Psychological injury in victims of child sexual abuse: A meta-analytic review. *Psychosocial Intervention, 24*(1), 49–62. https://doi.org/10.1016/j.psi.2015.03.002

Amankwaa, B. (2017). Informal caregiver stress. *ABNF journal, 28*(4), 92–95.

Amano, T., & Toichi, M. (2014). Effectiveness of on-the-spot EMDR method for the treatment of behavioral symptoms in patients with severe dementia. *Journal of EMDR Practice and Research, 8*(2), 50–65.

Amegbor, P. M., & Pascoe, L. (2021). Variations in emotional, sexual, and physical intimate partner violence among women in Uganda: A multilevel analysis. *Journal of Interpersonal Violence, 36*(15–16), NP7868–NP7898. https://doi.org/10.1177/0886260519839429

American Association of Suicidology. (1991). *Postvention guidelines for the schools*.

American Counseling Association. (1995). *Code of ethics and standards of practice*.

American Counseling Association. (2014). *ACA code of ethics*. https://www.counseling.org/knowledge-center/ethic#2014code?

American Foundation for Suicide Prevention. (n.d.). *Project 2025 | American Foundation for Suicide Prevention*. https://project2025.afsp.org/

American Psychiatric Association. (n.d.). *Stigma, prejudice and discrimination against people with mental illness*. https://www.psychiatry.org/patients-families/stigma-and-discrimination

American Psychiatric Association. (1974). *Clinical aspects of the violent individual*. American Psychiatric Association Press.

American Psychiatric Association. (1980). *Diagnostic and statistical manual of mental disorders* (3rd ed.). American Psychiatric Publishing.

American Psychiatric Association. (2000). *Diagnostic and statistical manual of mental disorders* (4th ed., rev.). American Psychiatric Publishing.

American Psychiatric Association. (2013). *Diagnostic and statistical manual of mental disorders* (5th ed.). American Psychiatric Publishing.

American Psychiatric Association. (2020). *Practice guidelines for the treatment of patients with acute stress disorder and posttraumatic stress disorder.* http://www.psychiatryonline.org/pb/assets/raw/sitewide/practice_guidelines/guidelines/acutestressdisorderptsd.pdf. American Psychiatric Publishing.

American Psychiatric Association. (2022). *Diagnostic and statistical manual of mental disorders: DSM-5-TR* (5th ed., text rev.). American Psychiatric Association.

American Psychological Association. (2002). Ethical principles of psychologists and code of conduct. *American Psychologist, 57,* 1060–1073.

American Psychological Association. (2010). *Strategies for reducing the risk of patient violence toward clinicians.* www.apa.org/divisions/div12/sections/div12/sections/section7/tfreport.html

American Psychological Association. (2014). Incarceration nation. *Monitor on Psychology, 45*(9), 56.

American Psychological Association. (2015). *Review confirms link between playing violent video games and aggression.* https://www.apa.org/news/press/releases/2015/08/violent-video-games

American Psychological Association. (2017). *Clinical practice guideline for the treatment of posttraumatic stress disorder (PTSD) in adults.* https://www.apa.org/ptsd-guideline

American Psychological Association. (2020a). *Warning signs of youth violence.* https://www.apa.org/topics/physical-abuse-violence/youth-warning-signs

American Psychological Association. (2020b). *APA reaffirms position on video games and violent behavior.* https://www.apa.org/news/press/releases/2020/03/violent-video-games-behavior

American Psychological Association (2020c). *APA resolution on violent video games: February 2020 revision to the 2015 resolution.* https://www.apa.org/about/policy/resolution-violent-video-games.pdf

American Psychological Association. (2023). *Burnout.* PsychInfo search. https://psycnet.apa.org/search/results?type=direct&db=pi,pb,pa,pe,pt,pbc&fields=AnyField&term=burnout

American Psychological Association Zero Tolerance Task Force. (2008). *Are zero tolerance policies effective in schools? American Psychologist, 63*(9), 852–862.

American School Counselor Association. (1998). *Ethical standards for school counselors.*

American School Counselor Association. (2022). The school counselor and trauma-informed practice. https://www.schoolcounselor.org/Standards-Positions/Position-Statements/ASCA-Position-Statements/The-School-Counselor-and-Trauma-Informed-Practice

American School Counselor Association. (2023) Disasters. https://www.schoolcounselor.org/search?query=disaster#?wst=a42c66d97e1d628d3967c283a48d695b

Americans with Disabilities Act. (1990). PL 110-325.

Amiri, S. (2022). Unemployment and suicide mortality, suicide attempts, and suicide ideation: A meta-analysis. *International Journal of Mental Health, 51*(4), 294–318. https://doi.org/10.1080/00207411.2020.1859347

An, Y., Zhao, J., & Hou, W. K. (2022). Network analysis of posttraumatic stress disorder symptoms among adolescent survivors of a major disaster in China. *Psychological Trauma: Theory, Research, Practice, and Policy, 14*(1), 132–140. http://doi.org/10.1037/tra0001053

Anderson, A., & West, S. G. (2011). Violence against mental health professionals: When the treater becomes the victim. *Innovations in Clinical Neuroscience 8*(3), 34–39.

Anderson, C. A. (2001). Heat and violence. *Current Directions in Psychological Science, 10*(1), 33–38.

Anderson, C. A., Shibuya, A., Ihori, N., Swing, E., Bushman, B., Sakamoto, A., Rothstein, H. R., & Saleem, M. (2010). Violent video game effects on aggression, empathy, and prosocial behavior in Eastern and Western countries: A meta-analytic review. *Psychological Bulletin, 136*(2), 151–173.

Anderson, E. J., Krause, K. C., Meyer Krause, C., Welter, A., McClelland, D. J., Garcia, D. O., Ernst, K., Lopez, E. C., & Koss, M. P. (2021). Web-based and mHealth interventions for intimate partner violence victimization prevention: A systematic review. *Trauma, Violence, & Abuse, 22*(4), 870–884. https://doi.org/10.1177/1524838019888889

Anderson, K., Danis, F., & Havig, K. (2011). Adult daughters of battered women: Recovery and posttraumatic growth following childhood adversity. *Families in Society, 92*(2), 154–160.

Anderson, L. J., Flynn, A., & Pilgrim, J. L. (2017). A global epidemiological perspective on the toxicology of drug-facilitated sexual assault: A systematic review. *Journal of Forensic and Legal Medicine, 47,* 46–54. https://doi.org/10.1016/j.jflm.2017.02.005

Anderson, M. A., Kaufman, J., & Simon, T. R. (2001). School-associated violent deaths in the United States, 1994–1999. *Journal of the American Medical Association, 286,* 2695–2702.

Ando, M. (2005). A case study of usefulness of cognitive therapy based on reminiscence method for cancer patients. *Japanese Journal of Health Psychology, 18*(2), 53–64.

Andriessen, K., Krysinska, K., Dransart, D. A. C., Dargis, L., & Mishara, B. L. (2020). Grief after euthanasia and physician-assisted suicide. *Crisis, 41*(4), 255–272. https://doi.org/10.1027/0227-5910/a000630

Angelini, G. (2023). Big five model personality traits and job burnout: A systematic literature review. *BMC Psychology, 11*(1), 49. https://doi.org/10.1186/s40359-023-01056-y

Annis, L. V., McClaren, H. A., & Baker, C. A. (1984). Who kills us? In J. T. Turner (Ed.), *Violence in the medical care setting: A survival guide* (pp. 19–31). Aspen Systems.

Ansbacher, H. L., & Ansbacher, R. R. (1956). *The individual psychology of Alfred Adler.* Greenberg.

Anthony, K., & Nagel, D. M. (2010). *Therapy online: A practical guide.* SAGE.

Antonovsky, A. (1980). *Health, stress, and coping.* Jossey-Bass.

Antonovsky, A. (1991). The structural sources of salutogenic strengths. In C. Cooper & R. Payne (Eds.), *Personality and stress: Individual differences in the stress process* (pp. 67–104). Wiley.

APA Task Force. (2015). *Technical report on the review of violent game literature.* American Psychological Association. https://www.apa.org/pi/families/review-video-games.pdf

Archibald, H. C., Long, D. M., Miller, C., & Tuddenham, R. D. (1962). Gross stress reaction in combat—A 15-year follow-up. *American Journal of Psychiatry, 119,* 317–322.

Arditte Hall, K. A., & Mitchell, K. S. (2022). The Affective Control Scale: Factor structure and associations with posttraumatic stress symptoms in trauma-exposed male veterans.

Psychological Trauma: Theory, Research, Practice, and Policy, 14(5), 812–820. https://doi.org/10.1037/tra0000575

Arditti, J. A. (2016). A family stress-proximal process model for understanding the effects of parental incarceration on children and their families. *Couple and Family Psychology: Research and Practice, 5*(2), 65–88. http://dx.doi.org/10.1037/cfp0000058

Arkin, M., Lowe, S. R., Poon, C. Y., & Rhodes, J. E. (2022). Association between religious coping and long term mental health in survivors of Hurricane Katrina. *Psychology of Religion and Spirituality.* https://doi.org/10.1037/rel0000483

Armenti, N. A., & Babcock, J. C. (2016). Conjoint treatment for intimate partner violence: A systematic review and implications. *Couple and Family Psychology: Research and Practice, 5*(2), 109–123. https://doi.org/10.1037/cfp0000060

Armistead-Jehle, P., Johnston, S. L., Wade, N. G., & Ecklund, C. J. (2011). Posttraumatic stress in U.S. Marines: The role of unit cohesion and combat exposure. *Journal of Counseling & Development, 89*(1), 81–88.

Armitage, D., Rice, D., James, R., & Groenendyk, P. (2007, July). *Triage for psychological disorders.* [Paper presentation]. Association of College and University Housing Officers Convention, Seattle, WA, the United States.

Armour, C., Fried, E. I., Deserno, M. K., Tsai, J., & Pietrzak, R. H. (2017). A network analysis of DSM-5 posttraumatic stress disorder symptoms and correlates in U.S. military veterans. *Journal of Anxiety Disorders, 45,* 49–59. https://doi.org/10.1016/j.janxdis.2016.11.008

Armstrong, D., & Shakespeare-Finch, J. (2011). Relationship to the bereaved and perceptions of severity of trauma differentiate elements of posttraumatic growth. *Omega: Journal of Death and Dying, 63*(2), 125–140.

Armstrong, K., O'Callahan, W., & Marmar, C. (1991). Debriefing Red Cross disaster personnel: The multiple stressor debriefing model. *Journal of Traumatic Stress, 4,* 581–593.

Armsworth, M. W., & Holaday, M. (1993). The effects of psychological trauma on children and adolescents. *Journal of Counseling and Development, 72*(1), 49–56.

Arnold, D., Calhoun, L. G., Tedeschi, R., & Cann, A. (2005). Vicarious posttraumatic growth in psychotherapy. *Journal of Humanistic Psychology, 45*(2), 239–263.

Aron, L., Honberg, R., Duckworth, K., Kimball, A., Edgar, E., Carolla, B., Meltzer, K., Usher, L., Gay, K., Giliberti, M., Carrasco, M. J., Pandya, A., & Fitzpatrick, M. (2009). *Grading the states: A report on America's health care system for adults with serious mental illness.* National Alliance for Mental Illness.

Aronin, L., & Ransdell, J. (1994). *A handbook for crisis intervention.* Los Angeles Unified School District.

Arroyo, K., Lundahl, B., Butters, R., Vanderloo, M., & Wood, D. S. (2017). Short-term interventions for survivors of intimate partner violence: A systematic review and meta-analysis. *Trauma, Violence, & Abuse, 18*(2), 155–171. https://doi.org/10.1177/1524838015602736

Arvay, M. J., & Uhlemann, M. R. (1996). Counselor stress in the field of trauma: A preliminary study. *Canadian Journal of Counselling, 30*(3), 193–210.

Arvidsson, M., & Caman, S. (2022). Treatment experiences among intimate partner violence perpetrators: A qualitative analysis. *International Journal of Offender Therapy and Comparative Criminology,.* https://doi.org/10.1177/0306624X221102846

Ashley, C. S., & Wicks, S. J. (2022). The feasibility and utility of the Terrorist Radicalization Assessment Protocol (TRAP-18): A review and recommendations. *Journal of Threat Assessment and Management, 9*(4), 218–159. https://doi.org/10.1037/tam0000179

Association of Threat Assessment Professionals. (2006). *Risk assessment guideline elements for violence (RAGE-V): Considerations for assessing the risk of future violent behavior.*

Association of Threat Assessment Professionals. (2023). *Become a certified threat manager.* https://www.atapworldwide.org/

Astor, R. (1999). Unknown places and times. *American Educational Research Journal, 36*(1), 3–42.

Astroem, S., Bucht, G., Eisemann, M., Norberg, A., & Saveman, B. (2002). Incidence of violence towards staff caring for the elderly. *Scandinavian Journal of Caring Services, 16*(1), 66–72.

Astur, R. S., Germain, S., Tolin, D., Ford, J., Russell, D., & Stevens, S. (2006). Hippocampus function predicts severity of posttraumatic stress disorder. *Cyber Psychology & Behavior, 9*(2), 234–240.

Aten, J. D., Leavell, K., Gonzalez, R., Luke, T., Defee, J., & Harrison, K. (2011). Everyday technologies for extraordinary circumstances: Possibilities for enhancing disaster communication. *Psychological Trauma, Theory, Research, and Practice, 3*(1), 16–20.

Aten, J. D., O'Grady, K., Milsten, G., Boan, D., Smigelsky, M., Schruba, A., & Weaver, I. (2015). Providing spiritual and emotional care in response to a disaster. In D. F. Walker, C. A. Courtois, & J. D. Aten (Eds.), *Spiritually oriented psychotherapy for trauma.* (pp. 189–210). American Psychological Association.

Aten, J. D., Smith, W. R., Davis, E. B., Van Tongeren, D. R., Hook, J. N., Davis, D. E., Shannonhouse, L., DeBlaere, C., Ranter, J., O'Grady, K., & Hill, P. C. (2019). The psychological study of religion and spirituality in a disaster context: A systematic review. *Psychological Trauma: Theory, Research, Practice, and Policy, 11*(6), 597–613. https://doi.org/10.1037/tra0000431

Atkinson, D., Bui, U., & Mori, S. (2001). Multiculturally sensitive empirically supported treatments: An oxymoron? In J. G. Ponterotto, J. M. Casas, L. A. Suzuki, & C. M. Alexander (Eds.), *Handbook of multicultural counseling* (2nd ed., pp. 542–574). SAGE

Atkinson, D., Morten, G., & Sue, D. W. (1998). *Counseling American minorities.* McGraw Hill.

Atkinson, R. M., Sparr, L. F., & Sheff, A. G. (1984). Diagnosis of posttraumatic stress disorder in Vietnam veterans: Preliminary findings. *American Journal of Psychiatry, 141,* 694–696.

Atteraya, M. S., Gnawali, S., & Song, I. H. (2015). Factors associated with intimate partner violence against married women in Nepal. *Journal of Interpersonal Violence, 30*(7), 1226–1246. https://doi.org/10.1177/0886260514539845

Attig, T. (2000). *The heart of grief: Death and the search for lasting love.* Oxford University Press.

Audate, T. S. (2021). The pandemic within the pandemic of 2020. In T. Sonone (Ed.), *Shared trauma, shared resilience during a pandemic: Social work in the time of COVID-19.* (pp. 271–278). Springer. http://doi.org/10.1007/978-3-030-61442-3

Augsburger, D. W. (1992). *Conflict mediation across cultures.* Westminster/John Knox Press.

Austin, S. (2003). Multiple lessons from multiple suicides. *ASCA School Counselor, 41*(2), 22–27.

Australian Center for Posttraumatic Mental Health. (2007). *Australian guidelines for the treatment of adults with acute stress disorder and posttraumatic stress disorder.*

AuthoraCare (2019). *How play therapy helps grieving children.* Authrora Care Collective. https://authoracare.org

Avanzi, L., Fraccaroli, F., Castelli, L., Marcionetti, J., Crescentini, A., Balducci, C., & van Dick, R. (2018). How to mobilize social support against workload and burnout: The role of organizational identification. *Teaching and Teacher Education, 69,* 154–167. https://doi.org/10.1016/j.tate.2017.10.001

Avery, A., & Orner, R. (1998a, Summer). First report of psychological debriefing abandoned—The end of an era? *Traumatic Stress Points, 12*(3), 1112.

Avery, A., & Orner, R. (1998b, July). More on debriefing: Report of psychological debriefing abandoned—The end of an era? *Australian Traumatic Stress Points,* 4–6.

Ayadi, N., Dargahi, S., Ghamari Givi, H., & Abbasi, M. (2016). The impact of job stress on subjective well-being, marital stress and empathy of nurses. *Iranian Journal of Medical Ethics and History of Medicine, 9*(2), 67–79.

Ayalon, O. (1983). Coping with terrorism. In D. Meichenbaum & M. Jaremko (Eds.), *Stress reduction and prevention.* Plenum Press.

Aymer, S. R. (2008). Beyond power and control: Clinical interventions with men engaged in partner abuse. *Clinical Social Work Journal, 36*(4), 323–332.

Azar, B. (2010). Virtual violence. *Monitor on Psychology. 41*(11), 36–39.

Babcock, J., Armenti, N., Cannon, C., Lauve-Moon, K., Buttell, F., Ferreira, R., Cantos, A., Hamel, J., Kelly, D., Jordan, C., Lehmann, P., Leisring, P. A., Murphy, C., O'Leary, K. D., Bannon, S., Salis, K. L., & Solano, I. (2016). Domestic violence perpetrator programs: A proposal for evidence-based standards in the United States. *Partner Abuse, 7*(4), 355–460. https://doi.org/10.1891/1946-6560.7.4.355

Bach y Rita, G., Lion, J. R., & Climent, C. E. (1971). Episodic dyscontrol: A study of 630 violent patients. *American Journal of Psychiatry, 128,* 1473–1478.

Bagge, C., Nickell, A., Stepp, S., Durrett, C., Jackson, K., & Trull, T. J. (2004). Borderline personality disorder features predict negative outcomes 2 years later. *Journal of Abnormal Psychology, 113*(2), 279–288.

Bahora, M., Hanafi, S., Chien, V. H., & Compton, M. T. (2008). Preliminary evidence of effects of crisis intervention team training on self-efficacy and social distance. *Administration and Policy in Mental Health and Mental Health Services Research, 35*(3), 159–167.

Bailey, K. A. (2001). Legal implications of profiling students for violence. *Psychology in the Schools, 38,* 141–155.

Bailey, K. A., West, R., & Anderson, C. A. (2011). The association between chronic exposure to video game violence and affective picture processing: An ERP study. *Cognitive, Affective, & Behavioral Neuroscience, 11*(2), 259–276.

Bailey, R., Dugard, J., Smith, S. F., & Porges, S. W. (2023). Appeasement: Replacing Stockholm syndrome as a definition of a survival strategy. *European Journal of Psychotraumatology, 14*(1), 2161038. https://doi.org/10.1080/20008066.2022.2161038

Bain, S. F. (2011). Itinerant counseling services for rural communities: A win/win opportunity. *Journal of Rural Community Psychology 13*(1). http://www.aabri.com/OC2010Manuscripts/OC10046.pdf

Baird, B. N., Bossett, S. B., & Smith, B. J. (1994). A new technique for handling sexually abusive calls to telephone crisis lines. *Community Mental Health Journal, 30,* 55–60.

Baird, S. L., Tarshis, S., Messenger, C., & Falla, M. (2022). Virtual support and intimate partner violence services: A scoping review. *Research on Social Work Practice, 32*(8), 878–897. https://doi.org/10.1177/10497315221087232

Baird, S., & Jenkins, S. R. (2003). Vicarious traumatization, secondary traumatic stress, and burnout in sexual assault and domestic violence agency staff. *Violence and Victims, 18*(1), 71–86.

Baker, D. G., Risbrough, V. B., & Schork, N. J. (2008). Posttraumatic stress disorder: Genetic and environmental risk factors. In B. J. Lukey & V. Tepe (Eds.), *Biobehavioral resilience to stress* (pp. 177–218). CRC Press, Taylor & Francis Group.

Baker, L. R., & Cormier, L. A. (2015). *Disaster and vulnerable populations: Evidence-based practice for the helping professions.* Springer.

Baker, N. J. (1985). Reminiscing in group therapy for self-worth. *Journal of Gerontological Nursing, 11,* 21–24.

Bakker, A. B., Demerouti, E., & Schaufeli, W. B. (2002). Validation of the Maslach Burnout Inventory—General survey: An Internet study. *Anxiety, Stress, and Coping: An International Journal, 15*(3), 245–260.

Bakker, A. B., Demerouti, E., & Schaufeli, W. B. (2005). The crossover of burnout and work engagement among working couples. *Human Relations, 58*(5), 661–689.

Balasubramaniam, M. (2018). Rational suicide in elderly adults: A clinician's perspective. *Journal of the American Geriatrics Society, 66*(5), 998–1001. https://doi.org/10.1111/jgs.15263

Balk, D. E. (1990, August). *The many faces of bereavement on the college campus.* Paper presented at the annual meeting of the American Psychological Association, Boston, MA, the United States.

Balk, D. E. (2009). Adolescent development: The back story to adolescent encounters with death and bereavement. In D. E. Balk & C. A. Corr (Eds.), *Adolescent encounters with death, bereavement, and coping* (pp. 3–20). Springer.

Balk, D. E., & Corr, C. A. (2001). Bereavement during adolescence: A review of research. In M. S. Stroebe, R. O. Hansson, H. Schut, & W. Stroebe (Eds.), *Handbook of bereavement research: Consequences, coping and care* (pp. 199–218). American Psychological Association.

Balk, D. E., Zaengle, D., & Corr, C. A. (2011). Strengthening grief support for adolescents coping with a peer's death. *School Psychology International, 32*(2), 144–162.

Ball, J. S., & Links, P. S. (2009). Borderline personality disorder and childhood trauma: Evidence for a causal relationship. *Current Psychiatry Reports, 11*(1), 63–68. https://doi.org/10.1007/s11920-009-0010-4

Ballan, M. S., Freyer, M. B., Marti, C. N., Perkel, J., Webb, K. A., & Romanelli, M. (2014). Looking beyond prevalence: A demographic profile of survivors of intimate partner violence with disabilities. *Journal of Interpersonal Violence, 29*(17), 3167–3179. https://doi.org/10.1177/0886260514534776

Balson, P., & Dempster, C. (1980). Treatment of war neurosis from Vietnam. *Comprehensive Psychiatry, 21,* 167–176.

Bandura, A. (1999). Moral disengagement in the perpetration of inhumanities. *Personality and Social Psychology Review, 3*(3), 193–209. http://doi.org/10.1207/s15327957pspr0303_3

Baradell, J. G. (1985, February). Humanistic care of the patient in seclusion. *Journal of Psychosocial Nursing and Mental Health Services, 23,* 9–14.

Barak, Y., Fortune, S., Hobbs, L., Cheung, G., Johari, N., & Zalsman, G. (2022). Strategies to prevent elderly suicide: A Delphi consensus study. *Australasian Psychiatry, 30*(3), 298–302. https://doi.org/10.1177/10398562211064256

Baranowsky, A. B. (2002). The silencing response in clinical practice: On the road to dialogue. In C. R. Figley (Ed.), *Treating compassion fatigue* (pp. 155–170). Brunner/Routledge.

Bard, M., & Sangrey, D. (1986). *The crime victim's book* (2nd ed.). Brunner/Mazel.

Bardhoshi, G., Erford, B. T., & Jang, H. (2019). Psychometric synthesis of the Counselor Burnout Inventory. *Journal of Counseling & Development, 97*(2), 195–208. https://doi.org/10.1002/jcad.12250

Barnes, V. A., Davis, H. M., & Treiber, F. A. (2007). Perceived stress, heart rate, and blood pressure among adolescents with family members deployed in Operation Iraqi Freedom. *Military Medicine, 172*, 40–43.

Barnett, E. R., Pittman, C. R., Ragan, C., & Salus, M. K. (1980). *Family violence: Intervention strategies* (DHHS Publication No. OHD 580-30258). U.S. Government Printing Office.

Baron, A., Jr., & Cohen, R. B. (1982). Helping telephone counselors cope with burnout: A consciousness-raising workshop. *Personnel and Guidance Journal, 60*, 508–510.

Barr, N., Keeling, M., & Castro, C. (2019). Associations between mindfulness, PTSD, and depression in combat deployed post-9/11 military veterans. *Mindfulness, 10*, 1–12. https://doi.org/10.1007/s12671-019-01212-9

Barret, K. E., Riggar, T. F., & Flowers, C. R. (1997). Violence in the workplace. Preparing for the age of rage. *Journal of Rehabilitation Administration, 21*(3), 171–188.

Barrick, A. L., Rader, J., Hoeffer, B., Sloane, P. D., & Biddle, S. (2008). General guidelines for bathing persons with dementia. In A. L. Barrick, J. Rader, J. B. Hoeffer, P. D. Sloane, & S. Biddle (Eds.), *Bathing without a battle: Person-directed care of individuals with dementia* (2nd ed., pp. 17–21). Springer.

Bartik, W., Maple, M., & McKay, K. (2020) Youth suicide bereavement and the continuum of risk. *Crisis: The Journal of Crisis Intervention and Suicide Prevention, 41*(6), 483–489. https://doi.org/10.1027/0227-5910/a000653

Barton, A. M. (1969). *Communities in disaster.* Doubleday.

Basile, K. C., Smith, S. G., Kresnow, M. J., Khatiwada, S., & Leemis, R. W. (2022). *The National Intimate Partner and Sexual Violence Survey: 2016/2017 report on sexual violence.* National Center for Injury Prevention and Control, Centers for Disease Control and Prevention. https://www.cdc.gov/violenceprevention/pdf/nisvs/nisvsReportonSexualViolence.pdf?ACSTrackingID=DM83944&ACSTrackingLabel=CDC%20Releases%20NISVS%202016%2F2017%20Report%20on%20Sexual%20Violence&deliveryName=DM83944

Basile, K. C., Swahn, M. H., Chen, J., & Saltzman, L. E. (2006). Stalking in the United States: Recent national prevalence estimates. *American Journal of Preventive Medicine, 31*(2), 172–175. https://doi.org/10.1016/j.amepre.2006.03.028

Basocak, R., Nargundkar, A., & Warren, L. J. (2021). The duality of risk from threats: Are homicidal threats a novel determinant for suicide risk? *Behavioral Sciences & the Law, 39*(3), 358–368. https://doi.org/10.1002/bsl.2526

Bass, D. D., & Yep, R. (2002). *Terrorism, trauma, and tragedies: A counselor's guide to preparing and responding.* American Counseling Association.

Bateman, A., & Fonagy, P. (2006). *Mentalization-based treatment for borderline personality disorder.* Oxford University Press.

Bathje, G., & Pryor, J. (2011). The relationships of public and self-stigma to seeking mental health services. *Journal of Mental Health Counseling, 33*(2), 161–176. https://doi.org/10.17744/mehc.33.2.g6320392741604l1

Battaglia, T., Finley, E., & Liebschutz, J. (2003). Survivors of intimate partner violence speak out: Trust in the patient-provider relationship. *Journal of General Internal Medicine, 18*, 617–623.

Battle, C. L., Shea, M., Johnson, D. M., Yen, S., Zlotnik, C., Zanarini, M. C., Sanislow, C. A., Skodol, A. E., Gunderson, J. G., Grilo, C. M., McGlashan, T. H., & Morey, L. C. (2004). Childhood maltreatment associated with adult personality disorders: Findings from the collaborative longitudinal personality disorders study. *Journal of Personality Disorders, 18*, 193–211.

Bauer, C. C. C., Caballero, C., Scherer, E., West, M. R., Mrazek, M. D., Phillips, D. T., Whitfield-Gabrieli, S., & Gabrieli, J. D. E. (2019). Mindfulness training reduces stress and amygdala reactivity to fearful faces in middle-school children. *Behavioral Neuroscience, 133*(6), 569–585. https://doi.org/10.1037/bne0000337

Baum, N., Rahav, G., & Sharon, M. (2014). Heightened susceptibility to secondary traumatization: A meta-analysis of gender differences. *American Journal of Orthopsychiatry, 84*(2), 111–122.

Bauman, S. (2011). *Cyberbullying: What counselors need to know.* American Counseling Association.

Bayramzadeh, S. (2016). An assessment of levels of safety in psychiatric units. *HERD: Health Environments Research & Design Journal, 10*(2), 66–80. https://doi.org/10.1177/1937586716656002

Beamish, P. M. (2005). Introduction to the special section—Severe and persistent mental illness on college campuses: Consideration for service provision. *Journal of College Counseling, 8*(2), 138–139.

Beane, A. L. (1999). *Bully-free classroom.* Free Spirit Press.

Beauchamp, T. L., & Childress, J. F. (2019). *Principles of biomedical ethics* (8th ed.). Oxford University Press.

Beck, A. T. (1976). *Cognitive therapy and the emotional disorders.* International Universities Press.

Beck, A. T. (1979). *Cognitive Therapy of Depression.* Guilford Press.

Beck, A. T. (1993). *Beck Hopelessness Scale.* Pearson Assessments. https://www.pearsonassessments.com/store/usassessments/en/Store/Professional-Assessments/Personality-%26-Biopsychosocial/Beck-Hopelessness-Scale/p/100000105.html

Beck, A. T., Steer, R. A., & Brown, G. (1996). *Beck Depression Inventory 2.* https://www.pearsonassessments.com/store/usassessments/en/Store/Professional-Assessments/Personality-%26-Biopsychosocial/Beck-Depression-Inventory/p/100000159.html

Beck, A., & Freeman, A. (1990). *Cognitive therapy of personality disorders.* Guilford Press.

Beck, J. C. (1988). The therapist's legal duty when the patient may be violent. *Psychiatric Clinics of North America, 11*, 665–679.

Becker, W. C. (1971). *Parents are teachers.* Research Press.

Beckwith, M. (2023). Brazilian President blasts video games as "violent" and teaching kids to kill. https://metro.co.uk/2023/04/19/brazilian-president-blasts-video-games-for-teaching-kids-to-kill-18640716/

Becvar, D. S. (2001). *In the presence of grief.* Guilford Press.

Bedikian, S. (2008). The death of mourning: From Victorian crepe to the little black dress. *Omega: Journal of Death and Dying, 57*(1), 35–52.

Beebe, L., Smith, K., & Phillips, C. (2014). A comparison of telephone and texting interventions for persons with schizophrenia spectrum disorders. *Issues in Mental Health Nursing, 35*(5), 323–329.

Belak, A. G., & Busse, D. (1993). Legal issues. In P. E. Blumenreich & S. Lewis (Eds.), *Managing the violent patient: A clinician's guide* (pp. 137–149). Brunner-Mazel.

Belkin, G. S. (1984). *Introduction to counseling* (2nd ed.). William C. Brown.

Bell, S. C. (2016). *The relationship between the effects of rape, Posttraumatic Stress Disorder, complex trauma, and post-attack victim-perpetrator interaction in female college students* (2016-16234-010; Issues 10-B(E)). ProQuest Information & Learning.

Bellet, B. W. (2022). The Social Meaning in Life Events Scale (SMILES) In B. Neimeyer (Ed.). *New techniques of grief therapy* (pp.80–85) https://doi.org/10.4324/9781351069120-10

Bellet, B. W., Holland, J. M., & Neimeyer, R. A. (2018). The Social Meaning in Life Events Scale (SMILES): A preliminary psychometric evaluation in a bereaved sample. *Death Studies, 43*(2), 103–112 https://doi.org/10.1080/07481187.2018.1456008

Bellet, B. W., LeBlanc, N. J., Nizzi, M.-C., Carter, M. L., van der Does, F. H. S., Peters, J., Robinaugh, D. J., & McNally, R. J. (2020). Identity confusion in complicated grief: A closer look. *Journal of Abnormal Psychology, 129*(4), 397–407. https://doi.org/10.1037/abn0000520

Belling, S., Bozzatello, P., De Grandi, E., & Bogetto, F. (2014). Interpersonal psychotherapy: A model of intervention for borderline personality disorder. *Rivista di Psichiatria, 49*(4), 158–163.

Bemak, F., & Keys, S. (2000). *Violent and aggressive youth: Intervention and prevention strategies for changing times.* SAGE.

Bender, M. G. (1986). Young adult chronic patients: Visibility and style of interaction in treatment. *Hospital and Community Psychiatry, 37,* 265–268.

Bengelsdorf, H., Church, J. O., & Kaye, R. A. (1993). The cost effectiveness of crisis intervention: Admission diversion savings can offset the high cost of service. *Journal of Nervous Mental Disorders, 181,* 757–762.

Benjamin, L., & Walz, G. R. (1983). *Violence in the family: Child and spouse abuse* (Report No. EDN00001). National Institute of Education (ERIC Document Reproduction Service No. ED 226-309).

Bennett, L. W., & Vincent, N. V. (2001). Standards for batterer programs: A formative evaluation of the Illinois protocol. *Journal of Aggression, Maltreatment, & Trauma, 5,* 181–197.

Ben-Porath, Y. S. & Tellegen, A. (2008). *Minnesota Multiphasic Personality Inventory-2–Restructured Form.* https://www.pearsonassessments.com/store/usassessments/en/Store/Professional-Assessments/Personality-%26-Biopsychosocial/Minnesota-Multiphasic-Personality-Inventory-2-Restructured-Form/p/100000631.html

Benson, H. U. (2012). *Neurobiological foundations for EMDR practice.* Springer.

Bent-Goodley, T. B., Rice, J., Williams, O., & Pope, M. (2011). Treatment for perpetrators of domestic violence. In M. P. Koss, J. White, & A. Kazdin (Eds.), *Violence against women and children: Vol. 2. Navigating solutions* (pp. 199–213). American Psychological Association.

Bentley, K. H., Franklin, J. C., Ribeiro, J. D., Kleiman, E. M., Fox, K. R., & Nock, M. K. (2016). Anxiety and its disorders as risk factors for suicidal thoughts and behaviors: A meta-analytic review. *Clinical Psychology Review, 43,* 30–46. https://doi.org/10.1016/j.cpr.2015.11.008

Benton, S. A., Robertson, J. M., Tseng, W., Newton, F., & Benton, S. L. (2003). Changes in counseling center client problems across 13 years. *Professional Psychology: Research and Practice, 34*(1), 66–72.

Bercier, M., & Maynard, B. (2015). Interventions for secondary traumatic stress with mental health workers: A systematic review. *Research on Social Work Practice, 25*(1), 81–89.

Bergmans, Y., Gordon, E., & Eynan, R. (2017). Surviving moment to moment: The experience of living in a state of ambivalence for those with recurrent suicide attempts. *Psychology and Psychotherapy, 90*(4), 633–648. https://doi.org/10.1111/papt.12130

Berman, A. L., & Canning, R. D. (2022). Proximal risk for suicide in correctional settings: A call for priority research. *Psychological Services, 19*(3), 407–412. https://doi.org/10.1037/ser0000516

Berman, A. L., & Jobes, D. A. (1991). *Adolescent suicide: Assessment and intervention.* American Psychological Association.

Berman, A. L., & Jobes, D. A. (1994). Treatment of the suicidal adolescent [Special Issue: Suicide assessment and intervention]. *Death Studies, 18,* 375–389.

Berman, A. L., & Silverman, M. M. (2022). Hospital-based suicides: Challenging existing myths. *Psychiatric Quarterly, 93*(1), 1–13. https://doi.org/10.1007/s11126-020-09856-w

Berman, A. L., Jobes, D. A., & Silverman, M. M. (Eds.). (2006). *Adolescent suicide: Assessment and intervention* (2nd ed.). American Psychological Association.

Bernal, G., & Domenech Rodriguez, M. M. (Eds.). (2012). *Cultural adaptations: Tools for evidence-based practice with diverse populations.* American Psychological Association.

Bernardy, N. C., & Friedman, M. J. (2015). Antidepressant strategies for managing PTSD. In N. C. Bernardy and M. J. Friedman (Eds.), *A practical guide to treatment: Pharmacological and psychotherapeutic approaches* (pp. 55–70). American Psychological Association.

Bernardy, N. C., Souter, T., & Friedman, M. J. (2015). The use of anxiolytics in the management of PTSD. In N. C. Bernardy and M. J. Friedman (Eds.), *A practical guide to treatment: Pharmacological and psychotherapeutic approaches* (pp. 71–88). American Psychological Association.

Bernstein, A. (1986). The treatment of noncompliance in patients with posttraumatic stress disorder. *Psychosomatic Medicine, 27,* 37–40.

Bernstein, J. R. (1997). *When the bough breaks: Forever after the death of a son or daughter.* Andrews & McKeel.

Berrouiguet, S., Gravey, M., Le Galudec, M., Alavi, Z., & Walter, M. (2014). Post-acute crisis text messaging outreach for suicide prevention: A pilot study. *Psychiatry Research, 217*(3), 154–157. https://doi.org/10.1016/j.psychres.2014.02.034

Best, P., Foye, U., Taylor, B., Hazlett, D., & Manktelow, R. (2013). Online interactive suicide support services: Quality and accessibility. *Mental Health Review Journal, 18*(4), 226–239. https://doi.org/10.1108/MHRJ-03-2013-0009

Bethel, B. I., & Oates, J. (2007, March). *The untold story of the Beverly Hillbillies.* Thirty-first Annual Convening of Crisis Intervention Personnel and the CONTACT USA Conference. Chicago, the United States.

Betz, G., & Thorngren, J. M. (2006). Ambiguous loss and the family grieving process. *Family Journal, 14*(4), 359–365.

Beyer, K., Wallis, A. B., & Hamberger, L. K. (2015). Neighborhood environment and intimate partner violence: A systematic review. *Trauma, Violence, & Abuse, 16*(1), 16–47. https://doi.org/10.1177/1524838013515758

Bhuptani, P. H., & Messman-Moore, T. L. (2019). Blame and shame in sexual assault. In W. T. O'Donohue & P. A. Schewe (Eds.), *Handbook of sexual assault and sexual assault prevention.* (2019-79354-019; pp. 309–322). Springer Nature Switzerland AG. https://doi.org/10.1007/978-3-030-23645-8_18

Bianchi, R., & Laurent, E. (2015). Emotional information processing in depression and burnout: An eye tracking study. *European Archives of Psychiatry and Clinical Neuroscience, 265*(1), 27–34.

Bianchi, R., Schoenfield, I., & Laurent, E. (2015). Burnout-depression overlap. *Clinical Psychology Review, 36,* 28–41.

Bianchi, R., Truchot, D., Laurent, E., Brisson, R., & Schonfeld, S. (2014). Is burnout solely job related: A critical comment. *Scandinavian Journal of Psychology, 55*(4), 357–361.

Bierens de Haan, B. (1998). Le débriefing émotionnel collectif des intervenants humanitaires: L'expérience du CICR. *Schweizer Archiv für Neurologie und Psychiatrie, 149*(5), 218–228.

Biernesser, C., Ohmer, M., Nelson, L., Mann, E., Frzan, R., Schwanke, B., & Radovic, A. (2023). Middle school students' experiences with cyberbullying and perspectives toward prevention and bystander intervention in schools. *Journal of School Violence.* Advance online publication. https://doi.org/10.1080/15388220.2023.2186417

Bigot, T., & Ferrand, I. (1998). Individualologie de la prise d'oage: Etude auprès de 29 individuelles. *Annales Médico Psychologiques, 156*(1), 22–27.

Bilchik, S. (1998, May). Serious and violent juvenile offenders. *Office of Justice Bulletin.* Office of Juvenile Justice and Delinquency Prevention.

Billig, M., & Tajfel, H. (1973). Social categorization and similarity in intergroup behaviour. *European Journal of Social Psychology, 3*(1), 27–52. https://doi.org/10.1002/ejsp.2420030103

Bingham, R. (2010). My life is a balance between . . . In J. G. Ponterotto, J. M. Casas, L. A. Suzuki, & C. M. Alexander (Eds.), *Handbook of multicultural counseling* (3rd ed., pp. 19–25). SAGE.

Birrell, P. J., & Bruns, C. M. (2016). Ethics and relationship: From risk management to relational engagement. *Journal of Counseling & Development, 94*(4), 391–397. https://doi.org/10.1002/jcad.12097

Birrell, P. J., & Freyd, J. J. (2006). Betrayal trauma: Relational models of harm and healing. *Journal of Trauma Practice, 5,* 49–63.

Bishop, J. B. (2006). College and university counseling centers: Questions in search of answers. *Journal of College Counseling, 9*(1), 6–19.

Biskin, R., & Paris, J. (2012). Diagnosing borderline personality disorder. *Canadian Medical Journal, 184*(16), 1789–1794. http://doi.org/10.1503/cmag.090618

Bisson, J. I., & Deahl, M. P. (1994). Psychological debriefing and prevention of post-traumatic stress—More research is needed. *British Journal of Psychiatry, 165,* 717–720.

Bisson, J. I., Jenkins, J. A., & Bannister, C. (1997). Randomized controlled trial of psychological debriefing for victims of acute burn trauma. *British Journal of Psychiatry, 171,* 78–81.

Bjelopera, J. P., Bagalman, E., Caldwell, S. W., Finklea, K. M., & McCallion, G. (2013). *Public mass shootings in the United States: Selected implications for federal public health and safety policy.* Congressional Research Service.

Björklund, K., Häkkänen-Nyholm, H., Sheridan, L., & Roberts, K. (2010). The prevalence of stalking among Finnish university students. *Journal of Interpersonal Violence, 25*(4), 684–698. https://doi.org/10.1177/0886260509334405

Black, M. C. (2011). Intimate partner violence and adverse health consequences: Implications for clinicians. *American Journal of Lifestyle Medicine, 5*(5), 428–439. https://doi.org/10.1177/1559827611410265

Blair, D. T. (1991). Assaultive behavior: Does provocation begin in the front office? *Journal of Psychosocial Nursing and Mental Health Services, 29,* 21–24.

Blair, D. T., & New, S. A. (1991). Assaultive behavior: Know the risks. *Journal of Psychosocial Nursing and Mental Health Services, 29,* 25–29.

Blake, D. D., Weathers, F., Nagy, L. M., Kaloupek, D. G., Klauminzer, G., & Charney, D. S. (1990). A clinician rating scale for assessing current and lifetime PTSD: The CAPS-1. *Behavior Therapist, 13,* 187–188.

Blancett, J. (2008). *A reliability and validity study of the Triage Assessment System for Students in Learning Environments.* Unpublished doctoral dissertation. University of Memphis, Memphis, TN.

Blanchard, E. A., & Jones, M. (1997). Care of clinicians doing trauma work. In M. Harris & C. L. Landis (Eds.), *Sexual abuse in the lives of women diagnosed with serious mental illness: New direction in therapeutic interventions* (Vol. 2, pp. 303–319). Harwood Academic.

Blauvelt, P. D. (1998). *Blauvelt . . . on making our schools safe* (2nd rev. ed.). National Alliance for Safe Schools.

Bloch, D. A., Silber, E., & Perry, S. E. (1956). Some factors in the emotional reaction of children to disaster. *American Journal of Psychiatry, 113,* 416–422.

Blocher, D. H. (2000). *Counseling: A developmental approach* (4th ed.). John Wiley & Sons.

Bloom, B. L. (1984). *Community mental health: A general introduction* (2nd ed.). Brooks/Cole.

Blore, D. (2014). EMDR for mining and related trauma. In M. Luber (Ed.), *Implementing EMDR early mental health interventions for man-made and natural disasters: Models, scripted protocols, and summary sheet.* (pp. 451–466). Springer.

Blumenreich, P. E. (1993a). Assessment. In P. E. Blumenreich & S. Lewis (Eds.), *Managing the violent patient: A clinician's guide* (pp. 35–40). Brunner/Mazel.

Blumenreich, P. E. (1993b). Etiology. In P. E. Blumenreich & S. Lewis (Eds.), *Managing the violent patient: A clinician's guide* (pp. 21–33). Brunner/Mazel.

Boehm-Tabib, E., & Gelkopf, M. (2023, March 13). *The role of the timing of previous traumatic events in moderating the relationship between acute stress disorder and posttraumatic stress. Traumatology.* Advance online publication. https://dx.doi.org/10.1037/trm0000436

Boelen, P. A., & Prigerson, H. G. (2007). The influence of symptoms of prolonged grief disorder, depression, and anxiety on quality of life among bereaved adults: A prospective study. *European Archives of Psychiatry and Clinical Neuroscience, 257*(8), 442–452.

Boelen, P. A., de Keijser, J., & Smid, G. (2015). Cognitive-behavioral variables mediate the impact of violent loss on post-loss psychopathology. *Psychological Trauma, Theory, Research, Practice and Policy, 7*(4), 382–390.

Boelen, P. A., van de Schoot, R., van den Hout, M. A., de Keijser, J., & van den Bout, J. (2010). Prolonged grief disorder, depression, and posttraumatic stress disorder are distinguishable syndromes. *Journal of Affective Disorders, 125*(1-3), 374–378.

Bograd, M. (2005). Strengthening domestic violence theories: Intersections of race, class, sexual orientation, and gender. In N. Sololoff & C. Pratt (Eds.), *Domestic violence at the margins: Reading on race, class, gender, and culture* (pp. 25–38). Rutgers University Press.

Boin, A., McConnell, A., & Hart, P. (2021). Governing the pandemic: The politics of navigating a mega-crisis. Palgrave MacMillan. https://doi.org/10.1007/978-3-030-72680-5

Bolton, J., Palmer, L., & Cawdron, R. (2016). Survey of psychiatric assessment rooms in UK emergency departments. *British Journal of Psychiatry Bulletin, 40*(2), 64–67. https://doi.org/10.1192/pb.bp.114.049742

Bonanno, G. A., Papa, A., Lalande, K., Zhang, N., & Noll, J. G. (2005). Grief processing and deliberate grief avoidance: A prospective comparison of bereaved spouses and parents in the United States and the People's Republic of China. *Journal of Consulting and Clinical Psychology, 73*(1), 86–98.

Bonanno, G. A., Westphal, M., & Mancini, A. D. (2011). Resilience to loss and potential trauma. *Annual Review of Clinical Psychology, 7*, 511–535.

Bondu, R., & Scheithauer, H. (2015). Leaking and death threats by students: A study in German schools. *School Psychology International, 35*(6), 592–608.

Bonfine, N., Ritter, C., & Munetz, M. R. (2014). Police officer perceptions of the impact of crisis intervention team (CIT) programs. *International Journal of Law and Psychiatry, 37*(4), 341–350.

Bongar, B., & Sullivan, G. R. (2013). *The suicidal patient: Clinical and legal standards of care* (3rd ed.). American Psychological Association.

Bonnefil, M., & Jacobson, G. F. (1979). Family crisis intervention. *Clinical Social Work Journal, 7*, 200–213.

Bonomi, A. E., Anderson, M. L., Nemeth, J., Bartle-Haring, S., Buettner, C., & Schipper, D. (2012). Dating violence victimization across the teen years: Abuse frequency, number of abusive partners, and age at first occurrence. *BMC Public Health, 12*(1), 637. https://doi.org/10.1186/1471-2458-12-637

Bonynge, E. R., & Thurber, S. (2008). Development of clinical ratings for crisis assessment in community mental health. *Brief Treatment and Crisis Intervention, 8*, 304–312. https://doi.org/10.1093/brief-treatment/mhn017

Bordow, S., & Porritt, D. (1979). An experimental evaluation of crisis intervention. *Social Science & Medicine. Part A: Medical Psychology & Medical Sociology, 13*, 251–256. https://doi.org/10.1016/0271-7123(79)90042-7

Borritz, M., Bültmann, U., Rugulies, R., Christensen, K., Viladsen, E., & Kristensen, T. S. (2005). Psychosocial work characteristics as predictors for burnout: Findings from 3-year follow up of the PUMA study. *Journal of Occupational and Environmental Medicine, 47*(10), 1015–1025.

Borschmann, R., & Moran, P. (2011). Crisis management in borderline personality disorder. *International Journal of Social Psychiatry, 57*(1), 18–20.

Borschmann, R., Barret, B., Hellier, J., Byford, S., Henderson, C., Rose, D., Slade, M., Sutherby, K., Szmukler, G., Thornicroft, G., Hogg, J., & Moran, P. (2013). Joint crisis plans for people with borderline personality disorder: Feasibility and outcomes in a randomized controlled trial. *The British Journal of Psychiatry, 202*(5), 357–364.

Borum, R. (2000). Improving high risk encounters between people with mental illness and the police. *Journal of the American Academy of Law and Psychiatry, 28*, 332–337.

Borum, R., Lodewijks, H., Bartel, P., & Forth, A. (2010). Structured Assessment of Violence Risk in Youth (SAVRY). In R. Oyyo & K. Douglas (Eds.), *Handbook of violence risk assessment* (pp. 63–80). Routledge.

Borumandnia, N., Khadembashi, N., Tabatabaei, M., & Alavi Majd, H. (2020). The prevalence rate of sexual violence worldwide: A trend analysis. *BMC Public Health, 20*(1), 1835. https://doi.org/10.1186/s12889-020-09926-5

Boschen, M. J. (2009). Mobile telephones and psychotherapy: Capability and applicability. *Behavior Therapist, 32*(8), 168–175.

Bosquet, M. (2004). How research informs clinical work with traumatized young children. In J. D. Osofsky (Ed.), *Young children and trauma: Intervention and treatment* (pp. 301–325). Guilford Press.

Boss, P. (2002). *Family stress management: A contextual approach* (2nd ed.). SAGE.

Boss, P. (2006). *Loss, trauma, and resilience: Therapeutic work with ambiguous loss.* W. W. Norton & Company.

Bostwick, J. M., Pabbati, C., Geske, J. R., & McKean, A. J. (2016). Suicide attempt as a risk factor for completed suicide: Even more lethal than we knew. *American Journal of Psychiatry, 173*(11), 1094–1100. https://doi.org/10.1176/appi.ajp.2016.15070854

Bosworth, K., Espelage, D., Dubay, T., Dahlberg, L., & Daytner, G. (1996). Using multi-media to teach conflict-resolution skills to young adolescents. *American Journal of Preventive Medicine, 12*(suppl), 65–74.

Bott, S., Guedes, A., Ruiz-Celis, A. P., & Mendoza, J. A. (2019). Intimate partner violence in the Americas: A systematic review and reanalysis of national prevalence estimates. *Revista Panamericana de Salud Pública, 43*, e26. https://doi.org/10.26633/RPSP.2019.26

Bottini, S., Wiseman, K., & Gillis, J. (2020). Burnout in providers serving individuals with ASD: The impact of the workplace. *Research in Developmental Disabilities, 100*, 103616. https://doi.org/10.1016/j.ridd.2020.103616

Bottomley, J. S. & Neimeyer, R. A. (2022). Quality of Relationships Inventory-Bereavement Version (QRI-B). In R. A. Neimeyer (Ed.). *New Techniques of Grief Therapy* (pp. 87–93). http://doi.org/10.4324/9781351069120-11

Bottomley, J. S., Smigelsky, M. A., Floyd, R. G., & Neimeywer, R. A. (2017). Closeness and conflict with the deceased: Exploring the factor structure of the quality of relationships inventory in a bereaved student sample. *OMEGA-Journal of Death and Dying, 79*(4), 25–37. https://doi.org/10.1177/0030222817718959

Bourbonais, A., Goulet, M., Landreville, P., Elefsen, E., Larue, C., Lalonde, M., & Gendreau, P. (2019). Physically aggressive behaviors in older people living with cognitive disorders: A national collaboration center of mental health, systematic scoping review protocol. *Systematic Reviews, 8*, article 164. https://doi.org/10.1186/s13643-019-1091-8

Bower, G. H. (1981). Mood and memory. *American Psychologist, 36*, 129–148.

Bowlby, J. (1969). *Attachment and loss: Vol. 1. Attachment.* Basic Books.

Bowlby, J. (1973). *Attachment and loss: Vol. 2. Separation, anxiety, and anger.* Basic Books.

Bowlby, J. (1980). *Attachment and loss: Vol. 3. Loss, sadness, and depression.* Basic Books.

Bowlby, J. (1982). *Attachment and loss: Vol. 1. Attachment* (2nd ed.). Basic Books.

Bowlby, J. (1988). *A secure base: Parent-child attachment and healthy human development.* Basic Books.

Bowman, R. P. (1987). Approaches for counseling children through music. *Elementary School Guidance & Counseling, 21*, 284–291.

Boyd, B., Quevillon, R. P., & Engdahl, R. M. (2010). Working with rural and diverse communities after disasters. In P. Dass-Braillsford (Ed.), *Crisis and disaster counseling: Lessons learned from Hurricane Katrina and other disasters* (pp. 149–163). SAGE.

Boyd, J. E., O'Connor, C., Protopopescu, A., Jetly, R., Lanius, R. A., & McKinnon, M. C. (2020). The contributions of emotion regulation difficulties and dissociative symptoms to functional impairment among civilian inpatients with posttraumatic stress symptoms. *Psychological Trauma: Theory, Research, Practice, and Policy, 12*(7), 739–749. https://doi.org/10.1037/tra0000576

Boyd-Franklin, N. (2010). Families affected by Hurricane Katrina and other disasters: Learning from the experiences of African-American survivors. In P. Dass-Braillsford (Ed.), *Crisis and disaster counseling: Lessons learned from Hurricane Katrina and other disasters* (pp. 67–82). SAGE.

Bozgeyikli, H. (2012). Self efficacy as a predictor of compassion satisfaction, burnout, compassion fatigue: A study on psychological counselors. *African Journal Of Business Management, 6*(2). https://doi.org/10.5897/AJBM11.2167

Bradley v. *State of Mississippi*, 1 Miss. 156 (1824).

Bradley, R. G., Green, J., Russ, E., Dutra, L., & Westen, D. (2005). A multidimensional analysis of psychotherapy for PTSD. *American Journal of Psychiatry, 162*, 214–227.

Brainerd, A. M. (2002). Tragic events and the effects on all of us. In D. D. Bass & R. Yep (Eds.), *Terrorism, trauma, and tragedies: A counselor's guide to preparing and responding* (pp. 111–112). American Counseling Association.

Brammer, L. M. (1985). *The helping relationship: Process and skills* (3rd ed.). Prentice Hall.

Brammer, L. M., Abrego, P., & Shostrom, E. (1993). *Therapeutic counseling and psychotherapy* (6th ed.). Prentice Hall.

Brand, A. G. (1987). Writing as counseling. *Elementary School Guidance & Counseling, 21*, 266–275.

Brandt, M. R. (2014). War, trauma and technologies of the self: The making of virtual reality exposure therapy. *Dissertation Abstracts International Section A: Humanities and Social Sciences, 74*(10-A(E)), 1231.

Braun, M. J., & Berg, D. H. (1994). Meaning reconstruction in the experience of parental bereavement. *Death Studies, 18*, 105–129.

Braverman, M. (1999). *Preventing workplace violence: A guide to employers and practitioners.* SAGE.

Bray, B. (2018, March 28). The battle against burnout. *Counseling Today.* https://ct.counseling.org/2018/03/the-battle-against-burnout/

Bray, B. (2019, September). Making it safe to talk about suicidal ideation. *Counseling Today.* 20–26.

Bray, B. (2019, November 21). Multicultural encounters. *Counseling Today.* https://ct.counseling.org/2019/11/multicultural-encounters/

Bray, B. (2021). Crisis counseling: A blend of safety and compassion. *Counseling Today, 64*(2), 22–27.

Bray, B. (2021, March 25). Finding balance in counseling private practice. *Counseling Today.* https://ct.counseling.org/2021/03/finding-balance-in-counseling-private-practice/

Breet, E., Seedat, S., & Kagee, A. (2019). Posttraumatic stress disorder and depression in men and women who perpetrate intimate partner violence. *Journal of Interpersonal Violence, 34*(10), 2181–2198. https://doi.org/10.1177/0886260516660297

Breiding, M. J. (2014). Prevalence and characteristics of sexual violence, stalking, and intimate partner violence victimization—National intimate partner and sexual violence survey, the United States, 2011. *Morbidity and Mortality Weekly Report. Surveillance Summaries, 63*(8), 1–18. https://www.ncbi.nlm.nih.gov/pmc/articles/PMC4692457/

Breiding, M. J. (2015). Prevalence and characteristics of sexual violence, stalking, and intimate partner violence. National Intimate Partner and Sexual Violence Survey, the United States, 2011. *American Journal of Public Health, 105*(4), e11–e12.

Bremner, J. D., Randall, P. K., Vermetten, E., Staib, L., Mazure, C., Capelli, S., McCarthy, G., Innis, R. B., & Charney, D. S. (1997). Magnetic resonance imaging based measurement of hippocampal volume in posttraumatic stress disorder related to childhood physical and sexual abuse: A preliminary report. *Biological Psychiatry, 41*(1), 23–32.

Brende, J. O., & Parson, E. R. (1985). *Vietnam veterans: The road to recovery.* Plenum Press.

Brenner, L. A., Vanderploeg, R. D., & Terro, H. (2009). Assessment and diagnosis of mild traumatic brain injury, posttraumatic stress disorder, and other polytrauma conditions: Burden of adversity hypothesis. *Rehabilitation Psychology, 54*, 239–246.

Brent, D., & Brown, C. (2015). Effectiveness of school-based suicide prevention programmes. *The Lancet, 385*(9977), 1489–1491.

Brent, D., McMakin, F., Kennard, B., Goldstein, T., Mayes, T., & Douaihy, A. (2013). Protecting adolescents from self-harm: A critical review of intervention studies. *Journal of the American Academy of Child & Adolescent Psychiatry, 52*(12), 1260–1271.

Brethren Disaster Ministries (2023). Disaster Recovery. https://www.brethren.org/bdm/rebuild/#:~:text=Brethren%20Disaster%20Ministries%E2%80%99%20Rebuilding%20Program%20engages%20volunteers%20to,restore%20damaged%20homes%2C%20volunteers%20also%20restore%20broken%20lives

Breuer, J., & Freud, S. (1955). Studies on hysteria. In J. Strachey (Ed. & Trans.), *The standard edition of the complete psychological works of Sigmund Freud* (Vol. 2, pp. 1–10). Hogarth Press. (Original work published 1895)

Brewi, B. (Speaker). (1986). *Crisis intervention with the Vietnam veteran* (Cassette recording No. 9). Department of Counseling and Personnel Services, Memphis State University, the United States.

Brewin, C. (2005). Risk factor effect sizes in PTSD: What this means for intervention. *Journal of Trauma & Dissociation, 6*(2), 123–130.

Brewington, J. O., Nassar-McMillan, S., Flowers, C. P., & Furr, S. R. (2004). A preliminary investigation of factors associated with job loss grief. *Career Development Quarterly, 53*(1), 78–83.

Brewster, M. P. (2002). Domestic violence theories, research, and practice implications. In A. R. Roberts (Ed.), *Handbook of domestic violence: Intervention strategies* (pp. 23–48). Oxford University Press.

Bridges by Epoch. (2023). *The benefits of reminiscence therapy.* https://www.bridgesbyepoch.com/2020/10/28/benefits-reminiscence-therapy-dementia-1603905506/

Briere, J. (1995). *Trauma Symptom Inventory.* Psychological Assessment Resources.

Briere, J. (1996). *Trauma Checklist for Children.* Psychological Assessment Resources.

Briere, J. (2005). *Trauma Checklist for Young Children.* Psychological Assessment Resources.

Briere, J., & Scott, C. (2006). *Principles of trauma therapy: A guide to symptoms, evaluation, and treatment.* SAGE.

Brock, S. E., Nickerson, A. B., Reeves, M. A., Jimerson, S. R., Lieberman, R. A., & Feinberg, T. A. (2009). *School crisis prevention and intervention: The PREPaRE model.* National Association of School Psychologists.

Brock, S. E., Sandoval, J., & Lewis, S. (2001). *Preparing for crisis in the schools* (2nd ed.). Clinical Psychology.

Brock, S., Nickerson, M., Lovar Reeves, L., Conolly, S., Jimerson, R., Pesce, R., & Lazzaro, B. (2016). *School crisis prevention + intervention: The PREPaRE Model* 2nd ed. National Association of School Psychologists.

Brock, S., Sandoval, J., & Hart, S. (2006). Suicidal ideation and behaviors. In G. Bear & K. Minke (Eds.), *Children's needs III: Development, prevention and intervention* (pp. 225–238). National Association of School Psychologists.

Brockian, N. R. (2002). *New hope for people with borderline personality disorder: Your friendly, authoritative guide to the latest in traditional and complementary solutions.* Prima Publishing.

Brockopp, G. W. (1973a). The covert cry for help. In D. Lester & G. W. Brockopp (Eds.), *Crisis intervention and counseling by telephone* (pp. 193–198). Charles C. Thomas.

Brockopp, G. W. (1973b). The nuisance caller. In D. Lester & G. W. Brockopp (Eds.), *Crisis intervention and counseling by telephone* (pp. 206–210). Charles C. Thomas.

Brockopp, G. W. (2002a). The therapeutic management of the chronic caller. In D. Lester & G. W. Brockopp (Eds.), *Crisis intervention and counseling by telephone* (2nd ed., pp. 159–164). Charles C. Thomas.

Brockopp, G. W. (2002b). Working with the silent caller. In D. Lester & G. W. Brockopp (Eds.), *Crisis intervention and counseling by telephone* (2nd ed., pp. 182–186). Charles C. Thomas.

Brockopp, G. W., & Lester, D. (2002). The chronic caller. In D. Lester & G. W. Brockopp (Eds.), *Crisis intervention and counseling by telephone* (2nd ed., pp. 154–167). Charles C. Thomas.

Brom, D., & Kleber, R. J. (1989). Prevention of posttraumatic stress disorders. *Journal of Traumatic Stress, 2,* 335–351.

Brom, D., Kleber, R. J., & Defares, P. B. (1989). Brief psychotherapy for posttraumatic stress disorders. *Journal of Consulting and Clinical Psychology, 57,* 607–612.

Bromet, E. J. (1995). Methodological issues in designing research on community-wide disasters with special reference to Chernobyl. In S. E. Hobfoll & M. W. de Vries (Eds.), *Extreme stress and communities: Impact and intervention* (pp. 307–324). Kluwer.

Bronfenbrenner, U. (1981). *The ecology of human development: Experiments by nature and design.* Harvard University Press.

Bronfenbrenner, U. (1986). Ecology of the family as a context for human development: Research perspectives. *Developmental Psychology, 22,* 723–742.

Bronfenbrenner, U. (1995). Developmental ecology through space and time: A future perspective. In P. Moen, G. H. Elder, Jr., & K. Luscher (Eds.), *Examining lives in context: Perspectives on the ecology of human development* (pp. 619–647). American Psychological Association.

Bronfenbrenner, U., & Morris, P. A. (1998). The ecology of developmental processes. In W. Damon & R. M. Lerner (Eds.), *Handbook of child psychology* (5th ed., Vol. 1, pp. 993–1028). Wiley.

Bronson J., & Berzofsky, M. (2017, June). *Indicators of mental health problems reported by prisoners and jail inmates, 2011-12.* U.S. Department of Justice.

Brooker, D., & Duce, L. (2000). Well-being and activity in dementia: A comparison of group reminiscence therapy, structured goal-directed group activity and unstructured time. *Aging & Mental Health, 4*(4), 354–358.

Brooks, J. D., & Martinez, C. (1999). Animals as neglected members of the family in studies of death and dying. In B. De Vries (Ed.), *End of life issues: Interdisciplinary and multidimensional perspectives* (pp. 167–179). Springer.

Brown v. Entertainment Merchants Association. (2011). 564 U.S. 768 (2011), 131 S. Ct 2729, 180 L.Ed. 2d 708.

Brown, D. (2009). Assessment of attachment and abuse history, and adult attachment style. In C. A. Courtois & J. D. Ford (Eds.), *Treating complex traumatic stress disorders* (pp. 124–144). Guilford Press.

Brown, E. B. (1988). *Sunrise tomorrow: Coping with a child's death.* Baker Bookhouse.

Brown, E. B. (1999). *Loss, change and grief: An educational perspective.* David Fulton.

Brown, E. J., & Bobrow, A. L. (2004). School entry after a community-wide trauma: Challenges and lessons learned from September 11, 2001. *Clinical Child and Family Psychology Review, 7*(4), 211–221.

Brown, G. K., Have, T. T., Henriques, G. R., Xie, S. X., Hollander, J. E., & Beck, A. T. (2005). Cognitive therapy for the prevention of suicide attempts: A randomized controlled trial. *JAMA: Journal of the American Medical Association, 294*(5), 563–570. https://doi.org/10.1001/jama.294.5.563

Brown, J., James, K., & Taylor, A. (2010). Caught in the rejection abuse cycle: Are we really treating perpetrators of domestic abuse effectively? *Journal of Family Therapy, 32*(3), 280–307.

Brown, L. (2008). *Cultural competence in trauma therapy: Beyond the flashback.* American Psychological Association.

Brown, L. (2009). Cultural competence. In C. A. Courtois & J. Ford (Eds.), *Treating complex traumatic stress disorders: An evidence-base guide* (pp. 166–182). Guilford Press.

Brown, R. (2012, October 10). New Orleans limits hurricane themed excursions. New York Times. https://www.nytimes.com/2012/10/12/us/new-orleans-limits-hurricane-themed-tours.html?searchResultPosition=1

Brown, R. (2016) What are Tier 1, Tier 2, and Tier 3 interventions in education. *Renaissance.* https://www.renaissance.com/2016/11/03/blog-what-are-tier-1-tier-2-and-tier-3-interventions-in-education

Brown, S. (2023). *The real campus mental-health crisis and new models for well-being: Manage demand for counseling and stem students' rising rates of distress by focusing on prevention.* Chronicle of Higher Education

Brown, S., & Manning, W. (2009). Family boundary ambiguity and the measurement of family structure. *Demography, 46,* 85–102.

Browne, A. (1997). Violence in marriage: Until death do us part? In A. P. Cardarelli (Ed.), *Violence between intimate partners: Patterns, causes, and effects* (pp. 48–69). Allyn & Bacon.

Bruce, E. J., & Schultz, C. L. (2001). *Nonfinite loss and grief: A psychoeducational approach.* Paul H. Brookes Publishing.

Bruce, M. L., & Kim, K. M. (1992). Differences in the effects of divorce on major depression in men and women. *American Journal of Psychiatry, 149,* 914–917.

Brucia, E. F., Cordova, M., & Ruzek, J. (2020). Application and integration of psychological first aid in first responder organizations. IGI Global. https://doi.org/10.4018/978-1-5225-9803-9.ch008

Brummert-Lennings, H., & Warburton, W. A. (2011). The effect of auditory versus visual violent media exposure on aggressive behavior. *Journal of Experimental Social Psychology, 47*(4), 794–799.

Bryan, C. J. (2019). Cognitive behavioral therapy for suicide prevention (CBT-SP): Implications for meeting standard of care expectations with suicidal patients. *Behavioral Sciences & the Law, 37*(3), 247–258.

Bryan, C. J., & Rudd, M. D. (2006). Advances in the assessment of suicide risk. *Journal of Clinical Psychology, 62*(2), 185–200. https://doi.org/10.1002/jclp.20222

Bryant, R. A., & Harvey, A. G. (2000). Telephone crisis intervention skills: A simulated caller paradigm. *Crisis, 21*(2), 90–94.

Bryant, R., & Harvery, A. (2000). *Acute stress disorder: A handbook of theory, assessment and treatment*. American Psychological Association.

Bryant, R., Moulds, M., Guthrie, R., Dang, S., & Nixon, R. (2003). Imaginal exposure alone and imaginal exposure with cognitive restructuring in treatment of posttraumatic stress disorder. *Journal of Consulting & Clinical Psychology 71*(4), 706–712.

Brymer, M. J., Steinberg, A. M., Vernberg, E. M., Laynes, C. M., Watson, P. J., Jacobs, S. A., Ruzek, J. I, & Pynoos, R. S. (2009). Acute interventions for children and adolescents. In E. Foa, T. Keane, M. Friedman, & J. Cohen (Eds.), *Effective treatments for PTSD* (2nd ed., pp. 106–116). Oxford University Press.

Buchanan, D., Moorhouse, A., Cabaico, L., Krock, M., Campbell, H., & Spevakow, D. (2002). A critical review and synthesis of literature on reminiscing with older adults. *Canadian Journal of Nursing Research/Revue, 34*(3), 123–139.

Buchbinder, E., & Eisikovits, Z. (2003). Battered women's entrapment in shame: A phenomenological study. *American Journal of Orthopsychiatry, 73*(4), 355–366.

Bucich, M., Steel, Z., & Berle, D. (2022). Posttraumatic stress disorder (PTSD) symptom profiles among people who have experienced abuse: Findings from the NESARC-III study. *Psychological Trauma: Theory, Research, Practice, and Policy*. Advance online publication. https://doi.org/10.1037/tra0001193

Buckley, T., McKinley, S., Tofler, G., & Bartrop, R. (2010). Cardiovascular risk in early bereavement: A literature review and proposed mechanisms. *International Journal of Nursing Studies, 47*(2), 229–238.

Bucolo, D. (2011). Violent video game exposure and physical aggression in adolescence: Test of the general aggression model. *Dissertation Abstracts International: Section B The Sciences and Engineering*, 5180.

Buhr, G. T., Kuchibhatla, M., & Clipp, E. C. (2006). Caregivers' reasons for nursing home placement: Clues for improving discussions with families prior to the transition. *The Gerontologist, 46*, 52–61.

Burelomova, A. S., Gulina, M. A., & Tikhomandritskaya, O. A. (2018). Intimate partner violence: An overview of the existing theories, conceptual frameworks, and definitions. *Psychology in Russia, 11*(3), 128–144. https://doi.org/10.11621/pir.2018.0309

Burgess-Watson, I. P., Hoffman, L., & Wilson, G. V. (1988). The neuropsychiatry of post-traumatic stress disorder. *British Journal of Psychiatry, 152*, 164–173.

Burke, A. K., Galfalvy, H., Everett, B., Currier, D., Zelazny, J., Oquendo, M. A., Melhem, N. M., Kolko, D., Harkavy-Friedman, J. M., Birmaher, B., Stanley, B., Mann, J. J., & Brent, D. A. (2010). Effect of exposure to suicidal behavior on suicide attempt in a high-risk sample of offspring of depressed parents. *Journal of the American Academy of Child & Adolescent Psychiatry, 49*(2), 114–121. https://doi.org/10.1016/j.jaac.2009.10.008

Burnham, B. (2011). School wide bully prevention. *ASCA School Counselor, 48*(6), 13–17.

Burns, M., Griese, B., King, S., & Talmi, A. (2020). Childhood bereavement: Understanding prevalence and related adversity in the United States. *American Journal of Orthopsychiatry, 90*(4), 391–405. http://dx.doi.org/10.1037/ort0000442

Burrow-Sanchez, J. J., Call, M. E., Zheng, R., & Drew, C. (2011). How school counselors can prevent online victimization. *Journal of Counseling & Development, 89*(1), 3–10.

Burry, C. L. (2002). Working with potentially violent clients in their homes: What child welfare professionals need to know. *Clinical Supervisor, 21*(1), 145–153.

Busch, I., Scott, S., Connors, C., Story, A., Acharya, B., & Wu, A. (2021). The role of institution-based peer support for health care workers emotionally affected by workplace violence. *The Joint Commission on Quality and Patient Safety, March, (47)*3, 146–156. http://doi.org/10.1016/j.jcjq.2020.11.005

Busch, K. G., Zagar, R., Hughes, J. R., Arbit, J., & Bussell, R. E. (1990). Adolescents who kill. *Journal of Clinical Psychology, 46*(4), 472–485.

Bushman, B., Newman, K., Calver, S., Downey, G., Dredze, M., Gottfredson, M., Jablonski, N., Masten, A., Morrill, C., Neill, D., Romer, D., & Webster, D. (2016). Youth violence: What we know and need to know. *American Psychologist, 71*(1), 17–39. https://doi.org/10.1037/a0039687

Butcher, J. N., Hass, G. A., Greene, R. L., & Nelson, L. D. (2015). The MMPI-2 in cases of intimate partner violence. In *Using the MMPI-2 in forensic assessment.* (pp. 191–204). American Psychological Association. https://doi.org/10.1037/14571-011

Butler, C. S., & Lagoni, L. S. (1996). Children and pet loss. In C. A. Corr & D. M. Corr (Eds.), *Handbook of childhood death and bereavement* (pp. 179–200). Springer.

Butler, R. (1963). The life review: An interpretation of reminiscence in the aged. *Psychiatry, 26*, 65–76.

Butters, R. P., Droubay, B. A., Seawright, J. L., Tollefson, D. R., Lundahl, B., & Whitaker, L. (2021). Intimate partner violence perpetrator treatment: Tailoring interventions to individual needs. *Clinical Social Work Journal, 49*(3), 391–404. https://doi.org/10.1007/s10615-020-00763-y

Butts, S. (1996). *Therapeutic techniques, marriage and family therapy* (Cassette Recording No. 7640-96). Department of Counseling, Educational Psychology and Research, University of Memphis.

Butz, M. R. (1995). Chaos theory, philosophically old, scientifically new. *Counseling and Values, 39*, 84–98.

Butz, M. R. (1997). *Chaos and complexity: Implications for psychological theory and practice*. Taylor & Francis.

Buydens, S. L., Wilensky, M., & Hensley, B. J. (2014). Effects of the EMDR protocol for recent traumatic events on acute stress disorder: A case series. *Journal of EMDR Practice and Research, 8*(1), 2–12.

Cable, D. G. (1996). Grief counseling for survivors of traumatic loss. In K. J. Doka (Ed.), *Living with grief after sudden loss: Suicide, homicide, accident, heart attack, stroke* (pp. 117–126). Hospice Foundation of America.

Caetano, R., Vaeth, P. A. C., & Ramisetty-Mikler, S. (2008). Intimate partner violence victim and perpetrator characteristics among couples in the United States. *Journal of Family Violence, 23*(6), 507–518. https://doi.org/10.1007/s10896-008-9178-3

Calhoun, L. G., & Tedeschi, R. G. (1998). *Posttraumatic growth: Future directions*. Erlbaum Inc.

Calhoun, L. G., & Tedeschi, R. G. (2001). Posttraumatic growth: The positive lessons of loss. In R. A. Neimeyer (Ed.), *Meaning reconstruction & the experience of loss* (pp. 157–172). American Psychological Association.

Calhoun, L. G., & Tedeschi, R. G. (2014). *Handbook of posttraumatic growth: Research and practice*. Routledge.

Calhoun, V. (1975). *The effectiveness of remotivation therapy with socially withdrawn nursing home patients*. Unpublished master's thesis, University of Arizona. https://www.semanticscholar.org/paper/The-effectiveness-of-remotivation-therapy-wih-home-Calhoun/8d325bf4875f138f6c80a3f6b64f68f308ece2cf

California Department of Education. (2002). *Safe Schools: A planning guide for action*.

California Occupational Safety and Health Administration. (1998). *Guidelines of security and safety of health care and community service workers*.

California Occupational Safety and Health Administration. (2018). California Code of Regulations, Title 8, Section 3342. Violence Prevention in Health Care. [Cal/OSHA - Title 8 regulations]. https://www.dir.ca.gov/Title8/3342.html

California State Auditor. (2006). *Batterer intervention program: County probation departments could improve compliance with state law, but progress in batterer accountability also depends on the courts*.

Calkins, B. C., & Swetz, K. M. (2019). Physician aid-in-dying and suicide prevention in psychiatry: A moral imperative over a crisis. *American Journal of Bioethics, 19*(10), 68–70. https://doi.org/10.1080/15265161.2019.1653398

Callahan, C. J. (2001). Protecting and counseling gay and lesbian students. *Journal of Humanistic Counseling, Education and Development, 40*(1), 5–10.

Callahan, J. (1998). Crisis theory and crisis intervention in emergencies. In P. M. Kleespies (Ed.), *Emergencies in mental health: Evaluation and management* (pp. 22–40). Guilford Press.

Callahan, J. (2009). Emergency intervention and crisis intervention. In P. M. Kleespies (Ed.), *Behavioral emergencies: An evidence-based resource for evaluating and managing risk of suicide, violence, and victimization* (pp. 13–32). American Psychological Association.

Callahan, R. (2011, September 16). Sept. 11 panelists still see threats. *Memphis Commercial Appeal*, A3.

Camelley, K. B., Wortman, C. B., Bolger, N., & Burke, D. T. (2006). The time course of grief reactions to spousal loss: Evidence from a national probability sample. *Journal of Personality and Social Psychology. 91*(3), 476–492.

Campbell, C. L., McCoy, S., Burg, M. A., & Hoffman, N. (2014). Enhancing home health care staff safety through reducing client aggression and violence in non situational care settings: A systematic review. *Home Health Care Management & Practice, 26*(1), 3–10.

Campbell, J. C. (1989). A test of two explanatory models of women's responses to battering. *Nursing Research, 38*, 18–24.

Campbell, J. C., & Messing, J. T. (2017). *Assessing dangerousness* (3rd ed.). Springer. https://doi.org/10.1891/9780826133274

Campbell, J. C., Webster, D. W., & Glass, N. (2009). The danger assessment: Validation of a lethality risk assessment instrument for intimate partner femicide. *Journal of Interpersonal Violence, 24*(4), 653–674. https://doi.org/10.1177/0886260508317180

Campbell, M. (2021). Clients' experience of the therapeutic relationship and a counselor's way of being on the resolution of religious and spiritual struggles: A hermeneutical phenomenological study. *Dissertation Abstracts International Section B: The Sciences and Engineering. 82*(3-B).

Campbell, R., Javorka, M., Gregory, K., & Vollinger, L. (2021). Supporting sexual assault survivors with disabilities: Tracing disclosure and referral pathways to postassault health care services. *American Journal of Orthopsychiatry, 91*(6), 751–762. https://doi.org/10.1037/ort0000576

Cann, A., Calhoun, L., Tedeschi, R., Taku, K., Vishnevsky, T., Triplett, K., Danhauer, S. C. (2011a). A short form of the Posttraumatic Growth Inventory. *Anxiety, Stress, & Coping: An International Journal, 23*(2), 127–137.

Cann, A., Calhoun, L., Tedeschi, R., Triplett, K., Vishnevsky, T., & Lindstrom, C. (2011b). Assessing posttraumatic cognitive processes: The Event-Related Rumination Inventory. *Anxiety, Stress, & Coping: An International Journal, 24*(2), 137–156.

Cannon, C. (2020). On the importance of feminist theories: Gender, race, sexuality and IPV. In B. Russell (Ed.), *Intimate Partner Violence and the LGBT+ Community: Understanding Power Dynamics* (pp. 37–52). Springer International Publishing. https://doi.org/10.1007/978-3-030-44762-5_3

Cannon, C., Lauve-Moon, K., & Buttell, F. (2015). Retheorizing intimate partner violence through post-structural feminism, queer theory, and the sociology of gender. *Social Sciences, 4*(3), Article 3. https://doi.org/10.3390/socsci4030668

Canter, L., & Canter, E. (1982). *Assertive discipline for parents*. Canter Associates.

Capellan, J. A., Silva, J., Mills, C., & Schmuhl, M. (2023). Who lives, who dies, who decides: Differences between mass public shooters who survive, are killed, and commit suicide. *Journal of Investigative Psychology and Offender Profiling, 20*(1), 80–96. https://doi.org/10.1002/jip.1608

Caplan, G. (1961). *An approach to community mental health*. Grune & Stratton.

Caplan, G. (1964). *Principles of preventive psychiatry*. Basic Books.

Cappeliez, P., & Watt, L. (2005). L'integrazione della retrospettiva di vita e della terapia cognitiva della depressione con le persone anziane. *Pisicoterpaia Cognitiva e Comportamentale, 11*(2), 151–164.

Capps, M. (1982, April). *The co-optive and repressive state versus the battered women's movement*. Paper presented at annual meeting of Southern Sociological Society, Memphis, TN, the United States.

Captari, L. E., Riggs, S. A., & Stephen, K. (2021). Attachment processes following traumatic loss: A mediation model examining identity distress, shattered assumptions, prolonged grief, and posttraumatic growth. *Psychological Trauma: Theory, Research, Practice, and Policy, 13*(1), 94–103. https://doi.org/10.1037/tra0000555

Capuzzi, D. (2002). Legal and ethical challenges in counseling suicidal students. *Professional School Counselor, 6*(1), 36–45.

Capuzzi, D. (2009). *Suicide prevention in the schools: guidelines for middle and high school settings*. American Counseling Association.

Capuzzi, D., & Gross, D. R. (Eds.). (1995). *Counseling and psychotherapy: Theories and interventions*. Prentice Hall.

Carden, A. D. (1994). Wife abuse and the wife abuser: Review and recommendations. *Counseling Psychologist, 22*(4), 539–582.

Cardenas, I. (2023). Advancing intersectionality approaches in intimate partner violence research: A social justice approach. *Journal of Ethnic & Cultural Diversity in Social Work, 32*(1), 1–11. https://doi.org/10.1080/15313204.2020.1855494

Cares, A. C., Banyard, V. L., Moynihan, M. M., Williams, L. M., Potter, S. J., & Stapleton, J. G. (2015). Changing attitudes about being a bystander to violence: Translating an in-person sexual violence prevention program to a new campus. *Violence Against Women, 21*(2), 165–187. https://doi.org/10.1177/1077801214564681

Carey, K. B., Durney, S. E., Shepardson, R. L., & Carey, M. P. (2015). Incapacitated and forcible rape of college women: Prevalence across the first year. *Journal of Adolescent Health, 56*(6), 678–680. https://doi.org/10.1016/j.jadohealth.2015.02.018

Carkhuff, R. R. (1987). *The art of helping* (6th ed.). Human Resource Development Press.

Carkhuff, R. R., & Berenson, B. G. (1977). *Beyond counseling and therapy* (2nd ed.). Holt, Rinehart & Winston.

Carl Perkins Center. (2023). *Client Satisfaction Survey.*

Carney, J. (2008). Perceptions of bullying and associated trauma in adolescence. *Professional School Counseling, 11*(3), 179–187.

Carney, J., Hazler, R., Higgins, J., & Danser, S. (1999, April). *Peer-on-peer violence.* Poster session at the American Counseling Association World Conference, San Diego, CA, the United States.

Carpenter, R. W., & Trull, T. J. (2013). Components of emotion dysregulation in borderline personality disorder: A review. *Current Psychiatry Reports, 15*, 335. https://doi.org/10.1007/s11920-012-0335-2

Carroll, J. F. X., & White, W. L. (1982). Theory building: Integrating individual and environmental factors within an ecological framework. In W. S. Paine (Ed.), *Job stress and burnout* (pp. 41–60). SAGE.

Carroll, J. S., Olson, C. D., & Buckmiller, N. (2007). Family boundary ambiguity: A 30-year review of theory, research, and measurement. *Family Relations, 56*, 2120–2130.

Carter, S. R. (1987). Use of puppets to treat traumatic grief. *Elementary School Guidance & Counseling, 21*, 210–215.

Carthy, N., Best, D., Heckels, V., Weber, L., & Eberhardt, J. (2023). Complex posttraumatic stress disorder symptoms among midlife to older female survivors of intimate partner violence. *Psychological Trauma: Theory, Research, Practice, and Policy, 15*(2), 331–339. https://doi.org/10.1037/tra0001238

Casanovas, M., Kramer, T., Clarke, V., Goddard, A. M., Elena, G., & Khadr, S. (2022). Somatic symptoms following sexual assault in adolescents: A prospective longitudinal study. *Psychology, Health & Medicine, 27*(3), 546–558. https://doi.org/10.1080/13548506.2021.1874437

Casas, J. B., & Benuto, L. T. (2022). Work-related traumatic stress spillover in first responder families: A systematic review of the literature. *Psychological Trauma: Theory, Research, Practice, and Policy, 14*(2), 209–217. https://doi.org/10.1037/tra0001086

Caserta, M., Lund, D., Utz, R., & de Vries, B. (2009). Stress-related growth among the recently bereaved. *Aging & Mental Health, 13*(3), 463–476.

Casey, G. W. (2011). Comprehensive soldier fitness: A vision for psychological resilience in the U.S. Army. *American Psychologist, 66*(1), 1–3.

Caspi, E. (2022). *Understanding and preventing harmful interactions between residents with dementia.* Health Professional Press.

Cass, A., & Mallicoat, S. (2015). College student perceptions of victim action: Will targets of stalking report to police? *American Journal of Criminal Justice, 40*(2), 250–269.

Cassinerio, C., & Lane-Garon, P. (2006). Changing school climate one mediator at a time: Year-one analysis of a school-based mediation program. *Conflict Resolution Quarterly, 23*(4), 447–460.

Castelnuovo, G., Gaggioli, A., Mantovani, F., & Riva, G. (2003). New and old tools in psychotherapy: The use of technology for the integration of traditional clinical treatments. *Psychotherapy: Theory, Research, Practice, Training, 40*(1/2), 33–44.

Castro, Á., Ibáñez, J., Maté, B., Esteban, J., & Barrada, J. R. (2019). Childhood sexual abuse, sexual behavior, and revictimization in adolescence and youth: A mini review. *Frontiers in Psychology, 10.* https://www.frontiersin.org/articles/10.3389/fpsyg.2019.02018

Castro, W., Sanchez, M., Gonzalez, C., Bethencourt, J., de la Fuente Portero, J., & Marco, R. (2014). Cognitive behavioral treatment and anti-depressants combined with virtual reality exposure for patients with chronic agoraphobia. *International Journal of Clinical and Health Psychology, 14*(1), 9–17.

Cattanach, A. (2008). Working creatively with children and their families after trauma: The storied life. In C. A. Malchiodi (Ed.), *Creative interventions with traumatized children* (pp. 211–225). Guilford Press.

Cautela, J. R. (1976). The present status of covert modeling. *Journal of Behavior Therapy and Experimental Psychiatry, 6*, 323–326.

Cavanaugh, C. E., Messing, J. T., Del-Colle, M., O'Sullivan, C., & Campbell, J. C. (2011). Prevalence and correlates of suicidal behavior among adult female victims of intimate partner violence. *Suicide & Life-Threatening Behavior, 41*(4), 372–383. https://doi.org/10.1111/j.1943-278X.2011.00035.x

Cavanaugh, M. M., & Gelles, R. J. (2005). The utility of male domestic violence offender typologies: New directions for research, policy, and practice. *Journal of Interpersonal Violence, 20*(2), 155–165.

Cavezza, C., & McEwan, T. (2014). Cyberstalking versus off-line stalking in a forensic sample. *Psychology, Crime, & Law, 20*(10), 955–970.

Cawood, J. S., & Corcoran, M. H. (2009). *Violence assessment and intervention: The practitioner's handbook* (2nd ed.). CRC Press/Taylor & Francis.

Center for Collegiate Mental Health. (2021). *2021 annual report.* Penn State.

Centers for Disease Control and Prevention. (2022). *Prioritizing minority mental health.*

Centers for Disease Control and Prevention (CDC). (n.d.). *Podcasts at CDC.* www.cdc.gov/podcasts

Centers for Disease Control, Violence Prevention Injury Center. (2023, January 27). *Fast facts: Preventing teen dating violence.* https://www.cdc.gov/violenceprevention/intimatepartnerviolence/teendatingviolence/fastfact.html

Centers for Disease Control and Prevention. (2002). *Adolescent health survey.* U.S. Department of Health and Human Services, Public Health Service.

Centers for Disease Control and Prevention. (2020). Suicidal ideation and behaviors among high school students—Youth risk behavior survey, the United States, 2019. *Center for Disease Control Morbidity and Mortality Weekly report.* https://www.cdc.gov/mmwr/volumes/69/su/su6901a6.htm

Centers for Disease Control and Prevention. (2021). *School associated violent death.*

Centers for Disease Control and Prevention. (2022). *Suicide, suicide attempt, or self harm clusters.* https://www.cdc.gov/suicide/resources/suicide-clusters.html

Centers for Disease Control and Prevention. (2023). *Prioritizing minority mental health.* https://www.cdc.gov/healthequity/features/minority-mental-health/index.html

Centers for Homeland Security (2015). *Colleges and universities offering homeland security programs.* www.chds.us/?partners/institutions

Centers for Prevention Programs and Partnerships-Homeland Security. (n.d.). *Threat assessment and management teams.*

Centre for Research on the Epidemiology of Disasters. (2014). *Executive summary.* https://www.cred.be/sites/default/files/ADSR_2014.pdf

Cerel, J., Jordan, J. R., & Duberstein, P. R. (2008). The impact of suicide on the family. *Crisis, 29*(1), 38–44. https://doi.org/10.1027/0227-5910.29.1.38

Cerel, J., Moore, M., Brown, M. M., van de Venne, J., & Brown, S. L. (2015). Who leaves suicide notes? A six-year population-based study. *Suicide and Life-Threatening Behavior, 45*(3), 326–334. https://doi.org/10.1111/sltb.12131

CERT. (2011). *Community Emergency Response Team training manual module 7: Psychological First Aid.*

Chalk, R., & King, P. A. (Eds.). (1998). *Violence in families: Assessing prevention and treatment programs.* National Academy Press.

Chamberlain, L. (1993, August). *Strange attractors in patterns of family interactions.* [Paper presentation]. Annual Convention of the American Psychological Association, Toronto, Canada

Chamberlain, L. (1994, August). *Is there a chaotician in the house? Chaos and family therapy.* [Paper presentation]. Annual Convention of the American Psychological Association, Los Angeles, CA, the United States.

Chamberlin, J. (2006). Cyberbullies increasingly target peers online. *Monitor on Psychology, 37*(9), 17.

Chandra, A., Burns, R. M., Tanielian, T., Jaycox, L. H., Tanielian, T., & Scott, M. M. (2008). *Understanding the impact of deployment on children and families: Findings from a pilot study of Operation Purple Camp participants* (Working paper Rand Corporation.)

Chapman, A. (2018). *Phone coaching in Dialectal Behavior Therapy.* The Guilford Press.

Chapman, L., Morabito, D., Ladakakos, C., Schreier, H., & Knudson, M. (2001). The effectiveness of art therapy interventions in reducing posttraumatic stress disorder (PTSD) symptoms in pediatric trauma patients. *Art Therapy, 18*(2), 100–104.

Charach, A., Pepler, D., & Zeigler, S. (1995). Bullying at school—A Canadian perspective: A survey of problems and suggestions for intervention. *Education Canada, 35*(1), 12–18.

Chard, K. M., & Gilman, R. (2014). Cognitive processing therapy with adolescents. In R. M. Reece, R. F. Hanson, & J. Sargents (Eds.), *Treatment of child abuse: Common ground for mental health, medical and legal practitioners* (2nd ed.). (pp. 148–153). Johns Hopkins University Press.

Charles-Edwards, D. (2009). Introduction to the special section on death, loss, and work. *Death Studies, 33*(5), 399–401.

Charlton, P. F. C., & Thompson, J. A. (1996). Ways of coping with psychological distress after trauma. *British Journal of Psychology, 35*, 517–530.

Charney, A. M., & Pearlman, L. A. (1998). The ecstasy and the agony: The impact of disaster and trauma work on the self of the clinician. In P. M. Kleespies (Ed.), *Emergencies in mental health practice: Evaluation and management* (pp. 418–435). Guilford Press.

Chatham, P. M. (1989). *Treatment of the borderline personality.* Aronson.

Chattoraj, T. (2022). Critical review of theories evaluating stay and leave decisions in intimate partner violence: Implications for research. *International Journal of Indian Psychology, 10*(1), Article 1. https://doi.org/10.25215/1001.082

Chavez, L. (1999). *Workplace violence awareness for managers and supervisors.* Internet course.

Chemtob, C. M. (2000). Delayed debriefing after a disaster. In B. Raphael & J. P. Wilson (Eds.), *Psychological debriefing: Theory, practice, and evidence* (pp. 227–240). Cambridge University Press.

Chemtob, C. M., Nakashima, J. P., & Hamada, R. S. (2002). Psychosocial intervention for postdisaster trauma symptoms in elementary school children: A controlled community field study. *Archives of Pediatric and Adolescent Medicine, 156*, 211–216.

Chemtob, C., Nakashima, J., & Carlson, J. (2002). Brief treatment for elementary school children with disaster-related posttraumatic stress disorder: A field study. *Journal of Clinical Psychology, 58*(1), 99–112.

Chen, J., Walters, M. L., Gilbert, L. K., & Patel, N. (2020). Sexual violence, stalking, and intimate partner violence by sexual orientation, the United States. *Psychology of Violence, 10*(1), 110–119. https://doi.org/10.1037/vio0000252

Chermack, S. T., Fuller, B., & Blow, F. (2000). Predictors of expressed partner and non-partner violence among patients in substance abuse treatment. *Drug and Alcohol Dependence, 58*(1–2), 43–54.

Chiles, J. A., & Strosahl, K. D. (1995). *The suicidal patient: Principles of assessment, treatment, and case management* (pp. xi, 282). American Psychiatric Association.

Chirico, F., Afolabi, A. A., Ilesanmi, O. S., Nucera, G., Ferrari, G., Sacco, A., Szarpak, L., Crescenzo, P., Magnavita, N., & Leiter, M. (2021). Prevalence, risk factors and prevention of burnout syndrome among healthcare workers: An umbrella review of systematic reviews and meta-analyses. *Journal of Health and Social Sciences, 6*(4), 465–491. https://doi.org/10.19204/2021/prvl3

Chisholm, C. A., Bullock, L., & Ferguson, J. E. (2017). Intimate partner violence and pregnancy: Epidemiology and impact. *American Journal of Obstetrics and Gynecology, 217*(2), 141–144. https://doi.org/10.1016/j.ajog.2017.05.042

Chiu, L., Stewart, K., Woo, C., Yatham, L., & Lam, R. (2015). The relationship between burnout and depressive symptoms in patients with depressive disorders. *Journal of Affective Disorders, 172*(1), 361–366.

Christensen, D. R., Landes, R. D., Jackson, L., Marsch, L. A., Mancino, M., Chopra, M., & Bickel, W. K. (2014). Adding an Internet-delivered treatment to an efficacious treatment package for opioid dependence. *Journal of Consulting and Clinical Psychology, 82*(6), 964–972.

Christogiorgos, S., Vassilopoulou, V., Florou, A., Xydou, V., Douvou, M., & Vgenopoulou, S. (2010). Telephone counseling with adolescents and counter-transference phenomena: Particularities and challenges. *British Journal of Guidance & Counseling, 38*(3), 313–325.

Chu, J. (1999). Trauma and suicide. In D. G. Jacobs (Ed.), *The Harvard Medical School guide to suicide assessment and intervention* (pp. 332–354). Jossey-Bass.

Chuemchit, M., Chernkwanma, S., Rugkua, R., Daengthern, L., Abdullakasim, P., & Wieringa, S. E. (2018). Prevalence of intimate partner violence in Thailand. *Journal of Family Violence, 33*(5), 315–323. https://doi.org/10.1007/s10896-018-9960-9

Chung, D. T., Ryan, C. J., Hadzi-Pavlovic, D., Singh, S. P., Stanton, C., & Large, M. M. (2017). Suicide rates after discharge from psychiatric facilities. *JAMA Psychiatry, 74*(7), 694–702. https://doi.org/10.1001/jamapsychiatry.2017.1044

Chung, M. C., Easthope, Y., Farmer, S., Werrett, J., & Chung, C. (2003). Psychological sequelae: Post-traumatic stress reactions and personality factors among community residents as secondary victims. *Scandinavian Journal of Caring Science, 17*(3), 265–270.

Çimke, S., & Yildirim Gürkan, D. (2023). Psychological stress experienced by parents and posttraumatic emotional stress experienced by children during the COVID-19 pandemic. *Psychological Trauma: Theory, Research, Practice, and Policy, 15*(5), 888–894. https://doi.org/10.1037/tra0001391

CIT International. (2014, October). *Report presented to the general assembly.* CIT International Conference, Monterey, CA, the United States.

Clark, C. J., Renner, L. M., & Logeais, M. E. (2020). Intimate partner violence screening and referral practices in an outpatient care setting. *Journal of Interpersonal Violence, 35*(23–24), 5877–5888. https://doi.org/10.1177/0886260517724253

Clark, O. E., Fortney, C. A., Dunnells, Z. D. O., Winning, A. M., Gerhardt, C. A., & Baughcum, A. E. (2021). Parents' own words: Adjustment and coping following infant death in the NICU. *Clinical Practice in Pediatric Psychology, 9*(3), 261–271. https://doi.org/10.1037/cpp0000418

Clark, P., Holden, C., Russell, M., & Downs, H. (2022). The impostor phenomenon in mental health professionals: Relationships among compassion fatigue, burnout, and compassion satisfaction. *Contemporary Family Therapy: An International Journal, 44*(2), 185–197. https://doi.org/10.1007/s10591-021-09580-y

Clark, S. C., & McKiernan, W. (1981). Contacts with a Canadian "street level" drug and crisis centre, 1975–1978. *Bulletin on Narcotics, 33*, 23–31.

Clay, R. C. (2010). Treating traumatized children. *Monitor on Psychology, 41*(7), 36–39.

Clearinghouse for Military Family Readiness. (2017). *IPV Programs for Female Perpetrators.* Clearinghouse for Military Family Readiness at Penn State. https://militaryfamilies.psu.edu/wp-content/uploads/2019/10/IPV_Programs_for_Female_Perpetrators.pdf

Clemente, M., Reiq-Botella, A., & Coloma, R. (2015). The occupational health of correctional officers in Peru: The impact of length of work experience. *The Prison Journal, 95*(2), 244–263.

Cleveland Clinic (2023). *Sundown syndrome.* https://my.clevelandclinic.org/health/articles/22840-sundown-syndrome

Clow, S., Olafson, E., Ford, J., Moser, M., Slivinsky, M., & Kaplow, J. (2023). Addressing grief reactions among incarcerated adolescents and young adults using trauma and grief component therapy. *Psychological Trauma: Theory, Research, Practice, and Policy, 15*(Suppl 1), S192–S200. https://doi.org/10.1037/tra0001364

Cluss, P. A., Chang, J. C., Hawker, L., Hudson Scholle, S., Dado, D., Buranosky, R., & Goldstrohm, S. (2006). The process of change for victims of intimate partner violence: Support for a psychosocial readiness model. *Women's Health Issues, 16*(5), 262–274. https://doi.org/10.1016/j.whi.2006.06.006

Coaston, S. C. (2017). Self-care through self-compassion: A balm for burnout. *Professional Counselor, 7*(3), 285–297.

Coates, D., & Howe, D. (2014, October). *The design and development of staff well being initiatives: Staff stressors, burnout and emotional exhaustion at children and young people's mental health in Australia.* Administration and Policy in Mental Health Services Research.

Cochran, M., & Niego, S. (2002). Parenting and social networks. In M. H. Bornstein (Ed.). *Handbook of parenting: Vol. 4, Social conditions and applied parenting* (2nd ed., pp. 393–418). Erlbaum.

Cochran, S. (2014). Basic plays. *Memphis Police Department: Crisis intervention team training manual* (pp. 45–48). Memphis Police Department.

Coetzee, S. K., & Laschinger, H. K. S. (2018). Toward a comprehensive, theoretical model of compassion fatigue: An integrative literature review. *Nursing & Health Sciences, 20*(1), 4–15. https://doi.org/10.1111/nhs.12387

Cohen, A. (2002). Gestalt therapy and post-traumatic stress disorder: The potential and its (lack of) fulfillment. *Gestalt!, 6*(1), 21–28.

Cohen, A. (2003). Gestalt therapy and post traumatic stress disorder: The irony and the challenge. *Gestalt Review, 7*(1), 42–55.

Cohen, J. A., & Mannarino, A. P. (2011). Supporting children with traumatic grief: What educators need to know. *School Psychology International, 32*(2), 117–131. https://doi.org/10.1177/0143034311400827

Cohen, J. A., & Mannarino, A. P. (2015). Trauma-focused cognitive behavior therapy for traumatized children and families. *Child and Adolescent Psychiatric Clinics, 24*(3), 557–570. https://doi.org/10.1016/j.chc.2015.02.005

Cohen, J. A., Mannarino, A. P., & Deblinger, E. (2003). Child and parent trauma-focused cognitive behavioral therapy treatment manual. *Unpublished Manuscript.*

Cohen, J. A., Mannarino, A. P., & Deblinger, E. (2006). *Treating trauma and traumatic grief in children and adolescents.* Guilford Press.

Cohen, J. A., Mannarino, A. P., & Knudsen, K. (2004). Treating childhood traumatic grief: A pilot study. *Journal of the American Academy of Child and Adolescent Psychiatry, 43*, 1225–1233.

Cohen, J. A., Mannarino, A. P., Greenberg, T., Padlo, S., & Shipley, C. (2002). Childhood trauma and grief: Concepts and controversies. *Trauma, Violence, & Abuse, 3*, 307–327.

Cohen, J. A., Mannarino, A., & Deblinger, E. (2017). *Treating trauma and traumatic grief in children and adolescents* (2nd ed.). Guilford Press.

Cohen, O., Sharar, G., & Brunstein-Klomek, A. (2020). Peer victimization, coping strategies, depression, and suicidal ideation among young adolescents. *Crisis: The Journal of Crisis Intervention and Suicide Prevention, 41*(3), 156–162. https://doi.org/10.1027/0227-5910/a000614

Cohen, P. A., Kulik, J. A., & Kulik, C. C. (1982). Educational outcomes of tutoring. A meta-analysis of findings. *American Educational Research Journal, 19*, 237–248.

Cohen, P., Kasen, S., Chen, H., Gordon, K., Berenson, K., Brook, J., & White, T. (2006). Current affairs and the public psyche: American anxiety in the post 9/11 world. *Social Psychiatry and Psychiatric Epidemiology, 41*(4), 251–260.

Cohen, S. (2004). Social relationships and health. *American Psychologist, 59*, 676–684.

Coke-Weatherly, A. (2005). *An analysis of where and how crisis intervention is taught and learned.* Unpublished doctoral dissertation, University of Memphis.

Colgrove, M., Bloomfield, H. H., & McWilliams, P. (1991). *How to survive the loss of a love.* Prelude Press.

Collins, B. G., & Collins, T. M. (2005). *Crisis and trauma: Developmental-ecological intervention.* Lahaska Press.

Collins, B. G., & Collins, T. M. (2006). *Crisis and trauma: Developmental-ecological.* Cengage Learning.

Collins, C. J. & Clark, J. J. (2021). Using the TRAP-18 to identify an incel lone-actor terrorist. *Journal of Treat Assessment and Management, 8*(4), 159–173. https://doi.org/10.1037/tam0000167

Collins, S., & Long, A. (2003). Working with the psychological effects of trauma: Consequences for mental health care workers. *Journal of Psychiatric and Mental Health Nursing, 10*(4), 417–424.

Collins, W. L. (2005). Embracing spirituality as an element of professional self-care. *Social Work and Christianity, 32*(3), 263–274.

Collins, W. L., & Doolittle, A. (2006). Personal reflections of funeral rituals and spirituality in a Kentucky African American family. *Death Studies, 30*(10), 957–969.

Collison, K. L., & Lynam, D. R. (2021). Personality disorders as predictors of intimate partner violence: A meta-analysis. *Clinical Psychology Review, 88*, 102047. https://doi.org/10.1016/j.cpr.2021.102047

Coloroso, B. (2003). *The bully, the bullied, and the bystander.* HarperCollins.

Comans, T., Visser, V., & Scuffham, P. (2013). Cost effectiveness of a community-based crisis intervention program for people bereaved by suicide. *Crisis: The Journal of Crisis Intervention and Suicide Prevention, 34*(6), 390–397. https://doi.org/10.1027/0227-5910/a000210

Compassionate Friends (2023a). *Chapter locator.* http://www.compassionatefriends.org/Find_Support/Chapters/Chapter_Locator.aspx

Compassionate Friends. (2023b). *Compassionate Friends credo.* https://www.compassionatefriends.org/about_us.aspx

Compton, M. T., Bahore, M., Watson, A. C., & Oliva, J. R. (2008). A comprehensive review of extant research on CIT programs. *American Academy of Psychiatry and the Law, 36*, 47–55.

Compton, M. T., Bakeman, R., Broussard, B., Hankerson-Dyson, D., Husbands, L., Krishan, S., Stewart-Hutto, T., D'Orio, B. M., Oliva, J. R., Thompson, N. J., & Watson, A. C. (2014a). The police-based crisis intervention team (CIT) model: I. Effects on officers' knowledge, attitudes, and skills. *Psychiatric Services, 65*(4), 517–522.

Compton, M. T., Bakeman, R., Broussard, B., Hankerson-Dyson, D., Husbands, L., Krishan, S., Stewart-Hutto, T., D'Orio, B. M., Oliva, J. R., Thompson, N. J., & Watson, A. C. (2014b). The police-based crisis intervention team (CIT) model: II. Effects on level of force and resolution, referral and arrest. *Psychiatric Services, 65* (4), 523–529.

Compton, M. T., Esterberg, M. L., McGee, R., Kotwicki, R. J., & Oliva, J. R. (2006). Crisis Intervention Team training: Changes in knowledge, attitudes, and stigma related to schizophrenia. *Psychiatric Services 57*(8), 1199–1202.

Congress, E. P. (1996). Family crisis: Life cycle and bolts from the blue: Assessment and treatment. In A. R. Roberts (Ed.). *Crisis management and brief treatment: Theory, technique, and practice* (pp. 142–159). Nelson-Hall Publisher

Congress, E. P. (2000). Crisis intervention with culturally diverse families. In A. E. Roberts (Ed.), *Crisis intervention handbook: Assessment, treatment and research.* Oxford University Press.

Conoley, J. C., & Goldstein, A. P. (Eds.). (2004). *School violence intervention: A practical handbook* (2nd ed.). Guilford Press.

Conrad, D., & Kellar-Guenther, Y. (2006). Compassion fatigue, burnout, and compassion satisfaction among Colorado child protection workers. *Child Abuse and Neglect, 30*(10), 1071–1080.

Conroy, K. (1982). Long-term treatment issues with battered women. In J. P. Flanzer & B. Star (Eds.), *The many faces of violence* (pp. 53–75). Charles C Thomas.

Conte, C. (2005). *Examination of the reliability and validity of the Triage Assessment Survey: Organizations. Unpublished doctoral dissertation.* Duquesne University.

Conyne, R. K., & Cook, E. P. (2003, March). *Understanding persons within environment: An introduction to ecological counseling.* Program and paper presented at the annual meeting of the American Counseling Association, Anaheim, CA, the United States.

Conyne, R. K., Cook, E. P., Wilson, R. F., Tang, M., O'Connell, W. P., McWhirter, B. T., et al. (2003, March). *Ecological counseling: An approach for the 21st century.* Program and paper presented at the annual meeting of the American Counseling Association, Anaheim, CA, the United States.

Cook, E. P. (2012). *Understanding people in context: The ecological perspective in counseling.* American Counseling Association.

Cook, J. M., Naseem, A., & Thorp, S. R. (2015). Treating PTSD in older adults. Post traumatic stress disorder: Patient interview, clinical assessment, and diagnosis. In N. C. Bernardy and M. J. Friedman (Eds.), *A practical guide to treatment: Pharmacological and psychotherapeutic approaches* (pp. 151–161). American Psychological Association.

Cook, R. M., Fye, H. J., Jones, J. L., & Baltrinic, E. B. (2021). Self-reported symptoms of burnout in novice professional counselors: A content analysis. *The Professional Counselor, 11*(1). https://tpcjournal.nbcc.org/self-reported-symptoms-of-burnout-in-novice-professional-counselors-a-content-analysis/

Cook, S. W., Aten, J. D., Moore, M., Hook, J. N. & Davis, D. E. (2013). Resource loss, religiousness, health, and posttraumatic growth following Hurricane Katrina. *Mental Health, Religion & Culture, 16*, 352–366.

Cook, S., Pinazzola, J., Ford, J. D., Lanktreee, C., Blaustein, M., & Cloitre, M. (2005). Complex trauma in children and adolescents. *Psychiatric Annals, 35*, 390–398.

Cooley, E. J., & Keesey, J. C. (1981). Relationship between life change and illness in coping versus sensitive persons. *Psychological Reports, 48*, 711–714.

Cools, S., & Kotsadam, A. (2017). Resources and intimate partner violence in Sub-Saharan Africa. *World Development, 95*, 211–230. https://doi.org/10.1016/j.worlddev.2017.02.027

COPS. (n.d.) *Supporting safe schools.* U.S. Department of Justice. https://cops.usdoj.gov/supportingsafeschools

Corder, B. F., Ball, B. C., Haizlip, T. M., Rollins, R., & Beaumont, R. (1976). Adolescent parricide: A comparison with other adolescent murder. *American Journal of Psychiatry, 133*(8), 957–961.

Corey-Souza, P. (2007). Compassion fatigue in members of the Florida Crisis Response Team: A consequence of caring. *Dissertation Abstracts International: Section B. The Sciences and Engineering, 2695.*

Cormier, L. S., & Hackney, H. (1987). *The professional counselor: A process guide to helping.* Prentice Hall.

Cormier, W. H., & Cormier, L. S. (1985). *Interviewing strategies for helpers: Fundamental skills and cognitive behavioral interventions* (2nd ed.). Brooks/Cole.

Cormier, W. H., & Cormier, L. S. (1991). *Interviewing strategies for helpers: Fundamental skills and cognitive behavioral interventions* (3rd ed.). Brooks/Cole.

Corneil, W., Beaton, R., Murphy, S., Johnson, C., & Pike, K. (1999). Exposure to traumatic incidents and prevalence of posttraumatic stress symptomatology in urban firefighters in two countries. *Journal of Occupational Health Psychology, 4*(2), 131–141.

Cornille, T. A., & Boroto, D. R. (1992). The family distress model: A conceptual and clinical application of Reiss strong bonds finding. *Contemporary Family Therapy, 14*, 181–198.

Cornille, T. A., Meyer, A. S., Mullis, A. K., Mullis, R. L., & Boroto, D. (2008). The family outreach model: Tools for engaging and working with families in distress. *Journal of Family Social Work, 11*(2), 185–201.

Corr, C. A., & Corr, D. M. (1996). *Handbook of childhood death and bereavement*. Springer.

Correa, N. P., Cain, C. M., Bertenthal, M., & Lopez, K. K. (2020). Women's experiences of being screened for intimate partner violence in the health care setting. *Nursing for Women's Health, 24*(3), 185–196. https://doi.org/10.1016/j.nwh.2020.04.002

Correia-Santos, P., Ford, J. D., Maia, Â. C., & Pinto, R. J. (2023). Posttraumatic stress disorder symptoms and dissociation as serial mediators of the relationship between cumulative victimization and adjustment problems among poly-victimized at-risk youth. *Psychological Trauma: Theory, Research, Practice, and Policy, 15*(Suppl 1), S11–S19. https://doi.org/10.1037/tra0001383

Coryell, W., Fiedorowicz, J., Solomon, D., Endicott, J., & Keller, M. (2019). Anxiety symptom severity and long-term risk for suicidal behavior in depressive disorders. *Suicide & Life-Threatening Behavior, 49*(6), 1621–1629. https://doi.org/10.1111/sltb.12555

Costa, L., & Holliday, D. (1994). Helping children cope with the death of a parent. *Elementary School Guidance & Counseling, 28*, 206–213.

Costa, M., Reis, G., Pavlo, A., Bellamy, C., Ponte, K., & Davidson, L. (2021). Tele-mental health utilization among people with mental illness to access care during the COVID-19 pandemic. *Community Mental Health Journal, 57*(4), 720–726. https://doi.org/10.1007/s10597-021-00789-7

Costa, Y. R. de S., Lavorato, S. N., & Baldin, J. J. C. M. de C. (2020). Violence against women and drug-facilitated sexual assault (DFSA): A review of the main drugs. *Journal of Forensic and Legal Medicine, 74*, 102020. https://doi.org/10.1016/j.jflm.2020.102020

Counce, C., & Sommer, L. (2003, June). *Gentle guidance eases grief*. Paper presented at the American School Counselor Conference, St. Louis, MO, the United States.

Council for Accreditation of Counseling & Related Educational Programs. (2009). *CACREP 2009 standards and procedures manual*. http://www.cacrep.org/template/page

Courtois, C. A. (2015). First, do no harm: Ethics of attending to spiritual issues in trauma treatment. In D. F. Walker, C. A. Courtois, & J. Aten (Eds.), *Spiritually oriented psychotherapy for trauma* (pp. 55–76). American Psychological Association.

Courtois, C. A., & Ford, J. D. (Eds.). (2009). *Treating complex traumatic stress disorder*. Guilford Press.

Courtois, C. A., & Ford, J. D. (Eds.). (2020). *Treating complex traumatic stress disorders: An evidence-based guide*. Telemachus Press.

Courtois, C. A., & Gold, S. N. (2009). The need for inclusion of psychological trauma in the professional curriculum: A call to action. *Psychological Trauma: Theory, Research, Practice, and Policy, 1*, 3–25.

Courtois, C. A., Ford, J. D., & Cloitre, M. (2009). Best practices in psychotherapy for adults. In C. A. Courtois & J. D. Ford (Eds.), *Treating complex traumatic stress disorders: An evidence-based guide* (pp. 82–103). Guilford Press.

Covington, M. W., Huff-Corzine, L., & Corzine, J. (2014). Battered police: Risk factors for violence against law enforcement officers. *Violence and Victims, 29*(1), 34–52. https://doi.org/10.1891/0886-6708.VV-D-12-00022

Cowan, D. S. (2010). Death of a friend during childhood. In C. A. Corr, D. E. Balk (Eds.), *Children's encounters with death, bereavement, and coping* (pp. 219–236). Springer.

Cowan, K., & Paine, C. (2015). School safety: What really works. *Principal Leadership, 13*(7), 12. http://www.nasponline.org/resources/principals/March_13_School_Safety

Cowan, P. A., & Cowan, C. P. (2012). Normative family transitions, couple relationships, and healthy child development. In S. J. Price, C. A. Price, & P. C. McKenny (Eds.). *Families and change: Coping with stressful events and transitions* (pp. 428–451). SAGE.

Cowman, S., Björkdahl, A., Clarke, E., Gethin, G., & McGuire, J. (2017). A descriptive survey study of violence management and priorities among psychiatric staff in mental health services, across seventeen European countries. *BMC Health Services Research, 17*, 59–69. https://doi.org/10.1186/s12913-017-1988-7

Craig, C. D., & Sprang, G. (2010). Compassion satisfaction, compassion fatigue, and burnout in a national sample of trauma treatment therapists. *Anxiety, Stress & Coping, 23*(3), 319–339. https://doi.org/10.1080/10615800903085818

Cramer, R. J., Kaniuka, A. R., Yada, F. N., Diaz-Garelli, F., Hill, R. M., Bowling, J., Macchia, J. M., & Tucker, R. P. (2022). An analysis of suicidal thoughts and behaviors among transgender and gender diverse adults. *Social Psychiatry and Psychiatric Epidemiology, 57*(1), 195–205. https://doi.org/10.1007/s00127-021-02115-8

Cramer, S. H., Keitel, M. A., & Zevon, M. A. (1990). Spouses of cancer patients: A review of the literature. *Journal of Counseling and Development, 69*, 163–166.

Crane, C. A., & Easton, C. J. (2017). Integrated treatment options for male perpetrators of intimate partner violence. *Drug and Alcohol Review, 36*(1), 24–33. https://doi.org/10.1111/dar.12496

Crane, C. A., Oberleitner, L. M. S., Devine, S., & Easton, C. J. (2014). Substance use disorders and intimate partner violence perpetration among male and female offenders. *Psychology of Violence, 4*(3), 322–333. https://doi.org/10.1037/a0034338

Crase, D. (1994). Important consumer issues surrounding death. *Thanatos, 19*(1), 22–26.

Crenshaw, D. A., & Lee, J. (2010). The disenfranchised grief of children. In N. B. Webb (Ed.), *Helping bereaved children: A handbook for practitioners* (3rd ed., pp. 91–108). Guilford Press.

Crews, W. (1998). *Memphis Police Department procedures manual for school police officers*. Memphis Police Department.

Cross, D., Fani, N., Powers, A., & Bradley, B. (2017). Neurobiological development in the context of childhood trauma. *Clinical Psychology Science and Practice, 24*(2), 111–124. http://doi:10.1111/cpsp.12198

Cross, D., Vance, L. A., Kim, Y. J., Ruchard, A. L., Fox, N., Jovanovic, T., & Bradley, B. (2018). Trauma exposure, PTSD, and parenting in a community sample of low-income, predominantly African American mothers and children. *Psychological Trauma: Theory, Research, Practice, and Policy, 10*(3), 327–335. https://doi.org/10.1037/tra0000264

Crothers, L. M., & Levinson, E. M. (2004). Assessment of bullying. *Journal of Counseling and Development, 82*(4), 496–503.

Crow, G. A. (1977). *Crisis intervention: A social interaction approach*. Association Press.

Cryder, C. H., Kilmer, R. P., Tedeschi, R. G., & Calhoun, L. G. (2006). An exploratory study of posttraumatic growth in children following a natural disaster. *American Journal of Orthopsychiatry, 76*(1), 65–69.

Cukrowicz, K. C., Wingate, L. R., Driscoll, K. A., & Joiner, T. E. (2004). A standard of care for the assessment of suicide risk and associated treatment: The Florida State University Psychology Clinic as an example. *Journal of Contemporary Psychotherapy, 34*(1), 87–100. https://doi.org/10.1023/B:JOCP.0000010915.77490.71

Cullen, C. (2023). Method matters: The underreporting of intimate partner violence. *The World Bank Economic Review, 37*(1), 49–73. https://doi.org/10.1093/wber/lhac022

Culliford, L. (2002). Spirituality and clinical care. *British Medical Journal, 325*, 1413–1435.

Cully, J., LaVoie, D., & Gfeller, J. D. (2001). Reminiscence, personality, and psychological functioning in older adults. *Gerontologist, 41*(1), 89–95.

Cummock, V. (1996). Journey of a young widow. In K. J. Doka (Ed.), *Living with grief after sudden loss: Suicide, homicide, accident, heart attack, stroke* (pp. 1–10). Hospice Foundation of America.

Cunningham, M. (2000). Spirituality, cultural diversity and crisis intervention. *Crisis Intervention & Time-Limited Treatment, 6*(1), 65–77. https://doi.org/10.1080/10645130008951297

Cunningham, N. J., & Davis, B. (1999, April). *A study of middle school bullying using a framework for violence prevention.* Poster session at the American Counseling Association World Conference, San Diego, California, CA, the United States.

Cunradi, R. C., John Schafer, Carol B. (2007). Alcohol-related intimate partner violence among White, Black, and Hispanic couples in the United States. In *Domestic Violence*. Routledge.

Curran, D. K. (1987). *Adolescent suicidal behavior.* Hemisphere.

Curran, L. A. (2013). *101 trauma–informed interventions: Activities, exercises and assignments to move the client and therapy forward.* Pesi Publishing and Media.

Currier, J. M., Holland, J. M., & Neimeyer, R. A. (2007). The effectiveness of bereavement interventions with children: A meta-analytic review of controlled outcome research. *Journal of Clinical Child and Adolescent Psychology, 36*(2), 253–259.

Currier, J. M., Neimeyer, R. A., & Berman, J. S. (2008). The effectiveness of psychotherapeutic interventions for bereaved persons: A comprehensive quantitative review. *Psychological Bulletin, 134*(5), 648–661.

Cusack, K., Jonas, D. E., Forneris, C. A., Wines, C., Sonis, J., Middleton, J. C., Feltner, C., Brownley, K. A., Olmsted, K. R., Greenblatt, A., Weil, A., & Gaynes, B. N. (2016). Psychological treatments for adults with posttraumatic stress disorder: A systematic review and meta-analysis. *Clinical Psychology Review, 43*, 128–141. https://doi.org/10.1016/j.cpr.2015.10.003

Cusack, S. E., Ridings, L. E., Davidson, T. M., Espeleta, H. C., Wilson, D. A., & Ruggiero, K. J. (2023). Social support in relation to posttraumatic stress disorder symptoms among patients with violent versus nonviolent injury. *Psychological Trauma: Theory, Research, Practice, and Policy.* Advance online publication. https://dx.doi.org/10.1037/tra0001509

Cutajar, M. C., Ogloff, J. R. P., & Mullen, P. E. (2011). Child sexual abuse and subsequent offending and victimisation: A 45 year follow-up study. *Trends & Issues in Crime and Criminal Justice, 440*.

Cutler, D. L., Yeager, K. R., & Nunley, W. (2013). Crisis intervention and support. In K. R. Yeager, D. L. Cutler, D. Svendsen, & G. M. Sills (Eds.). *Modern community mental health: An interdisciplinary approach.* (pp. 243–255). Oxford.

Cybulski, L., Ashcroft, D. M., Carr, M. J., Garg, S., Chew-Graham, C. A., Kapur, N., & Webb, R. T. (2022). Risk factors for nonfatal self-harm and suicide among adolescents: Two nested case–control studies conducted in the U.K. Clinical Practice Research Datalink. *Journal of Child Psychology & Psychiatry, 63*(9), 1078–1088. https://doi.org/10.1111/jcpp.13552

Cypress, S., & Green, R. (2002). Preventing fatal shooting attacks in schools. *Global Visions for Counseling Professionals, 6*(1), 43–49.

Cyr, M., Frappier, J.-Y., Hébert, M., Tourigny, M., McDuff, P., & Turcotte, M.-E. (2018). Impact of child sexual abuse disclosure on the health of nonoffending parents: A longitudinal perspective. *Journal of Child Custody, 15*(2), 147–167. https://doi.org/10.1080/15379418.2018.1460649

Dagastino, A. (1984). *Crisis intervention series: Helping abused women in abuse centers and shelters* (Cassette Recording No. 4-1). Memphis State University Department of Counseling and Personnel Services.

Daggett, L. M. (2002). Living with loss: Middle-aged men face spousal bereavement. *Qualitative Health Research, 12*(5), 625–639.

Dahlenberg, C. J. (2000). *Countertransference and the treatment of trauma.* American Psychological Association.

Daigle, J. (2022), The school counselor's role in tier 3. *ASCA School Counselor, 60*(1), 26–29.

Dallos, R., & Vetere, A. (2009). *Systemic therapy and attachment narrative: Applications in a range of clinical settings.* Routledge/Taylor & Francis Group.

Dang, S. (1990). When the patient is out of control. *RN, 59*, 57–58.

Daniel, C. O. (2019). Effects of job stress on employee's performance. *International Journal of Business Management and Social Research, 6*(2), 375–382. https://doi.org/10.18801/ijbmsr.060219.40

Daniels, J. K., Lamke, J., Gaebler, M., Walter, H., & Scheel, M. (2013). White matter integrity and its relationship to PTSD and childhood trauma–A systematic review and meta-analysis. *Depression and Anxiety, 30*(3), 207–216.

Danielson, C. K., Hahn, A. M., Bountress, K. E., Adams, Z. W., Calhoun, C., Amstadter, A. B., & Thomas, S. (2021). Associations of subjective and objective stress responses with interpersonal trauma, PTSD, stress-induced drinking, and drinking to cope in young adults. *Psychology of Addictive Behaviors, 35*(1), 29–41. https://doi.org/10.1037/adb0000700

Danish, S. J. (1977). Human development and human services: A marriage proposal. In I. Iscoe, B. L. Bloom, & C. C. Speilberger (Eds.). *Community psychology in transition* (pp. 44–77). Halstead.

Dass-Brailsford, P. (2008). After the storm: Recognition, recovery and reconstruction. *Professional Psychology Research and Practice, 39*(1), 24–30.

Dass-Brailsford, P. (Ed.). (2010). *Crisis and disaster counseling: Lessons learned from Hurricane Katrina and other disasters.* SAGE.

Daugherty, L. M., Bolger, J. P., Preston, D. G., Jones, S. S., & Paynes, H. C. (1992). Effects of exposure to aggressive behavior on job satisfaction of healthcare staff. *Journal of Applied Gerontology, 11*, 160–172.

David-Ferdon, C., Vivolo-Kantor, A., Dahlberg, L., Marshall, L., Rainford, N., & Hall, J. (2016). *A comprehensive technical package for the prevention of youth violence and associated risk behaviors.* Division of Violence Prevention: Centers for Disease Control.

Davidson, J. R., & van der Kolk, B. A. (1996). The psychopharmacological treatment of posttraumatic stress disorder. In B. A. van der Kolk, A. C. McFarlane, & L. Weisaeth (Eds.), *Traumatic stress* (pp. 510–524). Guilford Press.

Davis, D. L. (2004). *Your angry child: A guide for parents.* Haworth Press.

Davis, E. B., Kimball, C. N., Aten, J. D., Andrews, B., Van Tongeren, D. R., Hook, J. N., Don, E. D., Granqvist, P., & Park, C. L. (2019). Religious meaning making and attachment in a disaster context: A longitudinal qualitative study of flood survivors. *The Journal of Positive Psychology, 14*(5), 659–671. https://doi.org/10.1080/17439760.2018.1519592

Davis, H. T., & Salasin, S. E. (1975). The utilization of evaluation. In E. L. Struening & M. Guttentag (Eds.), *Handbook of evaluation research* (Vol. 1, pp. 621–666). SAGE.

Davis, S., & Davis, L. (2003). *Schools where everyone belongs: Practical strategies for reducing bullying.* Stop Bullying Now.

Davis, W., Petrovic, L., Whalen, K., Danna, L., Zeigler, K., Brewton, A., Joseph, M., Baker, C. N., & Overstreet, S. (2022). Centering trauma-informed approaches in schools within a social justice framework. *Psychology in the Schools.* Wiley Online Library. https://doi.org/10.1002/pits.22664

Day, R. (2009). Counseling victims of intimate partner violence: Listening to the voices of clients—excerpts from a qualitative study. *Trauma Psychology Newsletter, 4*(3), 5–6.

Day, S. X., & Schneider, P. L. (2002). Psychotherapy using distance technology: A comparison of face-to-face, video, and audio treatment. *Journal of Counseling Psychology, 49*(4), 499–503.

Dayan, K., Fox, S., & Morag, M. (2013). Validation of spouse violence risk assessment inventory for police purposes. *Journal of Family Violence, 28*(8), 811–822.

Day-Vines, N. L., Wood, S. M., Grothaus, T., Craigen, L., Holman, A., Dotson-Blake, K., & Douglass, M. J. (2007). Broaching the subject of race, ethnicity, and culture during the counseling process. *Journal of Counseling & Development, 85*, 401–409.

Day-Vines, N., Day-Hairston, B. O., Carruthers, W. L., Wall, J. A., & Lupton-Smith, H. (1996). Conflict resolution: The value of diversity in the recruitment, selection, and training of peer mediators. *School Counselor, 43*, 393–410.

De Angelis, T. (2022, October). Helping children grieve, then thrive. *Monitor on Psychology,* 69–74.

De Diego-Cordero, R., Iglesias-Romo, M., Badanta, B., Lucchetti, G., & Vega-Escaño, J. (2022). Burnout and spirituality among nurses: A scoping review. *Explore, 18*(5), 612–620.

de Figueiredo, S., Yetwin, A., Shere, S., Radzik, M., & Iverson, E. (2014). A cross-disciplinary comparison of perceptions of compassion fatigue and satisfaction among service providers of highly traumatized children and adolescents. *Traumatology, 20*(4), 286–295.

De Moss, C. (2003, April). *Forgiveness—What's the secret?* Twenty-Seventh Convening of Crisis Intervention Personnel, Chicago, IL, the United States.

De Schrijver, L., Vander Beken, T., Krahé, B., & Keygnaert, I. (2018). Prevalence of sexual violence in migrants, applicants for international protection, and refugees in Europe: A critical interpretive synthesis of the evidence. *International Journal of Environmental Research and Public Health, 15*(9), Article 9. https://doi.org/10.3390/ijerph15091979

De Shazer, S. (1985). *Keys to solutions in brief therapy.* Norton.

De Shazer, S. (1994). *Words were originally magic.* Norton.

De Silva, S., Parker, A., Purcell, R., Callahan, P., Liu, P., & Hetrick, S. (2013). Mapping the evidence of prevention and intervention studies for suicidal and self-harming behaviors in young people. *The Journal of Crisis Intervention and Suicide Prevention, 34*(4), 223–232.

Deahl, M. (1999). Debriefing and body recovery: War grave soldiers. In B. Raphael & J. P. Wilson (Eds.), *Psychological debriefing: Theory, practice, and evidence* (pp. 108–117). Cambridge University Press.

DeAngelis, T. (2007). A new diagnosis for childhood trauma. *Monitor on Psychology, 38*(3), 32–33.

DeAngelis, T. (2009). Can Second Life therapy help with autism? *Monitor on Psychology, 40*(9), 40.

DeAngelis, T. (2011). Helping kids cope in an uncertain world. *Monitor on Psychology, 42*(8), 67–70.

DeAngeis, T. (2014). What every psychologist should know about disaster. *Monitor on Psychology, 45*(7), 62–65.

deArellano, M. A., Lyman, D., Jobes-Shields, L., George, P., Doougherty, R., Delphin-Rittmon, M. (2014). Trauma-focused cognitive behavioral therapy for children and adolescents: Assessing the evidence. *Psychiatric Services, 65*(5), 591–602.

Deaton, J., Wymer, B., & Carlson, R. (2021). Supervision strategies to facilitate vicarious post traumatic growth among trauma counselors. *Journal of Counselor Preparation and Supervision, 14*(4). https://digitalcommons.sacredheart.edu/jcps/vol14/iss4/12

Deblinger, E., Mannarino, A. P., Cohen, J. A., Runyon, M. K., & Heflin, A. H. (2015). *Child sexual abuse: A primer for treating children, adolescents, and their nonoffending parents.* Oxford University Press.

Deblinger, E., Pollio, E., & Dorsey, S. (2016). Applying trauma-focused cognitive–behavioral therapy in group format. *Child Maltreatment, 21*(1), 59–73. https://doi.org/10.1177/1077559515620668

deBont, P. A., van Minnen, A., & deJongh, A. (2013). Treating PTSD in patients with psychosis: A within group controlled feasibility study examining the efficacy and safety of evidence-based PE and EMDR protocols. *Behavior Therapy, 44*(4), 717–730.

Decker, J. T., Bailey, T. L., & Westergaard, N. (2002). Burnout among child care workers. *Residential Treatment for Children and Youth, 19*(4), 61–77.

Decker, J. T., Constantine, J. L., Ong, J., & Stiney-Ziskind, C. (2015). Mindfulness, compassion fatigue and compassion satisfaction among social work interns. *Social Work and Christianity, 42*(1), 28–42

DeCou, C. R., & Lynch, S. M. (2019). Emotional reactivity, trauma-related distress, and suicidal ideation among adolescent inpatient survivors of sexual abuse. *Child Abuse & Neglect, 89*, 155–164. https://doi.org/10.1016/j.chiabu.2019.01.012

Deisinger, E., & Scalora, M. (2016). Threat assessment and management in higher education in the United States: A review of the 10 years since the mass casualty incident at Virginia Tech. *Journal of Threat Assessment and Management 3*(3-4), 186v199. https://doi.org/10.1037/tam0000074

Deiter, P. J., & Pearlman, L. A. (1998). Responding to self-injurious behavior. In P. M. Kleespies (Ed.), *Emergencies in mental health practice: Evaluation and management* (pp. 235–257). Guilford Press.

Dejong, S. (2014). *Blogs and tweets, texting and friending: Social media and online professionalism in health care.* Elsevier Academic Press.

Delta Society (2023). Pet loss counselor directory. https://integrativeveterinaryhealthcenter.com/files/2016/10/Pet_Grief.pdf.

deMello, R. A. F., Coimbra, B. M., Pedro, B. D. M., Benvenutti, I. M., Yeh, M. S. L., Mello, A. F., Mello, M. F., & Poyares, D. R. (2023). Peri-traumatic dissociation and tonic immobility as severity predictors of posttraumatic stress disorder after rape.

Journal of Interpersonal Violence, 38(3–4), 4240–4266. https://doi.org/10.1177/08862605221114151

Dennis, H. (1978). Remotivation therapy groups. In I. M. Burnside (Ed.), *Working with the elderly: Group process and techniques* (pp. 219–235). Duxbury Press.

Dennis, H. (2013). Remotivation therapy for the elderly: A surprising outcome. *Journal of Gerontological Nursing, 2*(6), 28–30. https://doi.org/10.3928/0098-9134-19761101-07

Department of Homeland Security. (2008). *FEMA's crisis counseling assistance and training program: State of Florida Project Hope.* https://www.documentcloud.org/documents/241082-oig-08-96-femas-crisis-counseling-assistance-and.html

Department of Veterans Affairs & Department of Defense (2010). *VA/DoD clinical practice guideline for management of post-traumatic stress.* https://www.healthquality.va.gov/guidelines/mh/ptsd/cpg_ptsd-full-201011612.pdf

DePierro, J., D'Andrea, W., Spinazzola, J., Stafford, E., van Der Kolk, B., Saxe, G., Stolbach, B., McKernan, S., & Ford, J. D. (2022). Beyond PTSD: Client presentations of developmental trauma disorder from a national survey of clinicians. *Psychological Trauma: Theory, Research, Practice, and Policy, 14*(7), 1167–1174. https://doi.org/10.1037/tra0000532

Derkx, H., Rethans, J., Maiburg, B., Winkens, R., Muitiens, A., & van Rooii, H. (2009). Quality of communication during telephone triage at Dutch after-hours centres. *Patient Education and Counseling, 74*(2), 174–178.

Dershimer, R. A. (1990). *Counseling the bereaved.* Pergamon Press.

Deutsch, A.-M., & Lande, R. G. (2017). The reasons for living scale-military version: Assessing protective factors against suicide in a military sample. *Military Medicine, 182*(7), e1681–e1686. https://doi.org/10.7205/MILMED-D-16-00382

Devine, I. (1984). Organizational crisis and individual response: New trends for human service professionals (Special issue: Education and training in Canadian human services). *Canadian Journal of Community Mental Health, 3,* 63–72.

Devoe, E. R., Klein, T. P., Bannon, W. Jr., & Miranda-Julian, C. (2011). Young children in the aftermath of the World Trade Center attacks. *Psychological Trauma, Theory, Research, Practice, and Policy, 3,* 1–7.

deVries, F. (1998). To make a drama out of trauma is fully justified. *Lancet, 351,* 1579–1580.

deVries, M. W. (1996). Trauma in cultural perspective. In B. A. van der Kolk, A. C. McFarlane, & L. Weisaeth (Eds.). *Traumatic stress: The effects of overwhelming experience on mind, body, and society,* (pp. 398–413). Guilford Press.

Dewar, M., Paradis, A., & Brillon, P. (2023, May 1). Posttraumatic stress symptom profiles of aid workers: Identifying risk and protective factors. *Psychological Trauma: Theory, Research, Practice, and Policy.* Advance online publication. https://dx.doi.org/10.1037/tra0001512

Dewey, L., Allwood, N., Fava, J., Arias, E., Pinizzotto, A., & Schlesinger, L. (2013). Suicide by cop: Clinical risks and subtypes. *Archives of Suicide Research, 17*(4), 448–461.

Dewitt, M. (2019). Gang-associated youth avoid violence by acting tough online. *Stanford News.* https://news.stanford.edu/2019/05/01/gangs-use-social-media/

DeWolfe, D. J. (2000). *Training manual for mental health and human service workers in major disasters* (2nd ed.). DHHS Publication No. ADM 90-538. http://www.mentalhealth.org/publications/allpubs;ADM90-538/index.htm

Diamond, G., Diamond, G. M., & Levy, S. (2021). Attachment-based family therapy: Theory, clinical model, outcomes, and process research. *Journal of Affective Disorders, 294,* 286–295. https://doi.org/10.1016/j.jad.2021.07.005

Diamond, L. (2021) Recognize and address. *ASCA School Counselor, 59*(1), 10–13.

Diamond-Smith, N., Conroy, A. A., Tsai, A. C., Nekkanti, M., & Weiser, S. D. (2019). Food insecurity and intimate partner violence among married women in Nepal. *Journal of Global Health, 9*(1), 010412. https://doi.org/10.7189/jogh.09.010412

Dias, N., Friebert, S., Donelan, J., Schoemann, A. M., Morris, A., Guard, K., & Grossoehme, D. H. (2021). Bereaved parents' health outcomes following the death of their child. *Clinical Practice in Pediatric Psychology, 9*(3), 272–282. https://doi.org/10.1037/cpp0000414

Dickson, A., O'Brien, G., Ward, R., Allan, D., & O'Carroll, R. (2010). The impact of assuming the primary caregiver role following traumatic spinal cord injury: An interpretative phenomenological analysis of the spouse's experience. *Psychology & Health, 25*(9), 1101–1120.

DiClemente, C. C., & Prochaska, J. O. (1998). Toward a comprehensive, transtheoretical model of change: Stages of change and addictive behaviors. In W. R. Miller & N. Heather (Eds.), *Treating addictive behaviors* (pp. 3–24). Plenum Press. https://doi.org/10.1007/978-1-4899-1934-2_1

Diehl, J., Opmeer, B., Boer, F., Mannarino, A., & Lindauer, R. (2014, June). Trauma focused cognitive behavior therapy or eye movement desensitization and reprocessing: What works in children with posttraumatic stress symptoms? A randomized controlled trial. *European Child and Adolescent Psychiatry,* 5–15.

Dierkhising, C. B., Lane, A., & Natsuaki, M. N. (2014). Victims behind bars: A preliminary study of abuse during juvenile incarceration and post-release social and emotional functioning. *Psychology, Public Policy, and Law, 20*(2), 181–190. https://doi.org/10.1037/law0000002

Dillenburger, K., & McKerr, L. (2009). "40 years is an awful long time": Parents caring for adult sons and daughters with disabilities. *Behavior and Social Issues, 18,* 155–174.

DiMarco, D., Mizzoni, J., & Savitz, R. (2022). On the sexual assault of men. *Sexuality & Culture, 26*(2), 465–473. https://doi.org/10.1007/s12119-021-09901-1

Dingfelder, S. F. (2006). New needs in New Orleans schools. *Monitor on Psychology, 37*(6), 28–29.

Dingfelder, S. F. (2013). Predicting and preventing violence. *Monitor on Psychology 44*(3), 68.

Dinkmeyer, D. C., Pew, W. L., & Dinkmeyer, D. C., Jr. (1979). *Adlerian counseling and psychotherapy.* Brooks/Cole.

Distler, B. J. (1990, April). *Reducing the potential for burnout.* Paper presented at the Fourteenth Annual Convening of Crisis Intervention Personnel, Chicago, IL, the United States.

Doan, N., Patte, K., Ferro, M., & Leatherdale, S. (2020). Reluctancy towards help-seeking for mental health concerns at secondary schools among students in the COMPASS Study. *International Journal of Environmental Research & Public Health. 17*(19), 7128. http://doi.org/10.3390/ijerph17197128

Dodaj, A. (2020). Children witnessing domestic violence. *Journal of Children's Services, 15*(3), 161–174. https://doi.org/10.1108/JCS-04-2019-0023

Dodgen, D., & Meed, J. (2010). The federal government in disaster mental health response: An ever-evolving role.

In P. Dass-Brailsford (Ed.), *Crisis and disaster counseling: Lessons learned from Hurricane Katrina and other disasters* (pp. 181–195). SAGE.

Dogutas, C. (2008). Reactive vs. proactive strategies: The effectiveness of school resource officers to prevent violence in schools. *Section A: Humanities and Social Sciences 68*(10-A), 4470.

Doka, K. J. (1989). *Disenfranchised grief: Recognizing hidden sorrow.* D. C. Heath.

Doka, K. J. (1994). Disenfranchised grief. In L. A. DeSpelder & A. L. Strickland (Eds.), *The path ahead* (pp. 271–275). Mayfield.

Doka, K. J., & Davidson, J. D. (Eds.). (1998). *Living with grief: Who we are, how we grieve.* Hospice Foundation of America.

Dollard, J., Doob, L. W., Miller, N. E., Mower, O. H., & Sears, R. R. (1939). *Frustration and aggression.* Yale University Press.

Dollarhide, C. T. & Saginak, K. A. (2017). *Comprehensive school counseling programs: K-12 delivery systems in action.* Pearson.

Domenech Del Rio, I., & Sirvent Garcia Del Valle, E. (2017). The consequences of intimate partner violence on health: A further disaggregation of psychological violence—Evidence from Spain. *Violence Against Women, 23*(14), 1771–1789. https://doi.org/10.1177/1077801216671220

Domestic Abuse Intervention Programs. (n.d.). Duluth Family Visitation Center. *Domestic Abuse Intervention Programs.* https://www.theduluthmodel.org/duluth-family-visitation-center/

Domino, J. L., Whiteman, S. E., Davis, M. T., Witte, T. K., & Weathers, F. W. (2021). Sudden unexpected death as a traumatic stressor: The impact of the *DSM–5* revision of Criterion A for posttraumatic stress disorder. *Traumatology, 27*(2), 168–176. https://doi.org/10.1037/trm0000272

Doms, R. W. (1984). Personal distress devices for health care personnel. In J. T. Turner (Ed.), *Violence in the medical care setting: A survival guide* (pp. 225–229). Aspen Systems.

Donahue, H. H. (1965). Expanding the program. *Hospital and Community Psychiatry, 17*, 117–118.

Donahue, M. (2010). Investigating the grief process related to job loss. *Dissertation Abstracts International: Section B. The Sciences and Engineering,* 7850.

Donaldson, M. A., & Gardner, R., Jr. (1985). Diagnosis and treatment of traumatic stress among women after childhood incest. In C. R. Figley (Ed.), *Trauma and its wake: The study of post-trauma stress disorder* (pp. 356–377). NeBrunner/Mazel.

Donigan, R. (2017). *Bullying and cyberbullying.* Microsoft.NET

Doran, G., & Hansen, N. D. (2006). Constructions of Mexican American family grief after the death of a child: An exploratory study. *Cultural Diversity and Ethnic Minority Psychology, 12*(2), 199–211.

Dorn, F. J. (Ed.). (1986). *The social influence process in counseling and psychotherapy.* Charles C. Thomas.

Dorn, M., & Dorn, C. (2005). *Innocent targets when terrorism comes to school.* Safe Haven International.

dos Reis, S., Barnett, S. R., Love, L. C., Riddle, M. A., & Maryland Youth Practice Improvement Committee. (2003). A guide for managing acute aggression among youths. *Psychiatric Services, 54*(10), 1357–1363.

dos Santos, M. C. L., Giusti, B. B., Yamamoto, C. A., Ciosak, S. I., & Szylit, R. (2021). Suicide in the elderly: An epidemiologic study. *Revista Da Escola de Enfermagem Da USP, 55.* https://doi.org/10.1590/s1980-220x2019026603694

Doughty, E. A. (2009). Investigating adaptive grieving styles: A Delphi study. *Death Studies, 33*(5), 462–480.

Douglas, K. S., Nicholls, T. L., & Brink, J. (2009). Reducing the risk of violence among people with serious mental illness: A critical analysis of treatment approaches. In P. M. Kleespies (Ed.), *Behavioral emergencies: An evidence-based resource for evaluating and managing risk of suicide, violence, and victimization.* (pp. 351–376). American Psychological Association.

Douglas, K. S., Ogloff, J. R., & Hart, S. D. (2003). Evaluation of a model of violence risk assessment among forensic psychiatric patients. *Psychiatric Services, 54*(10), 1372–1379.

Douglas, K. S., Webster, C., Hart, S., Eaves, D., & Ogloff, J. (2001). *HCR-20 violence risk assessment companion guide.* Simon Fraiser University Mental Health, Law, and Policy Institute.

Doumas, D. M., Pearson, C. L., Elgin, J. E., & McKinley, L. L. (2008). Adult attachment as a risk factor for intimate partner violence: The "mispairing" of partners' attachment styles. *Journal of Interpersonal Violence, 23*(5), 616–634. https://doi.org/10.1177/0886260507313526

Dowgwillo, E. A., Ménard, K. S., Krueger, R. F., & Pincus, A. L. (2016). DSM-5 pathological personality traits and intimate partner violence among male and female college students. *Violence and Victims, 31*(3), 416–437. https://doi.org/10.1891/0886-6708.VV-D-14-00109

Drabek, T. E. (1986). *Human systems response to disaster: An inventory of sociological findings.* Springer.

Drapeau, M., & Perry, J. C. (2004). Interpersonal conflicts in borderline personality disorder: An exploratory study using the CCRT-LU. *Swiss Journal of Psychology, 63*(1), 53–57.

Draper, J., Murphy, G., Vega, E., Covington, D. W., & McKeon, R. (2015). Helping callers to the National Suicide Prevention Lifeline who are at imminent risk of suicide: The importance of active engagement, active rescue, and collaboration between crisis and emergency services. *Suicide and Life-Threatening Behavior, 45*, 261–270.

Draper, K., Siegel, C., White, J., Solis, C. M., & Mishna, F. (2009). Preschoolers, parents, and teachers (PPT): A preventive intervention with an at risk population. *International Journal of Group Psychotherapy, 59*(2), 221–242. https://doi.org/10.1521/ijgp.2009.59.2.221

Dreisbach, V. (2003). Post-traumatic stress disorder in fire and rescue personnel. *Journal of American Academy of Psychiatry & Law, 31*(1), 120–123.

Drescher, K., & Foy, D. W. (2010). When horror and loss intersect: Traumatic experience and traumatic bereavement. *Pastoral Psychology, 59*(2), 147–158.

Drogin, E. Y. (2019). *Ethical conflicts in psychology* (5th ed.). American Psychological Association. https://doi.org/10.1037/0000125-002

Drucker, K. (2001). Why can't she control herself? A case study. In J. Murphy (Ed.), *Art therapy with young survivors of sexual abuse: Lost for words* (pp. 101–125). Brunner-Routledge.

Dryden, W. (1984). *Rational emotive therapy: Fundamentals and innovations.* Croom Helm.

Dryden, W., & Neenan, W. M. (2004). *Counselling individuals: A rational emotive behavioural handbook* (4th ed.). Wiley.

Dubin, W. R. (1981). Evaluating and managing the violent patient. *Annals of Emergency Medicine, 10*, 481–484.

Dublin, L. I. (1969). Suicide prevention. In E. S. Shneidman (Ed.), *On the nature of suicide.* Jossey-Bass.

Ducharme, F., Couture, M., & Lamontange, J. (2012). Decision-making process of family caregivers regarding placement of a cognitively impaired elderly relative. *Home Health Care Services Quarterly, 31,* 197–218.

Duffey, T., & Haberstroh, S. (2020). Introduction to crisis and trauma counseling. In *Introduction to crisis and trauma counseling.* American Counseling Association.

Duffey, T., & Haberstroh, S. (2022). Multicultural and social justice counseling through relational-cultural theory. In D. Capuzzi & M. D. Stauffer (Eds.), *Counseling and Psychotherapy: Theories and Interventions* (7th ed.). (2022-40403-002, pp. 29–50). American Counseling Association.

Duffey, T., & Haberstroh, S. (Eds.). (2020). *Introduction to crisis and trauma counseling.* American Counseling Association.

Duncan, J. W., & Duncan, G. M. (1971). Murder in the family: A study of some homicidal adolescents. *American Journal of Psychiatry, 127*(11), 74–78.

Durivage, A. (1989). Assaultive behavior: Before it happens. *Canadian Journal of Psychiatry, 34*(5), 393–397.

Dutheil, F., Aubert, C., Pereira, B., Dambrun, M., Moustafa, F., Mermillod, M., Baker, J. S., Trousselard, M., Lesage, F.-X., & Navel, V. (2019). Suicide among physicians and healthcare workers: A systematic review and meta-analysis. *PLOS ONE, 14*(12), e0226361. https://doi.org/10.1371/journal.pone.0226361

Dutra, K., Preis, L. C., Caetano, J., dos Santos, J. L. G., & Lessa, G. (2018). Experiencing suicide in the family: From mourning to the quest for overcoming. *Revista Brasileira de Enfermagem, 71*(suppl 5), 2146–2153. https://doi.org/10.1590/0034-7167-2017-0679

Dutro, K. R. (1994, April). *A dynamic, structural model of grief.* Paper presented at the Eighteenth Annual Convening of Crisis Intervention Personnel, Chicago, IL, the United States.

Dutton, D. G. (1985). An ecologically nested theory of male violence towards intimates. *International Journal of Women's Studies, 8,* 404–413.

Dutton, D. G. (1995). *The domestic assault of women.* University of British Columbia Press.

Dutton, D. G., & Painter, S. (1993). Emotional attachments in abusive relationships: A test of traumatic bonding theory. *Violence and Victims, 8*(2), 105–120. https://doi.org/10.1891/0886-6708.8.2.105

Dutton, D. G., & Starzomski, A. (1993). Borderline personality organization in perpetrators of psychological and physical abuse. *Violence and Victims, 8*(4), 327–338.

Dutton, D. G., & White, K. R. (2012). Attachment insecurity and intimate partner violence. *Aggression and Violent Behavior, 17*(5), 475–481. https://doi.org/10.1016/j.avb.2012.07.003

Duval, A., Lanning, B. A., & Patterson, M. S. (2020). A systematic review of dating violence risk factors among undergraduate college students. *Trauma, Violence, & Abuse, 21*(3), 567–585. https://doi.org/10.1177/1524838018782207

Dwyer, K., Osher, D., & Warger, C. (1998). *Early warning, timely response: A guide to safe schools.* U.S. Department of Education.

Dyckman, J. (2011). Exposing the gloss in Seligman and Fowler's (2011) straw-man arguments. *American Psychologist, 66,* 644–645.

Dyer, J., & Stotts, M (Eds.). (2005). *Handbook of remotivation therapy.* Haworth Press.

Dyer, K. F. W., & Corrigan, J. P. (2021). Psychological treatments for complex PTSD: A commentary on the clinical and empirical impasse dividing unimodal and phase-oriented therapy

positions. *Psychological Trauma: Theory, Research, Practice, and Policy, 13*(8), 869–876. https://doi.org/10.1037/tra0001080

Dyer, W. O., Murrell, D. S., & Wright, D. (1984). Training for hospital security: An alternative to training negligence suits. In J. T. Turner (Ed.), *Violence in the medical care setting: A survival guide* (pp. 1–18). Aspen Systems.

Dykeman, C. (1999, June). *Preventing school-based violence: Practical steps for school counselors.* Paper presented at the American School Counselor Association Convention, Phoenix, AZ, the United States.

Dyregrov, A. (1997). The process in psychological debriefings. *Journal of Traumatic Stress, 10,* 589–605.

Dyregrov, A., Gupta, L., Gjestad, R., & Raundalen, M. (2002). Is the culture always right? *Traumatology, 8,* 1–10.

Dyregrov, K., & Dyregrov, A. (2008). *Effective grief and bereavement support: Friends, colleagues, schools, and support professionals.* Jessica Kingsley.

Dziegielewski, S. F., & Powers, G. T. (2005). Designs and procedures for evaluating crisis intervention. In A. R. Roberts (Ed.), *Crisis intervention handbook* (3rd ed., pp. 742–773). Oxford University Press.

Dziegielewski, S. F., & Sumner, K. (2005). An examination of the U.S. response to bioterrorism: Handling the threat and aftermath through crisis intervention. In A. R. Roberts (Ed.), *Crisis intervention handbook* (3rd ed., pp. 262–290). Oxford University Press.

East, T. W., James, R. K., & Keim, J. (2001, April). *The best little vicarious trauma prevention program in Tennessee.* Paper presented at the Twenty-Fifth Annual Convening of Crisis Intervention Personnel, Chicago, IL, the United States.

Eastwood, C. D. (2007). Compassion fatigue risk and self-care practices among residential treatment center childcare workers. *Dissertation Abstract International: Section B. The Sciences and Engineering, 67*(10), 2645.

Ebersole, P. P. (1978a). A theoretical approach to the use of reminiscence. In I. M. Burnside (Ed.), *Working with the elderly: Group process and techniques* (pp. 139–154). Duxbury Press.

Ebersole, P. P. (1978b). Establishing reminiscence groups. In I. M. Burnside (Ed.), *Working with the elderly: Group process and techniques* (pp. 236–254). Duxbury Press.

Echterling, L. G., & Stewart, A. (2008). Creative crisis intervention techniques with children and families. In C. A. Malchiodi (Ed.), *Creative interventions with traumatized children* (pp. 189–210). Guilford Press.

Echterling, L. G., & Wylie, M. L. (1999). In the public arena: Disaster as a socially constructed problem. In R. Gist & B. Lubin (Eds.), *Response to disaster: Psychosocial, community, and ecological approaches* (pp. 327–352). Brunner/Mazel.

Echterling, L. G., McKee, E. J., & Presbury, J. (2000, March). *Resolution-focused crisis debriefing for traumatized groups.* Paper presented at the American Counseling Association Conference, Washington, D.C., the United States.

Eck, J. E., & Spelman, W. (1987). *Problem-solving: Problem-oriented policing in Newport News.* Police Executive Research Forum.

Eckardt, M. H. (2011). The use of the telephone to extend our therapeutic availability. *Journal of the American Academy of Psychoanalysis Dynamic Psychiatry, 39*(1), 151–154.

Eckhardt, C. I., Samper, R. E., & Murphy, C. M. (2008). Anger disturbances among perpetrators of intimate partner violence: Clinical characteristics and outcomes of court-mandated treatment. *Journal of Interpersonal Violence, 23*(11), 1600–1617. https://doi.org/10.1177/0886260508314322

Ecks, S. (2016). The strange absence of things in the "culture" of the DSM-V. *CMAJ : Canadian Medical Association Journal, 188*(2), 142–143. https://doi.org/10.1503/cmaj.150268

ECNP. (2022). Ukraine crisis. Network for Traumatic Stress. https://www.ecnp.eu

Ectherling, L. G., Presbury, J. H., & McKee, J. E. (2005). *Crisis intervention: Promoting resilience and resolution in troubled times.* Pearson.

Eddy, S. (1998). Risk management with the violent patient. In P. M. Kleespies (Ed.), *Emergencies in mental health practice: Evaluation and management* (pp. 217–231). Guilford Press.

Edelstein, L. (1984). *Maternal bereavement: Coping with the unexpected death of a child.* Praeger.

Edelwich, J., & Brodsky, A. (1982). Training guidelines: Linking the workshop experience to needs on and off the job. In W. S. Paine (Ed.), *Job stress and burnout* (pp. 133–154). SAGE.

Edwards, S. M. (1989). *Policing domestic violence: Women, the law, and the state.* SAGE.

EdWeek Research Center. (2018, June). School policing: Results of a national survey of school resource officers. https://www.edweek.org/research-center/research-center-reports/school-policing-results-of-a-national-survey-of-school-resource-officers

Efrid, D. M. (2013). Address anger management. *ASCA School Counselor, 51*(2), 22–27.

Egan, G. (1975). *The skilled helper: A model for systematic helping and interpersonal relating.* Wadsworth Publishing Company.

Egan, G. (1982). *The skilled helper: Model, skills, and methods for effective helping* (2nd ed.). Brooks/ Cole.

Egan, G. (1986). *The skilled helper: A systematic approach to effective helping* (3rd ed.). Brooks/Cole.

Egan, G. (1990). *The skilled helper: A systematic model for effective helping* (4th ed.). Thomson Brooks/Cole Publishing Co.

Egan, S. J., van Noort, E., Chee, A., Kane, R. T., Hoiles, K. J., Shafan, R., & Wade, T. D. (2014*).* A randomized controlled trial of face to face versus pure online self-help cognitive behavioural treatment for perfectionism. *Behavior Research and Therapy, 63,* 107–113.

Egendorf, A. (1975). A Vietnam veteran rap group and themes of post-war life. *Journal of Social Issues, 31,* 111–124.

Ehrensaft, M. K., Knous-Westfall, H., & Cohen, P. (2017). Long-term influence of intimate partner violence and parenting practices on offspring trauma symptoms. *Psychology of Violence, 7*(2), 296–305. https://doi.org/10.1037/a0040168

Eidelson, R. J., & Eidelson, J. I. (2003). Dangerous ideas: Five beliefs that propel groups toward conflict. *American Psychologist, 58,* 182–192.

Eidelson, R. J., D'Alessio, G. R., & Eidelson, J. I. (2003). The impact of September 11 on psychologists. *Professional Psychology: Research and Practice, 34*(2), 144–150.

Eidelson, R., Pilisuk, M., & Soldz, S. (2011). The dark side of Comprehensive Soldier Fitness. *American Psychologist, 66,* 643–644.

Eisel v. Board of Education of Montgomery County, 597 A.2d 447 (Maryland, 1991).

El Frenn, V., Halit, S. Obeid, S., & Soufia, M. (2022, May). Association of the time spent on social media news with depression and suicide ideation among a sample of Lebanese adults during the COVID-19 pandemic and the Lebanese economic crisis. *Current Psychology: A Journal for Diverse Perspectives on Diverse Psychological Issues,* 1–13. http://doi.org/10.1007/s12144-022-03148-1

El Ghaziri, M., Zhu, S., Lipscom, J., & Smith, B. (2014). Work schedule and client characteristics associated with workplace violence experience among nurses and midwives in sub-Sahara Africa. *JANAC: Journal of the Association of Nurses in AIDS Care, 25*(1,Suppl), S79–S89.

Elbaz, S., Richards, J. B., & Provost Savard, Y. (2022, May 23). Teleworking and work-life balance during the COVID-19 pandemic: A scoping review. *Canadian Psychology/Psychologie.* Advance online publication. http://dx.doi.org/10.1037/cap0000330

Eliason, G., LaPore, M., & Myer, R. A., (2008). The historical advancement of grief counseling. In A. Tomer, G. Eliason, & T. P. Wong. (Eds.). *Existential and spiritual issues in death attitudes* (pp. 417–438). Lawrence Earlbaum.

Ellis, A. (1971). *Growth through reason.* Wilshire Books.

Ellis, A. (1973). *Humanistic psychology: The rational-emotive approach.* Julian.

Ellis, A. (1974). *Humanistic psychotherapy: The rational-emotive approach.* McGraw Hill.

Ellis, A. E. (1962). *Reason and emotion in psychotherapy.* Lyle Stuart.

Ellis, A. E. (1982). Major systems. *Personnel and Guidance Journal, 61,* 6–7.

Ellis, A., & Abrahms, E. (1978). *Brief psychotherapy in medical and health practice.* Springer.

Ellis, A., & Dryden, W. (1977). *The practice of rational emotive behavior therapy.* Springer

Ellis, A., & Grieger, R. (1977). *Handbook of rational-emotive therapy.* Springer.

Ellis, A., & Harper, R. A. (1975). *A new guide to rational living* (rev. ed.). Wilshire Books.

Ellis, H. A. (2014). Effects of a Crisis Intervention Team (CIT) training program upon police officers before and after Crisis Intervention Team training. *Archives of Psychiatric Nursing, 28*(1), 10–18.

Elwert, F., & Christakis, N. A. (2006). Widowhood and race. *American Sociological Review, 71*(1), 16–41.

Elwert, F., & Christakis, N. A. (2008). The effect of widowhood on mortality by the causes of death of both spouses. *American Journal of Public Health, 98*(11), 2092–2098.

Emanuel, L., Taylor, L., Hain, A., Combes, J., Hatline, M., Karsh, B., Law, P., Shalowitz, J., Shaw, T., & Walton, M (Eds.). (2013). *The patient safety education program module 13: Mental health care- An introduction to patient safety issues.* Canadian Patient Safety Institute. https://www.patientsafetyinstitute.ca/en/education/PatientSafetyEducationProgram/PatientSafetyEducationCurriculum/MentalHealthModules/Pages/Mental-Health-Care-An-Introduction-to-Patient-Safety-Issues.aspx

Engel, J. L., & Follette, V., (2012). Acceptance and commitment therapy for trauma related problems. In R. A. McMackin, E. Newman, J. M. Fogler, & T. M. Keane (Eds.), *Trauma therapy in context: the science and craft of evidence – based practice.* (pp. 353–372). American Psychological Association.

Engel, R. C., Gallagher, L. B., & Lyle, D. S. (2010). Military deployments and children's academic achievement: Evidence from Department of Defense education activity schools. *Economics of Education Review, 29,* 73–82.

Englehardt, C. R., Bartholow, B. D., Kerr, G., & Bushman, B. (2011). This is your brain on violent video games: Neural desensitization to violence predicts increased aggression following violent video game exposure. *Journal of Experimental Social Psychology, 31*(4), 35–47.

Epstein, M., & Carter, L. (1988). *Training manual for Headquarters staff*. Headquarters.

Epstein, M., & Carter, L. (1991). *Headquarters training manual*. Lawrence, KS: Headquarters Crisis Center.

Epstein, R., Fullerton, C., & Ursano, R. (1998). Posttraumatic stress disorder following an air disaster: A prospective study. *American Journal of Psychiatry, 155*(7), 934–938.

Erbacher, T., Singer, J., & Poland, S. (2015). *Suicide in schools*. Routledge. https://doi.org/10.4324/9780203702970

Erdmann, A., & Schnepp, W. (2016). Conditions, components, and outcomes of Integrative Validation Therapy in a long-term care facility for people with dementia. A qualitative evaluation study. *Dementia. 15*(5), 1184–1204. https://doi.org/10.1177/1471301214556489

Erdur-Baker, O., Aberson, C., Barrow, J., & Draper, M. (2006). Nature and severity of college students' psychological concerns: A comparison of clinical and nonclinical national samples. *Professional Psychology: Research and Practice, 37*(3), 317–323.

Erickson, K. A., Jonnson, M., Langille, J. I., & Walsh, Z. (2017). Victim gender, rater attitudes, and rater violence history influence perceptions of intimate partner violence. *Violence and Victims, 32*(3), 533–544. https://doi.org/10.1891/0886-6708.VV-D-15-00086

Erikson, E. (1968). *Identity, youth, and crisis*. Norton.

Erikson, E. H. (1963). *Childhood and society* (2nd ed.). Norton.

Erikson, K. T. (1976). *Everything in its path: Destruction of community in the Buffalo Creek flood*. Simon & Schuster.

Erstling, S. (2006). Police and mental health collaborative outreach. *Psychiatric Services, 57*(3), 417–418.

Espelage, D., & Swearer, S. (2003). Research on school bullying and victimization: What have we learned and where do we go from here? *School Psychology Review, 32*(3), 365–384.

Espelage, D., Bosworth, K., & Simon, T. R. (2000). Examining the social context of bullying behaviors in early adolescence. *Journal of Counseling & Development, 78*(3), 326–333.

ESTSS. (2022). *European Society for Traumatic Stress Studies: Join now*. https://est.org/member

Eth, S., & Pynoos, R. S. (1985). Developmental perspective on psychic trauma in childhood. In C. R. Figley (Ed.), *Trauma and its wake: The study of post-trauma stress disorder* (pp. 36–52). Brunner/Mazel.

Evans, B. (2003). Hypnosis for post-traumatic stress disorders. *Australian Journal of Clinical & Experimental Hypnosis, 31*(1), 54–73.

Evans, R. E., & Petter, S. (2012). Identifying mitigating and challenging beliefs in dealing with threatening patients: An analysis of experiences of clinicians working in a psychiatric intensive care unit. *Journal of Psychiatric Intensive Care 8*(2), 113–119.

Everly, G. S., Jr. (1989). *A clinical guide to the treatment of the human stress response*. Plenum.

Everly, G. S., & Flynn, B. W. (2005). Principles and procedures of acute psychological first aid training for personnel without mental health experience. *International Journal of Emergency Mental Health, 8*(2), 93–100.

Everstine, D. S., & Everstine, E. (2006). *Strategic interventions for people in crisis, trauma, and disaster-revised edition*. Routledge.

Everstine, L. (1998). *The anatomy of suicide: Silence of the heart*. Charles C. Thomas.

Fairbank, J. A., & Keane, T. M. (1982). Flooding for combat-related stress disorders: Assessment of anxiety reduction across traumatic memories. *Behavior Therapy, 13*(4), 499–510.

Fairbank, J. A., Briggs, E. C., Carmody, K .A., Greeson, J., & Woods, B. A. (2014). Children. In L. A. Zoellner & N. C. Feeny (Eds.), *Facilitating resilience and recovery following trauma.* (pp. 91–112). Guilford Press.

Falco, A., Piccirelli, A., Girardi, D., Di Sipio, A., & De Carlo, N. (2014). "The best or nothing": The mediating role of workaholism in the relationship between perfectionism and burnout. *TMP—Testing, Psychometrics, Methodology in Applied Psychology, 21*(2), 213–232.

Falcus, C., & Johnson, D. (2018). The violent accounts of men diagnosed with comorbid antisocial and borderline personality disorders. *International Journal of Offender Therapy and Comparative Criminology, 62*(9), 2817–2830. https//doi.org/10.1177/0306624X17735254

Fanany, R., & Fananay, I. (2013). Post-disaster coping in Aceh: Sociocultural factors and emotional response. In C. Banwell, S. Uijaszek, & J. Dixon (Eds.), *When culture impacts health: Global lessons for effective health research* (pp. 225–235). Elsevier Academic Press

Farber, B. A. (Ed.). (1983). *Stress and burnout in the human service professions*. Pergamon Press.

Farberow, N. L., & Frederick, C. J. (1978). *Training for human service workers in major disasters*. National Institute of Mental Health.

Fareta, G. (1981). A profile of aggression from adolescence to adulthood: An 18-year follow-up of psychiatrically disturbed and violent adolescents. *American Journal of Orthopsychiatry, 51*, 439–453.

Farina, A. (2000). The few gains and many losses for those stigmatized by psychiatric disorder. In J. H. Harvey & E. D. Miller (Eds.), *Loss and trauma: General and close relationship perspectives* (pp. 183–207). Brunner-Routledge.

Fariña, F., Arce, R., Vilariño, M., & Novo, M. (2014). Assessment of the standard forensic procedure for the evaluation of psychological injury in intimate-partner violence. *The Spanish Journal of Psychology, 17*, 1–10. https://doi.org/10.1017/sjp.2014.30

Farm Family Resource Initiative. (April, 2023). https://www.siumed.edu/farm

Farmani, A., Rahimianbougar, M., Mohammadi, Y., Faramarzi, H., Khodarahimi, S., & Nahaboo, S. (2023). Psychological, structural, social and economic determinants of suicide attempt: Risk assessment and decision making strategies. *Omega: Journal of Death & Dying, 86*(4), 1144–1166. https://doi.org/10.1177/00302228211003462

Farrell, A. D., & Camou, S. (2006). School-based interventions for youth violence prevention. In J. R. Lutzker (Ed.), *Preventing violence: Research and evidence-based intervention strategies* (pp. 125–146). American Psychological Association.

Faschingbauer, T., Zisook, S., & DeVaul, R. (1987). *The Texas Revised Inventory of Grief*. In S. Zisook (Ed.), *Biopsychosocial aspects of bereavement* (pp. 111–124). American Psychiatric Press.

Fatum, W. R., & Hoyle, J. C. (1996). Is it violence? School violence from the student perspective: Trends and interventions. *School Counselor, 44*(1), 28–34.

Fauteux, K. (2010). De-escalating angry and violent clients. *American Journal of Psychotherapy, 64*(2), 195–213.

FBI. (n.d.). Gangs. https://www.fbi.gov/investigate/violent-crime/gangs

Feather, K. & Bordonada, T. (2019, January). Leading an anti-bullying intervention for students with disabilities. *Counseling Today*. 38–43.

Federal Bureau of Investigation. (2002, June). *Workplace violence symposium.* www.fbi.gov/stats-services/publications/workplace-violence

Federal Bureau of Investigation. (2009, February 6). The gang threat. www.fbi.gov/news/stories/2009/february/ngta_020609

Federal Emergency Management Agency. (n.d.). *History of FEMA.* www.fema.gov

Federal Emergency Management Agency (2023). *Introduction to Community Emergency Response Team.* https://training.fema.gov/is/courseoverview.aspx?code=IS-317.a&lang=en

Feeny, N., Hembree, E., & Zoellner, L. (2003). Myths regarding exposure therapy for PTSD. *Cognitive & Behavioral Practice, 10*(1), 85–90.

Feil, N. (1982). *Validation: The Feil method.* Edward Feil Productions.

Feil, N. (1999). Current concepts and techniques in validation therapy. In M. Duffy (Ed.), *Handbook of counseling and psychotherapy with older adults.* (pp. 590–613). John Wiley & Sons.

Feil, N., & Altman, R. (2004). Validation theory and the myth of the therapeutic lie. *American Journal of Alzheimer's Disease and Other Dementias, 19*(2), 77–78.

Feil, N. & deKlerk-Rubin, V. (2012). *The validation breakthrough: Simple communication techniques with people with Alzheimer's and other dementias* (3rd ed.). U.S. Health Professions.

Fein, A. H., Carlisle, C. S., & Issacson, N. S. (2008). School shootings and counselor leadership: Four lessons from the field. *Professional School Counseling, 11*(4), 246–252.

Fein, R. A., Vossekuil, B., Pollack, W. S., Borum, M., Modzeleski, W., & Reddy, M. (2002). *Threat assessment in schools: A guide to managing threatening situations and creating safe school climates.* U.S. Secret Service and U.S. Department of Education.

Feinberg, M. E., Mogle, J. A., Lee, J. K., Tornello, S. L., Hostetler, M. L., Cifelli, J. A., Bai, S., & Hotez, E. (2022). Impact of the COVID-19 pandemic on parent, child, and family functioning. *Family Process, 61*(1), 361–374. https://doi.org/10.1111/famp.12649

Feindler, E. L., & Scalley, M. (1998). Adolescent anger management for violence reduction. In K. C. Stoiber & T. R. Kratochwill (Eds.), *Handbook of group intervention for children and families* (pp. 100–119). Allyn & Bacon.

Feindler, E. L., & Weisner, S. (2006). Youth anger management treatments for school violence prevention. In S. R. Jimerson & M. Furlong (Eds.), *Handbook of school violence and school safety: From research to practice* (pp. 353–363). Erlbaum.

Feldman, G., Hayes, A., Kumar, S., Greeson, J., & Laurenceau, J. P. (2006). Mindfulness and emotion regulation: The development and initial validation of the Cognitive and Affective Mindfulness Scale- Revised (CAMS-R). *Journal of Psychopathology and Behavioral Assessment, 29,* 177–190. http://dx.doi.org/10.1007/s10862-006-9035-8

Feldman, T. R., Carlson, C. L., Rice, L. K., Kruse, M. I., Beevers, C. G., Telch, M. J., & Josephs, R. A. (2021). Factors predicting the development of psychopathology among first responders: A prospective, longitudinal study. *Psychological Trauma: Theory, Research, Practice, and Policy, 13*(1), 75–83. https://doi.org/10.1037/tra0000957

Felix, E. D., Meskunas, H. M., Jaramillo, N., & Quirk, M. (2020). Measuring media exposure to acute mass violence. *Psychological Trauma: Theory, Research, Practice, and Policy, 12*(4), 397–404. https://doi.org/10.1037/tra0000514

Felix, E., Afifi, T., Kia-Keating, M., Brown, L., Afifi, W., & Reyes, G. (2015). Family functioning and posttraumatic growth among parents and youth following wildfire disasters. *American Journal of Orthopsychiatry, 85,* 191–200.

Felthous, A. R. (1987). Liability of treaters for injuries to others: Erosion of three immunities. *Bulletin of the American Academy of Psychiatry and the Law, 15,* 115–125.

Felthous, A. R., & Kellert, S. (1986). Violence against animals and people: Is aggression against living creatures generalized? *Bulletin of the American Academy of Psychiatry and Law, 14*(1), 55–69.

Felton, T., Coates, L., & Christopher, J. (2015). Impact of mindfulness training on counseling students' perceptions of stress. *Mindfulness, 6*(2), 159–169.

Fenelon, D. A. (1990, April). *Recognizing and dealing with the bogus sex caller.* Paper presented at the Fourteenth Annual Convening of Crisis Intervention Personnel, Chicago, IL, the United States.

Ferguson, C. E., & Malouff, J. M. (2016). Assessing police classifications of sexual assault reports: A meta-analysis of false reporting rates. *Archives of Sexual Behavior, 45*(5), 1185–1193. https://doi.org/10.1007/s10508-015-0666-2

Ferguson, C. J. (2011). Video games and youth violence: A prospective analysis in adolescents. *Journal of Youth and Adolescence, 40*(4), 377–391.

Ferguson, C. J., & Kilburn, J. (2009). The public health risks of media violence: A meta-analytic review. *Journal of Pediatrics, 154*(5), 759–763.

Ferguson, C. J., & Kilburn, J. (2010). Much ado about nothing: The misestimation and overinterpretation of violent video game effects in Eastern and Western nations: Comment on Anderson et al., 2010. *Psychological Bulletin, 136*(2), 174–178.

Ferguson, C. J., Colwell, J., Mlacic, B., Milas, G., & Miklousic, I. (2011). Personality and media influences on violence and depression in a cross-national sample of young adults: Data from Mexican-Americans, English and Croatians. *Computers in Human Behavior, 27*(3), 1195–1200.

Ferguson, C. J., Copenhaver, A., & Markey M. P. (2020). Reexamining the findings of the American Psychological Association's 2015 task force on violent media: A meta-analysis. *Perspectives on Psychological Science, 15*(6), 22–33. https://doi.org/10.1177/1745691620927666

Fernández-Cabana, M., Ceballos-Espinoza, F., Mateos, R., Alves-Pérez, M. T., & García-Caballero, A. A. (2015). Suicide notes: Clinical and linguistic analysis from the perspective of the interpersonal theory of suicide. *The European Journal of Psychiatry, 29*(4), 293–308. https://doi.org/10.4321/S0213-61632015000400006

Fernández-Planells, A., Orduña-Malea, E., & Feixa Pàmpols, C. (2021). Gangs and social media: A systematic literature review and an identification of future challenges, risks and recommendations. *New Media & Society, 23*(7), 2099–2124. https://doi.org/10.1177/1461444821994490

Ferraro, K. J. (2017). *Current research on batterer intervention programs and implications for policy.* The Battered Women's Justice Project. https://bwjp.org/assets/batterer-intervention-paper-final-2018.pdf

Fidan, A., & Bui, H. N. (2016). Intimate partner violence against women in Zimbabwe. *Violence Against Women, 22*(9), 1075–1096. https://doi.org/10.1177/1077801215617551

Fields, L., Young, D. A., Patel, A. R., Munroe, C., Shumway, M., Bell, S., & Richer, L. A. (2022). Drug-facilitated sexual assault, impaired trauma memory, and implications for mental health treatment: *European Journal of Psychotraumatology, 13*(1), 1–16. https://doi.org/10.1080/20008198.2022.2057165

Fiese, B., Celano, M., Deater-Deckard, K. Joouriles, E., & Whisman, M. (Eds.). (2019). *APA handbook of contemporary family psychology: Foundations, methods, and contemporary issues across the lifespan.* American Psychological Association. https://doi.org/10.1037/0000099-000

Figley, C. R. (Ed.). (1978). *Stress disorder among Vietnam veterans.* Brunner/Mazel.

Figley, C. R. (Ed.). (1985). *Trauma and its wake: The study of post-trauma stress disorder.* Brunner/Mazel.

Figley, C. R. (1985). From individual to survivor: Social responsibility in the wake of catastrophe. In C. R. Figley (Ed.), *Trauma and its wake: The study of post-trauma stress disorder* (pp. 398–416). Brunner/Mazel.

Figley, C. R. (1988). Post-traumatic family therapy. In F. M. Ochberg (Ed.), *Posttraumatic therapy and individuals of violence* (pp. 83–113). Brunner/Mazel.

Figley, C. R. (1989) *Helping traumatized families.* Jossey-Bass.

Figley, C. R. (1990). *Posttraumatic stress disorder: Managing bad memories in individuals and family systems* (National teleconference). Tallahassee, Florida State University, School of Social Work.

Figley, C. R. (1995). Compassion fatigue: Toward a new understanding of the costs of caring. In *Secondary traumatic stress: Self-care issues for clinicians, researchers, and educators* (pp. 3–28). The Sidran Press.

Figley, C. R. (Ed.). (1995). *Compassion fatigue: Coping with secondary traumatic stress disorder in those who treat the traumatized.* Brunner-Mazel.

Figley, C. R. (1996). Traumatic death: Treatment implications. In K. J. Doka (Ed.), *Living with grief after sudden loss: Suicide, homicide, accident, heart attack, stroke* (pp. 91–102). Hospice Foundation of America.

Figley, C. R. (2002). Compassion fatigue: Psychotherapists' chronic lack of self care. *Journal of Clinical Psychology, 58*(11), 1433–1441. https://doi.org/10.1002/jclp.10090

Fine, R. (1973). Psychoanalysis. In R. J. Corsini (Ed.), *Current psychotherapies* (pp. 1–33). F. E. Peacock.

Fink, D. S., Santaella-Tenorio, J., & Keyes, K. M. (2018). Increase in suicides the months after the death of Robin Williams in the US. *PLOS ONE, 13*(2), e0191405. https://doi.org/10.1371/journal.pone.0191405

Finkbeiner, A. K. (1998). *After the death of a child: Living with loss through the years.* Johns Hopkins University Press.

Finkelhor, D., Gelles, R. J., Hotaling, G. T., & Straus, A. A. (Eds.). (1983). *The dark side of families.* SAGE.

Finkelhor, D., Shattuck, A., Turner, H. A., & Hamby, S. L. (2014). The lifetime prevalence of child sexual abuse and sexual assault assessed in late adolescence. *Journal of Adolescent Health, 55*(3), 329–333. https://doi.org/10.1016/j.jadohealth.2013.12.026

Finn, P. (2006). School resource officer programs: Finding the funding, reaping the benefits. *Law Enforcement Bulletin, 75*(8), 1–7.

Finn, P., Townsend, M., Shiveley, M., & Rich, T. (2005). *A guide to developing, maintaining, and succeeding with your school resource officer program: Practices from the field for law enforcement and school administration.* A report submitted to the U.S. Department of Justice Office of Community Oriented Policing Services. Abt Associates.

Fisch, R., Weakland, J. H., & Segal, L. (1983). *The tactics of change.* Jossey-Bass.

Fishbain, D. A., Cutler, R. B., Rosomoff, H. L., & Steele-Rosomoff, R. (2000). Risk for violent behavior in patients with chronic pain: Evaluation and management in the pain facility setting. *Pain Medicine, 1*(2), 140–155.

Fisher, B., Mowen, T., & Boman, J. (2020). School security measures and longitudinal trends in adolescents' experiences of victimization. *Journal of Youth and Adolescence, 49*(9), 1940–1941. https://doi.org/ 10.1007/s10964-020-01286-y

Fisher, C. B., & Fried, A. L. (2003). Internet-mediated psychological services and the American Psychological Association Ethics Code. *Psychotherapy: Theory, Research, Practice, Training, 40*(1/2), 86–93.

Fisher, E. M., & Stylianou, A. M. (2019). To stay or to leave: Factors influencing victims' decisions to stay or leave a domestic violence emergency shelter. *Journal of Interpersonal Violence, 34*(4), 785–811. https://doi.org/10.1177/0886260516645816

Fitzpatrick, S. J. (2022). The moral and political economy of suicide prevention. *Journal of Sociology, 58*(1), 113–129. https://doi.org/10.1177/14407833211001112

Flack, W., Litz, B., Weathers, F., & Beaudreau, S. (2002). Assessment and diagnosis of PTSD in adults: A comprehensive psychological approach. In M. Williams & J. Sommer (Eds.), *Simple and complex post-traumatic stress disorder: Strategies for comprehensive treatment in clinical practice* (pp. 9–22). Haworth Press.

Flake, E. M., Davis, B. E., Johnson, P. L., & Middleton, L. S. (2009). The psychosocial effects of deployment on military children. *Journal of Developmental and Behavioral Pediatrics, 30,* 271–278.

Flannery, M. (2020). Are you thinking about suicide? *NEA Today, 38*(3), 34–37.

Flannery, M.E. (2023). The mental health crisis on college campuses. *NEA Today,* 24.

Flannery, R. (2009). *The violent person: Professional risk management strategies for safety and care.* American Mental Health Foundation Books.

Flannery, R. B. Jr. & Everly, G. S. (2000). Crisis intervention: A review. *International Journal of Emergency Mental Health, 2*(2), 119–125.

Flannery, R., Fulton, P., Tausch, J. M., & DeLoffi, A. (1991). A program to help staff cope with psychological sequelae of assaults by patients. *Hospital and Community Psychiatry, 42,* 935–938.

Flannery, R., Le Vitre, V., Rego, S., & Walker, P. (2011). Characteristics of staff victims of psychiatric patient assaults: 20-year analysis of the Assaulted Staff Action Program. *Psychiatric Quarterly, 82*(1), 11–21.

Flemons, D., & Grainik, L. (2013). *Relational suicide assessment: Risks, resources, and possibilities for safety.* W. W. Norton.

Florida Emergency Preparedness Association (2023). *Certification requirements.* https://www.fepa.org/certification

Flynn, B. W. (1998, April). *Terrorist events using weapons of mass destruction: Confronting the mental health consequences.* Paper presented at the Third Harvard Symposium on Complex Humanitarian Disasters, Disaster Medical Response: Current Challenges and Strategies, Boston, MA, the United States.

Flynn, B. W. (2003). *Mental health all-hazards planning guide.* National Technical Assistance Center of the National Association of State Mental Health Directors.

Foa, E. B., McLean, C. P., Zang, Y., Zhong, J., Rauch, S., Porter, K., Knowles, K., Powers, M. B., & Kauffman, B. Y. (2016). Psychometric properties of the Posttraumatic Stress Disorder Symptom Scale Interview for *DSM–5* (PSSI-5). *Psychological Assessment, 28*(10), 1159–1165. https://doi.org/10.1037/pas0000259

Foa, E., Johnson, K., Feeny, N., & Treadwell, K. (2001). The Child PTSD Symptom Scale: A preliminary examination of its psychometric properties. *Journal of Clinical Child Psychology, 30*(3), 376–384.

Foa, E., Zoellner, L., Feeny, N., Hembree, E., & Alvarez-Conrad, J. (2002). Does imaginal exposure exacerbate PTSD symptoms? *Journal of Consulting & Clinical Psychology, 70*(4), 1022–1028.

Foley, C., & Murphy, M. (2015). Burnout in Irish teachers: Investigating the role of individual differences, work environment, and coping factors. *Teaching and Teacher Education, 50*, 46–55.

Follette, V. M., Iverson, K. M., & Ford, J. D. (2009). Contextual behavior trauma therapy. In C. A. Courtois & J. D. Ford (Eds.), *Treating complex traumatic stress disorders: An evidence-based guide* (pp. 264–285). Guilford Press.

Fonagy, P., Luyten, P., & Strathearn, L. (2011). Borderline personality disorder, mentalization, and the neurobiology of attachment. *Infant Mental Health Journal, 32*, 47–69.

Forbes, D., Creamer, M., Bisson, J., Cohen, J., Crow, B. E., Foa, E. B., Ursano, R. J. (2010). A guide to the guidelines for the treatment of PTSD and related conditions. *Journal of Traumatic Stress, 23*(5), 537–552. https://doi.org/10.1002/jts.20565

Forbes, D., Phelps, A., McHugh, A., Debenham, P., Hopwood, M., & Creamer, M. (2003). Imagery rehearsal in the treatment of posttraumatic nightmares in Australian veterans with chronic combat-related PTSD: 12-month follow-up data. *Journal of Traumatic Stress, 16*(5), 509–513.

Ford, J. D. (2009). Neurobiological and developmental research: Clinical implications. In C. A. Courtois & J. D. Ford (Eds.), *Treating complex traumatic stress disorders: An evidence-based guide* (pp. 31–58). Guilford Press.

Ford, J. D. (2017). Complex trauma and complex posttraumatic stress disorder. In S. N. Gold, J. M. Cook, & C. J. Dalenberg (Eds.), APA handbook of trauma psychology: Foundations in knowledge (pp. 281–305). American Psychological Association. https://doi.org/10.1037/0000019-015

Ford, J. D. (2018). Complex trauma and developmental trauma disorder in adolescence. *Adolescent Psychiatry, 7*(4), 220–235. https://doi.org/10.2174/2210676608666180112160419

Ford, J. D., & Courtois, C. A. (2020). *Treating complex traumatic stress disorders in adults* (2nd ed.). Guilford Press.

Ford, J. D., & Courtois, C A. (2021). Complex PTSD and borderline personality disorder. *Borderline Personality Disorder and Emotion Dysregulation, 8*(1). https://doi.org/10.1186/s40479-021-00155-9

Ford, J. S. (2021). *Crisis in the psychotherapy session: Transforming critical moments into turning points.* American Psychological Association. https://doi.org/10.1037/0000225-000

Ford, J., Thomas, F., Byng, R., & McCabe, R. (2021). Asking about self-harm and suicide in primary care: Moral and practical dimensions. *Patient Education and Counseling, 104*(4), 826–835. https://doi.org/10.1016/j.pec.2020.09.037

Forney, D. S., Wallace-Schutzman, F., & Wiggers, T. T. (1982). Burnout among career development professionals: Preliminary findings and implications. *Personnel and Guidance Journal, 60*, 435–439.

Forrest, L. N., Velkoff, E. A., Johnson, C. J., Luebbe, A., & Smith, A. R. (2019). Establishing the psychometric properties and construct validity of the Painful and Provocative Events Scale-Revised. *Journal of Affective Disorders, 253*, 438–448. https://doi.org/10.1016/j.jad.2019.04.074

Forster, P. (2006, October). "Beslan: Counter-terrorism incident command: Lessons learned." *Homeland Security Affairs, 2*, Article 3. https://www.hsaj.org/articles/162

Fortin, M., Fortin, C., Savard-Kelly, P., Guay, S., & El-Baalbaki, G. (2021). The effects of psychotherapies for posttraumatic stress disorder on quality of life in the civilian population: A meta-analysis of RCTs. *Psychological Trauma: Theory, Research, Practice, and Policy, 13*(6), 673–683. https://doi.org/10.1037/tra0000992

Fortinet. (2023). *What is catfishing online: Signs & how to tell.* https://www.fortinet.com/resources/cyberglossary/catfishing

Fosha, D., Paivio, S. C., Gleiser, K., & Ford, J. D. (2009). Experiential and emotion-focused therapy. In C. A. Courtois & J. D. Ford (Eds.), *Treating complex traumatic stress disorders: An evidence-based guide* (pp. 286–310). Guilford Press.

Foster, J. M. (2017). It happened to me: A qualitative analysis of boys' narratives about child sexual abuse. *Journal of Child Sexual Abuse, 26*(7), 853–873. https://doi.org/10.1080/10538712.2017.1360426

Foulkes, S. H. (1948). *Introduction to group analytic psychotherapy.* Heineman.

Fowler, J. W. (1991). Stages in faith consciousness. *New Directions for Child Development, 52*, 27–45.

Fowler, K., & Western, D. (2011). Subtyping perpetrators of intimate partner violence. *Journal of Interpersonal Violence, 26*(4), 607–639.

Fox, R., & Cooper, M. (1998). The effects of suicide on the private practitioner: A professional and personal perspective. *Clinical Social Work Journal, 26*(2), 143–157.

Frankl, V. (1969). *The will to meaning: Foundations and applications of logotherapy.* World.

Frankl, V. (2006). *Man's search for meaning.* Beacon Press.

Fraus, K., Dominick, W., Walenski, A., & Taku, K. (2023). The impact of multiple stressful life events on posttraumatic growth in adolescence. *Psychological Trauma: Theory, Research, Practice, and Policy, 15*(1), 10–17. https://doi.org/10.1037/tra0001181

Frazier, P., Nguyen-Feng, V., & Baker, M. (2017). Chapter 7—Reconstructing meaning after sexual assault. In E. M. Altmaier (Ed.), *Reconstructing meaning after trauma* (pp. 103–116). Academic Press. https://doi.org/10.1016/B978-0-12-803015-8.00007-3

Frederick, C. (1980). Effects of natural versus human induced violence upon individuals. *Evaluation and Change* (Special Issue), 71–75.

Freedy, J. R., & Hobfoll, S. E. (Eds.). (1995). *Traumatic stress: From theory to practice.* Plenum Press.

Freeman, L. (1978). *The sorrow and the fury: Overcoming hurt and loss from childhood to old age.* Prentice Hall.

Freeman, N. (Speaker). (2003, May 28). *Ecological disaster crisis management* (Cassette Recording No. 052803). Nassau County Emergency Management Department.

Freidel, R. O. (2004). *Borderline personality disorder demystified: An essential guide for understanding and living with BPD.* Marlowe & Company.

Frei-Landau, R., Tuval-Mashiach, R., Silberg, T., & Hasson-Ohayon, I. (2020). Attachment to God as a mediator of the relationship between religious affiliation and adjustment to child loss. *Psychological Trauma: Theory, Research, Practice, and Policy 12*(2), 165–174. http://dx.doi.org/10.1037/tra0000499

Freuchen, A., Kjelsberg, E., & Grøholt, B. (2012). Suicide or accident? A psychological autopsy study of suicide in youths under the age of 16 compared to deaths labeled as accidents. *Child and Adolescent Psychiatry and Mental Health, 6*(1), 30. https://doi.org/10.1186/1753-2000-6-30

Freud, S. (1959). Introduction to psychoanalysis and the war neurosis. In J. Strachey (Ed. & Trans.), *The standard edition of the complete psychological works of Sigmund Freud* (Vol. 5). Hogarth Press. (Original work published 1919)

Freud, S. (1963). Introductory lectures on psychoanalysis XVII. In J. Strachey (Ed. & Trans.), *The standard edition of the complete psychological works of Sigmund Freud* (Vol. 16). Hogarth Press. (Original work published 1917)

Freudenberger, H. J. (1974). Staff burn-out. *Journal of Social Issues, 30,* 159–165.

Freudenberger, H. J. (1975). The staff burnout syndrome in alternative institutions. *Psychotherapy: Theory, Research, and Practice, 12,* 73–82.

Freudenberger, H. J. (1977). Burn-out: Occupational hazard of child care workers. *Child Care Quarterly, 6,* 90–99.

Freudenberger, H. J., & Robbins, A. (1979). The hazards of being a psychoanalyst. *Psychoanalytic Review, 66,* 275–296.

Frey, M. (2021). The best exercises for when you are angry. *Very Well Fit.* https://www.verywellfit.com/the-best-exercises-for-when-you-re-feeling-angry-5120367

Frick, M. G., Butler, S. A., & deBoer, D. S. (2021). Universal suicide screening in college primary care. *Journal of American College Health, 69*(1), 17–22. https://doi.org/10.1080/07448481.2019.1645677

Frick, R., & Bogart, M. L. (1982). Transference and countertransference in group therapy with Vietnam veterans. *Bulletin of the Menninger Clinic, 46,* 429–444.

Fridel, E. E., & Zimmerman, G. M. (2019). Examining homicide-suicide as a current in the stream analogy of lethal violence. *Social Forces, 97*(3), 1177–1204. https://doi.org/10.1093/sf/soy071

Friedman, M. J. (2015). The human stress response. In N. C. Bernardy and M. J. Friedman (Eds.), *A practical guide to treatment: Pharmacological and psychotherapeutic approaches* (pp. 9–20). American Psychological Association.

Friedman, M. J., Ritchie, E. C., & Watson, P. J. (2006). Overview. In E. C. Ritchie, P. J. Watson, & M. J. Friedman (Eds.), *Interventions following mass violence and disasters: Strategies for mental health practice* (pp. 3–15). Guilford Press.

Friedman, M., & Rosenman, R. (1974). *Type A behavior and your heart.* Fawcett.

Friedman, R., & James, J. W. (2009, March). The myth of the stages of grieving, death, and grief. *Counseling Today,* 48–52.

Frueh, B. C., Monnier, J., Yim, E., Grubaugh, A. L., Hamner, M. B., & Knapp, R. G. (2007). A randomized trial of telepsychiatry for posttraumatic stress disorder. *Journal of Telemedicine and Telecare, 13,* 142–147.

Fujimura, L. E., Weis, D. M., & Cochran, J. R. (1985). Suicide: Dynamics and implications for counseling. *Journal of Counseling & Development, 63,* 612–615. https://doi.org/10.1002/j.1556-6676.1985.tb00643.x

Fukkink, R., & Hermanns, J. (2009). Counseling children at a helpline: Chatting or calling. *Journal of Community Psychology, 37*(8), 938–948.

Fuller, G. (2016). Non-offending parents as secondary victims of child sexual assault. *Trends and Issues in Crime and Criminal Justice.* https://search.informit.org/doi/abs/10.3316/ielapa.905268405558459

Fulton, L. (2015). Mean girls and rough boys. *ASCA School Counselor, 52*(5), 18–21.

Fuqua, D. S. (2008). *Safe @ last: The evaluation of a child sexual abuse prevention program for elementary students - ProQuest* [Tennessee State University]. https://www.proquest.com/docview/304338987

Furqan, Z., Sinyor, M., Schaffer, A., Kurdyak, P., & Zaheer, J. (2019). "I can't crack the code": What suicide notes teach us about experiences with mental illness and mental health care. *The Canadian Journal of Psychiatry, 64*(2), 98–106. https://doi.org/10.1177/0706743718787795

Fusick, L., & Bordeau, W. (2004). Counseling at-risk Afro-American youth: An examination of contemporary issues and effective school-based strategies. *Professional School Counseling, 8*(2), 102–115.

Gabe, J., & Elston, M. (2009). "We don't have time to take this." Zero tolerance of violence against health care workers in a time of insecurity. In D. Denney (Ed.), *Living in dangerous time: Fear, insecurity, risk and social policy* (pp. 131–149). Wiley-Blackwell.

Galai-Gat, T. (2004, April). *Early interventions with survivors of terrorist attacks in Jerusalem.* Paper presented at the 28th Annual Convening of Crisis Intervention Personnel and 2nd Collaborative Crisis Centers Conference, Chicago, IL, the United States.

Galatzen-Levy, A. (1993). Adolescent violence and the adolescent self. *Adolescent Psychiatry, 19,* 418–441.

Gallo, E. A. G., Munhoz, T. N., Loret de Mola, C., & Murray, J. (2018). Gender differences in the effects of childhood maltreatment on adult depression and anxiety: A systematic review and meta-analysis. *Child Abuse & Neglect, 79,* 107–114. https://doi.org/10.1016/j.chiabu.2018.01.003

Galvin, K. M., Grill, L. H., Arnston, P. H., & Kinahan, K. E. (2012). Beyond the crisis: Communication between parents and children who survived cancer. In F. C. Dickson, & L. M. Webb (Eds.), *Communication for families in crisis: Theories, research, and strategies* (pp. 229–248). Peter Lang.

Garber, R. S. (1965). A psychiatrist's view of remotivation. *Mental Hospitals, 16,* 219–221.

García de la Garza, Á., Blanco, C., Olfson, M., & Wall, M. M. (2021). Identification of suicide attempt risk factors in a national US survey using machine learning. *JAMA Psychiatry, 78*(4), 398–406. http://doi.org/10.1001/jamapsychiatry.2020.4165

Garcia v. City of New York, 646 N.Y.S. 2d 508 (App. Div., 1996).

Garfield, P. (1984). *Your child's dreams.* Ballantine Books.

Garza, A. D., & Franklin, C. A. (2021). The effect of rape myth endorsement on police response to sexual assault survivors. *Violence Against Women, 27*(3–4), 552–573. https://doi.org/10.1177/1077801220911460

Gascon, S., Leiter, M., Andres, E., Santed, M., Pereira, J., Cunha, M., Albesa, A., Montero-Marín, J., García-Campayo, J., & Martinez-Jarreta, B. (2013). The role of aggression suffered by health care workers as predictors of burnout. *Journal of Clinical Nursing, 22*(21–22), 3120–2129.

Gately, L. A., & Stabb, S. D. (2005). Psychology students' training in the management of potentially violent clients. *Professional Psychology: Research and Practice, 36*(6), 681–687.

Gates, D., Fitzwater, E., & Succop, P. (2005). Reducing assaults against nursing home caregivers. *Nursing Research, 54*(2), 119–127.

Gebrezgi, B. H., Badi, M. B., Cherkose, E. A., & Weldehaweria, N. B. (2017). Factors associated with intimate partner physical violence among women attending antenatal care in Shire Endaselassie town, Tigray, northern Ethiopia: A cross-sectional study, July 2015. *Reproductive Health, 14*(1), 76. https://doi.org/10.1186/s12978-017-0337-y

Geffner, R. A., & Rosenbaum, A. (2002). Domestic violence offenders: Treatment and intervention standards. *Journal of Aggression, Maltreatment, and Trauma, 5*(2), 1–9.

Gelles, R. J., & Cornell, C. P. (1985). *Intimate violence in families.* SAGE.

Gentry, J. E., Baranowsky, A. B., & Dunning, K. (2002). ARP: The accelerated recovery program (ARP) for compassion fatigue. In C. R. Figley (Ed.), *Treating compassion fatigue* (pp. 123–137). Brunner/Routledge.

George, J., & Stith, S. M. (2014). An updated feminist view of intimate partner violence. *Family Process, 53*(2), 179–193. https://doi.org/10.1111/famp.12073

Gerler, E. R., Jr. (Ed.). (2004). *Handbook of school violence.* Haworth Press.

Gewirtz-Meydan, A., & Finkelhor, D. (2020). Sexual abuse and assault in a large national sample of children and adolescents. *Child Maltreatment, 25*(2), 203–214. https://doi.org/10.1177/1077559519873975

Ghafournia, N. (2017). Muslim women and domestic violence: Developing a framework for social work practice. *Journal of Religion & Spirituality in Social Work: Social Thought, 36*(1–2), 146–163. https://doi.org/10.1080/15426432.2017.1313150

Gharakhani, D., & Zaferanchi, A. (2019). The effect of job burnout on turnover intention with regard to the mediating role of job satisfaction. *Journal of Health, 10*(1), 109–117. https://doi.org/10.29252/j.health.10.1.109

Ghelani, A., Douglin, M., & Diebold, A. (2022). Effectiveness of Canadian police and mental health co-response teams: A scoping review. *Social Work in Mental Health.* Advance online publication. http://doi.org/10.1080/15332985.2022.2074283

Gheytanchi, A., Joseph, L., Gierlach, E., Kimpara, S., Housley, J., Franco, Z., & Beutler, L. E. (2007). The dirty dozen: Twelve failures of the Hurricane Katrina response and how psychology can help. *American Psychologist, 62*(2), 118–130.

Gho, K. K., Jou, S., Lu, M., & Yeh, L. (2020). Younger, more senior, and most vulnerable? Interaction effects of age and job seniority on psychological distress and quality of life among firefighters. *Psychological Trauma: Theory, Research, Practice, and Policy, 13*(1), 56–65. http://dx.doi.org/10.1037/tra0000662

Ghosh, S., Ghosh, K., Ganguly, D., Chakraborty, T., Jones, G. J., Moens, M. F., & Imran, M. (2018). Exploitation of social media for emergency relief and preparedness: Recent research and trends. *Information Systems Frontiers, 20*, 901–907.

Ghuman, S. J., Brackbill, R. M, Stellman, S. D., Farfel, M. R., & Cone, J. E. (2014). Unmet mental health care need 10-11 years after the 9/11 terrorist attacks: 2011–2012 results from the World Trade Center Health Registry. *BMC Public Health.* (14), 491. https://doi.org/10.1186/1471-2458-14-491

Gibbons, P., Collins, M., & Reid, C. (2011). How useful are indices of personality pathology when assessing domestic violence perpetrators? *Psychological Assessment, 23*(1), 164–173.

Gibby, J. G., & Whiting, J. B. (2023). Insecurity, control, and abuse: What attachment theory can teach us about treating intimate partner violence. *Contemporary Family Therapy, 45*(1), 93–105. https://doi.org/10.1007/s10591-021-09623-4

Gibson, L. (2015). *Acute stress disorder.* U.S. Department of Veterans Affairs, National Center for PTSD. https://www.ptsd.va.gov/professional/treat/essentials/acute_stress_disorder.asp

Giduck, J. (2005). *Terror at Beslan.* Archangel Group.

Gidycz, C. A., Orchowski, L. M., Probst, D. R., Edwards, K. M., Murphy, M., & Tansill, E. (2015). Concurrent administration of sexual assault prevention and risk reduction programming: Outcomes for women. *Violence Against Women, 21*(6), 780–800. https://doi.org/10.1177/1077801215576579

Giebels, E., & Janssen, O. (2005). Conflict stress and reduced well-being at work: The buffering effect of third-party help. *European Journal of Work and Organizational Psychology, 14*(2), 137–155.

Giel, R. (1990). Psychosocial process in disaster. *International Journal of Mental Health, 19*, 7–20.

Gielkens, E. M. J., Sobczak, S., Rossi, G., & van Alphen, S. P. J. (2022). The feasibility of eye movement desensitization and reprocessing (EMDR) for older adults with posttraumatic stress disorder (PTSD) and comorbid psychiatric and somatic disorders. *Psychological Trauma: Theory, Research, Practice, and Policy.* Advance online publication. https://doi.org/10.1037/tra0001402

Gijzen, M., Rasing, S., Creemers, D., Engels, R., & Smit, F. (2022). Effectiveness of school-based preventive programs in suicidal thoughts and behaviors: A meta-analysis, *Journal of Affective Disorders, 298, Part A*, 408–420 https://doi.org/10.1016/j.jad.2021.10.062

Gil, E. (2016). *Posttraumatic play in children: What clinicians need to know.* Guilford Publications.

Gil, E., & Shaw, J. A. (2009). Prescriptive play therapy. In K. J. O'Connor & L. D. Braverman (Eds.), *Play therapy theory and practice: Comparing theories and techniques* (pp. 451–487). John Wiley & Sons.

Gil-Gonzalez, D., Vives-Cases, C., Ruiz, M. T., Carrasco-Portino, M., & Alvarez-Dardet, C. (2008). Childhood experiences of violence in perpetrators as a risk factor of intimate partner violence: A systematic review. *Journal of Public Health, 30*(1), 14–22. https://doi.org/10.1093/pubmed/fdm071

Gillies, J., & Neimeyer, R. A. (2006). Loss, grief, and the search for significance: Toward a model of meaning reconstruction in bereavement. *Journal of Constructivist Psychology, 19*, 31–65.

Gillig, P. M., Dumaine, M., Stammer, J. W., Hillard, J. R., & Grubb, P. (1990). What do police officers really want from the mental health system? *Hospital and Community Psychiatry, 41*, 663–665.

Gilliland, B. E. & James, R. K. (1988). *Crisis intervention strategies.* Brooks-Cole.

Gilliland, B. E., & James, R. K. (1998). *Theories and strategies in counseling and psychotherapy* (4th ed.). Allyn & Bacon.

Gil-Rivas, V., Kilmer, R. P., Hypes, A. W., & Roof, K. A. (2010). The caregiver–child relationship and children's adjustment following hurricane Katrina. In R. P Kilmer, V. Gil-Rivas, R. G. Tedeschi, & L. G. Calhoun (Eds.), *Helping families and communities recover from disaster: Lessons learned from Hurricane Katrina and its aftermath.* (pp. 55–76). American Psychological Association.

Gil-Rivas, V., Silver, R. C., Holman, E. A., McIntosh, D., & Poulin, M. (2007). Parental response and adolescent adjustment to the September 11 terrorist attacks. *Journal of Traumatic Stress, 20*, 1063–1068.

Gimenez-Diez, D., Maldonado-Alia, R., Torrent-Sola, L., Branel, N., & Bernabeu-Tamayo, M. (2022). Nurses' experiences of care at crisis resolution home treatment teams: A case study research. *Journal of Psychiatric and Mental Health Nursing, 29*(1), 48–56. https://doi.org/10.1111/jpm.12738

Giovannetti, M. (2023). Artificial intelligence and mental health. *Counseling Today, 65*(10), 21–22.

Girgenti, M. J., & Duman, R. S. (2018). Transcriptome alterations in post-traumatic stress disorder. *Biological Psychiatry, 83*(10), 840–848. https://doi.org/10.1016/j.biopsych.2017.09.023

Gist, R., & Lubin, B. (Eds.). (1989). *Psychological aspects of disaster.* Wiley.

Gist, R., & Lubin, B. (Eds.). (1999). *Response to disaster: Psychosocial, community and ecological responses.* Brunner/Mazel.

Gist, R., Lubin, B., & Redburn, B. (1999). Psychosocial, ecological and community perspectives on disaster response. In R. Gist & B. Lubin (Eds.), *Response to disaster: Psychosocial, community, and ecological approaches* (pp. 1–20). Brunner/Mazel.

Gist, R., Woodall, S. J., & Magenheimer, L. K. (1999). And then you do the Hokey Pokey and you turn yourself around . . . In R. Gist & B. Lubin (Eds.), *Response to disaster: Psychosocial, community and ecological responses* (pp. 269–290). Brunner/Mazel.

Giunta, R., & Giunta, C. (2002). *Grief recovery workbook.* Integrity Publishers.

Gladding, S. T. (1987). Poetic expressions: A counseling art in elementary schools. *Elementary School Guidance & Counseling, 21,* 307–311.

Gladding, S. T. (2002). From Pier 94, near Ground Zero, New York City. In D. D. Bass & R. Yep (Eds.), *Terrorism, trauma, and tragedies: A counselor's guide to preparing and responding* (pp. 7–9). American Counseling Association.

Glanz, J., Singhvi A., & Baker, M. (2021, July). Possible failure point emerges in Miami-area building collapse. *New York Times.*

Glass, V. Q., & Bickler, A. (2021). Cultivating the therapeutic alliance in a telemental health setting. *Contemporary Family Therapy: An International Journal, 43,* 189–198. https://doi.org/10.1007/s10591-021-09570-0

Glasser, W. (1965). *Reality therapy.* Harper & Row.

Glasser, W. (1969). *Schools without failure.* Harper & Row.

Glasser, W. (1976). *Positive addiction.* Harper & Row.

Glasser, W. (1985). *Control theory: A new explanation about how we control our lives.* Harper & Row.

Glasser, W. (2000, May 28). Invited address at the Evolution of Psychotherapy Conference, Anaheim, CA, the United States.

Glazer, H. R. (2010). Filial play therapy for grieving preschool children. In C. E. Schaefer (Ed.), *Play therapy for preschool children* (pp. 89–105). American Psychological Association.

Glazer, H. R., Clark, M. D., Thomas, R., & Haxton, H. (2010). Parenting after the death of a spouse. *American Journal of Hospice & Palliative Medicine, 27*(8), 532–536.

Gleick, J. (2008). *Chaos: Making a new science.* Penguin Books.

Glezer, A., & Brendel, R. W. (2010). Beyond emergencies: The use of physical restraints in medical and psychiatric settings. *Harvard Review of Psychiatry, 18*(6), 353–358.

Glueckauf, R. L., Drude. P., Wang, Y., Gustafson, D. J., Maheu, M. M., Wells, B. A., & Nelson, E. (2018). Survey of psychologists' telebehavioral health practices: Technology use, ethical issues, and training needs. *Professional Psychology: Research and Practice, 49*(3), 205–219. http://dx.doi.org/10.1037/pro0000188

Godbout, N., Daspe, M., Runtz, M., Cyr, G., & Briere, J. (2019). Childhood maltreatment, and borderline personality related symptoms: Gender-specific structural equation models. *Psychological Trauma: Theory, Research, Practice, and Policy, 11*(1), 90–96. https://doi.org/10.1037/tra0000403

Godbout, N., Vaillancourt-Morel, M.-P., Bigras, N., Briere, J., Hébert, M., Runtz, M., & Sabourin, S. (2019). Intimate partner violence in male survivors of child maltreatment: A meta-analysis. *Trauma, Violence, & Abuse, 20*(1), 99–113. https://doi.org/10.1177/1524838017692382

Golan, N. (1978). *Treatment in crisis situations.* Free Press.

Golan, N. (1987). Crisis intervention. In A. Minahan (Ed.), *Encyclopedia of social work, 18* (pp. 360–372). National Association of Social Workers.

Gold, S. N. (2009). Contextual therapy. In C. A. Courtois & J. D. Ford (Eds.), *Treating complex traumatic stress disorders: An evidence-based guide* (pp. 227–242). Guilford Press.

Goldbach, J., Rhoades, H., Green, D., Fuginiti, A., & Marshal, M. (2019). Is there a need for LGBT-specific suicide crises services? *Crisis: The Journal of Crisis Intervention and Suicide Prevention, 40*(3), 203–208. https://doi.org/10.1027/0227-5910/a000542

Goldbeck, L., Muche, R., Sachser, C., Tutus, D., & Rosner, R. (2016). Effectiveness of trauma-focused cognitive behavioral therapy for children and adolescents. A randomised controlled trial in eight German mental health clinics. *Psychotherapy and Psychosomatics, 85*(3), 159–170. https://doi.org/10.1159/000442824

Goldstein, A. P., & Kodluboy, D. W. (1998). *Gangs in schools: Signs, symbols, and solutions.* Research Press.

Golec, J. A. (1983). A contextual approach to the social psychological study of disaster recovery. *International Journal of Mass Emergencies and Disasters, 1,* 255–276.

Golembiewski, R. T., & Munzenrider, R. F. (1993). Health-related covariants of phases of burnout: A replication. *Organization Development Journal, 11,* 1–12.

Golembiewski, R. T., Munzenrider, R. F., & Stevenson, J. G. (1986). *Stress in organizations: Toward a phase model of burnout.* Praeger.

Golembiewski, R. T., Munzenrider, R. F., Scherb, K., & Billingsley, W. (1992). Burnout and "psychiatric" cases: Early evidence of an association. *Anxiety, Stress and Coping: An International Journal, 5,* 69–78.

Gölge, Z. B., Özgeldi, E. B., & Akdemir, S. (2021). Female perpetrators of sexual abuse. *Current Approaches in Psychiatry, 13*(3), 524–536. https://doi.org/10.18863/pgy.822224

Golomb, M. R., Warden, S. J., Fess, E., Rabin, B., Yonkman, J., & Shirley, B. (2011). Maintained hand function and forearm bone health 14 months after an in-home virtual reality videogame hand tele-rehabilitation intervention in an adolescent with hemiplegic cerebral palsy. *Journal of Child Neurology, 26*(3), 389–393.

Goncalves, R., Pedrozo, A. L., Coutinho, E., Figueria, I., & Ventura, P. (2012). Efficacy of virtual reality exposure therapy in the treatment of PTSD: A systematic review. *PLoS ONE, 7*(12), e48469.

Gondolf, E. (1984). *Men who batter: Why they abuse women and how they stop their abuse.* Domestic Violence Study Center, Indiana University of Pennsylvania.

Gondolf, E. (1985). Fighting for control: A clinical assessment of men who batter. *Social Casework, 65,* 48–54.

Gondolf, E., & Fisher, E. R. (1988). *Battered women as survivors: An alternative to treating learned helplessness.* Lexington Books.

Gonzalez, A. (2013). How do social workers in the ICU perceive their role in providing end-of-life care? What factors impede or help them in carrying out this role in end-of-life care and is social work education a contributing component? Unpublished dissertation. University of Pennsylvania.

Gonzalez, C. L., & Bell, H. (2016). Child-centered play therapy for Hispanic children with traumatic grief: Cultural implications for treatment outcomes. *International Journal of Play Therapy, 25*(3), 146–153. https://doi.org/10.1037/pla0000023

Gonzales, R., Ang, A., Murphy, D., Glik, D., & Anglin, D. (2014). Substance abuse recovery outcomes among a cohort of youth participating in a mobile-based texting aftercare pilot program. *Journal of Substance Abuse Treatment, 47*(1), 20-26.

Goode, S. (2022). Users in crisis response and recovery: Catharsis and social learning among social media users during and after a natural disaster. *Behaviour & Information Technology.* Advance online publication. https://doi.org/10.1080/01449 29x.2021.2016968

Goodman, L. A., & Epstein, D. (2011). The justice system response to domestic violence. In J. W. White, M. Koss, & A. E. Kazdin (Eds.), *Violence against women and children: Vol.1. Mapping the terrain* (pp. 215-235). American Psychological Association.

Goodman, R. D., Calderon, A. M., &Tate, K. A. (2014). Liberation focused community outreach: A qualitative exploration of peer group supervision during disaster response. *Journal of Community Psychology, 42*(2), 228-236.

Goodman-Williams, R., Clark, S. L., Campbell, R., & Ullman, S. E. (2022). Longitudinal patterns of posttraumatic stress disorder symptoms among sexual assault survivors: A latent transition analysis. *Psychological Trauma: Theory, Research, Practice, and Policy.* Advance online publication. http://dx.doi .org/10.1037/tra0001376

Gordon, N. S., Farberow, N. L., & Maida, C. A. (1999). *Children and disaster.* Brunner/Mazel.

Gori, A., Topino, E., & Musetti, A. (2023). Pathways towards posttraumatic stress symptomatology: A moderated medication model including perceived stress, worry, and defense mechanisms. *Psychological Trauma: Theory, Research, Practice, and Policy.* Advance online publication. https://dx.doi.org/10.1037 /tra0001435

Gorter, R., Albrecht, G., Hoostraten, J., & Eijkman, M. (1999). Factor validity of the Maslach Burnout Inventory—Dutch version (MBI-NL) among dentists. *Journal of Organizational Behavior, 20*(2), 209-217.

Gottfredson, D. C., Gottfredson, G. D., & Skroban, S. (1998). Can prevention work where it is needed most? *Evaluation Review, 22*(3), 315-340.

Gottman, J. M., Gottman, J. S., & Atkins, C. L. (2011). The Comprehensive Soldier Fitness program: Family skills component. *American Psychologist, 66*(1), 52-57.

Gould, M. S., Pisani, A., Gallo, C., Ertefaie, A., Harrington, D., Kelberman, C., & Green, S. (2022). Crisis text-line interventions: Evaluation of texters' perceptions of effectiveness. *Suicide and Life-Threatening Behavior, 52*(3), 583-595. https://doi .org/10.1111/sltb.12873

Gould, M., & Shaffer, D. (1986). The impact of suicide in television movies: Evidence of imitation. *New England Journal of Medicine, 315,* 690-693.

Gould, M., Jamieson, P., & Romer, D. (2003). Media contagion and suicide among the young. *American Behavioral Scientist, 46*(9), 1269-1284.

Governale, A., McTighe, K., & Cechova, V. (2023, May 11). Psychological reactions to COVID-19: Ambiguous loss, posttraumatic growth, and coronavirus impact among college students. *Psychological Trauma: Theory, Research, Practice, and Policy.* Advance online publication. https://dx.doi.org/10.1037 /tra0001508

Govindu, M. (2023, April 6). Recognizing burnout and compassion fatigue among counselors. *Counseling Today.* https:// ct.counseling.org/2023/04/recognizing-burnout-and-compassion-fatigue-among-counselors/

Gracia, E. (2004). Unreported cases of domestic violence against women: Towards an epidemiology of social silence, tolerance, and inhibition. *Journal of Epidemiology & Community Health, 58*(7), 536-537. https://doi.org/10.1136/jech.2003.019604

Gracia, E. (2014). Intimate partner violence against women and victim-blaming attitudes among Europeans. *Bulletin of the World Health Organization, 92,* 380-381. https://doi.org/10.2471 /BLT.13.131391

Gradus, J. L., Suvak, M. K., Wisco, B., Marx, B. P., & Resick, P. A. (2013). Treatment of posttraumatic stress disorder reduces suicidal ideation. *Depression and Anxiety 30*(10), 1046-1053.

Grady, M. D., Levenson, J. S., & Bolder, T. (2017). Linking adverse childhood effects and attachment: A theory of etiology for sexual offending. *Trauma, Violence, & Abuse, 18*(4), 433-444. https://doi.org/10.1177/1524838015627147

Graham, L. K. (2014). Political dimensions of pastoral care in community disaster responses. *Pastoral Psychology, 63*(4), 471-488.

Graham, L. M., Sahay, K. M., Rizo, C. F., Messing, J. T., & Macy, R. J. (2021). The validity and reliability of available intimate partner homicide and reassault risk assessment tools: A systematic review. *Trauma, Violence, & Abuse, 22*(1), 18-40. https:// doi.org/10.1177/1524838018821952

Gramaglia, C., Calati, R., & Zeppegno, P. (2019). Rational suicide in late life: A systematic review of the literature. *Medicina, 55*(10), 656-656. https://doi.org/10.3390/medicina55100656

Granello, D. H., & Granello, P. F. (2007). *Suicide: An essential guide for helping professionals and educators.* Pearson/Allyn & Bacon.

Grassi, L., Peron, L., Mafangoni, C., Zanchi, P., & Vanni, A. (2001). Characteristics of violent behavior in acute psychiatric inpatients: A 5-year Italian study. *Acta Psychiatrica Scandinavica, 104*(4), 273-279.

Gray, M. J., & Litz, B. T. (2005). Behavioral interventions for recent trauma: Empirically informed practice guidelines. *Behavior Modification, 29,* 189-215.

Gray, R. E. (1988). The role of the school counselor with bereaved teenagers: With and without peer support groups. *School Counselor, 35,* 185-192.

Grayson, P. A., & Meilman, M. W. (Eds.). (2006). *College mental health practice.* Routledge.

Graziano, R. C., LoSavio, S. T., White, M. A., Beckham, J. C., & Dillon, K. H. (2023). Examination of PTSD symptom networks over the course of cognitive processing therapy. *Psychological Trauma: Theory, Research, Practice, and Policy.* Advance online publication. https://doi.org/10.1037/tra0001464

Green, B. L., & Solomon, S. D. (1995). The mental health impact of natural and technological disasters. In J. R. Freedy & S. E. Hobfoll (Eds.), *Traumatic stress: From theory to practice* (pp. 163-180). Plenum Press.

Green, J. W. (2008). *Beyond the good death: The anthropology of modern dying.* University of Pennsylvania Press.

Greene, C. A., McCoach, D. B., Ford, J. D., McCarthy, K., Randall, K. G., & Lang, J. M. (2023). Bidirectional effects of parental and adolescent symptom change in trauma-focused cognitive behavioral therapy. *Psychological Trauma: Theory, Research, Practice, and Policy, 15*(Suppl 1), S172-S182. https://doi .org/10.1037/tra0001445

Greene, D. B. (1994). Childhood suicide and myths surrounding it. *Social Work, 39,* 230-233.

Greene-Cramer, B. J., Hulland, E. N., Russell, S. P., Eriksson, C. B., & Lopes-Cardozo, B. (2021). Patterns of posttraumatic stress symptoms among international humanitarian aid workers. *Traumatology, 27*(2), 177–184. https://doi.org/10.1037/trm0000286

Greenfield, T. K., McNeil, D. E., & Binder, R. L. (1989). Violent behavior and length of psychiatric hospitalization. *Hospital and Community Psychiatry, 40*, 809–814.

Greenspan, M. (2003). *Healing through the dark emotions: The wisdom of grief, fear, and despair.* Shambhala.

Greenstone, J. L., & Leviton, S. C. (1993). *Elements of crisis intervention.* Brooks/Cole.

Greenstone, J. L., & Leviton, S. C. (2011). *Elements of crisis intervention: Crises and how to respond to them* (3rd ed.). Cengage.

Greenwald, B. (1985a). *In-Touch Hotline training materials: Coping.* University of Illinois at Chicago Circle Campus, Counseling Center.

Greenwald, B. (1985b). *In-Touch Hotline training materials: The disturbed caller.* Chicago: University of Illinois at Chicago Circle Campus, Counseling Center.

Gregory, K., Nnawulezi, N., & Sullivan, C. M. (2021). Understanding how domestic violence shelter rules may influence survivor empowerment. *Journal of Interpersonal Violence, 36*(1–2), NP402–NP423. https://doi.org/10.1177/0886260517730561

Gressard, C. F. (1986). Self-help groups for Vietnam veterans experiencing post-traumatic stress disorder. *Journal for Specialists in Group Work, 11*(2), 74–79.

Griffith, J. L. (2010). *Religion that heals: Religion that harms: A guide for clinical practice.* Guilford Press.

Griffith, T. (2003). Assisting with the "big hurts, little tears" of the youngest grievers: Working with three-, four-, and five-year-olds who have experienced loss and grief because of death. *Illness, Crisis, & Loss, 11*(3), 217–225.

Griffiths, M., Allen, J., Patel, K., & Bell, V. (2020). Promoting family inclusive practice in home treatment teams. *The Journal of Mental Health Training, Education, and Practice, 15*(5), 261–273. https://doi.org/10.1108/JMHTEP-11-2019-0058

Grills, C. (2004). African-centered psychology: Basic principles. In T. Parham (Ed.), *Counseling persons of African descent: Raising the bar of practitioner competence* (pp. 32–56). SAGE.

Grinker, R. R., & Spiegel, J. P. (1945). *Men under stress.* Blakiston.

Grollman, E. A. (1996). Spiritual support after a sudden loss. In K. J. Doka (Ed.), *Living with grief after sudden loss: Suicide, homicide, accident, heart attack, stroke* (pp. 185–188). Hospice Foundation of America.

Gross, S., & Anthony, K. (Eds.). (2003). *Technology in counseling and psychotherapy: A practitioner's guide.* Palgrave Macmillan.

Grossi, G., Perski, A., Ekstedt, M., Johansson, T., Lindstrom, M., & Holm, K. (2005). The morning salivary cortisol response in burnout. *Journal of Psychosomatic Research, 59*(2), 103–111.

Grossman, D. (1995). *On killing: The psychological cost of learning to kill in war and society.* Little, Brown.

Grossmann, J., Shor, R., Schaefer, K., & Bennett Cattaneo, L. (2019). Development of a tool to assess client-centered practice on a domestic violence hotline. *Journal of Social Work, 19*(1), 102–120. https://doi.org/10.1177/1468017318757395

Groth, T., Hilsenroth, M., McMillen, K., Cersosimo, B., Bindon, M., Cain, L., & Katz, M. (2021). How are expert therapists similar, different, and integrative in the treatment of borderline personality disorder. *Psychotherapy, 58*(2), 310–323. htttp://doi.org/10.1037/pst0000352

Grouse, A. S. (1984). The effects of organizational stress on inpatient psychiatric medication patterns. *American Journal of Psychiatry, 141*, 878–881.

Grunsted, V. L., Cisneros, M. X., & Belen, D. V. (1991, April). *Working with the disturbed hotline caller.* Paper presented at the Fifteenth Annual Convening of Crisis Intervention Personnel, Chicago, IL, the United States.

Gryglewicz, K., Bozzay, M., Arthur-Jordan, B., Romero, G., Whitmeier, M., Chappie, R., & Karver, M. (2017). Silenced population: Uncovering correlates of suicidal-related behavior among def a and hard-of-hearing youth. *Crisis: The Journal of Crisis Intervention and Suicide Prevention, 38*(6), 433–442. https://doi.org/10.1027/0227-5910/a000470

Guarida, N., & Sippel, F. (2023). Retaliation against child abuse reporters. *Social Work Today (Spring).*

Gudas, L. (1990, August). *Children's reactions to bereavement: A developmental perspective.* Paper presented at the annual meeting of the American Psychological Association, Boston, MA, the United States.

Guerra, P. (1999, May). Counselors help victims of school shooting. *Counseling Today, 41*, 12–14.

Guerra, P., & Schmitt, S. M. (1999, June). Reactions to Littleton shooting. *Counseling Today, 41*, 26–27.

Guerriero-Austrom, M. G., & Fleming, S. J. (1990, August). *Effects of sibling death on adolescents' physical and emotional well-being: A longitudinal study.* Paper presented at the annual meeting of the American Psychological Association, Boston, MA, the United States.

Gühne, U., Weinmann, S., Katrin, A., Atav, E., Becker, T., & Riedel-Heller, S. (2011). Home treatment and systematic review and implementation in Germany. *Psychiatric Practice, 38*(2), 114–122.

Guida, A. (2001). Depression . . . or just the blues? *ASCA School Counselor, 39*(2), 10–13.

Gulati, P., & Guest, G. (1990). The community centered model: A garden-variety approach or a radical transformation of community practice? *Social Work, 35*, 63–68.

Gumaer, J. (1984). *Counseling and therapy for children.* Free Press.

Gumber, S., Gumber, L., & Gumber, A. (2020). Predictors of violent incidents among patients in psychiatric intensive care units: review of global evidence. Sheffield Hallam University Archive. http://shura.shu.ac.uk/26154/

Gurm, B., Salgado, G., Marchbank, J., & Early, S. D. (2020). *Making sense of a global pandemic: Relationship violence & working together towards a violence free society.* Kwantlen Polytechnic University. https://kpu.pressbooks.pub/nevr/chapter/why-do-survivors-not-report-to-police/

Gurvitz, T. V., Shenton, M. E., & Pittman, R. K. (1995). *Reduced hippocampal volume on magnetic resonance imagining in chronic post-traumatic stress disorder.* Paper presented at the International Society for Traumatic Stress Studies, Miami, FL, the United States.

Gurwitch, R. H., Nelson, M. M., Comer, J. S. (2020). Leveraging parent–child interaction therapy and telehealth capacities to address the unique needs of young children during the COVID-19 public health crisis. *Psychological Trauma: Public Health Theory, Research, Practice, and Policy, 50*(1), 82–84. http://dx.doi.org/10.1037/tra0000863

Gušic, S., Maleševic, A., Cardeña, E., Bengtsson, H., & Søndergaard, H. P. (2018). "I feel like I do not exist": A study of dissociative experiences among war-traumatized refugee youth. *Psychological Trauma: Theory, Research, Practice, and Policy, 10*(5), 542–550. https://doi.org/10.1037/tra0000348

Guterman, N. B., Jayaratme, S., & Bargal, D. (1996). Workplace violence and victimization experienced by social workers: A cross-national study of Americans and Israelis. In G. R. VandenBos & E. Q. Bulatao (Eds.), *Violence on the job: Identifying risks and developing solutions* (pp. 175–188). American Psychological Association.

Gutermman, J. T. (2013). *Mastering the art of solution focused counseling* (2nd ed.). American Counseling Association.

Gutheil, T. G. (1978). Observation on the theoretical basis for seclusion of the psychiatric inpatient. *American Journal of Psychiatry, 135*, 325–328.

Gutierrez, C. I., Arteaga, K., Schepis, T. S., & De Nadai, A. S. (2023). Posttraumatic stress disorder in diverse populations: Testing for assessment bias in a nationally representative sample. *Psychological Trauma: Theory, Research, Practice, and Policy.* Advance online publication. https://doi.org/10.1037/tra0001492

Gutner, C. A., Casement, M. D., Gilbert, K. S., & Resick, P. A. (2013). Change in sleep symptoms across Cognitive Processing Therapy and Prolonged Exposure: A longitudinal perspective. *Behaviour Research and Therapy, 51*(12), 817–822.

Guy, J. D., Brown, C. K., & Poelstra, P. L. (1990). Who gets attacked? A national survey of patient violence directed at psychologists in clinical practice. *Professional Psychology: Research and Practice, 21*, 493–495.

Haber, D. (2006). Life review: Implementation, theory, research, and therapy. *International Journal of Aging & Human Development, 63*(2), 153–171.

Hacker, K., Suglia, S., Fried, L., Rappaport, N., & Cabral, H. (2006). Developmental differences in risk factors for suicide attempts between ninth and eleventh graders. *Suicide and Life-Threatening Behavior, 36*(2), 154–166.

Hackney, H., & Bernard, J. M. (2017). *Professional counseling: A process guide to helping* (8th ed.). Pearson.

Haen, C. (2008). Vanquishing monsters: Drama therapy for treating childhood trauma in the group setting. In C. A. Malchiodi (Ed.), *Creative interventions with traumatized children* (pp. 225–246). Guilford Press.

Hafkenscheid, A. (2005). Event countertransference and vicarious traumatization: Theoretically valid and clinically useful concepts? *European Journal of Psychotherapy, Counseling and Health, 7*(3), 159–168.

Halbesleben, J. R. (2006). Sources of social support and burnout: Meta-analytic test of the Conservation of Resources model. *Journal of Applied Psychology, 91*(5), 1134–1145.

Halbsgut, J. L. (2011). Masculine gender role norms: Understanding the conformity of domestic violence perpetrators. *Dissertation Abstracts International: Section B. The Sciences and Engineering,* 7087.

Hale, A. C., Bremer-Landau, J., Wright, T. P., McDowell, J. E., & Rodriguez, J. L. (2021). Residential PTSD treatment outcomes during cognitive processing therapy for veterans with and without recent histories of cannabis use. *Psychological Services, 18*(4), 497–503. https://doi.org/10.1037/ser0000424

Haley, J. (1973). *Uncommon therapy.* Norton.

Haley, J. (1976). *Problem-solving therapy.* McGraw Hill.

Haley, W. E., Allen, R. S., Reynolds, S., Chen, H., Burton, A., & Gallagher-Thompson, D. (2002). Family issues in end-of-life decision making and end-of-life care. *American Behavioral Scientist, 46*, 284–298.

Haley, W. E., Bergman, E. J., Roth, D. L., McVie, T., Gaugler, J., & Mittleman, M. S. (2008). Long-term effects of bereavement and caregiver intervention on dementia caregiver depressive symptoms. *Gerontologist, 48*(6), 732–740.

Hallett, N., Huber, J., & Dickens, G. (2014). Violence prevention in inpatient psychiatric hospital settings: Systematic review of studies about the perceptions of care staff and patients. *Aggression and Behavior, 10*(5). 502–514. https://doi.org/10.1016/j.avb.2014.07.009

Hallinan, S., Shiyko, M., Volpe, R., & Molnar, B. E. (2021). On the back burner: Challenges experienced by change agents addressing vicarious trauma in first response and victim service agencies. *Traumatology, 27*(3), 316–325. https://doi.org/10.1037/trm0000291

Halpern, J., & Tramontin, M. (2007). *Disaster mental health theory and practice.* Cengage.

Hambrick, E. P., Brawner, T. W., & Perry, B. D. (2018). Examining developmental adversity and connectedness in child welfare-involved children. *Children Australia, 43*(2), 105–115. https://doi.org/10.1017/cha.2018.21

Hamilton, J., & Workman, R. (1998). Persistence of combat-related posttraumatic stress symptoms for 75 years. *Journal of Traumatic Stress, 11*(4), 763–768.

Hammond, L. C., & Gantt, L. (1998). Using art in counseling: Ethical considerations. *Journal of Counseling and Development, 76*(3), 271–275.

Hamois, D. A. (2015). The impact of coping strategies on work stress, burnout, and job satisfaction in school counselors. *Dissertation Abstracts International: Section B. The Sciences and Engineering, 75*(8-B(E)).

Hampton, R. L., Vandergriff-Avery, M., & Kim, J. (1999). Understanding the origins and incidence of spousal violence in North America. In T. P. Gullotta & S. J. McElhaney (Eds.), *Violence in homes and communities: Prevention, intervention and treatment* (pp. 39–70). SAGE.

Hamstra, B. (1986). Neurobiological substrates of violence: An overview for forensic clinicians. *Journal of Psychiatry and Law, 14*, 349–374.

Handford, H. A., Mayes, S. D., Mattison, R. E., Humphrey, F. J., Bahnato, S., Bixler, E. O., & Kales, J. D. (1986). Child and parent reactions to the Three Mile Island nuclear accident. *Journal of the American Academy of Child Psychiatry, 25*, 346–356.

Handran, J. (2014). Trauma-informed organizational culture: The prevention, reduction, and treatment of compassion fatigue. *Dissertation Abstracts International: Section A. Humanities and Social Sciences, 74*(10-A(E)).

Haney, K., LeBeau, K., Bodner, S., Czizik, A., Young, M. E., & Hart, M. (2020). Sex trafficking in the United States: A scoping review. *Journal of Evidence-Based Social Work, 17*(6), 714–748. https://doi.org/10.1080/26408066.2020.1765934

Hanna, D., & Romana, M., (2007). Debriefing after a crisis. *Nurse Management, 38*(8), 38–42. https://doi.org/10.1097/01.numa.0000286190.06433.0b

Hannan, S. M., Orcutt, H. K., Miron, L. R., & Thompson, K. L. (2017). Childhood sexual abuse and later alcohol-related problems: Investigating the roles of revictimization, PTSD, and drinking motivations among college women. *Journal of Interpersonal Violence, 32*(14), 2118–2138. https://doi.org/10.1177/0886260515591276

Hansen, J. C., & Frantz, T. T. (Eds.). (1984). *Death and grief in the family.* Aspen Systems.

Hanson, R. O., & Hayslip, B. (2000). Widowhood in later life. In J. H. Harvey & E. D. Miller (Eds.), *Loss and trauma: General and close relationship perspectives* (pp. 345–354). Brunner-Routledge.

Hanson, S., Kerkholt, T., & Bush, S. (2005). *Health care ethics for psychologists: A casebook* (pp. 9–37). American Psychological Association.

Hansson, K., & Cederblad, M. (2004). Sense of coherence as a meta-theory for salutogenic family therapy. *Journal of Family Psychotherapy, 15,* 39–54.

Hansson, R. O., & Stroebe, M. S. (2007). *Bereavement in late life: Coping, adaptation, and developmental influences.* American Psychological Association.

Hao, S., Hong, W., Xu, H., Zhou, L., & Xie, Z., (2015). Relationship between resilience, stress, and burnout among civil servants in Beijing, China: Mediating and moderating effect analyses. *Personality and Individual Differences, 83,* 65–71.

Happell, B., Sundram, S., Wortans, J., Johnstone, S., Ryan, R., & Lakshmana, R. (2009). Assessing nurse-initiated care in a mental health crisis assessment and treatment team in Australia. *Psychiatric Services, 60*(11), 1527–1531.

Hardiman, P., & Simmonds, J. (2013). Spiritual well-being, burnout, and trauma in counsellors and psychotherapists. *Mental Health, Religion, & Culture, 16*(10), 1044–1055.

Hardwick, P. J., & Rowton-Lee, M. A. (1996). Adolescent homicide: Toward assessment of risk. *Journal of Adolescence, 19*(3), 263–276.

Hardy, K. V. (1997). *Family systems therapy* (Videotape No. 0-205-32931-4, T. Labriola, Producer). In J. Carlson & D. Kjos (Eds.), *Family systems with Hardy: Psychotherapy with the experts.* Allyn & Bacon.

Hare, R. (1991). *Manual for the Hare Psychopathy Checklist-Revised.* Multi-health Systems.

Harker, R., Pidgeon, A. M., Klaassen, F., & King, S. (2016). Exploring resilience and mindfulness as preventative factors for psychological distress burnout and secondary traumatic stress among human service professionals. *Work, 54*(3), 631–637. https://doi.org/10.3233/WOR-162311

Harms, P. D., Herian, M. N., Krasikova, D. V., Vanhove, A., & Lester, D. B. (2013). *The Comprehensive Soldier Fitness Program evaluation report #4: Evaluation of resilience training mental and behavioral health outcomes.* U.S. Army. https://digitalcommons.unl.edu/cgi/viewcontent.cgi?article=1009&context=pdharms

Harned, M., & Sloan, C. (2022). Treating PTSD and borderline personality disorder. In U. Schnyder & M. Cloitre (Eds.). *Evidence based treatments for trauma-related psychological disorder: A practical guide for clinicians* (pp. 389–404) Springer Nature Switzerland AG. https://doi.org/10.1007/978-3-030-97802-0_18

Harpoth, T. S., Kongerslev, M., Moeyaert, M., Bo, S., Bateman, A. W., & Simonson, E. (2020). Evaluating "mentalizing positive affect" as an intervention for enhancing positive affectivity in borderline personality using a single case multiple baseline design. *Psychotherapy, 57*(4), 580–586. https://doi.org/10.1037/pst0000251

Harris, B., & Leather, P. (2012). Levels and consequences of exposure to service user violence: Evidence from a sample of UK social care staff. *British Journal of Social Work, 42*(5), 851–869.

Harris, D. L. (2011). Navigating intimate relationship loss: When the relationship dies but the person is still living. In D. L. Harris (Ed.), *Counting our losses: Reflecting on change, loss, and transition in everyday life* (pp. 65–74). Routledge/Taylor & Francis Group.

Harris, D. L. (2020). *Nondeath loss and grief.* Routledge.

Harris, D. L., & Isenor, J. (2011). Loss of employment. In D. L. Harris (Ed.), *Counting our losses: Reflecting on change, loss, and transition in everyday life* (pp. 163–170). Routledge/Taylor & Francis Group.

Harrison, R. L., & Westwood, M. J. (2009). Preventing vicarious traumatization of mental health therapists: Identifying protective practices. *Psychotherapy: Theory, Research, Practice, Training, 46*(2), 203–219.

Hart, C. L., Hole, D. J., Lawlor, D. A., Smith, G., & Lever, T. F. (2007). Effect of conjugal bereavement on mortality of the bereaved spouse in participants of the Renfrew/Paisley study. *Journal of Epidemiology and Community Health, 61*(5), 455–460.

Harte, J. M., van Leeuwen, M. E., & Theuws, R., (2013). The nature, extent, and judicial response to aggression and violence directed against care workers in psychiatry. *Tijdschrift vooor Psychiatrie, 55*(5), 325–335.

Hartel, J. A. (1993). The prosecution of assaultive clients. *Perspectives in Psychiatric Care, 29,* 7–14.

Hartsough, D. (1982). Planning for disaster: A new community outreach program for mental health centers. *Journal of Community Psychology, 10,* 255–264.

Harvey, M. R, Tummala-Narra, P., & Hamm, B. (2012). An ecological view of recovery and resilience in trauma survivors: Implications for clinical and community intervention. In R. A. McMackin, E. Newman, J. M. Fogler, & T. M. Keane (Eds.), *Trauma therapy in context: The science and craft of evidence –based practice* (pp. 99–120) American Psychological Association.

Harvey, S. B., Modini, M., Joyce, S., Milligan-Saville, J. S., Tan, L., Mykletun, A., Bryant, R. A., Christensen, H., & Mitchell, P. B. (2017). Can work make you mentally ill? A systematic meta-review of work-related risk factors for common mental health problems. *Occupational and Environmental Medicine, 74*(4), 301–310. https://doi.org/10.1136/oemed-2016-104015

Hassellberg, N., Holgersen, K., Uverud, G., Siqveland, J., Lloyd-Evans, B., Johnson, S., & Rudd, T. (2021). Fidelity to an evidence-based model for crisis resolution teams: A cross-sectional multicentre study in Norway. *Psychiatry, 21,* article 231. https://doi.org/10.1186/s12888-021-03237-8

Hastings, J. E., & Hamberger, L. K. (1988). Personality characteristics of spouse abusers: A controlled comparison. *Violence and Victims, 3,* 31–47.

Havron, S., Freed, D., Chatterjee, R., McCoy, D., Dell, N., & Ristenpart, T. (2019). *Clinical Computer Security for Victims of Intimate Partner Violence.* 105–122. https://www.usenix.org/conference/usenixsecurity19/presentation/havron

Hayes, G. (2002). Intervening with school students after terrorist acts. In D. D. Bass & R. Yep (Eds.), *Terrorism, trauma, and tragedies: A counselor's guide to preparing and responding* (pp. 63–65). American Counseling Association.

Hayes, G., Goodwin, T., & Miars, B. (1990). After disaster: A crisis support team at work. *American Journal of Nursing, 2,* 61–64.

Hayes, J. L. (2011). *The historic tornadoes of April 2011.* The National Oceanic and Atmospheric Administration.

Hayes, L. M. (2010). *National study of jail suicide: 20 years later.* U.S. Department of Justice, National Institute of Corrections.

Hayes, S. C., Strosahl, K. D., & Wilson, K. G. (1999). *Acceptance and commitment therapy: An experiential approach to behavior change.* Guilford Press.

Haynes, R. A., & Henderson, C. L. (2001). *Essential strategies for school security: A practical guide for teachers and school administrators.* Charles C. Thomas.

Haynes, S. (1995). Introduction to the special section on chaos theory and psychological assessment. *Psychological Assessment, 7*(1), 3–4. https://doi.org/10.1037/h0092772

Hays, P. A. (2001). *Addressing cultural complexities in practice: A framework for clinicians and counselors* (pp. vii, 239). American Psychological Association. https://doi.org/10.1037/10411-000

Hays, P. A. (2022). *Addressing cultural complexities in counseling and clinical practice: An intersectional approach* (4th ed.). American Psychological Association.

Haywood, C., & Leuthe, J. (1980, September 8). *Crisis intervention in the 1980s: From networking to social influence.* [Paper presentation]. Annual Convention of the American Psychological Association, Montreal, Canada.

Hazen, M. (2009). Recognizing and responding to workplace grief. *Organizational Dynamics, 38*(4), 290–296.

Hazler, R. J. (1996). *Breaking the cycle of violence: Interventions for bullying and victimization.* Accelerated Development.

Healy, M. J., Smith, C., & O'Sullivan, C. (1998). *Batterer intervention: Program approaches and criminal justice strategies* (Report No. NCJ 168638). U.S. Department of Justice.

Heath, M. A., & Hudnall, G. (2011). Special issue on strengthening school-based support for bereaved students: Editors' introduction. *School Psychology International, 32*(2), 115–117.

Heath, M. A., & Sheen, D. (2005). *School-based crisis intervention: Preparing all personnel to assist.* Guilford Press.

Heath, N. M., Lynch, S. M., Fritch, A. M., & Wong, M. M. (2013). Rape myth acceptance impacts the reporting of rape to the police: A study of incarcerated women. *Violence Against Women, 19*(9), 1065–1078. https://doi.org/10.1177/1077801213501841

Heerema, E. (2022). Using reality orientation in Alzheimer's and dementia. *Very Well Health.* https://www.verywellhealth.com/treating-alzheimers-disease-with-reality-orientation-98682

Heilbrun, A. B. (1990). The measurement of criminal dangerousness as a personality construct: Further validation of a research index. *Journal of Personality Assessment, 54*, 141–148.

Heilbrun, A. B., & Heilbrun, M. R. (1989). Dangerousness and legal insanity. *Journal of Psychiatry and Law, 17*, 39–53.

Heise, L. L., & Kotsadam, A. (2015). Cross-national and multilevel correlates of partner violence: An analysis of data from population-based surveys. *The Lancet Global Health, 3*(6), e332–e340. https://doi.org/10.1016/S2214-109X(15)00013-3

Helby, E. M. (1995). Chaos theory, nonlinear dynamic models, and psychological assessment. *Psychological Assessment, 7*(1), 5–9. https://doi.org/10.1037/1040-3590.7.1.5

Hellman, D. S., & Blackman, S. (1966). Enuresis, fire setting, and cruelty to animals: A triad predictive of adult crime. *American Journal of Psychiatry, 122*, 1431–1435.

Helsloot, I. (2012). *Mega-crises: Understanding the prospects, nature, characteristics, and the effects of cataclysmic events.* Charles C Thomas.

Helsloot, I., Boin, A., Jacobs, B., & Comfort, L. (Eds.). (2014). *Mega-crisis: Understanding the prospects, nature, characteristics and effects of cataclysmic events.* Charles C. Thomas.

Hembree, E., Rauch, S., & Foa, E. (2003). Beyond the manual: The insider's guide to prolonged exposure therapy for PTSD. *Cognitive and Behavioral Practice, 10*(1), 22–30.

Hendrickson, K. C. (2009). Morbidity, mortality, and parental grief: A review of the literature on the relationship between the death of a child and the subsequent health of parents. *Palliative & Supportive Care, 7*(1), 109–119. https://doi.org/10.1017/S1478951509000133

Henebery, B. (2021). How effective are peer support programs? *The Educator: Australia.* https://www.theeducatoronline.com/k12/news/how-effective-are-school-peer-support-programs/276536

Henning, E., Germann, J. N., Holder, N., Nakonezny, P., Loftin, S., Redondo-Doan, B., Jones, L., Petty, L. A., Pratt, C., Garza-Saenz, M., Isaacs, T., Liu, K., & Winick, N. (2021). The impact of family bereavement interventions: Qualitative feedback identifies needs. *Clinical Practice in Pediatric Psychology, 9*(3), 283–295. https://doi.org/10.1037/cpp0000416

Henning, J. A., & Brand, B. L. (2019). Implications of the American Psychological Association's posttraumatic stress disorder treatment guideline for trauma education and training. *Psychotherapy, 56*(3), 422–430. https://doi.org/10.1037/pst0000237

Henning, K., & Connor-Smith, J. (2011). Why doesn't he leave? Relationship continuity and satisfaction among male domestic offenders. *Journal of Interpersonal Violence, 26*(7), 1366–1387.

Henry, V. E. (2004). *Death work: Police, trauma, and the psychology of survival.* Oxford University Press.

Henry, V. E. (2005). In A. E. Roberts (Ed.), *Crisis intervention handbook* (3rd ed., pp. 171–199). Oxford University Press.

Hensel, J., Lunsky, Y., & Dewa, C. (2012). Exposure to client aggression and burnout among community staff who support adults with intellectual disabilities in Ontario, Canada. *Journal of Intellectual Disability Research, 56*(9), 910–915.

Hensel, J., Ruiz, C., Finney, C., & Dewa, C. (2015). Meta-analysis of risk factors for secondary traumatic stress in therapeutic work with trauma victims. *Journal of Traumatic Stress, 28*(2), 83–91.

Henson, J. S. (2020). Burnout or compassion fatigue: A comparison of concepts—ProQuest. *Medsurg Nursing, 29*(2), 77.

Heppner, M. J. (1978). Counseling the battered wife: Myths, facts, and decisions. *Personnel and Guidance Journal, 56*, 522–525.

Heppner, P. P., Heppner, M. J., Lee, D., Wang, Y.-W., Park, H., & Wang, L. (2006). Development and validation of a collectivist coping styles inventory. *Journal of Counseling Psychology, 53*(1), 107–125. https://doi.org/10.1037/0022-0167.53.1.107

Herman, J. (1992). *Trauma and recovery.* Basic Books.

Herman, J. L. (1992a). Complex PTSD: A syndrome in survivors of prolonged and repeated trauma. *Journal of Traumatic Stress, 5*(3), 377–391. https://doi.org/10.1002/jts.2490050305

Herman, J. L. (1992b). *Trauma and recovery: The aftermath of violence—from domestic abuser to political terror.* Basic Books.

Herman, J. L. (1997). *Trauma and recovery.* Basic Books.

Herman, J. L., Perry, C., & van der Kolk, B. A. (1989). Childhood trauma in borderline personality disorder. *American Journal of Psychiatry, 146*, 490–494.

Hermann, C. F. (1963). Some consequences of crisis which limit the viability of organizations. *Administrative Science Quarterly, 8*, 61–81.

Hermann, M. A., & Finn, A. (2002). An ethical and legal perspective on the role of school counselors in preventing violence in schools. *Professional School Counselor, 6*(1), 46–54.

Hermann, M. A., & Remley, T. P., Jr. (2000). Guns, violence, and schools: The results of school violence litigation against educators and students shedding more constitutional rights at the school house gate. *Loyola Law Review, 46*, 389–439.

Hernández, P., Gangsei, D., & Engstrom, D. (2007). Vicarious resilience: A new concept in work with those who survive trauma. *Family Process, 46*(2), 229–241. https://doi .org/10.1111/j.1545-5300.2007.00206.x

Herpertz-Dahlmann, B., Hahn, F., & Hempt, A. (2005). Clinical assessment and therapy of post-traumatic stress disorder in childhood and adolescence: Responsibilities of an outpatient clinic for traumatized children. *Nervenarzt, 76*(5), 546–556.

Herrera, V. M., Wiersma, J. D., & Cleveland, H. H. (2008). The influence of individual and partner characteristics on the perpetration of intimate partner violence in young adult relationships. *Journal of Youth and Adolescence, 37*(3), 284–296. https:// doi.org/10.1007/s10964-007-9249-4

Herringa, R. J., Phillips, M. L. Fournier, J. C., Kronhaus, D. M., & Germain, A. (2013). Childhood and adult trauma both correlate with dorsal anterior cingulate activation to threat in combat veterans. *Psychological Medicine, 43*(7), 1533–1542.

Hersh, J. B. (1985). Interviewing college students in crisis. *Journal of Counseling and Development, 63*, 286–289.

Hersh, M. A. (2022). Spiritual and religious beliefs. In M. A. Hersh (Ed.). *The thriving therapist: Sustaining self-care to prevent burnout and enhance well-being* (pp. 161–167). American Psychological Association.

Hersh, S. P. (1996). After heart attack and stroke. In K. J. Doka (Ed.), *Living with grief after sudden loss: Suicide, homicide, accident, heart attack, stroke* (pp. 17–24). Hospice Foundation of America.

Hertlein, K. M., & Teichert, R. (2023). The association between technology-mediated intimate partner violence and Stockholm syndrome. *Journal of Couple & Relationship Therapy, 22*(3), 1–15. https://doi.org/10.1080/15332691.2023.2165583

Hewnsel, J., Lunsky, Y., & Dewa, C. (2012). Exposure to client aggression and burnout among community staff who support adults with intellectual disabilities in Ontario, Canada. *Journal of Intellectual Disability Research, 56*(9), 910–915.

Hibberd, R., Elwood, L. S., & Galovski, T. E. (2010). Risk and protective factors for posttraumatic stress disorder, prolonged grief and depression in survivors of the violent death of a loved one. *Journal of Loss and Trauma, 15*(5), 426–447.

Hickman, R. I., & Douglas, S. L. (2010). Impact of chronic critical illness on the psychological outcomes of family members. *AACN Advanced Critical Care, 21*, 80–91.

Hicks, J. F. (2015). Empowering youth victimized by cyber bullying. *Counseling Today, 57*(9), 48–53.

Hicks, T. A., Bountress, K. E., Resnick, H. S., Ruggiero, K. J., & Amstadter, A. B. (2022). Caregiver support buffers posttraumatic stress disorder symptoms following a natural disaster in relation to binge drinking. *Psychological Trauma: Theory, Research, Practice, and Policy, 14*(7), 1142–1148. https://doi .org/10.1037/tra0000553

Hill, R. (1949). *Families under stress: Adjustment to the crisis of war separation and reunion.* Harper & Row.

Hill, R. (1965). Generic features of families under stress. In H. J. Parad (Ed.). *Crisis intervention: Selected readings* (pp. 32–52). Family Service Association of America.

Hill, R. M., Oosterhoff, B., Layne, C. M., Rooney, E., Yudovich, S., Pynoos, R. S., & Kaplow, J. B. (2019). Multidimensional grief therapy: Pilot open trial of a novel intervention for bereaved children and adolescents. *Journal of Child and Family Studies, 28*(11), 3062–3074. https://doi.org/10.1007/ s10826-019-01481-x

Hilliard, R. E. (2008). Music and grief work with children. In C. A. Malchiodi (Ed.), *Creative interventions with traumatized children* (pp. 63–80). Guilford Press.

Hillman, J., Flicker, S., LeGendre, L., & Traczuk, K. (2005). The pervasiveness of patient aggression among elderly residents in long-term care: Implications for intervention and prevention. In J. P. Morgan (Ed.), *Psychology of aggression* (pp. 69–85). Nova Science Publishers.

Hindley, N., & Gordon, H. (2000). The elderly, dementia, aggression and risk management. *International Journal of Geriatric Psychiatry, 15*(3), 254–259.

Hines, D. A., Brown, J., & Dunning, E. (2007). Characteristics of callers to the domestic abuse helpline for men. *Journal of Family Violence, 22*(2), 63–72. https://doi.org/10.1007/ s10896-006-9052-0

Hinrichsen, G. A., & Clougherty, K. F. (2006). *Interpersonal psychotherapy for depressed older adults.* American Psychological Association.

Hirsch, J. K., & Cukrowicz, K. C. (2014). Suicide in rural areas: An updated review of the literature. *Journal of Rural Mental Health, 38*, 65–78. https://doi.org/10.1037/rmh0000018

Ho, S., Lo, R., & Pau, N. (2013). Roles of intra- and extra-organizational support, coping strategies, and perceived control in combating burnout among health care workers after workplace violence. In B. R. Doolittle (Ed.), *Psychology of burnout: New research, psychology of emotions, motivations and actions* (pp. 85–106). Nova Science Publishers.

Hobfoll, S. E. (1988). *The ecology of stress.* Wiley.

Hobfoll, S. E., & deVries, M. W. (Eds.). (1995). *Extreme stress and communities: Impact and intervention.* Kluwer.

Hobfoll, S. E., Watson, P. J., Bell, C. C., Bryant, R. A., Brymer, M. J., Friedman, M. J., Friedman M, Gersons, B.P., de Jong, J. T, Layne, C. M., Maguen, S., Neria, Y., Norwood, A. E., Pynoos, R. S., Reissman, D., Ruzek, J. I., Shalev, A. Y., Solomon, Z., Steinberg, A. M., & Ursano, R. J. (2007). Five essential elements for immediate and mid-term crisis in mass trauma intervention: Empirical evidence. *Psychiatry, 70*, 283–315.

Hoeksma, J. H., Guy, J. D., Brown, C. K., & Brady, J. L. (1993). The relationship between psychotherapist burnout and satisfaction with leisure activities. *Psychotherapy in Private Practice, 12*, 51–57.

Hoff, I. A., Hallisey, B. J., & Hoff, M. (2009). *People in crisis: Clinical and diversity perspectives.* Routledge, Taylor, & Francis Group.

Hoffberg A.S., Stearns-Yoder K.A., & Brenner L.A. (2020). The effectiveness of crisis line services: A systematic review. *Front Public Health, 7*, 399. http://doi.org/10.3389/fpubh.2019.00399

Hogan, N. S., Greenfield, D. B., & Schmidt, L. A. (2001). Development and validation of the Hogan Grief Reaction Checklist. *Death Studies, 25*(1), 1–32.

Hoge, C. W., Auchterlonie, J. L., & Milliken, C. S. (2006). Mental health problems, use of mental health services and attrition from military service after returning from deployment to Iraq or Afghanistan. *Journal of the American Medical Association, 295*, 1023–1035.

Hoge, R. (2008). Serious and violent juvenile offenders. *Resource Material no. 78.* United Nations Asia and Far East Institute for the Prevention of Crime and the Treatment of Offenders. https://www.unafei.or.jp/english/publications/Resource _Material_78.html

Holgerson, K., Pedersen, S., Brattland, H., & Hynnekleiv, T. (2022). A scoping review into crisis resolution teams in community mental health services. *Nordic Journal of Psychiatry.* Advance online publication. https://doi.org/10.1080/08039488.2002.2029941

Holladay, J. (2010, Fall). Cyberbullying. *Teaching Tolerance,* 43–46.

Holland, J. M., & Neimeyer, R. A. (2011). Separation and traumatic distress in prolonged grief: The role of cause of death and relationship to the deceased. *Journal of Psychopathology and Behavioral Assessment, 33*(2), 254–263.

Holt, H., & Beutler, L. E. (2014). Concerns about the dissemination of evidence-based psychotherapies in the Veterans Affairs Health care system. *American Psychologist, 69*(7), 705.

Holt, H., Beutler, L. A., Castonguay, L. G., Silberchutz, G., Forrester, B., Temkin, R. S., & Miller, T. W. (2013). A critical examination for the movement towards evidence based mental health in the U.S. Department of Veterans Affairs health care system. *The Clinical Psychologist, 664,* 8–14.

Holtzworth-Munroe, A., & Stuart, G. L. (1994). Typologies of male batterers: Three subtypes and the differences among them. *Psychological Bulletin, 116*(3), 476–497.

Holtzworth-Munroe, A., Meehan, J., Herron, K., & Stuart, G. (1999). A typology of batterers: An initial examination. In X. B. Ariagapa & S. Oskamp (Eds.), *Violence in intimate relationships* (pp. 45–72). SAGE.

Holtzworth-Munroe, A., Meehan, J., Herron, K., Rehman, U., & Stuart, G. (2003). Do subtypes of maritally violent men continue to differ over time? *Journal of Consulting & Clinical Psychology, 71*(4), 728–740.

Homeland Security Administration (2015). *School safety.* www.dhs.gov/school-safety

Homeyer, L. E., & Sweeney, D. S. (2022). *Sandtray therapy: A practical manual.* Taylor & Francis.

Hong, S., Lu, N., Wu, D., Jimenez, D. E., & Milanaik, R. L. (2020). Digital sextortion: Internet predators and pediatric interventions. *Current Opinion in Pediatrics, 32*(1), 192. https://doi.org/10.1097/MOP.0000000000000854

Hooven, C. (2013). Parents-CARE: A suicide prevention program for parents of at-risk youth. *Journal of Child and Adolescent Psychiatric Nursing, 26*(1), 85–95. https://doi.org/10.1111/jcap.12025

Hoover, J. H., & Hazler, R. J. (1991). Bullies and victims. *Elementary School Guidance & Counseling, 25,* 212–219.

Hopkins, O., & King, N. (1994). PTSD in children and adolescents. *Behavior Change, 11,* 110–120.

Hoppe, M. (2019). The top qualities to look for when hiring a school resource officer. *RAVE Mobile Safety.* https://www.ravemobilesafety.com/blog/top-qualities-look-for-when-hiring-school-resource-officer/

Horn, J. (2002). Law enforcement and trauma. In M. Williams & J. Sommer (Eds.), *Simple and complex post-traumatic stress disorder: Strategies for comprehensive treatment in clinical practice* (pp. 311–323). Haworth Press.

Horne, A. M., Bartolomucci, C. L., & Newman-Carson, D. (2003). *Bully busters: A teacher's manual for helping bullies, victims, and bystanders.* Research Press.

Hornor, G. (2010). Child sexual abuse: Consequences and implications. *Journal of Pediatric Health Care, 24*(6), 358–364. https://doi.org/10.1016/j.pedhc.2009.07.003

Horowitz, M. J. (1976). *Stress response syndromes.* Aronson.

Horowitz, M. J. (1986). *Stress response syndromes* (2nd ed.). Jason Aronson.

Horowitz, M. J., & Solomon, G. F. (1975). A prediction of delayed stress response syndromes in Vietnam veterans. *Journal of Social Issues, 31,* 67–80.

Horowitz, M. J., Siegel, B., Holen, A., Bonnanno, G., Milbrath, C., & Stinson, C. H. (1997). Diagnostic criteria for complicated grief disorder. *American Journal of Psychiatry, 154*(7), 904–910.

Horowitz, M. J., Wilner, N., & Alvarez, W. (1979). Impact of Events Scale: A measure of subjective stress. *Psychosomatic Medicine, 41,* 209–218.

Horowitz, M. J., Wilner, N., Kaltreider, N., & Alvarez, W. (1980). Signs and symptoms of post-trauma stress disorders. *Archives of General Psychiatry, 37,* 85–92.

Horton, A. L. (1995). Sex-related hotline calls. In A. R. Roberts (Ed.), *Crisis intervention and time-related cognitive treatment* (pp. 292–312). SAGE.

Hotaling, G. T., & Sugarman, D. B. (1986). An analysis of risk markers in husband to wife violence: The current state of knowledge. *Violence and Victims, 1,* 101–124.

Howard Sharp, K. M., Russell, C., Keim, M., Barrera, M., Gilmer, M. J., Foster Akard, T., Compas, B. E., Fairclough, D. L., Davies, B., Hogan, N., Young-Saleme, T., Vannatta, K., & Gerhardt, C. A. (2018). Grief and growth in bereaved siblings: Interactions between different sources of social support. *School Psychology Quarterly, 33*(3), 363–371. https://doi.org/10.1037/spq0000253

Howarth, R. A. (2011). Promoting the adjustment of parentally bereaved children. *Journal of Mental Health Counseling, 33*(1), 21–32.

Howell, J. C. (2015). *The history of street gangs in the United States.* Lexington Books.

Hsieh, H., & Wang, J. (2003). Effect of reminiscence therapy on depression in older adults: A systematic review. *International Journal of Nursing Studies, 40*(4), 335–345.

Hsieh, H., Lee, D., Zimmerman, M., Pomerantz, N., Cunningham, C., Messman, E., Stoddard, S., Grodzinski, A., & Heinze, J. (2022). The effectiveness of the say-something anonymous reporting system in preventing school violence: A cluster randomized control trial in 19 middle schools. *Journal of School Violence, 21*(4), 413–428, https://doi.org/10.1080/15388220.2022.2105858

Hsiung, R. C. (2002). *E-therapy: Case studies, guiding principles, and the clinical potential of the Internet.* W. W. Norton.

Hsu, M. V. (2010). Continuing bonds expressions in pet bereavement. *Dissertation Abstracts International: Section B. The Sciences and Engineering,* 2049.

Huang, X., Ribeiro, J. D., & Franklin, J. C. (2020). The differences between individuals engaging in nonsuicidal self-injury and suicide attempt are complex (vs. complicated or simple). *Frontiers in Psychiatry, 11.* https://www.frontiersin.org/articles/10.3389/fpsyt.2020.00239

Hubbard, J. A., Dodge, K. A., Cillessen, A. H. N., Coie, J. D., & Schwartz, D. (2001). The dyadic nature of social information processing in boys' reactive and proactive aggression. *Journal of Personality and Social Psychology, 80,* 268–280.

Hudspeth, E. F. (2016). Play therapy applications with diverse cultures. *International Journal of Play Therapy, 25*(3), 113. https://doi.org/10.1037/pla0000030

Huff, C. (2022). The stress of media overload. *Monitor on Psychology, 53*(8), 20–23.

Hughes, R. B. (1988). Grief counseling: Facilitating the healing process. *Journal of Counseling and Development, 67,* 77.

Humane Society (2023). *How to cope with the death of your pet*. The Humane Society. http://humanesociety.org

Humanitarian charter and minimum standards in disaster response. (1998). *Sphere Project*. World Health Organization.

Hummer, G. A., Wang, Y., Kronenberger, W., Mosier, K., Kalnin, A., Dunn, D., & Mathews, V. P. (2010). Short-term violent video game play by adolescents alters prefrontal activity during cognitive inhibition. *Media Psychology, 13*(2), 136–154.

Humphrey, K. M. (2009). *Counseling strategies for loss and grief*. American Counseling Association

Humphrey, N., & Brooks, A. (2006). An evaluation of a short cognitive-behavioural anger management intervention for pupils at risk of exclusion. *Emotional & Behavioural Difficulties, 11*(1), 5–23.

Hunt, R. D., Osten, C., & Teague, S. (1991). Youth suicide: Teachers should know. . . *Tennessee Teacher, 91*, 16–21, 29.

Husky, M., Olfson, M., He, J., Nock, M. K., Swanson, S., Alsemgeest, M., & Ries, K. (2012). Twelve-month suicidal symptoms and use of services among adolescents: Results from the National Comorbidity Survey. *Psychiatric Services, 63*(10), 989–996.

Hutchinson, M., Jackson, D, Haigh, C., & Hayter, M. (2013). Editorial: Five years of scholarship on violence, bullying and aggression towards nurses in the workplace: What have we learned? *Journal of Clinical Nursing, 22*(7-8), 903–905.

Hwang, W. (2012). Integrating top-down bottom-up approaches to culturally adapting psychotherapy application to Chinese Americans. In G. Bernal & M. M. Domenech-Rodriguez (Eds.), *Cultural adaptations: Tools for evidence–based practice with diverse populations.* (pp. 179–198). American Psychological Association.

Hyer, L., Sohnle, S., Mehan, D., & Ragan, A. (2002). Use of positive core memories in LTC: A review. *Clinical Gerontologist, 25*(1/2), 51–90.

Hymel, S., & Swearer, S. (2015). Four decades of research on school bullying. *American Psychologist, 70*(4), 293–299. https://doi.org/10.1037/a0038928

Ibrahim, F. A., & Herr, E. L. (1987). Battered women: A developmental life-career counseling perspective. *Journal of Counseling and Development, 65*, 244–248.

ICE. (2022). *Combatting gangs*. Department of Homeland Security. https://www.ice.gov/features/gangs

Ielmini, M., Lucca, G., Trabucchi, E., Aspesi, G. L., Bellini, A., Caselli, I., & Callegari, C. (2022). Assessing mental pain as a predictive factor of suicide risk in a clinical sample of patients with psychiatric disorders. *Behavioral Sciences (2076-328X), 12*(4), 111. https://doi.org/10.3390/bs12040111

Ilkevich, S. & Shlapak, V. (2014). The interdisciplinary approach to crisis management: Recent trends in international studies. *Servis Plus, 2*(1), 51–65. https://doi.org/10.12737/2797

Imber-Black, E. (2012). The value of rituals in family life. In F. Walsh (Ed.), *Normal family processes: Growing diversity and complexity* (4th ed., pp. 483–497). Guilford Press.

Institute of Medicine. (2015). *Healthy, resilient, and sustainable communities after disasters: Strategies, opportunities, and planning for recovery*. National Academies Press.

Inter-Agency Standing Committee (IASC). (2007). *IASC guidelines on mental health and psychosocial input support in emergency situations*.

Inter-Agency Standing Committee (IASC). (2023). *IASC guidelines on mental health and psychosocial input support in emergency situations*.

International Classification of Diseases. (2023). *ICD-10Z63.8- Other specified problems related to primary family support*. https://www.icd10data.com/ICD10CM/Codes/Z00-Z99/Z55-Z65/Z63-/Z63.8

International Federation of Red Cross and Red Crescent Societies (2022). *Psychosocial support*. http://www.ifrc.org/en/what-we-do/health/psychosocial-support/

International Society for the Study of Trauma and Dissociation (2015). Dissociation FAQs. http://www.isst-d.org/default.asp?contentID=76#diss

International Society for Traumatic Stress Studies. (2019). Posttraumatic stress disorder prevention and treatment guidelines: Methodology and recommendations. https://istss.org/clinical-resources/treating-trauma/new-istss-prevention-and-treatment-guidelines

Ironson, G., Hylton, E., Gonzalez, B., Small, B., Freund, B., Gerstein, M., Thurston, F., & Bira, L. (2021). Effectiveness of three brief treatments for recent traumatic events in a low-SES community setting. *Psychological Trauma: Theory, Research, Practice, and Policy, 13*(1), 123–132. https://doi.org/10.1037/tra0000594

Irwin, E. C. (1987). Drama: The play's the thing. *Elementary School Guidance & Counseling, 21*, 276–283.

Irwin, V., Wang, K., Thompson, A., & Cui, J. (2022). *Report on indicators of school crime and safety: 2021*. Bureau of Justice Statistics. https://bjs.ojp.gov/library/publications/report-indicators-school-crime-and-safety-2021

Isaksson, U., Graneheim, U. H., Ricter, J., Eisenmann, M., & Astrom, S. (2008). Exposure to violence in relation to personality traits, coping abilities and burnout among caregivers in nursing homes: A case-control approach. *Scandinavian Journal of Caring Sciences, 22*(4), 551–559.

Ishikawa, R. Z. (2020). I may never see the ocean again: Loss and grief among older adults during the COVID-19 pandemic. *Psychological Trauma: Theory, Research, Practice, and Policy, 12*(S1), S85–S86. https://doi.org/10.1037/tra0000695

Ishimoto, W. (1984). Security management for health care administrators. In J. T. Turner (Ed.), *Violence in the medical care setting: A survival guide* (pp. 209–223). Aspen Systems.

Iskamto, D. (2021). Stress and its impact on employee performance. *International Journal of Social and Management Studies, 2*(3), Article 3. https://doi.org/10.5555/ijosmas.v2i3.42

Issacs, J. S. (2004). Numerical distraction therapy: Initial assessment of a treatment for posttraumatic stress disorder. *Traumatology, 10*(1), 39–54

Italiano, F. (2001). Listening and learning at North Arlington High School. *Police Chief, 68*(9), 53–55.

Iverson, K. M., King, M. W., Cunningham, K. C., & Resick, P. A. (2015). Rape survivors' trauma–related beliefs before and after cognitive processing therapy: Associations with PTSD and depression symptoms. *Behaviour Research and Therapy, 66*, 49–55.

Iwakabe, S. (1999). Psychotherapy and chaos theory: The metaphoric relationship between psychodynamic therapy and chaos theory. *Psychotherapy: Theory, Research, Practice, Training, 36*(3) 274–286. https://doi.org/10.1037/h0087720

Jackson, K., & Harding, M. (2010, July). *Advocating for LGBTQ students*. Paper presented at American School Counselor Conference, Boston, MA, the United States.

Jackson, N. A., & Jabbi, M. M. (2022). Integrating biobehavioral information to predict mood disorder suicide risk. *Brain,*

Behavior, & Immunity - Health, 24. https://doi.org/10.1016/j. bbih.2022.100495

Jackson, T. (2019). Unified mental health teams. *ASCA School Counselor, 57*(1), 12–15.

Jacobs, J. (2010). Suicide prevention on the Golden Gate Bridge. *American Journal of Psychiatry, 167*(4), 473.

Jacobs, J., Horne-Moyer, H. L., & Jones, R. (2004). The effectiveness of critical incident stress debriefing with primary and secondary trauma victims. *International Journal of Emergency Mental Health, 6*, 5–14.

Jahoda, M., Lazarsfeld, P. F., & Zeisel, H. (1933/1971). *"Marienthal": The sociography of an unemployed community.* Aldine.

Jaime, M., McCauley, H., Tancredi, D., Nettiksimmons, J., Decker, M., Silverman, J., O'Connor, B., Stetkevich, N., & Miller, E. (2015). Athletic coaches as violence prevention advocates. *Journal of Interpersonal Violence, 30*(7), 1090–1111.

Jain, A., Mulvey, E. P. & Maruna, S. (2017). Risk assessment and violence: Implications of the interactionist perspective. In H. Toth (Ed.). *Violent men: An inquiry into the psychology of violence* (25th anniversary ed., pp. 277–293). American Psychological Association.

James, B. (1994). School violence and the law: The search for suitable tools. *School Psychology Review, 23*(2), 190–203.

James, B. (1997). FERPA and school violence: The silence that kills. In A. P. Goldstein & J. C. Conoley (Eds.), *School violence prevention: A practical handbook* (pp. 460–489). Guilford Press.

James, D. J., & Glaze, L. E., (2006, September 6). Mental health problems of prison and jail inmates. *Bureau of Justice Statistics.* http://www.bjs.gov/index.cfm?ty=pbdetail&iid=789

James, D. V., Allen, P., Wolfe, A., MacKenzie, R. D., Yang, J., De Silva, A., & Farnham, F. R. (2022). The CTAP, a threat assessment tool for the initial evaluation of concerning or threatening communications: Development and inter-rater reliability. *Journal of Threat Assessment and Management, 9*(3), 129–152. https://doi.org/10.1037/tam0000173

James, D. V., Farnham, F. R., Wilson, S. P., Meloy, J. R., & Hoffmann, J. (2013). The fixated threat assessment centre. *International handbook of threat assessment, 299.*

James, D. V., MacKenzie, R. D., & Farnham, F. R. (2014). *Communications Threat Assessment Protocol-25: Guidelines for the initial assessment of problematic communications.* Theseus.

James, D. V., MacKenzie, R. D., Allen, P., Wolfe, M., De Silva, A., Yang, J., & Farnham, F. (2023). Factors associated with approach and persistence in corporate threat assessment cases: The validity of the CTAP. *Journal of Threat Assessment and Management, 10*(1), 42–56. https://doi.org/10.1037/tam0000180

James, R. (1970). *Parent Effectiveness Training Manual.* Title III ESEA, Intensive Care Unit, Mattoon, Illinois, Community Unit #2 School District.

James, R. (1974). A study of the effects of parent participation in a parent group education program on seventh and eighth grade underachieving, socially maladjusted students. [Unpublished doctoral dissertation]. Indiana State University

James, R., & Crawford, R. (2002). The estranged, violent, juvenile offender: Profiling, screening, intervention, and legal considerations. *Global Visions for Counseling Professionals, 6*(1), 1–14.

James, R., & Dorner, K. (1999, June). *Profiling, screening, and counseling the estranged juvenile violent offender.* Paper presented at the American School Counselor Association Convention, Phoenix, AZ, the United States.

James, R., Kirchberg, T., Nobbman, K., & Skirius, M. (2013a, October). *Where and why are your social locations important?* Paper presented at Crisis Intervention Team International Convention, Hartford, CT, the United States.

James, R., Logan, J., & Davis, S. (2011). Including school resource officers in school-based crisis intervention: Strengthening student support. *School Psychology International, 32*(2), 210–224.

James, R., Myer, R., Skirius, M., & Nobbman, K. (2013b, October). *Crisis intervention and diversity: A story of social locations.* Paper presented at American Counselor Education and Supervision Conference, Denver, CO, the United States.

James, R. K. & Gilliland, B. E. (2017). *Crisis intervention strategies.* (8th ed.). Cengage Learning.

James, R. K. & Myer, R. A. (2022). Evaluation de la violence dans les malades mentaux. (Evaluation of violence in the mentally ill). In M. Bibeau (Ed.). *Evaluation de la menace et du risqué: Dans different contextes.* Thomas Reuter.

James, R. K. (1994). Commentary to "Dial 911: Schizophrenia and the Police Response." In P. Backlar (Ed.), *The family face of schizophrenia* (pp. 182–200). Jeremy Tarcher/Putnam.

James, R. K. (2003, April). *Drawing out the trauma.* Paper presented at the Twenty-seventh Annual Convening of Crisis Intervention Personnel, Chicago, IL, the United States.

James, R. K. (2006, May). *Four hundred miles from landfall: Lesson learned from Katrina.* Paper presented at the Thirtieth Annual Convening of Crisis Intervention Personnel and the Contact USA Conference, Chicago, IL, the United States.

James, R. K. (2014). Basic verbal practicum techniques. In Memphis Police Department, *Crisis intervention team training manual* (pp. 56–60). Memphis Police Department.

James, R. K., & Crews, W. (2009). Systems consultation: Working with a metropolitan police department. In A. M. Dougherty (Ed.), *Psychological consultation and collaboration in schools and community settings: A casebook* (5th ed., pp. 93–114). Brooks/Cole.

James, R. K., & Crews, W. (2014). Systems consultation: Working with a metropolitan police department. In A. M. Dougherty (Ed.), *Psychological consultation and collaboration in schools and community settings: A casebook* (6th ed., pp. 93–114). Brooks/Cole.

James, R. K., & Gilliland, B. E. (2003). *Theories and strategies in counseling and psychotherapy* (5th ed.). Allyn & Bacon.

James, R. K., & Myer, R. (1987). Puppets: The elementary counselor's right or left arm. *Elementary School Guidance & Counseling, 21*, 292–299.

James, R. K., Blancett, J., & Addy, C. (2007, March). *Adapting the TACKLE form to civilian use: The Triage Assessment Severity Checklist for Civilians.* [Paper presentation]. Thirty-First Convening of Crisis Intervention Personnel and Contact USA, Chicago, IL, the United States.

James, R. K., Cogdal, P., & Gilliland, B. E. (2003, April). *An ecological theory of crisis intervention.* [Paper presentation]. American Counseling Association convention, Kansas City, MO, the United States.

James, R. K., Cogdal, P., & Gilliland, B. E. (2003, April). *Crisis intervention in the ecosystem.* [Paper presentation]. American Counseling Association Convention, Kansas City, MO, the United States

James, R. K., Davis, S., & Myer, R. A. (2014, October). *Triage checklist for Law Enforcement: TACKLE.* [Paper presentation]. Crisis

Intervention Team International Convention. Monterey, CA, the United States.

James, R. K., Myer, R., & Moore, H. (2006). *Triage Assessment Checklist for Law Enforcement (TACKLE) manual and CD*. Crisis Intervention and Prevention Solutions.

Jankowski, J., & Frey, A. (2012). Students connecting with the elderly: Validation as a tool. *Educational Gerontology, 38*(7), 486–490.

Janoff-Bulmal, R (1992). *Shattered assumptions*. Free Press.

Janosik, E. H. (1984). *Crisis counseling: A contemporary approach*. Wadsworth Health Sciences Division.

Janosik, S. M. (2004). Parents' views on the Clery Act and campus safety. *Journal of College Student Development, 45*(1), 43–56.

Janssen, J., & Giberson, D. (2013). Remotivation therapy. *Journal of Gerontological Nursing, 4*(6), 31–34. https://doi.org/10.3928/0098-9134-19880601-10

Jarero, I., & Ureibe, S. (2012). The EMDR protocol for recent critical incidents: Follow-up report of an application in a human massacre situation. *Journal of EMDR Practice and Research, 6*(2), 50–61.

Jasinski, J. L., & Williams, L. M. (Eds.). (1998). *Partner violence: A comprehensive review of 20 years of research*. SAGE.

Jeanne Clery Disclosure of Campus Security Policy and Campus Crime Statistics Act (1990). P.L.101-542 (20 U.S.C. 1092(f))

Jeffreys, M. D., Reinfeld, C., Nair, P. V., Garcia, H. A., Mata-Galan, E. & Rentz, T. O. (2014). Evaluating treatment of posttraumatic stress disorder with cognitive processing therapy and prolonged exposure therapy in a VHA specialty clinic. *Journal of Anxiety Disorders, 28*(1), 108–114.

Jennicus, M. (2013). Manners on the internet. *Counseling Today 56*(3), 16–17.

Jennings, K. (2011). Federal action to stop bullying. *ASCA School Counselor, 48*(6), 14–15.

Jensen, D., & Absher, J. (1994, April). *Assaultive behavior, the crisis is over: Preventing another crisis*. Paper presented at the Eighteenth Annual Convening of Crisis Intervention Personnel, Chicago, IL, the United States.

Jensen, D., & Absher, J. (1998, April). *Predicting/managing violence in crisis situations: Ensuring provider safety*. Paper presented at the Twenty-Second Annual Convening of Crisis Intervention Personnel, Chicago, IL, the United States.

Jensen, T. K., Holt, T., Ormhaug, S., Egeland, K., Granly, L., Hoaas, L. C., & Wentzel-Larsen, T. (2014). A randomized effectiveness study of trauma-focused cognitive behavioral therapy with therapy as usual for youth. *Journal of Clinical Child and Adolescent Psychology, 43*(3), 356–369.

Jetelina, K. K., Beauchamp, A. M., Reingle Gonzalez, J. M., Molsberry, R. J., Bishopp, S. A., & Lee, S. C. (2020). Cumulative, high-stress calls impacting adverse events among law enforcement and the public. *BMC Public Health, 20*(1), 1–9. https://doi.org/10.1186/s12889-020-09219-x

Jimenez, X. F. (2013). Patients with borderline personality disorder who are chronically suicidal: Therapeutic alliance and therapeutic limits. *American Journal of Psychotherapy, 67*(2), 185–201.

Jimerson, S. R., & Furlong, M. J. (Eds.). (2006). *Handbook of school violence and school safety: From research to practice*. Erlbaum.

Jin, L., Keegan, F. S., Weiss, N. H., Alghraibeh, A. M., Aljomaa, S. S., Almuhayshir, A. R., & Contractor, A. A. (2022). Examining indirect effects of emotion dysregulation between PTSD symptom clusters and reckless/self-destructive behaviors.

Psychological Trauma: Theory, Research, Practice, and Policy, 14(4), 688–695. https://doi.org/10.1037/tra0001118

Jo, H., & Song, E., (2015). The effect of reminiscence therapy on depression, quality of life, ego-integrity, social behavior function, and activities of daily living in elderly patients with mild dementia. *Educational Gerontology, 41*(1), 1–13.

Jobes, D. A. (2006). *Managing suicidal risk: A collaborative approach*. Guilford Press.

Jobes, D. A., Gregorian, M. J., & Colborn, V. A. (2018). A stepped care approach to clinical suicide prevention. *Psychological Services, 15*(3), 243–250. https://doi.org/10.1037/ser0000229

Jobes, D. A., Wong, S. A., Conrad, A. K., Drozd, J. F., & Neal-Walden, T. (2005). The collaborative assessment and management of suicidality versus treatment as usual: A retrospective study with suicidal outpatients. *Suicide & Life-Threatening Behavior, 35*(5), 483–497. https://doi.org/10.1521/suli.2005.35.5.483

Joffrion, L. P., & Douglas, D. (1994). Grief resolution: Facilitating transcendence in the bereaved. *Journal of Psychosocial Nursing and Mental Health Services, 32*(3), 13–19.

Johnson, C. N. E., & Hunter, M. (1997). Vicarious traumatization in counsellors working in the New South Wales Sexual Assault Service: An exploratory study. *Work and Stress, 11*(4), 319–328.

Johnson, D. R. (2000a). Creative therapies. In E. Foa & T. Keane (Eds.), *Effective treatments for PTSD: Practice guidelines from the International Society for Traumatic Stress Studies* (pp. 356–358). Guilford Press.

Johnson, D. R. (2000b). Creative therapies. In E. Foa & T. Keane (Eds.), *Effective treatments for PTSD: Practice guidelines from the International Society for Traumatic Stress Studies* (pp. 302–314). Guilford Press.

Johnson, D. R., Feldman, S. C., & Southwick, S. M. (1994). The concept of the second-generation program in the treatment of PTSD among Vietnam veterans. *Journal of Traumatic Stress, 7*, 217–235.

Johnson, I. M. (1999). School violence: The effectiveness of a school resource officer program in a southern city. *Journal of Criminal Justice, 27*(2), 173–192.

Johnson, K. (2000). *School crisis management: A hands-on guide to training crisis response teams* (2nd ed.). Hunter House.

Johnson, M. (1995). Patriarchal terrorism and common couple violence: Two forms of violence against women. *Journal of Marriage and Family, 57*, 283–294.

Johnson, M., & Leone, J. (2005). The differential effects of intimate terrorism and situational couple violence: Findings from the National Violence Against Women Survey. *Journal of Family Issues, 26*(3), 322–349.

Johnson, R. G. (1987). Using computer art in counseling children. *Elementary School Guidance & Counseling, 21*, 262–265.

Johnson, R. R. (2017). How dangerous are domestic violence calls to officer safety? *Dolan Consulting Group*.

Johnson, S. M. (1977). *First person singular: Living the good life alone*. Lippincott.

Joiner, T. E. Jr., Orden, K. A. V., Witte, T. K., & Rudd, M. D. (2009). *The interpersonal theory of suicide: Guidance for working with suicidal clients* (1st ed.). American Psychological Association.

Joiner, T. E. Jr., Walker, R. L., Rudd, M. D., & Jobes, D. A. (1999). Scientizing and routinizing the assessment of suicidality in outpatient practice. *Professional Psychology: Research and Practice, 30*(5), 447–453. https://doi.org/10.1037/0735-7028.30.5.447

Joiner, T., Jr. (2010). *Myths about suicide*. Harvard University Press.

Jones Farrelly, M., & Robles-Fernandez, R. (2011, April). *Counseling skills and issues in gay straight alliance advisement and LGBTQ youth*. Paper presented at the American Counseling Association Conference, New Orleans, Louisiana.

Jones, G., & Stokes, A. (2009). *Online counseling: A handbook for practitioners*. Palgrave Macmillan.

Jones, J. (1984). *Counseling in correctional settings* (Cassette Recording No. 25-6611). Memphis, TN: Memphis State University, Department of Counseling and Personnel Services.

Jones, J. S., Alexander, C., Wynn, B. N., Rossman, L., & Dunnuck, C. (2009). Why women don't report sexual assault to the police: The influence of psychosocial variables and traumatic injury. *The Journal of Emergency Medicine, 36*(4), 417–424. https://doi.org/10.1016/j.jemermed.2007.10.077

Jones, M. K. (1985, June). Patient violence: Report of 200 incidents. *Journal of Psychosocial Nursing and Mental Health, 23*, 12–17.

Jonson, R. (2016). *What effects do school resource officers have on schools?* Dolan Consulting Group.

Jordan, J. (2000). The role of mutual empathy in relational/cultural therapy. *Journal of Clinical Psychology, 56*(8), 1005–1016.

Jordan, J. V. (2017). Relational-Cultural Theory: The power of connection to transform our lives. *Journal of Humanistic Counseling, 56*(3), 228–243. https://doi.org/10.1002/johc.12055

Jordan, J. V. (2018). *Relational-cultural therapy* (2nd ed.). American Psychological Association. https//doi.org/10.1037/0000063-000

Jordan, K. (2002). Providing crisis counseling to New Yorkers after the terrorist attack on the World Trade Center. *The Family Journal, 10*(2), 139–144.

Jordans, M., Upadhaya, N., Tol, W., Shrestha, P., Doucet, J., Gurung, R., Aguettant, J., Mahat, P., Shah, S., Shrestha, K. P., Sherchan, S., Maharjan, R., Kunwar, A., Regmi, I. R., Shyangwa, P., Melville, A., van Ommeren, M. (2010). Introducing the IASC mental health and psychosocial support guidelines in emergencies in Nepal: A process description. *Intervention, 8*(1), 52–63.

Journal of Threat Assessment and Management. (2023). *Scope statement*. American Psychological Association. https://www.apa.org/pubs/journals/tam

Jovanovic, A., Aleksandric, B. V., Dunjic, D., & Todorovic, V. (2004). Family hardiness and social support as predictors of posttraumatic stress disorder. *Psychiatry and Law, 11*(2), 263–268.

Jozkowski, K. N. (2015). On social determinants of sexual assault among college students. *Violence Against Women, 21*(7), 848–874.

Juhnke, G. A. (2002). Intervening with school students after terrorist attacks. In D. D. Bass & R. Yep (Eds.), *Terrorism, trauma, and tragedies: A counselor's guide to preparing and responding* (pp. 55–58). American Counseling Association.

Jurgersen, T. S., Dailey, S., Uhernik, J., & Smith, C. M. (2013). All trauma is not the same. *Counseling Today, 55*(9), 47–50.

Kaehler, L. A., & Freyd, J. F. (2009). Borderline personality characteristics: A betrayal approach. *Psychological Trauma: Theory, Research, Practice, and Policy, 1*(4), 261–268.

Kagan, R., & Schlosberg, S. (1989). *Families in perpetual crisis*. W. W. Norton & Company.

Kahn, W. A. (2005). *Holding fast: The struggle to create resilient caregiving organizations*. Brunner/Routledge.

Kaiser-Permanente. (2022). *Warning signs of suicide in children and teens*. https://healthy.kaiserpermanente.org/health-wellness/health-encyclopedia/he.warning-signs-of-suicide-in-children-and-teens.ty6090

Kalafat, J. (1990). Adolescent suicide and the implications for school response programs. *School Counselor, 37*(5), 359–369.

Kalafat, J. (2003). School approaches to youth suicide prevention. *American Behavioral Scientist, 46*(9), 1211–1223.

Kalafat, J., Gould, M. S., Munfakh, J. L. H., & Kleinman, M. (2007). An evaluation of crisis hotline outcomes. Part 1: Nonsuicidal crisis callers. *Suicide and Life-Threatening Behavior, 37*(3), 322–337. https://doi.org/10.1521/suli.2007.37.3.322

Kalaitzaki, A. (2020). Cyberstalking victimization and perpetration among young adults: Prevalence and correlates. In M. F. Wright (Ed.), *Advances in Human and Social Aspects of Technology* (pp. 22–38). IGI Global. https://doi.org/10.4018/978-1-7998-1063-6.ch002

Kammer, J., Rahman, M., Finnerty, M., Layman, D., Vega, K., Galfalvy, H., Labouliere, C., Brown, G. K., Green, K., Cummings, A., Vasan, P., & Stanley, B. (2021). Most individuals are seen in outpatient medical settings prior to intentional self-harm and suicide attempts treated in a hospital setting. *Journal of Behavioral Health Services & Research, 48*(2), 306–319. https://doi.org/10.1007/s11414-020-09717-1

Kandt, V. E. (1994). Adolescent bereavement: Turning a fragile time into acceptance and peace. *School Counselor, 41*, 203–211.

Kanel, K. (1999). *A guide to crisis intervention*. Brooks/Cole.

Kanel, K. (2011). *A guide to crisis intervention* (4th ed.). Cengage.

Kanel, K. (2018). *A guide to crisis intervention* (6th ed.). Cengage.

Kanel, P., Koeppe, R. A., Kotagal, V., Roytman, S., Muller, M. L. T. M., Bohnen, N. I., & Albin, R. L. (2023). Regional serotonin terminal density in aging human brain: A [11C] DASB PET study. *Neurobiology of Aging Science, 3*. https://doi.org/10.1016/j.nbas.2023.100071

Kaniasty, K., & Norris, F. (1999). The experience of disaster: Individuals and communities sharing trauma. In R. Gist & B. Lubin (Eds.), *Response to disaster: Psychosocial, community and ecological approaches* (pp. 25–62). Brunner/Mazel.

Kaniasty, K., Norris, F., & Murrell, S. A. (1990). Received and perceived social support following natural disaster. *Journal of Applied Social Psychology, 20*, 85–114.

Kaplan, C. P., & Gallagher-Thompson, D. (1995). Treatment of clinical depression in caregivers of spouses with dementia. *Journal of Cognitive Psychotherapy, 9*, 35–44.

Kaplan, H. B. (1996). *Psychosocial stress: Perspectives on structure, theory, life course and methods*. Academic Press.

Kaplan, R. L., Van Damme, I., Levine, L. J., & Loftus, E. F. (2016). Emotion and false memory. *Emotion Review, 8*(1), 8–13. https://doi.org/10.1177/1754073915601228

Karaffa, K., Openshaw, L., Koch, J., Clark, H., Harr, C., & Stewart, C. (2015). Perceived impact of police work on marital relationships. *The Family Journal, 23*(2), 120–131. https://doi.org/10.1177/1066480714564381

Karakurt, G., Koç, E., Çetinsaya, E. E., Ayluçtarhan, Z., & Bolen, S. (2019). Meta-analysis and systematic review for the treatment of perpetrators of intimate partner violence. *Neuroscience & Biobehavioral Reviews, 105*, 220–230. https://doi.org/10.1016/j.neubiorev.2019.08.006

Karatzias, T., Hyland, P., Bradley, A., Fyvie, C., Logan, K., Easton, P., Thomas, J., Philips, S., Bisson, J. I., Roberts, N. P., Cloitre, M., & Shevlin, M. (2019). Is self-compassion a worthwhile therapeutic target for ICD-11 Complex PTSD (CPTSD)? *Behavioural and Cognitive Psychotherapy, 47*(3), 257–269. https://doi.org/10.1017/S1352465818000577

Kardiner, A. (1941). *The traumatic neurosis of war*. Hoover.

Karkazis, J. L., & Lazaneo, S. L. (2000). Unyielding custody disputes: Tempering loss and courting disaster. In J. H. Harvey

& E. D. Miller (Eds.), *Loss and trauma* (pp. 375–385). Brunner/Mazel.

Karl, A., Malta, L. S., & Maercker, A. (2006). Meta-analytic review of event-related potential studies in post-traumatic stress disorder. *Biological Psychology, 71*(2), 123–147.

Karpman, S. (1968). Fairy tales and script drama analysis. *Transactional Analysis Bulletin 26*(7), 39–43.

Kasick, D. P., & Bowling, C. D. (2013). Crisis intervention teams: A boundary spanning collaboration between the law enforcement and mental health communities. In K. R. Yeager, D. L. Cutler, D. E. Svendsen, & G. M. Sills (Eds), *Modern community mental health: An interdisciplinary approach* (pp. 304–315). Oxford University Press.

Katafiasz, H. (2020). A systemic conceptualization of intimate partner violence: Attachment and differentiation. *The Family Journal, 28*(3), 306–312. https://doi.org/10.1177/1066480720929697

Kataoka, S., Langley, A. K., Wong, M., Baweja, S., & Stein, B. D. (2012). Responding to students with posttraumatic stress disorder in schools. *Child Adolescent Psychiatric Clinics of North America, 21*(1), 119–133. https://doi.org/ 10.1016/j.chc.2011.08.009

Katiti, V., Sigalla, G. N., Rogathi, J., Manongi, R., & Mushi, D. (2016). Factors influencing disclosure among women experiencing intimate partner violence during pregnancy in Moshi Municipality, Tanzania. *BMC Public Health, 16*(1), 715. https://doi.org/10.1186/s12889-016-3345-x

Kato, P. M., & Mann, T. (1999). A synthesis of psychological interventions for the bereaved. *Clinical Psychology Review, 19*(3), 275–296.

Katz, C. L. (2011). Needs assessment. In F. J. Stoddard, A. Pandya, & C. Katz (Eds.), *Disaster psychiatry: Readiness, evaluation, and treatment* (pp. 49–68). American Psychiatric Publishing.

Katz, C., Bolton, S., Katz, L., Isaak, C., Tilston-Jones, T., & Sareen, J. (2013). Swampy Cree Suicide Prevention Team. *Depression and Anxiety, 30*(10), 1030–1045.

Katz, C., Randall, J. R., Sareen, J., Chateau, D., Walld, R., Leslie, W. D., Wang, J., & Bolton, J. M. (2017). Predicting suicide with the SAD PERSONS scale. *Depression and Anxiety, 34*(9), 809–816. https://doi.org/10.1002/da.22632

Kaufman, B., & Wohl, A. (1992). *Casualties of childhood: A developmental perspective on sexual abuse using projective drawings.* Brunner/Mazel.

Kaul, R. E., & Welzant, V. (2005). Disaster mental health: A discussion of best practices applied after the Pentagon attack. In A. R. Roberts (Ed.), *Crisis intervention handbook* (3rd ed., pp. 200–220). Oxford University Press.

Kaur, P., Dhir, A., Tandon, A., Alzeiby, E. A., & Abohassan, A. A. (2021). A systematic literature review on cyberstalking. An analysis of past achievements and future promises. *Technological Forecasting and Social Change, 163*, 120426. https://doi.org/10.1016/j.techfore.2020.120426

Kaut, K. P. (2006). End-of-life assessment within a holistic bio-psycho-social-spiritual framework. In J. L. Werth & D. Blevins (Eds.). *Psychosocial issues near the end of life: A resource for professional care providers* (pp. 111–135). American Psychological Association.

Kay, W. J., Neiburg, H. A., Kutscher, A. H., Grey, R. M., & Fudin, C. E. (Eds.). (1984). *Pet loss and human bereavement.* Iowa State University Press.

Kazdin, A. E. (1975). Covert modeling, imagery assessment, and assertive behavior. *Journal of Consulting and Clinical Psychology, 43*, 716–724.

Kazdin, A. E. (2008). Trauma in children: How can we communicate what we know? *Monitor on Psychology, 39*(9), 5.

Keane, T. M. (1976). *State dependent retention and its relationship to psychopathology.* Unpublished manuscript, State University of New York at Binghamton.

Keane, T. M., & Kaloupek, D. G. (1982). Imaginal flooding in the treatment of a posttraumatic stress disorder. *Journal of Consulting and Clinical Psychology, 50*, 138–140.

Keane, T. M., Caddell, J., & Taylor, K. (1988). Mississippi Scale for Combat-Related Posttraumatic Stress Disorder: Three studies in reliability and validity. *Journal of Consulting and Clinical Psychology, 56*, 85–90.

Keane, T. M., Fairbank, J. A., Caddell, J. M., & Zimmering, R. T. (1989). Implosive (flooding) therapy reduces symptoms of PTSD in Vietnam veterans. *Behavior Therapy, 20*, 245–260.

Keane, T. M., Fairbank, J. A., Caddell, J. M., Zimmering, R. T., & Bender, M. E. (1985). A behavioral approach to assessing and treating posttrauma stress disorder in Vietnam veterans. In C. R. Figley (Ed.), *Trauma and its wake: The study of post-traumatic stress disorder* (pp. 257–294). Brunner/Mazel.

Keane, T. M., Malloy, P. F., & Fairbank, J. A. (1984). Empirical development of an MMPI subscale for the assessment of combat-related posttraumatic stress disorder. *Journal of Consulting and Clinical Psychology, 52*(5), 888–891.

Keasar, V., Sznitman, S., & Baumel, A. (2022). Suicide prevention outreach on social media delivered by trained volunteers: A qualitative study. *Crisis: The Journal of Crisis Intervention and Suicide Prevention* Advance online publication. http://dx.doi.org/10.1027/0227-5910/a000864

Keene, J. R., & Prokos, A. H. (2008). Widowhood and the end of spousal caregiving: Relief or wear and tear? *Ageing & Society, 28*(4), 551–570.

Kelly, G. A. (1955). *The psychology of personal constructs.* Routledge.

Kelly, L., Meeker, E., Zajac, K., Bryan, R., & O'Connor, B. (2020). Interactive effect of adverse child experiences and suicidal thoughts and behaviors on adolescent alcohol and cannabis use frequency. *Psychology of Addictive Behaviors.* Advance online publication. https://doi.org/10.1037/adb0000947

Kenardy, J., Webster, R., Lewin, T., Carr, V., & Carter, G. (1996). Stress debriefing and patterns of recovery following natural disaster. *Journal of Traumatic Stress, 9*, 37–49.

Kennedy, A. (2006, November). Know when to say "no" and let go. *Counseling Today, 1*, 22–23.

Kennedy, A. (2007, July). Responding to the call. *Counseling Today.*

Kenny, M. C., Abreu, R. L., Marchena, M. T., Helpingstine, C., Lopez-Griman, A., & Matthews, B. (2017). Legal and clinical guidelines for making a child maltreatment report. *Professional Psychology: Research and Practice, 48*, 469–480. https://doi.org/10.1037/pro0000166

Kerig, P. K., & Modrowski, C. A. (2018). Testing gender-differentiated models of the mechanisms linking polyvictimization and youth offending: Numbing and callousness versus dissociation and borderline traits. *Journal of Trauma & Dissociation, 19*(3), 347–361. https://doi.org/10.1080/15299732.2018.1441355

Kerr, M. M. (2009). *School crisis prevention and intervention.* Pearson.

Kersting, A., & Kroker, K. (2010). Prolonged grief as a distinct disorder, specifically affecting female health. *Archives of Women's Mental Health, 13*(1), 27–28.

Kersting, A., Brahler, E., Glaesmer, H., & Wagner, B. (2011). Prevalence of complicated grief in a representative population-based sample. *Journal of Affective Disorders, 131*(13), 339–343.

Keshet, H., Foa, E. B., & Gilboa-Schechtman, E. (2019). Women's self-perceptions in the aftermath of trauma: The role of trauma-centrality and trauma-type. *Psychological Trauma: Theory, Research, Practice, and Policy, 11*(5), 542–550. https://doi.org/10.1037/tra0000393

Kesler, K. D. (1990). Burnout: A multimodal approach to assessment and resolution. *Elementary School Guidance and Counseling, 24*, 303–311.

Kessler, R. C., Sonnega, A., Bromer, E., Hughes M., & Nelson, C. B. (1995). Posttraumatic stress disorder in the National Comorbidity Survey. *Archives of General Psychiatry, 52*, 1048–1060.

Khalsa, H. M., Denens, A., Pasini-Hill, D., Santelli, J., & Baklessarini, R. (2021). Specialized police-based mental health crisis response: The first ten years of Colorado's crisis intervention team implementation. *Psychiatric Services, 69*(2), 239–241. https://doi.org/10.1176/appi.ps.201700055

Khaw, L., & Hardesty, J. L. (2007). Theorizing the process of leaving: Turning points and trajectories in the stages of change. *Family Relations, 56*(4), 413–425. https://doi.org/10.1111/j.1741-3729.2007.00470.x

Khayyat-Abuaita, U., Paivio, S., Pascual-Leone, A., & Harrington, S. (2019). Emotional processing of trauma narratives is a predictor of outcome in emotion-focused therapy for complex trauma. *Psychotherapy, 56*(4), 526–536. https://doi.org/10.1037/pst0000238

Khosravan, S., Salehi, S., Ahmadi, F., Sharif, F., & Zamani, A. (2010). Experiences of widows with children: A qualitative study about spousal death in Iran. *Nursing & Health Sciences, 12*(2), 205–211.

Khosravi, M., & Kasaelyan, R. (2023). A current challenge in classification and treatment of DSM-5-TR prolonged grief disorder. *Psychological Trauma: Research, Practice, and Policy.* Advance online publication. https://doi.org/10.1037/tra0001510

Khoury, B., Barbarin, O., Gutierrez, G., Klicperova-Baker, M., Padakannaya, P., & Thompson, A. (2022). Complicated grief during COVID-19. *International Perspectives in Psychology (2022), 11*(3), 214–221. https://doi.org/10.1027/2157-3891/a000055

Kilijanek, T., & Drabek, T. E. (1979). Assessing long-term impacts of a natural disaster: A focus on the elderly. *Gerontologist, 19*(6), 555–566.

Killian, K. D. (2008). Helping till it hurts? A multi-method study of compassion fatigue, burnout, and self-care in clinicians working with trauma survivors. *Traumatology, 14*(2), 32–44.

Killian, K., Hernandez-Wolfe, P., Engstrom, D., & Gangsei, D. (2017). Development of the Vicarious Resilience Scale (VRS): A measure of positive effects of working with trauma survivors. *Psychological Trauma: Theory, Research, Practice, and Policy, 9*(1), 23–31. https://doi.org/10.1037/tra0000199

Kilmer, R. P, & Gil-Rivas, V. (2010). Responding to the needs of children and families after a disaster: Linkages between unmet needs and caregiver functioning. *American Journal of Orthopsychiatry, 80*, 135–142.

Kilmer, R. P., Gil-Rivas, V., & MacDonald, J. (2010). Implications of major disaster for educators, administrators, and school-based mental health professionals: Needs, actions, and the example of Mayfair Elementary. In R. P. Kilmer, V. Gil-Rivas, R. G. Tedeschi, & L. G. Calhoun (Eds.), *Helping families and communities recover from disaster: Lessons learned from hurricane Katrina and its aftermath* (pp. 167–191). American Psychological Association.

Kilmer, R. P., Gil-Rivas, V., Tedeschi, R. G., & Calhoun, L. G. (Eds.). (2010). *Helping families and communities recover from disaster: Lessons learned from Hurricane Katrina and its aftermath.* American Psychological Association.

Kilmer, R. P., Gil-Rivas, V., Tedeschi, R. G., Cann, A., Calhoun, L., Buchanan, T., & Taku, K. (2009). Use of the revised Post-traumatic Growth Inventory for Children. *Journal of Traumatic Stress, 22*(3), 248–253.

Kim, H. S., Sherman, D. K., & Taylor, S. E. (2008). Culture and social support. *American Psychologist, 63*(6), 518–526.

Kim, S., Lee, H. -K., & Lee, K. (2020). Assessment of suicidal risk using Minnesota multiphasic personality inventory-2 restructured form. *BMC Psychiatry, 20*, 1–10. https://doi.org/10.1186/s12888-020-02495-2

King, C. A., Foster, C., & Rogalski, K. (2013). *Teen suicide risk: A practitioner guide to screening, assessment, and management.* Guilford Press.

King, C. A., Kramer, A., Preuss, L., Kerr, D., Weisse, L., & Venkataraman, S. (2006). Youth-nominated support team for suicidal adolescents (Version 1): A randomized controlled test. *Journal of Consulting and Clinical Psychology, 74*(1), 199–206.

King, K. A. (2000). Preventing adolescent suicide: Do high school counselors know the risk factors? *Professional School Counseling, 3*, 255–263.

King, L. A., King, D. W., Leskin, G., & Foy, D. W. (1995). The Los Angeles Symptom Checklist: A self-report measure of posttraumatic stress disorder. *Assessment, 2*(1), 1–17.

King, R. & Schindler, M. (2021). *A better path forward for criminal justice: Reconsidering police in schools.* Brookings. https://www.brookings.edu/articles/a-better-path-forward-for-criminal-justice-reconsidering-police-in-schools/

Kingsbury, S. J. (1988). Hypnosis in the treatment of posttraumatic stress disorder: An isomorphic intervention. *American Journal of Clinical Hypnosis, 31*(2), 81–90.

Kinney, J. A. (1995). *Violence at work.* Prentice Hall.

Kinnunen, S., Puolakanaho, A., Tolvane, A., Makikangas, A., & Lappalainen, R. (2020). Improvement in mindfulness facets mediate the alleviation of burnout dimensions. *Mindfulness, 11*(12), 2779–2792. https://doi.prg/10.1007/s12671-020-1490-8

Kinzie, J., & Goetz, R. (1996). A century of controversy surrounding posttraumatic stress-spectrum syndromes: The impact of DSM III and DSM IV. *Journal of Traumatic Stress, 9*(2), 159–179.

Kious, B. M., & Battin, M. (Peggy). (2019). Physician aid-in-dying and suicide prevention in psychiatry: A moral crisis? *American Journal of Bioethics, 19*(10), 29–39. https://doi.org/10.1080/15265161.2019.1653397

Kira, I. A., Arıcı Özcan, N., Shuwiekh, H., Kucharska, J., Al-Huwailah, A. H., & Kanaan, A. (2020). The compelling dynamics of "will to exist, live, and survive" on effecting posttraumatic growth upon exposure to adversities: Is it mediated, in part, by emotional regulation, resilience, and spirituality? *Traumatology, 26*(4), 405–419. https://doi.org/10.1037/trm0000263

Kira, I., Aljakoub, J., Ibraheem, B. A., & Shuwiekh, H. (2023). The effects of Type III traumatic stressors of the protracted conflict and prolonged COVID-19 on Syrians internally displaced: A validation study of Type III continuous traumatic stressors and their impact. *International Perspectives in Psychology, 12*(1), 1–15. https://doi.org/10.1027/2157-3891/a000054

Kirchberg, T. M., James, R. K., Dupont, R., & Cochran, S. (2014, October 6). *Something old, something new, something borrowed for the blue.* [Paper presentation]. Crisis Intervention Team International convention, Hartford, CT, the United States.

Kirchberg, T., James, R., Cochran, S., & Dupont, R. (2013, October). *Something old, something new, something borrowed for the blue.* [Paper presentation]. Crisis Intervention Team International Conference, Hartford, CT, the United States.

Kirk, A. (1989). The prediction of violent behavior during short-term civil commitment. *Bulletin of the American Academy of Psychiatry and the Law, 17,* 345–353.

Kirk, W. (1993). *Adolescent suicide: A school-based approach to assessment and intervention.* Research Press.

Kiselica, M. S. (1998). Preparing Anglos for the challenges and joys of multiculturalism. *The Counseling Psychologist, 26*(1), 5–21. https://doi.org/10.1177/0011000098261001

Kisely, S., Campbell, L. A., Peddle, S., Hare, S., Pyche, M., Spicer, D., & Moore, M. (2010). A controlled before-and-after evaluation of a mobile crisis partnership between mental health and police services in Nova Scotia. *Canadian Journal of Psychiatry, 55*(10), 662–668.

Kisiel, C., Fehrenbach, T., Liang, L.-J., Stolbach, B., McClelland, G., Griffin, G., Maj, N., Briggs, E. C., Vivrette, R. L., Layne, C. M., & Spinazzola, J. (2014). Examining child sexual abuse in relation to complex patterns of trauma exposure: Findings from the National Child Traumatic Stress Network. *Psychological Trauma: Theory, Research, Practice, and Policy, 6,* S29–S39. https://doi.org/10.1037/a0037812

Kitchener, K. S. (1984). Intuition, critical evaluation, and ethical principles: The foundation for ethical decision in counseling psychology. *The Counseling Psychologist, 12*(3), 43–55.

Kitchingman, T. A., Wilson, C. J., Caputi, P., Wilson, I., & Woodward, A. (2018). Telephone crisis support workers' psychological distress and impairment. *Crisis, 39*(1), 13–26. https://doi.org/10.1027/0227-5910/a000454

Kitzman, K. M., & Gaylord, N. K. (2001). Divorce counseling. In E. R. Welfel & R. E. Ingersoll (Eds.), *The mental health desk reference* (pp. 32–37). Wiley.

Kivimäki, M., & Kawachi, I. (2015). Work stress as a risk factor for cardiovascular disease. *Current Cardiology Reports, 17*(9), 74. https://doi.org/10.1007/s11886-015-0630-8

Klassen, D., & O'Connor, W. A. (1988). A prospective study of predictors of violence in adult male mental health admissions. *Law and Human Behavior, 12,* 143–158.

Kleespies, P. M. (2009). *Behavioral emergencies: An evidence-based resource for evaluating and managing risk of suicide, violence, and victimization.* American Psychological Association. https://doi.org/10.1037/11865-000

Kleespies, P. M. (2014). *Decision making in behavioral emergencies: Acquiring skill in evaluating and managing high-risk patients* (pp. x, 210). American Psychological Association. https://doi.org/10.1037/14337-000

Kleespies, P. M., & Ponce, A. N. (2009). The stress and emotional impact of clinical work with the patient at risk. In P. Kleespies (Ed.), *Behavioral emergencies: An evidence-based resource for evaluating and managing risk of suicide, violence and victimization*

(pp. 431–448). American Psychological Association. https://doi.org/10.1037/11865-000

Kleespies, P. M., & Richmond, J. (2009). Evaluating behavioral emergencies: The clinical interview. In P. Kleespies (Ed.), *Behavioral emergencies: An evidence-based resource for evaluating and managing risk of suicide, violence and victimization* (pp. 33–55). American Psychological Association. https://doi.org/10.1037/11865-000

Klein, C. (2019). *Stockholm Syndrome: The true story of hostages loyal to their captor.* History Channel. https://www.history.com/news/stockholm-syndrome

Kleindienst, N., Steil, R., Priebe, K., Müller-Engelmann, M., Biermann, M., Fydrich, T., Schmahl, C., & Bohus, M. (2021). Treating adults with a dual diagnosis of borderline personality disorder and posttraumatic stress disorder related to childhood abuse: Results from a randomized clinical trial. *Journal of Consulting and Clinical Psychology, 89*(11), 925–936. https://doi.org/10.1037/ccp0000687

Kleinman, S. B., & Stewart, L. (2004). Psychiatric legal considerations in providing mental health assistance to disaster survivors. *Psychiatric Clinics of North America, 27*(3), 559–570.

Klevan, T., Karlson, B., Ness, O., Grant, A., & Rudd, T. (2018). Between a rock and a softer place: A discourse analysis of helping cultures in Crisis Resolution teams. *Research and Practice, 17*(2), 252–267. https://doi.org/10.1177/1473325016668962

Klever, S. (2013). Reminiscence therapy. Finding meaning in memories. *Nursing 43*(4) pp. 36–37. http://doi.org/10.1097/01. https://doi.org/NURSE.0000427988.23941.51

Kliman, A. S. (1978). *Crisis: Psychological first aid for recovery and growth.* Holt, Rinehart & Winston.

Klotz, J. M. (2003). *Welcome to ecological counseling.org.*

Knipe, J. (2015). *EMDR toolbox: Theory and treatment of complex PTSD and dissociation.* Springer.

Knott, T., & Fabre, A. (2014). Maternal response to the disclosure of child sexual abuse: Systematic review and critical analysis of the literature. *Institute for Psychological Therapies, 20*(1). https://doi.org/10.1023/A:1014274311428

Knowles, R., Sasser, D. D., & Besty Garrison, M. E. (2010). Family resilience and resiliency following Hurricane Katrina. In R. P. Kilmer, V. Gil-Rivas, R. G. Tedeschi, & L. G. Calhoun (Eds.). *Helping families and communities recover from disaster* (pp. 97–116). American Psychological Association.

Knox, K., & Roberts, A. R. (2005). Crisis intervention with stalking victims. In A. R. Roberts (Ed.), *Crisis intervention handbook* (3rd ed., pp. 483–498). Oxford University Press.

Knudson, M. (1991, April). *Chronic and abusive callers: Appropriate responses and interventions.* Paper presented at the Fifteenth Annual Convening of Crisis Intervention Personnel, Chicago, IL, the United States.

Kobasa, S. (1979). Stressful life events, personality, and health: An inquiry into hardiness. *Journal of Personality and Social Psychology, 37,* 1–11.

Kocmur, M., & Zavasnik, A. (1993). Problems with borderline patients in a crisis intervention unit: A case history. *Crisis, 14,* 71–75, 89.

Koeske, G. F., & Kelly, T. (1995). The impact of over involvement on burnout and job satisfaction. *American Journal of Orthopsychiatry, 65,* 282–292.

Koeske, G. F., Kirk, S. A., & Koeske, R. D. (1993). Coping with job stress: Which strategies work best? *Journal of Occupational and Organizational Psychology, 66,* 319–335.

Kokou-Kpolou, C. K., Fernández-Alcántara, M., & Cénat, J. M. (2020). Prolonged grief related to COVID-19 deaths: Do we have to fear a steep rise in traumatic and disenfranchised griefs? *Psychological Trauma: Theory, Research, Practice, and Policy, 12*(S1), S94–S95. https://doi.org/10.1037/tra0000798

Kolb, L. C., & Mutalipassi, L. R. (1982). The conditioned emotional response: A subclass of the chronic and delayed stress disorder. *Psychiatric Annals, 12,* 969–987.

Kolbe, V., & Büttner, A. (2020). Domestic violence against men—Prevalence and risk factors. *Deutsches Ärzteblatt International, 117*(31–32), 534–541. https://doi.org/10.3238/arztebl.2020.0534

Kolski, T. D., Jongsma Jr., A. E, .& Myer, R. A. (2012). *The crisis counseling and trauma event treatment planner, with DSM V updates.* Wiley & Sons, Inc.

Komar, A. A. (1994). Adolescent school crises: Structures, issues, and techniques for postventions. *International Journal of Adolescence and Youth, 5*(1/2), 35–46.

Konanur, S., Muller, R. T., Cinamon, J. S., Thornback, K., & Zorzella, K. P. M. (2015). Effectiveness of trauma-focused cognitive behavioral therapy in a community-based program. *Child Abuse & Neglect, 50,* 159–170. https://doi.org/10.1016/j.chiabu.2015.07.013

Kongshøj, I. L. L., & Berntsen, D. (2023). Is young age a risk factor for PTSD? Age differences in PTSD-symptoms after Hurricane Florence. *Traumatology, 29*(2), 211–223. https://doi.org/10.1037/trm0000389

Konigsberg, R. D. (2011). *The truth about grief: The myth of its five stages and the new science of loss.* Simon & Schuster.

Koocher, G. (1975). Why isn't the gerbil moving? Discussing death in the classroom. *Children Today, 4,* 18–36.

Koon, L. M., Greiman, L., Schulz, J. A., Goddard, K. S., Nzuki, I. M., & Hall, J. P. (2022). Examining the effects of the COVID-19 pandemic on community engagement for people with mobility disabilities. *Disability and Health Journal, 15*(1S), 101212. https://doi.org/10.1016/j.dhjo.2021.101212

Koraan, R., & Geduld, A. (2015). Corrective rape of lesbians in the era of transformative constitutionalism in South Africa. *Potchefstroom Electronic Law Journal, 18*(5), 1931–1953.

Koritsas, S., Coles, J., & Boyle, M. (2010). Workplace violence towards social workers: The Australian experience. *British Journal of Social Work, 40*(10), 257–271.

Kornblum, R. (2002). *Disarming the playground: Violence prevention through movement and prosocial skills.* Woods and Barnes.

Koss, M. P., Swartout, K. M., Lopez, E. C., Lamade, R. V., Anderson, E. J., Brennan, C. L., & Prentky, R. A. (2022). The scope of rape victimization and perpetration among national samples of college students across 30 years. *Journal of Interpersonal Violence, 37*(1–2), NP25–NP47. https://doi.org/10.1177/08862605211050103

Kottman, T. (2014). *Play therapy: Basics and beyond.* John Wiley & Sons.

Koutsimani, P., Montgomery, A., & Georganta, K. (2019). The relationship between burnout, depression, and anxiety: A systematic review and meta-analysis. *Frontiers in Psychology.* https://www.frontiersin.org/articles/10.3389/fpsyg.2019.00284/full?fbclid=IwAR2a7Cpq9sEcWK6z-Pv7QZzox3fUAp5vsLo_fLTKzMKEfAOEn_1s-1K28uQ

Koverola, C., & Panchanadeswaran, S. (2004). Domestic violence interventions with women of color: The intersection of victimization and cultural diversity. In K. Kendall-Tackett (Ed.), *Health consequences of abuse in the family: A clinical guide for evidence-based practice. Application and practice in health psychology* (pp. 45–61). American Psychological Association.

Kovess-Masfety, V., Pilowsky, D., Goelitz, D., Kuijpers, R., Otten, R., Moro, M., Bitfoi, A., Koç, C., Lesinskiene, S., Mihova, Z., Hanson, G., Fermanian, C., Pez, O., & Carta, M. (2015, May). Suicidal ideation and mental health disorders in young school children across Europe. *Journal of Affective Disorders, 177,* 28–35. https://doi.org/10.1016/j.jad.2015.02.008

Kowalchuk, K. (2021). *Older people grieve differently.* Center for Grief and Trauma Therapy. http://centerforgrieftherapy.com

Koziarski, J., O'Connor, C., & Frederick, T. (2021). Policing mental health: The composition and perceived challenges of co-response teams and crisis intervention teams in the Canadian context. *Police Practice and Research: An International Journal, 22*(1), 977–995. https://doi.org/10.1080/15614263.2020.1786689

Kraanen, F. L., Scholing, A., & Emmelkamp, P. M. G. (2014). Prediction of intimate partner violence by type of substance use disorder. *Journal of Substance Abuse Treatment, 46*(4), 532–539. https://doi.org/10.1016/j.jsat.2013.10.010

Kraft, S. G. (2003). Sudden unexpected deaths create unique challenges when counseling children. *Counseling Today, 46*(1), 12.

Krahe, B., & Moller, I. (2011). Links between self-reported media violence exposure and teacher ratings of aggression and prosocial behavior among German adolescents. *Journal of Adolescence, 34*(2), 279–287.

Krahe, B., Moller, I., Huesmann, L., Kirwil, L., Felber, J., & Berger, A. (2011). Desensitization to media violence: Links with habitual media violence exposure, aggressive cognitions, and aggressive behavior. *Journal of Personality and Social Psychology, 100*(4), 630–646.

Kramer, B. J., Kavanaugh, M., Trentham-Dietz, A., Walsh, M., & Yonker, J. A. (2010). Complicated grief symptoms in caregiver of persons with lung cancer: The role of family conflict, intrapsychic strains, and hospice utilization. *Omega: Journal of Death and Dying, 62*(3), 210–220.

Kramer, L. B., Whiteman, S. E., Witte, T. K., Silverstein, M. W., & Weathers, F. W. (2020). From trauma to growth: The roles of event centrality, posttraumatic stress symptoms, and deliberate rumination. *Traumatology, 26*(2), 152–159. https://doi.org/10.1037/trm0000214

Kreisman, J. J., & Straus, H. (2004). *Sometimes I act crazy: Living with borderline personality disorder.* John Wiley & Sons.

Kreisman, J. J., & Straus, H. (2010). *I hate you—Don't leave me: Understanding the borderline personality* (rev. ed.). Perigee/Penguin Group.

Kress, V. E., Haiyasoso, M., Zoldan, C. A., Headley, J. A., & Trepal, H. (2018). The use of Relational-Cultural Theory in counseling clients who have traumatic stress disorders. *Journal of Counseling & Development, 96*(1), 106–114. https://doi.org/10.1002/jcad.12182

Kroger, C., Roepke. S., & Kliem, S. (2014). Reasons for premature termination of dialectical behavior therapy for inpatients with borderline personality disorder. *Behavior Research and Therapy, 60*(1), 46–52.

Kroll, J. (2003). Posttraumatic symptoms and the complexity of response to trauma. *Journal of the American Medical Association, 290*(5), 667–670.

Kropp, R. P., & Hart, S. D. (2004). *The development of the brief spousal assault form for the evaluation of risk (B-SAFER): A tool for criminal justice professionals.* Department of Justice Canada. https://www.justice.gc.ca/eng/rp-pr/fl-lf/famil/rr05_fv1-rr05_vf1/rr05_fv1.pdf

Krueger, J. I. (2011). Shock without awe. *American Psychologist, 66,* 642–643.

Krysinska, K., Andriessen, K., Ozols, I., Reifels, L., Robinson, J., & Pirkis, J. (2022). Effectiveness of psychosocial interventions for family members and other informal support persons of individuals who have made a suicide attempt: A systematic review. *Crisis, 43*(3), 245–260 https://doi.org/10.1027/0227-5910/a000776

Kübler-Ross, E. (1969). *On death and dying.* Macmillan.

Kübler-Ross, E. (1975). *Death: The final stage of growth.* Prentice Hall.

Kübler-Ross, E. (1983). *On children and death.* Macmillan.

Kübler-Ross, E. (1987). *AIDS: The ultimate challenge.* Macmillan.

Kübler-Ross, E., & Kessler, D. (2005). *On grief and grieving: Finding the meaning of grief through the five stages of loss.* Scribner.

Kuhn, K., Wagner, A., & Velioza, J. (2019). Estimating the magnitude of the relation between bullying, E-bullying, and suicidal behaviors among United States youth, 2015. *Crisis: The Journal of Crisis Intervention and Suicide Prevention, 40*(3), 157–165. https://doi.org/10.1027/0227-5910/a000544

Kuhn, T. S. (1962). *The structure of scientific revolutions.* The University of Chicago Press.

Kukla, R. A., Schlenger, W. E., Fairbank, J. A., Hough, R. L., Jordan, B. K., & Marmar, C. R. (1990). *Trauma and the Vietnam War generation: Report of findings from the National Vietnam Veterans' Readjustment Study.* Brunner/Mazel.

Kulkami, S., Bell, H., Hartman, J., & Herman-Smith, R. (2013). Exploring individual and organizational factors contributing to compassion satisfaction, secondary traumatic stress, and burnout in domestic violence service providers. *Journal of the Society for Social Work Research, 4*(2), 114–130.

Kulkarni, S. J., Stylianou, A. M., & Wood, L. (2019). Successful rules reduction implementation process in domestic violence shelters: From vision to practice. *Social Work, 64*(2), 147–156. https://doi.org/10.1093/sw/swz010

Kumar, S. A., Brand, B. L., & Courtois, C. A. (2022). The need for trauma training: Clinicians' reactions to training on complex trauma. *Psychological Trauma: Theory, Research, Practice, and Policy, 14*(8), 1387–1394. https://doi.org/10.1037/tra0000515

Kumble, S., & McSherry, B. (2010). Seclusion and restraint: Rethinking regulation from a human rights perspective. *Psychiatry, Psychology and Law, 17*(4), 551–561.

Kurlowicz, L. H. (1990). Violence in the emergency department. *American Journal of Nursing, 90,* 35–40.

Kushner, H. S. (1983). *When bad things happen to good people.* Avon.

Kvarstein, E. H., Pedersen, G., Umes, Ø., Hummelem, B., Wilberg, T., & Karterud, S. (2015). Changing from a traditional psychodynamic treatment programme to mentalization-based treatment for patients with borderline personality disorder. *Psychology and Psychotherapy: Theory, Research and Practice, 88*(1), 71–86.

La Greca, A. M., & Prinstein, M. J. (2002). Hurricanes and earthquakes. In A. M. LaGreca, W. K. Silverman, E. M. Vernberg, & M. C. Roberts (Eds.). *Helping children cope with disasters and terrorism* (pp. 107–138). American Psychological Association.

La Greca, A. M., Tarlow, N., Brodar, K. E., Danzi, B. A., & Comer, J. S. (2022). The stress before the storm: Psychological correlates of hurricane-related evacuation stressors on mothers and children. *Psychological Trauma: Theory, Research, Practice, and Policy, 14*(S1), S13–S22. https://doi.org/10.1037/tra0001052

Lacey, K. K., Parnell, R., Mouzon, D. M., Matusko, N., Head, D., Abelson, J. M., & Jackson, J. S. (2015). The mental health of US Black women: The roles of social context and severe intimate partner violence. *BMJ Open, 5*(10), e008415. https://doi.org/10.1136/bmjopen-2015-008415

Lachkar, J. (2011). *How to talk to a borderline.* Routledge & Taylor.

LaFauci Schutt, J. M. (2009). Personal and environmental predictors of posttraumatic stress in emergency management professionals. *Dissertation Abstracts International: Section A. Humanities and Social Sciences, 69*(1), 483.

Lagadec, P. (2009). The mega-crisis: Unknown territory: In search of conceptual and strategic breakthroughs. *National Safety & Security and Crisis Management: Special Mega-crisis.* https://www.researchgate.net/publication/46479033_THE_MEGACRISIS_UNKNOWN_TERRITORY_-_In_Search_of_Conceptual_and_Strategic_Breakthroughs

Lagadec, P. (2012). The unknown territory of mega-crisis in search of conceptual and strategic break throughs. In I. Helsloot, A. Boin, B. Jacobs, & L. Comfort (Eds.), *Mega-crisis: Understanding the prospects, nature, characteristics and effects of cataclysmic events.* (pp. 12–24). Charles C. Thomas.

Lagoni, L., Butler, C., & Hetts, S. (1994). *The human–animal bond and grief.* PhiSaunders.

Lakeside Hospital, Memphis, TN. (1988). *Verbal techniques for deescalating violent behavior.*

Lakey, M. J. (2023). Mental health-medical crisis team impact on first responder outcomes on persons with mental illness. *Dissertation Abstracts International Section B; The Sciences and Engineering, 84*(5-B).

Lam, J., McNeil, D. E., & Binder, R. L. (2000). The relationship between patients' gender and violence leading to staff injuries. *Psychiatric Services, 51*(9), 1167–1170.

Lamb, D., Lloyd-Evans, B., Fullarton, K., Kelly, K., Goater, N., Mason, O., Gray, R., Osborn, D., Nolan, F., Piling, S., Sullivan, S., Henderson, C., Milton, A., Burgess, E., Churchard, A., Davidson, M., Freidichs, J., Hindle, D., Paterson, B., . . . Johnson, S. (2020). Crisis resolution and home treatment in the UK: A survey of model fidelity using a novel review methodology. *Informational Journal of Mental Health Nursing, 29*(2), 187–201. https://doi.org/10.1111/inm.12658

Lamb, H. R., Weinberger, L. E., & DeCuir, W. J. (2002). The police and mental health. *Psychiatric Services, 53*(10), 1266–1271.

Lamb, H. R., Weinberger, L. E., & Gross, B. H. (2004). Mentally ill persons in the criminal justice system: Some perspectives. *Psychiatric Quarterly, 75*(2), 107–126.

Lancman, S., Mangia, E., & Muramoto, M., (2013). Impact of conflict and violence on workers in a hospital emergency room. *Journal of Prevention, Assessment, & Rehabilitation, 45*(4), 519–527.

Lanctot, N., & Guay, S., (2014). The aftermath of workplace violence among healthcare workers: A systematic literature review of the consequences. *Aggression and Violent Behavior, 19*(5), 492–501.

Landreth, G. L. (1987). Play therapy: Facilitative use of child's play in elementary school counseling. *Elementary School Guidance & Counseling, 21*, 253–261.

Landreth, G. L. (2012). *Play therapy: The art of the relationship.* Routledge.

Landy, J. F., & Shah, P. (2022). What drives opposition to suicide? Two exploratory studies of normative judgments. *Judgment and Decision Making, 17*(1), 164–188.

Lane, J. (2003). *Ecological crisis management* (Cassette Recording No. 082803). University of Memphis.

Laney, C., & Loftus, E. F. (2008). Emotional content of true and false memories. *Memory, 16*(5), 500–516. https://doi.org/10.1080/09658210802065939

Laney, C., & Loftus, E. F. (2013). Recent advances in false memory research. *South African Journal of Psychology, 43*(2), 137–146. https://doi.org/10.1177/0081246313484236

Lang, W. A., Ramsay, R. F., Tanney, B. L., Kinzel, T., Turley, B., Tayler, D., Tierney, R. J., & Schmidt, R. J. (2020). *ASIST trainer manual.* LivingWorks Education Incorporated.

Langenderfer-Magruder, L., Whitfield, D. L., Walls, N. E., Kattari, S. K., & Ramos, D. (2016). Experiences of intimate partner violence and subsequent police reporting among lesbian, gay, bisexual, transgender, and queer adults in Colorado: Comparing rates of cisgender and transgender victimization. *Journal of Interpersonal Violence, 31*(5), 855–871. https://doi.org/10.1177/0886260514556767

Langer, N. (2011). Who did you *used* to be? Loss for older adults. In D. L. Harris (Ed.), *Counting our losses: Reflecting on change, loss, and transition in everyday life* (pp. 215–221). Routledge/Taylor & Francis Group.

Langman, P. (2009). *Why kids kill: Inside the minds of school shooters.* Palgrave MacMillan.

Langreo, L. (2022, August 9). How many teachers have been assaulted by students or parents? We asked educators. *Education Week.* https://www.edweek.org/leadership/how-many-teachers-have-been-assaulted-by-students-or-parents-we-asked-educators/2022/08

Lanius, R. A., Bluhm, R., & Frewen, P. A. (2013). Childhood trauma, brain connectivity and the self. In J. Ford, & C. A. Courtois (Eds.), *Treating complex stress disorders in children and adolescents: Scientific foundations and therapeutic models.* (pp. 24–38). Guilford Press.

Lankford, A., Silver, J., & Cox, J. (2021). An epidemiological analysis of public mass shooters and active shooters: Quantifying key differences between perpetrators and the general population, homicide offenders, and people who die by suicide. *Journal of Threat Assessment and Management, 8*(4), 125–144. https://doi.org/10.1037/tam0000166

Lanza, M. L. (1984). A follow-up study of nurses' reactions to physical assault. *Hospital and Community Psychiatry, 35*, 492–494.

Lanza, M. L. (1985, June). How nurses react to patient assault. *Journal of Psychosocial Nursing and Mental Health, 23*, 6–11.

Lapierre, C. B., Schwegler, A. F., & LaBauve, B. J. (2007). Posttraumatic stress and depression symptoms in solders returning from combat operations in Iraq and Afghanistan. *Journal of Traumatic Stress, 20*(6), 933–943.

Lapierre, S., Erlangsen, A., Waern, M., Leo, D. D., Oyama, H., Scocco, P., Gallo, J., Szanto, K., Conwell, Y., Draper, B., & Quinnett, P. (2011). A systematic review of elderly suicide prevention programs. *Crisis.* https://econtent.hogrefe.com/doi/10.1027/0227-5910/a000076

Larson, D. G. (1993). *The helper's journey: Working with people facing grief, loss, and life-threatening illness.* Research Press.

Larson, J. (1994). Violence prevention in the schools: A review of selected programs and procedures. *School Psychology Review, 23*(2), 151–164.

Laskey, P. (2016). Systematic review of female perpetrators of intimate partner violence and their treatment. *Journal of Applied Psychology and Social Science, 2*(1), Article 1.

Laskey, P., Bates, E. A., & Taylor, J. C. (2019). A systematic literature review of intimate partner violence victimisation: An inclusive review across gender and sexuality. *Aggression and Violent Behavior, 47*, 1–11. https://doi.org/10.1016/j.avb.2019.02.014

Lating, J. M., & Everly, G. S. (1995). Psychophysiological assessment of PTSD. In G. S. Everly, Jr., & J. M. Lating (Eds.), *Psychotraumatology* (pp. 129–146). Plenum Press.

Lau, M. (2022). What should I do if my child is thinking about suicide? *American Academy of Pediatrics.* https://www.healthychildren.org/English/tips-tools/ask-the-pediatrician/Pages/what-should-i-do-if-my-child-is-thinking-about-suicide.aspx

Laufer, R., Yager, T., & Grey-Wouters, E. (1981). Postwar trauma: Social and psychological problems of Vietnam veterans in the aftermath of the Vietnam War. In A. Egendorf, C. Kadushin, & R. S. Laufer (Eds.), *Legacies of Vietnam* (Vol. 1). U.S. Government Printing Office.

Laughout, R., & Annear, L. (2011). Safe and unsafe school spaces: Comparing elementary school student perceptions to common ecological interventions and operationalizations. *Journal of Community and Applied Psychology, 21*(1), 71–86.

Lau-Zhu, A., Henson, R. N., & Holmes, E. A. (2019). Intrusive memories and voluntary memory of a trauma film: Differential effects of a cognitive interference task after encoding. *Journal of Experimental Psychology: General, 148*(12), 2154–2180. https://doi.org/10.1037/xge0000598

Lavine v. Blaine School District, 257 F.3d 981 (9th Cir. 2001).

Lavoie, J. A., Alvarez, N., & Kandil, Y. (2022). Developing community co-designed scenario-based training for police mental health crisis response: A relational policing approach to deescalation. *Journal of Police and Criminal Psychology, 37*(3), 587–601. https://doi.org/10.1007/s11896-022-09500-2

Lawrence, K. A., Allen, J., & Chanen, A. (2011). A study of maladaptive schema and borderline personality disorder in young people. *Cognitive Therapy and Research, 35*(1), 30–39.

Lawson, D. M. (2013). *Family violence: Explanations and evidence based practice.* American Counseling Association.

Lawson, G., & Myers, J. E. (2011). Wellness, professional quality of life, and career-sustaining behaviors: What keeps us well? *Journal of Counseling and Development, 89*(2), 163–171.

Lawson, G., Bodenhorn, N., & Welfare, L. (2010). Virginia Tech: A campus and a community respond. In J. Webber & J. B. Mascari (Eds.), *Terrorism, trauma, and tragedies: A counselor's guide to preparing and responding* (3rd ed., pp. 73–76). American Counseling Association Foundation.

Lawson, G., Venart, E., Hazler, R. J., & Kottler, J. A. (2007). Toward a culture of counselor wellness. *Journal of Humanistic Counseling, Education, and Development, 46*, 5–19.

Lazarus, A. (1977). *In the mind's eye: The powers of imagery for personal enrichment.* Guilford Press.

Lazarus, A. (1989). *The practice of multimodal therapy.* Johns Hopkins University Press.

Lazarus, A. A. (1976). *Multimodal behavior therapy.* Springer.

Lazarus, R. S., & Folkman, S. (1984). *Stress, appraisal, and coping.* Springer-Verlag.

Leadbetter, D. (1993). Trends in assault on social work staff: The experience of one Scottish department. *British Journal of Social Work, 23,* 613–628.

Leahy, M. J. (1993). A comparison of depression in women bereaved of a spouse, child, or parent. *Omega: Journal of Death and Dying, 26*(3), 207–215.

Lebow, J. & Stroud, C. B. (2012). Assessment of effective couple and family functioning. In S. J. Price, C. A. Price, & P. C. McKenny (Eds.). *Families and change: Coping with stressful events and transitions* (pp. 501–528). SAGE.

LeCroy, C. W. (1988). Anger management or anger expression: Which is most effective? *Residential Treatment for Children and Youth, 5,* 29–39.

Ledingham, M. D., Standen, P., Skinner, C., & Busch, R. (2019). "I should have known." The perceptual barriers faced by mental health practitioners in recognising and responding to their own burnout symptoms. *Asia Pacific Journal of Counselling and Psychotherapy, 10*(2), 125–145. https://doi.org/10.1080/215076 86.2019.1634600

Lee, C., & Cuijpers, P. (2013). A meta-analysis of eye movements in processing emotional memories. *Journal of Behavior Therapy and Experimental Psychiatry, 44*(2), 231–239.

Lee, C., Slade, P. & Lygo, V. (1996). The influence of psychological debriefing on emotional adaption in women following early miscarriage: A preliminary study. *British Journal of Medical Psychology, 69,* 37–49.

Lee, C., Taylor, G., & Drummond, P. (2006). The active ingredient of EMDR: Is it traditional exposure or dual focus of attention? *Clinical Psychology & Psychotherapy, 13*(2), 97–107.

Lee, H., Aldwin, C. M., & Kang, S. (2022). Do different types of war stressors have independent relations with mental health? Findings from the Korean Vietnam Veterans Study. *Psychological Trauma: Theory, Research, Practice, and Policy, 14*(5), 840–848. https://doi.org/10.1037/tra0000557

Lee, H., Aldwin, C. M., Kang, S., & Ku, X. (2022). Vulnerability and resilience among older South Korean Vietnam war veterans: A latent profile analysis. *Psychological Services, 19*(Suppl 1), 95–105. https://doi.org/10.1037/ser0000568

Lee, M., Raitt, J., Hong, B., Diduck, A., Nyguyen, A. M., Villareal, A., Moden, M., Turner, B., North, C. S., & Pollio, D. (2022). Making meaning of disaster experience in highly trauma-exposed survivors of the Oklahoma City bombing. *Traumatology, 26*(2), 202–210. https://doi.org/10.1037/trm0000326

Lee, R. T., & Ashforth, B. E. (1993). A longitudinal study of burnout among supervisors and managers: Comparisons between the Leiter and Maslach and Golembiewski models. *Organizational Behavior and Human Decision Processes, 54,* 369–398.

Lee, R. T., & Ashforth, B. E. (1996). A meta-analytic examination of the correlates of the three dimensions of job burnout. *Journal of Applied Psychology, 81*(2), 123–133.

Lee, S. A. (2015). The persistent Complex Bereavement Inventory: A measure based on the DSM-5. *Death Studies, 39,* 399–410. https://doi.org/10.1080/07481187.2015.1029144

Lee, S. A., & Milman, E., (2021). The Persistent Complex Bereavement Inventory (PCBI). In R. Neimeyer (Ed.)., *New techniques of grief therapy* (pp. 79–86). Routledge. http://doi .org/10.4324/9781351069120-9

Lee, S. M., Baker, C. R., Cho, S. H., Heckathorn, D. E., Holland, M. W., & Newgent, R. A. (2007). Development and initial psychometrics of the Counselor Burnout Inventory. *Measurement and Evaluation in Counseling and Development, 40*(2), 142–154.

Lee, S. M., Cho, S. H., Kissinger, D., & Ogle, N. (2010). A typology of burnout in professional counselors. *Journal of Counseling and Development, 88*(2), 131–138.

Leemis, R. W., Friar, N., Khatiwada, S., Chen, M. S., Kresnow, M., Smith, S. G., Caslin, S., & Basile, K. C. (2022). *The National Intimate Partner and Sexual Violence Survey: 2016/2017 report on intimate partner violence.* National Center for Injury Prevention and Control, Centers for Disease Control and Prevention. https://www.cdc.gov/violenceprevention/pdf/nisvs /NISVSReportonIPV_2022.pdf

Leffler, C. T., & Dembert, M. L. (1998). Posttraumatic stress symptoms among U.S. Navy divers recovering TWA Flight 800. *Journal of Nervous & Mental Disease, 186,* 574–577.

Lehmann, P., & Rabenstein, S. (2002). Children exposed to domestic violence: The role of impact, assessment, and treatment. In A. R. Roberts (Ed.), *Handbook of domestic violence: Intervention strategies* (pp. 343–364). Oxford University Press.

Lehmann, P., & Simmons, C. (Eds.). (2009). *Strengths-based batterer intervention: A new paradigm in ending family violence.* Springer.

Leibert, T. W., & Dunne-Bryant, A. (2015). Do common factors account for counseling outcome? *Journal of Counseling & Development, 93*(2), 225–235. https://doi.org/10.1002/j.1556-6676 .2015.00198.x

Leichsenring, F., Leibing, E., Kruse, J., New, A., & Leweke, F. (2011). Borderline personality disorder. *Lancet, 377,* 74–84.

Leiter, M. P., & Maslach, C. (1999). Six areas of worklife: A model of the organizational context of burnout. *Journal of Health and Human Services Administration, 21*(4), 472–489.

Leiter, M. P., & Maslach, C. (2005). *Banishing burnout: Six strategies for improving your relationship with work.* Jossey-Bass.

Leitner, L. A. (1974). Crisis counseling may save a life. *Journal of Rehabilitation, 40,* 19–20.

Lempp, R. C. (1990). To the diagnostic of "incomprehensible" offenses of adolescents and juveniles. *Acta Paedopsychiatrica, 53,* 173–175.

Lenehan, G. P., & Turner, J. T. (1984). Treatment of staff victims of violence. In J. T. Turner (Ed.), *Violence in the medical setting: A survival guide* (pp. 251–260). Aspen Systems.

Lenferink, L. I. M., de Keijser, J., Smid, G. E., & Boelen, P. A. (2020). Cognitive therapy and EMDR for reducing psychopathology in bereaved people after the MH17 plane crash: Findings from a randomized controlled trial. *Traumatology, 26*(4), 427–437. https://doi.org/10.1037/trm0000253

Lenferink, L. I. M., Eisma, M. C., Smid, G. E., de Keijser, J., & Boelen, P. A. (2022). Valid measurement of DSM-5 persistent complex bereavement disorder and DSM-5-TR and ICD-11 prolonged grief disorder: The Traumatic Grief Inventory-Self Report Plus (TGI-SR+). *Comprehensive Psychiatry, 112.* https:// doi.org/10.1016/j.comppsych.2021.152281

Lenihan, G. O., & Kirk, W. (1999, April). *Rural community level crisis intervention.* Paper presented at the Twenty-Third Annual Convening of Crisis Intervention Personnel, Chicago, IL, United States.

Lent, J. (2010). *The impact of work setting, demographic factors, and personality factors on burnout of professional counselors.* University of Akron. https://etd.ohiolink.edu/apexprod/rws_olink/ r/1501/10?clear=10&p10_accession_num=akron1270138348

Lenton-Brym, A. P., Landy, M. S. H., Whitfield, K. M., Burdo, J., & Monson, C. M. (2023). Considerations in adapting cognitive-behavioral conjoint therapy for posttraumatic stress disorder to a family setting. *Journal of Psychotherapy Integration*. Advance online publication. https://dx.doi.org/10.1037/int0000305

Lenz, A. S., & Hollenbaugh, K. M. (2015). Meta-analysis of trauma-focused cognitive behavioral therapy for treating PTSD and co-occurring depression among children and adolescents. *Counseling Outcome Research and Evaluation, 6*(1), 18–32. https://doi.org/10.1177/2150137815573790

Lenz, S., Bruijn, B., Serman, N., & Bailey, L. (2014). Effectiveness of cognitive processing therapy for treating posttraumatic stress disorder. *Journal of Mental Health Counseling, 36*(4), 360–376.

Leo, J. (2010, Fall). Let the hot air out of bullies! *Teaching Tolerance*, 12.

Lerner, M. J. (2000). The human cost of organizational downsizing: The irrational effects of the justice motive on managers, dismissed workers, and survivors. In J. H. Harvey & E. D. Miller (Eds.), *Loss and trauma: General and close relationship perspectives* (pp. 208–224). Brunner-Routledge.

Lerner, S. (2020). Crisis-prevention mini lessons. *ASCA School Counselor 57* (5), 15–23.

Lerner, S. (2021). Build trauma informed practices. *ASCA School Counselor, 58*(4), 10–14.

LeRoy, A. S., Robles, B., Kilpela, L. S., & Garcini, L. M. (2020). Dying in the face of the COVID-19 pandemic: Contextual considerations and clinical recommendations. *Psychological Trauma: Theory, Research, Practice, and Policy, 12*(S1), S98–S99. https://doi.org/10.1037/tra0000818

Leskin, G. A., Huleatt, W., Jerrmann, J., Ladue, L., & Gusman, F. (2006). Rapid development of family assistance centers: Lessons learned following the September 11 terrorist attacks. In E. C. Ritchie, P. J. Watson, & M. J. Friedman (Eds.), *Interventions following mass violence and disasters: Strategies for mental health practice* (pp. 257–277). Guilford Press.

Lester, D. (2002). *Crisis intervention and counseling by telephone*. Charles C. Thomas.

Lester, D. (2002). When things go wrong. In D. Lester & G. W. Brockopp (Eds.), *Crisis intervention and counseling by telephone* (2nd ed., pp. 167–170). Charles C. Thomas.

Lester, D. (Ed.). (2001). *Suicide prevention: Resources for the millennium*. Brunner-Routledge.

Lester, D. & Rogers, J. R. (2012). *Crisis intervention and counseling by telephone and the internet* (3rd ed.). Charles C. Thomas.

Lester, D., & Brockopp, G. W. (Eds.). (1973). *Crisis intervention and counseling by telephone*. Charles C. Thomas.

Lester, P. B., McBride, S., & Cornum, R. L. (2013). Building psychological resilience in military personnel: Theory and practice. In R.R. Sinclair & T.W. Britt (Eds.), *Building psychological resilience in military personnel: Theory and Practice* (pp. 193–220).

Levinson, D. J. (1986). A concept of adult development. *American Psychologist, 41*(1), 3–133.

Levinson, D. J., & Levinson, J. D. (1996). *The seasons of a woman's life*. Knopf.

Levinson, J. D. (1986). A conception of adult development. *American Psychologist, 41*(1), 3–13.

Levis, D. O. (1992). From abuse to violence: Psychophysiological consequences of maltreatment. *Journal of American Academy Child and Adolescent Psychiatry, 142*(10), 1161–1166.

Lewellyn, A. (1985). *Counseling emotionally disturbed high school students: The Mattoon, Illinois, TLC program* (Cassette Recording No. 12-6611). Memphis, TN: Memphis State University, Department of Counseling and Personnel Services.

Lewis, S. (1993). Restraint and seclusion. In P. E. Blumenreich & S. Lewis (Eds.), *Managing the violent patient: A clinician's guide* (pp. 101–109). Brunner-Mazel.

Lewitzka, U., Sauer, C., & Bauer, M. (2019). Are national suicide prevention programs effective? A comparison of 4 verum and 4 control countries over 30 years. *BMC Psychiatry, 19*(158). https://doi.org/10.1186/s12888-019-2147-y

Li, A., Early, S., Mahrer, N., Klaristenfeld, J., & Gold, J. (2014). Group cohesion and organizational commitment: Protective factors for nurse residents' job satisfaction, compassion fatigue, compassion satisfaction and burnout. *Journal of Professional Nursing, 30*(1), 89–99.

Li, J., Theng, Y., & Foo, S. (2014). Game-based digital interventions for depression therapy: A systematic review and meta-analysis. *Cyberpsychology, Behavior, and Social Networking, 17*(8), 519–527.

Li, S., Zhao, F., & Yu, G. (2019). Childhood maltreatment and intimate partner violence victimization: A meta-analysis. *Child Abuse & Neglect, 88*, 212–224. https://doi.org/10.1016/j.chiabu.2018.11.012

Li, S., Zhao, F., & Yu, G. (2020). A meta-analysis of childhood maltreatment and intimate partner violence perpetration. *Aggression and Violent Behavior, 50*, 101362. https://doi.org/10.1016/j.avb.2019.101362

Li, W., Dorstyn, D. S., & Jarmon, E. (2020). Identifying suicide risk among college students: A systematic review. *Death Studies, 44*(7), 450–458. https://doi.org/10.1080/07481187.2019.1578305

Li, Z., Gao, S., Chen, M. Gourley, J. J., Liu, C., Prein, A. F., & Hong, Y. (2022). The conterminous United States are projected to become more prone to flash floods in a high-end emissions scenario. *Community Earth Environment, 3*, 86. https://doi.org/10.1038/s43247-022-00409-6

Liao Siling, J., Truss, K., Philips, L., Eastwood, O., & Bendall, S. (2021). Young people's journeys of recovery from trauma: A qualitative study of narratives from Internet forums. *Psychological Trauma: Theory, Research, Practice, and Policy, 13*(3), 293–301. https://doi.org/10.1037/tra0000990

Liese, B. S. (1994). Brief therapy, crisis intervention, and the cognitive therapy of substance abuse. *Crisis Intervention, 1*, 11–29.

Lifton, R. J. (1973). *Home from the war: Vietnam veterans—neither individuals nor executioners*. Simon & Schuster.

Lifton, R. J. (1974). "Death imprints" on youth in Vietnam. *Journal of Clinical Child Psychology, 3*, 47–49.

Lifton, R. J. (1975). The postwar war. *Journal of Social Issues, 31*, 181–195.

Lifton, R. J. (1983). *The broken connection: On death and the continuity of life*. Basic Books.

Ligon, J. (2000). Mobile crisis units: Frontline community mental health services. In A. R. Roberts (Ed.), *Contemporary perspectives on crisis intervention and prevention* (pp. 357–372). Prentice Hall.

Lim, M., Lee, S., & Park, J.-I. (2016). Differences between impulsive and non-impulsive suicide attempts among individuals treated in emergency rooms of South Korea. *Psychiatry Investigation, 13*(4), 389–396. https://doi.org/10.4306/pi.2016.13.4.389

Linaker, O. M., & Busch-Iversen, H. (1995). Predictors of imminent violence in psychiatric inpatients. *Acta Psychiatrica Scandinavica, 92*(4), 250–254.

Lindebø Knutsen, M., Sachser, C., Holt, T., Goldbeck, L., & Jensen, T. K. (2020). Trajectories and possible predictors of treatment outcome for youth receiving trauma-focused cognitive behavioral therapy. *Psychological Trauma: Theory, Research, Practice, and Policy, 12*, 336–346. https://doi.org/10.1037/tra0000482

Lindemann, E. (1944). Symptomatology and management of acute grief. *American Journal of Psychiatry, 101*, 141–148.

Lindemann, E. (1956). The meaning of crisis in individual and family. *Teachers College Record, 57*, 310.

Lindsay, J., & Brady, D. (2002). "Nurturing fragile relationships": Early reflections on working with victims of domestic violence on the National Probation Service's Duluth Pathfinder research programme. *Issues in Forensic Psychology, 3*, 59–71.

Lindsay, M., & Lester, D. (2004). *Suicide-by-cop: Committing suicide by provoking police to shoot you*. Baywood Publishing.

Lindstrom, C. M., Cann, A., Calhoun, L. G., & Tedeschi, R. G. (2013). The relationship of core belief challenge, rumination, disclosure, and sociocultural elements to posttraumatic growth. *Psychological Trauma: Theory, Research, Practice and Policy, 5*(1), 50–55.

Lindy, J. D. (1996). Psychoanalytic psychotherapy of posttraumatic stress disorder: The nature of the therapeutic relationship. In B. A. van der Kolk, A. C. McFarlane, & L. Weisaeth (Eds.), *Traumatic stress* (pp. 525–536). Guilford Press.

Lindy, J. D. (2012). Listening to what the trauma patient teaches us: A 35-year perspective. In R. A. McMackin, E. Newman, J. M. Fogler, & T. M. Keane (Eds.), *Trauma therapy in context: The science and craft of evidence–based practice.* (pp. 15–28). American Psychological Association.

Linehan, M. (1993). *Dialectical behavior therapy for borderline personality disorder*. Guilford Press.

Linehan, M. (2014). *DBT? Skills Training Manual, Second Edition*. Guilford Publications.

Linehan, M. M., Comtois, K. A., Murray, A. M., Brown, M. Z., Gallop, R. J., Heard, H. L., Korslund, K. E., Tutek, D. A., Reynolds, S. K., & Lindenboim, N. (2006). Two-year randomized controlled trial and follow-up of dialectical behavior therapy vs therapy by experts for suicidal behaviors and borderline personality disorder. *Archives of General Psychiatry, 63*(7), 757–766. https://doi.org/10.1001/archpsyc.63.7.757

Linehan, M. M., Goodstein, J. L., Nielsen, S. L., & Chiles, J. A. (1983). Reasons for staying alive when you are thinking of killing yourself: The Reasons for Living Inventory. *Journal of Consulting and Clinical Psychology, 51*, 276–286. https://doi.org/10.1037/0022-006X.51.2.276

Ling, J., Hunter, S., & Maple, M. (2014). Navigating the challenges of trauma counseling: How counsellors thrive and sustain their engagement. *Australian Social Work, 67*(2), 297–310.

Linley, A., Joseph, S., & Loumidis, K. (2005). Trauma work, sense of coherence and positive and negative changes in therapists. *Psychotherapy and Psychosomatics, 74*(3), 185–188.

Linzer, M., & Harwood, E. (2018). Gendered expectations: Do they contribute to high burnout among female physicians? *Journal of General Internal Medicine, 33*(6), 963–965. https://doi.org/10.1007/s11606-018-4330-0

Lion, J. R., & Pasternak, S. A. (1973). Countertransference reactions to violent patients. *American Journal of Psychiatry, 130*, 207–210.

Lippard, E. T. C., & Nemeroff, C. B. (2020). The devastating clinical consequences of child abuse and neglect: Increased disease vulnerability and poor treatment response in mood disorders. *American Journal of Psychiatry, 177*, 20–36. http://dx.doi.org/10.1176/appi.ajp.2019.19010020

Lipsey, M. W. (1992). Juvenile delinquency treatment: A meta-analytic inquiry into the variability of effects. In T. D. Cook (Ed.), *Meta-analysis for explanation* (pp. 67–89). SAGE.

Littlechild, B. (1995). Violence against social workers. *Journal of Interpersonal Violence, 10*, 123–131.

Littlechild, B. (2002). The effects of client violence on child protection networks. *Trauma, Violence, & Abuse, 3*, 144–158.

Litz, B. T., & Gibson, L. E. (2006). Conducting research on mental health interventions. In E. C. Ritchie, P. J. Watson, & M. J. Friedman (Eds.), *Interventions following mass violence and disasters: Strategies for mental health practice* (pp. 387–404). Guilford Press.

Liu, S., Duan, M., Sun, Y., Wang, L., An, L., & Ming, D. (2023). Neural responses to social decision-making in suicide attempters with mental disorders. *BMC Psychiatry, 23*(1), 1–13. https://doi.org/10.1186/s12888-022-04422-z

Livingston, J. (2016). Contact between police and people with mental disorders: A review of rates. *Psychiatric Services, 67*(8), 850–857. https://doi.org/10.1176/appi.ps.201500312

Lizano, E. L., Godoy, A. J., & Allen, N. (2019). Spirituality and worker well-being: Examining the relationship between spirituality, job burnout, and work engagement. *Journal of Religion & Spirituality in Social Work: Social Thought, 38*(2), 197–216. https://doi.org/10.1080/15426432.2019.1577787

Lloyd-Evans, B., Paterson, B., Onyett, S., Brown, E., Istead, H., Gray, A., Henderson, C., & Johnson, S. (2018). National implementation of a mental health service model: A survey of Crisis Resolution teams in England. *Informational Journal of Mental Health Nursing, 27*(1), 214–226. https://doi.org/10.1111/inm.12311

Loeber, R. (1990). Development and risk factors of juvenile antisocial behavior and delinquency. *Clinical Psychology Review, 10*(1), 1–41.

Loeber, R., & Farrington, D. P. (1999). *Serious and violent juvenile offenders: Risk factors and successful interventions*. SAGE. https://doi.org/10.4135/9781452243740

Loeber, R., Farrington, D. P., Rumsey, C. A., & Allen-Hagen, B. (1998, May). Serious and violent juvenile offenders. *Juvenile Justice Bulletin*. U.S. Department of Justice.

Loftus, E. F. (1997). Creating false memories. *Scientific American, 277*(3), 70–75. https://doi.org/10.1038/scientificamerican0997-70

Logan, J., Myer, R., & James, R. (2006). *How to TACKLE an excessive force complaint.* [Paper presentation]. Second Annual Crisis Intervention Team Conference, Orlando, FL, the United States.

Logie, R. (2014). EMDR-more than just a therapy for PTSD. *The Psychologist, 27*(7) 512–516.

Lohr, J. M., Montgomery, R. W., Lilienfeld, S. O., & Tolin, D. F. (1999). Pseudoscience and the commercial promotion of trauma treatments. In R. Gist & B. Lubin (Eds.), *Response to disaster: Psychosocial, community and ecological approaches* (pp. 291–321). Brunner/Mazel.

Loinaz, I., (2014). Typologies, risk and recidivism in partner-violent men with the B-SAFER: A pilot study. *Psychology, Crime, & Law, 20*(2), 183–198.

Lopata, H. Z. (1996). *Current widowhood: Myths and realities*. SAGE.

Lord, J. H. (1996). America's number one killer: Vehicle crashes. In K. J. Doka (Ed.), *Living with grief after sudden loss: Suicide, homicide, accident, heart attack, stroke* (pp. 25–41). Hospice Foundation of America.

Lord, V. (2015). *Suicide by cop: A comprehensive examination of this phenomenon and its aftermath* (2nd ed.). Looseleaf Publications.

Lorenz, E. N. (1993). *The essence of chaos*. University of Washington Press.

Loumeau-May, L. V. (2008). Grieving in the public eye: Art therapy with children who lost parents in the World Trade Center attacks. In C. A. Malchiodi (Ed.), *Creative interventions with traumatized children* (pp. 112–131). Guilford Press.

Louvre, C. (2002). Helping students grieve a friend's death. *School Counselor, 39*(5), 10–11.

Louvre, C. (2008). Weaving the community tapestry. *School Counselor, 45*(5), 28–31.

Lovell v. *Poway Unified School District,* 90 F.3d. 367 (9th Cir. 1996).

Lovell, D., Allen, D., Johnson, C., & Jemelka, R. (2001). Evaluating the effectiveness of residential treatment for prisoners with mental illness. *Criminal Justice and Behavior, 28*, 83–104.

Lövestad, S., Löve, J., Vaez, M., & Krantz, G. (2017). Prevalence of intimate partner violence and its association with symptoms of depression; a cross-sectional study based on a female population sample in Sweden. *BMC Public Health, 17*(1), 335. https://doi.org/10.1186/s12889-017-4222-y

Lovre, C. (2013). Student threat assessment. *ASCA School Counselor, 51*(2), 17–21.

Lu, S., Gao, W., Wei, Z., Wei, W., Liao, M., Ding, Y., Zhang, Z., & Li, L. (2013). Reduced cingulate gyrus volume associated with enhanced cortisol awakening response in young healthy adults reporting childhood trauma. *PLos ONE, 8*(7), e69350.

Lubell, K. M., & Vetter, J. B. (2006). Suicide and youth violence prevention: The promise of an integrated approach. *Aggression and Violent Behavior, 11*(2), 167–175.

Luciano, M. T., Acuff, S. F., Olin, C. C., Lewin, R. K., Strickland, J. C., McDevitt-Murphy, M. E., & Murphy, J. G. (2022). Posttraumatic stress disorder, drinking to cope, and harmful alcohol use: A multivariate meta-analysis of the self-medication hypothesis. *Journal of Psychopathology and Clinical Science, 131*(5), 447–456. https://doi.org/10.1037/abn0000764

Luckett, J. B., & Slaikeu, K. A. (1990). Crisis intervention by police. In K. A. Slaikeu (Ed.), *Crisis intervention: A handbook for practice and research* (2nd ed., pp. 227–242). Allyn & Bacon.

Lui, Z., Yang, F., Yifan, L., Zhou, W., & Tong, F. (2021). The effectiveness of reminiscence therapy on alleviating depressive symptoms in older adults: A systematic review. *Frontiers in Psychology, 12*, 12–24. https://doi.org/10.3389/fpsyg.2021.709853

Luna, J. T., & Hoffman, R. M. (1999, June). *The counselor as catalyst: Forming partnerships for school violence reduction.* Paper presented at the American School Counselor Convention, Phoenix, AZ, the United States.

Lupton-Smith, H., Carruthers, W. L., Flythe, R., Goette, E., & Modest, K. H. (1996). Conflict resolution as peer mediation: Programs for elementary, middle, and high school students. *School Counselor, 43*, 375–391.

Lussier, P., & Cale, J. (2016). Understanding the origins and the development of rape and sexual aggression against women: Four generations of research and theorizing. *Aggression and Violent Behavior, 31*, 66–81. https://doi.org/10.1016/j.avb.2016.07.008

Luther, L., Gearhart, T., Fukui, S., Morse, G., Rollins, A. L., & Salyers, M. P. (2017). Working overtime in community mental health: Associations with clinician burnout and perceived quality of care. *Psychiatric Rehabilitation Journal, 40*, 252–259. https://doi.org/10.1037/prj0000234

Lutz, B. J., Young, M. E., Cox, K. J., Martz, C., & Creasy, K. R. (2011). The crisis of stroke: Experiences of patients and their family caregivers. *Top Stroke Rehabilitation, 18*, 1–16.

Lutz, J., Edelstein, B., Katz, E., & Gallegos, J. V. (2019). A shortened version of the Reasons for Living-Older Adults Scale for clinical and research utility. *The Gerontologist, 59*(4), e241–e247. https://doi.org/10.1093/geront/gny009

Luyten, P., Campbell, C., & Fonagy, P. (2020). Borderline personality disorder, complex trauma, and problems with self and identity: A social-communicative approach. *Journal of Personality, 88*(1), 88–105. https://doi.org/10.1111/jopy.12483

Lyndall, D., & Bicknell, J. (2001). Trauma and the therapist: The experience of therapists working with the perpetrators of sexual abuse. *Australasian Journal of Disaster and Trauma Studies, 5*(1), 1–12.

Lyons, J. A., & Keane, T. M. (1989). Implosive therapy for the treatment of combat-related PTSD. *Journal of Traumatic Stress, 2*, 137–152.

Lysova, A., Dim, E. E., & Dutton, D. (2019). Prevalence and consequences of intimate partner violence in Canada as measured by the National Victimization Survey. *Partner Abuse, 10*(2), 199–221. https://doi.org/10.1891/1946-6560.10.2.199

MacDonald, C. M. (2003). Evaluation of stress debriefing interventions with military populations. *Military Medicine, 168*, 961–967.

MacDonald, G., & Sirotich, F. (2001). Reporting client violence. *Social Work, 46*, 107–114.

Macfarlane, A. (2018). Gangs and adolescent mental health: A narrative review. *Journal of Child and Adolescent Trauma. 12*(3), 411–420. https://doi.org/10.1007/s40653-018-0231-y

MacIntosh, H. B., Godbout, N., & Dubash, N. (2015). Borderline personality disorder: Disorder of trauma or personality, a review of the empirical literature. *Canadian Psychology/Psychologie canadienne, 56*(2), 227–241. https://doi.org/10.1037/cap0000028

MacIsaac, M. B., Bugeja, L. C., & Jelinek, G. A. (2017). The association between exposure to interpersonal violence and suicide among women: A systematic review. *Australian and New Zealand Journal of Public Health, 41*(1), 61–69. https://doi.org/10.1111/1753-6405.12594

Mack, D. A., Shannon, C., Quick, J. D., & Quick, J. C. (1998). Stress and the preventative management of workplace violence. In R. W. Griffin, A. O'Leary-Kelly, & J. M. Collins (Eds.), *Dysfunctional behavior in organizations: Violent and deviant behavior,* (pp. 119–141). Jai Press.

Maclean, G. (1977). Psychic trauma and traumatic neurosis: Play therapy with a four-year-old boy. *Canadian Psychiatric Association Journal, 22*, 71–76.

MacMullin, K., Jerry, P., & Cook, K. (2020). Psychotherapist experiences with telepsychotherapy: Pre COVID-19 lessons for a post COVID-19 world. *Journal of Psychotherapy Integration, 30*(2), 248–264. https://doi.org/10.1037/int0000213

MacPherson, M. (1984). *Long time passing: Vietnam and the haunted generation.* Doubleday.

Macy, R. J., Rizo, C. F., Johns, N. B., & Ermentrout, D. M. (2013). Directors' opinions about domestic violence and sexual assault service strategies that help survivors. *Journal of Interpersonal Violence, 28*(5), 1040–1066. https://doi.org/10.1177/0886260512459375

Madden, D. J., Lion, J. R., & Penna, M. W. (1976). Assaults on psychiatrists by patients. *American Journal of Psychiatry, 133*, 422–425.

Madnick, D., & Spokas, M. (2022). Reporting and inclusion of specific sociodemographic groups in the adult PTSD treatment outcome literature within the United States: A systematic review. *Clinical Psychology: Science and Practice, 29*(3), 311–321. https://doi.org/10.1037/cps0000067

Magaletta, P. R., Glynn, S. M., & Goodie, J. L. (2022). Responding to individuals and communities after disasters and other traumatic events: An introduction. *Psychological Services, 19*(Suppl 2), 1–4. https://doi.org/10.1037/ser0000640

Maheu, M. M. (2001). Practicing psychotherapy on the Internet: Risk management challenges and opportunities. *Register Report, 27,* 23–28.

Maheu, M. M. (2003). The online clinical practice management model. *Psychotherapy: Theory, Research, Practice, Training, 40*(1/2), 20–32.

Mahon, J., Packman, J., & Liles, E. (2023). Preservice teachers' knowledge about bullying: Implications for teacher education. *International Journal of Qualitative Studies in Education, 36*(4), 642–654. https://doi.org/10.3102/00346543221094081

Main, B. (2008). The effects of treating sex offenders on treatment providers who have a history of child sexual abuse. *Dissertation Abstracts International: Section B. The Sciences and Engineering, 68*(12), 1960.

Main, M. (1996). Introduction to the special section on attachment and psychopathology: Overview of the field of attachment. *Journal of Consulting and Clinical Psychology, 64*(2), 237–243.

Main, M. (2000). Attachment theory. In A. Kazdin (Ed.), *Encyclopedia of Psychology* (Vol. 1, pp. 289–293). American Psychological Association.

Malchiodi, C. A. (Ed.). (2003). *Handbook of art therapy.* Guilford Press.

Malchiodi, C. A. (Ed.). (2008). *Creative interventions with traumatized children.* Guilford Press.

Malchiodi, C. A., & Ginns-Gruenberg, D. (2008). Trauma, loss, and bibliotherapy: The healing process of stories. In C. A. Malchiodi (Ed.), *Creative interventions with traumatized children* (pp. 167–188). Guilford Press.

Malchiodi, C., Steele, W., & Kuban, C. (2008). Resilience and posttraumatic growth in traumatized children. In C. Malchiodi (Ed.), *Creative interventions with traumatized children* (pp. 285–301). Guilford Press.

Maldonado, A. I., & Murphy, C. M. (2021). Does trauma help explain the need for power and control in perpetrators of intimate partner violence? *Journal of Family Violence, 36*(3), 347–359. https://doi.org/10.1007/s10896-020-00174-0

Maldonado, R. C., Watkins, L. E., & DiLillo, D. (2015). The interplay of trait anger, childhood physical abuse, and alcohol consumption in predicting intimate partner aggression. *Journal of Interpersonal Violence, 30*(7), 1112–1127. https://doi.org/10.1177/0886260514539850

Malet-Karas, A., Bernard, D., Piet, E., & Bertin, E. (2022). Disordered eating as a repercussion of sexual assault: A consequence to consider. *Eating and Weight Disorders: EWD, 27*(6), 2095–2106. https://doi.org/10.1007/s40519-021-01356-5

Malizia, A., & Nutt, D. (2000). Human brain imaging and post-traumatic stress disorder. In D. Nutt, J. Davidson, & J. Zohar (Eds.), *Post-traumatic stress disorder: Diagnosis, management, and treatment* (pp. 41–52). Martin Dunitz.

Malkinson, R. (2007). *Cognitive grief therapy: Constructing a rational meaning to life following loss.* Norton.

Malley, P. B., Kush, F., & Bogo, R. J. (1994). School-based adolescent suicide prevention and intervention programs. *School Counselor, 42*(2), 1301–1336.

Malloy, P. F., Fairbank, J. A., & Keane, T. M. (1983). Validation of a multimodal assessment of posttraumatic stress disorders in Vietnam veterans. *Journal of Consulting and Clinical Psychology, 51,* 488–494.

Malone, P. (2011). The impact of peer death on adolescent girls: An efficacy study of the adolescent grief and loss group. *Dissertation Abstracts International Section A: Humanities and Social Sciences,* 4568.

Mancinelli-Hough, K., Lucas Breda, K., Karl, C., & Wentland, B. A. (2022). Don't ask, won't tell: Suicide screening in the pediatric perioperative setting. *Comprehensive Child & Adolescent Nursing, 45*(4), 395–402. https://doi.org/10.1080/24694193.2022.2060376

Mandatory Treatment of Mental Health Patients. (2007). Virginia Codes 37.2-817.1 through 37.2-817.3.

Maneta, E. K., Cohen, S., Schulz, M. S., & Waldinger, R. J. (2013). Two to tango: A dyadic analysis of links between borderline personality traits and intimate partner violence. *Journal of Personality Disorders, 27*(2), 233–243. https://doi.org/10.1521/pedi_2013_27_082

Manly, J., Kim, J., Rogosch, F., & Cicchetti, D. (2001). Dimensions of child maltreatment and children's adjustment: Contributions of developmental timing and subtype. *Development and Psychopathology, 13*(4), 759–782.

Maples, M. F., Packman, J., Abney, P., Daughtery, R., Casey, J., & Pirtle, L. (2005). Suicide by teenagers in middle school: A postvention team approach. *Journal of Counseling & Development, 83*(4), 397–405.

Maran, D., Varetto, A., Zedda, M., & Munai, J. (2014). Stalking victimization among Italian university students. *Gender & Behavior, 12*(1), 6070–6079.

Marcus, N., & Stergiopoulos, V. (2022). Re-examining mental health crisis intervention: A rapid review comparing outcomes across police, co-responder and nonpolice models. *Health and Social Care, 30*(5), 1665–1679. https://doi.org/10.1111/hsc.13731

Markey, P., & Markey, C. (2010). Vulnerability to violent video games: A review and integration of personality research. *Review of General Psychology, 14*(2), 82–91. http://doi.org/10.1037/a0019000

Marlasca, M. (2014). Tracking violence against health care workers in Spain. *The Lancet, 384*(9947), 955.

Marohn, R. C. (1982). Adolescent violence: Causes and treatment. *Journal of the American Academy of Child Psychiatry, 21*(4), 354–360.

Marohn, R., Locke, E., Rosenthal, R., & Curtis, G. (1982). Juvenile delinquents and violent deaths. *Adolescent Psychiatry, 10,* 147–170.

Marshall, E. M., Karantzas, G. C., Romano, D., Lee, J., Feeney, J. A., Mullins, E. R., McCabe, M. P., & Simpson, J. A. (2023). Older adults' support seeking from their adult children: The Support-Seeking Strategy Scale. *Journal of Family Psychology.* Advance online publication. https://dx.doi.org/10.1037/fam0001063

Marshall, R. D., Bryant, R. A., Amsel, L., Suh, E. J. Cook, J. M., & Neria, Y. (2007). The psychology of ongoing threat: Relative risk appraisal, the September 11 attacks and terrorism related fears. *American Psychologist, 62*(4), 304–316.

Marteens, T. (2023). How drugs and alcohol can fuel violence. *American Addiction Centers*. https://americanaddictioncenters. org/rehab-guide/addiction-and-violence

Martin, L., Francisco, E., Nichol, C., & Schweiger, J. L. (1991). A hospital-wide approach to crisis control: One inner-city hospital's experience. *Journal of Emergency Nursing, 17*, 395–401.

Martin, T., & Doka, K. (2000). *Men don't cry . . . Women do: Transcending gender stereotypes of grief*. Brunner/Mazel.

Martin-Cuellar, A., Atencio, D. J., Kelly, R. J., & Lardier, D. T. (2018). Mindfulness as a moderator of clinician history of trauma on compassion satisfaction. *The Family Journal, 26*(3), 358–368. https://doi.org/10.1177/1066480718795123

Martinez, R., Williams, R., & Green, J. (2020). The role of school counselors delivering a trauma-informed care approach to supporting youth in foster care. *Professional School Counseling, 23*(1), https://doi.org/10.1177/2156759X20947747

Martinez-Prather, K. (2020). *Proper planning is critical for school safety*. National Institute of Justice. https://nij.ojp.gov/topics/ articles/proper-planning-critical-school-safety

Martín-Fernández, M., Gracia, E., & Lila, M. (2019). Psychological intimate partner violence against women in the European Union: A cross-national invariance study. *BMC Public Health, 19*(1), 1739. https://doi.org/10.1186/s12889-019-7998-0

Martin-Ingo, L., Ortiz, S., Urbqo, D., Teb Perez, S., Contaldo, S., Alvaros, J., Baladon, L., Parody-Rua., E, & Rubio-Valera, M. (2022). Assessment of the efficacy of crisis intervention team: Experiences in the Esplugues Mental Health Center (Barcelona). *Social Psychiatry and Psychiatric Epidemiology: The International Journal of Research and Genetic Epidemiology and Mental Health Services*. Advance online publication. https://doi .org/10.1007/s00127-022-02250-w

Marx, B. P., & Gutner, C. A. (2015). Post traumatic stress disorder: Patient interview, clinical assessment, and diagnosis. In N. C. Bernardy & M. J. Friedman (Eds.), *A practical guide to treatment: Pharmacological and psychotherapeutic approaches* (pp. 35–51). American Psychological Association.

Masino, T., & Norman, S. (2015). Challenging presentations in PTSD. Post traumatic stress disorder: Patient interview, clinical assessment, and diagnosis. In N. C. Bernardy & M. J. Friedman (Eds.), *A practical guide to treatment: Pharmacological and psychotherapeutic approaches* (pp. 163–178). American Psychological Association.

Maslach, C. (1976). Burned-out. *Human Behavior, 5*, 16–22.

Maslach, C. (1982a). *Burnout: The cost of caring*. Prentice Hall.

Maslach, C. (1982b). Understanding burnout: Definitional issues in analyzing a complex phenomenon. In W. S. Paine (Ed.), *Job stress and burnout* (pp. 29–40). SAGE.

Maslach, C., & Goldberg, J. (1998). Prevention of burnout: New perspectives. *Applied and Preventive Psychology, 7*(1), 63–74. https://doi.org/10.1016/S0962-1849(98)80022-X

Maslach, C., & Jackson, S. E. (1981a). The measurement of experienced burnout. *Journal of Organizational Behavior, 2*(2), 99–113. https://doi.org/10.1002/job.4030020205

Maslach, C., & Jackson, S. E. (1981b). *The Maslach Burnout Inventory*. Consulting Psychologists Press.

Maslach, C., & Leiter, M. P. (2016). Understanding the burnout experience: Recent research and its implications for psychiatry. *World Psychiatry, 15*(2), 103–111. https://doi.org/10.1002 /wps.20311

Maslach, C., Jackson, S. E., & Leiter, M. P. (1996). *Maslach Burnout Inventory—GS manual*. Consulting Psychologist's Press.

Maslach, C., Schaufeli, W., & Leiter, M. (2001). Job burnout. *Annual Review of Psychology, 52*, 397–422.

Maslow, A. H. (1954). *Motivation and personality*. Harpers.

Massachusetts Coalition of Battered Women Service Groups. (1981). *For shelter and beyond: An educational manual for working with women who are battered*. Red Sun Press.

Massazza, A., Joffe, H., Hyland, P., & Brewin, C. R. (2021). The structure of peritraumatic reactions and their relationship with PTSD among disaster survivors. *Journal of Abnormal Psychology, 130*(3), 248–259. https://doi.org/10.1037/abn0000663

Mather, L., Blom, V., & Svedberg, P. (2014). Stressful and traumatic life events are associated with burnout: A cross-sectional twin study. *International Journal of Behavioral Medicine, 21*(6), 899–907.

Matos, M., Grangeia, H., Ferreira, C., Azevedo, V., Gonçalves, M., & Sheridan, L. (2019). Stalking victimization in Portugal: Prevalence, characteristics, and impact. *International Journal of Law, Crime and Justice, 57*, 103–115. https://doi.org/10.1016/j. ijlcj.2019.03.005

Matter, D., & Matter, R. (1982). Developmental sequences in children's understanding of death with implications for counselors. *Elementary School Guidance and Counseling, 17*, 112–118.

Matthews, M. D. (2009). *Self-report knowledge of posttraumatic stress disorder and posttraumatic growth among West Point cadets*. Unpublished raw data, United States Military Academy, West Point, NY.

Mattson, M. R., & Sacks, M. H. (1978). Seclusion: Uses and implications. *American Journal of Psychiatry, 135*, 1210–1212.

Maurer, C. M., & Sheets, T. E. (Eds.). (1999). *Encyclopedia of associations* (34th ed., Vol. I, Parts 1–3). Gale Research.

May, C. L., & Wisco, B. E. (2016). Defining trauma: How level of exposure and proximity affect risk for posttraumatic stress disorder. *Psychological Trauma: Theory, Research, Practice, and Policy, 8*(2), 233–240. https://doi.org/10.1037/tra0000077

Mazza, J., & Reynolds, W. M. (1998). A longitudinal investigation of depression, hopelessness, social support, and major and minor life events and their relation to suicidal ideation in adolescents. *Journal of Suicide and Life-Threatening Behavior, 28*, 358–374.

Mazzer, K., O'Riordan, M., Woodward, A., & Rickwood, D. (2021). A systematic review of user expectations and outcomes of crisis support services. *Crisis, 42*(6), 465–473. https://doi .org/10.1027/0227-5910/a000745

McAdams, C. R., & Schmidt, C. (2007). How to help a bully: Recommendation for counseling the proactive aggressor. *Professional School Counseling, 11*(2), 121–127.

McCabe, J. A., Banasik, C. S., Jackson, M. G., Postlethwait, E. M., Steitz, A., & Wenzel, A. R. (2023). Exploring perceptions of cognitive load and mental fatigue in pandemic-era Zoom classes. *Scholarship of Teaching and Learning in Psychology*. Advance online publication. https://doi.org/10.1037/stl0000347

McCann, I. L., & Pearlman, L. A. (1990). Vicarious traumatization: A framework for understanding the psychological effects of working with victims. *Journal of Traumatic Stress, 3*(1), 131–149.

McCart, M. R., Chapman, J. E., Zajac, K., & Rheingold, A. (2020). Community-based randomized controlled trial of psychological first aid with crime victims. *Journal of Consulting and Clinical Psychology, 88*(8), 681–695. https://doi.org/10.1037/ ccp0000588

McCarthy, J. J. (2002). How a school district crisis response team can help. In D. D. Bass & R. Yep (Eds.), *Terrorism, trauma, and tragedies: A counselor's guide to preparing and responding* (pp. 53–54). American Counseling Association.

McCaskie, M., Ward, S., & Rasor, L. (1990, April). *Short-term crisis counseling and the regular caller.* Paper presented at the Fourteenth Annual Convening of Crisis Intervention Personnel, Chicago, IL, the United States.

McCollum, E. E. (2015). *Mindfulness for therapists: Practice for the heart.* Routledge.

McCollum, S. (2010, Fall). Country outposts. *Teaching Tolerance,* 33–35.

McCown, C. (1986). *Counseling in an adolescent psychiatric treatment facility* (Cassette Recording No. 7). Memphis, TN: Memphis State University, Department of Counseling and Personnel Services.

McCown, D. E., & Davies, B. (1995). Patterns of grief in young children following the death of a sibling. *Death Studies, 19,* 41–53.

McCubbin, H. I., & Patterson, J. M. (1983). The family stress process: The Double ABCX Model of adjustment and adaptation. *Marriage and Family Review, 6*(1-2), 1–37.

McCutcheon, K. A., & Fleming, S. J. (2001–2002). Grief resulting from euthanasia and natural death of companion animals. *Omega: Journal of Death & Dying, 44*(2), 169–188.

McDonald, H. Z., Franz, M., R., & Vasterling, J. J. (2012). Assessment and treatment of neuropsychological deficits in post-traumatic stress disorder. In R.A. McMackin, E. Newman, J. M. Fogler, & T. M. Keane (Eds.), *Trauma therapy in context: The science and craft of evidence–based practice.* (pp. 331–352). American Psychological Association.

McFarlane, A. C., & Yehuda, R. (1996). Resiliency, vulnerability, and the course of posttraumatic reactions. In B. A. van der Kolk, A. C. McFarlane, & L. Weisaeth (Eds.), *Traumatic stress* (pp. 155–181). Guilford Press.

McGhie, S. F., Bellet, B. W., Mellen, E. J., & McNally, R. J. (January, 2022). Self-triggering: Does function determine pathogenesis? *Psychological Trauma: Theory, Research, Practice, and Policy.* Advance online publication. http://dx.doi.org/10.1037/tra0001195

McGilloway, C., Smith, D., & Galvin, R. (2020). Barriers faced by adults with intellectual disabilities who experience sexual assault: A systematic review and meta-synthesis. *Journal of Applied Research in Intellectual Disabilities, 33*(1), 51–66. https://doi.org/10.1111/jar.12445

McGlothlin, J. M. (2008). *Developing clinical skills in suicide assessment, prevention, and treatment.* American Counseling Association.

McGoldrick, M., & Ashton, D. (2010). Culture: A challenge to concepts of normality. In S. J. Price, C. A. Price, & P. C. McKenny (Eds.). *Families and change: Coping with stressful events and transitions* (pp. 249–272). SAGE.

McGoldrick, M. & Ashton, D. (2012). Culture: A challenge to concepts of normality. In F. Walsh (Ed.). *Spiritual resources in family therapy* (2nd ed, pp. 249–272). Guilford Press.

McGoldrick, M., & Shisbusawa, T. (2010). The family life cycle. In S. J. Price, C. A. Price, & P. C. McKenny (Eds.). *Families and change: Coping with stressful events and transitions* (pp. 375–398). SAGE.

McGuire, A., Steele, R. G., & Singh, M. N. (2021). Systematic review on the application of trauma-focused cognitive behavioral therapy (TF-CBT) for preschool-aged children. *Clinical Child and Family Psychology Review, 24*(1), 20–37. https://doi.org/10.1007/s10567-020-00334-0

McGuire, T. M., Lee, C., & Drummond, P. (2014). Potential of eye movement desensitization and reprocessing therapy in the treatment of post-traumatic stress disorder. *Psychology Research and Behavior Management, 7,* 273–283.

McHenry, S. (1994). When the therapist needs therapy: Characterological countertransference issues and failures in the treatment of the borderline personality disorder. *Psychotherapy, 31,* 557–570.

McIntosh, K., Kauffman, A., Carter, D., Dickey, C., & Horner, R. (2009). Differential effects of a direct behavior rating intervention based on function of problem behavior. *Journal of Positive Behavioral Interventions, 11*(2), 15–27. https://doi.org/10.1177/1098300708319127

McKee, K. J., Wilson, F., Chung, M., Hinchliff, S., Goudie, F., & Elford, H., (2005). Reminiscence, regrets and activity in older people in residential care: Associations with psychological health. *British Journal of Clinical Psychology, 44*(4), 543–561.

McKenna, J., & Petrosino, A. (2022, February). School policing program: Where we have been and where we need to go next. *National Institute of Justice.* https://nij.ojp.gov/library/publications/school-policing-programs-where-we-have-been-and-where-we-need-go-next

McKenna, S. (1999, September 28). *Stages of grieving.* www.thirdage.com/features/family/alone/sb01.html

McKeon, B., McEwan, T., & Luebbers, S. (2015). It's not really stalking if you know the person: Measuring community attitudes that normalize, justify, and minimize stalking. *Psychiatry, Psychology, and Law, 22*(2), 291–306.

McLay, R. N., Graap, K., Spira, J., Perlman, K., Johnson, S., Rothbaum, B., Rizzo, J. M. (2012). Development and testing of virtual reality exposure therapy for post-traumatic stress disorder in active service members who served in Iraq and Afghanistan. *Military Medicine, 177*(6), 635–642.

McLendon, D., & Petr, C. G. (2005). Family-direct structural therapy. *Journal of Marital and Family Therapy, 31,* 327–339.

McLeod, A. L., Hays, D. G., & Chang, C. Y. (2010). Female intimate partner violence survivors' experiences with accessing resources. *Journal of Counseling and Development, 88*(3), 303–310.

McLeod, D. A. (2015). Female offenders in child sexual abuse cases: A national picture. *Journal of Child Sexual Abuse, 24*(1), 97–114. https://doi.org/10.1080/10538712.2015.978925

McLeod, P. (September 2022). Puerto Rico's recovery from Hurricane Maria was years behind schedule. Then Fiona hit. *Vanity Fair.*

McMahon, A., & Rhudick, P. (1964). Reminiscing: Adaptational significance in the aged. *Archives of General Psychiatry, 10,* 292–298.

McMahon, M., Neville-Sorvilles, J., & Schubert, L. (1999). Undoing harm to children: The Duluth Family Visitation Center. In M. F. Shepard & E. L. Pence (Eds.), *Coordinating community responses to domestic violence: Lessons from Duluth and beyond* (pp. 151–167). SAGE.

McMahon, S., Anderman, E., Astor, R., Espelage, D., Eddy, L., & Worrell, F. (2022). *Violence against educators and school personnel: Crisis During COVID.* Policy Brief. American Psychological Association.

McNeil,,D. (2009). Assessment and management of acute risk of violence in adult patients. In P. M. Kleespies (Ed.), *Behavioral emergencies: An evidence-based resource for evaluating and managing risk of suicide, violence, and victimization.* (pp. 125–146). American Psychological Association.

McNeil, D. E., Binder, M. R., & Greenfield, T. L. (1988). Predictors of violence in civilly committed acute psychiatric patients. *American Journal of Psychiatry, 8*, 965–970.

McNeil, D. E., Gregory, A. L., Lam, J. L. M., Binder, R. L., & Sullivan, G. R. (2003). Utility of decision support tools for assessing acute risk of violence. *Journal of Consulting and Clinical Psychology, 71*, 945–953.

McNeil, D. E., Hatcher, C., Zeiner, H., Wolfe, H. L., & Myers, R. S. (1991). Characteristics of persons referred by police to the psychiatric emergency room. *Hospital and Community Psychiatry, 42*, 425–427.

McNeil, D., & Binder, R. L. (1994). The relationship between acute psychiatric symptoms, diagnosis, and short-term risk of violence. *Hospital and Community Psychiatry, 45*, 133–137.

McVey, L., Gurrieri, L., & Tyler, M. (2021). The structural oppression of women by markets: The continuum of sexual violence and the online pornography market. *Journal of Marketing Management, 37*(1/2), 40–67. https://doi.org/10.1080/02672 57X.2020.1798714

McWhirter, E. H., & Linzer, M. (1994). The provision of critical incident services by EAPs: A case study. *Journal of Mental Health Counseling, 16*, 403–414.

McWhirter, J. J., McWhirter, B. T., McWhirter, E. H., & McWhirter, R. J. (2013). *At risk youth: A comprehensive response for counselors, teachers, psychologists, and human services professionals.* Cengage.

Meadows, E. A., & Foa, E. B. (1999). Cognitive behavioral treatment for traumatized adults. In P. A. Saigh & J. D. Bremner (Eds.), *Posttraumatic stress disorder: A comprehensive text.* Allyn & Bacon.

Meagher, D. K. (2009). *Zach and his dog: A story of bonding, love, and loss for children and adults to share together.* Authorhouse.

Meckes, S. J., McDonald, M. A., & Lancaster, C. L. (2021). Association between physical activity and mental health among first responders with different service roles. *Psychological Trauma: Theory, Research, Practice, and Policy, 13*(1), 66–74. https://doi .org/10.1037/tra0000971

Mederos, F. (1999). Batterer intervention programs: The past and future prospects. In M. F. Shepard & E. L. Pence (Eds.), *Coordinating community response to domestic violence: Lessons from Duluth and beyond* (pp. 127–150). SAGE.

Meehan, T., Brack, J., Mansfield, Y.,& Stedman, T. (2019). Do police-mental health co-responder programmes reduce emergency department presentations or simply delay the inevitable? *Australasian Psychiatry, 27*(1), 18–20. http://doi .org/10.1177/1039856218797424

Meehan, T., de Alwis, A., & Stedman, T. (2016). Identifying patients at risk of inpatient aggression at time of admission to acute mental healthcare. What factors should clinicians consider? *Advances in Mental Health: Promotion, Prevention, and Early Intervention, 15*(2), 161–171. https://doi.org/10.1080/183 87357.2016.1259001

Meehl, P. (1954). *Clinical versus statistical prediction: A theoretical analysis and review of the evidence.* University of Minnesota Press.

Megan's Law. Violent Crime Control and Law Enforcement Act of 1994. Pub.L. 104-145, 42 U.S.C. § 14071 et seq., U.S.C. § 13701.

Mehrabian, A. (1971). Nonverbal betrayal of feeling. *Journal of Experimental Research in Personality, 5*, 64–73.

Meichembaum, D. (1985). *Stress inoculation training.* Pergamon Press.

Meichenbaum, D. (1985, May). Cognitive behavior modification: Perspectives, techniques, and applications. Two-day workshop, St. Louis, MO, the United States, presented by Evaluation Research Associates.

Meichenbaum, D. (2017). Thirty-five years of working with suicidal patients: Lessons learned. In *The Evolution of Cognitive Behavior Therapy.* Routledge.

Meichenbaum, D. H. (1977). *Cognitive behavior modification: An integrative approach.* Plenum.

Meichenbaum, D. H. (2005). Thirty-five years working with suicidal patients: Lessons learned. *Canadian Psychology, 46*(2), 64–72. https://doi.org/10.1037/h0087006

Mejías-Martín, Y., Martí-García, C., Rodríguez-Mejías, Y., Esteban-Burgos, A. A., Cruz-García, V., & García-Caro, M. P. (2023). Understanding for prevention: Qualitative and quantitative analyses of suicide notes and forensic reports. *International Journal of Environmental Research and Public Health, 20*(3). https://doi.org/10.3390/ijerph20032281

Melamed, S., Meir, E. I., & Samson, A. (1995). The benefits of personality–leisure congruence: Evidence and implications. *Journal of Leisure Research, 27*(1), 25–40.

Melamed, S., Shirom, A., Toker, S., Berliner, S., & Shapira, I. (2006). Burnout and risk of cardiovascular disease: Evidence, possible causal paths, and promising research directions. *Psychological Bulletin, 132*(3), 327–353.

Melchior, M., van der Berg, A., Halfens, R., & Abu-Saad, H. (1997). Burnout and the work environment of nurses in psychiatric long-stay care settings. *Social Psychiatry and Psychiatric Epidemiology, 32*(3), 158–164.

Melendez-Moral, J. C., Charco-Ruiz, L., Mayordomo-Rodriguez, T., & Sales-Galan, A. (2013). Effects of a reminiscence program among institutionalized elderly adults. *Psicothema, 25*(3), 319–322.

Mellish, S., Ryan, J. C., & Litchfield, C. A. (2022). Short-term psychological outcomes of Australia's 2019/20 bushfire season. *Psychological Trauma: Theory, Research, Practice, and Policy.* Advance online publication. https://doi.org/10.1037 /tra0001323

Meloy, J. R. (2017). *The TRAP-18 manual.* Global Institute of Forensic Research.

Meloy, J. R. (2018). The operational development and empirical testing of the terrorist radicalization assessment protocol (TRAP-18). *Journal of Personality Assessment.* https://doi.org/ 10.1080/00223891.2018.1481077

Meloy J. R., & Gill, P. (2016). The lone actor terrorist and the TRAP-18. *Journal of Threat Assessment and Management, 3*(1), 37–52. https://doi.org/10.1037/tam0000061

Meloy, J. T., & O'Toole, M. E. (2011). The concepts of leakage in threat assessment. *Behavioral Sciences and the Law, 29*(4), 513–527

Melton, B. (2001). Seeing the unseen. *ASCA School Counselor, 39*, 21–25.

Memphis Police Department. (2010). *Crisis intervention training manual.*

Memphis Vietnam Veterans Center. (1985). *The nonveteran helper* (Pamphlet).

Mental Health Advisory Team V. (2008, February 14). *Mental Health Advisory Team (MHAT) V Operation Iraqi Freedom 06-08* (Report chartered by the Office of the Surgeon Multi-National Force-Iraq and the Office of the Surgeon General United States Army Medical Command).

Mereish, E., Peters, J., Brick, L., Killam, M., & Yen, S. (2023). A daily diary study of minority stressors, suicidal ideation, nonsuicidal self-injury ideation, and affective mechanisms among sexual and gender minority youth. *Journal of Psychopathology and Clinical Science, 132*(4) 372–384. https://doi.org/10.1037/abn0000813

Merlino, J. P. (2011). Rescuing ourselves: Self-care in the disaster response community. In F. J. Stoddard, A. Pandya, & C. Katz (Eds.), *Disaster psychiatry: Readiness, evaluation, and treatment* (pp. 35–48). American Psychiatric Publishing.

Messinger, A. M., & Koon-Magnin, S. (2019). Sexual violence in LGBTQ communities. In W. T. O'Donohue & P. A. Schewe (Eds.), *Handbook of sexual assault and sexual assault prevention* (pp. 661–674). Springer International Publishing. https://doi.org/10.1007/978-3-030-23645-8_39

Metha, A., Cohen, R., & Chan, L. S. (2009). Palliative care: A need for family systems approach. *Palliative and Supportive Care, 7,* 235–243.

Meyers, T. W., & Cornille, T. A. (2002). The trauma of working with traumatized children. In C. R. Figley (Ed.), *Treating compassion fatigue* (pp. 39–55). Brunner/Routledge.

Michaelis, D. (2019). *The value of threat assessment teams.* Virginia Center for School and Campus Safety, Virginia Department of Criminal Justice Services. https://nij.ojp.gov/topics/articles/value-threat-assessment-teams

Michaels, K. (2009, November). Recession depression: Coping and survival techniques. *Counseling Today,* 48–50.

Michaelsis, D. (2019). *The value of threat assessment teams.* National Institute of Justice. https://nij.ojp.gov/topics/articles/value-threat-assessment-teams

Middleton, A. M., Gunn, J., Bassilios, B., & Pirkis, J. (2014). Systematic review of research into frequent callers to crisis helplines. *Journal of Telemedicine and Telecare, 20*(2), 89–98.

Middleton, W., Raphael, B., Burnett, P., & Martinek, N. (1998). A longitudinal study comparing bereavement phenomena in recently bereaved spouses, adult children and parents. *Australian & New Zealand Journal of Psychiatry, 32*(2), 235–241.

Midgett, A. (2016). Bullying: How counselors can intervene. *Counseling Today, 58*(12), 39–43

Millen, D. H., Kennedy, T. D., Black, R. A., Detullio, D., & Walker, L. E. (2019). Battered Woman Syndrome Questionnaire (BWSQ) subscales: Development, reliability, and validity. *Journal of Aggression, Maltreatment & Trauma, 28*(7), 848–869. https://doi.org/10.1080/10926771.2019.1627684

Miller, G. (2015). Healing and trauma: Response. In T. E. Robert & V. A. Kelly, *Critical incidents in integrating spirituality into counseling.* (pp. 11–114). American Counseling Association.

Miller, J. B. (1976). *Toward a new psychology of women.* Beacon Press.

Miller, J., Martin, I., & Schamess, G. (2003). *School violence and children in crisis: Community and school interventions for social workers and counselors.* Love Publishing.

Miller, L. (2006). *Practical police psychology: Stress management and crisis intervention for law enforcement.* Charles C. Thomas.

Miller, L. (2010). On-scene crisis intervention: Psychological guidelines and communication strategies for first responders. *International Journal of Emergency Mental Health, 12*(1), 11–19.

Miller, M. (1986). *Counseling geriatric clients* (Cassette Recording No. 14). Memphis, TN: Memphis State University, Department of Counseling and Personnel Services.

Miller, M. L. (1999). Chaos, complexity, and psychoanalysis. *Psychoanalytic Psychology, 16*(3), 355–379. http://doi.org/10.1037/0736-9735.16.3.355

Miller, M. W., Wolf, E. J., Martin, E., Kaloupek, D. G., & Keane, T. M. (2008). Structural equation modeling of associations among combat exposure, PTSD symptom factors, and global assessment of functioning, *Journal of Rehabilitation Research and Development, 45,* 359–370.

Miller, S. (Ed.). (2010). Discussing the Duluth curriculum: Creating a process of change for men who batter. *Violence Against Women, 16*(9), 1007–1021.

Miller, W. R., & Rollnick, S. (2013). *Motivational interviewing: Helping people change* (3rd ed.). Guilford Press.

Milner, A., Spittal, M. J., Pirkis, J., & LaMontagne, A. D. (2013). Suicide by occupation: Systematic review and meta-analysis. *The British Journal of Psychiatry, 203*(6), 409–416. https://doi.org/10.1192/bjp.bp.113.128405

Minayo, M. C. de S., & Cavalcante, F. G. (2015). Tentativas de suicídio entre pessoas idosas: Revisão de literatura (2002/2013). *Ciência & Saúde Coletiva, 20*(6), 1751–1762. https://doi.org/10.1590/1413-81232015206.10962014

Minihan, S., Songco, A., Fox, E., Ladouceur, C. D., Mewton, L., Moulds, M., Pfeifer, J. H., Van Harmelen, A.-L., & Schweizer, S. (2023, May 18). Affect and mental health across the lifespan during a year of the COVID-19 pandemic: The role of emotion regulation strategies and mental flexibility. *Emotion.* Advance online publication. https://dx.doi.org/10.1037/emo0001238

Minuchin, S. (1974). *Families and family therapy.* Harvard University Press.

Mirhashemi, S., Ghanjal, A., Mohebbi, H. A., & Moharamzad, Y. (2007). The 2003 Bam earthquake: Overview of first aid and transport of victims. *Prehospital and Disaster Medicine, 22,* 513–516.

Mirick, R. G., McCauley, J., & Bridger, J. (2023, May 1). Integrating trauma-informed principles into suicide prevention, intervention, and postvention. *Practice Innovations.* Advance online publication. https://dx.doi.org/10.1037/pri0000212

Mishara, B. L., Houle, J., & Lavoie, B. (2005). Comparison of the effects of four suicide prevention programs for family and friends of high-risk suicidal men who do not seek help themselves. *Suicide and Life-Threatening Behavior, 35*(3), 329–342. https://doi.org/10.1521/suli.2005.35.3.329

Mishara, L. B. L., Chagnon, F., Daigle, M., Balan, B., Raymond, S., & Marcous, I. (2005). *A silent monitoring of telephone help provided over the Hopeline network and its short-term effects.* Montreal: Center for Research and Intervention on Suicide and Euthanasia.

Mishna, F., Bogo, M., & Sawyer, J.-L. (2015). Cyber counseling: Illuminating benefits and challenges. *Clinical Social Work Journal, 43*(2), 169–178. https://doi.org/10.1007/s10615-013-0470-1

Missing Children. (2006). Missing Children: Getting home after disaster strikes. *Challenge, 14*(1), 1–2.

Missouri School Counselor Association. (2002). *Crisis manual.*

Mistry, D., Zhu, J., Tremblay, P., Wekerle, C., Lanius, R., Jetly, R., & Frewen, P. (2020). Meditating in virtual reality: Proof-of-concept intervention for posttraumatic stress. *Psychological Trauma: Theory, Research, Practice, and Policy, 12*(8), 847–858. https://doi.org/10.1037/tra0000959

Mitchell, A. M., Kim, Y., Prigerson, H. G., & Mortimer-Stephens, M. (2004). Complicated grief in survivors of suicide. *Crisis, 25*(1), 12–18. https://doi.org/10.1027/0227-5910.25.1.12

Mitchell, J. (1983). When disaster strikes: The critical incident stress debriefing process. *Journal of Emergency Medical Services, 8,* 36–39.

Mitchell, J. T., & Everly, G. S., Jr. (1995). *Critical incidents stress debriefing: The basic course workbook.* International Critical Incidents Stress Foundation.

Mitchell, J. T., & Everly, G. S., Jr. (1995a). *Advanced critical incidents stress debriefing.* International Critical Incidents Stress Foundation.

Mitchell, J. T., & Everly, G. S., Jr. (1995b). Critical incidents stress debriefing (CISD) and the prevention of work-related traumatic stress among high risk occupational groups. In G. S. Everly, Jr., & J. T. Lating (Eds.), *Psychotraumatology* (pp. 267–280). Plenum Press.

Mitchell, J. T., & Everly, G. S., Jr. (1999). Critical incident stress management and critical incident stress debriefings: Evolutions, effects, and outcomes. In B. Raphael & J. P. Wilson (Eds.), *Psychological debriefing: Theory, practice, and evidence* (pp. 71–90). Cambridge University Press.

Mitchell, L. L., Frazier, P. A., & Sayer, N. A. (2020). Identity disruption and its association with mental health among veterans with reintegration difficulty. *Developmental Psychology, 56*(11), 2152–2166. https://doi.org/10.1037/dev0001106

Mittelmark, M. B., Sagy, S., Eriksson, M., Bauer, G., Pelikan, J., Linstrom, B., & Espnes, G. (Eds.), (2017) *The Handbook of Salutogenesis.* Springer. https://doi.org/10.1007/978-3-319-04600-6

Mittendorfer-Rutz, E., Rasmussen, F., & Wasserman, D. (2008). Familial clustering of suicidal behaviour and psychopathology in young suicide attempters. *Social Psychiatry & Psychiatric Epidemiology, 43*(1), 28–36. https://doi.org/10.1007/s00127-007-0266-0

Mneine, M., Fleeson, W., Arnold, E., & Furr, R. (2018). Differentiating everyday emotion dynamics of borderline personality disorder from major depressive disorder and bipolar disorder. *Personality Disorder: Theory, Research, and Treatment, 9*(2), 192–196. https://doi.org/10.1037/per0000255

Modrak, R. (1992, January). Mass shootings and airplane crashes: Counselors respond to the changing face of community crisis. *Guidepost, 34,* 4.

Moffitt, P., Aujla, W., Giesbrecht, C. J., Grant, I., & Straatman, A.-L. (2022). Intimate partner violence and COVID-19 in rural, remote, and Northern Canada: Relationship, vulnerability and risk. *Journal of Family Violence, 37*(5), 775–786. https://doi.org/10.1007/s10896-020-00212-x

Mohr, W. K. (2010). Restraints and the code of ethics: An uneasy fit. *Archives of Psychiatric Nursing, 24*(1), 3–14.

Möller, A., Söndergaard, H. P., & Helström, L. (2017). Tonic immobility during sexual assault—a common reaction predicting post-traumatic stress disorder and severe depression. *Acta Obstetricia et Gynecologica Scandinavica, 96*(8), 932–938. https://doi.org/10.1111/aogs.13174

Möller, I., & Krahé, B. (2009). Exposure to violent video games and aggression in German adolescents: A longitudinal analysis. *Aggressive Behavior, 35*(1), 75–89. https://doi.org/10.1002/ab.20290

Møller, L., Meisner, M. W., Søgaard, U., Elklit, A., & Simonsen, E. (2021). Assessment of personality functioning in ICD-11 posttraumatic stress disorder and complex posttraumatic stress disorder. *Personality Disorders: Theory, Research, and Treatment, 12*(5), 466–474. https://doi.org/10.1037/per0000491

Molnar, B. E., Sprang, G., Killian, K. D., Gottfried, R., Emery, V., & Bride, B. E. (2017). Advancing science and practice for vicarious traumatization/secondary traumatic stress: A research agenda. *Traumatology, 23*(2), 129–142. https://doi.org/10.1037/trm0000122

Monahan, J. (1981). *The clinical prediction of violent behavior.* National Institute of Mental Health.

Monahan, J. (1984). The prediction of violent behavior: Toward a second generation of theory and policy. *American Journal of Psychiatry, 141,* 10–15.

Monahan, J. (1988). Risk assessment of violence among the mentally disordered: Generating useful knowledge. *International Journal of Law and Psychiatry, 11*(3), 249–257.

Monahan, J., Steadman, H. J., Silver, E., Applebaum, P. S., Robbins, P. C., & Mulvey, E. P. (2001). *Rethinking risk assessment: The McArthur Study of mental disorder and violence.* Oxford University Press.

Monk, G., Drewery, W., & Winslade, J. (2005). Using narrative ideas in group work: A new perspective. *Counseling and Human Development, 38*(1), 1–13.

Monk, G., Winslade, J., Crocket, K., & Epston, D. (Eds.). (1997). *Narrative therapy in practice: The archeology of hope.* Jossey-Bass.

Monson, C. M., & Shnaider, P. (2014). *Treating PTSD with cognitive-behavioral therapies: Interventions that work.* American Psychological Association.

Montano, R., & Dowdall-Thomae, C. (2003). *Are you ready for the crisis?* Paper presented at the American School Counselor Association Convention, St. Louis, MO, the United States.

Montgomery, A. P., Patrician, P. A., & Azuero, A. (2022). Nurse burnout syndrome and work environment impact patient safety grade. *Journal of Nursing Care Quality, 37*(1), 87–93. https://doi.org/10.1097/NCQ.0000000000000574

Moore, B. A., & Jongsma, A. E. (2009). *The veterans and active duty military psychotherapy treatment planner.* John Wiley & Sons.

Moos, R. H. (1981). *Work Environment Scale manual.* Consulting Psychologists Press.

Moos, R. H., & Moos, B. S. (1981). *Family Environment Scale.* Consulting Psychologists Press.

Moran, C. C. (2002). Humor as a moderator of compassion fatigue. In C. R. Figley (Ed.), *Treating compassion fatigue* (pp. 139–154). Brunner/Routledge.

Moran, J. F. (1984). Teaching the management of violent behavior to nursing staff: A health care model. In J. T. Turner (Ed.), *Violence in the medical care setting: A survival guide* (pp. 231–250). Aspen Systems.

Moran, M. (2022, February 24). Impact of culture, race, social determinants reflected throughout new DSM-5-TR. *Psychiatric News.* https://psychnews.psychiatryonline.org/doi/10.1176/appi.pn.2022.03.3.20

Moret, J. D., Todd, A., Rose, L., Pollitt, E., & Anderson, J. (2022). Mobile phone apps for intimate partner and sexual violence prevention and response: Systematic search on app stores. *JMIR Formative Research, 6*(2), e28959. https://doi.org/10.2196/28959

Morgan, J. D., & Laungani, L. (Eds.). (2002). *Death and bereavement around the world* (Vol. 1). Baywood.

Morgan, J. D., & Laungani, L. (Eds.). (2003). *Death and bereavement around the world* (Vol. 2). Baywood.

Morgan, J. D., & Laungani, L. (Eds.). (2004a). *Death and bereavement around the world* (Vol. 3). Baywood.

Morgan, J. D., & Laungani, L. (Eds.). (2004b). *Death and bereavement around the world* (Vol. 4). Baywood.

Morgan, J. D., Laungani, L., & Palmer, S. (Eds.). (2009). *Death and bereavement around the world* (Vol. 5). Baywood.

Morgan, M. C. (2009). The impact of traumatic brain injury on the survivor's partner or spouse: Implications for treatment. *Dissertation Abstracts International: Section B: The Sciences and Engineering, 3180.*

Morgan, R. E., & Oudekerk, B. A. (2019). *Criminal Victimization, 2018* (NCJ 253043). Bureau of Justice Statistics. https://bjs.ojp.gov/content/pub/pdf/cv18.pdf

Morgan, S. M. (1982). *Conjugal terrorism: A psychological and community treatment model of wife abuse.* R & E Research Associates.

Morgan, W., & Wells, M. (2016). 'It's deemed unmanly': Men's experiences of intimate partner violence (IPV). *The Journal of Forensic Psychiatry & Psychology, 27*(3), 404–418. https://doi.org/10.1080/14789949.2015.1127986

Morinaj, J., Scharf, J., Grecu, A., Hadjar, A. Hascher, T., & Marcin, K. (2017). School alienation: A construct validation study. *Frontline Learning Research, 5*(2), 36–59. https://doi.org/10.14786/flr.v5i2.298

Moritz, S., Voigt, M. K., Kother, U., Leighton, L., Kiahili, B., Babur, Z., Jungclaussen, D., & Grzella, K. (2014). Can virtual reality reduce reality distortion? Impact of performance feedback on symptom change in schizophrenia patients. *Journal of Behavior Therapy and Experimental Psychiatry, 45*(2), 267–271.

Mørkved, N., Hartmann, K., Aarsheim, L. M., Holen, D., Milde, A. M., Bomyea, J., & Thorp, S. R. (2014). A comparison of narrative exposure therapy and prolonged exposure therapy for PTSD. *Clinical Psychology Review, 34*(6), 453–467.

Morland, L. A., Knopp, K. C., Khalifian, C. E., Macdonald, A., Grubbs, K. M., Mackintosh, M.-A., Becker-Cretu, J. J., Sautter, F. J., Buzzella, B. A., Wrape, E. R., Glassman, L. H., Webster, K., Sohn, M. J., Glynn, S. M., Acierno, R., & Monson, C. M. (2022). A randomized trial of brief couple therapy for PTSD and relationship satisfaction. *Journal of Consulting and Clinical Psychology, 90*(5), 392–404. https://doi.org/10.1037/ccp0000731

Morris Trainor, Z., Jong, J., Bluemke, M., & Halberstadt, J. (2019). Death salience moderates the effect of trauma on religiosity. *Psychological Trauma: Theory, Research, Practice, and Policy, 11*(6), 639–646. https://doi.org/10.1037/tra0000430

Morris, A. J. (2011). Psychic aftershocks: Crisis counseling and disaster relief policy. *History of Psychology, 14*(3), 264–286.

Morris, M. C., Kouros, C. D., Janecek, K., Freeman, R., Mielock, A., & Garber, J. (2017). Community-level moderators of a school-based childhood sexual assault prevention program. *Child Abuse & Neglect, 63*, 295–306. https://doi.org/10.1016/j.chiabu.2016.10.005

Morrison, J. M. (1993). Physical techniques. In P. E. Blumenreich & S. Lewis (Eds.), *Managing the violent patient: A clinician's guide* (pp. 79–100). Brunner-Mazel.

Morrison, P. K., Burke, J., Cluss, P. A., Hawker, L., Miller, E., George, D., Bicehouse, T., Fleming, R., Wright, K., & Chang, J. C. (2018). The influence of batterer intervention programs on male perpetrators of intimate partner violence: Reports of change in beliefs and behaviors. *Journal of Offender Rehabilitation, 57*(5), 311–329. https://doi.org/10.1080/10509674.2018.1487900

Morrissey, M. (1994, June). ACA, Red Cross to work together to help disaster victims. *Guidepost, 36*, 1, 6.

Morse, G. A. (2000). On being homeless and mentally ill: A multitude of losses and the possibility of recovery. In J. H. Harvey & E. D. Miller (Eds.), *Loss and trauma: General and close relationship perspectives* (pp. 249–262). Brunner-Routledge.

Moshier, S. J., Bovin, M. J., Gay, N. G., Wisco, B. E., Mitchell, K. S., Lee, D. J., Sloan, D. M., Weathers, F. W., Schnurr, P. P., Keane, T. M., & Marx, B. P. (2018). Examination of posttraumatic stress disorder symptom networks using clinician-rated and patient-rated data. *Journal of Abnormal Psychology, 127*(6), 541–547. https://doi.org/10.1037/abn0000368

Moss, J. (2019). Burnout is about your workplace, not your people. *Harvard Business Review.*

Mott, J. M., Galovski, T. E., Walsh, R. M., & Elwood, L. S. (2015). Change in trauma narrative and perceived recall ability over a course of cognitive processing therapy for PTSD. *Traumatology, 21*(1), 47–54.

Mowbray, C. T. (1988). Post-traumatic therapy for children who are victims of violence. In F. M. Ochberg (Ed.), *Post-traumatic therapy and victims of violence* (pp. 196–212). Brunner/Mazel.

Mowen T., & Freng, A. (2019). Is more necessarily better? School security and perceptions of safety among students and parents in the United States. *American Journal of Criminal Justice, 44*(3), 376–394. https://doi.org/10.1007/s12103-018-9461-7

MST Services. (2018). *Youth detention centers.* https://info.mstservices.com/blog/violence-in-youth-detention-centers

Mullen, P. R., Blount, A. J., Lambie, G. W., & Chae, N. (2017). School counselors' perceived stress, burnout, and job satisfaction. *Professional School Counseling, 21*(1). https://doi.org/10.1177/2156759X18782468

Mulvey, E. P., & Cauffman, E. (2001). The inherent limits of predicting school violence. *American Psychologist, 56*(10), 797–802.

Mulvey, E. P., & Lidz, C. W. (1984). Clinical considerations on the prediction of dangerous mental patients. *Clinical Psychology Review, 4*, 379–401.

Munetz, M. R., & Griffin, P. (2006). Use of the Sequential Intercept Model as an approach to decriminalization of people with serious mental illness. *Psychiatric Services, 57*(4), 544–549. https://doi.org/10.1176/ps.2006.57.4.544

Munoz, M., Joaquin, C., Noval, D., Moringo, A., & Garcia de la Concha, J. A. (2000). Factores predictores de agresividad en esquizofrenicos hospitalizados. *Actas Espanolas de Psiquiatria, 28*(3), 151–155.

Munsey, C. (2006). Schools: A post-Katrina anchor for children. *Monitor on Psychology, 37*(9), 46–47.

Munsey, C. (2008). Stay safe in practice. *Monitor on Psychology, 39*(4), 37–39.

Munsey, C. (2009). Women and war. *Monitor on Psychology, 40*(8), 34–35.

Munsey, C. (2010). More students with serious psychological issues are showing up at campus counseling centers. *Monitor on Psychology, 41*(4), 10–11.

Munsey, C. (2011). APA is front and center at White House bullying conference. *Monitor on Psychology, 42*(5), 18–19.

Munsey, C. (2012). Anti-bullying efforts ramp up. *Monitor on Psychology, 43*(2), 55–57.

Murdach, A. D. (1993). Working with potentially assaultive clients. *Health and Social Work, 18*, 307–312.

Muro, J. J., & Kottman, T. (1995). *Guidance and counseling in the elementary and middle schools.* William C. Brown Communications.

Murray, C. I., Toth, K., Larson, B. L., & Moulton, S. (2010). Death, dying, and grief in families. In S. J. Price, C. A. Price, & P. C. McKenny (Eds.). *Families and change: Coping with stressful events and transitions* (pp. 73–96). SAGE.

Murray, G., & Snyder, J. C. (1991). When staff are assaulted. *Journal of Psychosocial Nursing, 29*, 24–29.

Muschalla, B., & Schönborn, F. (2021). Induction of false beliefs and false memories in laboratory studies—A systematic review. *Clinical Psychology & Psychotherapy, 28*(5), 1194–1209. https://doi.org/10.1002/cpp.2567

Myer, R. A. (1999, April). *Crisis intervention using the Internet.* Paper presented at the Twenty-third Annual Convening of Crisis Intervention Personnel, Chicago, IL, the United States.

Myer, R. A. (2001). *Assessment for crisis intervention: A triage assessment model.* Thomson Brooks/Cole.

Myer, R. A. (2014). *A reliability study of the modified TAF using an earthquake disaster scenario.* Attilian University.

Myer, R. A. (2014). Practical guide to disaster counseling. Cengage.

Myer, R. A. (2015). *Practical issues for disaster counseling.* Brooks-Cole/Cengage

Myer, R. A. (2015). Triage Assessment Form for Family Therapy (TAFFT). In R. K. James & B. E. Gilliland (Eds.), *Crisis intervention strategies* (8th ed.). Brooks-Cole/Cengage.

Myer, R. A., & James, R. K. (2005). *Crisis intervention workbook and CD-ROM.* Thomson: Brooks/Cole.

Myer, R. A., & Moore, H. (2006). Crisis in context theory: An ecological model. *Journal of Counseling & Development, 84*(2), 139–147.

Myer, R. A., James, R. K., & Moulton, P. (2011). *This is not a fire drill: Crisis intervention and prevention on college campuses.* John Wiley & Sons.

Myer, R. A., Lewis, J. S., James, R. K. (2013). The introduction of a task model for crisis intervention. *Journal of Mental Health Counseling, 35*(2), 95–107.

Myer, R. A., Moore, H., & Hughes, T. (2003). September 11th survivors and the refugee model. *Journal of Mental Health Counseling, 25,* 245–258.

Myer, R. A., Moulton, P., Cogdal, P. C., Rice, N. D., James, R. K., & Allen, S. (2007). *Triage Assessment System Training Manual: Higher education: Instructor's manual.* CIPS-Solutions Inc.

Myer, R. A., Rice, D., Moulton, P., Cogdal, P., Allen, S., & James, R. (2007). *Triage Assessment System for Students in Learning Environments (TASSLE) manual and CD.* Crisis Intervention and Prevention Solutions.

Myer, R. A., Whisenhunt, J. L., & James, R. K. (2022). *Crisis intervention ethics case book.* American Counseling Association.

Myer, R. A., Williams, R. C., Haley, M., Brownfield, J., Austin, K., & Pribozie, N. (2014). Crisis intervention with families: Assessing changes in family characteristics, *The Family Journal, 22,* 179–185.

Myer, R. A., Williams, R. C., Ottens, A. J., & Schmidt, A. E. (1991). *Three-dimensional crisis assessment model.* Unpublished manuscript, Department of Educational Psychology, Counseling, and Special Education, Northern Illinois University.

Myer, R. A., Williams, R. C., Ottens, A. J., & Schmidt, A. E. (1992). A three-dimensional model for triage. *Journal of Mental Health Counseling, 14,* 137–148.

Myers, D., & Wee, D. F. (2005). *Disaster mental health services.* Brunner-Routledge.

Myers, D., & Zunin, L. (1994). Debriefing and grief: Easing the pain. *Today's Supervisor, 6*(12), 14–15.

Myers, J. E., & Sweeney, T. J. (Eds.). (2005). *Counseling for wellness.* American Counseling Association.

Myers, J. E., Sweeney, T. J., & Witmer, J. E. (2000). The wheel of wellness counseling for wellness: A holistic model for treatment planning. *Journal of Counseling and Development, 78*(3), 251–266.

Myers, L. (2021). Working our way through a pandemic, *Counseling Today, 63*(9), 30–34.

Myers, W. C., & Mutch, P. J. (1992). Language disorders in disruptive behavior-disordered homicidal youth. *Journal of Forensic Sciences, 37*(3), 919–992.

Na, C. & Gottfredson, D. (2013). Police officers in schools: Effects on school crime and the processing of criminal behaviors. *Justice Quarterly, 30*(4), 619–650.

Nadel, B. (2004). *Security: Handbook for architectural planning and design.* McGraw Hill.

Nader, K. O. (1997). Assessing traumatic experiences in children. In J. P. Wilson & T. M. Keane (Eds.), *Assessing psychological trauma and PTSD* (pp. 291–348). Guilford Press.

Nader, K. O., Kreigler, J. A., Blake, D. D., & Pynoos, R. S. (1994). *Clinician Administered PTSD Scale, Child and Adolescent Version (CAPS-C).* National Center for PTSD.

Nagata, J. M., Trompeter, N., Singh, G., Raney, J., Ganson, K. T., Testa, A., Jackson, D. B., Murray, S. B., & Baker, F. C. (2023). Adverse childhood experiences and early adolescent cyberbullying in the United States. *Journal of Adolescence, 95*(3), 609–616. https://onlinelibrary.wiley.com/doi/abs/10.1002/jad.12124

Nagel, D. M., & Anthony, K. (2011a). Ethical framework for the use of technology in disaster mental health. *Online Therapy Institute.* www.onlinetherapyinstitute.com/disaster-mental-health/

Nagel, D. M., & Anthony, K. (2011b). Ethical framework for the use of technology in mental health. *Online Therapy Institute.* www.onlinetherapyinstitute.com/ethical-training

Nagy, S. M., Pickett, S. M., & Hunsanger, J. A. (2022). The relationship between mindfulness, PTSD-related sleep disturbance, and sleep quality: Contributions beyond emotion regulation difficulties. *Psychological Trauma: Theory, Research, Practice, and Policy, 14*(7), 1073–1079. https://doi.org/10.1037/tra0000572

Naifeh, J. A., Gonzalez, O. I., Mash, H. B. H., Fullerton, C. S., & Ursano, R. J. (2021). The cost of anger: Suicide in the U.S. Army. In A. B. Adler & D. Forbes (Eds.), *Anger at work: Prevention, intervention, and treatment in high-risk occupations* (pp. 201–246). American Psychological Association. https://doi.org/10.1037/0000244-008

Namnyak, M., Tufton, N., Szekely, R., Toal, M., Worboys, S., & Sampson, E. L. (2008). 'Stockholm syndrome': Psychiatric diagnosis or urban myth? *Acta Psychiatrica Scandinavica, 117*(1), 4–11. https://doi.org/10.1111/j.1600-0447.2007.01112.x

NASRO. (n.d.). About NASAO. *National Association of School Resource Officers.* https://www.nasro.org/main/about-nasro/

Nassau County Emergency Management Department. (2003). *Storm time and event schedule.*

Nassau County Florida Emergency Management Department (2023).

NASSP. (2023), School resource officer and law enforcement in schools. *National Association of Secondary School Principals.* https://www.nassp.org/school-resource-officers-and-law-enforcement-in-schools

National Alliance on Mental Illness. (2011). Crisis Intervention Team resource center. https://www.nami.org/Advocacy/Crisis-Intervention/Crisis-Intervention-Team-(CIT)-Programs

National Alliance on Mental Illness. (n.d.). *Never be ashamed of seeking help.* https://www.nami.org/Personal-Stories/Never-Be-Ashamed-of-Seeking-Help

National Association of School Psychologists. (2010). *NASP Professional Standards (2010).* http://www.nasponline.org/standards/2010standards.aspx

National Association of School Psychologists (2015). *Threat assessmentatschool*.https://www.nasponline.org/resources-and-publications/resources-and-podcasts/school-safety-and-crisis/systems-level-prevention/threat-assessment-at-school

National Association of School Psychologists. (2015). *School violence prevention*.https://www.nasponline.org/resources-and-publications/resources-and-podcasts/school-safety-and-crisis/school-violence-resources/school-violence-prevention

National Association of School Psychologists. (2023). https://apps.nasponline.org/search-results.aspx?q=disaster

National Association of School Resource Officers. (2011). *NASRO Training*. https://www.nasro.org/training/training-courses/

National Association of School Resource Officers. (2022). *NASRO basic school resource officer course outline and objectives*.

National Center for Education Statistics. (2004). *Indicators of School Crime and Safety: 2004*. https://nces.ed.gov/pubsearch/pubsinfo.asp?pubid=2005002

National Center for Education Statistics. (2010). *Indicators of school crime and safety: 2010*. https://nces.ed.gov/pubs2011/2011002.pdf

National Center for Education Statistics. (2022). Criminal incidents at postsecondary institutions. *Condition of Education*. U.S. Department of Education, Institute of Education Sciences. https://nces.ed.gov/programs/coe/pdf/2022/a21_508.pdf

National Center for Education Statistics. (2022). Criminal incidents recorded by public schools and those reported to sworn law enforcement. *Condition of Education*. U.S. Department of Education, Institute of Education Sciences. https://nces.ed.gov/programs/coe/indicator/a06

National Center for Education Statistics. (2022). Incidence of victimization at school and away from school. *Condition of Education*. U.S. Department of Education, Institute of Education Sciences. https://nces.ed.gov/programs/coe/indicator/a02

National Center for Education Statistics. (2022). Marijuana use and illegal drug availability. *Condition of Education*. U.S. Department of Education, Institute of Education Sciences. https://nces.ed.gov/programs/coe/indicator/a15

National Center for Education Statistics. (2022). Safety and security practices at public schools. *Condition of Education*. U.S. Department of Education, Institute of Education Sciences. https://nces.ed.gov/programs/coe/indicator/a19

National Center for Education Statistics. (2022). Students' perceptions of personal safety at school and away from school. *Condition of Education*. U.S. Department of Education, Institute of Education Sciences. https://nces.ed.gov/programs/coe/indicator/a16

National Center for Education Statistics. (2022). Violent deaths at school and away from school and school shootings. *Condition of Education*. U.S. Department of Education, Institute of Education Sciences. https://nces.ed.gov/programs/coe/indicator/a01?tid=200

National Center for Health Statistics. (1992). Advance report of final mortality statistics. *NCHS Monthly Vital Statistics Report, 45*(Suppl. 3).

National Center for Health Statistics. (2012). *First marriages in the United States: Data from the 2006-2010 National Survey of Family Growth*. https://www.cdc.gov/nchs/data/nhsr/nhsr049.pdf

National Center for Health Statistics, & Heron, M. (2021). *Deaths: leading causes for 2019*. https://doi.org/10.15620/cdc:104186

National Center for PTSD. (2011, July). *PTSD in children and teens*. U.S. Department of Veterans Affairs. https://www.ptsd.va.gov/professional/treat/specific/ptsd_child_teens.asp

National Center for PTSD (2014). *Mental health effects from serving in Afghanistan and Iraq*. http://www..ptsd.va.gov/public/PTSD-overview/reintegration/overview-mental-health-effects.asp

National Center for PTSD. (2023). *PTSD in Children and Adolescents*. https://www.ptsd.va.gov/professional/treat/specific/ptsd_child_teens.asp#one

National Center for School Crisis and Bereavement. (2020). *Guidelines for responding to the death of a student or school staff*. https://www.schoolcrisiscenter.org/wp-content/uploads/2020/08/Guidelines-Death-Student-or-Staff-Booklet-Format.pdf

National Crime Victimization Survey. (2022). *2022 school crime supplement to the national crime victimization survey*. https://omb.report/omb/1121-0184

National Child Traumatic Stress Network and National Center for PTSD (NCTSN/NCPTSD). (2006). *Psychological first aid: Field operations guide* (2nd ed.).

National Child Traumatic Stress Network. (2017, August 28). *Trauma-focused cognitive behavioral therapy*. https://www.nctsn.org/interventions/trauma-focused-cognitive-behavioral-therapy

National Child Traumatic Stress Network. (2018, January 30). *Creating trauma-informed systems*. What Is a Trauma- Informed Child and Family Service System? https://www.nctsn.org/trauma-informed-care/creating-trauma-informed-systems

National Collaborating Centre for Mental Health (UK). (2015). *Violence and aggression: Short-term management in mental health, health and community settings: Updated edition*. https://www.ncbi.nlm.nih.gov/books/NBK356346/

National Gang Center. (2017). *Gang violence protocols for medical facilities*. https://nationalgangcenter.ojp.gov/insights/34/gang-violence-protocols-for-medical-facilities

National Gang Center (2021). *Comprehensive gang intervention, prevention, and suppression model*. U.S. Department of Justice. https://nationalgangcenter.ojp.gov/spt/Programs/53

National Incident Management System. (2011). *About the National Incident Management System*.

National Incident Management System. (2023). *About the National Incident Management System*. https://www.fema.gov/emergency-managers/nims

National Institute for Clinical Excellence (NICE). (2018). *Posttraumatic stress disorder*. www.nice.org.uk/guidance/ng116

National Institute for Health and Care Excellence. (2005). *Clinical guideline 26: Posttraumatic stress disorder (PTSD): The management of PTSD in adults and children in primary and secondary care*. National Collaborating Centre for Mental Health.

National Institute for Occupational Safety and Health. (1992, October). *Epidemiology of workplace violence*. Centers for Disease Control and Prevention.

National Institute for Occupational Safety and Health. (2002). *Violence: Occupational hazards in hospitals*. Centers for Disease Control and Prevention.

National Institute for Occupational Safety and Health. (2020). *Be attuned to patient behaviors*. Centers for Disease Control and Prevention.

National Institute of Corrections (n.d.) *Module 5: Section 2. The Risk-Need-Responsivity Model for assessment and rehabilitation*. https://info.nicic.gov/tjc/module-5-section-2-risk-need-responsivity-model-assessment-and-rehabilitation

National Institute of Justice. (1998). *Crime in the schools: A problem-solving approach*. Summary of a Presentation by Dennis Kenney, Police Executive Research Forum.

National Institute of Justice. (2015). *Program profile: Bully proofing your school.* https://crimesolutions.ojp.gov/ratedprograms/403

National Institute of Mental Health. (2002). *Mental health and mass violence: Evidence-based early psychological intervention for victims/survivors of mass violence* (NIH Publication No. 02-5138). U.S. Government Printing Office.

National Institute of Mental Health. (2021). *Understanding the characteristics of suicide in young children.* https://www.nimh.nih.gov/news/science-news/2021/understanding-the-characteristics-of-suicide-in-young-children

National Organization for Victim Assistance. (n.d.). *NOVA's mission, purposes, accomplishments, and organizational structure.* www.trynova.org/about-us/overview

National Organization for Victim Assistance. (1997). *Community crisis response team training manual* (2nd ed.).

National Parenting Helpline. (April, 2023). https://www.national-parenthelpline.org/

National Runaway Safeline. (2023). *National Runaway Safeline: Keeping America's runaway, homeless, and at-risk youth safe and off the streets.* www.1800runaway.org

National School Safety and Security Services. (2013). *Schools & terrorism: School terrorism preparedness.* http://www.schoolsecurity.org/terrorist_response.html

National School Safety Center. (1998). *Checklist of characteristics of youth who have caused school-associated violent deaths.*

National Suicide Prevention Lifeline. (2023). www.suicidepreventionlifeline.org

National Terrorism Advisory System. (2023, May). Summary of terrorism-related threat to the United States. *National Terrorism Advisory System Bulletin.* https://www.dhs.gov/ntas/advisory/national-terrorism-advisory-system-bulletin-may-24-2023

Naz, I., Suri, S., & Parveen, S. (2012, October). *Spirituality, self-efficacy and burnout: A study of health professionals.* [Paper presentation]. 2nd Indian Psychological Science Congress. Chandigarh, India.

Negash, S., Carlson, S. H., & Linder, J. N. (2018). Emotionally focused therapy and eye movement desensitization and reprocessing: An integrated treatment to heal the trauma of infidelity. *Couple and Family Psychology: Research and Practice, 7*(3-4), 143–157. https://doi.org/10.1037/cfp0000107

Neil, M., & Barton Wright, P. (2003). Validation therapy for dementia. *Cochrane Library.* https://doi.org/10.1002/14651858.CD001394

Neimeyer, R. A. (1993). Constructivism and the problem of psychotherapy integration. *Journal of Psychotherapy Integration, 3,* 133–137.

Neimeyer, R. A. (1995). *Constructivism in Psychotherapy* (M. J. Mahoney, Ed.; 1st edition). American Psychological Association.

Neimeyer, R. A. (1996). Process intervention in psychotherapy. In H. Rosen & R. T. Kuehlwein (Eds.), *Constructing realities.* Jossey Bass.

Neimeyer, R. A. (2000). Searching for the meaning of meaning: Grief therapy and the process of reconstruction. *Death Studies, 24,* 541–558.

Neimeyer, R. A. (2004). Fostering post traumatic growth. *Psychological Inquiry, 15,* 53–59.

Neimeyer, R. A. (2009). *Constructivist psychology.* Routledge.

Neimeyer, R. A. (2010a). Reconstructing the continuing bond: A constructivist approach to grief therapy. In J. D. Raskin, S. K. Bridges, & R. Neimeyer (Eds.), *Studies in meaning 4: Constructivist perspective on theory, practice, and social justice* (pp. 65–91). Pace University Press.

Neimeyer, R. A. (2010b). Reconstructing life out of loss: Reorganizing the continuing bond. In M. Kerman (Ed.), *Clinical pearls of wisdom: Twenty-one leading therapists offer their key insights* (pp. 104–117). Norton.

Neimeyer, R. A. (2018). *The goal of grief therapy and how it works.* https://www.youtube.com/watch?v=VuAILCclSHA

Neimeyer, R. A. (Ed.). (2001). *Meaning reconstruction and the experience of loss.* American Psychological Association.

Neimeyer, R. A., & Currier, J. M. (2009). Grief therapy: Evidence of efficacy and emerging directions. *Current Directions in Psychological Science, 18*(6), 352–356. https://doi.org/10.1111/j.1467-8721.2009.01666.x

Neimeyer, R. A., & Kosminsky, P. (2014). Bereavement. In L. Grossman & S. Walfish (Eds.), *Translating psychological research into practice* (pp. 132-139). Springer Publishing.

Neimeyer, R. A., & Levitt, H. M. (2000). What's narrative got to do with it? Construction and coherence in accounts of loss. In J. H. Harvey & E. D. Miller (Eds.), *Loss and trauma: General and close relationship perspectives* (pp. 401–413). Brunner-Routledge.

Neimeyer, R. A., & Sands D. C. (2011). Meaning reconstruction in bereavement: From principles to practice. In R. A. Neimeyer, D. L. Harris, H. R. Winokuer, & G. F. Thornton (Eds.), *Grief and bereavement in contemporary society: Bridging research and practice* (pp. 9–22). Routledge. https://doi.org/10.4324/9780203840863

Neimeyer, R. A., & Vaughans, D. C. (2022). *New techniques of grief therapy.* Routledge. https://doi.10.4324/9781351069120-71

Neimeyer, R. A., Burke, L. A., & Mackay, M. M. (2010). Grief therapy and the reconstruction of meaning: From principles to practice. *Journal of Contemporary Psychotherapy, 40,* 73–83. https://doi.org/10.1007/s10879-009-9135-3

Neimeyer, R. A., Holland, J. M., Currier, J. M., & Mehta, T. (2007). Meaning reconstruction in later life: Toward a cognitive-constructivist approach to grief therapy. In D. Gallagher-Thompson, A. M. Steffen, & L. W. Thompson (Eds.), *Handbook of behavioral and cognitive therapies with older adults* (pp. 264–277). Springer.

Nelson, E. R., & Slaikeu, K. A. (1990). Crisis intervention in schools. In K. A. Slaikeu (Ed.), *Crisis intervention: A handbook for research and practice* (2nd ed., pp. 329–347). Allyn & Bacon.

Nelson, G. (2022). Helping students grieve. *ASCA School Counselor, 60*(1), 14–17.

Nelson, R. E., & Galas, J. (1994). *The power to prevent suicide: A guide to helping teens.* Free Spirit.

Nelson, R. J. (2013). Is virtual reality exposure therapy effective for service members and veterans experiencing PTSD? *Traumatology, 19*(3), 171–178.

Nelson, W. M., Finch, A., & Ghee, A. (2006). Anger management with children and adolescents: Cognitive-behavior therapy. In P. C. Kendall (Ed.), *Child and adolescent therapy: Cognitive-behavioral procedures* (3rd ed., pp. 114–165). Guilford Press.

Neubauer, F., Deblinger, E., & Sieger, K. (2007). Trauma-focused cognitive-behavioral therapy for child sexual abuse and exposure to domestic violence: Case of Mary, age 6. In N. B. Webb (Ed.), *Play therapy with children in crisis: Individual, group, and family treatment* (3rd ed., pp. 107–132). Guilford Press.

Newgass, S., & Schonfeld, D. J. (2005). School crisis intervention, crisis prevention, and crisis response. In A. R. Roberts (Ed.), *Crisis intervention handbook* (pp. 499–518). Oxford University Press.

Newhill, C. E. (2003). *Client violence in social work practice: Prevention, intervention, and research*. Guilford Press.

Newman, C. F. (1994). Understanding client resistance: Methods for enhancing motivation to change. *Cognitive and Behavioral Practice, 1*, 47–69.

Newman, C. J. (1976). Children of disaster: Clinical observations at Buffalo Creek. *American Journal of Psychiatry, 133*, 306–312.

Newman, D. A., Horne, A. M., & Bartolomucci, C. L. (2000). *Bully busters: A teacher's manual for helping bullies, victims, and bystanders, grades 6–8*. Research Press.

Newman, K. S. (1993). *Declining fortunes: The withering of the American dream*. Basic Books.

NFL Lifeline. (2023). www.NFLlifeline.org/about/

Ng, A. T. (2006). Mobile crisis teams. In P. M. Gillette & H. L. McQuistion (Eds.), *Clinical guide to the treatment of the mentally ill homeless person* (pp. 73–82). American Psychiatric Publishing.

Nicholas, A., Niederkrotenthaler, T., Reavley, N., Pirkis, J., Jorm, A., & Spittal, M. J. (2020). Belief in suicide prevention myths and its effect on helping: A nationally representative survey of Australian adults. *BMC Psychiatry, 20*(1), 1–12. https://doi.org/10.1186/s12888-020-02715-9

Nichter, B., Holliday, R., Monteith, L. L., Na, P. J., Hill, M. L., Kline, A. C., Norman, S. B., & Pietrzak, R. H. (2022). Military sexual trauma in the United States: Results from a population-based study. *Journal of Affective Disorders, 306*, 19–27. https://doi.org/10.1016/j.jad.2022.03.016

Nichter, M. (2010). Idioms of distress revisited. *Culture, Medicine & Psychiatry, 34*(2), 401–416. https://doi.org/10.1007/s11013-010-9179-6

Nickerson, A., Brock, S., & Reeves, M. (2006). School crisis teams with an incident command system. *California School Psychologist, 11*, 63–72.

Nickerson, R. S. (2011). Roles of human factors and ergonomics in meeting the challenge of terrorism. *American Psychologist, 66*(6), 555–566. https://doi.org/10.1037/a0024474

Nicoletti, J., & Spooner, K. (1996). Violence in the workplace: Response and intervention strategies. In G. R. VandenBos & E. Q. Bulatao (Eds.), *Violence on the job: Identifying risks and developing solutions* (pp. 267–282). American Psychological Association.

Nieburg, H. A., & Fischer, A. (1982). *Pet loss: A thoughtful guide for adults and children*. Harper & Row.

Niederkrotenthaler, T., Voracek, M., Herberth, A., Till, B., Strauss, M., Etzersdorfer, E., & Sonnec, G. (2010). Role of media reports in completed and prevented suicide: Werther v. Papageno effects. *The British Journal of Psychiatry, 197*(3), 234–243.

Nielsen, M. K., Neergaard, M. A., Jensen, A. B., Bro, F., & Guldin, M. B. (2016). Psychological distress, health, and socio-economic factors in caregivers of terminally ill patients: A nationwide population-based cohort study. *Supportive Care in Cancer, 24*, 3057–3067. http://dx.doi.org/10.1007/s00520-016-3120-7

Nijdam-Jones, A., Chen, Y., & Rosenfeld, B. (2020). Detection of feigned posttraumatic stress disorder: A meta-analysis of the Minnesota Multiphasic Personality Inventory-2 (MMPI-2). *Psychological Trauma: Theory, Research, Practice, and Policy, 12*(7), 790–798. https://doi.org/10.1037/tra0000593

Niles, B. L., Klun-Gillis, J., Ryngala, D. J., Silberbogen, A. K., & Paysnick, E. J. (2012). Comparing mindfulness and psychoeducation treatments for combat-related PTSD using a telehealth approach. *Psychological trauma: Theory, research, practice and trauma, 4*(5), 538–547.

Nisbett, R. E. (1993). Violence and U.S. regional culture. *American Psychologist, 48*, 441–449.

Nisivoccia, D., & Lynn, M. (2007). Helping forgotten victims: Using activity groups with children who witness violence. In N. B. Webb (Ed.), *Play therapy with children in crisis: Individual, group, and family treatment* (pp. 294–321). Guilford Press.

Noonan, J. H., & Vavra, M. C. (2007). *Crime in schools and colleges: A study of offenders and arrestees reported via national incident-based reporting system data*. http://www.fbi.gov/about-us/cjis/ucr/nibrs/crime-in-schools-and-colleges-pdf

Noonan, P. (2007, April 21–22). Cold standard. *Wall Street Journal*, p. 16.

Norcross, J. C., Pfund, R. A., & Cook, D. M. (2022). The predicted future of psychotherapy: A decennial e-Delphi Poll. *Professional Psychology: Research and Practice, 53*(2), 109–115. https://doi.org/10.1037/pro0000431

Norcross, J. C., Zimmerman, B., Greenberg, R., & Swift, J. (2017). Do all therapists do that when they say goodbye? A study of commonalities in termination behaviors. *Psychotherapy, 54*(1), 66–75. http://doi.org/10.1037/pst0000097

Norlander, B., & Eckhardt, C. (2005). Anger, hostility, and male perpetrators of intimate partner violence: A meta-analytic review. *Clinical Psychology Review, 25*(2), 119–152. https://doi.org/10.1016/j.cpr.2004.10.001

Norris, F. H. (2006). Disaster research methods: Past progress and future directions. *Journal of Traumatic Stress, 19*(2), 173–184.

Norris, F. H., & Alegria, M. (2006). Promoting disaster recovery in ethnic-minority individuals and communities. In E. C. Ritchie, P. J. Watson, & M. J. Friedman (Eds.), *Interventions following mass violence and disasters: Strategies for mental health practice* (pp. 319–342). Guilford Press.

Norris, F. H., Hamblen, J., Watson, P., Ruzek, J., Gibson, L., & Pfefferbaum, B. (2006). Toward understanding and creating systems of postdisaster care. In E. C. Ritchie, P. J. Watson, & M. J. Friedman (Eds.), *Interventions following mass violence and disasters: Strategies for mental health practice* (pp. 343–364). Guilford Press.

North, C. S. (2004). Approaching disaster mental health research after the 9/11 World Trade Center terrorist attacks. *Psychiatric Clinics of North America, 27*(3), 589–602.

North, C. S. (2010). A tale of two studies of two disasters: Comparing psychosocial responses to disaster among Oklahoma City bombing survivors and Hurricane Katrina evacuees. *Rehabilitation Psychology, 55*(3), 241–246.

Notman, M., & Nadelson, C. (1976). The rape individual: Psychodynamic considerations. *American Journal of Psychiatry, 133*, 408–412.

NOVA. (2015). *Crisis response team training*. http://www.trynova.org/help-crisis-victims/crisis-training/

NOVA. (2016). *Nova's crisis intervention model*. http://www.gocit.org/information/-novas-crisis-intervention-model

NOVA. (2023). *Crisis response team training overview*. https://www.trynova.org/crisis-response-program/overview/

Novella, E. J. (2010). Mental health care in the aftermath of deinstitutionalization: A retrospective and prospective view. *Health Care Analysis, 18*, 222–238. https://doi.org/10.1007/s10728-009-0138-8

Nurius, P. S. (1984). Stress: A pervasive dilemma in psychiatric emergency care. *Comprehensive Psychiatry, 25*, 345–354.

O'Brien, C., Keith, J., & Shoemaker, L. (2015). Don't tell: Military culture and male rape. *Psychological Services, 12*, 357–365. https://doi.org/10.1037/ser0000049

O'Connor, K., Neff, D. M., & Pitman, S. (2018). Burnout in mental health professionals: A systematic review and meta-analysis of prevalence and determinants. *European Psychiatry, 53*, 74–99. https://doi.org/10.1016/j.eurpsy.2018.06.003

O'Connor, M., Nickerson, A., Aderka, I., & Bryant, R. (2015). The temporal relationship between change in symptoms of prolonged grief and posttraumatic stress following old age spousal bereavement. *Depression and Anxiety, 32*(5), 335–340.

O'Donnell, O., House, A., & Waterman, M. (2015). The co-occurrence of aggression and self-harm: Systematic literature review. *Journal of Affective Disorders, 175*, 325–350. https://doi.org/10.1016/j.jad.2014.12.051

O'Donohue, W. T., & Fanetti, M. (Eds.). (2016). *Forensic interviews regarding child sexual abuse: A guide to evidence-based practice*. Springer International Publishing. https://doi.org/10.1007/978-3-319-21097-1

O'Gorman, K., Pilkinton, V., Seidler, Z., Oliffe, J., Peters, W., Bendall, S., & Price, S. (2023). Childhood sexual abuse in boys and men: The case for gender sensitive interventions. *Psychological Trauma: Theory, Research, Practice and Policy*. Advance online publication. https://doi.org/10.1037/tra0001520

O'Leary, E., & Nieuwstraten, I. M. (2001). The exploration of memories in Gestalt reminiscence therapy. *Counseling Psychology Quarterly, 14*(2), 165–180.

O'Reilly, J. T., Hagan, P., & de la Cruz, P. (2001). *Environmental and workplace safety: A guide for university, hospital, and school management*. Wiley.

O'Rourke, M., Wrigley, C., & Hammond, S. (2018). Violence within mental health services: How to enhance risk management. *Risk Management Health Policy, 11*, 159–167. http://doi.org/10.2147/RMHP.S131834

O'Toole, M. E. (2003). *The school shooter: A threat assessment perspective*. Federal Bureau of Investigation.

Ober, C., Peeters, L., Archer, R., & Kelly, K. (2000). Debriefing in different cultural frameworks: Responding to acute trauma in Australian Aboriginal contexts. In B. Raphael & J. P. Wilson (Eds.), *Psychological debriefing: Theory, practice, and evidence* (pp. 241–253). Cambridge University Press.

Obhu, S., Yamashina, A., Takasu, N., Yamaguchi, T., Murai, T., Naknbao, K., Matsui, R., Mikami, R., Sakurai, K., & Hinohora, S. (1997). Sarin poisoning on the Tokyo subway. *Southern Medical Journal, 90*, 587–593.

Occupational Safety and Health Administration. (2003). *Guidelines for preventing workplace violence for healthcare and social service workers*. OSHA 3148. U.S. Department of Labor.

Occupational Safety and Health Administration. (2015). *Guidelines for preventing workplace violence for healthcare and social service workers*. OSHA 3148. U.S. Department of Labor.

Ochberg, F. M. (Ed.). (1988). *Post-traumatic therapy and individuals of violence*. Brunner/Mazel.

Oerlemans, W., & Bakker, A. (2014). Burnout and daily recovery: A day reconstruction study. *Journal of Occupational Health Psychology, 19*(3), 302–314.

Office for Victims of Crime. (2002). *Strengthening anti-stalking statutes* (NCJ Publication No. 189192). U.S. Department of Justice.

Office of Elementary & Secondary Education. (2023a). *Safe and supportive schools*. U.S. Department of Education. https://oese.ed.gov/offices/office-of-formula-grants/safe-supportive-schools

Office of Elementary & Secondary Education. (2023b). *Readiness and Emergency Management for Schools (REMS) Technical Assistance (TA) Center, U.S. Department of Education*. https://rems.ed.gov/

Office of the Surgeon General (2001). *Youth violence: A report of the surgeon general*. National Institute of Mental Health. https://www.ncbi.nlm.nih.gov/books/NBK44293/

Office of Victims of Crime. (2003). *A model for school-based crisis preparedness and response*. https://ovc.ojp.gov/sites/g/files/xyckuh226/files/publications/bulletins/schoolcrisis/pg3.html

Office on Women's Health. (2023). *Caregiver stress*. https://womenshealth.gov

Ogloff, J. R., & Daffern, M. (2006). The dynamic appraisal of situational aggression: An instrument to assess risk for imminent aggression in psychiatric inpatients. *Behavioral Sciences & the Law, 24*, 799–813.

Okuda, M., Olfson, M., Wang, S., Rubio, J. M., Xu, Y., & Blanco, C. (2015). Correlates of intimate partner violence perpetration: Results from a national epidemiologic survey. *Journal of Traumatic Stress, 28*(1), 49–56. https://doi.org/10.1002/jts.21986

Okun, B., & Nowinski, J. (2011). *Saying goodbye: How families can find renewal through loss*. Berkley Books/Penguin Group.

Okun, L. (1986). *Woman abuse: Facts replacing myths*. State University of New York Press.

Olashore, A. A., Akanni, O.O., & Ogundipe, R.M. (2018). Physical violence against health staff by mentally ill patients at a psychiatric hospital in Botswana. *BMC Health Services Research, 18*, 362. https://doi.org/10.1186/s12913-018-3187-6

Olden, M., Mello, B., Cukor, J., Wyka, K., Jayasinghe, N., & Difede, J. (2015). Implementation of evidence-based assessment, treatment, and research programs following the World Trade Center disaster on September 11, 2001. In M. Safir, J. Wallach, & A. Rizzo (Eds.), *Future directions in post-traumatic stress disorder: Prevention, diagnosis, and treatment* (pp. 367–387). Springer Science+Business Media.

Olfson, M., Cosgrove, C. M., Altekruse, S. F., Wall, M. M., & Blanco, C. (2022). Living alone and suicide risk in the United States, 2008–2019. *American Journal of Public Health, 112*(12), 1774–1782. https://doi.org/10.2105/ajph.2022.307080

Oliffe, J. L., Han, C., Sta Maria, E., Lohan, M., Howard, T., Stewart, D. E., & MacMillan, H. (2014). Gay men and intimate partner violence: A gender analysis. *Sociology of Health & Illness, 36*(4), 564–579. https://doi.org/10.1111/1467-9566.12099

Olivares-Faundez, V., Gil-Monte, P., Mena, L., Jelvez -Wilke, C., & Figueiredo-Ferraz, H. (2014). Relationships between burnout and role ambiguity, role conflict and employee absenteeism among health workers. *Terapia Psicologicaa, 32*(2), 111–120.

Olmstead v. United States, 277 U.S. 438 (1928).

Olson, D. H. (2000). Circumplex model of marital and family systems. *Journal of Family Therapy, 22,* 144–167.

Onder, G., Zanetti, O., Giacobini, E., Frisoni, G., Bartorelli, L., Carbone, G., Lamertucci, P. Silveri, M. & Bernabei, R. (2018). Reality orientation therapy combined with cholinesterase inhibitors in Alzheimer's disease: A randomized controlled trial. *The British Journal of Psychiatry, 187*(5), 450–455. http://doi.org/10.1192/bjp.187.5.450

Oosterhoff, B., Kaplow, J. B., & Layne, C. M. (2018). Links between bereavement due to sudden death and academic functioning: Results from a nationally representative sample of adolescents. *School Psychology Quarterly, 33*(3), 372–380. https://doi.org/10.1037/spq0000254

Oras, R., de Ezpeleta, S., & Ahmad, A. (2004). Treatment of traumatized refugee children with Eye Movement Desensitization and Reprocessing in a psychodynamic model. *Nordic Journal of Psychiatry, 58*(3), 199–203.

Orchowski, L. M., Barnett, N. P., Berkowitz, A., Borsari, B., Oesterle, D., & Zlotnick, C. (2018). Sexual assault prevention for heavy drinking college men: Development and feasibility of an integrated approach. *Violence Against Women, 24*(11), 1369–1396. https://doi.org/10.1177/1077801218787928

Orchowski, L. M., Edwards, K. M., Hollander, J. A., Banyard, V. L., Senn, C. Y., & Gidycz, C. A. (2020). Integrating sexual assault resistance, bystander, and men's social norms strategies to prevent sexual violence on college campuses: A call to action. *Trauma, Violence, & Abuse, 21*(4), 811–827. https://doi.org/10.1177/1524838018789153

Organista, K. C., & Munoz, R. F. (1996). Cognitive behavior therapy with Latinos. *Cognitive Behavioral Practice, 3*(2), 255–270.

Ørner, J. R. J., Kent, A., Pfefferbaun, B., Raphael, B., & Watson, P. (2006). The context of providing immediate postevent intervention. In E. C. Ritchie, P. J. Watson, & M. J. Friedman (Eds.), *Interventions following mass violence and disasters: Strategies for mental health practice* (pp. 121–133). Guilford Press.

Oro, P., Esquerda, M., Mas, B., Vinas, J., Yuguero, O., & Pifarre, J. (2021). Effectiveness of a mindfulness-based programme on perceived stress: Psychopathological symptomatology and burnout in medical students. *Mindfulness, 12*(5), 1138–1147. https://doi.org/10.1007/s12671-020-01582-5

Oropeza, B. A., Clark, F., Fitzgibbon, M., & Baron, A. (1991). Managing mental health crises of foreign college students. *Journal of Counseling and Development, 69*, 280–283.

Osborn, C. L. (1991). Reminiscence: When the past eases the present. *Journal of Gerontological Nursing, 15*, 6–11.

Osher, D., Poirier, J., Jarjoura, G., Brown, R., & Kendziora, K. (2014). Avoid simple solutions and quick fixes: Lessons learned from a comprehensive district wide approach to improving student behavior and school safety. *Journal of Applied Research on Children, 5*(2). https://files.eric.ed.gov/fulltext/EJ1188500.pdf

Oshodi, Y., Macharia, M., Lachman, A., & Seedat, S. (2020). Immediate and long-term mental health outcomes in adolescent female rape survivors. *Journal of Interpersonal Violence, 35*(1–2), 252–267. https://doi.org/10.1177/0886260516682522

Osofsky, J. D. (1995). The effects of exposure to violence on young children. *American Psychologist, 50*(9), 781–788.

Osterweis, M., Solomon, F., & Green, M. (Eds.). (1984). *Bereavement: Reactions, consequences, and care.* National Academy Press.

Otgaar, H., Howe, M. L., Dodier, O., Lilienfeld, S. O., Loftus, E. F., Lynn, S. J., Merckelbach, H., & Patihis, L. (2021). Belief in unconscious repressed memory persists. *Perspectives on Psychological Science, 16*(2), 454–460. https://doi.org/10.1177/1745691621990628

Ott, C. H., Sanders, S., & Kelber, S. T. (2007). Grief and personal growth experience of spouses and adult-child caregivers of individuals with Alzheimer's disease and related dementias. *Gerontologist, 47*(6), 798–809.

Ouimette, P., & Read, J. P. (2014). *Trauma and substance abuse: Causes, consequences, and treatment of comorbid disorders.* American Psychological Association.

Outlaw, F. H., & Lowery, B. J. (1992). Seclusion: The nursing challenge. *Journal of Psychosocial Nursing, 30*, 13–17.

Ovenstad, K. S., Ormhaug, S. M., Shirk, S. R., & Jensen, T. K. (2020). Therapists' behaviors and youths' therapeutic alliance during trauma-focused cognitive behavioral therapy. *Journal of Consulting and Clinical Psychology, 88*(4), 350–361. https://doi.org/10.1037/ccp0000465

Owens, K. A., Haddock, G., & Berry, K. (2013). The role of the therapeutic alliance in the regulation of emotion in psychosis: An attachment perspective. *Clinical Psychology & Psychotherapy, 20*(6), 523–530. https://doi.org/10.1002/cpp.1793

Oyserman, D., Coon, H. M., & Kemmelmeier, M. (2002). Rethinking individualism and collectivism: Evaluation of theoretical assumptions and meta-analyses. *Psychological Bulletin, 128*(1), 3–72. https://doi.org/10.1037/0033-2909.128.1.3

Pachankis, J. E., Clark, K., Jackson, S., Pereira, K., & Levine, D. (2021). Current capacity and human implementation of mental health services in U.S. LGBTQ community centers. *Psychiatric Services, 72*(6), 669–676. https://doi.org/10.1176/appi.ps.202000575

Packman, W., Andalibian, H., Eudy, K., Howard, B., & Bongar, B. (2009). Legal and ethical risk management with behavioral agencies. In P. M. Kleespies (ed.). *Behavioral emergencies: An evidence-based resource for evaluating and managing risk of suicide, violence, and victimization* (pp. 405–430). American Psychological Association.

Padach, K. M. (1984). Long-term telephone counseling. In F. W. Kaslow (Ed.), *Counseling with psychotherapists* (pp. 173–190). Haworth Press.

Padmanathan, P., Biddle, L., Carroll, R., Derges, J., Potokar, J., & Gunnell, D. (2018). Suicide and self-harm related internet use: A cross sectional study and clinician focus groups. *Crisis: The Journal of Crisis Intervention and Suicide Prevention, 39*(6), 469–476. https://doi.org/10.1027/0227-5910/a000522

Page, J. M., Daniels, J., & Craig, S. (2015). *Violence in schools.* Springer International Publishing.

Pagelow, M. D. (1981). *Woman battering: Victims and their experiences.* SAGE.

Paine, W. S. (1982). Overview of burnout stress syndromes and the 1980s. In W. S. Paine (Ed.), *Job stress and burnout* (pp. 11–25). SAGE.

Palgi, Y., Shrira, A., & Shmotkin, D. (2015). Aging with trauma across the lifetime and experiencing trauma in old age: Vulnerability and resilience intertwined. In K. Cherry (Ed.), *Traumatic Stress and Long-Term Recovery* (pp. 293–308). Springer. https://doi.org/10.1007/978-3-319-18866-9_16

Palmstierna, T., & Wistedt, B. (1990). Risk factors for aggressive behaviour are of limited value in predicting the violent behaviour of acute involuntarily admitted patients. *Acta Psychiatrica Scandinavica, 81*, 152–155.

Pargament, K. I. (2007). *Spiritually integrated psychotherapy: Understanding and addressing the sacred.* Guilford Press.

Pargament, K. I., & Sweeney, P. J. (2011). Building spiritual fitness in the Army. *American Psychologist, 66*(1), 58–64.

Parikh, M. R., O'Dell, S. M., Cook, L. A., Corlis, M., Sun, H., & Gass, M. (2021). Integrated care is associated with increased behavioral health access and utilization for youth in crisis. *Families,*

Systems, & Health, 39(3), 426–433. https://doi.org/10.1037/fsh0000620

Paris, J. (2008). Treatment of borderline personality disorder: A guide to evidence-based practice. Guilford Press.

Paris, J. (2018). Differential diagnosis of borderline personality disorder. Psychiatric Clinics of North America 41(4), 575–582. http://doi.org/10.1016/j.psc.2018.07.001

Park, C. L., Sacco, S. J., & Mills, M. A. (2019). Do religious habits and coping help in the immediate aftermath of a crisis? Relations with Hurricane Katrina evacuees' acute stress symptoms and functional impairment. Psychological Trauma: Theory, Research, Practice, and Policy, 11(6), 563–570. https://doi.org/10.1037/tra0000426

Park, C., Park, S., Gwak, A., Sohn, B., Lee, J., Jung, H., Choi, S., Kim, D., & Choi, J. (2015). The effect of repeated exposure to virtual gambling cues on the urge to gamble. Addictive Behaviors, 41(1), 61–64.

Parker, B., McFarlane, J., Soeken, K., Torres, T., & Campbell, D. (1993). Physical and emotional abuse in pregnancy: A comparison of adult and teenage women. Nursing Research, 42, 173–177.

Parker, C., Barnett, D., Everly, G., & Links, J. (2006). Establishing evidence-informed core intervention competencies in Psychological First Aid for public health personnel. International Journal of Emergency Mental Health, 8(2), 83–92.

Parker, J. G., & Gottman, H. J. M. (1989). Social and emotional development in a relational context. In T. J. Berndt & G. W. Ladd (Eds.), Peer relationships in child development (pp. 95–131). Wiley.

Parkes, C., & Prigerson, H. A. (2010). Bereavement: Studies of grief in adult life (4th ed.). Routledge/Taylor-Francis Group.

Parra-Uribe, I., Blasco-Fontecilla, H., Garcia-Parés, G., Martínez-Naval, L., Valero-Coppin, O., Cebrià-Meca, A., Oquendo, M. A., & Palao-Vidal, D. (2017). Risk of re-attempts and suicide death after a suicide attempt: A survival analysis. BMC Psychiatry, 17(1), 163. https://doi.org/10.1186/s12888-017-1317-z

Parrott, B. (2020). The American mega-crisis: COVID-19 and beyond. Challenge, 63(5). https://doi.org/10.1080/05775132.2020.1804756

Parsons, S. (2011). Long term impact of childhood bereavement: Preliminary analysis of the 1970 British cohort study. Childhood Welfare Research Center. https://www.gov.uk/government/publications/long-term-impact-of-childhood-bereavement-preliminary-analysis-of-the-1970-british-cohort-study-bcs70

Pastel, B. H., & Ritchie, E. C. (2006). Mitigation of psychological weapons of mass destruction. In E. C. Ritchie, P. J. Watson, & M. J. Friedman (Eds.), Interventions following mass violence and disasters: Strategies for mental health practice (pp. 300–318). Guilford Press.

Paterson, J. (2010). Bullies with byte. Counseling Today, 53(12), 44–47.

Paterson, J. (2011). Young and depressed. Counseling Today, 54(1), 32–35.

Path, Ä. M. (2002). Surviving stalking. Cambridge University Press.

Patihis, L., Ho, L. Y., Tingen, I. W., Lilienfeld, S. O., & Loftus, E. F. (2014). Are the "memory wars" over? A scientist-practitioner gap in beliefs about repressed memory. Psychological Science, 25(2), 519–530. https://doi.org/10.1177/0956797613510718

Patros, P. G., & Shamoo, T. K. (1989). Depression and suicide in children and adolescents: Prevention, intervention, and postvention. Allyn & Bacon.

Patterson, C. H. (1980). Theories of counseling and psychotherapy (3rd ed.). Harper & Row.

Patterson, J. (2002). Integrating family resilience and family stress theory. Journal of Marriage and Family, 64, 349–360.

Patterson, W. M., Dohn, H. H., Bird, J., & Patterson, G. A. (1983). Evaluation of suicidal patients: The SAD PERSONS scale. Psychosomatics: Journal of Consultation and Liaison Psychiatry, 24(4), 343–349. https://doi.org/10.1016/S0033-3182(83)73213-5

Patterson, Z. R., Gabrys, R. L., Prowse, R. K., Abizaid, A. B., Hellemans, K. G. C., & McQuaid, R. J. (2021). The influence of COVID-19 on stress, substance use, and mental health among postsecondary students. Emerging Adulthood, 9(5), 516–530. https://doi.org/10.1177/21676968211014080

Paunovic, N. (2002). Prolonged exposure counterconditioning (PEC) as a treatment for chronic posttraumatic stress disorder and major depression in an adult survivor of repeated child sexual and physical abuse. Clinical Case Studies, 1(2), 148–169.

Paunovic, N. (2003). Prolonged exposure counterconditioning as a treatment for chronic posttraumatic stress disorder. Journal of Anxiety Disorders, 17(5), 479–499.

Paunovic, N., & Ost, L. (2001). Cognitive-behavior therapy vs. exposure therapy in the treatment of PTSD in refugees. Behavior Research & Therapy, 39(10), 1183–1197.

Payne, J. S., Galvan, F. H., Williams, J. K., Prusinski, M., Zhang, M., Wyatt, G. E., & Myers, H. F. (2014). Impact of childhood sexual abuse on the emotions and behaviours of adult men from three ethnic groups in the USA. Culture, Health & Sexuality, 16(3), 231–245. https://doi.org/10.1080/13691058.2013.867074

Pazar, J. (2005). A reliability study of the triage assessment scale. Unpublished doctoral dissertation. University of Memphis.

Pearlman, L. A., & Mac Ian, P. S. (1995). Vicarious traumatization: An empirical study of the effects of trauma work on trauma therapists. Professional Psychology, 26(6), 558–565.

Pearlman, L. A., & Saakvitne, K. W. (1995). Trauma and the therapist: Countertransference and vicarious traumatization in psychotherapy with incest survivors. (pp. xix, 451). W. W. Norton & Company.

Pearlman, L. A., & Saakvitne, K. W. (1995a). Treating therapists with vicarious traumatization and secondary traumatic stress disorders. In C. R. Figley (Ed.), Compassion fatigue: Coping with secondary traumatic stress disorder in those who treat the traumatized (pp. 150–177). Brunner-Mazel.

Pearlman, M. Y., Schwalbe, K. D., & Cloitre, M. (2010). Grief in childhood: Fundamentals of treatment in clinical practice. American Psychological Association.

Pearsons, L. (1965). The use of written communications in psychotherapy. Charles C Thomas.

Pedersen, P. (Ed.). (1999). Multiculturalism as a fourth force. Brunner/Mazel.

Pedersen, P. B., & Marsella, A. (1982). The ethical crisis for cross-cultural counseling and therapy. Professional Psychology, 13, 492–500.

Peitzmeier, S. M., Malik, M., Kattari, S. K., Marrow, E., Stephenson, R., Agénor, M., & Reisner, S. L. (2020). Intimate partner violence in transgender populations: Systematic review and meta-analysis of prevalence and correlates. American Journal of Public Health, 110(9), e1–e14. https://doi.org/10.2105/AJPH.2020.305774

Pellerin, C. (2017, April 28). Service experts discuss progress in recognizing, treating PTSD and TBI. Department of Defense News.

Pence, E. L., & McDonnell, C. (2000). Developing policies and pro-tocols in Duluth, Minnesota. In J. Hanmer & C. Itzin (Eds.), *Home truths about domestic violence: Feminist influences on policy and practice: A reader* (pp. 249–268). Routledge.

Pence, E. L., & Shepard, M. F. (1999). An introduction: Develop-ing a coordinated community response. In M. F. Shepard & E. L. Pence (Eds.), *Coordinating community response to domestic violence: Lessons from Duluth and beyond* (pp. 3–24). SAGE.

Pender, D. A., & Prichard, K. K. (2008). Group process research and emergence of therapeutic factors in critical incident stress debriefing. *International Journal of Emergency Mental Health, 10*, 39–48.

Pender, D. A., & Prichard, K. K. (2009). AGSW best practices guide-lines as a research tool: A comprehensive examination of criti-cal incident stress debriefing. *Journal of Specialists in Group Work, 34*(2), 175–192.

Pengpid, S., & Peltzer, K. (2014). Sexual assault and other type of intimate partner violence in women with protection orders in Vhembe district, South Africa. *Violence and Victims 29*(5), 857–871.

Pennebaker, J. W., & Harber, K. D. (1993). A social stage model of collective coping: The Loma Prieta earthquake and the Per-sian Gulf War. *Journal of Social Issues, 49*, 125–146.

Pereira-Morales, A. J., Adan, A., Camargo, A., & Forero, D. A. (2017). Substance use and suicide risk in a sample of young Colombian adults: An exploration of psychosocial factors. *American Journal on Addictions, 26*(4), 388–394.

Perez, Z., & Erwin, B. (2020). A turning point: School resource officers and state policy. *ED Note: Education Commission of the States.* https://ednote.ecs.org/a-turning-point-school-resource-officers-and-state-policy/

Pérez-Sales, P., Vergara-Campos, M., Eiroa-Orosa, F. J., Olivos-Jara, P., Fernández-Liria, A., Barbero-Val, E., & Galán-Santama-rina, A. (2022). Perceived resistance to experiences of trauma and crisis: A study comparing multiple life events. *Traumatol-ogy, 28*(1), 109–119. https://doi.org/10.1037/trm0000339

Perilla, J., Norris, F., & Lavizzo, E. (2002). Ethnicity, culture, and disaster response: Identifying and explaining ethnic differ-ences in PTSD six months after Hurricane Andrew. *Journal of Social and Clinical Psychology, 21*, 28–45.

Perilloux, C., Duntley, J. D., & Buss, D. M. (2012). The costs of rape. *Archives of Sexual Behavior, 41*(5), 1099–1106. https://doi.org/10.1007/s10508-011-9863-9

Perloe, A., & Pollard, J. (2016). University counseling centers' role in campus threat assessment and management. *Journal of Threat Assessment and Management, 3*(1). https://doi.org/10.1037/tam0000051

Perrone, F., Player, D., & Youngs, P. (2019). Administrative cli-mate, early career teacher burnout, and turnover. *Journal of School Leadership, 29*(3), 191–209. https://doi.org/10.1177/1052684619836823

Perrou, B. (2019). *Suicide by cop: Fifteen warning signs that you might be involved.* Caliber Press. https://mpitraining.com/wp-content/uploads/Suicide-by-cop

Perry, N. S., Goetz, D. B., & Shea, M. T. (2021). Longitudinal associations of PTSD and social support by support func-tions among returning veterans. *Psychological Trauma: Theory, Research, Practice, and Policy.* Advance online publication. https://doi.org/10.1037/tra0001190

Perski, O., Grossi, G., Perski, A., & Niemi, M. (2017). A systematic review and meta-analysis of tertiary interventions in clinical

burnout. *Scandinavian Journal of Psychology, 58*, 551561. https://doi.org/10.1111/sjop.12398

Peterman, A., Pereira, A., Bleck, J., Palermo, T. M., & Yount, K. M. (2017). Women's individual asset ownership and experience of intimate partner violence: Evidence from 28 international surveys. *American Journal of Public Health, 107*(5), 747–755. https://doi.org/10.2105/AJPH.2017.303694

Peters, W., Rice, S., Cohen, J., Murray, L., Schley, C., Alvarez-Jimenez, M., & Bendall, S. (2021). Trauma-focused cognitive-behavioral therapy (TF-CBT) for interpersonal trauma in transitional-aged youth. *Psychological Trauma: Theory, Research, Practice, and Policy, 13*(3), 313–321. https://doi.org/10.1037/tra0001016

Petersen, J. V. (2008). The role of the Chandler Police Department resource officers as law-related educational leaders. *Disserta-tion Abstracts International, 69*(6-A), 2078.

Petersen, S. (1999, April). *School crisis planning.* Workshop at the American Counseling Association World Conference, San Diego, CA, the United States.

Petersen, S., & Straub, R. L. (1992). *School crisis survival guide: Man-agement techniques and materials for counselors and administrators.* Center for Applied Research in Education.

Peterson, C., DeGue, S., Florence, C., & Lokey, C. N. (2017). Life-time economic burden of rape among U.S. adults. *Ameri-can Journal of Preventive Medicine, 52*(6), 691–701. https://doi.org/10.1016/j.amepre.2016.11.014

Peterson, C., Park, N., & Castro, C. A. (2011). Assessment for the U.S. Army Comprehensive Soldier Fitness program: The Global Assessment Tool. *American Psychologist, 66*(1), 10–18.

Peterson, G. W., Hennon, C. B., & Knox, T. (2010). Conceptualizing parental stress with family stress theory. In S. J. Price, C. A. Price, & P. C. McKenny (Eds.). *Families and change: Coping with stressful events and transitions* (pp. 25–50). SAGE.

Petersson, J., & Strand, S. J. M. (2020). Family only perpetrators of intimate partner violence: A systematic review. *Trauma, Violence, & Abuse, 21*(2), 367–381. https://doi.org/10.1177/1524838018770410

Petrie, W. M. (1984). Violence: The geriatric patient. In J. T. Turner (Ed.), *Violence in the medical care setting: A survival guide* (pp. 107–122). Aspen Systems.

Pew Research Center. (2022). *Older teen girls more likely than younger girls or boys of any age to have faced false rumor spreading, constant monitoring online, as well as cyberbullying overall.* https://www.pewresearch.org/internet/2022/12/15/teens-and-cyberbullying-2022/pi_2022-12-13_teens-cyberbullying_0-02a/

Pfeffer, C. R. (2006). Suicide and suicidality. In M. K. Dulcan & J. M. Wiener (Eds.), *Essentials of child and adolescent psychiatry* (pp. 621–632). American Psychiatric Publishing.

Pfefferbaum, B. (2021). Challenges for child mental health raised by school closure and home confinement during the COVID-19 pandemic. *Current Psychiatry Rep, 23*, 65. https://doi.org/10.1007/s11920-021-01279-z

Pfefferbaum, B., & North, C. S. (2020). Mental health and the Covid-19 pandemic. *The New England Journal of Medicine, 383*(6), 510–512. https://doi.org/10.1056/NEJMp2008017

Pfefferbaum, B., Flynn, B. W., Schonfeld, D,. Brown, L. M., Jacobs, G. A., Dodgen, D., Donato, D., Kaul, R. E., Stone, B., Norwood, A. E., Reissman, D. B., Herrmann, J., Hobfoll, S., Jones, R. T., Ruzek, J. I., Ursano, R. J., Taylor, R. J., & Lindley, D. (2012). The integration of mental and behavioral health into disas-ter preparedness, response, and recovery. *Disaster Medicine and*

Public Health Preparedness, 6(1), 60–66. http://doi.org/10.1001/dmp.2012.1

Pfefferbaum, B., Houston, B., Reyes, G., Steinberg, A. M., Pynoos, R, S., Fairbank, J. A., Brymer, M. J., & Maida, C. A. (2010). Building national capacity for child and family disaster mental health research. *Professional Psychology Research and Practice, 41*(1), 26–33. https://doi.org/10.1037/a0017056

Pfefferbaum, B., Nitiéma, P., Newman, E., & Patel, A. (2019). The benefit of interventions to reduce posttraumatic stress in youth exposed to mass trauma: A review and meta-analysis. *Prehospital and Disaster Medicine, 34*(5), 540–551. https://doi.org/10.1017/S1049023X19004771

Phillips, B., & Jenkins, P. (2010). The roles of faith-based organizations after Hurricane Katrina. In R. P. Kilmer, V. Gil-Rivas, R. G. Tedeschi, & L. G. Calhoun (Eds.). *Helping families and communities recover for disaster* (pp. 215–238). American Psychological Association.

Phillips, J. A., & Luth, E. A. (2020). Beliefs about suicide acceptability in the United States: How do they affect suicide mortality? *Journals of Gerontology Series B: Psychological Sciences & Social Sciences, 75*(2), 414–425. https://doi.org/10.1093/geronb/gbx153

Phillips, L. (2019). Learning to love (or at least leverage) technology. *Counseling Today, 61*(12), 21–28.

Phipps, A., Byrne, M., & Deane, F. (2007). Can volunteer counselors help prevent psychological trauma? A preliminary communication on volunteers' skill using the "Orienting Approach" to trauma counseling. *Stress and Health: Journal of the International Society of the Investigation of Stress, 23*(1), 15–21.

Phipps, S. (2011). Positive psychology and war: An oxymoron. *American Psychologist, 66,* 641–642.

Piedmont, R. L. (1993). A longitudinal analysis of burnout in the health care setting: The role of personal dispositions. *Journal of Personality Assessment, 61,* 457–473.

Pierce, G. R., Sarason, B. R., & Sarason, I. G. (Eds.). (1996). *Handbook of social support and the family.* Plenum Press.

Piercy, D. (1984). Violence: The drug and alcohol patient. In J. T. Turner (Ed.), *Violence in the medical care setting: A survival guide* (pp. 123–152). Aspen Systems.

Pinciotti, C. M. (2023). Adapting and integrating exposure therapies for obsessive–compulsive disorder and posttraumatic stress disorder: Translating research into clinical implementation. *Clinical Psychology: Science and Practice.* Advance online publication. https://doi.org/10.1037/cps0000143

Pine, V. R. (1996). Social psychological aspects of disaster death. In K. J. Doka (Ed.), *Living with grief after sudden loss: Suicide, homicide, accident, heart attack, stroke* (pp. 103–116). Hospice Foundation of America.

Pines, A. (1983). On burnout and the buffering effects of social support. In B. A. Farber (Ed.), *Stress and burnout in the human service professions* (pp. 155–173). Pergamon Press.

Pines, A., & Aronson, E. (1988). *Career burnout: Causes and cures.* Free Press.

Pingley, T. (2017). *The impact of witnessing domestic violence on children: A systematic review.* St. Catherine University. https://sophia.stkate.edu/ msw_papers/776

Pinkhasov, A., Hallo, C., Avishi, A., Akerman, M., & Brand, D. (2020). Towards prevention of behavioral emergencies in a general hospital insights from a one year series. *General Hospital Psychiatry, 66,* 54–58. https://doi.org/10.1016/j.genhosppsych.2020.06.008

Pinto e Silva, T., Cunha, O., & Caridade, S. (2022). Motivational interview techniques and the effectiveness of intervention programs with perpetrators of intimate partner violence: A systematic review. *Trauma, Violence, & Abuse, 24*(4), 2691–2710. https://doi.org/10.1177/15248380221111472

Piper, W. E., Ogrodniczuk, J. S., Joyce, S. S., & Weideman, R. (2011). Risk factors for complicated grief. In W. E. Piper, J. S. Ogrodniczuk, S. S. Joyce, & R. Weideman (Eds.), *Short-term group therapies for complicated grief: Two research-based models* (pp. 193–202). American Psychological Association.

Pirkis, J., Currier, D., Too, L. S., Bryant, M., Bartlett, S., Sinyor, M., & Spittal, M. J. (2020). Calls to helplines in Australia following media reports of Robin Williams' suicide. *Suicide and Life-Threatening Behavior, 50*(6), 1115–1120. https://doi.org/10.1111/sltb.12661

Pisarick, G. (1981, September). The violent patient. *Nursing,* pp. 63–65.

Pitcher, G. D., & Poland, S. (1992). *Crisis intervention in the schools.* Guilford Press.

Pittman, F. S. (1987). *Turning points: Treating families in transition and crisis.* W. W. Norton and Company.

Pizarro, J., Silver, R. C., & Prause, J. (2006). Physical and mental health costs of traumatic war experiences among Civil War veterans. *Archives of General Psychiatry, 63*(2), 193–200.

Pizzetti, P., & Manfredini, M. (2008). "The shock of widowhood": Evidence from an Italian population (Parma 1989–2000). *Social Indictors Research, 85*(3), 499–513.

Pizzey, E. (1974). *Scream quietly or the neighbors will hear.* Penguin Books.

Planchon, L. A., Templer, D. I., Stokes, S., & Keller, J. (2002). Death of a companion cat or dog and human bereavement. *Society & Animals, 10*(3), 327.

Pleck, E. (1987). *The making of societal policy against family violence from colonial times to the present.* Oxford University Press.

Pledge, D. S. (2003). *When something feels wrong: A survival guide about abuse.* Free Spirit.

Pledge, D. S., Lapan, R., Heppner, P., Kivlighan, D., & Roehlke, H. (1998). Stability and severity of presenting problems at a university counseling center: A 6-year analysis. *Professional Psychology: Research and Practice, 29*(4), 386–389.

Plouffe, R. A., Wilson, C. A., & Saklofske, D. H. (2022). The role of dark personality traits in intimate partner violence: A multi-study investigation. *Current Psychology, 41*(6), 3481–3500. https://doi.org/10.1007/s12144-020-00871-5

Plough, A., Fielding, J., Chandra, A., Williams, M., Eisenman, D., Wells, K ., Law, G., Fogleman, S., & Magana, A. (2013). Building community disaster resilience: Perspectives from a large urban county department of public health. *American Journal of Public Health, 103*(7), 1190–1197.

Poijula, S., Dyregrov, A., Wahleberg, K., & Jokelainen, J. (2001). Reactions to adolescent suicide and crisis intervention in three secondary schools. *International Journal of Emergency Mental Health, 3*(2), 97–106.

Poland, S. (1989). *Suicide intervention in the schools.* Guilford Press.

Poland, S. (1994). The role of school crisis intervention team to prevent and reduce school violence and trauma. *School Psychology Review, 239*(2), 175–189.

Poland, S. (1999). *School crisis & youth violence: Lessons learned.* Cypress-Fairbanks Independent School District, Department of Psychological Services.

Poland, S. (2004). School crisis teams. In J. Conoley & A. P. Goldstein (Eds.), *School violence intervention: A practical handbook* (2nd ed., pp. 131–163). Guilford Press.

Poland, S., & McCormick, J. S. (1999). *Coping with crisis: Lessons learned*. Sophris West.

Poliak, O., Cheek, S., Rudolph, P., Hastings, P., Nock, M., & Prinstein, M. (2023). Social problem solving and suicidal behavior in adolescent girls: A prospective examination of proximal and distal stress-related factors. *Oliak, 5*, 610–620. https://doi.org/10.1037/abn0000836

Poliks, O. (1999, April). *The noble victim: Survival, self-care and spirituality*. Paper presented at the Twenty-Third Annual Convening of Crisis Intervention Personnel, Chicago, IL, the United States.

Polster, E., & Polster, M. (1973). *Gestalt therapy integrated*. Brunner/Mazel.

Polusny, M. A., Ries, B. J., Meis, L. A., DeGarmo, D., McCormick-Deaton, C. M., Thuras, P., & Erbes, C. R. (2011). Effects of parents' experiential avoidance and PTSD on adolescent disaster-related posttraumatic stress symptomatology. *Journal of Family Psychology, 25*, 220–229.

Ponterotto, J. G., Utsey, S. O., & Pedersen, P. (2006). *Preventing prejudice: A guide for counselors, educators, and parents* (2nd ed) SAGE Publications.

Pope, K. S. & Vasquez, M. J. T. (2016). *Ethics in counseling and psychotherapy: A practical guide* (5th ed.). John Wiley & Sons, Inc.

Pope, R. (2015). *Crisis counseling of the walk-in* (Videotape Recording No. 6731-2015D). Memphis, TN: Memphis State University, Department of Counseling and Personnel Services.

Popova, N. K., Tsybko, A. S., & Naumenko, V. S. (2022). The implication of 5-HT receptor family members in aggression, depression and suicide: Similarity and difference. *International Journal of Molecular Sciences, 23*(15), 8814–8814. https://doi.org/10.3390/ijms23158814

Portnoy, G. A., Colon, R., Gross, G. M., Adams, L. J., Bastian, L. A., & Iverson, K. M. (2020). Patient and provider barriers, facilitators, and implementation preferences of intimate partner violence perpetration screening. *BMC Health Services Research, 20*(1), 746. https://doi.org/10.1186/s12913-020-05595-7

Posner, K., Brown, G. K., Stanley, B., Brent, D. A., Yershova, K. V., Oquendo, M. A., Currier, G. W., Melvin, G. A., Greenhill, L., Shen, S., & Mann, J. J. (2011). The Columbia–Suicide Severity Rating Scale: Initial validity and internal consistency findings from three multisite studies with adolescents and adults. *American Journal of Psychiatry, 168*(12), 1266–1277. https://doi.org/10.1176/appi.ajp.2011.10111704

Postrel, V. (1998). *The future and its enemies: The growing conflict over creativity, enterprise, and progress*. Free Press.

Potter, S., Howard, R., Murphy, S., & Moynihan, M. M. (2018). Long-term impacts of college sexual assaults on women survivors' educational and career attainments. *Journal of American College Health, 66*(6), 496–507. https://doi.org/10.1080/07448481.2018.1440574

Poursadeghiyan, M., Abbasi, M., Mehri, A., Hami, M., Raei, M., & Ebrahimi, M. H. (2016). Relationship between job stress and anxiety, depression and job satisfaction in nurses in Iran. *The Social Sciences, 11*(9), 2349–2355

Powell, W. E. (1994). The relationship between feelings of alienation and burnout in social work. *Families in Society, 75*, 229–235.

Powers, R., & Griffith, J. (1987). *Understanding life-style: The psychoclarity process*. American Institute of Adlerian Studies.

Pratt-Eriksson, D., Bergbom, I., & Lyckhage, E. D. (2014). Don't ask don't tell: Battered women living in Sweden encounter with healthcare personnel and their experience of the care given. *International Journal of Qualitative Studies on Health and Well-Being, 9*(1), 23166. https://doi.org/10.3402/qhw.v9.23166

Preziosa, A., Grassi, A., Gaggioli, A., & Riva, G. (2009). Therapeutic applications of the mobile phone. *British Journal of Guidance & Counselling, 37*(3), 313–325.

Price, C. A., Bush, K. R., Price, S. J., & McKenry, P. C. (2021). Families coping with change: A conceptual overview. In K. R. Bush & C. A. Price (Eds.), *Families and change: Coping with stressful events and transitions* (6th ed., pp. 3–24).

Price, J. L. (2011). Findings from the National Vietnam Veterans' Readjustment Study. *United States Department of Veterans Affairs*. https://www.research.va.gov/topics/vietnam.cfm

Price, M. (2007). TV violence harms children, APA member testifies to Congress. *Monitor on Psychology, 38*(8), 16.

Price, M. (2010). Suicide among preadolescents. *Monitor on Psychology, 41*(9), 52–53.

Price, M., Legrand, A., Brier, Z., van Stolk-Cooke, K., Peck, K., Dodds, P., Danforth, C., & Adams, Z. (2022). Doomscrolling during COVID-19: The negative association between daily social and traditional media consumption and mental health symptoms during the COVID-19 pandemic. *Psychological Trauma: Theory, Research, Practice, and Policy, 14*(8), 1336–1346. https://doi.org/10.1037/tra0001202

Price, R. H., Friedland, D. S., & Vinokur, A. D. (1998). Job loss: Hard times and eroded identity. In J. H. Harvey (Ed.), *Perspective on loss: A sourcebook* (pp. 303–316). Brunner/Mazel.

Price, S. J., Price, C. A., & McKenry, P. C. (2010). Families coping with change. In S. J. Price, C. A. Price, & P. C. McKenny (Eds.). *Families and change: Coping with stressful events and transitions* (pp. 1–24). SAGE.

Prigerson, H. G., & Jacobs, S. (2001). Traumatic grief as a distinct disorder: A rationale, consensus criteria, and a preliminary empirical test. In M. S. Stroebe, R. O. Hansson, & H. Schut (Eds.), *Handbook of bereavement research and practice: Consequences, coping, and caring* (pp. 613–641). American Psychological Association.

Prigerson, H. G., Maciewjewski, P. K., Reynolds, C. F., Bierhals, A. J., Newsom, J. T., & Fasiczka, A. (1995). Inventory of Complicated Grief: A scale to measure maladaptive symptoms of loss. *Psychiatry Research, 59*(1/2), 65–79.

Prigerson, H. G., Vanderwerker, L. C., & Maciejewski, P. K. (2008). A case for inclusion of prolonged grief disorder in DSM-V. In M. S. Stroebe, R. O. Hansson, H. Schut, & W. Stroebe (Eds.), *Handbook of bereavement research and practice: Advances in theory and intervention* (pp. 165–186). American Psychological Association.

Prison Policy Initiative. (2022). *Mental health*. https://www.prisonpolicy.org/research/mental_health/

Prochaska, J. O., DiClemente, C. C., & Norcross, J. C. (1992). In search of how people change: Applications to addictive behaviors. *American Psychologist, 47*, 1102–1114.

Prochuk, A. (2018). *We are here: Women's experiences of the barriers to reporting sexual assault*. West Coast LEAF. http://tld-documents.llnassets.com.s3.amazonaws.com/0008000/8350/west-coast-leaf-dismantling-web-final.pdf

Progoff, I. (1975). *At a journal workshop*. Dialogue House Library.

Pronk, R., Willems, D. L., & van de Vathorst, S. (2021). Do doctors differentiate between suicide and physician-assisted death? A qualitative study into the views of psychiatrists and general practitioners. *Culture, Medicine and Psychiatry, 45*(2), 268–281. https://doi.org/10.1007/s11013-020-09686-2

Prothrow-Stith, D. (1987). *Violence prevention curriculum for adolescents.* Education Development Center

Prudenzi, A., Graham, C., Clancy, F., Hill, D., O'Driscoll, R., Day, F. & O'Connor, D. (2021) Group based acceptance and commitment therapy interventions for improving general distress and work related distress in health care professionals: A systematic review and meta-analysis. *Journal of Affective Disorders, 295*(4), 192–202. https://doi.org/10.1016/j.jad.2021.07.084

Puiu, T. (2022). Nursing home violence among patients is a problem of neglect, not mental illness. *ZME Science.* https://www.zmescience.com/science/nursing-home-violence

Purves, B. A., Phinney, A., Hulko, W., Puurveen, G., & Astell, A. (2015). Developing CIRCA-BC and exploring the role of the computer as a third participant in conversation. *American Journal of Alzheimer's Disease and Other Dementias. 30(1),* 101–107.

Pynoos, R. S., & Eth, S. (1986). Witness to violence: The child interview. *Journal of the American Academy of Child Psychiatry, 25*(3), 306–319.

Pynoos, R. S., & Nader, K. (1988). Psychological first aid and treatment approach to children exposed to community violence: Research implications. *Journal of Traumatic Stress, 1,* 445–473.

Pynoos, R. S., Steinberg, A. M., & Goenjian, A. (1996). Traumatic stress in childhood and adolescence: Recent developments and current controversies. In B. A. van der Kolk, A. C. McFarlane, & L. Weisaeth (Eds.), *Traumatic stress* (pp. 331–358). Guilford Press.

Pynoos, R. S., Steinberg, A. M., Layne, C. M., Liang, L.-J., Vivrette, R. L., Briggs, E. C., Kisiel, C., Habib, M., Belin, T. R., & Fairbank, J. A. (2014). Modeling constellations of trauma exposure in the National Child Traumatic Stress Network Core Data Set. *Psychological Trauma: Theory, Research, Practice, and Policy, 6*(Suppl 1), S9–S17. https://doi.org/10.1037/a0037767

Pyszczynski, T., Solomon, S., & Greenberg, J. (2002). *In the wake of 9/11: The psychology of terror.* American Psychological Association.

Quero, S., Pererz-Ara, M., Breton-Lopez, J., Garcia-Palacios, A., Banos, R., & Botella, C. (2014). Acceptability of virtual reality interoceptive exposure for the treatment of panic disorder and agoraphobia. *British Journal of Guidance & Counselling, 42*(2), 123–137.

Rabin, R. F., Jennings, J. M., Campbell, J. C., & Bair-Merritt, M. H. (2009). Intimate partner violence screening tools: A systematic review. *American Journal of Preventive Medicine, 36*(5), 439–445.e4. https://doi.org/10.1016/j.amepre.2009.01.024

Rach-Beisel, J. M., Scott, J., & Dixon, L. (1999). Co-occurring severe mental illness and substance use disorders: A review of recent research. *Psychiatric Services, 50,* 1427–1434.

Racine, C., & Billick, S. (2014). Classification systems for stalking behavior. *Journal of Forensic Sciences, 59*(1), 250–254. https://doi.org/10.1111/1556-4029.12262

Rada, R. T. (1981). The violent patient: Rapid assessment and management. *Psychosomatics, 22,* 101–109.

Rainone, G. A., Schmeidler, J., Frank, B., & Smith, R. (2006). Violent behavior, substance use, and other delinquent behaviors among middle and high school students. *Youth Violence and Juvenile Justice, 4*(3), 247–265.

Ram, V., Webb-Murphy, J., McLay, R. N., Baird, A. R., Nebeker, B. J., & Johnson, S. (2014, August). *Interim analysis of head-to-head comparison of virtual reality exposure treatment for PTSD.* Paper presented at American Psychological Association 122nd conference. Washington, D. C., the United States.

Ramos Silva, H. F., & Pucci, S. H. M. (2021). Mental disorders as a risk factor for suicide and suicidal ideation: Trastornos mentales como fator de riesgo de suicidio e ideación suicida. *Saúde Coletiva (Barueri), 11*(68), 7235–7242. https://doi.org/10.36489/saudecoletiva.2021v11i68p7227-7242

Ramsey, J. L., & Blieszner, R. (2000). Transcending a lifetime of losses: The importance of spirituality in old age. In J. H. Harvey & E. D. Miller (Eds.), *Loss and trauma: General and close relationship perspectives* (pp. 225–236). Brunner-Routledge.

Ramshaw, E. J. (2010). The personalization of postmodern postmortem rituals. *Pastoral Psychology, 59*(2), 171–178.

Rando, T. A. (1984). *Grief, dying, and death: Clinical intervention for caregivers.* Research Press.

Rando, T. A. (1993). *Treatment of complicated mourning.* Research Press.

Rando, T. A. (1996). Complications in mourning traumatic death. In K. J. Doka (Ed.), *Living with grief after sudden loss: Suicide, homicide, accident, heart attack, stroke* (pp. 139–160). Hospice Foundation of America.

Rando, T. A. (Ed.). (1986). *Parental loss of a child.* Research Press.

Raphael, B. (1977). Preventive intervention with the recently bereaved. *Archives of General Psychiatry, 34*(12), 1450–1454.

Raphael, B. (1983). *The anatomy of bereavement.* Harper & Row/Basic Books.

Raphael, B. (1986). *When disaster strikes: How individuals and communities cope with catastrophe.* Basic Books.

Raphael, B. (1999). Conclusion: Debriefing—Science, belief, and wisdom. In B. Raphael & J. P. Wilson (Eds.), *Psychological debriefing: Theory, practice, and evidence* (pp. 351–359). Cambridge University Press.

Raphael, B. (2000). *Disaster mental health response handbook: An educational resource for mental health professionals involved in disaster management.* New South Wales Institute of Psychiatry.

Raphael, B., & Dobson, M. (2000). Bereavement. In J. H. Harvey & E. D. Miller (Eds.), *Loss and trauma: General and close relationship perspectives* (pp. 45–61). Brunner-Routledge.

Raphael, B., & Minkov, C. (1999). Abnormal grief. *Current Opinion in Psychiatry, 12,* 99–102.

Raphael, B., & Wilson, J. (2000). *Psychological debriefing: Theory, practice, and evidence.* Cambridge University Press.

Raphael, B., Meldrum, L., & McFarland, A. C. (1995). Does debriefing after psychological trauma work? *British Medical Journal, 310,* 1479–1480.

Rapoport, L. (1967). Crisis-oriented short-term case work. *Social Services Review, 41,* 31–44.

Raskin, N. J., & Rogers, C. R. (1995). Person-centered therapy. In R. J. Corsini & D. Wedding (Eds.), *Current psychotherapies* (5th ed.). F. E. Peacock.

Rasnayake, S., & Navratil, P. (2022). Warning signs of elderly suicide and factors affecting professional help-seeking: Case of Sri Lanka. *Journal of Population & Social Studies, 1–19.* https://doi.org/10.25133/JPSSv312023.001

Ratnarajah, D., & Schofield, M. J. (2008). Survivors' narrative of the impact of parental suicide. *Suicidal and Life-Threatening Behavior, 38,* 618–630.

Ratts, M. J., & Pedersen, P. B. (2014). *Counseling for multiculturalism and social justice: Integration, theory, and application.* American Counseling Association.

Ratts, M., Ayers, L., & Bright, M. (2009). Sticks and stones. *ASCA School Counselor, 47*(1), 20–25.

Rauvola, R. S., Vega, D. M., & Lavigne, K. N. (2019). Compassion fatigue, secondary traumatic stress, and vicarious traumatization: A qualitative review and research agenda. *Occupational Health Science, 3*(3), 297–336. https://doi.org/10.1007/s41542-019-00045-1

Ray, C. M., Tyler, K. A., & Gordon Simons, L. (2021). Risk factors for forced, incapacitated, and coercive sexual victimization among sexual minority and heterosexual male and female college students. *Journal of Interpersonal Violence, 36*(5–6), 2241–2261. https://doi.org/10.1177/0886260518758332

Ray, S. L., Wong, C., White, D., & Heaslip, K. (2013). Compassion satisfaction, compassion fatigue, work life conditions, and burnout among frontline mental health care professionals. *Traumatology, 19*(4), 255–267. https://doi.org/10.1177/1534765612471144

Reaves, B. (2017). *Police Response to Domestic Violence, 2006–2015.*

Rebmann, T., Carrico, R., & English, J. F. (2008). Lessons public health professionals learned from past disasters. *Public Health Nursing, 25,* 344–352.

Rector, M. (2021). Examination of counselor crisis intervention competencies in a mobile crisis team program: A sequential explanatory mixed methods study. *Dissertation Abstracts International Section B: The Sciences and Engineering 82(12-B).*

Red Cross. (2023). Mission Statement. https://www.redcross.org/about-us/who-we-are/mission-and-values.html

Reddy, M., Borum, R., Berglund, J., Vossekuil, B., Fen, R., & Modzeleski, W. (2001). Evaluating risk for targeted violence in schools: Comparing risk assessment, threat assessment, and other approaches. *Psychology in the Schools, 38,* 157–173.

Redmon, L. M. (1996). Sudden violent death. In K. J. Doka (Ed.), *Living with grief after sudden loss: Suicide, homicide, accident, heart attack, stroke* (pp. 53–72). Hospice Foundation of America.

Reed, R. A., Pamlanye, J. T., Truex, H. R., Murphy-Neilson, M. C., Kunaniec, K. P., Newins, A. R., & Wilson, L. C. (2020). Higher rates of unacknowledged rape among men: The role of rape myth acceptance. *Psychology of Men & Masculinities, 21*(1), 162–167. https://doi.org/10.1037/men0000230

Reese, M. T. (2009). Compassion fatigue and spirituality with emergency health care providers. *Dissertation Abstracts International: Section B. The Sciences and Engineering, 69*(12), 7843.

Reese, R. J., Conoley, C. W., & Brossart, D. F. (2002). Effectiveness of telephone counseling: Field-based investigation. *Journal of Counseling Psychology, 49*(2), 233–242.

Reese, R. J., Conoley, C. W., & Brossart, D. F. (2006). The attractiveness of telephone counseling: An empirical investigation of client perceptions. *Journal of Counseling & Development, 84*(1), 54–60.

Reeves, N. C. (2011). Death acceptance through ritual. *Death Studies, 35*(5), 408–419.

Reger, G. M., Rizzo, A. A., & Gahm, D. A. (2015). Initial development and dissemination of virtual reality exposure therapy for combat-related PTSD. In M.P. Safir, H. S. Wallach, & A. Rizzo (Eds.), *Future directions in post-traumatic stress disorder: Prevention, diagnosis and treatment* (pp. 289–302). Springer.

Reger, G., Holloway, K., Candy, C., Rothbaum, B., Difede, J., Rizzo, A., & Gahm, G. (2011). Effectiveness of virtual reality exposure therapy for active duty soldiers in a military mental health clinic. *Journal of Traumatic Stress 24*(1), 93–96.

Reich, W., Shayka, J. J., & Taibleson, C. (1991). *Diagnostic Interview for Children and Adolescents (DICA).* Washington University.

Reichel, D. (2017). Determinants of intimate partner violence in Europe: The role of socioeconomic status, inequality, and partner behavior. *Journal of Interpersonal Violence, 32*(12), 1853–1873. https://doi.org/10.1177/0886260517698951

Reichle, B., Schneider, A., & Montada, L. (1998). How do observers of victimization preserve their belief in a just world cognitively or actionally? Findings from a longitudinal study. In L. Montanda & J. Lerner (Eds.), *Responses to victimizations and belief in a just world* (pp. 55–87). Plenum Press.

Reim Ifrach, E., & Miller, A. (2016). Social action art therapy as an intervention for compassion fatigue. *The Arts in Psychotherapy, 50,* 34–39. https://doi.org/10.1016/j.aip.2016.05.009

Reinecke, A., Thilo, K., Filippini, N., Croft, A., & Hamer, C. (2014). Predicting rapid response to cognitive-behavioural treatment for panic disorder: The role of hippocampus, insula, and dorsolateral prefrontal cortex. *Behaviour Research and Therapy, 62,* 120–128.

Reinke, B., Mahlke, C., Bolros, C., Klaring, A., Reyes, G., Elhai, J. D., & Ford, J. D. (Eds.). (2008). *The encyclopedia of psychological trauma.* John Wiley & Sons.

Reinke, B., Mahlke, C., Botros, C., Klaring, A., Lambert, M., Karow, A., Gallinat, J., Zapf, A., Ozga, A., Baumgardt, J., Spiegel, J., Hardt, O., & Becker, T. (2022). Study protocol of a randomized control evaluating treatment outcome with peer support for acute mental health crises. *BMC Psychiatry, 22,* Article 619. https://doi.org/10.1186/s12888-022-04247-w

Reis, C., & Cornell, D. (2008). An evaluation of suicide gatekeeper training for school counselors and teachers. *Professional School Counseling, 11*(6), 386–394.

Reitmeyer, R. (2000). Dog gone? From cats to snakes, counselors help heal human hearts following a pet loss. *Counseling Today, 42*(9), 1, 26–27.

Reivich, K. J., Seligman, M. P., & McBride, S. (2011). Master resilience training in the U.S. Army. *American Psychologist, 66*(1), 25–34.

Remboldt, C. (1994). *Violence in schools: The enabling factor.* Johnson Institute.

Remley, T. P., & Herlihy, B. (2020). *Ethical, legal, and professional issues in counseling.* Pearson.

Remley, T. R., & Herlihy, B. (2020). *Ethical, legal, and professional issues in counseling.* Pearson.

Ren, C. H. (2000). Understanding and managing the dynamics of linked crisis events. *Disaster Prevention and Management, 9*(1), 12–17.

Repetti, R., & Wang, S. (2017). Effects of job stress on family relationships. *Current Opinion in Psychology, 13,* 15–18. https://doi.org/10.1016/j.copsyc.2016.03.010

Reporting on suicide. (2022). *Best practices and recommendations for reporting on suicide.* https://reportingonsuicide.org/recommendations/

Resick, P. A. (2014). *Stress and trauma.* Psychology Press. http://dx.doi.org/10.4324/9781315820125

Resick, P. A., & Schnicke, M. K. (1993). *Cognitive processing therapy for rape victims: A treatment manual.* SAGE.

Resick, P. A., Monson, C. M., & Chard, K. M. (2008). *Cognitive processing therapy: Veterans/Military version.* Department of Veterans' Affairs.

Resick, P. A., Monson, C. M., & Chard, K. M. (2017). *Cognitive processing therapy for PTSD. A comprehensive manual.* Guilford Press.

Resick, P. A., Monson, C. M., & Gutner, C. (2007). Psychological treatments for PTSD. In N. J. Friedman, T. M. Keane, & P. A. Resick (Eds.), *Handbook of PTSD: Science and practice* (pp. 330–358). Guilford Press.

Reyes, G., Elhai, J. D., & Ford, J. D. (Eds.). (2008). *The encyclopedia of psychological trauma*. John Wiley & Sons.

Rhee, W. K., Merbaum, M., Strube, M. J., & Self, S. (2005). Efficacy of brief telephone psychotherapy with callers to a suicide hotline. *Suicide and Life-Threatening Behavior, 35*(3), 317–328.

Rhodes, L. R. (2023). The impact of telebehavioral health on clinical practice. *Counseling Today, 65*(10), 23–30.

Ribeiro, J. D., Witte, T. K., Van Orden, K. A., Selby, E. A., Gordon, K. H., Bender, T. W., & Joiner, T. E. Jr. (2014). Fearlessness about death: The psychometric properties and construct validity of the revision to the Acquired Capability for Suicide Scale. *Psychological Assessment, 26*(1), 115–126. https://doi.org/10.1037/a0034858

Rice, M. & Harris, G. (1995). Violent recidivism: Assessing predictive validity. *Journal of Consulting and Clinical Psychology, 63,* 737–748.

Richards, P. S., Hardman, R. K., Lea, T., & Berrett, M. E. (2015). Religious and spiritual assessment of trauma survivors. In D. F. Walker, C. A. Courtois, & J. Aten, J. (Eds.). *Spiritually oriented psychotherapy for trauma* (pp. 77–102). American Psychological Association.

Richards, T. N., Nix, J., Mourtgos, S. M., & Adams, I. T. (2021). Comparing 911 and emergency hotline calls for domestic violence in seven cities: What happened when people started staying home due to COVID-19? *Criminology & Public Policy, 20*(3), 573–591. https://doi.org/10.1111/1745-9133.12564

Richardson, C. M. E., Trusty, W. T., & George, K. A. (2020). Trainee wellness: Self-critical perfectionism, self-compassion, depression, and burnout among doctoral trainees in psychology. *Counselling Psychology Quarterly, 33*(2), 187–198. https://doi.org/10.1080/09515070.2018.1509839

Riding-Malon, R., & Werth, J. L., Jr. (2014). Psychological practice in rural settings: At the cutting edge. *Professional Psychology: Research and Practice, 45*(2), 85–91. https://doi.org/10.1037/a0036172

Ridley, C. R. (2005). *Overcoming unintentional racism in counseling and therapy: A practitioner's guide to intentional intervention* (2nd ed). SAGE Publications.

Riethmayer, J. (2002a). Dealing with the impact of trauma. In D. D. Bass & R. Yep (Eds.), *Terrorism, trauma, and tragedies: A counselor's guide to preparing and responding* (pp. 107–109). American Counseling Association.

Riethmayer, J. (2002b). Explaining terrorism to children. In D. D. Bass & R. Yep (Eds.), *Terrorism, trauma, and tragedies: A counselor's guide to preparing and responding* (pp. 27–31). American Counseling Association.

Riggar, T. F. (1985). *Stress burnout: An annotated bibliography*. Southern Illinois University Press.

Rija, A., Islam, Z., Bilal, W., Qamar, K., Gangat, S., Abbas, S., Mirha, H., Mohanana, P., Rahmat, Z., Shaeen, S., Djedid, S., Essar, M., & Kashyap, R. (2022). The impact of violence on health care workers' mental health in conflict based settings amidst COVID-19 pandemic, and potential interventions: A narrative review. *Health Science Reports, 5*(6), e920. https://doi.org/10.1002/hsr2.920

Ringenbach, R. (2009). A comparison between counselors who practice meditation and those who do not on compassion fatigue, compassion satisfaction, burnout, and self-compassion. *Dissertation Abstracts International: Section B. The Science and Engineering, 69*(6), 3820.

Riordan, R. J., & Allen, L. (1989). Grief counseling: A funeral home-based model. *Journal of Counseling and Development, 67,* 424–425.

Ritter, C., Teller, J., Marcussen, K., Munetz, M., & Teasdale, B. (2011). Crisis Intervention Team officer dispatch, assessment, and disposition: Interactions with individuals with severe illness. *International Journal of Law and Psychiatry, 34*(1), 30–38.

Rizzo, A., Difede, J., Rothbaum, B., Buckwater, J., Daughtry, J., & Reger, G. M. (2015). Update and expansion of the virtual Iraq /Afghanistan PTSD exposure therapy system. In M. P. Safir, H. S. Wallach, & A. Rizzo (Eds.), *Future directions in post-traumatic stress disorder: Prevention, diagnosis and treatment* (pp. 303–328). Springer.

Robbins, S., & Bell, M. (2008). *Second life for dummies*. Wiley.

Robert, T. E., & Kelly, V. A. (2015). *Critical incidents in integrating spirituality into counseling*. American Counseling Association.

Roberts, A. R. (1991). Crisis intervention units and centers in the United States. In A. R. Roberts (Ed.), *Contemporary perspectives on crisis intervention and prevention* (pp. 18–31). Prentice Hall.

Roberts, A. R. (2002). Myths, facts, and realities regarding battered women and their children: An overview. In A. R. Roberts (Ed.), *Handbook of domestic violence: Intervention strategies* (pp. 3–22). Oxford University Press.

Roberts, A. R. (2005a). Bridging the past and present to the future of crisis intervention and crisis management. In A. R. Roberts, (Ed.). *Crisis intervention handbook: Assessment, treatment, and research* (3rd ed., pp. 3–34). Oxford University Press.

Roberts, A. R. (2005b). The ACT model: Assessment, crisis intervention, and trauma treatment in the aftermath of community disaster and terrorism attacks. In A. R. Roberts (Ed.), *Crisis intervention handbook* (3rd ed., pp. 143–170). Oxford University Press.

Roberts, A. R. (Ed.). (1991). *Contemporary perspectives on crisis intervention and prevention*. Prentice Hall.

Roberts, A. R. (Ed.). (2005). *Crisis intervention handbook* (3rd ed.). Oxford University Press.

Roberts, A. R., & Kurst-Swanger, K. (2002). Police responses to battered women: Past, present, and future. In A. R. Roberts (Ed.), *Handbook of domestic violence: Intervention strategies* (pp. 101–126). Oxford University Press.

Roberts, A. R., & Roberts, B. S. (2002). A comprehensive model for crisis intervention with battered women and their children. In A. R. Roberts (Ed.), *Handbook of domestic violence: Intervention strategies* (pp. 365–395). Oxford University Press.

Roberts, A. R., & Roberts, B. S. (2005). A comprehensive model for crisis intervention with battered women and their children. In A. R. Roberts (Ed.), *Crisis intervention handbook* (3rd ed., pp. 441–482). Oxford University Press.

Robertson, E. L., Walker, T. M., & Frick, P. J. (2020). Intimate partner violence perpetration and psychopathy: A comprehensive review. *European Psychologist, 25*(2), 134–145. https://doi.org/10.1027/1016-9040/a000397

Robertson, H. (2013). Common crises. *ASCA School Counselor, 50*(4), 40–45

Robinson, H. M., Sigman, M. R., & Wilson, J. P. (1997). Duty-related stressors and PTSD symptoms in suburban police officers. *Psychological Reports, 81,* 835–845.

Robinson-Whelen, S., Hughes, R. B., Taylor, H. B., Holmes, S. A., Rodriquez, J., & Manohar, S. (2023). Impacts of the COVID-19 pandemic on people with spinal cord injury. *Rehabilitation Psychology, 68*(1), 1–11. https://doi.org/10.1037/rep0000480

Rodesch, C. K. (1994, April). *Keeping the counselor sane.* Paper presented at the Eighteenth Annual Convening of Crisis Intervention Personnel, Chicago, IL, the United States.

Rodriguez, D., & Bernal, G. (2012). Frameworks, models, and guidelines for cultural adaption. In G. Bernal & D. Rodriguez (Eds), *Cultural adaptions: Tools for evidence-based practice with diverse populations.* (pp. 23–44). American Psychological Association.

Rodriguez, L., & Read, J. P. (2020). Momentary emotional responding and emotion regulation in PTSD-related drinking urge. *Experimental and Clinical Psychopharmacology, 28*(1), 99–111. https://doi.org/10.1037/pha0000292

Rofman, E. S., Askinazi, C., & Fant, E. (1980). The prediction of dangerous behavior in emergency civil commitment. *American Journal of Psychiatry, 137*, 1061–1064.

Rogel, A., Loomis, A. M., Hamlin, E., Hodgdon, H., Spinazzola, J., & van der Kolk, B. (2020). The impact of neurofeedback training on children with developmental trauma: A randomized controlled study. *Psychological Trauma: Theory, Research, Practice, and Policy, 12*(8), 918–929. https://doi.org/10.1037/tra0000648

Rogers, C. R. (1961). *On becoming a person.* Houghton Mifflin.

Rogers, C. R. (1969). *Freedom to learn: A view of what education might become.* Merrill.

Rogers, C. R. (1977). *Carl Rogers on personal power: Inner strength and its revolutionary impact.* Delacorte.

Rogers, L. L. (2019, November 1). *Transitional housing programs and empowering survivors of domestic violence.* U.S. Department of Justice. https://www.justice.gov/archives/ovw/blog/transitional-housing-programs-and-empowering-survivors-domestic-violence

Rogers, M. S., McNeil, D. E., & Binder, R. L. (2019). Effectiveness of police crisis intervention training program. *The Journal of the American Academy of Psychiatry and Law. 44*(4), 414–421. https://doi.org/10.29158/jaapl.003863-19

Rohland, B. M., Saleh, S. S., Rohrer, J. E., & Romitti, P. A. (2000). Acceptability of telepsychiatry to a rural population. *Psychiatric Services, 51*(5), 672–674.

Rolland, J. S. (2012). Mastering family challenges in serious illness and disability. In F. Walsh (Ed.), *Normal family processes: Growing diversity and complexity* (4th ed., pp. 452–482). Guildford Press.

Rollero, C., & De Piccoli, N. (2020). Myths about intimate partner violence and moral disengagement: An analysis of sociocultural dimensions sustaining violence against women. *International Journal of Environmental Research and Public Health, 17*(21), Article 21. https://doi.org/10.3390/ijerph17218139

Romanoff, B. (1993). When a child dies: Special consideration for providing mental health counseling for bereaved parents. *Journal of Mental Health Counseling, 15*, 384–393.

Romero-Sánchez, M., Krahé, B., Moya, M., & Megías, J. L. (2018). Alcohol-related victim behavior and rape myth acceptance as predictors of victim blame in sexual assault cases. *Violence Against Women, 24*(9), 1052–1069. https://doi.org/10.1177/1077801217727372

Romig, C. A., & Gruenke, C. (1991). The use of metaphor to overcome inmate resistance to mental health counseling. *Journal of Counseling & Development, 69*(4), 414–418.

Ronan, G. F., Dreer, L., Maurelli, K., Wollerman-Ronan, D., & Gerhart, J. (2014). *Practitioner's guide to empirically supported measures of anger, aggression, and violence: ABCT clinical assessment series.* Springer.

Rosenbaum, A., & Kunkel, T. S. (2009). Group interventions for intimate partner violence. In K. D. O'Leary & E. Woodin (Eds.), *Psychology and physical aggression in couples: Causes and interventions* (pp. 191–210). American Psychological Association.

Rosenberg, S. (2004). Inoculation effect in prevention of increased verbal aggression in schools. *Psychological Reports, 95*(2), 1219–1226.

Rosenblatt, P. C. (2010). Shame and death in cultural context. In J. Kauffman (Ed.), *The shame of death, grief, and trauma* (pp. 113–137). Routledge/Taylor & Francis Group.

Rosencrans, P. L., Zoellner, L. A., & Feeny, N. C. (2021). A network approach to posttraumatic stress disorder: Comparing interview and self-report networks. *Psychological Trauma: Theory, Research, Practice, and Policy.* Advance online publication. https://doi.org/10.1037/tra0001151

Rosenfeld, L. B., Caye, J. S., Lahad, M., & Gurwitch, R. H. (2010). *When their world falls apart: Helping families and children manage the effects of disasters* (2nd ed.). National Social Workers Press.

Rosenfeld, S., Newell, M., Zwolski, S., & Benmishek, L. (2018). Evaluating problem solving teams in K–12 schools: Do they work? *American Psychologist, 73*(4), 407–419. https://doi.org/10.1037/amp0000254

Rosenheck, R., & Fontana, A. (1998). Warrior fathers and warrior sons: Intergenerational aspects of trauma. In Y. Danieli (Ed.), *International handbook of multigenerational legacies of trauma* (pp. 225–242). Plenum Press.

Rosenrthal, L., Byerly, A., Taylor, A., & Martinovich, Z. (2018). Impact and prevalence of physical and verbal violence toward health care workers. *Psychosomatics, 59*(6), 584–590. https://doi.org/10.1016/j.psym.2018.04.007

Rosino, M. (2016). ABC-X model of family stress and coping. *Encyclopedia of Family Studies, 1*–6.

Rosner, R., Kruse, J., & Hagl, M. (2010). A meta-analysis of interventions for bereaved children and adolescents. *Death Studies, 34*(2), 99–136.

Ross, J. M. (2011). Personality and situational correlates of self-reported reasons for intimate partner violence among women versus men referred for batterers' intervention. *Behavioral Sciences & the Law, 29*(5), 711–727.

Roth, L. (2000, April). *Preventing school violence through community organization.* Paper presented at Proceedings of the Twenty-Fourth Annual Convening of Crisis Intervention Personnel, Chicago, IL, the United States.

Rothschild, B. (2000). *The body remembers: The psychophysiology of trauma and trauma treatment.* Norton.

Rothschild, B. (2010). *8 keys to safe recovery.* Norton.

Rottman, J., Kelemen, D., & Young, L. (2014). Tainting the soul: Purity concerns predict moral judgments of suicide. *Cognition, 130*(2), 217–226. https://doi.org/10.1016/j.cognition.2013.11.007

Rouchy, E., Germanaud, E., Garcia, M., & Michel, G. (2020). Characteristics of homicide-suicide offenders: A systematic review. *Aggression and Violent Behavior, 55.* https://doi.org/10.1016/j.avb.2020.101490

Rouse, B. A. (1998). *Substance abuse and mental health statistics source book.* U.S. Government Printing Office.

Roux, N., & Benita, T. (2020). Best practices for burnout self-care. *Nursing Management, 51*(10), 30. https://doi.org/10.1097/01. NUMA.0000698116.82355.0d

Roysircar, G. (2013). Disaster counseling: A Haitian family case post January 12, 2010 earthquake. In S. Poyrazli & C.E. Thompson (Eds.), *International case studies in mental health* (pp. 155–180). SAGE.

Roysircar, G., Podkova, M., & Pignatiello, V. (2013). Crisis intervention, social class, and counseling: Macrolevel disaster effects. In W. Ming Liu (Ed.), *The Oxford handbook of social class in counseling, Oxford library of psychology* (pp. 144–163). Oxford University Press,

Ruane, M. E. (2007, April 22). Cho's bizarre behavior alarmed suite mate. *Memphis Commercial Appeal*, pp. 1A, 5A.

Ruben, I., Wolkon, G., & Yamamoto, J. (1980). Physical attacks on psychiatric residents by patients. *Journal of Nervous and Mental Disease, 168*, 243–245.

Rubin, R. (1999, June). *Crisis intervention.* Paper presented at the American School Counselor Association Convention, Phoenix, AZ, United States.

Rubin, S. (1999). The two-track model of bereavement: Overview, retrospect and prospect. *Death Studies, 23*(8), 681–714.

Rubin, S., & Yasien-Esmael, H. (2004). Loss and bereavement among Israel's Muslims: Acceptance of God's will, grief, and the relationship of the deceased. *Omega: Journal of Death and Dying, 49*(2), 149–162.

Rudd, M. D. (2004). University counseling centers: Looking more and more like community clinics. *Professional Psychology: Research and Practice, 35*(3), 316–317.

Rudd, M. D., Berman, A. L., Joiner, T. E., Nock, M. K., Silverman, M. M., Mandrusiak, M., Van Orden, K., & Witte, T. (2006). Warning signs for suicide: Theory, research, and clinical applications. *Suicide and Life-Threatening Behavior, 36*(3), 255–262. https://doi.org/10.1521/suli.2006.36.3.255

Rudd, M. D., Joiner Jr, T. E., & Rajab, M. H. (2004). *Treating suicidal behavior: An effective, time-limited approach* (1st ed.). The Guilford Press.

Rudd, M. D., Mandrusiak, M., & Joiner Jr., T. E. (2006). The case against no-suicide contracts: The commitment to treatment statement as a practice alternative. *Journal of Clinical Psychology, 62*(2), 243–251. https://doi.org/10.1002/jclp.20227

Ruderfer, D. M., Walsh, C. G., Aguirre, M. W., Tanigawa, Y., Ribeiro, J. D., Franklin, J. C., & Rivas, M. A. (2020). Significant shared heritability underlies suicide attempts and clinically predicted probability of attempting suicide. *Molecular Psychiatry, 25*(10), 2422–2430. https://doi.org/10.1038/s41380-018-0326-8

Rudolph, C. W., & Zacher, H. (2021). Family demands and satisfaction with family life during the COVID-19 pandemic. *Couple and Family Psychology: Research and Practice, 10*(4), 249–259. https://doi.org/10.1037/cfp0000170

Ruesch, J. (1973). *Therapeutic communication.* Norton.

Rufo, R. A. (Ed.). (2016). *Police suicide: Is police culture killing our officers?* CRC Press.

Ruhi, C. (2023). Broken windows theory of criminology. *Simply Psychology.* https://www.simplypsychology.org/broken-windows-theory.html

Rumsey, A. D., & Milsom, A. (2019). Supporting school engagement and high school completion through trauma-informed school counseling. *Professional School Counseling, 22*(1). https://doi.org/10.1177/2156759X19867254

Rupert, P. A., Miller, A. O., & Dorociak, K. E. (2015). Preventing burnout: What does the research tell us? *Professional Psychology: Research and Practice, 46*(3), 168–174. https://doi.org/10.1037/a0039297

Rural Health Hub. (2021). *Rural mental health.* http://www.rural-healthinfo.org

Russell, B., & Hamel, J. (2022). *Gender and domestic violence: Contemporary legal practice and intervention reforms.* Oxford University Press.

Russell, B., & Uhlemann, M. R. (1994). Women surviving an abusive relationship: Grief and the process of change. *Journal of Counseling and Development, 72*, 362–367.

Russell, S. T., Ryan, C., Toomey, R. B., Diaz, R. B., & Sanchez, J. (2011). Lesbian, gay, bisexual, and transgender adolescent school victimization: Implications for young adult health and adjustment. *Journal of School Health, 81*(5), 223–230

Russon, J., Morrissey, J., Dellinger, J., Jin, B., & Diamond, G. (2022). Implementing attachment-based family therapy for depressed and suicidal adolescents and young adults in LGBTQ+ services: Feasibility, acceptability, and preliminary effectiveness. *Crisis, 43*(6), 500–507. https://doi.org/10.1027/0227-5910/a000821

Rutherford, B. R., Zilcha-Mano, S., Chrisanthopolous, M., Salzman, C., Zhu, C., Cimino, N., Yehuda, R., Neria, Y., & Roose, S. P. (2021). Symptom profiles and treatment status of older adults with chronic post-traumatic stress disorder. *International Journal of Geriatric Psychiatry, 36*(8), 1216–1222. https://doi.org/10.1002/gps.5514

Ruzek, J. I. (2006). Models of early intervention following mass violence and other trauma. In E. C. Ritchie, P. J. Watson, & M. J. Friedman (Eds.), *Interventions following mass violence and disasters: Strategies for mental health practice* (pp. 16–36). Guilford Press.

Ryan, K., Lane, S. J., & Powers, D. (2017). A multidisciplinary model for treating complex trauma in early childhood. *International Journal of Play Therapy, 26*(2), 111–123. https://doi.org/10.1037/pla0000044

Rynearson, E. K. (2010). The clergy, the clinician, and the narrative of violent death. *Pastoral Psychology, 59*(2), 179–189.

Saakvitne, K. W. (2002). Shared trauma: The therapist's increased vulnerability. *Psychoanalytic Dialogues, 12*(3), 443–449.

Saakvitne, K. W., & Pearlman, L. A. (1996). *Transforming the pain: A workbook on vicarious traumatization.* W. W. Norton.

Sabella, R. A. (2010, July). *Cyberbullying.* Paper presented at the American School Counselor Conference, Boston, MA, the United States.

Sabina, C., Schally, J. L., & Marciniec, L. (2017). Problematic alcohol and drug use and the risk of partner violence victimization among male and female college students. *Journal of Family Violence, 32*(3), 305–316. https://doi.org/10.1007/s10896-017-9907-6

Safran, J., & Hunter, J. (2020). Summary. In J. Safran & J. Hunter, (Eds.), *Psychoanalysis and psychoanalytic therapies* (pp. 167–172). American Psychological Association. https://doi.org/10.1037/0000190-007

SAGE Publications, Inc. Public Broadcasting Service. (2002). Faith and doubt at ground zero. [VHS Tape]. Available from http://www.pbs.org/wgbh/pages/frontline/programs/.

Sage, R., & Dietz, W. (1994). Television viewing and violence in children: The pediatrician's agent for change. *Paediatrics, 94*(4), 600–607.

Saigh, P. A. (1987). In vitro flooding of childhood posttraumatic stress disorders: A systematic replication. *Professional School Psychology, 2*, 135–146.

Salinas, C. L. (2021). Playing to heal: The impact of bereavement camp for children with grief. *International Journal of Play Therapy, 30*(1), 40–49. https://doi.org/10.1037/pla0000147

Salloum, A., & Overstreet, S. (2008). Evaluation of individual and group grief and trauma interventions of children post disaster. *Journal of Clinical Child and Adolescent Psychology, 37*, 495–507.

Salloum, A., Kondraf, D., Johnco, C., & Olson, K. (2015). The role of self-care on compassion satisfaction, burnout, and secondary trauma among child welfare workers. *Children and Youth Services Review, 49*, 54–61.

Salston, M. D., & Figley, C. R. (2003). Secondary traumatic stress effects of working with survivors of criminal victimization. *Journal of Traumatic Stress, 16*(2), 167–174.

Saltzman, W. R., Babayan, T., Lester, P., Beardslee, W. R., & Pynoos, R. S. (2009). Family-based treatment for child traumatic stress. In D. Brom, R. Pat-Horenczyk, & J. D. Ford (Eds.). *Treating traumatized children: Risk, resiliency, and recovery* (pp. 240–254). Routledge.

Salvation Army Disaster Services. https://disaster.salvationarmy-usa.org

Salyers, M. P., Flanagan, M. E., Firmin, R., & Rollins, A. L. (2015). Clinicians' perceptions of how burnout affects their work. *Psychiatric Services, 66*(2), 204–207. https://doi.org/10.1176/appi.ps.201400138

Salyers, M. P., Fukui, S., Rollins, A. L., Firmin, R., Gearhart, T., Noll, J. P., Williams, S., & Davis, C. J. (2015). Burnout and self-reported quality of care in community mental health. *Administration and Policy in Mental Health and Mental Health Services Research, 42*(1), 61–69. https://doi.org/10.1007/s10488-014-0544-6

Salzer, M. S., & Bickman, L. (1999). The short- and long-term psychological impact of disasters: Implications for mental health interventions and policy. In R. Gist & B. Lubin (Eds.), *Response to disaster: Psychological, community, and ecological approaches* (pp. 63–82). Brunner/Mazel.

Samaritan Purse. (2023). https://www.samaritanspurse.org/what-we-do/international-crisis-response/

SAMHSA. (2003). *Tips for emergency and disaster response workers stress prevention and management approaches for rescue workers in the aftermath of terrorist acts.* http://search.usa.gov/search/docs?affiliate=samhsa-store&dc=1415&query=Tips%20%20for%20emergency%20and%20disaster%20response%20%20workers

SAMHSA (2020). *Treatment for suicidal ideation, self-harm, and suicide attempts among youths.*

SAMHSA. (2023, June 20). *Compassion fatigue and self-care for crisis counselors.* https://www.samhsa.gov/dtac/ccp-toolkit/self-care-for-crisis-counselors

SAMHSA. (2023). *SAMHSA's suicide prevention efforts.* http://www.samhsa.gov/suicide-prevention/samhsas-efforts

SAMHSA. (2022). *The Sequential Intercept Model.* https://www.samhsa.gov/criminal-juvenile-justice/sim-overview

SAMHSA. (2021). *Tap 34: Disaster planning handbook for behavioral health service programs.* https://store.samhsa.gov/product/tap-34-disaster-planning-handbook-for-behavioral-health-service-programs/pep21-02-01-001

Samide, L. L., & Stockton, R. (2002). Letting go of grief: Bereavement groups for children in the school setting. *Journal of Specialists in Group Work, 27*(2), 192–204.

San Roman, L., Mosher, D. K., Hook, J. N., Captari, L. E., Aten, J. D., Davis, E. B., Van Tongeren, D. R., Davis, D. E., Heinrichsen, H., & Campbell, C. D. (2019). Religious support buffers the indirect negative psychological effects of mass shooting in church-affiliated individuals. *Psychological Trauma: Theory, Research, Practice, and Policy, 11*(6), 571–577. https://doi.org/10.1037/tra0000448

Sandage, S., Rupert, D., Stavros, G., & Devor, N. (2020). *Relational spirituality in psychotherapy: Healing, suffering, and promoting growth.* American Psychological Association. https://doi.org/10.1037/0000174-013

Sanders, C. (2023, June 17). *Interview on burnout strategies for Carl Perkins Child Abuse Center.* [Speech recording]. Crisis Intervention & Prevention Solutions, Inc.

Sanders, C. M., Mauger, P. A., & Strong, P. N. (1985). *A manual for the Grief Experience Inventory.* Consulting Psychologists Press.

Sandhu, D. S. (2000, June). *Psycho-cultural profiles of violent students: Implications for counseling and therapy.* Paper presented at the American School Counselor Association Convention, Cherry Hill, NJ, the United States.

Sandler, I. N., Ayers, T. S., Wolchik, S. A., Tein, J.-Y., Kwok, O.-M., Haine, R. A., Twohey-Jacobs, J., Suter, J., Lin, K., Padgett-Jones, S., Weyer, J. L., Cole, E., Kriege, G., & Griffin, W. A. (2003). The Family Bereavement Program: Efficacy evaluation of a theory-based prevention program for parentally bereaved children and adolescents. *Journal of Consulting and Clinical Psychology, 71*(3), 587–600. https://doi.org/10.1037/0022-006X.71.3.587

Sandoval, J. (2013). *Crisis counseling, intervention, and prevention in schools.* (3rd ed.). Routledge.

Sansone, R. A., Chu, J., & Wiederman, M. (2011). Sexual behavior and borderline personality disorder among female psychiatric inpatients. *International Journal of Psychiatry in Clinical Practice, 15*(1), 69–73.

Santa Ana, E. J., Saladin, M. E., Back, S., Waldrop, A., Spratt, E., McRae, A., LaRowe, S. D., Timmerman, M. A., Upadhyaya, H., & Brady, K. T. (2006). PTSD and the HPA axis: Difference in response to the cold pressor task among individuals with child vs. adult trauma. *Psychoneuroendocrinology, 31*(4), 501–509.

Santilli, A., O'Connor Duffany, K., Carroll-Scott, A., Thomas, J., Greene, A., Arora, A., & Ickovics, J. (2017). Bridging the response to mass shootings and urban violence: Exposure to violence in New Haven, CT. *American Journal of Public Health, 107*, 374–379. http://dx.doi.org/10.2105/AJPH.2016.303613

Santrock, J. W. (2021). *Life-span development* (18th ed.). McGraw Hill.

Sanz-Barbero, B., Pereira, P. L., Barrio, G., & Vives-Cases, C. (2018). Intimate partner violence against young women: Prevalence and associated factors in Europe. *Journal of Epidemiology and Community Health, 72*(7), 611–616. https://doi.org/10.1136/jech-2017-209701

Sardinha, L., Maheu-Giroux, M., Stöckl, H., Meyer, S. R., & García-Moreno, C. (2022). Global, regional, and national prevalence estimates of physical or sexual, or both, intimate partner violence against women in 2018. *The Lancet, 399*(10327), 803–813. https://doi.org/10.1016/S0140-6736(21)02664-7

Sarri, S. (2005). *A bolt from the blue: Coping with disaster and acute trauma.* Jessica Kingsley.

Sato, M., Horner, P., Velez Ortiz, D., & Nelson, A. (2022). The role of spirituality in family adjustment and resilience among Puerto Rican families post-Hurricane Maria. *Journal of Religion & Spirituality in Social Work: Social Thought, 41*(1), 90–103. https://doi.org/10.1080/15426432.2021.2000553

Saturno, S. (2023). Violent crime and social worker safety. *Social Work Today Web Exclusive.* https://www.socialworktoday.com/archive/exc_032511.shtml

Satyen, L., Rogic, A. C., & Supol, M. (2019). Intimate partner violence and help-seeking behaviour: A systematic review of cross-cultural differences. *Journal of Immigrant and Minority Health, 21*(4), 879–892. https://doi.org/10.1007/s10903-018-0803-9

Saufler, C. (2010, July). *Bringing the brain to bullying prevention.* Paper presented at the American School Counselor Conference, Boston, MA, the United States.

Saulnier, K. G., Volarov, M., Velimirović, M., Bauer, B. W., Kolnogorova, K., Ashrafioun, L., Stecker, T., & Allan, N. P. (2023). Risk factors of suicidal behaviors in a high-risk longitudinal veteran sample: A network analysis. *Suicide and Life-Threatening Behavior, 53*(1), 4–15. https://doi.org/10.1111/sltb.12918

Saunders, C. L. (2012). The truth, the half-truth, and nothing like the truth: Reconceptualizing false allegations of rape. *The British Journal of Criminology, 52*(6), 1152–1171. https://doi.org/10.1093/bjc/azs036

Saunders, D. G. (1992). A typology of men who batter: Three types derived from cluster analysis. *American Journal of Orthopsychiatry, 62,* 264–275.

Saunders, M. (2010, Summer). CIT statistics. *The Team News.* CIT International. http://www.citinternational.org/news-letters/139-citintnewsletters.html

Savage, J., & Morabito, M. (2020). Police response to people with mental illness in a major US city: The Boston experience with the co-response model and mental health innovation. In J .L. McDaniel, K. Moss, & K. Pease (Eds.), *Policing and mental health: Theory, policy, practice.* (pp. 125–142). Routledge/Taylor & Francis Group.

Savicki, V. (2002). *Burnout across thirteen cultures: Stress and coping in child and youth care workers.* Praeger.

Savicki, V., & Cooley, E. J. (1982). Implications of burnout research and theory for counselor education. *Personnel and Guidance Journal, 60,* 415–419.

Savicki, V., & Cooley, E. J. (1987). The relationship of work environment and client contact to burnout in mental health professionals. *Journal of Counseling and Development, 65,* 249–252.

Saxe, G. N., Ellis, B. H., & Kaplow, J. B. (2007). *Collaborative treatment of traumatized children and teens: The trauma system therapy approach.* Guilford Press.

Saylor, C. F., Cowart, B. L., Lipovsky, J. A., Jackson, C., & Finch, A. (2003). Media exposure to September 11: Elementary school students' experiences and posttraumatic symptoms. *American Behavioral Scientist, 46*(12), 1622–1642.

Schaefer-Schiumo, K., & Ginsberg, A. (2003). The effectiveness of the warning signs program in high school youth about violence prevention: A study with urban high school students. *Professional School Counseling, 7*(1), 1–8.

Schafer, K. M., Daurio, A., French, J. E., Rogers, M. L., Meltzer, A. L., Cougle, J. R., & Joiner, T. E. (2022). The relationship between anger and suicidal ideation: Investigations in two samples. *Journal of Clinical Psychology, 78*(9), 1866–1877. https://doi.org/10.1002/jclp.23331

Schaufeli, W. B. (2006). The balance of give and take: Toward a social exchange model of burnout. *Revue Internationale de Psychologie Sociale, 19*(1), 87–131.

Schechter, S. (1982). *Women and male violence.* South End Press.

Scheer, J. R., Clark, K. A., Talan, A., Cabral, C., Pachankis, J. E., & Rendina, H. J. (2021). Longitudinal associations between childhood sexual abuse-related PTSD symptoms and passive and active suicidal ideation among sexual minority men. *Child Abuse & Neglect, 122.* https://doi.org/10.1016/j.chiabu.2021.105353

Scheffer Lindgren, M., & Renck, B. (2008). Intimate partner violence and the leaving process: Interviews with abused women. *International Journal of Qualitative Studies on Health & Well-Being, 3*(2), 113–124. https://doi.org/10.1080/17482620801945805

Scherer, L., Allen, J., & Harp, E. (2016). Grin and bear it: An examination of volunteers' fit with their organization, burnout and spirituality, *Burnout Research, 3*(1), 1–10.

Schliebner, C. T., & Peregoy, J. J. (1994). Unemployment effects on the family and the child: Interventions for counselors. *Journal of Counseling and Development, 72,* 368–372.

Schlosser, L. Z., Foley, P. F., Stein, E. P., & Holmwood, J. R. (2010). Why does counseling psychology exclude religion? A content analysis and methodological critique. In J. G. Ponterotto, J. M. Casas, L. A. Suzuki, & C. M. Alexander (Eds.), *Handbook of multicultural counseling* (3rd ed., pp. 453–466). SAGE.

Schmidt, C. K., & Welsh, A. C. (2010). College adjustment and subjective well-being when coping with a family member's illness. *Journal of Counseling and Development, 88,* 397–406.

Schneider, J. (1984). *Stress, loss, and grief: Understanding their origins and growth potential.* University Park Press.

Schneider, S., Rasul, R., Liu, B., Corry, D., Lieberman-Cribbin, W., Watson, A., Kerath, S. M., Taioli, E., & Schwartz, R. M. (2019). Examining posttraumatic growth and mental health difficulties in the aftermath of Hurricane Sandy. *Trauma: Theory, Research, Practice, and Policy, 11*(2), 127–136. https://doi.org/10.1037/tra0000400

Schniedman, E. S. (1987, March). At the point of no return: Suicide follows a predictable path. *Psychology Today,* 54–58.

Schoenberg, B. M. (Ed.). (1980). *Bereavement counseling: A multidisciplinary handbook.* Greenwood Press.

Schonfeld, D. J. (1989). Crisis intervention for bereavement support: A model of intervention in the children's school. *Clinical Pediatrics, 28,* 27–33.

Schonfeld, D., & Quackebush, A. (2017) Help for grieving students. *ASCA School Counselor, 54*(3), 21–24.

School Safety Advisory Council. (2015, July). *National School Safety Conference.* https://schoolsafety911.org/

School Violence Resource Center. (2003). *Weapons and schools: II. Fact sheet.* University of Arkansas System.

Schore, A. N. (2013). Relation trauma, brain development, and dissociation. In J. Ford, & C. A. Courtois (Eds.), *Treating complex stress disorders in children and adolescents: Scientific foundations and therapeutic models.* (pp. 3–23). Guilford Press.

Schouten, R., & Brennan, D. V. (2016). Targeted violence against law enforcement officers. *Behavioral Sciences & the Law, 34*(5), 608–621.

Schreier, H., Ladakakos, C., Morabito, D., Chapman, L., & Knudson, M. (2005). Posttraumatic stress symptoms in children after mild to moderate pediatric trauma: A longitudinal examination of symptom prevalence, correlates, and parent–child symptom reporting. *Journal of Trauma: Injury, Infection and Critical Care, 58*(2), 352–363.

Schriver, J. (2021). Campus police response to mental illness: Training, collaboration, and perceived effectiveness. *Journal of Police and Criminal Psychology, 36*(2), 307–313. https://doi.org/10.1007/s11896-020-09421-y

Schrumpf, F., Crawford, D. K., & Bodine, R. J. (1997). *Peer mediation: Conflict resolution in schools: Student manual* (Rev. ed.). Research Press.

Schueller, S. M., Hunter, J. F., Figueroa, C., & Aguilera, A. (2019). Use of digital mental health for marginalized and underserved populations. *Current Treatment Options in Psychiatry, 6*, 243–255. https://doi.org/10.1007/s40501-019-00181-z

Schutte, N. S., Bouleige, L., Fix, J. L., & Malouff, J. M. (1986). Returning to partner after leaving a crisis shelter: A decision faced by battered women. *Journal of Social Behavior and Personality, 1*, 295–298.

Schuurman, D. L., & DeCristofaro, J. (2007). After a parent's death: Group, family, and individual therapy to help children. In N. B. Webb (Ed.), *Play therapy with children in crisis* (pp. 173–196). Guilford Press.

Schuyler, A. C., Klemmer, C., Mamey, M. R., Schrager, S. M., Goldbach, J. T., Holloway, I. W., & Castro, C. A. (2020). Experiences of sexual harassment, stalking, and sexual assault during military service among LGBT and non-LGBT service members. *Journal of Traumatic Stress, 33*(3), 257–266. https://doi.org/10.1002/jts.22506

Schwab-Reese, L. M., Peek-Asa, C., & Parker, E. (2016). Associations of financial stressors and physical intimate partner violence perpetration. *Injury Epidemiology, 3*(1), 6. https://doi.org/10.1186/s40621-016-0069-4

Schwartz, A. J. (2006). Are college students more disturbed today? Stability in the acuity and qualitative character of psychopathology of college counseling center clients: 1992–1993 through 2001–2002. *Journal of American College Health, 54*(6), 327–337.

Schwiebert, V. L., Myers, J. E., & Dice, C. (2000). Ethical guidelines for counselors working with older adults. *Journal of Counseling & Development, 78*, 123–129.

Scott, A., Gavin, J., Sleath, E. & Sheridan, L. (2014). The attribution of responsibility in cases of stalking. *Psychology, Crime, & Law, 20*(7), 705–721.

Scruggs, T. E., Mastropieri, M. A., & Richter, L. (1985). Peer tutoring with behaviorally disordered students: Social and academic benefits. *Behavioral Disorders, 10*, 283–294.

Sculley, R. (1983). The work-setting support group: A means of preventing burnout. In B. A. Farber (Ed.), *Stress and burnout in the human service professions* (pp. 198–212). Pergamon Press.

Scurfield, R. M. (1985). Post-trauma stress assessment and treatment: Overview and formulations. In C. R. Figley (Ed.), *Trauma and its wake: The study of posttrauma stress disorder* (pp. 219–256). Brunner/Mazel.

Seely, M. F. (1997a). The discrete role of the hotline. *Crisis, 18*(2), 53–54.

Seely, M. F. (1997b). The role of hotlines in the prevention of suicide. In R. M. Maris & M. M. Silverman (Eds.), *Review of suicidology* (pp. 251–270). Guilford Press.

Segal, D. L., Chatman, C., Bogaards, J. A., & Becker, L. A. (2001). One-year follow-up of an emotional expression intervention for bereaved older adults. *Journal of Mental Health & Aging, 7*(4), 465–472.

Seligman, M. (1972). *Learned Helplessness.* 407–412.

Seligowski, A. V., Lee, D. J., Bardeen, J. R., & Orcutt, H. K. (2015). Emotion regulation and posttraumatic stress symptoms: A meta-analysis. *Cognitive Behaviour Therapy, 44*, 87–102. http://dx.doi.org/10.1080/16506073.2014.980753

Selye, H. (1956). *The stress of life.* McGraw Hill.

Selye, H. (1974). *Stress without distress.* Lippincott.

Selye, H. (1976). *The stress of life* (revised ed.). McGraw Hill.

Semiatin, J. N., Torres, S., LaMotte, A. D., Portnoy, G. A., & Murphy, C. M. (2017). Trauma exposure, PTSD symptoms, and presenting clinical problems among male perpetrators of intimate partner violence. *Psychology of Violence, 7*(1), 91–100. https://doi.org/10.1037/vio0000041

Semple, T., Tomlin, M., Bennett, C., & Jenkins, B. (2020). An evaluation of a community-based mobile crisis intervention team in a small Canadian police service. *Community Mental Health Journal.* Advance online publication. https://doi.org/10.1007/s10597-020-00683-8

Senger, H. L. (1999). Borderline mnemonic. *American Journal of Psychiatry 54*(9), 1321.

Seo, C., Kim, B., & Kruis, N. (2021). Validation across police response models for handling encounters with people with mental illnesses: A systematic review and meta-analysis. *Journal of Criminal Justice, 72*, Article 101752. https://doi.org/10.1016/j.jcrimjus.2020.101752

Sestir, M. A., & Bartholow, B. (2010). Violent and nonviolent video games produce opposing effects on aggressive and prosocial outcomes. *Journal of Experimental Social Psychology, 46*(6), 934–942.

Sexton-Radek, K. (Ed.). (2004). *Violence in schools: Issues, consequences, and expressions.* Praeger.

Seymour-Smith, S., & Kloess, J. A. (2021). A discursive analysis of compliance, resistance and escalation to threats in sexually exploitative interactions between offenders and male children. *British Journal of Social Psychology, 60*(3), 988–1011. https://doi.org/10.1111/bjso.12437

Shafer, C. (1989a, September). Counselors offer crisis intervention at Iowa crash site. *Guidepost,* pp. 1, 3, 6.

Shafer, C. (1989b, December). Recent disasters trigger NIMH response. *Guidepost,* pp. 1, 5.

Shaffer, D. (1988). The epidemiology of teen suicide: An examination of risk factors. *Journal of Clinical Psychiatry, 49*, 36–41.

Shaffer, D., Garland, A., Gould, M., Fisher, P., & Tratuman, P. (1988). Preventing teen suicide: A critical review. *Journal of the American Academy of Child and Adolescent Psychiatry, 27*, 675–687.

Shaffer, D., Vieland, V., & Garland, A. (1990). Adolescent suicide attempters: Response to suicide prevention programs. *Journal of the American Medical Association, 264*, 3151–3155.

Shah, A. K., Fineberg, N. A., & James, D. V. (1991). Violence among psychiatric in-patients. *Acta Psychiatrica Scandinavica, 84*, 305–309.

Shah, K., Bedi, S., Onyeaka, H., Singh, R., & Chaudhari, G. (2020). The role of psychological first aid to support public mental health in the COVID-19 pandemic. *Cureus, 12*(6), Article e8821. https://doi.org/10.7759/cureus.8821

Shahnaz, A., Bauer, B. W., Daruwala, S. E., & Klonsky, E. D. (2020). Exploring the scope and structure of suicide capability. *Suicide & Life-Threatening Behavior, 50*(6), 1230–1240. https://doi.org/10.1111/sltb.12686

Shalev, A., Sahar, T., Freedman, S., Peri, T., Lick, N., Brandes, D., Orr, S. P., & Pitman, R. K. (1998). A prospective study of heart rate response following trauma and the subsequent development of posttraumatic stress disorder. *Archives of General Psychiatry, 55*, 553–559.

Shallcross, L. (2009, September). Rewriting the "rules" of grief. *Counseling Today*, 28–31.

Shallcross, L. (2010). Treating trauma. *Counseling Today, 52*(10), 26–35.

Shallcross, L. (2011). A day that changed the nation and a profession. *Counseling Today, 54*(3), 36–40.

Shallcross, L. (2013). Bully pulpit. *Counseling Today, 55*(8), 30–38.

Shallcross, L. (2013, September). Multicultural competence: A continual pursuit. *Counseling Today*. https://ct.counseling.org/2013/09/multicultural-competence-a-continual-pursuit/

Shaluf, I. M. (2007). An overview of disasters. *Disaster Prevention and Management, 16*, 687–703.

Shanhinfar, A., Vishnevsky, T., Kilmaer, R. P., & Gil-Rivas, V. (2010). Service needs of children and families affected by Hurricane Katrina. In R. P. Kilmer, V. Gil-Rivas, R. G. Tedeschi, & L. G. Calhoun (Eds.). *Helping families and communities recover from disaster* (pp. 143–166). American Psychological Association.

Shao, Y., Fang, Y., Wang, M., Chang, C.-H. (D.), & Wang, L. (2021). Making daily decisions to work from home or to work in the office: The impacts of daily work- and COVID-related stressors on next-day work location. *Journal of Applied Psychology, 106*(6), 825–838. https://doi.org/10.1037/apl0000929

Shapiro, F. (1989a). Efficacy of the eye movement desensitization procedure in the treatment of traumatic memories. *Journal of Traumatic Stress, 2*, 199–223.

Shapiro, F. (1989b). Eye movement desensitization: A new treatment for posttraumatic stress disorder. *Journal of Behavior Therapy and Experimental Psychiatry, 20*, 211–217.

Shapiro, F. (1991). Eye movement desensitization and reprocessing procedure: From EMD to EMD/R—a new treatment model for anxiety and related traumata. *Behavior Therapist, 14*, 128, 133–135.

Shapiro, F. (1995). *Eye movement desensitization and reprocessing: Basic principles, protocols, and procedures.* Guilford Press.

Shapiro, F. (2014, Spring). EMDR therapy: Brief overview of trauma research, clinical practice, and proposed neurobiological mechanisms. *Trauma Psychology Newsletter*, 5–8.

Shapiro, F., & Maxfield, L. (2002). Eye movement desensitization and reprocessing (EMDR): Information processing in the treatment of trauma. *Journal of Clinical Psychology, 58*(8), 933–946.

Shapiro, R., & Brown, L. S. (2019). Eye movement desensitization and reprocessing therapy and related treatments for trauma: An innovative, integrative trauma treatment. *Practice Innovations, 4*(3), 139–155. https://doi.org/10.1037/pri0000092

Sharp, S. R., & McCallum, R. (2005). A rationalemotive behavior approach to improve anger management and reduce office referrals in middle school children: A formative investigation and evaluation. *Journal of Applied School Psychology, 21*(1), 39–66.

Sharples, L., Nguyen, C., Singh, B., & Lin, S. (2018). Identifying opportunities to improve intimate partner violence screening in a primary care system. *Family Medicine, 50*(9), 702–705. https://doi.org/10.22454/FamMed.2018.311843

Shaver, P. R., & Fraley, R. C. (2008). Attachment, loss, and grief: Bowlby's views and current controversies. In J. Cassidy & P. Shaver (Eds.), *Handbook of attachment: Theory, research, and clinical applications* (2nd ed., pp. 48–77). Guilford Press.

Shea, S. C. (1998). The chronological assessment of suicide events: A practical interviewing strategy for the elicitation of suicidal ideation. *The Journal of Clinical Psychiatry, 59*(Suppl 20), 58–72.

Shea, S. C. (2011). *The practical art of suicide assessment: A guide for mental health professionals and substance abuse counselors* (Illustrated edition). Mental Health Presses.

Shea, S. C. (2017). Uncovering a patient's hidden method of choice for suicide: Insights from the Chronological Assessment of Suicide Events (CASE Approach). *Psychiatric Annals, 47*(8), 421–427. https://doi.org/10.3928/00485713-20170708-01

Shear, K., & Frank, E. (2006). Treatment of complicated grief: Integrating cognitive-behavioral methods with other treatment approaches. In V. M. Follette & J. I. Ruzek (Eds.), *Cognitive-behavioral therapies for trauma* (2nd ed., pp. 290–320). Guilford Press.

Shear, M. K., & Mulhare, E. (2008). Complicated grief. *Psychiatric Annals, 38*(10), 662–670.

Sheehy, G. (1974). *Passages: Predictable crises of adult life.* Random House.

Sheehy, G. (1996). *New passages: Mapping your life across time.* Random House.

Sheerin, C. M., Bountress, K. E., Meyers, J. L., Saenz de Viteri, S. S., Shen, H., Maihofer, A. X., Duncan, L. E., & Amstadter, A. B. (2020). Shared molecular genetic risk of alcohol dependence and posttraumatic stress disorder (PTSD). *Psychology of Addictive Behaviors, 34*(5), 613–619. https://doi.org/10.1037/adb0000568

Sheftall, A. H., Vakil, F., Ruch, D. A., Boyd, R. C., Lindsey, M. A., & Bridge, J. A. (2022). Black youth suicide: Investigation of current trends and precipitating circumstances. *Journal of the American Academy of Child & Adolescent Psychiatry, 61*(5), 662–675. https://doi.org/10.1016/j.jaac.2021.08.021

Shelby, J. S., & Tredinnick, M. G. (1995). Crisis intervention with survivors of natural disaster: Lessons from Hurricane Andrew. *Journal of Counseling and Development, 73*, 491–497.

Sherman, L. W., & Berk, R. A. (1984). The specific deterrent effects of arrest for domestic assaults. *American Sociological Review, 49*, 1261–1272.

Sherman, L. W., Gottfredson, D., MacKenzie, D., Eck, J., Reuter, P., & Bushway, S. (1997). *Preventing crime: What works, what doesn't, what's promising* (Report to the United States Congress). University of Maryland, Department of Criminology and Criminal Justice, Office of Justice Program.

Shibuya, A., Sakamoto, A. Ihori, N., & Yukawa, S. (2008). The effects of the presence and contexts of video game violence in children: A longitudinal study in Japan. *Simulation & Gaming. 39*(4), 528–539. https://doi.org/10.1177/1046878107306670

Shifrin, A., Sharma, S., Zeifman, R. J., Roth, M. L., Gifford, S., & Monson, C. M. (2022). Posttraumatic stress disorder treatment preference: Prolonged exposure therapy, cognitive processing therapy, or medication therapy? *Psychological Services.* Advance online publication. https://doi.org/10.1037/ser0000688

Shinn, M., & Mørch, H. (1983). A tripartite model of coping with burnout. In B. A. Farber (Ed.), *Stress and burnout in the human service professions* (pp. 227–239). Pergamon Press.

Shnaider, P., Boyd, J. E., Cameron, D. H., & McCabe, R. E. (2022). The relationship between emotion regulation difficulties and PTSD outcomes during group cognitive processing therapy for PTSD. *Psychological Services, 19*(4), 751–759. https://doi.org/10.1037/ser0000546

Shneidman, E. (2001). *Comprehending suicide: Landmarks in 20th century suicidology.* American Psychological Association.

Shore, J. H., Tatum, E. L., & Vollmer, W. M. (1986). Evaluation of mental health effects of disaster: Mount St. Helen's eruption. *American Journal of Public Health, 76*(3), 76–86.

Shorey, R., Comelius, T., & Strauss, C. (2015). Stalking in college student dating relationships: A descriptive investigation. *Journal of Family Violence 40*(30), 1–2,

Short, E., Guppy, A., Hart, J. A., & Barnes, J. (2015). The impact of cyberstalking. *Studies in Media and Communication, 3*(2), 23–37. https://doi.org/10.11114/smc.v3i2.970

Shraberg, M. (2006, May). *Disaster planning for a crisis center.* Paper presented at the Thirtieth Convening of Crisis Intervention Personnel/Contact USA Conference, Chicago., IL, the United States

Shupe, A., Stacey, W. A., & Hazlewood, L. R. (1987). *Violent men, violent couples.* Lexington Books.

Sicafuse, L. L., & Miller, M. K. (2012). The effects of information processing and message quality on attitudes toward the AMBER alert system. *Applied Psychology in Criminal Justice, 8*(2), 69–86.

Siegel, D. J. (1995). Memory, trauma, and psychotherapy: A cognitive science view. *Journal of Psychotherapy Practice and Research, 4,* 93–122.

Sijtsema, J. J., Stolz, E. A., & Bogaerts, S. (2020). Unique risk factors of the co-occurrence between child maltreatment and intimate partner violence perpetration. *European Psychologist, 25*(2), 122–133. https://doi.org/10.1027/1016-9040/a000396

Silove, D. (1999). A conceptual framework for mass trauma: Implications for adaptation, intervention, and debriefing. In B. Raphael & J. P. Wilson (Eds.), *Psychological debriefing: Theory, practice, and evidence* (pp. 337–350). Cambridge University Press.

Silva, A., & Klotz, M. B. (2006, May). Culturally competent crisis response. *PL.* https://www.nasponline.org/Documents/Resources%20and%20Publications/Handouts/Families%20and%20Educators/cultcompcrisis.pdf

Silva, C., Smith, P. N., Rogers, M., Joiner, T. E., Foote, B., & Van Orden, K. A. (2023). Clinically significant scores for thwarted belonging and perceived burden from the Interpersonal Needs Questionnaire (INQ-15). *Crisis: The Journal of Crisis Intervention and Suicide Prevention.* https://doi.org/10.1027/0227-5910/a000898

Silver, T., & Goldstein, H. (1992). A collaborative model of a county intervention team: The Lake County experience. *Community Mental Health Journal, 28,* 249–253.

Silverman, P. R. (1986). The perils of borrowing: Role of the professional in mutual self-help groups. *Journal of Specialists in Group Work, 11,* 68–73.

Silverman, P. R. (2000). *Never too young to know: Death in children's lives.* Oxford University Press.

Silverman, W. K., Allen, A., & Ortiz, C. D. (2010). Lessons learned from Hurricane Katrina and other devastating hurricanes: Steps necessary for preparedness, response, and intervention. In R. P. Ryan, V. Gil-Rivas, R. G. Tedeschi, & L. G. Calhoun (Eds.), *Helping families and communities recover from disaster: Lessons learned from Hurricane Katrina and its aftermath* (pp. 289–311). American Psychological Association.

Simionato, G., Simpson, S., & Reid, C. (2019). Burnout as an ethical issue in psychotherapy. *Psychotherapy, 56,* 470–482. https://doi.org/10.1037/pst0000261

Simmons, J. (2000, October). FBI release study aimed at identifying dangerous students. *Counseling Today, 43*(4), 1, 22.

Simonds, J. F., & Kashani, J. (1980). Specific drug use and violence in delinquent boys. *American Journal of Drug and Alcohol Abuse, 7,* 305–322.

Simpson, L. R. (2006). Level of spirituality as a predictor of the occurrence of compassion fatigue among counseling professionals in Mississippi. *Dissertation Abstracts International: Section A. Humanities and Social Sciences, 66*(6), 3223.

Siner, L., Hoffman, Y., Littrell, M., Fry, M. W., Thornburgh, M. (2010). Supporting children after Hurricane Katrina: Reflections on psychosocial principles in practice. In R. P. Kilmer, V. Gil-Rivas, R. G. Tedeschi, & L. G. Calhoun (Eds.). *Helping families and communities recover from disaster,* (pp. 127–114). American Psychological Association.

Singer, J., Spiegel, J. A., & Papa, A. (2020). Preloss grief in family members of COVID-19 patients: Recommendations for clinicians and researchers. *Psychological Trauma: Theory, Research, Practice, and Policy, 12*(S1), S90–S93. https://doi.org/10.1037/tra0000876

Singer, V. I., Tracz, S. M., & Dworkin, S. H. (1991). Reminiscence group therapy: A treatment modality for older adults. *Journal for Specialists in Group Work, 16,* 167–171.

Singh, A., & Sharma, J. (2022). Marital rape: Causes and consequences. *IUP Law Review, 12*(1), 36–47.

Singh, J. P., Desmarais, S., Hurducas, C., Arbach-Lucioni, K., Condemarin, C., Dean, K., Doyle, M., Folino, J. O., Godoy-Cervera, V., Grann, M., Ho, R. M. Y., Large, M. M., Nielsen, L. H., Pham, T. H., Rebocho, M. F., Reeves, K. A., Rettenberger, M., de Ruiter, C., Seewald, K., & Otto, R. K. (2014). International perspectives on the practical application of violence risk assessment: A global survey of 44 countries. *International Journal of Forensic Mental Health, 13,* 193–206. http://dx.doi.org/10.1080/14999013.2014.922141

Singh, J. P., Grann, M., & Fazel, S. (2011). A comparative study of violence risk assessment tools: A systematic review and meta regression analysis of 68 studies involving 25,980 participants. *Clinical Psychology Review, 31,* 499–513.

Singh, V., Tolman, R., Walton, M., Chermack, S., & Cunningham, R. (2014). Characteristics of men who perpetrate intimate partner violence. *The Journal of the American Board of Family Medicine, 27*(5), 661–668. https://doi.org/10.3122/jabfm.2014.05.130247

Sinyor, M., Hartman, M., Zaheer, R., Williams, M., Pirkis, J., Heisel, M. J., Schaffer, A., Redelmeier, D. A., Cheung, A. H., Kiss, A., & Niederkrotenthaler, T. (2022). Differences in suicide-related Twitter content according to user influence. *Crisis: The Journal of Crisis Intervention and Suicide Prevention.* Advance online publication. https://doi.org/10.1027/0227-5910/a000865

Sitterle, K. A., & Gurwitch, R. H. (1999). The terrorist bombing in Oklahoma City. In E. S. Zinner and M. B. Williams (Eds.). *When a community weeps: Case studies in group survivorship* (pp. 161–189). Brunner/Mazel.

Skeem, J., & Bibeau, L. (2008). How does violence potential relate to crisis intervention team responses in emergencies? *Psychiatric Services, 59*(2), 201–204.

Sklare, G. (1997). *Brief counseling works: A solution focused approach for school counselors.* Corwin Press.

Slagel, L. (2009). *Examination of the reliability and validity of the Triage Assessment Survey: Families.* Unpublished doctoral dissertation. Duquesne University.

Slaikeu, K. A. (1990). *Crisis intervention: A handbook for practice and research* (2nd ed.). Allyn & Bacon.

Slaikeu, K. A., & Leff-Simon, S. I. (1990). Crisis intervention by telephone. In K. A. Slaikeu (Ed.), *Crisis intervention: A handbook for practice and research* (2nd ed., pp. 319–328). Allyn & Bacon.

Slattery, J. M., & Park, C. L. (2015). Spirituality and meaning making: Implications for therapy with trauma survivors. In D. F. Walker, C. A. Courtois, & J. D. Aten (Eds.), *Spiritually oriented psychotherapy for trauma.* (pp. 127–146). American Psychological Association.

Slattery, J. M., & Park, D. L. (2015). Spiritualty and making meaning: Implications for therapy with trauma survivors. In D. F. Walker, C. A. Courtois, & J. Aten (Eds.), *Spiritually oriented psychotherapy for trauma.* (pp. 147–168). American Psychological Association.

Sleek, S. (1998, August). Experts scrambling on school shootings: School violence in rural areas could worsen. *APA Monitor, 29*(1), 35–36.

Sloan, J. H. (1988). Handgun regulations, crime, assaults, and homicide. *New England Journal of Medicine, 319,* 1256–1262.

Sloore, H. (1988). Use of the MMPI in the prediction of dangerous behavior. *Acta Psychiatrica Belgica, 88,* 42–51.

Sloup, T. (2023, January 9). Illinois farm based programs connect farmers to mental health specialists. *Farm Week, 51*(2), 9.

Slovenko, R. (2006). Violent attacks in psychiatric and other hospitals. *Journal of Psychiatry & Law, 34*(2), 249–268.

Smart, D., English, A., James, J., Wilson, M., Darantha, K., Childers, B., & Magera, C. (2014). Compassion fatigue and satisfaction: A cross-sectional survey among US health care workers. *Nursing and Health Sciences, 16*(1), 3–10.

Smith, D. C., Larson, J., & Nuckles, D. (2006). A critical analysis of school-based anger management programs for youth. In S. R. Jimerson & M. Furlong (Eds.), *Handbook of school violence and school safety: From research to practice* (pp. 365–382). Erlbaum.

Smith, H. B. (2002). The American Red Cross: How to be a part of the solution, rather than a part of the problem. In D. D. Bass & R. Yep (Eds.), *Terrorism, trauma, and tragedies: A counselor's guide to preparing and responding* (pp. 37–38). American Counseling Association.

Smith, K. J., & Belgrave, L. L. (1995). The reconstruction of everyday life: Experiencing Hurricane Andrew. *Journal of Contemporary Ethnography, 24,* 244–269.

Smith, K. Z., Smith, P. H., & Grekin, E. R. (2014). Childhood sexual abuse, distress, and alcohol-related problems: Moderation by drinking to cope. *Psychology of Addictive Behaviors, 28,* 532–537. https://doi.org/10.1037/a0035381

Smith, L., Abdel-Salam, L., Scott-Mclaughlin, R. E., Baranowski, K., Madon, N., & Williams, M. (2022). Counseling psychology and participatory justice: "Sharing the university." *Counseling Psychology Quarterly.* Advance online publication. https://doi.org/10.1080/09515070.2022.2115459

Smith, P. N., Cukrowicz, K. C., Poindexter, E. K., Hobson, V., & Cohen, L. M. (2010). The acquired capability for suicide: A comparison of suicide attempters, suicide ideators, and non-suicidal controls. *Depression and Anxiety, 27*(9), 871–877. https://doi.org/10.1002/da.20701

Smith, S. (2009, September). Why does it hurt so much? Grieving the loss of a pet. *Your Mind Your Body.* American Psychological Association. www.yourmindyourbody.org/about-2

Smith, S. (2013). Could Comprehensive Soldier Fitness have iatrogenic consequences? A commentary. *The Journal of Behavioral Health Sciences & Research, 40*(2), 242–246.

Smith, T. C., Ryan, M. A., Wingard, D. L., Slymen, D. J., Sallis, J. F., & Kritz-Silverstein, D. (2008). New onset and persistent symptoms of post-traumatic stress disorder self reported after deployment and combat exposures: Prospect population based US military cohort study. *British Medical Journal, 336,* 366–371.

Snaman, J. M., Kaye, E. C., Levine, D. R., Cochran, B., Wilcox, R., Sparrow, C. K., Noyes, N., Clark, L., Avery, W., & Baker, J. N. (2017). Empowering bereaved parents through the development of a comprehensive bereavement program. *Journal of Pain and Symptom Management, 53*(4), 767–775. https://doi.org/10.1016/j.jpainsymman.2016.10.359

Snyder, D. J., Jordan, B. A., Aizvera, J., Innis, M., Mayberry, H., Raju, M., Lawrence, D., Dufek, A., Pao, M., & Horowitz, L. M. (2020). From pilot to practice: Implementation of a suicide risk screening program in hospitalized medical patients. *The Joint Commission Journal on Quality and Patient Safety, 46*(7), 417–426. https://doi.org/10.1016/j.jcjq.2020.04.011

Snyder, L. A., Chen, P., & Vacha-Haase, T. (2007). The underreporting gap in aggressive incidents from geriatric patients against certified nursing assistants. *Violence and Victims, 22*(3), 367–379.

Society of Clinical Psychology. (2012). *Reminiscence/life review therapy for depression.* American Psychological Association.

Sofka, C. J. (2004). What kind of funeral? Identifying and resolving family conflicts. *Generations, 28,* 21–25.

Softas-Nall, B. C., & Francis, P. C. (1998). A solution-focused approach to a family with a suicidal member. *The Family Journal, 6*(3), 227–230. https://doi.org/10.1177/1066480798063011

Sokol, L., & Fox, M. (2019). *The comprehensive clinician's guide to cognitive behavioral therapy.* Pesi Publishing & Media.

Sokolski, K., Denson, T., Lee, R., & Reist, C. (2003). Quetiapine for treatment of refractory symptoms of combat-related post-traumatic stress disorder. *Military Medicine, 168*(6), 486–489.

Solomon, R. M. (1995). Critical incidents stress management in law enforcement. In G. S. Everly (Ed.), *Innovations in disaster and trauma psychology: Applications in emergency services and disaster response* (pp. 123–157). Chevron.

Solomon, Z., Neria, Y., & Ram, A. (1998). Mental health professionals' responses to loss and trauma of holocaust survivors. In J. H. Harvey (Ed.), *Perspective on loss: A sourcebook* (pp. 221–231). Brunner/Mazel.

Sommers-Flanagan, J., & Sommers-Flanagan, R. S. (1997). *Tough kids, cool counseling: User-friendly approaches with challenging youth.* American Counseling Association.

Somohano, V. C., Vasquez, A., Shank, T., Irrgang, M., Newman, A. G., Evans, C., Wyse, J., Denneson, L., O'Neil, M., & Lovejoy, T. (2022). Perceptions of women with comorbid PTSD and substance use disorder on mechanisms underlying mindfulness-based interventions. *Cognitive and Behavioral Practice.* https://doi.org/10.1016/j.cbpra.2022.05.003

Sonkin, D. J., & Dutton, D. (2003). Treating assaultive men from an attachment perspective. *Journal of Aggression, Maltreatment, & Trauma, 7*(1/2), 105–133.

Sonkin, D. J., Martin, D., & Walker, L. E. (1985). *The male batterer: A treatment approach.* Springer.

Sopezki, D., Andreoni, S., Montero-Marin, J., Dias de Castro Fho, E., Fotes, S., de Lima, G., Pizutti, L., Girado, A., Silva, T., Garcia-Campayo, J., & Dearzo, M. (2020). Feasibility and effectiveness of a mindfulness-based program vs. relaxation in the treatment of burnout in Brazilian primary care providers: A mixed-methods pragmatic controlled study. *Mindfulness, 11*(1), 2573–2588. http://doi.org/10.1007/s12671-020-01472-w

Sorensen, L., Montserrrat, A., Engberg, J., & Bushway, S. (2021). *The thin blue line in schools: New evidence on school-based policing across the U.S.* Anneberg Institute at Brown University. https://eric.ed.gov/?id=ED616763

Soriano, M., Soriano, F., & Jimenez, E. (1994). School violence among culturally diverse populations: Sociocultural and institutional considerations. *School Psychology Review, 23*(2), 216–235.

Sorscher, N. (2022, December 22). The parallel pandemic: The impact of COVID-19 on the mental health of children with neurocognitive impairments. *Psychoanalytic Psychology.* Advance online publication. https://dx.doi.org/10.1037/pap0000436

Southern Baptist Conference. (2006). *On Southern Baptist Disaster Relief.* https://www.sbc.net/resource-library/resolutions/on-southern-baptist-disaster-relief/

Southwick, S. & Watson, P. (2015). The emerging scientific and clinical literature on resilience and psychological first aid. Post traumatic stress disorder: Patient interview, clinical assessment, and diagnosis. In N.C. Bernardy and M. J. Friedman (Eds.), *A practical guide to treatment: Pharmacological and psychotherapeutic approaches* (pp. 21–34). American Psychological Association.

Spangaro, J. M., Zwi, A. B., & Poulos, R. (2011). "Persist. Persist": A qualitative study of women's decisions to disclose and their perceptions of the impact of routine screening for intimate partner violence. *Psychology of Violence 1*(2), 150–162.

Spanno, T. K. (1990, April). *Eclipse of the self: The grief of the battered women.* Paper presented at Crisis Convening XIV, Chicago, IL, the United States.

Spar, J., & La Rue, A. (2006). *Clinical manual of geriatric psychiatry.* American Psychiatric Publishing.

Sparrow, K., Kwan, J., Howard, L., Fear, N., & MacManus, D. (2017). Systematic review of mental health disorders and intimate partner violence victimisation among military populations. *Social Psychiatry and Psychiatric Epidemiology, 52*(9), 1059–1080. https://doi.org/10.1007/s00127-017-1423-8

Spector, A., Thorgrimsen, L., & Woods, B. (2003) Efficacy of an evidence-based cognitive stimulation therapy programme for people with dementia: Randomised controlled trial. *British Journal of Psychiatry, 183,* 248–254.

Spencer, C., Mallory, A., Toews, M., Stith, S., & Wood, L. (2017). Why sexual assault survivors do not report to universities: A feminist analysis. *Family Relations, 66*(1), 166–179. https://doi.org/10.1111/fare.12241

Spencer, J., & Myer, R. A. (2007a). A population and economic overview of Cambria County, Pennsylvania following the 1977 Johnstown flood. *Disaster Prevention and Management, 16,* 259–264.

Spencer, J., & Myer, R. A. (2007b). A comparison of population and economies: Story County, Iowa, after the Great Flood of 1993 and Cambria County, Pennsylvania, after the 1977 Johnstown Flood. *Disaster Prevention and Management, 16,* 6–14.

Spencer, P., & Munch, S. (2003). Client violence toward social workers: The role of management in community mental health programs. *Social Work, 48,* 532–544.

Spidel, A., Greaves, C., Nicholls, T. L., Goldenson, J., & Dutton, D. G. (2013). Personality disorders, types of violence, and stress responses in females who perpetrate intimate partner violence. *Psychology, 4*(9B), 5–11. https://doi.org/10.4236/psych.2013.49A1002

Spiegel, D. (1981). Vietnam grief work under hypnosis. *American Journal of Clinical Hypnosis, 24,* 33–40.

Spiegel, D. (1989). Hypnosis in the treatment of victims of sexual abuse. *Psychiatric Clinics of North America, 12,* 295–305.

Spielberg, S. (Director). (1989). *Always* [Motion picture]. United Artists.

Spinazzola, J., van der Kolk, B., & Ford, J. D. (2018). When nowhere is safe: Trauma history antecedents of posttraumatic stress disorder and developmental trauma disorder in childhood. *Journal of Traumatic Stress, 31,* 631–642. http://dx.doi.org/10.1002/jts.22320

Spittal, M. J., Fedyszyn, I., Middleton, A., Bassilios, B., Gunn, J., Woodward, A., & Pirkis, J. (2015). Frequent callers to crisis helplines: Who are they and why do they call? *Australian and New Zealand Journal of Psychiatry, 49*(1), 54–64.

Spitzer, W. H., & Neely, M. K. (1992). Critical incident stress: The role of hospital-based social work in developing a statewide intervention system for first-responders delivering emergency services. *Social Work in Health Care, 18,* 39–58.

Spitzer, W. J., & Burke, L. (1993). A critical-incident stress debriefing program for hospital-based health care personnel. *Health & Social Work, 18*(2), pp. 149–156.

Sprague, S., Goslings, J. C., Hogentoren, C., de Milliano, S., Simunovic, N., Madden, K., & Bhandari, M. (2014). Prevalence of intimate partner violence across medical and surgical health care settings: A systematic review. *Violence Against Women, 20*(1), 118–136.

Sprang, G., & Steckler, Z. (2023). Traumatic stress symptom expression following indirect exposure: A multidisciplinary investigation. *Traumatology, 29*(2), 224–232. https://doi.org/10.1037/trm0000386

Sprang, G., Clark, J. J., & Whitt-Woosley, A. (2007). Compassion fatigue, compassion satisfaction, and burnout: Factors impacting a professional's quality of life. *Journal of Loss and Trauma, 12*(3), 259–280. https://doi.org/10.1080/15325020701238093

Sroufe, L., Egeland, B., Carlson, E., & Collins, W. (2005). *The development of the person: The Minnesota study of risk and adaptation from birth to adulthood.* Guilford Press.

Stalker, C. A., & Davies, F. (1995). Attachment organization and adaptation in sexually abused women. *Canadian Journal of Psychiatry, 40,* 234–240.

Stambor, Z. (2005). Responders must consider victim's culture, experts say. *Monitor on Psychology, 36*(11), 28.

Stamm, B. H. (2002). Measuring compassion satisfaction as well as fatigue: Developmental history of the Compassion Satisfaction and Fatigue Test. In C. R. Figley (Ed.), *Treating compassion fatigue* (pp. 107–119). Brunner/Routledge.

Stamm, B. H. (2005). *The ProQOL manual.* Sidran Press.

Stamm, B. H. (2010). *The concise ProQOL manual* (2nd ed.). ProQol.org. https://proqol.org/proqol-manual

Stampfl, T. G., & Levis, D. J. (1967). Essentials of implosive therapy: A learning-theory-based psychodynamic behavioral therapy. *Journal of Abnormal Psychology, 72*, 496–503.

Stanley, B., & Brown, G. K. (2012). Safety planning intervention: A brief intervention to mitigate suicide risk. *Cognitive and Behavioral Practice, 19*(2), 256–264. https://doi.org/10.1016/j.cbpra.2011.01.001

Stanley, I. H., & Marx, B. P. (2022). When a patient dies by suicide: A consideration of PTSD Criterion A and disentangling self-blame from medicolegal blame. *Clinical Psychology: Science and Practice, 29*(2), 121–123. https://doi.org/10.1037/cps0000087

Stanley, I. H., Hom, M. A., Marx, B. P., & Reger, M. A. (2020). Post-traumatic stress disorder and firearm ownership, access, and storage practices: A systematic review. *Clinical Psychology: Science and Practice, 27*(3), Article e12358. https://doi.org/10.1111/cpsp.12358

Star, K. L. (2015). The relationship between self-care practices, burnout, compassion fatigue, and compassion satisfaction among professional counselors and counselors-in-training. *Dissertation Abstracts International: Section A. Humanities and Social Sciences 75*(8-A(E)).

Stark, E., & Flitcraft, A. (1988). Personal power and institutional victimization: Treating the dual trauma of women battering. In F. M. Ochberg (Ed.), *Posttrauma therapy and victims of violence* (pp. 115–151). Brunner/Mazel.

State of North Carolina v. Oliver, 70 N. C. 60, 61–62 (1874).

Statista. (2023). Number of deaths from natural disaster events worldwide from 2000 to 2022. https://www.statista.com/statistics/510952/number-of-deaths-from-natural-disasters gloally/#:˜:text=In%202022%2C%20there%20were%20 roughly%2031%2C000%20reported,fatalities%20caused%20by%20natural%20disaster%20events%20worldwide

Steadman, H. J., Osher, F. C., Robbins, P. C., Case, B., & Samuels, S. (2009). Prevalence of serious mental illness among jail inmates. *Psychiatric Services, 60*, 761–765.

Steele, W., & Malchiodi, C. A. (2008). Interventions for parents of traumatized children. In C. A. Malchiodi (Ed.), *Creative interventions with traumatized children* (pp. 264–284). Guilford Press.

Steele, W., & Raider, M. (2001). *Structured sensory intervention for traumatized children, adolescents, and parents: Strategies to alleviate trauma.* Mellen Press.

Steenkamp, M. M., & Litz, B. T. (2014). One-size-fits-all approach to PTSD in the VA not supported by the evidence. *American Psychologist, 69*(7), 706.

Steenkamp, M. M., Nash, W. P., & Litz, B. T. (2013). Post-traumatic stress disorder: Review of the Comprehensive Soldier Fitness Program. *American Journal of Preventive Medicine, 44*(5), 507–512.

Steger, M. F., & Park, C. L. (2012). The creation of meaning following trauma: Meaning making and trajectories of distress and recovery. In R. A. McMackin, E. Newman, J. M. Fogler, & T. M. Keane (Eds.), *Trauma therapy in context: The science and craft of evidence–based practice.* (pp. 171–191). American Psychological Association.

Stein, M. B., Hannah, C., Koverola, C., Yehuda, R., Torchia, M., & McClarty, B. (1994, December). *Neuroanatomical and neuroendocrine correlates in adulthood of severe sexual abuse in childhood.* Paper presented at the 33rd Annual Meeting of the American College of Neuropsychopharmacology, San Juan, Puerto Rico.

Steinberg, A. M., Pynoos, R. S., Biggs, E. C., Gerrity, E. T., Layne, C. M., Vivrette, R. L., Beyerlein, B., & Fairbank, J. A. (2014). The National Child Traumatic Stress Network Core Data Set: Emerging findings, future directions, and implications for theory, research, practice, and policy. *Psychological Trauma: Theory Research and Practice, 6*(1), 50–57.

Steiner, E., Phillips, A., Moore, P., Jackson, B., & Augustine, C. (2021). *Challenges in implementing physical security measures in K–12 schools.* Rand Corporation. https://doi.org/10.7249/RR-A1077-2

Stephen Ministries, Saint Louis. (2023). *Transforming lives and equipping the saints for ministry since 1975.* stephenministries.org

Stephens, R. D. (1997). National trends in school violence: Statistics and prevention strategies. In A. P. Goldstein & J. C. Conoley (Eds.), *School violence prevention: A practical handbook* (pp. 72–90). Guilford Press.

Stern, A. (1938). Psychoanalytic investigation of and therapy in the borderline group of neuroses. *Psychoanalytic Quarterly, 7*, 467–489.

Steveson, S. (1991). Heading off violence with verbal de-escalation. *Journal of Psychosocial Nursing, 29*, 7–10.

Stewart, C., & MacNeil, G. (2005). Crisis intervention with chronic school violence and volatile situations. In A. R. Roberts (Ed.), *Crisis intervention handbook* (3rd ed., pp. 519–540). Oxford University Press.

Stewart, H. (2012). Regression post-Ferenczi. In J. Szekacs-Weisz & T. Keve (Eds.), *Ferenczi and his world: Rekindling the spirit of the Budapest school.* Karnac Books.

Stewart, R. W., Orengo-Aguayo, R. E., Cohen, J. A., Mannarino, A. P., & De Arellano, M. A. (2017). A pilot study of trauma-focused cognitive–behavioral therapy delivered via telehealth technology. *Child Maltreatment, 22*(4), 324–333. https://doi.org/10.1177/1077559517725403

Stewart-Sicking, J. A., & Mutai, W. W. (2012). Working with faith based communities in ecological counseling. In E.P. Cook (Ed.), *Understanding people in context: The ecological perspective in counseling.* (pp. 259–278). American Counseling Association.

Stilling, L. (1992). The pros and cons of physical restraints and behavior controls. *Journal of Psychosocial Nursing, 30*, 18–20.

Stöckl, H., & Penhale, B. (2015). Intimate partner violence and its association with physical and mental health symptoms among older women in Germany. *Journal of Interpersonal Violence, 30*(17), 3089–3111. https://doi.org/10.1177/0886260514554427

Stokols, D., Misra, S., Runnerstrom, J. M., & Hipp, J. A. (2009). Psychology in an age of ecological crisis: From personal angst to collective action. *American Psychologist, 64*(3), 181–193.

Stoltenborgh, M., Van IJzendoorn, M. H., Euser, E. M., & Bakermans-Kranenburg, M. J. (2011). A global perspective on child sexual abuse: Meta-analysis of prevalence around the world. *Child Maltreatment, 16*(2), 79–101. https://doi.org/10.1177/1077559511403920

Stone, C. (2013, May). Cyber bullying: Disruptive conduct or free speech? *ASCA School Counselor, 50*(5), 6–9.

Stone, C. (2015). Rural, suburban, or urban settings: Ethical behavior is context dependent. *ASCA School Counselor, 53*(2), 5–9.

Stone, C. (2017). *School counseling principles: Ethics and law.* American School Counselor Association.

Stone, C. (2020). Issues and lessons emerging from COVID-19. *ASCA School Counselor, 57*(5), 6–9.

Stone, D. A., & Conley, J. A. (2004). A partnership between Roberts' crisis intervention model and the multicultural competencies. *Brief Treatment & Crisis Intervention, 4*(4), 367–375. https://doi.org/10.1093/brief-treatment/mhh030

Stone, G. (2001). *Suicide and attempted suicide.* Da Capo Lifelong Books.

Stone, R., & Rothman, E. F. (2019). Opioid use and intimate partner violence: A systematic review. *Current Epidemiology Reports, 6*(2), 215–230. https://doi.org/10.1007/s40471-019-00197-2

Storer, H. L., Rodriguez, M., & Franklin, R. (2021). "Leaving was a process, not an event": The lived experience of dating and domestic violence in 140 characters. *Journal of Interpersonal Violence, 36*(11–12), NP6553–NP6580. https://doi.org/10.1177/0886260518816325

Stortch, D. D. (1991). Starting an in-hospital support group for victims of violence in the psychiatric hospital. *Psychiatric Hospital, 22*, 5–9.

Stosny, S. (1995). *Treating attachment abuse: A compassion approach.* Springer.

Straus, M. A., & Gelles, R. J. (1986). Societal change and change in family violence from 1975 to 1985 as revealed by two national surveys. *Journal of Marriage and Family, 48*, 465–479.

Straus, M. A., Gelles, R. J., & Steinmetz, S. (1980). *Behind closed doors: Violence in the American family.* Anchor/Doubleday.

Strawhun, J., Adams, N., & Huss, M. T. (2013). The assessment of cyberstalking: An expanded examination including social networking, attachment, jealousy, and anger in relation to violence and abuse. *Violence and Victims, 28*(4), 715–730. https://doi.org/10.1891/0886-6708.11-00145

Stroebe, M. S., Hansson, R. O., Schut, H., & Stroebe, W. (Eds.). (2008). *Handbook of bereavement research and practice: Advances in theory and intervention.* American Psychological Association.

Stroebe, M., Schut, H., & Stroebe, W. (2005). Attachment in coping with bereavement: A theoretical integration. *Review of General Psychology, 9*, 48–66.

Stroebe, W., & Schut, H. (1999). The dual process model of coping with bereavement: Rationale and description. *Death Studies, 23*, 197–224.

Stroebe, W., & Schut, H. (2001). Making meaning in the dual process model of coping with bereavement. In R. A. Neimeyer (Ed.), *Meaning reconstruction and the experience of loss* (pp. 55–69). American Psychological Association.

Stuart, G., Meehan, J., Moore, T., Morean, M., Hellmuth, J., & Follansbee, K. (2006). Examining a conceptual framework of intimate partner violence in men and women arrested for domestic violence. *Journal of Studies on Alcohol, 67*(1), 102–112.

Stuart-Maver, S. L., Foley Nicpon, M., Stuart-Maver, C. I. M., & Mahatmya, D. (2023). Trends and disparities in suicidal behaviors for heterosexual and sexual minority youth 1995–2017. *Psychology of Sexual Orientation and Gender Diversity, 10*(2), 279–291. https://doi.org/10.1037/sgd0000525

Stubenbort, K. M., Donnelly, G. R., & Cohen, J. (2001). Cognitive-behavioral group therapy for bereaved adults and children following an air disaster. *Group Dynamics: Theory, Research, and Practice, 5*, 261–176.

Stuhlmiller, C., & Dunning, C. (2000). Challenging the mainstream: From pathogenic to salutogenic models of post-trauma interventions. In J. M. Violanti, D. Paton, & C. Dunning (Eds.). *Posttraumatic stress intervention: Challenges, issues and perspectives* (pp. 10–42). Charles C. Thomas.

Stuhmiller, C., & Dunning, C. (2000). Concerns about debriefing: Challenging the mainstream. In B. Raphael & J. P. Wilson (Eds.), *Psychological debriefing: Theory, practice, and evidence* (pp. 305–320). Cambridge University Press.

Stuke, H., Priebe, K., Weilnhammer, V. A., Stuke, H., & Schoofs, N. (2023). Sparse models for predicting psychosocial impairments in patients with PTSD: An empirical Bayes approach. *Psychological Trauma: Theory, Research, Practice, and Policy, 15*(1), 80–87. https://doi.org/10.1037/tra0001279

Su, Y. & Chen, S. (2015). Emerging posttraumatic growth: A prospective study with pre- and posttraumatic psychological predictors. *Psychological Theory, Research, Practice and Policy, 7*(2),103–111.

Suarez, E., & Gadalla, T. M. (2010). Stop blaming the victim: A meta-analysis on rape myths. *Journal of Interpersonal Violence, 25*(11), 2010–2035. https://doi.org/10.1177/0886260509354503

Substance Abuse and Mental Health Services (Director). (2019, August 21). *Stress management techniques, healthy coping strategies, breathing exercises.* https://www.youtube.com/watch?v=IqpCCnmwNVY

Sue, D. W. (1992, Winter). The challenge of multiculturalism: The road less traveled. *American Counselor, 1*, 5–14.

Sue, D. W., & Torino, G. C. (2004). Racial-cultural competence: Awareness, knowledge, and skills. In *Handbook of racial-cultural psychology and counseling* (Vol. 2, pp. 3–18). John Wiley & Sons.

Sue, D. W., Sue, D., Neville, H. A., & Smith, L. (2022). *Counseling the culturally diverse: Theory and practice* (9th ed.). Wiley.

Sueki, H. (2022). Characteristics of train stations where railway suicides have occurred and locations within the stations. *Crisis: The Journal of Crisis Intervention and Suicide Prevention, 43*(1), 53–58. https://doi.org/10.1027/0227-5910/a000761

Suglia, S. F., Staudenmayer, J., Cohen, S., Enlow, M., Rice-Edwards, J., & Wright, R. (2010). Cumulative stress and cortisol disruption among Black and Hispanic pregnant women in an urban cohort. *Psychological Trauma: Theory, Research, Practice, and Policy, 2*(4), 326–334.

Suler, J. (2004). The online disinhibition effect. *Cyberpsychology and Behavior, 7*(3), 321–326.

Sullivan, C. M. (2018). Understanding how domestic violence support services promote survivor well-being: A conceptual model. *Journal of Family Violence, 33*(2), 123–131. https://doi.org/10.1007/s10896-017-9931-6

Sullivan, C. P., Smith, A. J., Lewis, M., & Jones, R. T. (2018). Network analysis of PTSD symptoms following mass violence. *Psychological Trauma: Theory, Research, Practice, and Policy, 10*(1), 58–66. https://doi.org/10.1037/tra0000237

Sullivan, J. (2002). How should HR and managers react in the aftermath of terrorism events? In D. D. Bass & R. Yep (Eds.), *Terrorism, trauma, and tragedies: A counselor's guide to preparing and responding* (pp. 67–68). American Counseling Association.

Sullivan, K. (2011). *The anti-bullying handbook.* SAGE.

Sullivan, L. (2004). Staff development and secondary traumatic stress among AIDS staff. *Dissertation Abstracts International: Section A. Humanities and Social Sciences, 64*(4), 2365.

Summerfield, D. (2005). What exactly is emergency or disaster "mental health"? *Bulletin of the World Health Organization, 83*(1), 76.

Suniti Bhat, C., Chang, S. H., & Linscott, J. A. (2010). Bullying as a media literacy issue. *New Horizons in Education, 58*(3), 44–57.

Swihart, J., Silliman, B., & McNeil, J. (1992). Death of a student: Implications for secondary school counselors. *School Counselor, 40*, 55–58.

Swirsky, J. M., Carfagno, L., Milligan, F., & Raiff, B. (2014, August). *A systematic review of studies utilizing serious games; 2014.* Paper presented at the American Psychological Association convention, Washington, D.C., the United States.

Synnott, J., Ioannou, M., Coyne, A., & Hemingway, S. (2018). A content analysis of online suicide notes: Attempted suicide versus attempt resulting in suicide. *Suicide and Life-Threatening Behavior, 48*(6), 767–778. https://doi.org/10.1111/sltb.12398

Szabo, Y. Z., Frankfurt, S., Kurz, A. S., Anderson, A., & McGuire, A. P. (2022). Resilience predicts posttraumatic cognitions after a trauma reminder task and subsequent positive emotion induction among veterans with PTSD. *Psychological Trauma: Theory, Research, Practice, and Policy, 14*(S1), S101–S108. https://doi.org/10.1037/tra0001143

Tabernero, C., Castillo-Mayén, R., Luque, B., & Cuadrado, E. (2020). Social values, self- and collective efficacy explaining behaviours in coping with Covid-19: Self-interested consumption and physical distancing in the first 10 days of confinement in Spain. *PLOS ONE, 15*(9), Article e0238682. https://doi.org/10.1371/journal.pone.0238682

Tak, S., Sweeney, M. H., Alterman, T., Baron, S., & Calvert, G. M. (2010). Workplace assaults on nursing assistants in US nursing homes: A multilevel analysis. *American Journal of Public Health, 100*(10), 1938–1945. https://doi.org/10.2105/AJPH.2009.185421

Taku, K., Cann, A, Calhoun, L. G., & Tedeschi, R. G. (2008). The factor structure of the Posttraumatic Growth Inventory: A comparison of five models using confirmatory factor analysis. *Journal of Traumatic Stress, 21*(2), 158–164.

Taku, K., Cann, A., Tedeschi, R. G., Calhoun, & L. G. (2015, May). Core beliefs shaken by an earthquake correlate with posttraumatic growth. *Psychological Trauma: Theory, Research, Practice, and Policy, 7*(6), 563–569. https://doi.org/10.1037/tra0000054

Talbot, A., Manton, M., & Dunn, P. J. (1995). Debriefing the debriefers: An intervention strategy to assist psychologists after a crisis. In G. S. Everly, Jr., & J. M. Lating (Eds.), *Psychotraumatology* (pp. 281–298). Plenum Press.

Tarasoff v. Regents of the University of California, 17 Cal. 3d 425, 551 P.2d 334, 131 Cal. Rptr. 14 (1976).

Tardiff, K. (1984a). Violence: The psychiatric patient. In J. T. Turner (Ed.), *Violence in the medical care setting: A survival guide* (pp. 33–55). Aspen Systems.

Tardiff, K. (1984b). *The psychiatric uses of seclusion and restraint.* American Psychiatric Association Press.

Tardiff, K. (1989). *Assessment and management of violent patients.* American Psychiatric Association Press.

Tardiff, K. (2003). Violence. In R. E. Hales, S. C. Yudofsky, & J. A. Talbot (Eds.), *Textbook of clinical psychiatry* (4th ed., pp. 1489–1509). American Psychiatric Press.

Tarrier, N., & Humphreys, A. L. (2003). PTSD and the social support of the interpersonal environment: The development of social cognitive behavior therapy. *Journal of Cognitive Psychotherapy, 17*(2), 187–198.

Tarvydas, V., & Ng, H. K. Y. (2012). Ethical perspectives on trauma work. In L. L. Levers (Ed.), *Trauma counseling: Theories and interventions.* (pp. 521–539). Springer.

Taulbee, L. R. (1978). Reality orientation: A therapeutic group activity for elderly persons. In I. M. Burnside (Ed.), *Working with the elderly: Group process and techniques* (pp. 206–218). Duxbury Press.

Taulbee, L. R., & Folsom, J. C. (2006). Reality orientation for geriatric patients. *Psychiatric Services.* https://doi.org/10.1176/ps.17.5.133

Taylor, D. H., Kuchibhatia, M., Østbye, T., Plassman, B. L., & Clipp, E. C. (2008). The effect of spousal caregiving and bereavement on depressive symptoms. *Aging & Mental Health, 12*(1), 100–107.

Taylor, F. (2003). Tiagabine for posttraumatic stress disorder: A case series of 7 women. *Journal of Clinical Psychiatry, 64*(12), 1421–1425.

Taylor, R. J., Chatters, L. M., & Levin, J. S. (2004). *Religion in the lives of African Americans: Social, psychological, and health perspectives.* SAGE.

Taylor, S. (2003). Outcome predictors for three PTSD treatments: Exposure therapy, EMDR, and relaxation training. *Journal of Cognitive Psychotherapy, 17*(2), 149–161.

Taylor, S. (2022). The psychology of pandemics: Lessons learned for the future. *Canadian Psychology/Psychologie canadienne, 63*(2), 233–246. https://doi.org/10.1037/cap0000303

Taylor, S. E. (2007). Social support. In H. S. Friedman & R. C. Silver (Eds.), *Foundations of health psychology* (pp. 145–171). Oxford University Press.

Taylor, Z. W. (2018). Unreadable and underreported: Can college students comprehend how to report sexual assault? *Journal of College Student Development, 59*(2), 248–253. https://doi.org/10.1353/csd.2018.0023

Taylor-Austin, L. (2023). *Counseling gang members.* Taylor-Austin Group. https://thetayloraustingroup.com/our-experts/counseling-gang-members/

Tayyib, N. M. (2022). An action plan to address the mental health impact of COVID-19 on communities: Five effective strategies. *Psychological Services, 19*(Suppl 2), 5–16. https://doi.org/10.1037/ser0000575

Tedeschi, R. G., & Calhoun, L. G. (1995). *Trauma & transformation: Growing in the aftermath of suffering.* SAGE.

Tedeschi, R. G., & Calhoun, L. G. (2003). Routes to posttraumatic growth through cognitive processing. In D. Paton, J. M. Volanti, & L. M. Smith (Eds.), *Promoting capabilities to manage posttraumatic stress: Perspective on resilience* (pp. 12–26). Charles C Thomas.

Tedeschi, R. G., & Calhoun, L. G. (2004). Posttraumatic growth: Conceptual foundations and empirical evidence. *Psychological Inquiry, 15*(1), 1–18.

Tedeschi, R. G., & Calhoun, L. G. (2006). Time of change? The spiritual challenges of bereavement and loss. *Omega: Journal of Death and Dying, 53*(1/2), 105–116.

Tedeschi, R. G., & Calhoun, L. G. (2009). The clinician as expert companion. In C. L. Park, S. C. Lechner, M. H. Antoni, & A. Stanton (Eds.), *Medical illness and positive life change: Can crisis lead to personal transformation?* (pp. 215–235). American Psychological Association.

Tedeschi, R. G., & Calhoun, L. G. (2010). A surprise attack, a surprise result: Posttraumatic growth through expert companionship. In G. W. Burns (Ed.), *Happiness, healing, enhancement: Your case book collection of applying positive psychology in therapy* (pp. 226–236). John Wiley & Sons.

Tedeschi, R. G., & Calhoun, L. G. (2012). Pathways to personal transformation: Theoretical and empirical developments. In P. T. Wong (Ed.). *The human quest for meaning: Theories, research, and applications* (2nd ed.). *Personality and clinical psychology series* (pp. 559–572). Routledge/Taylor & Francis Group.

Tedeschi, R. G., & Calhoun, L. G. (2021). Post traumatic growth and expert companionship in grief therapy. In R. A. Neimeyer & D. C. Vaughans (Eds.). *New techniques of grief therapy* (pp.68–72).Routledge.http://doi.org/10.4324/9781351069120-7

Tedeschi, R. G., & McNally, R. J. (2011). Can we facilitate posttraumatic growth in combat veterans? *American Psychologist, 66*(1), 19–24.

Tedeschi, R. G., Park, C. L., & Calhoun, L. G. (Eds.). (1998). *Posttraumatic growth: Positive changes in the aftermath of crisis.* Erlbaum.

Teller, J. L., Munetz, M. R., Gil, K. M., & Ritter, C. (2006). Crisis intervention team training for police officers responding to mental disturbance calls. *Psychiatric Services, 57*(2), 232–237.

Templeton, K., Bernstein, C. A., Sukhera, J., Nora, L. M., Newman, C., Burstin, H., Guille, C., Lynn, L., Schwarze, M. L., Sen, S., & Busis, N. (2019). Gender-based differences in burnout: Issues faced by women physicians. *NAM Perspectives.* https://doi.org/10.31478/201905a

TENTS. (2011). *TENTS–TP: The European Network for Traumatic Stress—Training and Practice.* www.estss.org/uploads/2011/07/146TENTS-TP_TTT_Trainers_manual_draft_1-18th_Jan.pdf

ter Kuile, H., & Ehring, T. (2014). Predictors of changes in religiosity after trauma: Trauma, religiosity, and posttraumatic stress disorder. *Psychological Trauma: Theory, Research, Practice, and Policy, 6,* 353–360. https://doi.org/10.1037/a0034880

Terr, L. C. (1979). Children of Chowchilla: Study of psychic trauma. *Psychoanalytic Study of the Child, 34,* 547–623.

Terr, L. C. (1981). "Forbidden games": Posttraumatic child's play. *Journal of the American Academy of Child Psychiatry, 22,* 221–230.

Terr, L. C. (1983). Chowchilla revisited: The effects of psychic trauma four years after a school-bus kidnapping. *American Journal of Psychiatry, 140,* 1543–1550.

Terr, L. C. (1995). Childhood traumas: An outline and overview. In G. S. Everly, Jr., & J. M. Lating (Eds.), *Psychotraumatology* (pp. 301–320). Plenum Press.

Tervalon, M., & Murray-García, J. (1998). Cultural humility versus cultural competence: A critical distinction in defining physician training outcomes in multicultural education. *Journal of Health Care for the Poor and Underserved, 9*(2), 117–125. https://doi.org/10.1353/hpu.2010.0233

Tesarz, J., Leisner, S., Gerhardt, A., Janke, S., Seidler, G., Eich, W., & Hartmann, M. (2014). Effect of eye movement desensitization and reprocessing (EMDR) treatment in chronic pain patients: A systematic review. *Pain Medicine, 15*(2), 247–263.

Thackrey, M. (1987). *Therapeutics for aggression.* Human Sciences Press.

The Joint Commission. (2018). Physical and verbal violence against healthcare workers. *Sentinel Event Alert, 59.* https://jointcommission.org

The National Domestic Violence Hotline. (2015). *We're here to listen.* www.thehotline.org

Theriot, M. T. (2009). School resource officers and criminalization of student behavior. *Journal of Criminal Behavior, 37,* 280–287.

Theuninck, A. C., Lake, N., & Gibson, S. (2010). HIV-related posttraumatic stress disorder: Investigating the traumatic stress. *AIDS Patient Care and STDS, 24*(8), 458–491.

Thoburn, J. W., Bentley, J. A., Ahman, Z. S., & Jones, K. C. (2012). International disaster psychology ethics: A social justice model embedded in a system paradigm. *Traumatology, 18*(4), 79–85. https://doi.org/10.1177/1534765612444880

Thomae, C. (2002). *The incident command system and standard operating procedures for a school crisis team.* Arizona School Counselor Association.

Thomas, A. M., & Levitt, D. (2010, August). Self-care: An ethical obligation and preventive tool. *Counseling Today,* 44–46.

Thomas, B. J. (2007). The relationship between affect balance, self-care behavior, and secondary traumatic stress reactions. *Dissertation Abstracts International: Section B. The Sciences and Engineering, 67*(8), 4145.

Thomas, C., Kitchen, D., & Smith, A. (2005). The management of aggression care plans: Implementation and efficacy in a forensic learning disability service. *British Journal of Forensic Science, 7*(2), 3–9.

Thomas, M., Kohli, V., & Choi, J. (2014). Correlates of job burnout among human services workers: Implications for workforce retention. *Journal of Sociology and Social Welfare, 41*(4), 69–90.

Thomas, R. B., & Wilson, J. P. (2004). Issues and controversies in the understanding and diagnosis of compassion fatigue, vicarious traumatization and secondary traumatic stress disorder. *International Journal of Emergency Mental Health, 6*(2), 81–92.

Thompson, C. L., & Rudolph, L. B. (1992). *Counseling children.* Brooks/Cole.

Thompson, I., Amatea, E., & Thompson, E. (2014). Personal and contextual predictors of mental health counselors' compassion fatigue and burnout. *Journal of Mental Health Counseling, 36*(1), 58–77. https://doi.org/10.17744/mehc.36.1.p61m73373m4617r3

Thompson, R. A. (2004). *Crisis intervention and crisis management: Strategies that work in schools and communities.* Brunner-Rutledge.

Thorne, F. C. (1973). Eclectic psychotherapy. In R. Corsini (Ed.), *Current psychotherapies* (pp. 445–486). F. E. Peacock.

Thorne, F. C. (Ed.). (1968). *Psychological case handling: Vol. 1. Establishing the conditions necessary for counseling and psychotherapy.* Clinical Psychology Publishing.

Thornton, P. T. (1992). The relation of coping, appraisal, and burnout in mental health workers. *Journal of Psychology, 126,* 261–271.

Threat assessment team formation. (2008). Virginia Code 23-31 9.2:3C.

Threat of violence. (2008). Virginia Code 23-31 92:10.

Tillman, K., & Rust, J. (2011). Kids supporting kids. *ASCA School Counselor, 49*(1), 18–23.

Tinnin, L., Bills, L., & Gantt, L. (2002). Short-term treatment of simple and complex PTSD. In M. Williams & J. Sommer (Eds.), *Simple and complex post-traumatic stress disorder: Strategies for comprehensive treatment in clinical practice* (pp. 99–118). Haworth Press.

Tjaden, P., & Thoennes, N. (2000). *Extent, nature, and consequences of intimate partner violence.* National Institute of Justice, and Centers for Disease Control and Prevention.

Tjersland, O. A., Mossige, S., Gulbrandsen, W., Jensen, T. K., & Reichelt, S. (2006). Helping families when child sexual abuse is suspected but not proven. *Child and Family Social Work, 11,* 297–306.

Toker, S., Shirom, A., Shapira, I., Berliner, S., & Melamed, S. (2005). The association between burnout, depression, anxiety, and inflammation biomarkers: C-reactive protein and fibrinogen in men and women. *Journal of Occupational Health Psychology, 10*(4), 344–362.

Tolmach, J. (1985). "There ain't nobody on my side." A new day treatment program for black urban youth. *Journal of Clinical Child Psychology, 14,* 214–219.

Tomine, S. (1986). Private practice in gerontological counseling. *Journal of Counseling and Development, 68,* 406–409.

Tomlinson-Clarke, S. M., & Georges, C. M. (2014). DSM-5: A commentary on integrating multicultural and strength-based considerations into counseling training and practice. *The Professional Counselor, 4*(3), 272–281. https://doi.org/10.15241/stc.4.3.272

Torres, A., Garcia-Esteve, L., Navarro, P., Tarragona, M. J., Imaz, M. L., Ascaso, C., Gelabert, E., Plaza, A., Subirà, S., Valdés, M., & Martín-Santos, R. (2013). Relationship between intimate partner violence, depressive symptomatology, and personality traits. *Journal of Family Violence, 28*(4), 369–379. https://doi.org/10.1007/s10896-013-9502-4

Torrey, E. F., Kennard, A. D., & Eslinger, D. (2010). *More mentally ill persons in jails and prisons than hospitals: A survey of the states.* Treatment Advocacy Center and National Sheriff's Association.

Torrey, E. F., Zdanowicz, M., & Kennard A. (2014). *The treatment of persons with mental illness in prisons and jails: A state survey.* Treatment Advocacy Center and National Sheriff's Association.

Tortella-Feliu, M., Botella, C., Llabres, J., Breton-Lopez, J., del Amo, A., Banos, R., & Gelabert, J. (2011). Virtual reality versus computer-aided exposure treatments for fear of flying. *Behavior Modification, 35*(1), 3–30.

Towey-Swift, K. D., Lauvrud, C., & Whittington, R. (2022). Acceptance and commitment therapy (ACT) for professional staff burnout: A systematic review and narrative synthesis of controlled trials. *Journal of Mental Health,* 1–13. https://doi.org/10.1080/09638237.2021.2022628

Tran, U.S., Birnbaum, L., Burzler, M. A., Hegewisch, U. J. C., Ramazanova, D., & Voracek, M. (2022). Self-reported mindfulness accounts for the effects of mindfulness interventions and nonmindfulness controls on self-reported mental health: A preregistered systematic review and three-level meta-analysis of 146 randomized controlled trials. *Psychological Bulletin, 148*(1-2), 86–106. https://doi.org/10.1037/bul0000359

Trauma-Focused Cognitive Behavioral Therapy & National Therapist Certification Program. (2021a, March 26). *About trauma-focused cognitive behavior therapy (TF-CBT)—TF-CBT certification program.* https://tfcbt.org/about/

Trauma-Focused Cognitive Behavioral Therapy & National Therapist Certification Program. (2021b, March 26). *TF-CBT implementation resources—TF-CBT certification program.* https://tfcbt.org/resources/implementation/

Treatment Advocacy Center. (2014). The treatment of persons with mental illness in prisons and jails. *Research from the Treatment Advocacy Center.* http://www.tacreports.org/treatment-behind-bars

Treatment Advocacy Center. (2014). *The treatment of persons with mental illness in prisons and jails.* Research from the Treatment Advocacy Center.: Author. http//: www.racreports.org/treatment-behind-bars.

Treworgy, S. L. (2010). *Supportive and strength-based supervision as predictive factors of compassion fatigue, burnout and compassion satisfaction among female sexual assault advocates.* University of La Verne. https://www.proquest.com/openview/b248263eed1e3373bd826e9ee797e45a/1?pq-origsite=gscholar&cbl=18750&casa_token=1e3mnTXUhA0AAAAA:iultzGQqZx3anjtXoxzQqAGiBpuN4uwI8jEvZZQlxd9ML74tTFzsTwMB0KAJnqTYESn3rahZP1At

Trimble, M. R. (1985). Post-traumatic stress disorder: History of a concept. In C. R. Figley (Ed.), *Trauma and its wake: The study of post-trauma stress disorder* (pp. 5–14). Brunner/Mazel.

Triplett, K., Tedeschi, R., Cann, A., Calhoun, L., & Reeve, C. (2011). Posttraumatic growth, meaning in life, and life satisfaction in response to trauma. *Psychological Trauma: Theory, Research, Practice, and Policy, 4*(4), 400–410.

Trotter, S. (2003, June). *Handling a crisis at school.* Paper presented at the American School Counselor Association Conference, St. Louis, MO, the United States.

Truscott, D., Evans, J., & Mansell, S. (2019). Outpatient psychotherapy with dangerous clients: A model for clinical decision making. In E. Y. Drogin (Ed.). *Ethical conflicts in psychology* (pp. 287–308). American Psychological Association.

Tsirimokou, A., Kloess, J. A., & Dhinse, S. K. (2022). Vicarious post-traumatic growth in professionals exposed to traumatogenic material: A systematic literature review. *Trauma, Violence, & Abuse, 24*(3), 1848–1866. https://doi.org/10.1177/15248380221082079

Ttofi, M., & Farrington, D. (2011). Effectiveness of school-based programs to reduce bullying: A systematic and meta-analytic review. *Journal of Experimental Criminology, 7,* 27–56. https://doi.org/10.1007/s11292-010-9109-1

Tuber, S., Boesch, K., Gorkin, J., & Terry, M. (2014). Chronic early trauma as a childhood syndrome and its relationship to play. In C. Malchiodi & D.A. Crenshaw (Eds.), *Creative arts and play therapy for attachment problems: Creative arts and play therapy* (pp. 215–226).

Tubesing, D. A., & Strosahl, S. G. (1976). *Wholistic health centers: Survey research report.* Society for Wholistic Medicine.

Tubesing, N. L., & Tubesing, D. A. (1982). The treatment of choice: Selecting stress skills to suit the individual and the situation. In W. S. Paine (Ed.), *Job stress and burnout* (pp. 155–172). SAGE.

Tucker, E. (2022, January 22). *Domestic incidents are highly dangerous for police officers, experts say.* CNN. https://www.cnn.com/2022/01/22/us/domestic-incidents-police-officers-danger/index.html

Tucker, P., Pfefferbaum, B., Nixon, S., & Foy, D. (1999). Trauma and recovery among adults highly exposed to a community disaster. *Psychiatric Annals, 29*(2), 78–83.

Tuckey, M. (2007). Issues in the debriefing debate for the emergency services: Moving research outcomes forward. *Clinical Psychology: Science and Practice, 14*(2), 106–116. https://doi.org/10.1111/j.1468-2850.2007.00069.x

Tuerk, P. W., Yoder, M., Ruggiero, K. J., Gros, D. F., & Acierno, R. (2010). A pilot study of prolonged exposure therapy for post-traumatic stress disorder delivered via telehealth technology. *Journal of Traumatic Stress, 23,* 116–123.

Tunick, R. A., Gavin, J. A., DeMaso, D. R., & Meyer, E. C. (2013). Pediatric psychology critical care consultation: An emerging subspecialty. *Clinical Practice in Pediatric Psychology, 1*(1), 42–54.

Turchik, J. A., & Hassija, C. M. (2014). Female sexual victimization among college students: Assault severity, health risk behaviors, and sexual functioning. *Journal of Interpersonal Violence, 29*(13), 2439–2457. https://doi.org/10.1177/0886260513520230

Turnbull, J., Aitken, I., Black, L., & Patterson, B. (1990, June). Turn it around: Short-term management for aggression and anger. *Journal of Psychosocial Nursing and Mental Health Services, 28,* 7–13.

Turner, J. (Ed.). (1984). *Violence in the medical care setting: A survival guide.* Aspen Systems.

Turner, S. F., & Shapiro, C. H. (1986). Battered women: Mourning the death of a relationship. *Social Work, 31,* 372–376.

Turner, S. W., McFarlane, A. C., & van der Kolk, B. A. (1996). The therapeutic environment and new explorations in the treatment of posttraumatic stress disorder. In B. A. van der Kolk, A. C. McFarlane, & L. Weisaeth (Eds.), *Traumatic stress* (pp. 537–558). Guilford Press.

Turns, D. M. (1993). Institutional response to violent incidents. In P. E. Blumenreich & S. Lewis (Eds.). *Managing the violent patient: A clinician's guide* (pp. 131–135). Brunner-Mazel.

Turns, D. M., & Blumenreich, P. E. (1993). Epidemiology. In P. E. Blumenreich & S. Lewis (Eds.), *Managing the violent patient: A clinician's guide* (pp. 5–20). Brunner-Mazel.

Tuttle, A. (1991). *Advantages and strategies of telephone crisis counseling* [audiotape]. Memphis, TN: The Crisis Center.

Tutty, L. M., & Rothery, M. A. (2002). Beyond shelters: Support groups and community-based advocacy for abused women. In A. R. Roberts (Ed.), *Handbook of domestic violence: Intervention strategies* (pp. 396–418). Oxford University Press.

Tutty, L. M., Bidgood, B. A., & Rothery, M. A. (1993). Support groups for battered women: Research on their efficacy. *Journal of Family Violence, 8,* 325–343.

21st Century Cures Act, pub. L114-255, Title XIV, Subtitle B Section 14021, codified as amended at 41 USC. 3797aa Title I, Section 2991.

Twomey, C., O'Reilly, G., Byrne, M., Bury, M., White, A., Kissane, S., McMahon, A., & Clancy, N. (2014). A randomized control trial of the computerized CBT programme, moodGYM, for public mental health service users waiting for intervention. *British Journal of Clinical Psychology, 53*(4), 433–450.

Tyrka, A. R., Burgers, D. E., Philip, N. S., Price, L. H., & Carpenter, L. (2013). The neurobiological correlates of childhood adversity and implications for treatment. *Acta Psychiatria Scandinavia, 128*(6), 434–447.

Tyson, R., Law, C., Reed, S., Johnsey, E., Aruna, O., & Hall, S. (2016). Preventing suicide and self-harm evaluating the efficacy of a helpline from a service user and helpline worker perspective. *Crisis, 37*(6), 353–360. https://doi.org/10.1027/0227-5910/a000390

U.S. Census Bureau. (2023). *Losing our parents: Recent statistics on parent mortality during the COVID-19 pandemic.*

U.S. Department of Education. (2003). *Practical information on crisis planning: A guide for schools and communities.* www2.ed.gov/admins/lead/safety/emergencyplan/crisisplanning.pdf

U.S. Department of Education. (2007). Practical information on crisis planning: A guide for schools and communities. https://www2.ed.gov/admins/lead/safety/crisisplanning.html

U.S. Department of Education. (2015a). *Anti-bully tool kit.* www.ed.gov/blog/tag/bullying/

U.S. Department of Education. (2015b). *Working in the community.* https://www.stopbullying.gov/prevention/in-the-community

U.S. Department of Education. (2020). *Guide for developing high quality school emergency operations plans.* https://www.fema.gov/sites/default/files/2020-07/guide-developing-school-emergency-operations-plans.pdf

U.S. Department of Health and Human Services, Public Health Service. (2021). *School-associated violent death study.* https://www.cdc.gov/violenceprevention/youthviolence/schoolviolence/SAVD.html

U.S. Department of Health and Human Services. (2003). *Developing cultural competence in disaster mental health programs: Guiding principles and recommendations.* DHHS Pub. No. SMA 3828. Center for Mental Health Services, Substance Abuse and Mental Health Services Administration.

U.S. Department of Health and Human Services. (2015). *Stop Bullying.* www.stopbullying.gov

U.S. Department of Justice, Bureau of Justice Statistics. (1998). *Data from the National Crime Victimization Survey 1992–1996.*

U.S. Department of Justice, Bureau of Justice Statistics. (2001). *Data from the National Crime Victimization Survey 1993–1999.*

U.S. Department of Justice. (2000). *Response to terrorism victims: Oklahoma City and beyond.*

U.S. Department of Justice. (2022). *School safety: Special feature.* Office of Justice Programs. https://www.ojp.gov/feature/school-safety/overview

U.S. Department of Labor, Bureau of Labor Statistics. (2015). *A look at violence in the workplace against psychiatric aides and psychiatric technicians.* https://www.bls.gov/opub/mlr/2015/article/a-look-at-violence-in-the-workplace-against-psychiatric-aides-and-psychiatric-technicians.htm#:~:text=Psychiatric%20aides%20and%20technicians%20are,it%20is%2038%20times%20higher

U.S. Department of Veterans Affairs. (2006). *Psychological first aid: Field operations guide.* http://ptsd.va.gov/professional/manuals/psych-first-aid.asp

U.S. Department of Veterans Affairs. (2014). Veterans crisis line. http://veteranscrisisline.net/

U.S. Department of Veterans Affairs: National Center for PTSD. (2014). *PTSD Coach.* https://www.va.gov/VHALEADERSHIPDEVELOPMENT/Programs/Leadership_Coaches_Mentors.asp

U.S. Department of Veterans Affairs: National Center for PTSD. (2023). *Clinician-Administered PTSD Scale for DSM-5 (CAPS-5).* https://www.ptsd.va.gov/professional/assessment/adult-int/caps.asp

U.S. Department of Veterans Affairs. (n.d.). *Types of debriefing following disasters.* https://www.ptsd.va.gov/professional/treat/type/debrief_after_disasters.asp

U.S. Office of Juvenile Justice and Delinquency Prevention. (1995). *A comprehensive response to America's youth gang problem.*

Ukpong, D., Owoeye, O., Udofia, O., Abasiubong, F., & Ukpong, S. (2018). *Violence against health staff: A survey in a Nigerian psychiatric hospital.* Cambridge University Press.

Ulibarri, M., Strathdee, S., Lozada, R., Maigs-Rodriquez, C., Amaro, H., O'Campo, P., & Pattterson, T. L. (2010). Intimate partner violence among female sex workers in two Mexico-U.S. border cities: Partner characteristics and HIV risk behaviors as correlates of abuse. *Psychological Trauma: Theory, Research, Practice, and Policy, 2*(4), 318–325.

Underwood, M. M., & Clark, C. (2002). Using metaphor to help children cope with trauma: An example from September 11th. In D. D. Bass & R. Yep (Eds.), *Terrorism, trauma, and tragedies: A counselor's guide to preparing and responding* (pp. 33–36). American Counseling Association.

University of Cincinnati Center for Police Research and Policy. (n.d.-a). *Assessing the impact of co-responder team programs: A review of the research.* http://theiacp.org

University of Cincinnati Center for Police Research and Policy. (n.d.-b). *Assessing the impact of resolution and home treatment teams: A review of the research.* http://theiacp.org

University of Denver. (2023). *Master's concentration: Emergency Planning and Response.* https://universitycollege.du.edu/smgt/degree/masters/emergency-planning-and-response-online/degreeid/420?gad=1&gclid=EAIaIQobChMIms_a38ORgAMVYijUAR3I9wirEAAYASAAEgI_qfD_BwE#curriculum

University of Nebraska-Lincoln. (n.d.) *Behavior and discipline briefs by tier.* Student Engagement Project. https://k12engagement .unl.edu/behavior-and-discipline-briefs-tier

University of South Dakota. (2023). *Disaster mental health.* https:// www.usd.edu/Academics/Graduate-Programs/Disaster -Mental-Health

Unterhitzenberger, J., Eberle-Sejari, R., Rassenhofer, M., Sukale, T., Rosner, R., & Goldbeck, L. (2015). Trauma-focused cognitive behavioral therapy with unaccompanied refugee minors: A case series. *BMC Psychiatry, 15*(1), 260. https://doi.org/10.1186 /s12888-015-0645-0

Urhausen, M. T. (2015). Eye movement desensitization and reprocessing and art therapy with traumatized children. In C. A. Malchiodi (Ed.), *Creative interventions with traumatized children* (2nd ed., pp. 45–74). Guilford Press.

Ursano, R., Fullerton, C., Vance, K., & Kao, T. (1999). Posttraumatic stress disorder and identification in disaster workers. *American Journal of Psychiatry, 156*(3), 353–359.

USA Facts. (2023). *Natural disaster deaths.* https://usafacts.org /data/topics/security-safety/fire-and-disaster/crisis-protection /natural-disaster-deaths/#:˜:text=In%202022%2C%20the%20 total%20number%20of%20deaths%20related,decrease%20 of%2035%25%20or%20250%20deaths%20from%202021

Ussery, C. (2022). The myth of the "ideal victim": Combatting misconceptions of expected demeanour in sexual assault survivors. *Appeal: Review of Current Law & Law Reform, 27*, 3–18.

Vahtera, J., Kivimäki, M., Väänänen, A., Linna, A., Pentti, J., Helenius, H., & Elovainio, M. (2006). Sex differences in health effects of family death or illness: Are women more vulnerable than men? *Psychosomatic Medicine, 68*(2), 283–291. https://doi .org/10.1097/01.psy.0000203238.71171.8d

Valecha, R. (2020). An investigation of interaction patterns in emergency management: A case study of the crash of Continental Flight 3407. *Information Systems Frontiers, 22*(8), 897–909. http://doi.org/10.1007/s10796-019-09896-z

Valentine, S. E., Peitzmeier, S. M., King, D. S., O'Cleirigh, C., Marquez, S. M., Presley, C., & Potter, J. (2017). Disparities in exposure to intimate partner violence among transgender/ gender nonconforming and sexual minority primary care patients. *LGBT Health, 4*(4), 260–267. https://doi.org/10.1089/ lgbt.2016.0113

Van Auken, S. (1979). Youth counselor burnout. *Personnel and Guidance Journal, 58*, 143–144.

Van Ballegoojien, W., Cuijpers, P., van Straten, A., Karvotaki, E., Andersson, G., Smit, J., & Riper, H. (2014). Adherence to internet-based and face-to-face cognitive behavioural therapy for depression: A meta-analysis. *PLOS One, 9*(7), e100674.

Van Brunt, B. (2015). *Harm to others: The assessment and treatment of dangerousness.* American Counseling Association.

van de Ven, P., Kleber, R. J., & van der Velden, P. G. (2022). Do initial mental health, somatic, and social problems predict post-disaster lack of social support in the medium term? A latent profile analysis. *Psychological Trauma: Theory, Research, Practice, and Policy, 14*(1), 124–131. https://doi.org/10.1037/tra0000919

van den Brink, R. H., Hooijschuur, A., van Os, T. W., Savenije, W., & Wiersma, D. (2010). Routine violence risk assessment in community forensic mental healthcare. *Behavioral Sciences & the Law, 28*(3), 396–410.

van den Eynde, J., & Veno, A. (1999). Coping with disastrous events: An empowerment model for community healing. In R. Gist & B. Lubin (Eds.), *Response to disaster: Psychosocial, community, and ecological approaches* (pp. 167–192). Brunner/Mazel.

Van der Heijden, I., & Swartz, S. (2010). Bereavement, silence, and culture within a peer-led HIV/AIDS-prevention strategy for vulnerable children in South Africa. *African Journal of AIDS Research, 9*(1), 41–50.

van der Kolk, B. A. (1996a). The body keeps the score: Approaches to the psychobiology of posttraumatic stress disorder. In B. A. van der Kolk, A. C. McFarlane, & L. Weisaeth (Eds.), *Traumatic stress* (pp. 214–241). Guilford Press.

van der Kolk, B. A. (1996b). Trauma and memory. In B. A. van der Kolk, A. C. McFarlane, & L. Weisaeth (Eds.), *Traumatic stress* (pp. 279–297). Guilford Press.

van der Kolk, B. A., & McFarlane, A. C. (1996). The black hole of trauma. In B. A. van der Kolk, A. C. McFarlane, & L. Weisaeth (Eds.), *Trauma stress: The effects of overwhelming experience on the mind, body, and society* (pp. 3–23). Guilford Press.

van der Kolk, B. A., McFarlane, A. C., & van der Hart, O. (1996). A general approach to treatment of posttraumatic stress disorder. In B. A. van der Kolk, A. C. McFarlane, & L. Weisaeth (Eds.), *Traumatic stress* (pp. 417–440). Guilford Press.

van der Kolk, B. A., van der Hart, O., & Burbridge, J. (2002). Approaches to the treatment of PTSD. In M. Williams & J. Sommer (Eds.), *Simple and complex post-traumatic stress disorder: Strategies for comprehensive treatment in clinical practice* (pp. 23–45). Haworth Press.

van der Kolk, B. A., Weisaeth, L., & van der Hart, O. (1996). History of trauma in psychiatry. In B. A. van der Kolk, A. C. McFarlane, & L. Weisaeth (Eds.), *Traumatic stress* (pp. 47–74). Guilford Press.

Van Dusen, S., & Courtois, C.A. (2015). Spirituality, religion, and complex developmental trauma. In D. F. Walker, C. A. Courtois, & J. D. Aten (Eds.), *Spiritually oriented psychotherapy for trauma* (pp. 189–210). American Psychological Association.

Van Emmerik, A. A., Kamphuis, J. H., Hulsbosch, A. M., & Emmelkamp, P. M. (2002). Single session debriefing after psychological trauma: A meta-analysis. *The Lancet, 360*(9335), 766–771. https://doi.org/10.1016/S0140-6736(02)09897-5

Van Ommeren, M., Saxena, S., & Saraceno, S. (2005). Mental and social health during and after acute emergencies: Emerging consensus? *Bulletin of the World Health Organization, 83*(1), 71–75.

Van Orden, K. A., Cukrowicz, K. C., Witte, T. K., & Joiner, T. E. Jr. (2012). Thwarted belongingness and perceived burdensomeness: Construct validity and psychometric properties of the Interpersonal Needs Questionnaire. *Psychological Assessment, 24*(1), 197–215. https://doi.org/10.1037/a0025358

Van Praagh, J. (2000). *Healing grief: Reclaiming life after any loss.* Random House.

Van Puyenbroeck, J., & Maes, B. (2006). Program development of reminiscence group work for aging people with intellectual disabilities. *Journal of Intellectual & Developmental Disability, 31*(3), 139–147.

Van Tongeren, D. R., Green, J. D., & Richmond, T. (2022). In the valley of the shadow of death: The existential benefits of imbuing life and death with meaning. *Psychology of Religion and Spirituality, 14*(3), 395–405. https://doi.org/10.1037/rel0000417

van Vuuren, C., van der Wal, M., Cuijpers, P., & Chinapaw, M. (2021). Are suicidal thoughts and behavior a temporary phenomenon in early adolescents? *Crisis: The Journal of Crisis Intervention and Suicide Prevention. 42*(1), 78–81. https://doi.org /10.1027/0227-5910/a000680

Vancleave, J. A. (2008). School resource officers: What high school teachers consider to be the most important tasks. *Dissertations Abstracts International: Section A. Humanities and Social Sciences, 69*(1-A), 389.

Vandenberg, N. (1992). Using critical incidents and debriefing to mediate organizational crisis, change, and loss. *Employee Assistance Quarterly, 8*, 35–55.

Vandentorren, S., Pirard, P., Sanna, A., Aubert, L., Motreff, Y., Dantchev, N., Lesieur, S., Chauvin, P., & Baubet, T. (2018). Healthcare provision and the psychological, somatic and social impact on people involved in the terror attacks in January 2015 in Paris: Cohort study. *The British Journal of Psychiatry, 212*(4), 207–214. https://doi.org/10.1192/bjp.2017.63

VanLeewen, M., & Harte, J. (2017). Violence against health care professionals: Prevalence, nature and consequences. *Forensic Psychiatry and Psychology, 28*(5), 581–598. https://doi.org/10.10 80/14789949.2015.1012533

Vanovermeire, R., Muysewinkel, E., Van Keer, R., Vesentini, L., & Bilsen, J. (2021). Victims of terrorist attacks in Belgium and barriers to professional mental health aid barriers: A qualitative study. *Frontiers in Psychiatry, 12.* https://doi.org/10.3389 /fpsyt.2021.638272

Vasquez, I., Tinto, A., Arjona, C., Martinez, M., & Diaz, A. (2023). Accompanying mental health problems at home: Preliminary data from a crisis resolution and home treatment team in Catalonia. *Journal of Psychiatric and Mental Health Nursing*, Advance online publication. http://doi.org/10.1111/jpm.12918

Velotti, P., Rogier, G., Beomonte Zobel, S., Chirumbolo, A., & Zavattini, G. C. (2022). The relation of anxiety and avoidance dimensions of attachment to intimate partner violence: A meta-analysis about perpetrators. *Trauma, Violence, & Abuse, 23*(1), 196–212. https://doi.org/10.1177/1524838020933864

Vermette, H. S., Pinals, D. A., & Applebaum, P. S. (2005). Mental health training for law enforcement professionals. *Journal of the American Academy of Psychiatry and the Law, 33*(1), 42–46.

Vermetten, E., & Bremner, J. (2002). Circuits and systems in stress: II. Applications to neurobiology and treatment in posttraumatic stress disorder. *Depression & Anxiety, 16*(1), 14–38.

Vernberg, E. M. (1999). Children's responses to disaster: Family and systems approaches. In R. Gist & B. Lubin (Eds.), *Response to disaster: Psychosocial, community and ecological approaches* (pp. 193–210). Brunner/Mazel.

Vickers, M. H. (2009). Journeys into grief: Exploring redundancy for a new understanding of workplace grief. *Journal of Loss and Trauma, 14*(5), 401–419.

Vilariño, M., González Amado, B., Vázquez, M. J., & Arce, R. (2018). Psychological harm in women victims of intimate partner violence: Epidemiology and quantification of injury in mental health markers. *Intervención Psicosocial*, 145–152. https://doi.org/10.5093/pi2018a23

Vilvens, H. L., Jones, D. E., & Vaughn, L. M. (2021). Exploring the recovery of non-offending parents after a child's sexual abuse event. *Journal of Child and Family Studies, 30*(11), 2690–2704. https://doi.org/10.1007/s10826-021-02082-3

Viner, J. (1982). Toward more skillful handling of acutely psychotic patients: Part I. Evaluation. *Emergency Room Report, 3*, 125–130.

Vinick, B. (1986). *Counseling in a state mental hospital* (Cassette Recording No. 13). Memphis State University, Department of Counseling and Personnel Services.

Vinturella, L., & James, R. K. (1987). Sand play: A therapeutic medium with children. *Elementary School Guidance & Counseling, 21*, 229–238.

Violanti, J. M. (2000). Scripting trauma: The impact of pathogenic intervention. In J. M. Violanti, D. Paton, & C. Dunning (Eds.).

Posttraumatic stress intervention: Challenges, issues and perspectives, (pp. 153–165). Charles C. Thomas.

Virupaksha, H. G., Muralidhar, D., & Ramakrishna, J. (2016). Suicide and suicidal behavior among transgender persons. *Indian Journal of Psychological Medicine, 38*(6), 505–509. https://doi .org/10.4103/0253-7176.194908

Vismara, M., Girone, N., Conti, D., Nicolini, D., & Dell'Osso, B. (2022). The current status of cyberbullying research: A short review of the literature, *Current Opinion in Behavioral Sciences, 46.* https://doi.org/10.1016/j.cobeha.2022.101152

Vitaro, F., & Brendgen, M. (2005). Proactive and reactive aggression: A developmental perspective. In R. E. Tremblay, W. W. Hartup, & J. Archer (Eds.), *Developmental origins of aggression* (pp. 178–201). Guilford Press.

Vitaro, F., Brendgen, M., & Tremblay, R. E. (2002). Reactively and proactively aggressive children: Antecedent and subsequent characteristics. *Journal of Child Psychology and Psychiatry, 43*, 495–505.

Vitas Healthcare (2023). *Experiencing grief as a teenager.* vitas.com

Voelkel, E., Pukay-Martin, N. D., Walter, K., & Chard, K. (2015). Effectiveness of cognitive processing therapy for male and female veterans with and without military sexual trauma. *Journal of Traumatic Stress, 28*(3), 174–182.

Voght, A. (2017). All my relations: Re-membering and honouring those who come before and after us. *The International Journal of Narrative Therapy and Community Work, (3)*, 17–20.

Volpe, U., Luciano, M., Palumbo, C., Sampogna, G., Del Vecchio, V., & Fiorillo, A. (2014). Risk of burnout among early career mental health professionals. *Journal of Psychiatric and Mental Health Nursing, 21*(9), 774–781

Vos, S. R., Clark-Ginsberg, A., Puente-Duran, S., Slas-Wright, C. P., Suque, M. C., Herra, I. C., Maldinado-Molina, M. M., Castillo, M. N., Lee, T. K., Garcia, M. F., Fernandez, C. A., Hanson, M., Scaramutti, C., & Schwartz, S. J. (2021). The family crisis migration stress framework: A framework to understand the mental health effects of crisis migration on children and families caused by disasters. *Child and Adolescent Development Online Library*, 41–59.

Vossekuil, B., Fein, R. A., Reddy, M., Borum, R., & Modzelski, W. (2002). *The final report and findings on the safe school initiative: Implications for the prevention of school attacks in the United States.* U.S. Secret Service and U.S. Department of Education.

Vossekuil, B., Reddy, M., Fein, R., Borum, R., & Modzeleski, W. (2000). *U.S. Safe School Initiative: An interim report on the prevention of targeted violence in schools.* Secret Service, National Threat Assessment Center.

Wachen, J., Jimenez, S., Smith, K., & Resick, P. A. (2014). Long-term functional outcomes of women receiving cognitive processing therapy and prolonged exposure. *Psychological Trauma: Theory, Research, Practice, and Policy, 6* (suppl 1), S58–S65.

Wachter, C. A. (2007, March). *Crisis in the schools: Crisis, crisis intervention training, and school counselor burnout.* Paper presented at the American Counseling Association Convention, Detroit, MI, United States.

Wagner, B. (1997). Family risk factors for child and adolescent suicidal behavior. *Psychological Bulletin, 121*, 246–298.

Wagner, S. L. (2005). Emergency response service personnel & the critical incident stress debriefing debate. *International Journal of Emergency Mental Health, 7*, 33–41.

Wakefield, J. C., Schmitz, M. F., & Baer, J. C. (2011). Did narrowing the major depression bereavement exclusion from DSM-III-R to DSM-IV increase validity? Evidence from a national comorbidity study. *Journal of Nervous and Mental Disease, 199*(2), 66–73.

Wakelee-Lynch, J. (1990, October). Florida crisis elicits aid from college officials and counselors. *Guidepost*, pp. 1, 3.

Walker, D. F., Courtois, C. A., & Aten, J. (Eds.). (2015). *Spiritually oriented psychotherapy for trauma*. American Psychological Association.

Walker, D. F., Courtois, C. A., & Aten, J. D. (2015). Basics of working on spiritual matters with traumatized individuals. In D. F. Walker, C. A. Courtois, & J. D. Aten (Eds.), *Spiritually oriented psychotherapy for trauma*. (pp. 15–28). American Psychological Association.

Walker, D. F., Gorusch, L., & Tan, S. Y. (2004). Therapists' integration of religion and spirituality in counseling: A meta-analysis. *Counseling and Values, 49*, 69–80.

Walker, D. F., McGregor, K. L., Quagliana, F., Stephens, R. L., & Knodel, K. (2015). Understanding and responding to changes in spirituality and religion after traumatic events. In D. F. Walker, C. A. Courtois, & J. Aten (Eds.), *Spiritually oriented psychotherapy for trauma*. (pp. 147–168). American Psychological Association.

Walker, G. (1990). Crisis-care in critical incident debriefing. *Death Studies, 14*, 121–133.

Walker, H. E., Freud, J. S., Ellis, R. A., Fraine, S. M., & Wilson, L. C. (2019). The prevalence of sexual revictimization: A meta-analytic review. *Trauma, Violence, & Abuse, 20*(1), 67–80. https://doi.org/10.1177/1524838017692364

Walker, J. I. (1983). Comparison of "rap" groups with traditional group therapy in the treatment of Vietnam combat veterans. *Group, 7*, 48–57.

Walker, L. E. (1979). How battering happens and how to stop it. In D. Moore (Ed.), *Battered women* (pp. 59–78). SAGE.

Walker, L. E. (1984). *The battered woman syndrome*. Springer.

Walker, L. E. (1989). *Terrifying love: Why battered women kill and how society responds*. Harper & Row.

Walker, L. E. (2000). *The battered woman syndrome* (2nd ed). Springer.

Walker, L. E. A. (2017). *The Battered Woman Syndrome* (4th ed.). Springer Publishing Company.

Walker, T. (2019, November). More schools are leveraging peer counseling and mentoring programs to supplement suicide prevention and trauma-informed strategies. *NEA Today*. https://www.nea.org/advocating-for-change/new-from-nea/peer-programs-helping-schools-tackle-student-depression-anxiety

Walker, Z., & Seifert, R. (1994). Violent incidents in a psychiatric intensive care unit. *British Journal of Psychiatry, 164*, 826–828.

Waller, R., Mahmood, T., Gandi, R., Delves, S., Humphreys, N., & Smith, D. (2005). Student mental health: How can psychiatrists better support the work of university medical centre and university counseling services? *British Journal of Guidance & Counseling, 33*(1), 117–128.

Wallerstein, J. S., & Kelly, J. B. (1975). The effects of parental divorce: Experiences of the preschool child. *Journal of the American Academy of Child Psychiatry, 14*, 600–616.

Walsh, A. R., & Stephenson, R. (2023). Intimate partner violence perpetration denial and underreporting in cisgender male couples: Negar y no informar el haber ejercido violencia de pareja en parejas de hombres cisgénero. *Psychosocial Intervention, 32*(2), 109–121. https://doi.org/10.5093/pi2023a8

Walsh, F. (2009a). Integrating spirituality and family therapy: Wellsprings for health, healing, and resilience. In F. Walsh (Ed.). *Spiritual resources in family therapy* (2nd ed, pp. 31–61). Guilford Press.

Walsh, F. (2009b). Spiritual resources in family adaptation to death and loss. In F. Walsh (Ed.), *Spiritual resources in family therapy* (2nd ed., pp. 81–102). Guilford Press.

Walsh, F. (2012a). Clinical views of family normality, health, and dysfunction: From a deficits to a strength perspective. In F. Walsh (Ed.), *Normal family processes: Growing diversity and complexity* (4th ed., pp. 28–54). Guilford Press.

Walsh, F. (2012b). Family resiliency: Strengths forged through adversity. In F. Walsh (Ed.), *Normal family processes: Growing diversity and complexity* (4th ed., pp. 399–428). Guilford Press.

Walsh, K., King, M., Jones, L., Tookman, A., & Blizard, R. (2002). Spiritual beliefs may affect outcome of bereavement: Prospective study. *British Medical Journal, 324*(7353), 1551.

Walsh, T. (2021). Family resilience. In M. Ungar (Ed.). *Multisystemic resilience: Adaptation and transformation in contexts of change* (pp. 250-270). Oxford University Press. https://doi.org/10.1093/oso/9780190095888.003.0015

Walter, J, L., & Peller, J. E. (1992). *Becoming solution–focused in brief therapy*. Routledge Taylor & Francis.

Wampold, B. E. (2010). The research evidence for the common factors models: A historically situated perspective. In B. L. Duncan, S. D. Miller, B. E. Wampold, & M. A. Hubble (Eds.), *The heart and soul of change: Delivering what works in therapy* (2nd ed., pp. 49–81). American Psychological Association. https://doi.org/10.1037/12075-002

Wampold, B. E. (2012). Humanism as a common factor in psychotherapy. *Psychotherapy, 49*(4), 445–449. https://doi.org/10.1037/a0027113

Wang Y. L., Zhao, X., Feng, G., & Luo, R. (2020). Using mobile phone data for emergency management: A systematic literature review. *Information System Frontiers. 22*(6), 1539–1559. https://doi.org/10.1007/s10796-020-10057-w

Wang, D. C., Aten, J. D., Boan, D., Jean-Charles, W., Griff, K. P., Valcin, V. C., Davis, E. B., Hook, J. N., Davis, D. E., Van Tongeren, D. R., Abouezzeddine, T., Sklar, Q., & Wang, A. (2016). Culturally adapted spiritually oriented trauma-focused cognitive-behavioral therapy for child survivors of Restavek. *Spirituality in Clinical Practice, 3*(4), 224–236. https://doi.org/10.1037/scp0000101

Wang, J. (2005). The effects of reminiscence on depressive symptoms and mood status of older institutionalized adults in Taiwan. *International Journal of Geriatric Psychiatry, 20*(1), 57–62.

Wang, Y., Gao, S., & Gao, W. (2022). Investigating dynamic relations between factual information and misinformation: Empirical studies of tweets related to prevention measures during COVID-19. *Journal of Contingencies and Crisis Management, 30*(4), 427–439. https://doi.org/10.1111/1468-5973.12385

Wark, V. (1982). A look at the work of the telephone counseling center. *Personnel and Guidance Journal, 61*, 110–112.

Wark, V. (1984). *The sex caller and the telephone counseling center*. Charles C. Thomas.

Warnath, C. F., & Shelton, J. L. (1976). The ultimate disappointment: The burned out counselor. *Personnel and Guidance Journal, 55*, 172–175.

Warren, J. I., South, S., Burnette, M., Rogers, A., Friend, R., Bale, R., & Van Patten, I. (2005). Understanding the risk factors for violence and criminality in women: The concurrent validity of the PCL-R and the HCR-20. *International Journal of Law and Psychiatry, 28*(3), 269–289.

Wasserman, D., Hoven, D., Wasserman, C., Wall, M., Eisenberg, R., Hadlaczky, G., Kelleher, I., Sarchiapone, M., Apter, A., Balazs,

J., Bobes, J., Brunner, R., Corcoran, P., Cosman, D., Guillemin, F., Haring, C., Iosue, M., Kaess, M., Kahn, J., Keeley, H.,... & Carli, V. (2015). School-based suicide prevention programmes: The SEYLE cluster-randomized controlled trial. *The Lancet, 3285*(9977), 1536–1544.

Waters, J. (2022). *Narrative therapy: Techniques.* Center for Family Transformation. http://familytransformation.com

Waters, J., & Finn, E. (1995). Handling crisis effectively on the telephone. In A. R. Roberts (Ed.), *Crisis intervention and time-limited cognitive treatment* (pp. 251–289). SAGE.

Watkins, A., & Taylor, T. (2016). The prevalence, predictors, and criminogenic effect of joining a gang among urban, suburban, and rural youth. *Journal of Criminal Justice, 47*(2), 133–142. https://doi.org/10.1016/j.jcrimjus.2016.09.001

Watkins, C. E. (1983). Burnout in counseling practice: Some potential professional and personal hazards of becoming a counselor. *Personnel and Guidance Journal, 61,* 304–308.

Watson, A. C., & Compton, M. (2019). What research on crisis intervention tells us and what we need to ask. *Journal of the American Academy of Psychiatry and Law, 47*(4), 422–426. https://doi.org/10.29158/JAAPL.003894-19

Watson, A. C., & Fulambarker, A. J. (2012). The crisis intervention team model of police response to mental health crises: A primer for mental health practitioners. *Best Practices in Mental Health: An International Journal, 8*(2), 71–81.

Watson, A. C., Ottai, V. C., Morabito, M., Draine, J., Kerr, A. N., & Angell, B. (2010). Outcomes of police contacts with persons with mental illness: The impact of CIT. *Administration and Policy in Mental Health and Mental Health Services Research, 37*(4), 302–317.

Watson, P. J., Brymer, M. J., & Bonanno, G. (2011). Postdisaster psychological intervention since 9/11. *American Psychologist, 66*(6), 482–494.

Watson, R. J., McDonald, J., & Pearce, D. (2006). An exploration of calls to Lifeline Australia: Social support or urgent suicide intervention? *British Journal of Guidance and Counselling, 34*(4), 471–482.

Watt, K. A., Storey, J. E., & Hart, S. D. (2018). Violence risk identification, assessment, and management practices in inpatient psychiatry. *Journal of Threat Assessment and Management, 5,* 155–172. https://doi.org/10.1037/tam0000099

Wattendorf, G. E. (2002). School threat decision demonstrates support for early action. *Police Chief, 69*(3), 11–12.

Watters, D. (1997). A study of the reliability of the Triage Severity Scale. (Doctoral dissertation, University of Memphis.) *Dissertation Abstracts International, 58-08A,* 3028.

Weathers, F. W., Blake, D. D., Schnurr, P. P., Kaloupek, D. G., Marx, B. P., & Keane, T. M. (2023). *The Life Events Checklist for DSM-5 (LEC-5).* https://www.ptsd.va.gov/professional/assessment/documents/LEC5_Standard_Self-report.PDF

Weathers, F.W., Blake, D.D., Schnurr, P.P., Kaloupek, D.G., Marx, B.P., & Keane, T.M. (2013). *The Life Events Checklist for DSM-5 (LEC-5).* National Center for PTSD. www.ptsd.va.gov

Webb, C., Hayes, A. M., Grasso, D., Kaurenceau, J., & Deblinger, E. (2014). Trauma-focused cognitive behavioral therapy for youth: Effectiveness in a community setting. *Psychological Trauma: Theory, Research, Practice and Policy, 6*(5), 555–562.

Webb, L. M., & Dickson, F. C. (2012). Effective family communication for coping with crises. In F. C. Dickson & L. M. Webb (Eds.), *Communication for families in crisis: Theory, research, strategies* (pp. 1–26). Peter Lang.

Webb, N. (Ed.). (2007). *Play therapy with children in crisis.* Guilford Press.

Webb, N. B. (2004). A developmental-transactional framework for assessment of children and families following a mass trauma. In N. B. Webb (Ed.), *Mass trauma and violence: Helping families and children cope.* (pp. 23–49). Guilford Press.

Webb, N. B. (2005). The impact of traumatic stress and loss on children and families. In C. B. Webb (Ed.), *Mass trauma and violence: Helping families and children cope* (pp. 3–22). Guilford Press.

Webb, N. B. (2007). *Play therapy with children in crisis: Individual, group, and family treatment* (3rd ed.). Guilford Press.

Webb, N. B. (2007). Sudden death of a parent in a terrorist attack: Crisis intervention conjoint therapy with a preschool boy and his mother. In N. B. Webb (Ed.), *Play therapy with children in crisis: Individual, group, and family treatment* (pp. 389–407). Guilford Press.

Webb, N. B. (2011). Play therapy for bereaved children: Adapting strategies to community, school, and home settings. *School Psychology International, 32*(2), 132–143.

Webb, N. B. (Ed.). (2007). *Play therapy with children in crisis: Individual, group, and family treatment* (3rd ed.). Guilford Press.

Webb, S. B., & Griffiths, F. (1998–1999). *Young people at risk of suicide: Part A. School facilitators' handbook; Part B. Supplementary resources.* College of Education, Massey University.

Webber, J., & Mascari, J. B. (Eds.). (2010). *Terrorism, trauma, and tragedies: A counselor's guide to preparing and responding* (3rd ed.). American Counseling Association Foundation.

Webber, J., Bass, D., & Yep, R. (Eds.). (2005). *Terrorism, trauma, and tragedies: A counselor's guide to preparing and responding.* American Counseling Association.

Webber, J., Mascari, J. B., & Runte, J. (2010). Psychological first aid: A new paradigm for disaster mental health. In J. Webber & J. B. Mascari (Eds.), *Terror, trauma, and tragedies: A counselor's guide to preparing and responding* (3rd ed., pp. 201–205). American Counseling Association Foundation.

Weber, J. G. (2011). *Individual and family stress and crises.* SAGE.

Weber, J. G. (2011). The abcx formula and the double abcx model. In *Individual and family stress and crises* (pp. 82–96). SAGE Publications, Inc.

Webersinn, A. L., Hollinger, C. L., & Delamatre, J. E. (1991). Breaking the cycle of violence: An examination of factors relevant to treatment follow-through. *Psychological Reports, 68,* 231–239.

Websdale, N., & Johnson, B. (2005). Reducing woman battering: The role of structural approaches. In N. Sololoff & C. Pratt (Eds.), *Domestic violence at the margins: Readings on race, class, gender, and culture* (pp. 389–415). Rutgers University Press.

Webster, C. D., Douglas, K. S., Eaves, D., & Hart, S. D. (1997). *HCR-20: Assessing risk of violence.* Simon Fraser University.

Webster, C. D., Haqu, Q., & Hucker, S. J. (2014). *Violence risk assessment and management: Advances through structured professional judgment and sequential redirections* (2nd ed.). Wiley-Blackwell.

Webster, D. W., & Wilson, M. (1994). Gun violence, angry youth and the pediatrician's role in primary prevention. *Paediatrics, 94*(4), 617–622.

Webster, J. D. (1993). Construction and validation of the Reminiscence Functions Scale. *Journal of Gerontology, 48*(5), 256–262. https://doi.org/10.1093/geronj/48.5.p256

Wee, D. F., & Myers, D. (2002). Stress response of mental health workers following disaster: The Oklahoma City bombing.

In C. R. Figley (Ed.), *Treating compassion fatigue* (pp. 57–83). Brunner/Routledge.

Wee, D. F., & Myers, D. (2003). Compassion satisfaction, compassion fatigue, and critical incidents stress management. *International Journal of Emergency Mental Health, 5*(1), 33–37.

Wei, Y., & Chen, S. (2021). Narrative exposure therapy for posttraumatic stress disorder: A meta-analysis of randomized controlled trials. *Psychological Trauma: Theory, Research, Practice, and Policy, 13*(8), 877–884. https://doi.org/10.1037/tra0000922

Weincourt, R. (1985). Never to be alone: Existential therapy for battered women. *Journal of Psychosocial Nursing, 23*, 24–29.

Weiner, M., & Mehrabian, A. (1968). *Language within language.* Appleton-Century-Croft.

Weinreb, M., & Groves, B. M. (2007). Child exposure to parental violence: Case of Amanda, age 4. In Nancy Webb (Ed.), *Play therapy with children in crisis: Individual, group, and family treatment* (3rd ed., pp. 73–90). Guilford Press.

Weinstock, R., Read, S., Leong, G. B., & Silvia, J. (2008). The elderly. In R. I. Simon & K. Tardiff (Eds.), *Textbook of violence assessment and management* (pp. 381–406). American Psychiatric Publishing.

Weis, C. N., Webb, E. K., Stevens, S. K., Larson, C. L., & deRoon-Cassini, T. A. (2022). Scoring the Life Events Checklist: Comparison of three scoring methods. *Psychological Trauma: Theory, Research, Practice, and Policy, 14*(4), 714–720. https://doi.org/10.1037/tra0001049

Weisaeth, L. (2000). Briefing and debriefing: Group psychological interventions in acute stressor situations. In B. Raphael & J. P. Wilson (Eds.), *Psychological debriefing: Theory, practice, and evidence* (pp. 43–57). Cambridge University Press.

Weisheit, R., & Wells, E. (2004). *Youth gangs in rural America.* Department of Justice, Office of Justice Programs. http://ojp.usdoj.gov

Weisman, A. D. (1990–1991). Bereavement and companion animals. *Omega: Journal of Death and Dying, 22*, 241–248.

Weisman, R. (2011). Workplace violence in mental and general healthcare settings. In M. Rivitera (Ed.), *Staff safety and workplace violence education* (pp. 151–162). Ed Jones and Bartlett LLC.

Weiss, D. S. (1997) The Impact of Event Scale-Revised. In J. P. Wilson & T. M. Keane (Eds.), *Assessing psychological trauma and PTSD: A practitioner handbook* (2nd ed., pp. 168–189). Guilford Press.

Weiss, D. S., & Marmar, C. R. (1997). The Impact of Event Scale-Revised. In J. P. Wilson, & T. M. Keane (Eds.), *Assessing Psychological Trauma and PTSD: A Practitioner's Handbook* (pp. 399–411). Guilford Press.

Weiss, K. J., & Alexander, J. C. (2013). Sex, lies, and statistics: Inferences from the child sexual abuse accommodation syndrome. *Journal of the American Academy of Psychiatry and the Law, 41*(3), 412–420.

Weiss, R. S. (1998). Issues in the study of loss and grief. In J. H. Harvery (Ed.), *Perspectives on loss: A sourcebook* (pp. 343–353). Brunner/Mazel.

Weitzman, S. (2000). *Not to people like us.* Basic Books.

Welfel, E. R. (2016). *Ethics in counseling and psychotherapy: Standards, research and emerging issues* (6th ed.). Cengage Learning.

Welsh, J. A., & Domitrovich, C. (2006). Safe schools, healthy students initiative in rural Pennsylvania. In S. R. Jimerson & M. Furlong (Eds.), *Handbook of school violence and school safety: From research to practice* (pp. 511–524). Erlbaum.

Weniger, J., Distelberg, B., & Vaswani, D. (2017). Depression and anger as risk factors for suicide with inpatient adolescents. *Suicidology Online, 8*(2), 1–10.

Wenzel, A., Brown, G. K., & Beck, A. T. (2008). *Cognitive therapy for suicidal patients: Scientific and clinical applications* (1st ed.). American Psychological Association.

Werner, P. D., Rose, T. L., Murdach, A. D., & Yesavage, J. A. (1989). Social workers' decision making about the violent client. *Social Work Research and Abstracts, 25*, 17–20.

Wessely, S. C., Bryant, R. A., Greenberg, N., Earnshaw, N., Shapley, J., & Hacker-Huges, J. (2008). Does psychoeducation help prevent post traumatic psychological distress? *Psychiatry, 71*(2), 287–302.

West, J., Liang, B., & Spinazzola, J. (2017). Trauma sensitive yoga as a complementary treatment for posttraumatic stress disorder: A qualitative descriptive analysis. *International Journal of Stress Management, 24*(2), 173–195. https://doi.org/10.1037/str0000040

Western Carolina University Emergency Management Institute. (2023). *Emergency and Disaster Management Program.* https://www.wcu.edu/learn/programs/emergency-disaster-management/index.aspx

Westervelt, E. (21 September, 2020). *Mental health and police violence: How crisis intervention teams are failing.* [Radio broadcast and manuscript]. All Things Considered. National Public Radio. https://www.npr.org.

Westheimer, K. (2017). Safe haven. *ASCA School Counselor, 54*(5). 22–25

Whaley, A. L., & Davis, K. E. (2007). Cultural competence and evidence-based practice in mental health services. *American Psychologist, 62*(6), 563–574.

What is The Duluth Model? (n.d.). *Domestic abuse intervention programs.* https://www.theduluthmodel.org/what-is-the-duluth-model/

Whealin, J. M., Ciro, D., Dasaro, C. R., Udasin, I. G., Crane, M., Moline, J. M., Harrison, D. J., Luft, B. J., Todd, A. C., Feder, A., & Pietrzak, R. H. (2022). Race/ethnic differences in prevalence and correlates of posttraumatic stress disorder in World Trade Center responders: Results from a population-based, health monitoring cohort. *Psychological Trauma: Theory, Research, Practice, and Policy, 14*(2), 199–208. https://doi.org/10.1037/tra0001081

Wheeler, A. (2023). HIPAA compliance after the COVID-19 public health emergency. *Counseling Today, 65*(10), 10–11.

Wheeler, A. M. (2023). Mental telehealth apps and client data privacy. *Counseling Today, 65*(11), 8–9.

Wheeler, A. M., & Bertram, B. (2019). *The counselor and the law* (8th ed.). American Counseling Association.

Wheeler, C., Lloyd-Evans, B., Churchard, A., Fitzgeralds, C. Fularton, K., Mosse, L., Paterson, B., Zugaro, C., & Johnson S. (2015). Implementation of the Crisis Resolution team model in adult mental health settings: A systematic review. *BMC Psychiatry, 15*, 74. http://doi.org/10.1186/s12888-015-0441-x

Wheeler, I. (2001). Parental bereavement: The crisis of meaning. *Death Studies, 25*(1), 51–66.

Wheeler, K. (2014). Inadequate treatment and research for PTSD at the VA. *American Psychologist, 69*(7), 706.

White, B. D., Martin C. S., Walk, R., Pollice, L., Weissfeld, L., Hong, S., Landefeld, C. S., & Arnold, R. M. (2012). Nurse-led intervention to improve surrogate decision making for patients with advanced critical illness. *American Journal of Critical Care, 21*, 396–409.

White, K. R., & Dutton, D. G. (2013). Perceptions of female perpetrators. In B. L. Russell (Ed.), *Perceptions of female offenders: How stereotypes and social norms affect criminal justice responses* (pp. 101–116). Springer. https://doi.org/10.1007/978-1-4614-5871-5_7

White, L. M., Aalsma, M. C., Holloway, E. D., Adams, E. L., & Salyers, M. P. (2015). Job-related burnout among juvenile probation officers: Implications for mental health stigma and competency. *Psychological Services, 12,* 291–302. https://doi.org/10.1037/ser0000031

White, M. (1989). *Selected papers.* Dulwich Centre.

White, M. (2005). *An outline of narrative therapy.* www.massey.ac.nz

White, M. B., Raitt, J. M., Pfefferbaum, B., & North, C. S. (2022). Postdisaster mental health assistance provision and utilization among employees of companies affected by the 9/11 attacks on New York City. *Traumatology.* Advance online publication. http://dx.doi.org/10.1037/trm0000392

Whitman, M. E., & Mattord, H. J. (2021). *Principles of incident response and disaster recovery* (3rd ed.). Cengage.

Widom, C. S., & Massey, C. (2015). A prospective examination of whether childhood sexual abuse predicts subsequent sexual offending. *JAMA Pediatrics, 169*(1), e143357. https://doi.org/10.1001/jamapediatrics.2014.3357

Wiederhold, B. K., & Wiederhold, M. D. (2005). *Virtual reality therapy for anxiety disorders: Advances in evaluation and treatment.* American Psychological Association.

Wijkman, M. D. S., & Da Silva, T. (2021). Multiple perpetrator rape committed by female offenders: A comparison of solo, duo, and 3+ group offenders. *Sexual Abuse, 33*(3), 321–338. https://doi.org/10.1177/1079063219897065

Wilkinson, C. B. (1983). Aftermath of a disaster: The collapse of the Hyatt Regency steel skywalk. *American Journal of Psychiatry, 140,* 1134–1139.

Wilks, C. R., Morland, L. A., Dillon, K. H., Mackintosh, M.-A., Blakey, S. M., Wagner, H. R., & Elbogen, E. B. (2019). Anger, social support, and suicide risk in U.S. military veterans. *Journal of Psychiatric Research, 109,* 139–144. https://doi.org/10.1016/j.jpsychires.2018.11.026

Willard, N. (2007). *Cyberbullying and cyberthreats: Responding to the challenge of online social aggression, threats, and distress.* Research Press.

Williams, C. C. (1983). The mental foxhole: The Vietnam veteran's search for meaning. *American Journal of Orthopsychiatry, 53,* 4–17.

Williams, C. M., Larsen, U., & McCloskey, L. A. (2008). Intimate partner violence and women's contraceptive use. *Violence Against Women, 14*(12), 1382–1396. https://doi.org/10.1177/1077801208325187

Williams, K., Fildes, D., Conrad, K., Grootemaat, G., Gradford, S., & Gordon, R. (2020). Evaluation of outcomes for help seekers accessing a pilot SMS-based crisis intervention service in Australia. *Crisis, 42*(1), 32–39. https://doi.org/10.1027/0227-5910/a000681

Williams, M. B. (2004). How schools respond to traumatic events: Debriefing interventions and beyond. In N. B. Webb (Ed.), *Mass trauma and violence: Helping families and children cope* (pp. 120–141) Guilford Press.

Williams, M. B. (2006). How schools respond to traumatic events: Debriefing interventions and beyond. *Journal of Aggression, Maltreatment & Trauma, 12*(1), 57–81.

Williams, R. L., & Long, J. D. (1979). *Toward a self-managed life style* (2nd ed.). Houghton Mifflin.

Williams, R. L., & Long, J. D. (1983). *Toward a self-managed life style* (3rd ed.). Houghton Mifflin.

Williams, T., & Douds, J. (2012). The unique contributions of telephone therapy. In D. Lester & J. R. Rogers (Eds.), *Crisis intervention and counseling by telephone* (2nd ed., pp. 41–47). Charles C. Thomas.

Williston, S. K., Grossman, D., Mori, D. L., & Niles, B. L. (2021). Mindfulness interventions in the treatment of posttraumatic stress disorder. *Professional Psychology: Research and Practice, 52*(1), 46–57. https://doi.org/10.1037/pro0000363

Willoughby, T., Heffer, T., & Hamza, C. A. (2015). The link between nonsuicidal self-injury and acquired capability for suicide: A longitudinal study. *Journal of Abnormal Psychology, 124*(4), 1110–1115. https://doi.org/10.1037/abn0000104

Wills, T., Kern, L., Hedden, B., Nelson, V., Comartin, E., & Kubiak, S. (2023). The impact of crisis intervention team training on police use of force. *Journal of Offender Rehabilitation.* Advance online publication. https://doi.org/10.1080/10509674.2023.2182863

Wilson J. P., Friedman, M. J., & Lindy, J. D. (2001). *Treating psychological trauma and PTSD.* Guilford Press.

Wilson, C., Sheridan, L., & Garratt-Reed, D. (2022). What is cyberstalking? A review of measurements. *Journal of Interpersonal Violence, 37*(11–12), NP9763–NP9783. https://doi.org/10.1177/0886260520985489

Wilson, G., & Lester, D. (2002). Crisis intervention by e-mail. In D. Lester & G. W. Brockopp (Eds.), *Crisis intervention and counseling by telephone* (2nd ed., pp. 212–219). Charles C. Thomas.

Wilson, J. P. (1980). Conflict, stress, and growth: Effects of the war on psychosocial development. In C. R. Figley & S. Leventman (Eds.), *Strangers at home.* Praeger.

Wilson, J. P., Smith, W. K., & Johnson, S. (1985). A comparative analysis of PTSD among various survivor groups. In C. R. Figley (Ed.), *Trauma and its wake: The study of post-trauma stress disorder* (pp. 142–172). Brunner/Mazel.

Wilson, S. (2017). *The shocking reality of violence in healthcare: And what we can do about it.* Stop Health Care Violence.

Wilson, S. M., Krenek, M., & Dennis, P. A. (2017). Daily associations between PTSD, drinking, and self appraised alcohol-related problems. *Psychology of Addictive Behaviors, 31*(1), 27–35. http://dx.doi.org/10.1037/adb0000238

Wilson, S. T., Chesin, M., Fertuck, E., Keilp, J., Brodsky, B., Mann, J. J., Sönmez, C. C., Benjamin-Phillips, C., & Stanley, B. (2016). Heart rate variability and suicidal behavior. *Psychiatry Research, 240,* 241–247. https://doi.org/10.1016/j.psychres.2016.04.033

Windmeyer, S. (2009). Helping LGBTQ & ally students find the right college fit. *ASCA School Counselor, 47*(1), 24.

Winslade, M. J., & Monk, F. (1999). *Narrative counseling in schools: Powerful and brief.* Corwin Press.

Wirth-Cauchon, J. (2001). *Women and borderline personality disorder.* Rutgers University Press.

WISQARS (2021). *Leading cause of death visualization tool.* Centers for Disease Control. https://wisqars.cdc.gov/data/lcd/home

Wittenberg, E., Goldsmith, J. V., Chen, C., Prince-Paul, M., & Johnson, R. R. (2021). Opportunities to improve COVID-19 provider communication resources: A systematic review. *Patient Education and Counseling.* Elsevier Ireland Ltd. https://doi.org/10.1016/j.pec.2020.12.031

Wolanin, M. O., & Phillips, L. R. (1981). *Confusion: Prevention and care.* Mosby.

Wolf, E. J., Hawn, S. E., Sullivan, D. R., Miller, M. W., Sanborn, V., Brown, E., Neale, Z., Fein-Schaffer, D., Zhao, X., Logue, M. W., Fortier, C. B., McGlinchey, R. E., & Milberg, W. P. (2023). Neurobiological and genetic correlates of the dissociative subtype of posttraumatic stress disorder. *Journal of Psychopathology and Clinical Science, 132*(4), 409–427. https://doi.org/10.1037/abn0000795

Wolfe, D. A., Crooks, C. C., Chiodo, D., & Jaffe, P. (2009). Child maltreatment, bullying, gender-based harassment, and adolescent dating violence: Making the connections. *Psychology of Women Quarterly, 33*(1), 21–24. https://journals.sagepub.com/doi/abs/10.1111/j.1471-6402.2008.01469.x

Wolpe, J. (1958). *Psychotherapy by reciprocal inhibition.* Stanford University Press.

Wolpe, J. (1982). *The practice of behavior therapy.* Pergamon Press.

Women Against Abuse. (n.d.). *Why it's so difficult to leave.* https://www.womenagainstabuse.org/education-resources/learn-about-abuse/why-its-so-difficult-to-leave

Wong, N., Hagan, M., & Holley, S. (2023). Childhood maltreatment and suicidal thoughts and behaviors in young adults: The role of limited access to emotional regulation strategies. *Crisis: The Journal of Crisis Intervention and Suicide Prevention.* Advance online publication. https://doi.org/10.1027/0227-5910/a000909

Wong, S., Gordon, A., & Gu, D. (2007). Assessment and treatment of violence-prone forensic clients: An integrated approach. *British Journal of Psychiatry, 190*(49), 66–74.

Wood, K. A., & Khuri, R. (1984). Violence: The emergency room patient. In J. T. Turner (Ed.), *Violence in the medical care setting: A survival guide* (pp. 57–84). Aspen Systems.

Woodard, N. (2023). Differentiating borderline personality disorder from bipolar disorder: A systematic review of current literature. *Dissertation Abstracts International: Section B. The Sciences and Engineering, 84*(5-B).

Woods, B., O'Philbin, L., Farrell, E.M., Spector, A. E., & Orrell, M. (2018). Reminiscence therapy for dementia. *Cochrane Database Systems Review. 3*(3), CD001120. http://doi.org/10.1002/14651858.CD001120

Worden, J. W. (1991). *Grief counseling and grief therapy: A handbook for the mental health practitioner* (2nd ed.). Springer.

Worden, J. W. (1996). *Children and grief: When a parent dies.* Guilford Press.

Worden, J. W. (2002). *Grief counseling and grief therapy: A handbook for the mental health practitioner* (3rd ed.). Springer.

Worden, W. (2018). *Grief counseling and grief therapy* (5th ed.). Springer. http://doi.org/10.1891/9780826134752

World Health Organization, I. T. (2022). *Intimate partner violence.* http://apps.who.int/violence-info/intimate-partner-violence

World Health Organization. (2018). *International classification of diseases, 11th revision (ICD-11).*

World Health Organization. (2021). *Suicide worldwide in 2019: Global healthestimates.*https://www.who.int/publications-detail-redirect/9789240026643

World Health Organization. (2021). *Suicide.* https://www.who.int/news-room/fact-sheets/detail/suicide

World Health Organization. (2022). *ICD 11.* ICD-11 2022 release.

World Health Organization. (2023). *Youth violence.* https://www.who.int/news-room/fact-sheets/detail/youth-violence

Wortman, C. B., & Lehman, D. R. (1985). Reactions to victims of life crises: Support attempts that fail. In I. G. Sarason & B. R. Sarason (Eds.), *Social support: Theory, research and application* (pp. 463–489). Martinus Nijhodff.

Wright, T., & Bonett, D. (1997). The contribution of burnout to work performance. *Journal of Organizational Behavior, 18*(5), 491–499.

Wright-Carrier, J. T. (1992). Evaluation of police crisis intervention in mental disturbance calls. Unpublished dissertation. University of Memphis. *Dissertation Abstract International Section A. Humanities and Social Sciences,* 538-A, 2686.

Wu, H., Lu, L., Qian, Y., Jin, X.-H., Yu, H.-R., Du, L., Fu, X.-L., Zhu, B., & Chen, H.-L. (2022). The significance of cognitive-behavioral therapy on suicide: An umbrella review. *Journal of Affective Disorders, 317,* 142–148. https://doi.org/10.1016/j.jad.2022.08.067

Wu, X., Kaminga, A. C., Dai, W., Deng, J., Wang, Z., Pan, X., & Liu, A. (2019). The prevalence of moderate-to-high posttraumatic growth: A systematic review and meta-analysis. *Journal of Affective Disorders, 243,* 408–415. https://doi.org/10.1016/j.jad.2018.09.023

Wuang, Y., Chiang, C., Su, C., & Wang, C. (2011). Effectiveness of virtual reality using Wii gaming technology in children with Down syndrome. *Research in Developmental Disabilities, 32*(1), 312–321.

Wykes, T., & Whittington, R. (1998). Prevalence and predictors of early traumatic stress reactions in assaulted psychiatric nurses. *Journal of Forensic Psychiatry, 9*(3), 643–658.

Wylie, M. S. (2004, September–October). Mindsight. *Psychotherapy Networker,* 29–39.

Xu, J., Murphy, S. L., Kochanek, K. D., & Arias, E. (2022). *Mortality in the United States. 202,* 456.

Xu, X., Jiang, J., Bai, H., & Tian, T. (2021). Effects of personality characteristics of different genders and quality of life analysis on risk factors for suicide in depressive patients. *Computational & Mathematical Methods in Medicine,* 1–7. https://doi.org/10.1155/2021/7850281

Yang, M., Wong, S.C., & Coid, J. (2010). The efficacy of violence prediction: A meta-analytic comparison of nine risk assessment tools. *Psychological Bulletin, 136*(5), 740–767. https://doi.org/10.1037/a0020473

Yang, S., Gill, C, Kanewske, L., & Thompson, P. (2018). Exploring police response to mental health calls in a nonurban area. A case study of Roanoke County, Virginia. *Victims & Offenders, 13*(8), 1132–1152. https://doi.org/10.1080/15564886.2018.1512540

Yang, Y., & Hayes, J. A. (2020). Causes and consequences of burnout among mental health professionals: A practice-oriented review of recent empirical literature. *Psychotherapy, 57,* 426–436. https://doi.org/10.1037/pst0000317

Yapp, E. J., & Quayle, E. (2018). A systematic review of the association between rape myth acceptance and male-on-female sexual violence. *Aggression and Violent Behavior, 41,* 1–19. https://doi.org/10.1016/j.avb.2018.05.002

Yarar, E. Z., Bulut, B. P., & Demirbaş, H. (2023). Does gender really matter: Childhood trauma, trait anger, and suicide risk in early adulthood. *Journal of Interpersonal Violence, 38*(1/2), NP1222–NP1238. https://doi.org/10.1177/08862605221087704

Yates, K., Kunz, M., Czobar, P., Rabinowitz, S., Lindenmayer, J. P., & Volavka, J. (2005). A cognitive, behaviorally based program for patients with persistent mental illness and a history of aggression, crime, or both: Structure and correlates of completers of the program. *Journal of the American Academy of Psychiatry and the Law, 33,* 214–222.

Yates, S., Axsom, S., & Tiedeman, K. (1999). The help-seeking process for distress after disasters. In R. Gist & B. Lubin (Eds.), *Response to disaster: Psychosocial, community, and ecological approaches* (pp. 133–166). Brunner/Mazel.

Ybarra, M. L., & Mitchell, K. J. (2013). Prevalence rates of male and female sexual violence perpetrators in a national sample of adolescents. *JAMA Pediatrics, 167*(12), 1125–1134. https://doi.org/10.1001/jamapediatrics.2013.2629

Yeater, E., Austin, J., Green, M., & Smith, J. E. (2011). Coping mediates the relations between posttraumatic stress disorder (PTSD) symptoms and alcohol use in homeless, ethnically diverse women: A preliminary study. *Psychological Trauma: Theory, Research, Practice, and Policy, 2*(4), 307–310.

Yeomans, F. (1993). When a therapist overindulges a demanding borderline patient. *Hospital and Community Psychiatry, 44,* 334–336.

Yerger, W., & Gehret, C. (2011). Understanding and dealing with bullying in schools. *The Educational Forum, 75*(4,) 315–326. https://doi.org/10.1080/00131725.2011.602468

Yesavage, J. A., & Zarcone, V. (1983). History of drug abuse and dangerous behavior in inpatient schizophrenics. *Journal of Clinical Psychiatry, 44,* 259–261.

Yin, C. W., Sien, N. Y., Ying, L. A., Chung, S., & Leng, D. T. (2014). Virtual reality for upper-extremity rehabilitation in early stroke: A pilot randomized control trial. *Clinical Rehabilitation, 28*(11), 1107–1114.

Yorgason, J. B. (2010). Illness and family stress. In S. J. Price, C. A. Price, & P. C. McKenny (Eds.). *Families and change: Coping with stressful events and transitions* (pp. 97–118). SAGE.

Yoshimura, S., Okamoto, Y., Onoda, K., Matsunaga, M., Okada, G., Kunisato, Y., & Yamawaka, S. (2014). Cognitive behavioral therapy for depression changes medial prefrontal and ventral anterior cingulate cortex activity associated with self-referential processing. *Social Cognitive and Affective Neuroscience, 9*(4), 487–493.

Young, B. H. (2006). The immediate response to disaster: Guidelines for adult psychological first aid. In E. C. Ritchie, P. J. Watson, & M. J. Friedman (Eds.), *Interventions following mass violence and disasters: Strategies for mental health practice* (pp. 134–154). Guilford Press.

Young, B. H., Ruzek, J. I., Wong, M., Salzer, M. S., & Naturale, A. J. (2006). Disaster mental health training: Guidelines, considerations, and recommendations. In E. C. Ritichie, P. J. Watson, & M. J. Friedman (Eds.), *Interventions following mass violence and disasters: Strategies for mental health practice* (pp. 54–79). Guilford Press.

Young, M. A. (1991). Crisis intervention and the aftermath of disaster. In A. R. Roberts (Ed.), *Contemporary perspectives on crisis intervention* (pp. 83–103). Prentice Hall.

Yule, W. (1998). PTSD in children. In T. W. Miller (Ed.), *Children of trauma: Stressful life events and their effects on children and adolescents* (pp. 219–244). International Universities Press.

Yung, M. (2013). Predictors of burnout and intentions to leave among staff that care for violence prone, court-dependent and emotionally disturbed youth in residential treatment facilities. *Dissertation Abstracts International: Section B. The Sciences and Engineering, 74*(2-B(E)).

Zagar, R., Arbit, J., Sylvies, R., Busch, K., & Hughes, J. (1990). Homicidal adolescent: A replication. *Psychological Reports, 67,* 1235–1242.

Zalaquett, C., Carrion, I., & Exum, H. (2010). Providing disaster services to culturally diverse survivors. In J. Webber & J. B. Mascari (Eds.), *Terrorism, trauma and tragedies: A counselor's guide to preparing and responding* (3rd ed., pp. 19–24). American Counseling Association Foundation.

Zalta, A. K., Tirone, V., Orlowska, D., Blais, R. K., Lofgreen, A., Klassen, B., Held, P., Stevens, N. R., Adkins, E., & Dent, A. L. (2021). Examining moderators of the relationship between social support and self-reported PTSD symptoms: A meta-analysis. *Psychological Bulletin, 147*(1), 33–54. https://doi.org/10.1037/bul0000316

Zanarini, M. C. (2000). Childhood experiences associated with the development of borderline personality disorder. *Psychiatric Clinics of North America, 23,* 89–101.

Zanskas, S., Myer, R. A., & James, R. K. (2017). Ethical and legal issues in crisis intervention. In R. K. James & B. E. Gilliland (Eds.). *Crisis intervention strategies* (8th ed., pp. 518–545). Cengage/Brooks/Cole.

Zapp, D., Buelow, R., Soutiea, L., Berkowitz, A., & DeJong, W. (2021). Exploring the potential campus-level impact of online universal sexual assault prevention education. *Journal of Interpersonal Violence, 36*(5–6), NP2324–NP2345. https://doi.org/10.1177/0886260518762449

Zarzaur, M. (2005, May). *Using a portable sandtray for crisis intervention.* Paper presented at the Twenty-ninth Annual Convening of Crisis Intervention Personnel, Chicago, IL, the United States.

Zdziarski, E. L., Dunkel, N. W., & Rollo, J. M. (2007). *Campus crisis management: A comprehensive guide to planning, prevention, response, and recovery.* John Wiley & Sons.

Zechenter, E. M. (2023). Uses of rape as a military weapon by Russian forces in Ukraine. *International Law News, 50*(2), 7–12.

Zeigler-Hill, V., & Abraham, J. (2006). Borderline personality features: Instability of self-esteem and affect. *Journal of Social and Clinical Psychology, 25*(6), 668–687.

Zenere, F. (1998, Fall). NASP/NEAT community crisis response. *Newsletter of the Florida Association of School Psychologists.*

Zenere, F. J., & Lazarus, P. J. (1997). The decline of youth suicidal behavior in an urban, multicultural public school system following the introduction of a suicide prevention and intervention program. *Suicide and Life-Threatening Behavior, 27*(4), 387–403.

Zetumer, S., Young, I., Sher, K., Skritskaya, N., Lebowitz, B., Simon, N., & Zisook, S. (2015). The impact of losing a child on the clinical presentation of complicated grief. *Journal of Affective Disorders, 170,* 15–21.

Zhang, B., El-Jawahri, A., & Prigerson, H. (2006). Update on bereavement research: Evidence-based guidelines for the diagnosis and treatment of complicated bereavement. *Journal of Palliative Medicine, 9,* 1188–1202.

Zhang, H., Hook, J. N., Hodge, A. S., Coomes, S. P., Davis, C. W., Van Tongeren, D. R., Davis, D. E., & Aten, J. D. (2021). Religious and spiritual struggles and coping amidst the COVID-19 pandemic: A qualitative study. *Spirituality in Clinical Practice, 8*(4), 245–261. https://doi.org/10.1037/scp0000272

Zhang, H., Hook, J. N., Van Tongeren, D. R., Davis, D. E., McElroy-Heltzel, S. E., Davis, E. B., & Aten, J. D. (2022). The role of spiritual fortitude in meaning and mental health symptoms following a natural disaster. *Psychology of Religion and Spirituality, 14*(3), 406–415. https://doi.org/10.1037/rel0000420

Zhao, L., & Jiang, G. (2010). Exposure to violent games: A research about aggression in middle school students. *Chinese Journal of Clinical Psychology, 18*(6), 765–768.

Zhong, S., Yu, R., & Fazel, S. (2020). Drug use disorders and violence: Associations with individual drug categories.

Epidemiology Review, 42(1), 103–116. https://doi.org/10.1093/epirev/mxaa006

Zhou, X., Wu, X., Fu, F., & An, Y. (2015). Core challenge and rumination as predictors of PTSD and PTG among adolescent survivors of the Wenchuan Earthquake. *Psychological Trauma: Theory, Research, Practice and Policy, 7*(4), 391–397.

Zhu, P., Luke, M., & Bellini, J. (2021). A grounded theory analysis of cultural humility in counseling and counselor education. *Counselor Education and Supervision, 60*(1), 73–89. https://doi.org/10.1002/ceas.12197

Zilberstein, K. (2014). Neurocognitive considerations in the treatment of attachment and complex trauma in children. *Clinical and Child Psychology and Psychiatry, 19*(3), 336–354.

Zimberhoff, A. K., & Brown, L. S. (2006). "Only the goyim beat their wives, right?" *Psychology of Women Quarterly, 30*, 422–424.

Zimmerman, J. L., & Dickerson, V. C. (1996). *If problems talked: Narrative therapy in action.* Guilford Press.

Zins, J. E., Travis, L., Brown, M., & Knighton, A. (1994). Schools and the prevention of interpersonal violence: Mobilizing and coordinating community resources. *Special Services in the Schools, 8*(2), 1–19.

Zlotnik, D. (2014). Predictors of revictimization following child sexual abuse: A meta-analytic review. *Dissertation Abstracts International: Section B: The Sciences and Engineering, 74*(12-B(E)), 515.

Zold, A. C., & Schilt, S. C. (1984). Violence: The child and the adolescent patient. In J. T. Turner (Ed.), *Violence in the medical care setting: A survival guide* (pp. 85–106). Aspen Systems.

Zuromski, K., Resnick, H., Price, M., Galea, S., Kilpatrick, D., & Ruggiero, K. (2019). Suicidal ideation among adolescents following natural disaster: The role of prior interpersonal violence. *Psychological Trauma: Theory, Research, Practice, and Policy, 11*(2), 184–188. https://doi.org/10.1037/tra0000365

Glossary

"I understand"   An owning statement that clearly conveys to the client that you do understand that what is happening right now is causing the client distress.

absence of community   One major source of burnout; needed for social support.

acceptance   Being open and aware of unpleasant emotions, thoughts, and experiences and just letting them be without making attempts to alter their frequency or form. Acceptance also means that the crisis worker feels an unconditional positive regard for the client.

acute stress disorder (ASD)   Symptoms mimic those of posttraumatic stress disorder (PTSD) but are time limited, usually dissipating within one month. The symptoms continue for a minimum of two days and a maximum of 4 weeks and occur within one month of the traumatic event; then those time frames will meet the criteria of ASD.

ADDRESSING model   The acronym encompasses Age, acquired and Developmental Disabilities, Religion, Ethnicity, Social class, Sexual orientation, Indigenous heritage, National origin, and Gender.

affect dysregulation   Alterations in impulse control, attention and consciousness, self-perception, perception of perpetrators, relationships to significant others, and systems of meaning.

alexithymia   A condition that develops in many survivors of childhood sexual abuse, which is the inability to recognize and label feelings.

altruistic suicide   Related to perceived or real social solidarity, such as the traditional Japanese hara-kiri or, to put it in a current context, the suicide attacks by members of Middle Eastern extremist groups.

ambiguous loss   This loss is of two types. The first is when a person is physically absent but psychologically present, as in the case of a missing person. The second is when a person is physically present but psychologically absent, as in the case of dementia or schizophrenia.

anger   One of four categories of rapists (mad at women).

animated guilt   Enables the individual to start taking responsibility for past actions and start to experience new degrees of personal liberation.

anomic suicide   Arises from a perceived or real breakdown in the norms of society, such as the financial and economic ruin of the Great Depression.

assertion statements   Owning statements that clearly and specifically ask for a specific action from the client.

assist first responders   Mental health personnel who may accompany or follow up first responders such as police, emergency medical technicians (EMTs), fire department, and disaster recovery workers.

autonomic hyperarousal   Affective, behavioral, and cognitive responses that occur when stimuli that may be associated with the original trauma, but present no threat, such as smells, clothing, settings, etc., cause a reaction in the individual as if the original threat were now present and imminent.

autonomic/intrusive rumination   The initial intrusion of unwanted thoughts that assails an individual after the trauma.

autonomy   Principle refers to a client's right to self-determination.

basic crisis theory   Focuses on helping people in crisis recognize and correct temporary affective, behavioral, and cognitive distortions brought on by traumatic events.

battered wife syndrome   A history of abuse with PTSD-like symptoms due to battering.

battered women syndrome   Lenore Walker's (1984, 1989, 2000) theory of learned helplessness that is applied to IPV and proposes that abused individuals stay in abusive relationships because they have been conditioned to believe that they cannot predict their own safety and nothing can be done to improve their circumstances.

behavioral emergency   Occurs when a crisis escalates to the point that the situation requires immediate intervention to avoid injury or death to oneself or others or the person is in imminent risk of serious injury or death by another.

bereavement   A period of sorrow following the death of a significant other and a common life transition rather than a clinical disorder.

body scanning   The individual monitors physical sensations throughout the body and gently allows himself or herself to feel, experience, and accept the physical sensations that emanate from various body parts.

bonadaptation   Successful adaptation in restoring balance to the family; considered to be good, useful, and healthy.

brief therapy theory   Typically attempts to remediate more or less ongoing emotional problems.

broaching   Refers to the crisis worker's consistent display of openness to invite the client to explore issues of diversity and a recognition that race, ethnicity, or some universal trait may be contributing to the crisis.

burnout   Total mental, physical, and emotional exhaustion caused by long-term involvement in emotionally demanding psychotherapy.

catfishing   When a person takes information and images, typically from other people, and uses them to create a new identity for themselves.

catharsis   Means simply letting clients talk, cry, swear, berate, rant, rave, mourn, or do anything else that allows them to ventilate feelings and thoughts; it may be one of the most therapeutic strategies the crisis worker can employ.

chronic callers   Callers who for various reasons are constant callers to crisis lines and because of this can tie up lines. Therefore, these callers are identified and time limits are usually set for them.

chronic suicide   A person who engages in repeated acts of suicidal behavior, eventually leading to suicide. Also characterized by people who engage in suicidal behavior to cope with and to achieve control over the psychic pain, hopelessness, and emptiness they feel.

closed-ended questions Seek specific, concrete information from the client; they are designed to elicit specific behavioral data and yes or no responses.

collective trauma One type of disaster trauma that affects the microsystem (the community) to the extent that the social bonds that connect people are torn apart and the community is rent asunder.

collectivism Based on the assumption that groups bind and mutually obligate individuals, that the personal is simply a component of the larger social group or context and subordinate to it.

combat fatigue Evolved from World War I term "Shell Shock." Now known as "PTSD."

Common Common" is used in place of "normal" because common is a better term to describe affective, behavioral, and cognitive aftershocks of a traumatic event...when reactions are anything but "normal."

comorbidity The presence of two diagnosable disorders such as major depression and substance abuse.

compassion fatigue (CF) Manifested in the continuous negative aspects of care provision for tough cases and customers in a demanding work environment that generally revolve around some type of trauma.

compassion satisfaction The positive feelings and intrinsic rewards one feels from helping others who have experienced a traumatic event.

conjugal or intimate terrorism Describes a tactic akin to brainwashing and political terrorism, whereby violence or the threat of violence is used to break the victim's resistance and bend her to the will of the terrorist (batterer).

conjunctive faith Wherein an individual can hold two differing beliefs and can deal with the paradoxes and polarities of those beliefs.

contagion suicide In a school the stimulus of one suicide or suicide attempt may cause a cluster of suicide attempts that occur a short time after the first attempt occurs.

contextual model Model of family stress that builds on the ABCX model and recognizes that families are unique and that events, the same or similar, will be experienced in distinctive ways.

control One major source of burnout; control issues from being micromanaged or having ineffective leaders or teams.

coping mechanisms Actions, behaviors, or environmental resources the client might use to help get through the present crisis.

core listening skills Empathy, genuineness, and acceptance or positive regard.

creating awareness The crisis worker attempts to bring to conscious awareness warded off, denied, shunted, and repressed feelings, thoughts, and behaviors that freeze clients' ability to act in response to the crisis.

creating order Used to help survivors rank order a list of what needs to be done and in what order these things should be worked on to promote stabilization.

crisis The perception or experiencing of an event or situation as an intolerable difficulty that exceeds the person's current resources and coping mechanisms.

Crisis Intervention Team Developed specifically to train patrol officers to deal with the mentally ill and emotionally disturbed people.

crisis management Refers to the act of planning a response to recurring suicidal behavior in collaboration with the client.

crisis therapy Second-order intervention that seeks to resolve the crisis and is generally provided by trained, licensed human services professionals.

cubic model Combines psychache, perturbation (how disturbed one is and degree of pain), and press (stress increased due to more negative factors piling up); when all three are combined, they create the critical mass necessary to activate a suicide.

cultural adaptation Adapting theories and techniques of counseling and psychotherapy to interface with nonwestern cultures.

culturally adaptive A culturally responsive approach that takes into account the client's diagnosis or treatment issues while honoring the "premise that race, ethnicity, and culture are powerful variables in influencing how people think, behave, and define events."

culturally responsive A multicultural counseling approach that takes into account the client's diagnosis or treatment issues while honoring the "premise that race, ethnicity, and culture are powerful variables in influencing how people think, behave, and define events."

culture specific A multicultural counseling approach in which the counselor adjusts their intervention to match the client's culture and, thereby, address the treatment issues.

culture-universal A counseling approach in which counselors focus on the treatment issue (i.e., diagnosis) and adjust their intervention to address the specific diagnosis or treatment issue without taking the client's culture into account.

cyberbullying Means using technology to harass, humiliate, or threaten someone.

cyberstalking A type of cyberbullying; the electronic version of pursuing a person who is not interested in the personal attention he or she is receiving, but receiving it anyway.

cyberthreats A type of cyberbullying; clearly meant to evoke fear and imply that danger is imminent.

death accepting A dominant belief within a culture that death is unavoidable and life is essentially transitory and usually involves movement in some manner to another plane of existence.

death defying A dominant cultural belief that through the miracle of modern medicine death can be defeated or at least postponed.

death denying A dominant belief within a culture that death is seen as defeat. The United States is generally seen as a death denying and defying culture to the point that the word itself is obscene.

decision support tools Understanding and knowing the observable risk factors for violence; these risk factors have been assessed to have high reliability and predictive ability in regard to violence risk.

deconstructing To analyze and break down into specific components that underlie assumptions or ideologies as a way of making sense of and moving forward from a loss.

defusion Focuses on decreasing the perceived literality (it is absolutely true and fact) of the avoidance language that debilitates and keeps sufferers of PTSD stuck in maladaptive value systems; the notion is that clients can be taught to detach from being fused with any idea (including the really bad ones that go with PTSD) by practicing acceptance and mindfulness when negative self and world attributions surface, and by continuous practice can come to believe that these are "just thoughts" that don't control one's behavior.

deliberate rumination   A process that issues out of a reflective state when a thorough reexamination of the traumatic event causes the individual to reframe his or her view of life and in fact grow from the experience.

denigration   A type of cyberbullying; sending or posting defaming information about someone.

developmental crises   Situations and events that occur during the life cycle of families that changes the families' structural integrity.

differential vulnerability   The degree to which people from different cultural backgrounds are vulnerable to and react to traumatic events.

directive intervention   Providing specific information and guidance clients need to make decisions, setting limits on behaviors that range from inappropriate to lethal, and apprising them of consequences of their affective, cognitive, and behavioral responses to the crisis based on the interventionist's expert clinical judgment and the self-same lack thereof in the client.

discordant values   One major source of burnout; these indicate the worker and the organization are severely at odds regarding the worker's belief in the validity and worth of the organization and the organization's belief about the worker's validity and worth.

disenfranchised grief   Occurs when a person has experienced a deep and meaningful attachment, experienced loss, and cannot openly acknowledge or grieve the loss or have it validated by others.

disequilibrium   Lack or destruction of emotional stability, balance, or poise in the organism.

disinhibition effect   A phenomenon in e-therapy; means that people tend to open up earlier with more distressing issues than they would normally do in a face-to-face therapy session.

disorganization of self   The first stage of trauma resolution that workers go through after a physical assault that includes feelings of shock. They may also dissociate from the experience as unreal, as if it didn't happen or they viewed it as a video of themselves. They may blame themselves and start having peritraumatic stress disorder symptoms involving sleep disturbances and emotional outbursts.

dissociation   Division of the personality into one component that attempts to function in the everyday world and another that regresses and is fixed in the trauma.

dissociative symptoms   Include memory loss, a sense of detachment from the world, belief that things and people are unreal, a blurred sense of identity, and a general disconnect from reality.

dissonant response   When a person's typical mode of grieving becomes compromised due to external pressures to adapt to a loss that does not fit the individual's grieving style and severe psychological conflict is the result.

duration   An identifying component in diagnosis of PTSD or treatment approach in terms of how chronic or transcrisis the problem is.

dysphoric/borderline batterer   Has a history of parental rejection and child abuse, delinquent acts, poor communication and social skills, violence-as-a-solution ideation, extreme fears of abandonment, and low remorse.

ecosystem   In crisis intervention the total system has interactive effects both on subsystems and individuals within those systems. The mesosystem (communication) and how effectively it operates is a key to understanding ecosystemic crisis intervention.

egoistic suicide   Related to one's lack of integration or identification with a group.

eliciting trust   A keystone that communicates that clients have the ability to get through tough times, recover, and grow. It is not cheerleading, but it is gentle encouragement and trust that the client can engage the grief and not avoid it.

emic   A cultural view that looks beyond physical features, race, and ethnicity to all of the social locations that make the individual distinct from others.

emotional dysregulated defense systems   When a person's normal ability to control emotions is overwhelmed by the traumatic event and subsequently he or she is unable to control his or her emotions. Even small trigger events may cause emotions to spiral out of control.

empathic presence   Involves listening, silence, and support through accepting and encouraging the expression of feelings, allowing pain to be expressed, and responding in a noncritical, nonjudgmental manner in allowing the grief-stricken to tell their story.

empathy   Means that the crisis worker accurately senses the inner feelings and meanings the client is experiencing and directly communicates to the client that the worker understands how it feels to be the client.

enticement   Used by child molesters and may include deceit, trickery, rewards, flattery, or the use of adult authority to tell the child in a matter-of-fact way that the child is expected to participate.

entrainment   A specific therapeutic technique that seeks to slow down the individual—whose thoughts, feelings, and acting may be spiraling out of control—through slow, measured responses and the use of calming techniques by the interventionist.

entrapment   Used by child molesters to manipulate the child into feeling obligated to participate through traps, blackmail, and so forth.

environment location   Refers to the physical and contextual setting in which the crisis occurs. At times changing the environment as opposed to changing the individual may de-escalate the crisis.

equilibrium   A state of mental or emotional stability, balance, or poise in the organism.

ergonomics   Profession that applies theory, principles, data, and methods to product design in order to optimize human well-being and overall system performance, which also applies to coordinating, collaborating, and allocating resources after a disaster.

etic   The traits and factors that are common to all persons within a particular ethnic or racial group.

exosystem   The experiences in another social setting in which the individual does not have an active role; does influence the individual's experiences in the immediate context.

expansion   When people in crisis are so locked into the crisis that they cannot see the bigger picture, and are paralyzed affectively, cognitively, and behaviorally, the crisis worker seeks to broaden their tunnel view of the crisis and thus start focusing on other aspects of the crisis.

expressive   Kinds of crime in which individuals pose a serious threat to themselves or others because of their own anger, fear, vulnerability, depression, or lack of emotional control.

externalize   Placement and projection of the origin of the crisis on some object, person, thing, or place external to the person without acceptance of the problem or owning any part of its origin.

face validity   Outward appearance of having substantial worth and content. In a person, he or she may "look like" he or she knows what he or she is doing whether he or she actually does.

facilitator role   By performing various physical activities and functions that help a person deal with a loss such as helping make organ donor rights or providing information about lawyers who handle wills.

fairness   One major source of burnout; lack of, with little justice and lots of arbitrary and secretive decision making and favoritism.

family communication model   Depicts an approach for families to cope with and prevail during crises using internal and external verbal interactions; the model makes the assumption that the root of family crises is communication.

family crisis   A crisis occurs when perceptions or experiencing of an event comes to bear on the family as a whole, testing the family's structural integrity, because the usual repertoire of problem-solving skills and communication styles are not adequate or have been exhausted. Unless relief is obtained the crisis jeopardizes family homeostasis and has the potential to strip family resilience.

family distress model (FDM)   The purpose for the model is to identify families' patterns of coping in order to develop interventions designed to support attempts at managing the situation. FDM states that when in distress, families use strategies that are different from their daily predictable patterns.

family only abuser   Abuse is isolated and contained within family unit. Typical of many batterers who are not violent outside the family unit.

family outreach model (FOM)   The family distress model was broadened by the formation of FOM that added a practical intervention component. FOM goes beyond traditional family intervention models based on conceptualizations of pathology that must be diagnosed or dysfunctional families that require expert assessment.

family transcrisis   Unresolved feelings, behaviors, and cognitions of a crises that lie dormant until situations or events occur that reactivate these reactions although not directly related to the current circumstances.

fatalistic suicide   Occurs when a person sees no way out of an intolerable or oppressive situation, such as being confined in a concentration camp.

first contact   Critical preliminary bonding techniques required when worker makes first contact with previously unknown person in crisis.

flaming   A type of cyberbullying; refers to angry offensive language.

focus   When people are so scattered in their thinking and behaving that they are paralyzed from taking action affectively, cognitively, and behaviorally, the crisis worker seeks to narrow their view and pick one component of the crisis to work on.

focused view   Looks at multicultural counseling in relation to visible and racial ethnic minorities. Based on physical features and defined racial groupings.

focusing   Helps families sort through what seems like a junk pile of responsibilities in order to focus on the most important ones at that moment.

friction location   Stimuli that trigger and escalate the crisis situation, whether they are intrapersonal, interpersonal, or systemic. Finding friction locations and easing them is critical to de-escalating and defusing a crisis.

gender inequality   Refers to the economic, political, and legal status of women in comparison to men.

general adaptation syndrome (GAS)   Overstimulation and excessive wear of target organs lead to stress-related dysfunction and disease.

generally violent/antisocial abuser   Type of abuser who is extremely aggressive and impulsive and views violence as appropriate to any provocation. This type of abuser may have no substantiating basis for their abuse, other than the pleasure it gives them.

gentle conversation   Allows for memory sharing, telling and retelling stories, and owning statements from the worker such as "I am sorry. I don't have words to begin to touch the feelings you must have, but I am here, and I will stay here and listen if you care to talk."

genuineness   Means that the worker is being completely open in the relationship: nothing is hidden, there are no facades, and there are no professional fronts.

goals   May be tangible, intangible, unspoken, or expressed; they motivate families in their desire to attain or achieve something.

grief   A psychic state or condition of mental anguish or emotional suffering and a result or anticipation of the bereavement.

grooming   Seduction phase wherein molesters successively approximate a child to accept that the sexual abuse is okay, appropriate, educational, acceptable, and even a duty.

grounding   A reality orientation technique that helps keep someone in the present and helps reorient a person to the here-and-now and in reality.

guidance   When the clients don't have the knowledge or resources available to make good decisions, the crisis worker provides information, referral, and direction in regard to clients' obtaining assistance from specific external resources and support systems.

harassment   A type of cyberbullying; the technology version of discriminatory or hostile behavior toward someone based on gender, race, religion, disability, or sexual orientation.

helplessness   Feminists see this pejorative term as casting women in a victim role with few resources or little empowerment.

hesitation wounds   One of multiple, usually superficial and parallel incisions that are self-inflicted in places where major vessels are near the skin surface, in an attempted suicide. Based on the notion that people are hesitant to kill themselves, so they inflict wounds that are superficial in nature.

hypervigilance   Being on constant guard for threats when there is no immediate threat.

hysterical neurosis   Concept formulated by Sigmund Freud to describe trauma cases of young Victorian women with whom he was working.

immobility   A state of physical being in which the person is not immediately capable of autonomously changing or coping in response to different moods, feelings, emotions, needs, conditions, influences; inability to adapt to the immediate physical and social world.

impact stage Occurs during the sexual assault and for approximately two weeks following it. During this time a kaleidoscope of emotions, thoughts, and behaviors may occur, or conversely the client may be in a state of shock and dissociation, with both physical pain associated with the sexual assault and dissociation, somatic reactions, hypervigilance, nightmares, and startle responses that are symptomatic of the acute stress disorder that often follows.

indirect and noncommissioned behavioral emergencies Indirect behavioral emergencies occur when people make bad decisions and wind up placing themselves in potentially lethal situations. Indirect and noncommissioned behavioral emergencies are crises that happen with no directed purpose or intentionality to do something harmful to oneself or others.

indirect suicide Suicide wherein suicidal persons may not have the courage to kill themselves, or they seek to publicize their deaths through the media by "going out in a blaze of glory."

individual trauma One type of disaster trauma that hammers the individual psyche and breaks through the person's defense so forcefully and suddenly that reaction is impossible.

individualism A worldview that centralizes the personal— personal goals, personal uniqueness, and personal control— and peripheralizes the social group or social context within which the individual operates.

individuative/reflective faith Where one is able to reflect critically on one's story and values and disregard personal myths about self, God, and one's relationship with the world.

inescapable One of the three I's and a major cause of perturbation: I can't get away from this pain no matter what I do.

instrumental acts of homicide Occur for some financial or other concrete gain.

instrumental crimes Crimes such as theft, robbery, and assault.

intensity Intensity is relevant in triaging a person in regard to both duration of negative responding in terms of time and degree of reaction.

interminable One of the three I's and a major cause of perturbation: "If I don't do something about this now, it'll go on forever." The person sees no relief in the future for the psychic pain he or she is suffering.

International Federation of Red Cross and Red Crescent Societies Helps individuals and communities heal the psychological wounds and rebuild social structures after an emergency or a critical event. Its mission is to change people into active survivors rather than passive victims.

intolerable One of the three I's and a major cause of perturbation: I've gone beyond what any human could endure.

intrusive rumination Unbidden terrifying thoughts entering the person's mind about the trauma.

large-scale crises Those crises that at a minimum affect whole communities or regions either directly or vicariously.

learned helplessness Means that battered women choose behavioral responses that have the highest predictability of causing them the least harm in the known situation, or what is called survivor hypothesis, wherein women become very active and resourceful in protecting themselves and their children.

legal The first step of the LASER protocol, which addresses legal considerations and responsibilities in determining ethical course of action.

legitimization of violence The support the culture gives to violence, as portrayed in the mass media (such as television programming), laws permitting corporal punishment in schools, violent sports, military exploits, and video games.

loss A universal human phenomenon, but people respond to it with varying degrees of grief and mourning. Any loss is some form of death. Death of a loved one, death of a relationship through the breakup of a marriage or a friendship, leaving a job, putting down a pet, repossession of a home, geographic moving away from friends and family, even the loss of precious keepsakes can constitute a loss that becomes a crisis. All losses produce some degree of grieving.

loss orientation One component of the dual process model that focuses on the affective, behavioral, and cognitive reactions that are typically experienced when a severe loss occurs.

low-level antisocial abuser Has antisocial behavior and moderate levels of domestic and general violence.

macrosystem Includes the national government and all its agencies, and national charitable, religious, service, professional, and benevolent organizations; encompasses the national rail, air, marine, and highway transportation modalities, and food, fuel, and energy transmission systems. It involves the total culture including beliefs, mores, legal constructs, and all the other artifacts, traits, and pursuits that define a group of people in the environment in which they live.

making contact/predispositioning A task with families in crises that involves placing yourself in a position of being helpful.

maladaptation Lack of balance in the family; considered to be negative, ineffective, and unhealthy.

masquerading A type of cyberbullying; using someone else's identity to send messages that are rude and inappropriate.

meaning making The attempt to restore the original global meaning system and not let it be driven by the one traumatic event that changed it; calls for reviewing and reframing the traumatic event in such a way that an acceptable appraisal of the event can be made.

megacrises Those crises that affect entire countries or the world, either directly or vicariously.

mentalization The process by which individuals interpret the actions of oneself and others as meaningful representations about what is going on both within themselves and between themselves and others. It is hypothesized that persons with borderline personality disorder have failed to develop this ability and thus cross intra- and interpersonal boundaries most people would not. The object of mentalization treatment is that borderline personality disorder clients increase mentalization capacity which should improve affect regulation and interpersonal relationships and give them better behavior control.

mesosystem The relationships, connections, and communication links between individuals and systems; everything from sign language for a deaf person to the most sophisticated wireless computer satellite uplinks to state and federal emergency management agencies.

metastasizing crises   Those crises that start small but, if not contained both physically and psychologically, can quickly turn into large-scale crises.

mobility   A state of physical being in which the person can autonomously change or cope in response to different moods, feelings, emotions, needs, conditions, influences; being flexible or adaptable to the physical and social world.

mobilization   The crisis worker gets the client moving behaviorally to take action on the crisis.

mobilized   When a client can take action to address the crisis without the further need for crisis intervention.

mourning   A social or cultural state or condition expressing grief or feeling because of bereavement; a communal rather than an individual reaction to loss, generally prescribed by cultural protocol and the time frame in which it occurs.

musturbatory behavior   Term used by Albert Ellis in defining debilitating dysfunctional cognitive behaviors that further and accelerate the crisis due to mistaken belief that "things" must be a certain way or the situation becomes intolerable.

mythical literal   Faith development model stage; a one-dimensional view of God as an entity that doles out rewards and punishment based on how rigorously one practices one's faith and follows its commandments (typical of children 8–12).

narrative therapy exposure   Through the use of either speaking or writing about the traumatic event, the trauma survivors reexpose themselves to the traumatic event. The purpose is to come to terms with the feared event by completely uncovering it, examining it as a now past event.

netiquette   Civil and appropriate rules of discourse when operating on the net, particularly in synchronous time with other netizens.

Neurasthenia   Presently referred to as Chronic Fatigue Syndrome, neurasthenia is characterized by various cognitive, musculoskeletal, and temperamental disturbances.

nonfinite losses   Loss experiences that are enduring in nature, usually precipitated by a negative life event or episode that retains a physical and/or psychological presence in an ongoing manner.

nostalgia   A nineteenth-century military term coined by physicians for combat soldiers with extreme homesickness.

off-time developmental crises   Occur when transitions are out of sequence, not happening in the expected order, and are particularly troublesome as they can be extremely disruptive to families' resilience and capacity to cope; examples include the untimely death of a parent, unplanned pregnancies, forced retirement, disability due to chronic illness, and so on.

open-ended questions   Usually start with what or how or ask for more clarification or details; they encourage clients to respond with full statements and at deeper levels of meaning.

order   What the crisis worker provides by methodically helping clients classify and categorize problems so as to prioritize and sequentially attack the crisis in a logical and linear manner.

outing or trickery   A type of cyberbullying; a way of getting people to reveal personal information that might then be used against them.

owning   Means communicating possession: "That's mine."

parallel processing   In a large-scale crisis when crisis workers as a group start to mimic (counter-transfer) their own thoughts, feelings, and actions such that they start to resemble the crisis clients with whom they are working.

parasuicide   Engaging in activities that are deliberately self-harming but where there is no result in death. It is a strong indicator for a future suicide attempt.

passive suicide   A variety of actions (or inactions) that tend to be self-destructive, but not actively, which are considered to depict suicidal intent. Instances of these actions include failing to feed oneself or to participate in basic self-care. Commonly seen in the elderly particularly after the passing of a spouse; they see their purpose in life as done, they become depressed, and they give up or fail to thrive.

period of struggle   The second stage of trauma resolution that workers go through after a physical assault, characterized by anxiety attacks, intrusive thoughts, hypervigilance, and psychosomatic symptoms, which are characteristic of acute stress disorder.

peritraumatic stress symptoms   Symptoms that mimic those of PTSD such as hypervigilance and startle response that occur immediately after a traumatic event is experienced, but disappear within two days.

perturbation   How disturbed one is and degree of psychic pain one is suffering.

pornography   Reduces women to sex objects, promotes male dominance, and encourages or condones sexual violence against women.

positive and constructive thinking patterns   Ways of reframing that might substantially alter the client's view of the problem and lessen the client's level of stress and anxiety.

positive traumatic growth   Comes out of any personal transformation that occurs as a result of trauma, or the ability to not just survive a traumatic incident, but grow from it.

posttraumatic stress disorder (PTSD)   A diagnosable personality disorder that occurs after experiencing or witnessing a traumatic event. It has specific affective, behavioral, and cognitive criteria that must be met according to the American Psychiatric Association DSM-5 before a diagnosis of PTSD may be given.

power distance   Means the amount of control that bosses feel they have over workers and vice versa.

power exploitative   One of four categories of rapists (show they have power over women).

power reassurance   One of four categories of rapists (continuously feel that they are powerful over women).

predispositioning   One important aspect of listening; the worker makes initial owning statements that express exactly what he or she is going to do. Also means getting ready to do something. It is usually the first step in a crisis model: placing oneself, or something, in a position to be of use in some future occurrence.

preloss grief   Is the reaction that occurs when an individual is diagnosed with an illness that will likely end in death.

Physicians Desk Reference (PDR)   A widely recognized reference for drug information.

primary losses   Death of a friend, child, parent, or spouse.

primary prevention   Stopping a problem before it starts.

procedural rules   Set the basis for family structure and provide consistency; when followed, they result in families maintaining a state of equilibrium. They determine internal and external interactions of family members as well as set the standard for topics for conversation.

protection   What the crisis worker provides by safeguarding clients from engaging in harmful, destructive, detrimental, and unsafe feelings, behaviors, and thoughts that may be psychologically or physically injurious or lethal to themselves or others.

providing available space   Has to do with what contemporary research and practice in the field of loss keep harping about—that is, helping the client find support, doing things clients can't do for themselves right now (pumping gas), but letting them tell us what they can and can't do so they have at least a modicum of control in their lives.

psychache   Refers to the hurt, anguish, soreness, and aching pain of the psyche or mind.

psychoeducation   Providing information to victims and survivors about what is happening and probably is going to happen to them psychologically in the aftermath of a traumatic event.

psychological anchor   Therapist who will act as advocate, support, and contact person for client.

psychological autopsy   Examines in detail the situation that led to a violent episode.

psychological first aid   First-order intervention that seeks to address the immediate crisis situation and provide immediate relief, possibly to a wide range of individuals.

psychosocial   Having mental distress as a result of social upheaval.

railway spine   A term used to describe the psychological symptoms of survivors of nineteenth-century train wrecks. It was thought that somehow these symptoms were related to injured spines.

rape   An unwanted act of oral, vaginal, or anal penetration committed though the use of force, threat of force, or when incapacitated.

Readiness and Emergency Management for Schools (REMS) Technical Assistance (TA) Center   A comprehensive planning tool for the establishment and implementation of school safety teams in developing comprehensive risk assessment and implementation plans.

readjustment of self   The third stage of trauma resolution that workers go through after a physical assault. If the worker is able to move forward, then the incident is integrated into the self and the worker becomes the wiser for it, comes to see that clients can be dangerous, and takes more precautions. However, if the worker does not integrate the incident, then the possibility of PTSD looms large.

reestablishing control   An essential, recurring task as families search, sometimes desperately, for ways to regain stable, predictable functioning.

relational markers   Shorten the psychological distance between the client and the worker through the use of such words as "this," "these," "we," "our," "here," and "now" as opposed to "that," "those," "mine," "there," and "then."

renewal   The third phase of crisis intervention. The crisis worker helps the family reformulate itself in a context of growth and movement beyond the suicide.

resiliency model   Represents a current focus of family crisis intervention and views families not as damaged, but rather challenged by adversities; concentrates on the potential for recovery and restoration functioning rather than pathologizing families' reactions while experiencing adversity.

RESPECTFUL   The acronym encompasses Religious/spiritual, Economic class, Sexual identity, Psychological development, Ethnic/racial identity, Chronological age, Trauma and threats to well-being, Family, Unique physical issues, and Language and location of residence.

restitutive play   Attempting to reenact the trauma through play and somehow resolve it.

restoration orientation   Occurs when grievers start to come to grips with the consequences of the loss and begin to form new roles and identities, develop new relationships, make life changes, and engage in new activities that distract their grief.

resuscitation   The first phase of crisis intervention. Within 24 hours, the crisis worker makes a supportive visit to assist the survivors of suicide in dealing with their initial shock, grief, anger, and most likely self-recrimination, guilt, and blame.

resynthesis   The second phase of crisis intervention. The crisis worker helps the survivors of suicide learn new ways of coping with their loss and prevents the development of pathological family responding.

reward   One major source of burnout; lack thereof, in the form of compensation, recognition, or pleasure.

risk-needs-responsivity (RNR) model   A procedure taken from the corrections field. The risk component proposes that high-risk individuals get more targeted, specific, and tailored therapeutic inputs before they go critical. The needs component focuses on the dynamic risk factors that when changed reduce recidivism. RNR usually incorporates cognitive-behavioral therapy, social skills training, anger management, and behavioral techniques that apply role rehearsal, modeling, and shaping to prosocial behavior.

ritualistic rules   Rules around rituals are ever present in families' lives and create meaning as they remember special times in their lives, such as kissing a partner as one leaves for work, tucking in children at bedtime, and celebrations at birthdays, anniversaries, and holidays.

role   A practical function taken on by someone within the family.

sadistic   One of four categories of rapists (take joy in hurting women).

safety   Refers to the physical and psychological safety of families and the crisis intervention worker.

SAFETY model   An acronym that is derived from social locations/trauma theory that is specifically applied to crisis intervention.

secondary intervention   Minimizing the harmful effects that have already occurred by follow-up therapy after the initial crisis has occurred and been stabilized.

secondary loss   A consequence of a primary loss. For example, death of a spouse (primary loss) may cause loss of status, social contacts, financial security, and sexual intimacy, which are secondary losses.

secondary traumatic stress (STS)   The transformation that occurs when an individual begins to change in a manner that mimics a client's trauma-related symptoms.

sexual assault   Refers to a broader range of sexual criminal offenses such as sexual battery and sexual coercion up to and including rape.

shell shock   The advent of modern warfare in World Wars I and II generated this term to explain the condition of traumatized soldiers who had no apparent physical wounds.

situational supports People known to the client in the present or past who might care about what happens to the client.

smart card A portable card that clients and counselors develop in collaboration, which contains information on coping skills, de-escalation techniques, and emergency resources for clients to use during times of heightened distress.

social disorganization Erodes social control and constraints and undermines freedom of individual behavior and self-determination.

social exclusion A type of cyberbullying; a means of deliberately excluding someone from a buddy list, chat room, discussion board, or game.

social locations The individual identifiers that go far beyond, race, sex, and skin tone that make us the specific and unique individuals that reside in a cultural group.

social norms theory Proposes that male peer aggression and female submission are part of the norm and justification for violent sexual interaction.

soldier's heart An archaic term used to describe behaviors associated with PTSD.

solicitation/traveling offenders Online offenders who will attempt to entice a child to meet with them to have sex or encourage them to run away with them.

somatization Physical problems, associated pain, and functional limitations.

spiritual crisis Occurs when a previously held religious or spiritual belief is called into question or completely abandoned.

stalking Generally defined as repeated harassment, following, and/or threats that are committed with the intent of causing the victim emotional distress, fear of bodily harm, and/or actual bodily harm.

Stigmatization The social process of shaming or disgracing someone based on a characteristic, trait, or action.

structured professional judgment (SPJ) Combining what professional crisis workers' experience tells them as they use verbal and visual assessments along with a reliable paper-and-pencil test—if time is available to make a decision on potential lethality.

suicide by legal intervention Coroner's verdict from suicide by cop.

summary clarification Ribbon-wraps the dialogue; that is, it packages the preceding dialogue and lets both client and crisis worker know they are on the same wavelength.

sundown syndrome Client disorientation and states of confusion that may arise during evening hours in geriatric settings and mental hospitals, due to the onset of darkness, change of shift, and decrease in staff.

support The crisis worker either finds or assumes temporary responsibility for providing a support system for the person or families in crisis. This support may be as a resource for information or for providing temporary emotional, behavioral, and cognitive support.

support group Deals with a variety of transcrisis issues that have to do with members' attempts to reintegrate themselves into a useful, functioning role in society.

synthetic-conventional Faith development model stage; conforms to the community's basic cultural standard of moral behavior, normative beliefs, values, and religious practices (typical of 12 years of age to early adulthood).

systemic crisis When a traumatic event occurs such that people, institutions, communities, and ecologies are overwhelmed and response systems are unable to effectively contain and control the event in regard to both physical and psychological reactions to it, the crisis has become systemic.

temperament location What the crisis worker and the client bring to a crisis situation based on both past personal and cultural experiences.

terroristic abuser Such people are extremely aggressive and impulsive, and view violence as appropriate to any provocation inside or outside the home.

transcrisis points Occur frequently in transcrisis states within the therapeutic intervention. These points are generally marked by the client's coming to grips with new developmental stages or other dimensions of the problem. Transcrisis points do not occur in regular, predictable, linear progression.

transcrisis state A continuous state of low grade crisis which has not been resolved and much like a sinus infection may flare up, given the right conditions, into a full blown crisis.

trauma metaphor The trauma survivor's use of metaphors that have literal meaning and relate specifically to the trauma, such as a Hurricane Katrina survivor saying "I was drowning in a tidal wave of responsibilities."

traumatic grief Generally subsumed under complicated or prolonged grief, with the additional requirement that the person witnessed or was in close proximity to the violent, sudden, unexpected, horrifying death of a loved one.

uncertainty avoidance principle The degree to which cultures feel threatened by uncertainty and ambiguous situations, so rules, procedures, rituals, and laws may be formulated to buffer uncertainties of individual judgment.

uncomplicated bereavement The process that occurs as the bereaved individual works through a variety of tasks to integrate the reality of moving forward in life without the person who died.

universal view Considers not only racial and ethnic minorities, but other minority or special populations as well.

values Arising out of families' belief system, they are those things deemed important for morale and drive families' perceptions.

veiled threats Circuitous statements that do not express a direct warning but contain a menacing message beyond the words.

vicarious traumatization (VT) A consequence for health care professionals who are frequently exposed to the stress and trauma of others in the course of treating them; also called secondary traumatic stress disorder (STSD).

war neurosis A term coined by Freud to describe psychological symptoms found in World War I soldiers that would later come to be known as PTSD.

witness role To observe, listen, and not do anything other than "be with" the client and allow the client to feel "felt."

working alliance A cooperative and trusting working relationship between interventionist and client.

workload One major source of burnout, when the work is too complex, too much, too urgent, or just too awful.

YAVIS clients Young, Attractive, Verbal, Intelligent, and Socially well-connected clients from higher socioeconomic backgrounds.

Index